Encyclopedia of Pain

Volume 2

H–O

With 713 Figures and 211 Tables

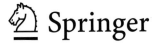
Springer

Professor em. Dr. Robert F. Schmidt
Physiological Institute
University of Würzburg
Röntgenring 9
97070 Würzburg
Germany
rfs@mail.uni-wuerzburg.de

Professor Dr. William D. Willis
Department of Neuroscience and Cell Biology
University of Texas Medical Branch
301 University Boulevard
Galveston
TX 77555-1069
USA
wdwillis@utmb.edu

ISBN-13: 978-3-540-43957-8 Springer Berlin Heidelberg New York

This publication is available also as:
Electronic publication under 978-3-540-29805-2 and
Print and electronic bundle under ISBN 978-3-540-33447-7
Library of Congress Control Number: 2006925866

Springer is part of Springer Science+Business Media

springer.com

Editor: Thomas Mager, Andrea Pillmann, Heidelberg
Development Editor: Michaela Bilic, Natasja Sheriff, Heidelberg
Production Editor: Frank Krabbes, Heidelberg
Cover Design: Frido Steinen-Broo, Spain

Printed on acid free paper   SPIN: 10877912 2109fk - 5 4 3 2 1 0

Preface

As all medical students know, pain is the most common reason for a person to consult a physician. Under ordinary circumstances, acute pain has a useful, protective function. It discourages the individual from activities that aggravate the pain, allowing faster recovery from tissue damage. The physician can often tell from the nature of the pain what its source is. In most cases, treatment of the underlying condition resolves the pain. By contrast, children born with congenital insensitivity to pain suffer repeated physical damage and die young (see Sweet WH (1981) Pain 10:275).

Pain resulting from difficult to treat or untreatable conditions can become persistent. Chronic pain "never has a biologic function but is a malefic force that often imposes severe emotional, physical, economic, and social stresses on the patient and on the family..." (Bonica JJ (1990) The Management of Pain, vol 1, 2nd edn. Lea & Febiger, Philadelphia, p 19). Chronic pain can be considered a disease in its own right.

Pain is a complex phenomenon. It has been defined by the Taxonomy Committee of the International Association for the Study of Pain as "An unpleasant sensory and emotional experience associated with actual or potential tissue damage, or described in terms of such damage" (Merskey H and Bogduk N (1994) Classification of Chronic Pain, 2nd edn. IASP Press, Seattle). It is often ongoing, but in some cases it may be evoked by stimuli. Hyperalgesia occurs when there is an increase in pain intensity in response to stimuli that are normally painful. Allodynia is pain that is evoked by stimuli that are normally non-painful.

Acute pain is generally attributable to the activation of primary afferent neurons called nociceptors (Sherrington CS (1906) The Integrative Action of the Nervous System. Yale University Press, New Haven; 2nd edn, 1947). These sensory nerve fibers have high thresholds and respond to strong stimuli that threaten or cause injury to tissues of the body. Chronic pain may result from continuous or repeated activation of nociceptors, as in some forms of cancer or in chronic inflammatory states, such as arthritis.

However, chronic pain can also be produced by damage to nervous tissue. If peripheral nerves are injured, peripheral neuropathic pain may develop. Damage to certain parts of the central nervous system may result in central neuropathic pain. Examples of conditions that can cause central neuropathic pain include spinal cord injury, cerebrovascular accidents, and multiple sclerosis.

Research on pain in humans has been an important clinical topic for many years. Basic science studies were relatively few in number until experimental work on pain accelerated following detailed descriptions of peripheral nociceptors and central nociceptive neurons that were made in the 1960's and 70's, by the discovery of the endogenous opioid compounds and the descending pain control systems in the 1970's and the application of modern imaging techniques to visualize areas of the brain that are affected by pain in the 1990's. Accompanying these advances has been the development of a number of animal models of human pain states, with the goal of using these to examine pain mechanisms and also to test analgesic drugs or non-pharmacologic interventions that might prove useful for the treatment of pain in humans. Basic research on pain now emphasizes multidisciplinary approaches, including behavioral testing, electrophysiology and the application of many of the techniques of modern cell and molecular biology, including the use of transgenic animals.

The "Encyclopedia of Pain" is meant to provide a source of information that spans contemporary basic and clinical research on pain and pain therapy. It should be useful not only to researchers in these fields but also to practicing physicians and other health care professionals and to health care educators and administrators. The work is subdivided into 35 Fields, and the Field Editor of each of these describes the areas covered in the Fields in a brief review chapter. The topics included in a Field are the subject of a series of short essays, accompanied by key words, definitions, illustrations, and a list of significant references. The number of authors who have contributed to the encyclopedia exceeds 550. The plan of the publisher, Springer-Verlag, is to produce both print and electronic versions of this encyclopedia. Numerous links within the electronic version should make comprehensive searches easy to manage. The electronic version will be updated at sufficiently short intervals to ensure that the content remains current.

The editors thank the staff at Springer-Verlag who have provided oversight for this project, including Rolf Lange, Thomas Mager, Claudia Lange, Natasja Sheriff, and Michaela Bilic. Working with these outstanding individuals has been a pleasure.

July 2006

ROBERT F. SCHMIDT   WILLIAM D. WILLIS
Würzburg, Germany   Galveston, Texas, USA

Editors-in-Chief

ROBERT R. SCHMIDT
Physiological Institute
University of Würzburg
Würzburg
Germany
rfs@mail.uni-wuerzburg.de

WILLIAM D. WILLIS
Department of Neuroscience and Cell Biology
University of Texas Medical Branch
Galveston, TX
USA
wdwillis@utmb.edu

Field Editors

A. VANIA APKARIAN
Department of Physiology
Northwestern University Feinberg School of Medicine
Chicago, IL
USA
a-apkarian@northwestern.edu

LARS ARENDT-NIELSEN
Laboratory for Experimental Pain Research
Center for Sensory-Motor Interaction
Aalborg University
Aalborg
Denmark
lan@hst.aau.dk

CARLOS BELMONTE
Instituto de Neurociencias de Alicante
Universidad Miguel Hernández-CSIC
San Juan de Alicante
Spain
carlos.belmonte@umh.es

PHILLIP BERRYHILL
PMG Cedar Neurosurgery
Albuquerque, NM
USA
phillip.berryhill@mac.com

NIELS BIRBAUMER
Institute of Medical Psychology and Behavioral
Neurobiology
University of Tübingen
Tübingen
Germany
niels.birbaumer@uni-tuebingen.de

NIKOLAI BOGDUK
Department of Clinical Research
Royal Newcastle Hospital Newcastle
University of Newcastle
Newcastle, NSW
Australia
michelle.gillam@newcastle.edu.au

SIR MICHAEL R. BOND
University of Glasgow
Glasgow
UK
m.bond@admin.gla.ac.uk

KIM J. BURCHIEL
Department of Neurological Surgery
The Oregon Health Sciences University
Portland, OR
USA
burchiek@ohsu.edu

KENNETH L. CASEY
Department of Neurology and
Department of Molecular and Integrative Physiology
University of Michigan
and
Consultant in Neurology
Veterans Administration Medical Center
Ann Arbor, MI
USA
kencasey@umich.edu

JIN MO CHUNG
Department of Neuroscience and Cell Biology
University of Texas Medical Branch
Galveston, TX
USA
jmchung@utmb.edu

MICHAEL J. COUSINS
Department of Anesthesia and Pain Management
Royal North Shore Hospital
University of Sydney
St. Leonards, NSW
Australia
mcousins@nsccahs.health.nsw.gov.au

MARSHALL DEVOR
Department of Cell and Animal Biology
Institute of Life Sciences and
Center for Research on Pain
Hebrew University of Jerusalem
Jerusalem
Israel
marshlu@vms.huji.ac.il

HANS-CHRISTOPH DIENER
Deptartment of Neurology
University of Duisburg-Essen
Essen
Germany
h.diener@uni-essen.de

JONATHAN O. DOSTROVSKY
Department of Physiology
Faculty of Medicine
University of Toronto
Toronto, ON
Canada
j.dostrovsky@utoronto.ca

RONALD DUBNER
Department of Biomedical Sciences
University of Maryland
Baltimore, MD
USA
rdubner@umaryland.edu

HERTA FLOR
Department of Neuropsychology at the
University of Heidelberg
Central Institute of Mental Health
Mannheim
Germany
flor@zi-mannheim.de

GERALD F. GEBHART
Department of Pharmacology
University of Iowa
Iowa City, IA
USA
gf-gebhart@uiowa.edu

GERD GEISSLINGER
Institute for Clinical Pharmacology
pharmazentrum frankfurt/ZAFES
Clinical Centre of the Johann Wolfgang Goethe
University Frankfurt am Main
Frankfurt
Germany
geisslinger@em.uni-frankfurt.de

GLENN J. GIESLER JR.
Department of Neuroscience
University of Minnesota
Minneapolis, MN
USA
giesler@mail.ahc.umn.edu

PETER J. GOADSBY
Institute of Neurology
The National Hospital for Neurology and
Neurosurgery
London
UK
peterg@ion.ucl.ac.uk

HERMANN O. HANDWERKER
Department of Physiology and Pathophysiology
University of Erlangen/Nürnberg
Erlangen
Germany
handwerker@physiologie1.uni-erlangen.de

WILFRID JÄNIG
Physiology Institute
Christian Albrechts University Kiel
Kiel
Germany
w.janig@physiologie.uni-kiel.de

MARTIN KOLTZENBURG
Institute of Child Health and Institute of Neurology
University College London
London
UK
m.koltzenburg@ich.ucl.ac.uk

FRED A. LENZ
Departments of Neurosurgery
Johns Hopkins University
Baltimore, MD
USA
flenz1@jhmi.edu

ROSS MACPHERSON
Department of Anesthesia and Pain Management
Royal North Shore Hospital
University of Sydney
St. Leonards, NSW
Australia
rmacpher@nsccahs.health.nsw.gov.au

PATRICIA A. MCGRATH
Department of Anaesthesia
Divisional Centre of Pain Management and Research
The Hospital for Sick Children
and
Brain and Behavior Program
Research Institute at The Hospital for Sick Children
and
Department of Anaesthesia
University of Toronto
Toronto, ON
Canada

FRANK PORRECA
Departments of Pharmacology and Anesthesiology
University of Arizona
Health Sciences Center
Tucson, AZ
USA
frankp@u.arizona.edu

RUSSELL K. PORTENOY
Department of Pain Medicine and Palliative Care
Beth Israel Medical Center
New York, NY
USA
rportenoy@chpnet.org

JAMES P. ROBINSON
Department of Anesthesiology
University of Washington School of Medicine
Seattle, WA
USA
jimrob@u.washington.edu

HANS-GEORG SCHAIBLE
Department of Physiology
University of Jena
Jena
Germany
hans-georg.schaible@mti.uni-jena.de

BARRY J. SESSLE
Department of Physiology
Faculty of Medicine
and
Faculty of Dentistry
University of Toronto
Toronto, ON
Canada
barry.sessle@utoronto.ca

BENGT H. SJÖLUND
Rehabilitation and Research Centre for Torture
Victims
South Danish University
Copenhagen
Denmark
bsj@rct.dk

DENNIS C. TURK
Department of Anesthesiology
University of Washington School of Medicine
Seattle, WA
USA
turkdc@u.washington.edu

URSULA WESSELMANN
Departments of Neurology
Neurological Surgery and Biomedical Engineering
The Johns Hopkins University School of Medicine
Baltimore, MD
USA
pain@jhmi.edu

GEORGE L. WILCOX
Department of Neuroscience
Pharmacology and Dermatology
University of Minnesota Medical School
Minneapolis, MN
USA
george@umn.edu

ROBERT P. YEZIERSKI
Department of Orthodontics
Comprehensive Center for Pain Research and
The McKnight Brain Institute
University of Florida
Gainesville, FL
USA
ryezierski@dental.ufl.edu

List of Contributors

TIPU AAMIR
The Auckland Regional Pain Service
Auckland Hospital
Auckland
New Zealand
bobl@adhb.govt.nz

CATHERINE ABBADIE
Department of Pharmacology
Merck Research Laboratories
Rahway, NJ
USA
catherine_abbadie@merck.com

FRANCES V. ABBOTT
Department of Psychiatry and Psychology
McGill University
Montreal, QC
Canada

HEATHER ADAMS
Department of Psychology
University of Montreal
Montreal, QC
Canada
heather.adams@umontreal.ca

ROLF H. ADLER
Prof. em. Medicine
Kehrsatz
Switzerland

CLAIRE D. ADVOKAT
Department of Psychology
Louisiana State University
Baton Rouge, LA
USA
cadvoka@lsu.edu

SHEFALI AGARWAL
Department of Anesthesiology and Critical Care
Medicine
The Johns Hopkins University School of Medicine
Baltimore, MD
USA

RETO M. AGOSTI
Headache Center Hirlsanden
Zürich
Switzerland
reto.agosti@kopfwww.ch

HUGO VAN AKEN
Clinic and Policlinic for Anaesthesiology and
operative Intensive Medicine
University Hospital Münster
Münster
Germany

ELIE D. AL-CHAER
Neurobiology and Developmental Sciences
College of Medicine
University of Arkansas for Medical Sciences
Center for Pain Research
Pediatrics
Little Rock, AR
USA
ealchaer@uams.edu

MARIE-CLAIRE ALBANESE
Department of Psychology
McGill University
Montreal, QC
Canada
mclaire@bic.mni.mcgill.ca

KATHRYN M. ALBERS
Department of Medicine
University of Pittsburgh School of Medicine
Pittsburgh, PA
USA
kaa2@pitt.edu

TERRY ALTILIO
Department of Pain Medicine and Palliative Care
Beth Israel Medical Center
New York, NY
USA
taltilio@chpnet.org

RAINER AMANN
Medical University Graz
Graz
Austria
rainer.amann@meduni-graz.at

RON AMIR
Institute of Life Sciences and
Center for Research on Pain
Hebrew University of Jerusalem
Jerusalem
Israel
ronamir@pob.huji.ac.il

PRAVEEN ANAND
Peripheral Neuropathy Unit
Imperial College London
Hammersmith Hospital
London
UK
p.anand@imperial.ac.uk

OLE K. ANDERSEN
Department of Health Science & Technology
Center for Sensory-Motor Interaction
Aalborg University
Aalborg
Denmark
oka@hst.aau.dk

STAN ANDERSON
Departments of Neurosurgery
Johns Hopkins University
Baltimore, MD
USA

WILLIAM S. ANDERSON
Department of Neurological Surgery
Johns Hopkins Hospital
Baltimore, MD
USA
wanderso@jhmi.edu

KARL-ERIK ANDERSSON
Departments of Clinical Pharmacology
Anesthesiology and Intensive Care
Lund University Hospital
Lund
Sweden

FRANK ANDRASIK
University of West Florida
Pensacola, FL
USA
fandrasik@uwf.edu

A. VANIA APKARIAN
Department of Physiology
Feinberg School of Medicine
Northwestern University
Chicago, IL
USA
a-apkarian@northwestern.edu

LARS ARENDT-NIELSEN
Laboratory for Experimental Pain Research
Center for Sensory-Motor Interaction
Aalborg University
Aalborg
Denmark
lan@hst.aau.dk

KIRSTEN ARNDT
CNS Pharmacology
Pain Research
Boehringer Ingelheim Pharma GmbH & Co. KG
Biberach/Riss
Germany
kirsten.arndt@bc.boehringer-ingelheim.de

ERIK ASKENASY
Health Science Center at Houston
Neurobiology and Anatomy
University of Texas
Houston, TX
USA

CHRISTOPH AUFENBERG
Functional Neurosurgery
Neurosurgical Clinic
University Hospital
Zürich
Switzerland

BEATE AVERBECK
Sanofi–Aventis Deutschland GmbH
Frankfurt
Germany
beate.averbeck@sanofi-aventis.com

QASIM AZIZ
Section of GI Sciences
Hope Hospital
University of Manchester
Salford
UK

F. W. BACH
Danish Pain Research Center and
Department of Neurology
Aarhus University Hospital
Aarhus
Denmark

S. K. BACK
Medical Science Research Center and Department of
Physiology
Korea University College of Medicine
Seoul
Korea

MISHA-MIROSLAV BACKONJA
Department of Neurology
University of Wisconsin-Madison
Madison, WI
USA
backonja@neurology.wisc.edu

CARSTEN BANTEL
Magill Department of Anaesthetics
Chelsea and Westminster Campus
Imperial College of Science
Technology and Medicine
London
UK
c.bantel@imperial.ac.uk

ALEX BARLING
Department of Neurology
Birmingham Muscle and Nerve Centre
Queen Elizabeth Hospital
Birmingham
UK
corisanderoad@aol.com

RALF BARON
Department of Neurological Pain Research and
Therapy
Department of Neurology
Christian Albrechts University Kiel
Kiel
Germany
r.baron@neurologie.uni-kiel.de

GORDON A. BARR
Department of Psychology
Hunter College
Graduate Center
City University of New York
and
Department of Developmental Psychobiology
New York State Psychiatric Institute
Department of Psychiatry
Medical Center
Columbia University
New York, NY
USA
gbarr@hunter.cuny.edu

JEFFREY R. BASFORD
Department of Physical Medicine and Rehabilitation
Mayo Clinic and Mayo Foundation
Rochester, MN
USA
basford.jeffrey@mayo.edu

HEINZ-DIETER BASLER
Institute of Medical Psychology
University of Marburg
Marburg
Germany
basler@med.uni-marburg.de

MICHELE C. BATTIÉ
Department of Physical Therapy
University of Alberta
Edmonton, AB
Canada
michele.critesbattie@ualberta.ca

ULF BAUMGÄRTNER
Institute of Physiology and Pathophysiology
Johannes Gutenberg University
Mainz
Germany

JOLENE D. BEAN-LIJEWSKI
Department of Anesthesiology
Scott and White Memorial Hospital
Temple, TX
USA
jbean-lijewski@swmail.sw.org

ALAIN BEAUDET
Montreal Neurological Institute
McGill University
Montreal, QC
Canada
abeaudet@frsq.gouv.gc.ca

LINO BECERRA
Brain Imaging Center
McLean Hospital-Harvard Medical School
Belmont, MA
USA
lbecerra@mclean.harvard.edu

YAAKOV BEILIN
Department of Anesthesiology and Obstetrics
Gynecology and Reproductive Sciences
Mount Sinai School of Medicine
New York, NY
USA
yaakov.beilin@mountsinai.org

ALVIN J. BEITZ
Department of Veterinary and Biomedical Sciences
University of Minnesota
St. Paul, MN
USA
beitz001@tc.umn.edu

MILES J. BELGRADE
Fairview Pain & Palliative Care
University of Minnesota Medical Center
and
Department of Neurology
University of Minnesota Medical School
Minneapolis, MN
USA
mbelgra1@fairview.org

CARLO VALERIO BELLIENI
Neonatal Intensive Care Unit
University Hospital
Siena
Italy
bellieni@iol.it

CARLOS BELMONTE
Instituto de Neurociencias de Alicante
Universidad Miguel Hernández-CSIC
San Juan de Alicante
Spain
carlos.belmonte@umh.es

ALLAN J. BELZBERG
Department of Neurosurgery
Johns Hopkins School of Medicine
Baltimore, MD
USA
abelzber@jhmi.edu

FABRIZIO BENEDETTI
Department of Neuroscience
Clinical and Applied Physiology Program
University of Turin Medical School
Turin
Italy
fabrizio.benedetti@unito.it

ROBERT BENNETT
Department of Medicine
Oregon Health and Science University
Portland, OR
USA
bennetrob1@comcast.net

DAVID BENNETT
Department of Neurology
King's College Hospital
London
UK
dlhbennett@talk21.com

MAURICE F. BENSIGNOR
Centre Catherine de Sienne
Reze
France
dr.ben@wanadoo.fr

EDWARD BENZEL
The Cleveland Clinic Foundation
Department of Neurosurgery
Cleveland Clinic Spine Institute
Cleveland, OH
USA
benzele@ccf.org

DAVID A. BEREITER
Department of Surgery
Brown Medical School
Providence, RI
USA
david_bereiter@brown.edu

ELMAR BERENDES
Clinic and Policlinic for Anaesthesiology and
operative Intensive Medicine
University Hospital Münster
Münster
Germany
berendes@klinikum-krefeld.de

KAREN J. BERKLEY
Program in Neuroscience
Florida State University
Tallahassee, FL
USA
kberkley@darwin.psy.fsu.edu

PETER BERLIT
Department of Neurology
Alfried Krupp Hospital
Essen
Germany
peter.berlit@krupp-krankenhaus.de

JEAN-FRANÇOIS BERNARD
Faculté de Médecine Pitié-Salpêtrière
Institut National de la Santé et de la Recherche
Médicale
INSERM U-677
Paris
France
jfbernar@ext.jussieu.fr

ANNE KJØRSVIK BERTELSEN
Department of Neurology
Haukeland University Hospital
Bergen
Norway
anne.kjorsvik@biomed.uib.no

MARCELO E. BIGAL
Department of Neurology
Albert Einstein College of Medicine
Bronx, NY
and
The New England Center for Headache
Stamford, CT
and
Montefiore Headache Unit,
Bronx, NY
USA

YITZCHAK M. BINIK
McGill University
Montreal, QC
Canada
binik@ego.psych.mcgill.ca

NIELS BIRBAUMER
Institute of Medical Psychology and Behavioral
Neurobiology
University of Tübingen
Tübingen
Germany
niels.birbaumer@uni-tuebingen.de

FRANK BIRKLEIN
Department of Neurology
University of Mainz
Mainz
Germany
birklein@neurologie.klinik.uni-mainz.de

THOMAS BISHOP
Centre for Neuroscience
King's College London
London
UK
thomas.bishop@kcl.ac.uk

HENNING BLIDDAL
The Parker Institute
Frederiksberg Hospital
Copenhagen
Denmark
hb@fh.hosp.dk

RONALD H. BLUM
Beth Israel Medical Center
New York, NY
USA
rblum@bethisraelny.org

JAMES A. BLUNK
Clinic for Anaesthesiology
University of Erlangen
Erlangen
Germany
blunk@physiologie1.uni-erlangen.de

NIKOLAI BOGDUK
Department of Clinical Research
Royal Newcastle Hospital
Newcastle, NSW
Australia
michelle.gillam@newcastle.edu.au

JÖRGEN BOIVIE
Department of Neurology
University Hospital
Linköping
Sweden
jorgen.boivie@lio.se

SIR MICHAEL R. BOND
University of Glasgow
Glasgow
UK
m.bond@admin.gla.ac.uk

RICHARD L. BOORTZ-MARX
Department of Neurosciences
Gundersen Lutheran Health Care System
La Crosse, WI
USA
rlboortz@gundluth.org

JAMES M. BOROWCZYK
Department of Orthopaedics and Musculoskeletal
Medicine
Christchurch Public Hospital
Christchurch Clinical School of Medicine and Health
Sciences
Christchurch
New Zealand
jmbor@clear.net.nz

DAVID BORSOOK
Brain Imaging Center
McLean Hospital-Harvard Medical School
Belmont, MA
USA

GEORGE S. BORSZCZ
Department of Psychology
Wayne State University
Detroit, MI
USA
borszcz@wayne.edu

JASENKA BORZAN
Department of Anesthesiology and
Critical Care Medicine
Johns Hopkins University
Baltimore, MD
USA
jborzan1@jhmi.edu

REGINA M. BOTTING
The William Harvey Research Institute
The John Vane Science Centre
Queen Mary University of London
St Bartholomew's and the London School of
Medicine and Dentistry
London
UK
r.m.botting@qmul.ac.uk

DAVID BOWSHER
Pain Research Institute
University Hospital Aintree
Liverpool
UK
pri@liv.ac.uk or bowsher@liv.ac.uk

EMMA L. BRANDON
Royal Perth Hospital and
University of Western Australia
Crawley, WA
Australia

HARALD BREIVIK
Rikshospitalet University Hospital
Rikshospitalet
Norway
harald.breivik@klinmed.uio.no

CHRISTOPHER R. BRIGHAM
Brigham and Associates Inc.
Portland, OR
USA
cbrigham@brighamassociates.com

STEPHEN C. BROWN
Department of Anesthesia
Divisional Centre of Pain Management and Pain
Research
The Hospital for Sick Children
Toronto, ON
Canada
stephen.brown@sickkids.ca

JEFFREY A. BROWN
Department of Neurological Surgery
Wayne State University
School of Medicine
Detroit and Neurological Surgery
NY, USA
jbrown@neurosurgery.wayne.edu

EDUARDO BRUERA
Department of Palliative Care and Rehabilitation
Medicine
The University of Texas M. D. Anderson Cancer
Center
Houston, TX
USA
ebruera@mdanderson.org

PABLO BRUMOVSKY
Department of Neuroscience
Karolinska Institute
Stockholm
Sweden
and
Neuroscience Laboratory
Austral University
Buenos Aires
Argentina

KAY BRUNE
Institute for Experimental and Clinical Pharmacology
and Toxicology
Friedrich Alexander University Erlangen-Nürnberg
Erlangen
Germany
kay.brune@pharmakologie.uni-erlangen.de

MARIA BURIAN
Pharmacological Center Frankfurt
Clinical Center Johann-Wolfgang Goethe University
Frankfurt
Germany
burian@em.uni-frankfurt.de

RICHARD BURSTAL
John Hunter Royal Hospital
Newcastle, NSW
Australia
richard.burstal@hnehealth.nsw.gov.au

DAN BUSKILA
Rheumatic Disease Unit
Faculty of Health Sciences
Soroka Medical Center
Ben Gurion University
Beer Sheva
Israel
dbuskila@bgumail.bgu.ac.il

CATHERINE M. CAHILL
Queen's University
Kingston, ON
Canada
cahillc@post.queensu.ca

BRIAN E. CAIRNS
Faculty of Pharmaceutical Sciences
University of British Columbia
Vancouver, BC
Canada
brcairns@interchange.ubc.ca

NIGEL A. CALCUTT
Department of Pathology
University of California San Diego
La Jolla, CA
USA
ncalcutt@ucsd.edu

KATHARINE ANDREWS CAMPBELL
Department of Anatomy and Developmental Biology
University College London
London
UK
k.campbell@ich.ucl.ac.uk

JAMES N. CAMPBELL
Department of Neurosurgery
The Johns Hopkins University School of Medicine
Baltimore, MD
USA
jcampbel@jhmi.edu

ADAM CARINCI
Department of Anesthesiology and Critical Care
Medicine
The Johns Hopkins University School of Medicine
Baltimore, MD
USA

GIANCARLO CARLI
Department of Physiology
University of Siena
Siena
Italy
carlig@unisi.it

CHRISTER P.O. CARLSSON
Rehabilitation Department
Lunds University Hosptial
Lund
Sweden
akusyd@swipnet.se

SUSAN M. CARLTON
Marine Biomedical Institute
University of Texas Medical Branch
Galveston, TX
USA
smcarlto@utmb.edu

KENNETH L. CASEY
Department of Neurology
University of Michigan
and
Neurology Research Laboratory
VA Medical Center
Ann Arbor, MI
USA
kencasey@umich.edu

CHRISTINE T. CHAMBERS
Departments of Pediatrics and Psychology
Dalhousie University and IWK Health Centre
Halifax, NS
Canada
christine.chambers@dal.ca

SANDRA CHAPLAN
Johnson & Johnson Pharmaceutical Research &
Development
San Diego, CA
USA
schaplan@prius.jnj.com

C. RICHARD CHAPMAN
Pain Research Center
Department of Anesthesiology
University of Utah School of Medicine
Salt Lake City, UT
USA
crc20@utah.edu

SANTOSH K. CHATURVEDI
National Institute of Mental Health & Neurosciences
Bangalore
India
chatur@nimhans.kar.nic.in

ANDREW C. N. CHEN
Human Brain Mapping and Cortical Imaging
Laboratory
Aalborg University
Aalborg
Denmark
ac@smi.auc.dk

ANDREA CHEVILLE
Department of Rehabilitation Medicine
University of Pennsylvania School of Medicine
Philadelphia, PA
USA
acheville@aol.com

NAOMI L. CHILLINGWORTH
Department of Physiology
School of Medical Sciences
University of Bristol
Bristol
UK

CATHERINE CHO
Clinical Neurophysiology Laboratories
Mount Sinai Medical Center
New York, NY
USA

EDWARD CHOW
Toronto Sunnybrook Regional Cancer Center
University of Toronto
Toronto, ON
Canada
edward.chow@sw.ca

JULIE A. CHRISTIANSON
University of Pittsburgh
Pittsburgh, PA
USA
jcc26+@pitt.edu

MACDONALD J. CHRISTIE
Pain Management Research Institute and Kolling
Institute
University of Sydney
Sydney, NSW
Australia
macc@med.usyd.edu.au

KYUNGSOON CHUNG
Department of Neuroscience and Cell Biology
University of Texas Medical Branch
Galveston, TX
USA
kchung@utmb.edu

JIN MO CHUNG
Department of Neuroscience and Cell Biology
University of Texas Medical Branch
Galveston, TX
USA
jmchung@utmb.edu

W. CRAWFORD CLARK
College of Physicians and Surgeons, Columbia
University
New York, NY
USA
USAclarkcr@pi.cpmc.columbia.edu

JUDY CLARKE
Institute for Work & Health
Toronto, ON
Canada
jclarke@iwh.on.ca

JAMES F. CLEARY
University of Wisconsin Comprehensive Cancer
Center
Madison, WI
USA
jfcleary@wisc.edu

CHARLES S. CLEELAND
The University of Texas M. D.
Anderson Cancer Center
Houston, TX
USA
ccleeland@mdanderson.org

JOHN DE CLERCQ
Department of Rehabilitation Sciences and
Physiotherapy
Ghent University Hospital
Ghent
Belgium

TERENCE J. CODERRE
Department of Anesthesia
Neurology, Neurosurgery and Psychology
McGill University
Montreal, QC
Canada
terence.coderre@mcgill.ca

ROBERT C. COGHILL
Department of Neurobiology and Anatomy
Wake Forest University School of Medicine
Winston-Salem, NC
USA
rcoghill@wfubmc.edu

ALAN L. COLLEDGE
Utah Labor Commission
International Association of Industrial Accident
Boards and Commissions
Salt Lake City, UT
USA
farmboyac@msn.com

BEVERLY J. COLLETT
University Hospitals of Leicester
Leicester
UK
beverly.collett@uhl.tr-nhs.uk

LESLEY A. COLVIN
Department of Anaesthesia
Critical Care and Pain Medicine
Western General Hospital
Edinburgh
UK
lesley.colvin@ed.ac.uk

KEVIN C. CONLON
Trinity College Dublin
University of Dublin
and
The Adelaide and Meath Hospital incorporating
The National Children's Hospital
Dublin
Ireland
profsurg@tcd.ie

BRIAN Y. COOPER
Department of Oral and Maxillofacial Surgery
University of Florida
Gainesville, FL
USA
bcooper@dental.ufl.edu

CHRISTINE CORDLE
University Hospitals of Leicester
Leicester
UK

MICHAEL J. COUSINS
Department of Anesthesia and Pain Management
Royal North Shore Hospital
University of Sydney
St. Leonards, NSW
Australia
mcousins@nsccahs.health.nsw.gov.au

VERNE C. COX
Department of Psychology
University of Texas at Arlington
Arlington, TX
USA

REBECCA M. CRAFT
Washington State University
Pullman, WA
USA
craft@wsu.edu

KENNETH D. CRAIG
Department of Psychology
University of British Columbia
Vancouver, BC
Canada
kcraig@psych.ubc.ca

GEERT CROMBEZ
Department of Experimental Clinical and
Health Psychology
Ghent University
Ghent
Belgium
geert.crombez@ugent.be

JOAN CROOK
Hamilton Health Sciences Corporation
Hamilton, ON
Canada

GIORGIO CRUCCU
Department of Neurological Sciences
La Sapienza University
Rome
Italy
cruccu@uniroma1.it

MICHELE CURATOLO
Department of Anesthesiology
Division of Pain Therapy
University Hospital of Bern
Inselspital
Bern
Switzerland
michele.curatolo@insel.ch

F. MICHAEL CUTRER
Department of Neurology
Mayo Clinic
Rochester, MN
USA
cutrer.michael@mayo.edu

NACHUM DAFNY
Health Science Center at Houston
Neurobiology and Anatomy
University of Texas
Houston, TX
USA
nachum.dafny@uth.tmc.edu

JØRGEN B. DAHL
Department of Anaesthesiology
Glostrup University Hospital
Herlev
Denmark
jbdahl@dadlnet.dk

YI DAI
Department of Anatomy and Neuroscience
Hyogo College of Medicine
Hyogo
Japan

STEFAAN VAN DAMME
Department of Experimental Clinical and
Health Psychology
Ghent University
Ghent
Belgium
stefaan.vandamme@ugent.be

ALEXANDRE F. M. DASILVA
Martinos Center for Biomedical Imaging
Massachusetts General Hospital
Harvard Medical School
Charlestown, MA
USA
alexandr@nmr.mgh.harvard.edu

BRIAN DAVIS
University of Pittsburgh
Pittsburgh, PA
USA
davisb@dom.pitt.edu

KAREN D. DAVIS
University of Toronto and the
Toronto Western Research Institute
University Health Network
Toronto, ON
Canada
kdavis@uhnres.utoronto.ca

RICHARD O. DAY
Department of Physiology and Pharmacology
School of Medical Sciences
University of New South Wales
and
Department of Clinical Pharmacology
St Vincent's Hospital
Sydney, NSW
Australia
r.day@unsw.edu.au

ISABELLE DECOSTERD
Anesthesiology Pain Research Group
Department of Anesthesiology
University Hospital (CHUV) and Department
of Cell Biology and Morphology
Lausanne University
Lausanne
Switzerland
isabelle.decosterd@chuv.ch

JOYCE A. DELEO
Dartmouth Hitchcock Medical Center
Dartmouth Medical School
Lebanon, NH
USA
joyce.a.deleo@dartmouth.edu

A. LEE DELLON
Johns Hopkins University
Baltimore, MD
USA
aldellon@starpower.net

MARSHALL DEVOR
Institute of Life Sciences and
Center for Research on Pain
Hebrew University of Jerusalem
Jerusalem
Israel
marshlu@vms.huji.ac.il

DAVID DIAMANT
Neurological and Spinal Surgery
Lincoln, NE
USA
ddiamant@neb.rr.com

ANTHONY H. DICKENSON
Department of Pharmacology
University College London
London
UK
anthony.dickenson@ucl.ac.uk

HANS-CHRISTOPH DIENER
Department of Neurology
University Hospital of Essen
Essen
Germany
h.diener@uni-essen.de

ADAM VAN DIJK
Department of Anesthesiology
Queen's University
Kingston General Hospital
Kingston, ON
Canada

NATALIA DMITRIEVA
Program in Neuroscience
Florida State University
Tallahassee, FL
USA
dmitrieva@darwin.psy.fsu.edu

REGINALD J. DOCHERTY
Wolfson Centre for Age-Related Diseases
King's College London
London
UK
reginald.docherty@kcl.ac.uk

LUCY F. DONALDSON
Department of Physiology
School of Medical Sciences
University of Bristol
Bristol
UK
lucy.donaldson@bris.ac.uk

HENRI DOODS
CNS Pharmacology
Pain Research
Boehringer Ingelheim Pharma GmbH & Co.
KG
Biberach/Riss
Germany

VICTORIA DORF
Social Security Administration
Baltimore, MD
USA
victoria.dorf@ssa.gov

MICHAEL J. DORSI
Department of Neurosurgery
Johns Hopkins School of Medicine
Baltimore, MD
USA

JONATHAN O. DOSTROVSKY
Department of Physiology
Faculty of Medicine
University of Toronto
Toronto, ON
Canada
j.dostrovsky@utoronto.ca

PAUL DREYFUSS
Department of Rehabilitation Medicine
University of Washington
Seattle, WA
USA
pauldspine@aol.com

PETER D. DRUMMOND
School of Psychology
Murdoch University
Perth, WA
Australia
p.drummond@murdoch.edu.au

RONALD DUBNER
University of Maryland
Department of Biomedical Sciences
Baltimore, MD
USA
rdubner@umaryland.edu

ANNE DUCROS
Headache Emergency Department and
Institute National de la Santé et de la Recherche
Médicale (INSERM)
Faculté de Médecine Lariboisière
Lariboisière Hospital
Paris
France
anne.ducros@lrb.ap-hop-paris.fr

GARY DUNCAN
Department of Psychology
McGill University
Montreal, QC
Canada

MARY J. EATON
Miller School of Medicine
University of Miami
Miami, FL
USA
meaton@miami.edu

ANDREA EBERSBERGER
Department of Physiology
Friedrich Schiller University of Jena
Jena
Germany
andrea.ebersberger@mti.uni-jena.de

CHRISTOPHER ECCLESTON
Pain Management Unit
University of Bath
Bath
UK
c.eccleston@bath.ac.uk

JOHN EDMEADS
Sunnybrook and Woman's College Health
Sciences Centre
University of Toronto
Toronto, ON
Canada
john.edmeads@sw.ca

ROBERT R. EDWARDS
Department of Psychiatry and Behavioral Sciences
The Johns Hopkins University School of Medicine
Baltimore, MD
USA
redwar10@jhmi.edu

EVAN R. EISENBERG
Department of Urology
Long Island Jewish Medical Center
New York, NY
USA

JANET W. M. ELLIS
Department of Anaesthesia
Divisional Centre for Pain Management
and
Pain Research
The Hospital for Sick Children
Toronto, ON
Canada
joostjanet@rogers.com

JOYCE M. ENGEL
Department of Rehabilitation Medicine
University of Washington
Seattle, WA
USA
knowles@u.washington.edu

MATTHEW ENNIS
Deptartment of Anatomy and Neurobiology
University of Tennessee Health Science Center
Memphis, TN
USA
mennis@utmem.edu

EDZARD ERNST
Complementary Medicine
Peninsula Medical School
Universities of Exeter and Plymouth
Exeter
UK
edzard.ernst@pms.ac.uk

LYDIA ESTANISLAO
Clinical Neurophysiology Laboratories
Mount Sinai Medical Center
New York, NY
USA

THOMAS EWERT
Department of Physical Medicine and Rehabilitation
Ludwig-Maximilians University
Munich
Germany

KERI L. FAKATA
College of Pharmacy and Pain Management Center
University of Utah
Salt Lake City, UT
USA
keri.fakata@hsc.utah.edu

MARIE FALLON
Department of Oncology
Edinburgh Cancer Center
University of Edinburgh
Edinburgh
Scotland
marie.fallon@ed.ac.uk

GILBERT J. FANCIULLO
Pain Management Center
Dartmouth-Hitchcock Medical Center
Lebanon, NH
USA
gilbert.j.fanciullo@hitchcock.org

ANDREW J. FARACI
Virginia Mason Medical Center
Seattle, WA
USA

CHARLOTTE FEINMANN
Eastman Dental Institute and Department if
Psychiatry and Behavioural Sciences
University College London
London
UK
rejucfe@ucl.ac.uk

ELIZABETH ROY FELIX
The Miami Project to Cure Paralysis
University of Miami Miller School of Medicine
Miami, FL
USA
efelix@miamiproject.med.miami.edu

YI FENG
Department of Anesthesiology
Peking University People's Hospital
Peking
P. R. China
yifeng65@263.net

ANDRES FERNANDEZ
Departments of Neurosurgery
Johns Hopkins University
Baltimore, MD
USA

ANTONIO VICENTE FERRER-MONTIEL
Institute of Molecular and Cell Biology
University Miguel Hernández
Elche
Alicante
Spain
aferrer@umh.es

MICHAEL FEUERSTEIN
Department of Medical and Clinical Psychology
Uniformed Services University of the Health
Sciences
Bethesda, MD
and
Department of Preventive Medicine & Biometrics
USUHS
Bethesda, MD
and
Georgetown University Medical Center
Washington, DC
USA
mfeuerstein@usuhs.mil

VERONIKA FIALKA-MOSER
Department of Physical Medicine and Rehabilitation
University Vienna
Vienna
Austria
Pmr.office@meduniwien.ac.at

PERRY G. FINE
Pain Management and Research Center
University of Utah
Salt Lake City, UT
USA
fine@aros.net

DAVID J. FINK
Department of Neurology
University of Michigan and VA Ann Arbor
Healthcare System
Ann Arbor, MI
USA
dfink@pitt.edu

NANNA BRIX FINNERUP
Department of Neurology and
Danish Pain Research Centre
Aarhus University Hospital
Aarhus
Denmark
finnerup@ki.au.dk

DAVID A. FISHBAIN
Department of Psychiatry and Department of
Neurological Surgery and Anesthesiology
University of Miami
School of Medicine and H. Rosomoff Pain
Center at South Shore Hospital
Miami, FL
USA
dfishbain@miami.edu

PER FLISBERG
Royal Perth Hospital
University of Western Australia
Perth, WA
Australia

HERTA FLOR
Department of Clinical and Cognitive Neuroscience
University of Heidelberg
Central Institute of Mental Health
Mannheim
Germany
flor@zi-mannheim.de

CHRISTOPHER M. FLORES
Drug Discovery
Johnson and Johnson Pharmaceutical Research and
Development
Spring House, PA
USA

WILBERT E. FORDYCE
Department of Rehabilitation
University of Washington School of Medicine
Seattle, WA
USA
wfordyce@msn.com

ROBERT D. FOREMAN
University of Oklahoma Health Sciences Center
Oklahoma City, OK
USA
robert-foreman@ouhsc.edu

GARY M. FRANKLIN
Department of Environmental and Occupational
Health Sciences
University of Washington
Seattle, WA
and
Washington State Department of Labor and Industries
Olympia, WA
USA
meddir@u.washington.edu

JAN FRIDÉN
Department of Hand Surgery
Sahlgrenska University Hospital
Göteborg
Sweden
jan.friden@orthop.gu.se

ALLAN H. FRIEDMAN
Division of Neurosurgery
Duke University Medical Center
Durham, NC
USA

PERRY N. FUCHS
Department of Psychology
University of Texas at Arlington
Arlington, TX
USA
fuchs@uta.edu

DEBORAH FULTON-KEHOE
Department of Health Services
University of Washington
Seattle, WA
USA

ARNAUD FUMAL
Departments of Neurology and Neuroanatomy
University of Liège
CHR Citadelle
Liege
Belgium

ANDREA D. FURLAN
Institute for Work & Health
Toronto, ON
Canada

VASCO GALHARDO
Institute of Histology and Embryology
Faculty of Medicine of Porto
University of Porto
Porto
Portugal
galhardo@med.up.pt

ANDREAS R. GANTENBEIN
Headache & Pain Unit
University Hospital Zurich
Zurich
Switzerland
andy.gantenbein@gmx.ch

ELVIRA DE LA PEÑA GARCÍA
Instituto de Neurociencias
Universidad Miguel Hernández-CSIC
Alicante
Spain
elvirap@umh.es

I. Garonzik
Johns Hopkins Medical Institutions
Department of Neurosurgery
Baltimore, MD
USA

Robert Gassin
Musculoskeletal Medicine Clinic
Frankston, VIC
Australia
rgassin@pen.hotkey.net.au

Robert J. Gatchel
Department of Psychology
College of Science
University of Texas at Arlington
Airlington, TX
USA
gatchel@uta.edu

Gerald F. Gebhart
Department of Pharmacology
University of Iowa
Iowa City, IA
USA
gf-gebhart@uiowa.edu

Gerd Geisslinger
Institute for Clinical Pharmacology
pharmazentrum frankfurt/ZAFES
Clinical Centre of the Johann Wolfgang Goethe
University Frankfurt am Main
Frankfurt
Germany
geisslinger@em.uni-frankfurt.de

Robert D. Gerwin
Department of Neurology
Johns Hopkins University
Bethesda, MD
USA
gerwin@painpoints.com

Maria Adele Giamberardino
Dipartimento di Medicina e Scienze
dell'Invecchiamento
University of Chieti
Chieti
Italy
mag@unich.it

Glenn J. Giesler Jr
Department of Neuroscience
University of Minnesota
Minneapolis, MN
USA
giesler@mail.ahc.umn.edu

Philip L. Gildenberg
Baylor Medical College
Houston, TX
USA
hsc@stereotactic.net

Myra Glajchen
Department of Pain Medicine and Palliative Care
Beth Israel Medical Center
New York, NY
USA
mglajchen@bethisraelny.org

Peter J. Goadsby
Institute of Neurology
The National Hospital for Neurology and
Neurosurgery
London
UK
peterg@ion.ucl.ac.uk

Hartmut Göbel
Kiel Pain Center
Kiel
Germany
hg@schmerzklinik.de

Philippe Goffaux
Faculty of Medicine
Neurochirurgy
University of Sherbrooke
Sherbrooke, QC
Canada
philippe.goffaux@chus.qc.ca

Ana Gomis
Instituto de Neurociencias de Alicante
Universidad Miguel Hernandez-CSIC
San Juan de Alicante
Spain
agomis@umh.es

Vivekananda Gonugunta
The Cleveland Clinic Foundation
Department of Neurosurgery
Cleveland, OH
USA

Gilbert R. Gonzales
Department of Neurology
Memorial Sloan-Kettering Cancer Center
New York, NY
USA

ALLAN GORDON
Wasser Pain Management Centre
Mount Sinai Hospital
University of Toronto
Toronto, ON
Canada
allan.gordon@utoronto.ca

LIESBET GOUBERT
Ghent University
Department of Experimental Clinical and
Health Psychology
Ghent
Belgium
liesbet.goubert@ugent.be

JAYANTILAL GOVIND
Pain Clinic
Department of Anaesthesia
University of New South Wales
Sydney, NSW
Australia
jaygovind@bigpond.com

RICHARD H. GRACELY
Ann Arbor Veterans Administration Medical Center
Departments of Medicine-Rheumatology and
Neurology
and Chronic Pain and Fatigue Research Center
University of Michigan Health System
Ann Arbor, MI
USA
rgracely@umich.edu

GARRY G. GRAHAM
Department of Physiology and Pharmacology
School of Medical Sciences
University of New South Wales
and
Department of Clinical Pharmacology
St. Vincent's Hospital
Sydney, NSW
Australia
ggraham@stvincents.com.au

DAVID K. GRANDY
Department of Physiology and Pharmacology
School of Medicine
Oregon Health and Science University
Portland, OR
USA
grandyd@ohsu.edu

THOMAS GRAVEN-NIELSEN
Laboratory for Experimental Pain Research
Center for Sensory-Motor Interaction (SMI)
Aalborg University
Denmark
tgn@hst.aau.dk

BARRY GREEN
Pierce Laboratory
Yale School of Medicine
New Haven, CT
USA
green@jbpierce.org

PAUL G. GREEN
NIH Pain Center (UCSF)
University of California
San Francisco, CA
USA
paul@itsa.ucsf.edu

JOEL D. GREENSPAN
Department of Biomedical Sciences
University of Maryland Dental School
Baltimore, MD
USA
jgreenspan@umaryland.edu

JOHN W. GRIFFIN
Department of Neurology
Departments of Neuroscience and Pathology
The Johns Hopkins University School of Medicine
Johns Hopkins Hospital
Baltimore, MD
USA
jgriffi@jhmi.edu

SABINE GRÖSCH
Pharmacological Center Frankfurt
Clinical Center Johann-Wolfgang Goethe University
Frankfurt
Germany
groesch@em.uni-frankfurt.de

DOUGLAS P. GROSS
Department of Physical Therapy
University of Alberta
Edmonton, AB
Australia
doug.gross@ualberta.ca

BLAIR D. GRUBB
Department of Cell Physiology and Pharmacology
University of Leicester
Leicester
UK
bdg1@leicester.ac.uk

RUTH ECKSTEIN GRUNAU
Centre for Community Child Health Research
Child and Family Research Institute
and
University of British Columbia
Vancouver, BC
Canada
rgrunau@cw.bc.ca

MICHEL GUERINEAU
Neurosurgery
Hotel Dieu
Nantes Cedex 1
France

CHRISTOPH GUTENBRUNNER
Department of Physical Medicine and Rehabilitation
Hanover Medical School
Hanover
Germany
gutenbrunner.christoph@mh-hannover.de

MAIJA HAANPÄÄ
Department of Anaesthesiology and Department of
Neurosurgery
Pain Clinic
Helsinki University Hospital
Helsinki
Finland

UTE HABEL
RWTH Aachen University
Department of Psychiatry and Psychotherapy
Aachen
Germany
uhabel@ukaachen.de

HEINZ-JOACHIM HÄBLER
FH Bonn-Rhein-Sieg
Rheinbach
Germany
heinz-joachim.haebler@fh-bonn-rhein-sieg.de

THOMAS HACHENBERG
Clinic for Anaesthesiology and Intensive Therapy
Otto-von-Guericke University
Magdeburg
Germany

NOUCHINE HADJIKHANI
Martinos Center for Biomedical Imaging
Massachusetts General Hospital
Harvard Medical School
Charlestown, MA
USA
nouchine@nmr.mgh.harvard.edu

OLE HAEGG
Department of Orthopedic Surgery
Sahlgren University Hospital
Goteborg
Sweden
ollehagg@hotmail.com

BRYAN C. HAINS
The Center for Neuroscience and Regeneration
Research
Department of Neurology
Yale University School of Medicine
West Haven, CT
USA
bryan.hains@yale.edu

DARRYL T. HAMAMOTO
University of Minnesota
Minneapolis, MN
USA

DONNA L. HAMMOND
Department of Anesthesiology
University of Iowa
Iowa, IA
USA
donna-hammond@uiowa.edu

H. C. HAN
Medical Science Research Center and
Department of Physiology
Korea University College of Medicine
Seoul
Korea

HERMANN O. HANDWERKER
Department of Physiology and Pathophysiology
University of Erlangen/Nürnberg
Erlangen
Germany
handwerker@physiologie1.uni-erlangen.de

JING-XIA HAO
Karolinska Institute
Stockholm
Sweden

ELENI G. HAPIDOU
Department of Psychiatry and
Behavioural Neurosciences
McMaster University and Hamilton Health Sciences
Hamilton, ON
Canada
hapidou@hhsc.ca

GEOFFREY HARDING
Sandgate, QLD
Australia
geoffharding@uq.net.au

LOUISE HARDING
Hospitals NHS Foundation Trust
University College London
London
UK
louise.harding@uclh.org

KENNETH M. HARGREAVES
Department of Endodontics
University of Texas Health Science Center
at San Antonio
San Antonio, TX
USA
hargreaves@uthscsa.edu

SARAH J. HARPER
Royal Perth Hospital and
University of Western Australia
Perth, WA
Australia

D. PAUL HARRIES
Pain Care Center
Samaritan Hospital Lexington
Lexington, KY
USA
pharries@kypain.com

S. E. HARTE
Department of Internal Medicine
Chronic Pain and Fatigue Research Center
Rheumatology University of Michigan Health System
Ann Arbor, MI
USA
seharte@umich.edu

SAMUEL J. HASSENBUSCH
The University of Texas M. D. Anderson Cancer
Center
Houston, TX
USA
samuel@neosoft.com

BRIDGET E. HAWKINS
Department of Anatomy and Neurosciences
University of Texas Medical Branch
Galveston, TX
USA
behawkin@utmb.edu

JENNIFER A. HAYTHORNTHWAITE
Johns Hopkins University
Baltimore, MD
USA
jhaytho1@jhmi.edu

JOHN H. HEALEY
Memorial Sloan Kettering Cancer Center and
Weill Medical College of Cornell University
New York, NY
USA
healeyj@mskcc.org

ALICIA A. HEAPY
VA Connecticut Healthcare System and Yale
University
Westhaven, CT
USA
alicia.heapy@va.gov

ANNE M. HEFFERNAN
The Adelaide and Meath Hospital incorporating
The National Children's Hospital
Dublin
Ireland

MARY M. HEINRICHER
Department of Neurological Surgery
Oregon Health Science University
Portland, OR
USA
heinricm@ohsu.edu

ROBERT D. HELME
Centre for Pain Management
St Vincent's Hospital
Melbourne, VIC
Australia
rhelme@bigpond.net.au

ROBERT D. HERBERT
School of Physiotherapy
University of Sydney
Sydney, NSW
Australia
r.herbert@fhs.usyd.edu.au

CHRISTIANE HERMANN
Department of Clinical and Cognitive Neuroscience
at the University of Heidelberg
Central Institute of Mental Health
Mannheim
Germany
chermann@zi-mannheim.de

JUAN F. HERRERO
Department of Physiology
Edificio de Medicina
University of Alcalá
Madrid
Spain
juanf.herrero@uah.es

AKI J. HIETAHARJU
Department of Neurology and Rehabilitation
Pain Clinic
Tampere University Hospital
Tampere
Finland
aki.hietaharju@pshp.fi

KARIN N. WESTLUND HIGH
Department of Neuroscience and Cell Biology
University of Texas Medical Branch
Galveston, TX
USA
kwhigh@utmb.edu

MARITA HILLIGES
Halmstad University
Halmstad
Sweden
marita.hilliges@set.hh.se

MAX J. HILZ
University of Erlangen-Nuernberg
Erlangen
Germany
max.hilz@neuro.imed.uni-erlangen.de

BURKHARD HINZ
Department of Experimental and Clinical
Pharmacology and Toxicology
Friedrich Alexander University Erlangen-Nürnberg
Erlangen
Germany
hinz@pharmakologie.uni-erlangen.de

ANTHONY R. HOBSON
Section of GI Sciences
Hope Hospital
University of Manchester
Salford
UK
ahobson@fs1.ho.man.ac.uk

TOMAS HÖKFELT
Department of Neuroscience
Karolinska Institutet
Stockholm
Sweden
tomas.hokfelt@neuro.ki.se

ANITA HOLDCROFT
Imperial College London
London
UK
aholdcro@imperial.ac.uk

SARAH V. HOLDRIDGE
Department of Pharmacology and Toxicology
Queen's University
Kinston, ON
Canada

KJELL HOLE
University of Bergen
Bergen
Norway
kjell.hole@fys.uib.no

GRAHAM R. HOLLAND
Department of Cariology
Restorative Sciences & Endodontics
School of Dentistry
University of Michigan
Ann Arbor, MI
USA
rholland@umich.edu

ULRIKE HOLZER-PETSCHE
Department of Experimental and Clinical
Pharmacology
Medical University of Graz
Graz
Austria
ulrike.holzer@meduni-graz.at

CHANG-ZERN HONG
Department of Physical Medicine and Rehabilitation
University of California Irvine
Irvine, CA
USA
czhong88@ms49.hinet.net

S. K. HONG
Medical Science Research Center and Department of
Physiology
Korea University College of Medicine
Seoul
Korea

MINORU HOSHIYAMA
Department of Integrative Physiology
National Institute for Physiological Sciences
Okazaki
Japan

FRED M. HOWARD
Department of Obstetrics and Gynecology
University of Rochester
Rochester, NY
USA
fred_howard@urmc.rochester.edu

SUNG-TSANG HSIEH
Department of Anatomy and Cell Biology
National Taiwan University
and
Department of Neurology
National Taiwan University Hospital
Taipei
Taiwan
sthsieh@ha.mc.ntu.edu.tw

JAMES W. HU
Faculty of Dentistry
University of Toronto
Toronto, ON
Canada
james.hu@utoronto.ca

CLAIRE E. HULSEBOSCH
Spinal Cord Injury Research
University of Texas Medical Branch
Galveston, TX
USA
cehulseb@utmb.edu

THOMAS HUMMEL
Department of Othorhinolaryngology
Smell and Taste Clinic
University of Dresden Medical School
Dresden
Germany
thummel@rcs.urz.tu-dresden.de

WALTER J. MEYER III
Department of Psychiatry and Behavioral Science
Shriners Hospitals for Children
Shriners Burns Hospital
Galveston, TX
USA
wmeyer@utmb.edu

ROSE-ANNE INDELICATO
Department of Pain and Palliative Care
Beth Israel Medical Center
New York, NY
USA

CHARLES E. INTURRISI
Department of Pharmacology
Weill Medical College of Cornell University
ceintur@med.cornell.edu

KOJI INUI
Department of Integrative Physiology
National Institute for Physiological Sciences
Okazaki
Japan

SUHAYL J. JABBUR
Neuroscience Program
Faculty of Medicine
American University of Beirut
Beirut
Lebanon

CAROL JAMES
Department of Neurological Surgery
Johns Hopkins Hospital
Baltimore, MD
USA

WILFRID JÄNIG
Institute of Physiology
Christian Albrechts University Kiel
Kiel
Germany
w.janig@physiologie.uni-kiel.de

NORA JANJAN
University of Texas M. D. Anderson Cancer Center
Houston, TX
USA

LUC JASMIN
Department of Anatomy
University of California San Francisco
San Francisco, CA
USA
ucpain@itsa.ucsf.edu

ANNE JAUMEES
Royal North Shore Hospital
St. Leonards, NSW
Australia

DANIEL JEANMONOD
Functional Neurosurgery
Neurosurgical Clinic
University Hospital
Zürich
Switzerland
daniel.jeanmonod@usz.ch

ANDREW JEFFREYS
Department of Anaesthesia
Western Health
Melbourne, NSW
Australia
andrew.jeffreys@wh.org.au

TROELS S. JENSEN
Danish Pain Research Center and
Department of Neurology
Aarhus University Hospital
Aarhus
Denmark
tsj@akhphd.au.dk

MARK P. JENSEN
Department of Rehabilitation Medicine
University of Washington
Seattle, WA
USA
mjensen@u.washington.edu

MARK JOHNSON
Musculoskeletal Physician
Hibiscus Coast Highway
Orewa
New Zealand
markjohn@ihug.co.nz

MARK I. JOHNSON
School of Health and Human Sciences
Faculty of Health
Leeds Metropolitan University
Leeds
UK
m.johnson@leedsmet.ac.uk

KURT L. JOHNSON
Department of Rehabilitation Medicine
School of Medicine
University of Washington
Seattle, WA
USA
kjohnson@u.washington.edu

MARK JOHNSTON
Musculoskeletal Physician
Hibiscus Coast Highway
Orewa
New Zealand
markjohn@ihug.co.nz

DAVID S. JONES
Division of Adolescent Medicine and Behavioral
Sciences
Vanderbilt University Medical Center
Nashville, TN
USA
david.s.jones@vanderbilt.edu

EDWARD JONES
Center for Neuroscience
University of California
Davies, CA
USA
ejones@ucdavis.edu

JEROEN R. DE JONG
Department of Rehabilitation and Department of
Medical Psychology
University of Maastricht
and
Department of Medical, Clinical and
Experimental Psychology
Maastricht University
Maastricht
The Netherlands
jdjo@smps.azm.nl

SVEN-ERIC JORDT
Department of Pharmacology
Yale University School of Medicine
New Haven, CT
USA
sven.jordt@yale.edu

ELLEN JØRUM
The Laboratory of Clinical Neurophysiology
Rikshospitalet University
Oslo
Norway
ellen.jorum@rikshospitalet.no

STEFAN JUST
CNS Pharmacology
Pain Research
Boehringer Ingelheim Pharma GmbH & Co. KG
Biberach/Riss
Germany

NOUFISSA KABLI
Department of Pharmacology and Toxicology
Queen's University
Kinston, ON
Canada

RYUSUKE KAKIGI
Department of Integrative Physiology
National Institute for Physiological Sciences
Okazaki
Japan
kakigi@nips.ac.jp

PETER C. A. KAM
Department of Anaesthesia
St. George Hospital
University of New South Wales
Kogorah, NSW
Australia
p.kam@unsw.edu.au

GIRESH KANJI
Wellington
New Zealand
dr.kanji@actrix.co.nz

Z. KARIM
Royal Perth Hospital and
University of Western Australia
Perth, WA
Australia

ZAZA KATSARAVA
Department of Neurology
University Hospital of Essen
Essen
Germany
zaza.katsarava@uni-essen.de

JOEL KATZ
Department of Psychology
McGill University
Montreal, QC
Canada

VALERIE KAYSER
NeuroPsychoPharmacologie Médecine
INSERM U677
Faculté de Medécine Pitié-Salpêtrière
Paris
France
kayser@ext.jussieu.fr

FRANCIS J. KEEFE
Pain Prevention and Treatment Research
Department of Psychiatry and Behavioral Sciences
Duke University Medical Center
Durham, NC
USA
keefe003@mc.duke.edu

LOIS J. KEHL
Department of Anesthesiology
University of Minnesota
Minneapolis, MN
USA
lois@mail.ahc.umn.edu

WILLIAM N. KELLEY
Department of Neurology
The University of Pennsylvania Medical School
Philadelphia, PA
USA

STEPHEN KENNEDY
Nuffield Department of Obstetrics and Gynaecology
University of Oxford
John Radcliffe Hospital
Oxford
UK
stephen.kennedy@obs-gyn.ox.ac.uk

ELIZABETH VAN DEN KERKHOF
Department of Community Health and Epidemiology
Queen's University
Kingston, ON
Canada
2anv1@qlink.queensu.ca

ROBERT D. KERNS
VA Connecticut Healthcare System and Yale
University
Westhaven, CT
USA
robert.kerns@med.va.gov

SANJAY KHANNA
Department of Physiology
National University of Singapore
Singapore
phsks@nus.edu.sg

KOK E. KHOR
Department of Pain Management
Prince of Wales Hospital
Randwick, NSW
Australia
kekhor@bigpond.net.au

H. J. KIM
Department of Life Science
Yonsei University Wonju Campus
Wonju
Korea

Y. I. KIM
Medical Science Research Center and Department
of Physiology
Korea University College of Medicine
Seoul
Korea

WADE KING
Department of Clinical Research
Royal Newcastle Hospital
University of Newcastle
Newcastle, NSW
Australia
wmbaking@tpg.com.au

K. L. KIRSH
Markey Cancer Center
University of Kentucky College of Medicine
Lexington, KY
USA

RICARDO J. KOMOTAR
Department of Neurological Surgery
Neurological Institute
Columbia University
New York, NY
USA

RHONDA K. KOTARINOS
Long Grove, IL
USA
rkotarinos@msn.com

KATALIN J. KOVÁCS
Department of Veterinary and Biomedical Sciences
University of Minnesota
St. Paul, MN
USA

MALGORZATA KRAJNIK
St. Elizabeth Hospice
Ipswich
Suffolk
UK

AJIT KRISHNANEY
The Cleveland Clinic Foundation
Department of Neurosurgery
Cleveland, OH
USA

GREGORY KROH
Utah Labor Commission
International Association of Industrial Accident
Boards and Commissions
Salt Lake City, UT
USA

M. M. TER KUILE
Department of Gynecology
Leiden University Medical Center
Leiden
The Netherlands

ALICE KVÅLE
Section for Physiotherapy Science
Department of Public Health and Primary
Health Care
Faculty of Medicine
University of Bergen
Bergen
Norway
alice.kvale@isf.uib.no

ANTOON F. C. DE LAAT
Department of Oral/Maxillofacial Surgery
Catholic University of Leuven
Leuven
Belgium
antoon.delaat@med.kuleuven.ac.be

JEAN-JACQUES LABAT
Neurology and Rehabilitation
Clinique Urologique
Nantes Cedex 1
France

GASTON LABRECQUE
Faculty of Pharmacy
Université Laval
Quebec City
Montreal, QC
Canada
gaston.labrecque@videotron.ca

MARCO LACERENZA
Scientific Institute San Raffaele
Pain Medicine Center
Milano
Italy

URI LADABAUM
Division of Gastroenterology
University of California
San Francisco, CA
USA
uri.ladabaum@ucsf.edu

MARIE ANDREE LAHAIE
McGill University
Montreal, QC
Canada

MIGUEL J. A. LÁINEZ-ANDRÉS
Department of Neurology
University of Valencia
Valencia
Spain
jlainez@meditex.es

TIMOTHY R. LAIR
Department of Anesthesiology
University of Vermont College of Medicine
Burlington, VT
USA

ROBERT H. LAMOTTE
Department of Anesthesiology
Yale School of Medicine
New Haven, CT
USA
robert.lamotte@yale.edu

JAMES W. LANCE
Institute of Neurological Sciences
Prince of Wales Hospital and University of
New South Wales
Sydney, NSW
Australia
jimlance@bigpond.com

ROBERT G. LARGE
The Auckland Regional Pain Service
Auckland Hospital
Auckland
New Zealand
boblarge@actrix.co.nz

ALICE A. LARSON
Department of Veterinary and Biomedical Sciences
University of Minnesota
St. Paul, MN
USA
larso011@umn.edu

PETER LAU
Department of Clinical Research
Royal Newcastle Hospital
University of Newcastle
Newcastle, NSW
Australia
petercplau@hotmail.com

STEFAN A. LAUFER
Institute of Pharmacy
Eberhard-Karls University of Tuebingen
Tuebingen
Germany
stefan.laufer@uni-tuebingen.de

GILES J. LAVIGNE
Facultés de Médecine Dentaire et de Médecine
Université de Montréal
Montréal, QC
Canada
gilles.lavigne@umontreal.ca

PETER G. LAWLOR
Our Lady's Hospice
Medical Department
Dublin
Ireland
plawlor@olh.ie

MICHEL LAZDUNSKI
Institut de Pharmacologie Moleculaire et Cellulaire
Valbonne
France

VINCENCO DI LAZZARO
FENNSI Group
National Hospital of Paraplejicos
SESCAM Finca "La Peraleda"
Toledo
Spain

MAAIKE LEEUW
Department of Medical
Clinical and Experimental Psychology
Maastricht University
Maastricht
The Netherlands
m.leeuw@dmkep.unimaas.nl

SIRI LEKNES
Pain Imaging Neuroscience (PaIN) Group
Department of Physiology, Anatomy and Genetics
and
Centre for Functional Magnetic Resonance Imaging of
the Brain
Oxford University
Oxford
UK
irene.tracey@anat.ox.ac.uk

TOBIAS LENIGER
Department of Neurology
University Essen
Essen
Germany
tobias.leniger@uni-essen.de

FREDERICK A. LENZ
Department of Neurosurgery
Johns Hopkins Hospital
Baltimore, MD
USA
flenz1@jhmi.edu

PAULINE LESAGE
Department of Pain Medicine and Palliative Care
Beth Israel Medical Center and
Albert Einstein College of Medicine
New York, NY
USA
plesage@bethisraelny.org

ISOBEL LEVER
Neural Plasticity Unit
Institute of Child Health
University College London
London
UK
i.lever@ich.ucl.ac.uk

KHAN W. LI
Department of Neurosurgery
Johns Hopkins Hospital
Baltimore, MD
USA

ALAN R. LIGHT
Department of Anesthesiology
University of Utah
Salt Lake City, UT
USA
alan.light@hsc.utah.edu

DEOLINDA LIMA
Instituto de Histologia e Embriologia
Faculdade de Medicina da Universidade do Porto
Porto
Portugal
limad@med.up.pt

VOLKER LIMMROTH
Department of Neurology
University of Essen
Essen
Germany
volker.limmroth@uni-essen.de

STEVEN J. LINTON
Department of Occupational and
Environmental Medicine
Department of Behavioral, Social and Legal Sciences
Örebro University Hospital
Örebro
Sweden
steven.linton@orebroll.se

CHRISTINA LIOSSI
School of Psychology
University of Southampton and Great Ormond
Street Hospital for Sick Children
London
UK
cliossi@soton.ac.uk

ARTHUR G. LIPMAN
College of Pharmacy and Pain Management
Center
University of Utah
Salt Lake City, UT
USA
arthur.lipman@hsc.utah.edu

RICHARD B. LIPTON
Departments of Neurology, Epidemiology and
Population Health
Albert Einstein College of Medicine
and Montefiore Headache Unit
Bronx
New York, NY
USA
rlipton@aecom.yu.edu

KENNETH M. LITTLE
Division of Neurosurgery
Duke University Medical Center
Durham, NC
USA
littl023@mc.duke.edu

SPENCER S. LIU
Virginia Mason Medical Center
Seattle, WA
USA
anessl@vmmc.org

ANNE ELISABETH LJUNGGREN
Section for Physiotherapy Science
Department of Public Health and Primary Health Care
Faculty of Medicine
University of Bergen
Bergen
Norway
elisabeth.ljunggren@isf.uib.no

JOHN D. LOESER
Department of Neurological Surgery
University of Washington
Seattle, WA
USA
jdloeser@u.washington.edu

PATRICK LOISEL
Disability Prevention Research and Training Centre
Université de Sherbrooke
Longueuil, QC
Canada
patrick.loisel@usherbrooke.ca

ELISA LOPEZ-DOLADO
FENNSI Group
National Hospital of Parapléjicos
SESCAM Finca "La Peraleda"
Toledo
Spain

JÜREGEN LORENZ
Hamburg University of Applied Sciences
Hamburg
Germany
juergen.lorenz@rzbd.haw-hamburg.de

JÖRN LÖTSCH
Institute for Clinical Pharmacology
Pharmaceutical Center Frankfurt
Johann Wolfgang Goethe University
Frankfurt
Germany
j.loetsch@em.uni-frankfurt.de

DAYNA R. LOYD
Center for Behavioral Neuroscience
Georgia State University
Atlanta, GA
USA

DAVID LUSSIER
McGill University
Montreal, QC
Canada
david.lussier@muhc.mcgill.ca

STEPHEN LUTZ
Blanchard Valley Regional Cancer Center
Findlay, OH
USA

BRUCE LYNN
Department of Physiology
University College London
London
UK
b.lynn@ucl.ac.uk

ROSS MACPHERSON
Department of Anesthesia and Pain Management
University of Sydney
Sydney, NSW
Australia
rmacpher@nsccahs.health.nsw.gov.au

MICHEL MAGNIN
INSERM
Neurological Hospital
Lyon
France

THORSTEN J. MAIER
Pharmacological Center Frankfurt
Clinical Center Johann-Wolfgang Goethe University
Frankfurt
Germany

STEVEN F. MAIER
Department of Psychology and the Center for
Neuroscience
University of Colorado at Boulder
Boulder, CO
USA

CHRIS J. MAIN
University of Manchester
Manchester
UK
cjm@fs1.ho.man.ac.uk

MARZIA MALCANGIO
Wolfson CARD King's College London
London
UK
marzia.malcangio@kcl.ac.uk

PAOLO L. MANFREDI
Essex Woodlands Health Ventures
New York, NY
USA
ggonzales@ewhv.com

KAISA MANNERKORPI
Department of Rheumatology and
Inflammation Research
Sahlgrenska Academy
Göteborg University
Göteborg
Sweden
kaisa.mannerkorpi@rheuma.gu.se

BARTON H. MANNING
Amgen Inc.
Thousand Oaks, CA
USA
bmanning@amgen.com

PATRICK W. MANTYH
Department Prevential Science
University of Minnesota
Minneapolis, MN
USA
manty001@umn.edu

JIANREN MAO
Pain Research Group
MGH Pain Center
and
Department of Anesthesia and Critical Care
Massachusetts General Hospital
Harvard Medical School
Boston, MA
USA
jmao@partners.org

SERGE MARCHAND
Faculty of Medicine
Neurochirurgy
University of Sherbrooke
Sherbrooke, QC
Canada
serge.marchand@usherbrooke.ca

PAOLO MARCHETTINI
Pain Medicine Center
Scientific Institute San Raffaele
Milano
Italy
marchettini.paolo@hsr.it

PEGGY MASON
Department of Neurobiology
Pharmacology and Physiology
University of Chicago
Chicago, IL
USA
p-mason@uchicago.edu

SCOTT MASTERS
Caloundra Spinal and Sports Medicine Centre
Caloundra, QLD
Australia
scotty1@ozemail.com.au

LAURENCE E. MATHER
Department of Anaesthesia and Pain Management
University of Sydney at
Royal North Shore Hospital
Sydney, NSW
Australia
lmather@med.usyd.edu.au

MERVYN MAZE
Magill Department of Anaesthetics
Chelsea and Westminster Campus
Imperial College of Science, Technology and
Medicine, London, UK
m.maze@imperial.ac.uk

BILL MCCARBERG
Pain Services
Kaiser Permanente and Univesrity of California
School of Medicine
San Diego, CA
USA
bill.h.mccarberg@kp.org

JOHN S. MCDONALD
Department of Anesthesiology
Obstetrics and Gynecology
Torrance, CA
USA
jsm5525@ucla.edu

PATRICIA A. MCGRATH
Department of Anaesthesia
Divisional Centre of Pain Management and Research
The Hospital for Sick Children
and
Brain and Behavior Program
Research Institute at The Hospital for Sick Children
and
Department of Anaesthesia
University of Toronto
Toronto, ON
Canada
patricia.mcgrath@sickkids.ca

BRIAN MCGUIRK
Occupational (Musculoskeletal) Medicine
Hunter Area Health Service
Newcastle, NSW
Australia
mgillam@mail.newcastle.edu.au

GREG MCINTOSH
Canadian Back Institute
Toronto, ON
Canada
gmcintosh@cbi.ca

PETER MCINTYRE
Department of Pharmacology
University of Melbourne
Melbourne, VIC
Australia
pmci@unimelb.edu.au

PETER A. MCNAUGHTON
Department of Pharmacology
University of Cambridge
Cambridge
UK
pam42@cam.ac.uk

J. MARK MELHORN
Section of Orthopaedics
Department of Surgery
University of Kansas School of Medicine
Wichita, KS
USA
melhorn@ctdmap.com

RONALD MELZACK
Department of Psychology
McGill University
Montreal, QC
Canada
rmelzack@ego.psych.mcgill.ca

LORNE M. MENDELL
Department of Neurobiology and Behavior
State University of New York at Stony Brook
Stony Brook, NY
USA
lorne.mendell@sunysb.edu

GEORGE MENDELSON
Department of Psychological Medicine
Monash University and Caulfield Pain Management &
Research Centre
Caulfield General Medical Centre
Caulfield, VIC
Australia
george.mendelson@med.monash.edu.au

DANIEL MENÉTREY
CNRS
Université René Descartes
Biomédicale
Paris
France
menetrey@biomedicale.univ-paris5.fr

SIEGFRIED MENSE
Institute for Anatomy and Cell Biology III
University Heidelberg
Heidelberg
Germany
mense@urz.uni-heidelberg.de

SEBASTIANO MERCADANTE
La Maddalena Cancer Pain Relief & Palliative
Care Unit Center
Palermo
Italy
terapiadeldolore@la-maddalena.it

SUSAN MERCER
School of Biomedical Sciences
University of Queensland
Brisbane, QLD
Australia
susan.mercer@stonebow.otago.ac.nz

HAROLD MERSKEY
Department of Psychiatry
University of Western Ontario
London, ON
Canada

KARL MESSLINGER
University of Erlangen-Nürnberg
Nürnberg
Germany
messlinger@physiologie1.uni-erlangen.de

RICHARD A. MEYER
Department of Neurosurgergy
School of Medicine
Johns Hopkins University
Baltimore, MD
USA
rmeyer@jhmi.edu

BJÖRN A. MEYERSON
Department of Clinical Neuroscience
Section of Neurosurgery
Karolinska Institute/University Hospital
Stockholm
Sweden
bjorn.meyerson@karolinska.se

MARTIN MICHAELIS
Sanofi-Aventis Deutschland GmbH
Frankfurt/Main
Germany
martin.michaelis@sanofi-aventis.com

JUDITH A. MIKACICH
Department of Obstetrics and Gynecology
University of California
Los Angeles Medical Center
Los Angeles, CA
USA
jmikacich@mednet.ucla.edu

KENSAKU MIKI
Department of Integrative Physiology
National Institute for Physiological Sciences
Okazaki
Japan

VJEKOSLAV MILETIC
School of Veterinary Medicine
University of Wisconsin-Madison
Madison, WI
USA
vam@svm.vetmed.wisc.edu

ERIN D. MILLIGAN
Department of Psychology and the
Center for Neuroscience
University of Colorado
Boulder, CO
USA
emilligan@psych.colorado.edu

ADRIAN MIRANDA
Division of Gastroenterology and Hepatology and
Pediatric Gastroenterology
Medical College of Wisconsin
Milwaukee, WI
USA

J. MOCCO
Department of Neurological Surgery
Neurological Institute
Columbia University
New York, NY
USA

JEFFREY S. MOGIL
Department of Psychology
McGill University
Montreal, QC
Canada
jeffrey.mogil@mcgill.ca

HARVEY MOLDOFSKY
Sleep Disorders Clinic
Centre for Sleep and Chronobiology
Toronto, ON
Canada
h.moldofsky@utoronto.ca

ROBERT M. MOLDWIN
Department of Urology
Long Island Jewish Medical Center
New York, NY
USA

DEREK C. MOLLIVER
Department of Medicine
University of Pittsburgh School of Medicine
Pittsburgh, PA
USA

LENAIC MONCONDUIT
INSERM
University of Clermont-Ferrand
Clermont-Ferrand
France

JACQUELINE MONTAGNE-CLAVEL
Inserm
Paris
France

ROBERT D. MOOTZ
Department of Environmental and Occupational
Health Sciences
Washington State Department of Labor and Industries
Olympia, WA
USA

ANNE MOREL
Functional Neurosurgery
Neurosurgical Clinic
University Hospital
Zürich
Switzerland

ANNE MORINVILLE
Montreal Neurological Institute
McGill University
Montreal, QC
Canada
annemorinville@yahoo.ca

STEPHEN MORLEY
Academic Unit of Psychiatry and Behavioral Sciences
University of Leeds
Leeds
UK
s.j.morley@leeds.ac.uk

DAVID B. MORRIS
University of Virginia
Charlottesville, VA
USA
dbm6e@virginia.edu

JOACHIM MÖSSNER
Medical Clinic and Policlinic II
University Clinical Center Leipzig AöR
Leipzig
Germany
moej@medizin.uni-leipzig.de

ERIC A. MOULTON
Program in Neuroscience
University of Maryland
Baltimore, MD
USA
emoulton@mclean.harvard.edu

ANNE Z. MURPHY
Center for Behavioral Neuroscience
Georgia State University
Atlanta, GA
USA
amurphy@gsu.edu

PAUL M. MURPHY
Department of Anaesthesia and Pain Management
Royal North Shore Hospital
St. Leonard's, NSW
Australia
drpmurphy@hotmail.com

ALISON MURRAY
Foothills Medical Center
Calgary, AB
Canada
amurray@ucalgary.ca

H. S. NA
Medical Science Research Center and
Department of Physiology
Korea University College of Medicine
Seoul
Korea
hsna@korea.ac.kr

DAISUKE NAKA
Department of Integrative Physiology
National Institute for Physiological Sciences
Okazaki
Japan

YOSHIO NAKAMURA
Pain Research Center
Department of Anesthesiology
University of Utah School of Medicine
Salt Lake City, UT
USA

MATTI V. O. NÄRHI
Department of Physiology
University of Kuopio
Kuopio
Finland
matti.narhi@uku.fi

H.J. W. NAUTA
University of Texas Medical Branch
Galveston, TX
USA
hjnauta@utmb.edu

LUCIA NEGRI
Department of Human Physiology and Pharmacology
University "La Sapienza" of Rome
Rome
Italy
lucia.negri@uniroma1.it

GARY NESBIT
Department of Radiology
Oregon Health and Science University
Portland, OR
USA
nesbitg@ohsu.edu

TIMOTHY NESS
Department of Anesthesiology
University of Alabama at Birmingham
Birmingham, AL
USA
loch@uab.edu

VOLKER NEUGEBAUER
Department of Neuroscience and Cell Biology
University of Texas Medical Branch
Galveston, TX
USA
voneugeb@utmb.edu

LAWRENCE C. NEWMAN
Albert Einstein College of Medicine
New York, NY
USA
lnewman@chpnet.org

CHARLES NG
Musculoskeletal Medicine Specialist
Australasian Faculty of Musculoskeletal Medicine
Auckland
New Zealand
cng@xtra.co.nz

MICHAEL K. NICHOLAS
Pain Management and Research Centre
Royal North Shore Hospital
University of Sydney
St. Leonards, NSW
Australia
miken@med.usyd.edu.au

ELLEN NIEDERBERGER
Pharmacological Center Frankfurt
Clinical Center Johann-Wolfgang Goethe University
Frankfurt
Germany
e.niederberger@em.uni-frankfurt.de

LONE NIKOLAJSEN
Department of Anaesthesiology
Aarhus University Hospital
Aarhus
Denmark
nikolajsen@dadlnet.dk

DONALD R. NIXDORF
Department of Diagnostic and Biological Sciences
School of Dentistry
University of Minnesota
Minneapolis, MN
USA
nixdorf@umn.edu

CARL E. NOE
Baylor University Medical Center
Texas Tech University Health Science Center
Lubbock, TX
USA

KOICHI NOGUCHI
Department of Anatomy and Neuroscience
Hyogo College of Medicine
Hyogo
Japan

RICHARD B. NORTH
Neurosurgery
The Johns Hopkins University School of Medicine
Baltimore, MD
USA
RNorth@jhmi.edu

TURO J. NURMIKKO
Department of Neurological Science and Pain
Research Institute
University of Liverpool
Liverpool
UK
tjn@liv.ac.uk

ANNE LOUISE OAKLANDER
Nerve Injury Unit
Departments of Anesthesiology, Neurology and
Neuropathology
Massachusetts General Hospital
Harvard Medical School
Boston, MA
USA
aoaklander@partners.org

KOICHI OBATA
Department of Anatomy and Neuroscience
Hyogo College of Medicine
Hyogo
Japan
noguchi@hyo-med.ac.jp

TIM F. OBERLANDER
Division of Developmental Pediatrics
Centre for Community Child Health Research and
The University of British Columbia
Vancouver, BC
Canada
toberlander@cw.bc.ca

BRUNO OERTEL
Institute for Clinical Pharmacology
Pharmaceutical Center Frankfurt
Johann Wolfgang Goethe University
Frankfurt
Germany

ALFRED T. OGDEN
Deptartment of Neurological Surgery
Neurological Institute
Columbia University
New York, NY
USA

PETER T. OHARA
Department of Anatomy
University of California San Francisco
San Francisco, CA
USA
pto@itsa.ucsf.edu

SHINJI OHARA
Departments of Neurosurgery
Johns Hopkins University
Baltimore, MD
USA

AKIKO OKIFUJI
Department of Anesthesiology, Psychology and
Clinical Pharmacy
University of Utah
Salt Lake City, UT
USA
akiko.okifuji@hsc.utah.edu

JEAN-LOUIS OLIVÉRAS
Inserm
Paris
France
jean-louis.oliveras@tolbiac.inserm.fr

ANTONIO OLIVIERO
FENNSI Group
National Hospital of Parapléjicos
SESCAM Finca "La Peraleda" Toledo
Toledo
Spain
antonioo@sescam.jccm.es

GUNNAR L. OLSSON
Pain Treatment Services
Astrid Lindgren Children's Hospital/Karolinksa
Hospital
Stockholm
Sweden
gunnar.olsson@ks.se

P. B. OSBORNE
Pain Management Research Institute and
Kolling Institute
University of Sydney
Sydney, NSW
Australia

MICHAEL H. OSSIPOV
Department of Pharmacology
University of Arizona
Health Sciences Center
Tucson, AZ
USA
michaelo@u.arizona.edu

SEAN O'MAHONY
Montefiore Medical Center and
Albert Einstein College of Medicine
Bronx
New York, NY
USA
somahony@montefiore.org

DEBORAH A. O'ROURKE
College of Nursing and Health Sciences
University of Vermont
Burlington, VT
USA
deborah.orourke@uvm.edu

JUDITH A. PAICE
Division of Hematology-Oncology
Northwestern University
Feinberg School of Medicine
Chicago, IL
USA
j-paice@northwestern.edu

JUAN A. PAREJA
Department of Neurology
Fundación Hospital Alcorcón
Madrid
Spain
jpg03m@saludalia.com

ANA M. PASCUAL-LOZANO
Clinical Hospital
University of Valencia
Valencia
Spain

STEVEN D. PASSIK
Markey Cancer Center
University of Kentucky College of Medicine
Lexington, KY
USA
spassik@uky.edu

GAVRIL W. PASTERNAK
Department of Neurology
Memorial Sloan-Kettering Cancer Center
New York, NY
USA
pasterng@mskcc.org

S. H. PATEL
Department of Neurosurgery
Johns Hopkins Hospital
Baltimore, MD
USA

ELLIOT M. PAUL
Department of Urology
Long Island Jewish Medical Center
New York, NY
USA
eliepaul@yahoo.com

KEVIN PAUZA
Tyler Spine and Joint Hospital
Tyler, TX
USA
kevinpauza@tyler.net

ERIC M. PEARLMAN
Pediatric Education
Mercer University School of Medicine
Savannah, GA
USA
pearlmane@aol.com

ELVIRA DE LA PEÑA
Instituto de Neurociencias de Alicante
Universidad Miguel Hernández-CSIC
Alicante
Spain
elvirap@umh.es

YUAN BO PENG
Department of Psychology
University of Texas at Arlington
Arlington, TX
USA

JOSE PEREIRA
Foothills Medical Center
Calgary, AB
Canada
pereiraj@ucalgary.ca

EDWARD PERL
Department of Cell and Molecular Physiology
School of Medicine
University of North Carolina
Chapel Hill, NC
USA
erp@med.unc.edu

ANTTI PERTOVAARA
Department of Physiology
University of Helsinki
Helsinki
Finland
antti.pertovaara@helsinki.fi

PRAMIT PHAL
Department of Radiology
Oregon Health and Science University
Portland, OR
USA

ISSY PILOWSKY
Emeritus Professor of Psychiatry
University of Adelaide
Adelaide, SA
Australia
issyp@med.usyd.edu.au

LEON PLAGHKI
Cliniques Universitaires St. Luc
Brussels
Belgium
plaghki@read.ucl.ac.be

MARKUS PLONER
Department of Neurology
Heinrich–Heine–University
Düsseldorf
Germany
ploner@neurologie.uni-duesseldorf.de

ESTHER M. POGATZKI-ZAHN
Department of Anesthesiology and Intensive Care
Medicine
University Muenster
Muenster
Germany
pogatzi@anit.uni-muenster.de

K. M. POLLOCK
Royal Perth Hospital and
University of Western Australia
Crawley, WA
Australia

MICHAEL POLYDEFKIS
Department of Neurology
The Johns Hopkins University School of Medicine
Baltimore, MD
USA
mpolyde@jhmi.edu

JAMES D. POMONIS
Algos Therapeutics Inc.
St. Paul, MN
USA
jpomonis@algosinc.com

DIETER PONGRATZ
Friedrich Baur Institute
Medical Faculty at the Neurological Clinic and
Policlinic
Ludwig Maximilians University
Munich
Germany
dieter.pongratz@fbs.med.uni-muenchen.de

FRANK PORRECA
Department of Pharmacology
College of Medicine
University of Arizona
Tucson, AZ
USA
frankp@u.arizona.edu

RUSSELL K. PORTENOY
Department of Pain and Palliative Care
Beth Israel Medical Center
New York, NY
USA
rportenoy@chpnet.org

IAN POWER
Anaesthesia Critical Care and Pain Medicine
University of Edinburgh
Edinburgh
UK
ian.power@ed.ac.uk

DONALD D. PRICE
Department of Oral and Maxillofacial Surgery
University of Florida
Gainesville, FL
USA
dprice@dental.ufl.edu

HERBERT K. PROUDFIT
Department of Anesthesiology
University of Iowa
Iowa, IA
USA
hk-proudfit@uiowa.edu

REBECCA W. PRYOR
Pain Prevention and Treatment Research
Department of Psychiatry and Behavioral Sciences
Duke University Medical Center
Durham, NC
USA

DARYL PULLMAN
Medical Ethics
Memorial University of Newfoundland
St. John's, NL
Canada
dpullman@mun.ca

CHAO QIN
Health Sciences Center
University of Oklahoma
Oklahoma City, OK
USA

YUNHAI QIU
Department of Integrative Physiology
National Institute for Physiological Sciences
Okazaki
Japan

MICHAEAL QUITTAN
Department of Physical Medicine and Rehabilitation
Kaiser-Franz-Joseph Hospital
Vienna
Austria
michael.quittan@wienkav.at

RAYMOND M. QUOCK
Department of Pharmaceutical Sciences
Washington State University
Pullman, WA
USA
quockr@wsu.edu

GABOR B. RACZ
Baylor University Medical Center
Texas Tech University Health Science Center
Lubbock, TX
USA
gabor.racz@ttuhsc.edu

LUKAS RADBRUCH
Department of Palliative Medicine
University of Aachen
Aachen
Germany
lradbruch@ukaachen.de

ROBERT B. RAFFA
Department of Pharmacology
Temple University School of Pharmacy
Philadelphia, PA
USA
robert.raffa@temple.edu

VASUDEVA RAGHAVENDRA
Algos Therapeutics Inc.
Saint Paul, MN
USA
rvasudeva@algosinc.com

FRANCINE RAINONE
Montefiore Medical Center and Albert Einstein
College of Medicine
Bronx
New York, NY
USA
frainone@montefiore.org

PIERRE RAINVILLE
Department of Stomatology
University of Montreal
Montreal, QC
Canada
pierre.rainville@umontreal.ca

SRINIVASA N. RAJA
Department of Anesthesiology and
Critical Care Medicine
The Johns Hopkins University School of Medicine
Baltimore, MD
USA
sraja@jhmi.edu

ALAN RANDICH
University of Alabama
Birmingham, AL
USA
arandich@uab.edu

ANDREA J. RAPKIN
Department of Obstetrics and Gynecology
University of California
Los Angeles Medical Center
Los Angeles, CA
USA
arapkin@mednet.ucla.edu

Z. HARRY RAPPAPORT
Department of Neurosurgery
Rabin Medical Center
Tel-Aviv University
Petah Tikva
Israel
zhr1@internet-zahav.net

MATTHEW N. RASBAND
University of Connecticut Health Center
Farmington, CT
USA
rasband@uchc.edu

DOUGLAS RASMUSSON
Department of Physiology and Biophysics
Dalhousie University
Halifax, NS
Canada

JAMES P. RATHMELL
Department of Anesthesiology
University of Vermont College of Medicine
Burlington, VT
USA
james.rathmell@vtmednet.org

K. RAVISHANKAR
The Headache and Migraine Clinic
Jaslok Hospital and Research Centre
Lilavati Hospital and Research Centre
Mumbai
India
dr_k_ravishankar@vsnl.com

KE REN
Department of Biomedical Sciences
University of Maryland
Baltimore, MD
USA
kren@umaryland.edu

CIELITO C. REYES-GIBBY
The University of Texas M. D. Anderson Cancer
Center
Houston, TX
USA
creyes@mdanderson.org

REBECCA PILLAI RIDDELL
York University and
The Hospital for Sick Kids
Toronto, ON
Canada
rpr@yorku.ca

MATTHIAS RINGKAMP
Department of Neurosurgery
School of Medicine
Johns Hopkins University
Baltimore, MD
USA
platelet@jhmi.edu

MARGARITA SANCHEZ DEL RIO
Neurology Department
Hospital Ruber Internacional
Madrid
Spain
msanchezdelrio@ruberinternacional.es

DANIEL RIRIE
Department of Radiology
Oregon Health and Science University
Portland, OR
USA

PIERRE J. M. RIVIÈRE
Ferring Research Institute
San Diego, CA
USA
pierre.riviere@ferring.com

ROGER ROBERT
Neurosurgery
Hotel Dieu
Nantes Cedex 1
France

JAMES P. ROBINSON
University of Washington Pain Center
University of Washington
Seattle, WA
USA
jimrob@u.washington.edu

JOHN ROBINSON
Pain Management Clinic
Burwood Hospital
Christchurch
New Zealand
jon.r@xtra.co.nz

HEATHER L. ROGERS
Department of Medical and Clinical Psychology
Uniformed Services University of the Health Sciences
Bethesda, MD
USA

DAVID ROSELT
Aberdovy Clinic
Bundaberg, QLD
Australia
droselt@aberdovy.com.au

SHLOMO ROTSHENKER
Department of Anatomy & Cell Biology
Faculty of Medicine
Hebrew University of Jerusalem
Jerusalem
Israel
rotsh@md.huji.ac.il

PAUL C. ROUSSEAU
VA Medical Center
Phoenix, AZ
USA
palliativedoctor@aol.com

RANJAN ROY
Faculty of Social Work and
Department of Clinical Health Psychology
Faculty of Medicine
University of Manitoba
Winnipeg, MB
Canada
rroy@cc.umanitoba.CA

CAROLINA ROZA
Institute of Neuroscience
University Miguel Hernández-CSIC
Alicante
Spain
croza@umh.es

TODD D. ROZEN
Michigan Head-Pain and Neurological Institute
Ann Arbor, MI
USA
tdrozmigraine@yahoo.com

ROMAN RUKWIED
Department of Anaesthesiology and Intensive Care
Medicine
Faculty of Clinical Medicine Mannheim
University of Heidelberg
Mannheim
Germany
roman.rukwied@anaes.ma.uni-heidelberg.de

I. JON RUSSELL
Division of Clinical Immunology and Rheumatology
Department of Medicine
The University of Texas Health Science Center
San Antonio, TX
USA
russell@uthscsa.edu

NAYEF E. SAADÉ
Neuroscience Program
Faculty of Medicine
American University of Beirut
Beirut
Lebanon
nesaade@aub.edu.lb

MARY ANN C. SABINO
Department Prevential Science
University of Minnesota
Minneapolis, MN
USA

THOMAS E. SALT
Institute of Ophthalmology
University College London
London
UK
t.salt@ucl.ac.uk

A. SAMDANI
Department of Neurosurgery
Johns Hopkins Medical Institutions
Baltimore, MD
USA

JÜRGEN SANDKÜHLER
Department of Neurophysiology
Center for Brain Research
Medical University of Vienna
Vienna
Austria
juergen.sandkuehler@meduniwien.ac.at

PETER S. SÁNDOR
Headache & Pain Unit
University Hospital Zurich
Zürich
Switzerland
peter.sandor@usz.ch

JOHANNES SARNTHEIN
Functional Neurosurgery
Neurosurgical Clinic
University Hospital
Zürich
Switzerland

SUSANNE K. SAUER
Department of Physiology and Pathophysiology
University of Erlangen
Erlangen
Germany
sauer@physiology1.uni-erlangen.de

JANA SAWYNOK
Department of Pharmacology
Dalhousie University
Halifax, NF
Canada

JOHN W. SCADDING
The National Hospital for Neurology and
Neurosurgery
London
UK
jwscadding@hotmail.com

M. SCHÄFER
Clinic for Anesthesiology and
Operative Intensive Medicine
Charité-University Clinical Center Berlin
Campus Benjamin Franklin
Berlin
Germany
mischaefer@zop-admin.ukbf.fu-berlin.de

HANS-GEORG SCHAIBLE
Department of Physiology
Friedrich Schiller University of Jena
Jena
Germany
hans-georg.schaible@mti.uni-jena.de

JÖRN SCHATTSCHNEIDER
Department of Neurology
University Hospital Schleswig-Holstein
Kiel
Germany
j.schattschneider@neurologie.uni-kiel.de

NEIL SCHECHTER
Department of Pediatrics
University of Connecticut School of Medicine and
Pain Relief Program
Connecticut Children's Medical Center
Hartford, CT
USA
nschecht@stfranciscare.org

STEVEN S. SCHERER
Department of Neurology
The University of Pennsylvania Medical School
Philadelphia, PA
USA
sscherer@mail.med.upenn.edu

MARTIN SCHMELZ
Institute of Anaesthesiology
Operative Intensive Medicine and Pain Research
Faculty for Clinical Medicine Mannheim
University of Heidelberg
Mannheim
Germany
martin.schmelz@anaes.ma.uni-heidelberg.de

ROBERT F. SCHMIDT
Institute of Physiology
University of Würzburg
Würzburg
Germany
rfs@mail.uni-wuerzburg.de

SUZAN SCHNEEWEISS
The Hospital for Sick Children and
The University of Toronto
Toronto, ON
Canada
suzan.schneeweiss@sickkids.ca

FRANK SCHNEIDER
RWTH Aachen University
Department of Psychiatry and Psychotherapy
Aachen
Germany
fschneider@ukaachen.de

ALFONS SCHNITZLER
Department of Neurology
Heinrich Heine University
Düsseldorf
Germany

JEAN SCHOENEN
Departments of Neurology and Neuroanatomy
University of Liège
CHR Citadelle
Liege
Belgium
jschoenen@ulg.ac.be

EVA SCHONSTEIN
School of Physiotherapy
Faculty of Health Science
The University of Sydney
Lidcombe
Sydney, NSW
Australia
e.schonstein@fhs.usyd.edu.au

JENS SCHOUENBORG
Section for Neurophysiology
Department of Physiological Sciences
Lund University
Lund
Sweden
Jens.Schouenborg@mphy.lu.se

STEPHAN A. SCHUG
Royal Perth Hospital and
University of Western Australia
Perth, WA
Australia
schug@cyllene.uwa.edu.au

ANTHONY C. SCHWARZER
Faculty of Medicine and Health Sciences
The University of Newcastle
Newcastle, NSW
Australia
msi5@ozemail.com.au

ZE'EV SELTZER
Centre for the Study of Pain
Faculty of Dentistry
University of Toronto
Toronto, ON
Canada

PETER SELWYN
Montefiore Medical Center and
Albert Einstein College of Medicine
Bronx
New York, NY
USA
selwyn@aecom.yu.edu

PATRICK B. SENATUS
Deptartment of Neurological Surgery
Neurological Institute
Columbia University
New York, NY
USA

JYOTI N. SENGUPTA
Division of Gastroenterology and Hepatology and
Pediatric Gastroenterology
Medical College of Wisconsin
Milwaukee, WI
USA
sengupta@mcw.edu

MARIANO SERRAO
Department of Neurology and Otorinolaringoiatry
University of Rome La Sapienza
Rome
Italy
victor.m@mclink.it

BARRY J. SESSLE
Department of Physiology
Faculty of Medicine
and
Faculty of Dentistry
University of Toronto
Toronto, ON
Canada
barry.sessle@utoronto.ca

VIRGINIA S. SEYBOLD
Department of Neuroscience
University of Minnesota
Minneapolis, MN
USA
vseybold@umn.edu

T. SHAH
Royal Perth Hospital and
University of Western Australia
Crawley, WA
Australia

REZA SHAKER
Division of Gastroenterology and Hepatology and
Pediatric Gastroenterology
Medical College of Wisconsin
Milwaukee, WI
USA

YAIR SHARAV
Department of Oral Medicine
School of Dental Medicine
Hebrew University-Hadassah
Jerusalem
Israel
sharav@cc.huji.ac.il

MARNIE SHAW
Brain Imaging Center
McLean Hospital-Harvard Medical School
Belmont, MA
USA

S. MURRAY SHERMAN
Department of Neurobiology
State University of New York
Stony Brook, NY
USA
s.sherman@sunysb.edu

YOSHIO SHIGENAGA
Department of Oral Anatomy and Neurobiology
Osaka University
Osaka
Japan
sigenaga@dent.osaka-u.ac.jp

EDWARD A. SHIPTON
Department of Anaesthesia
Christchurch School of Medicine
University of Otago
Christchurch
New Zealand
shiptonea@xtra.co.nz

YORAM SHIR
Pain Centre
Department of Anesthesia
McGill University Health Centre
Montreal General Hospital
Montreal, QC
Canada
yoram.shir@muhc.mcgill.ca

PETER SHRAGER
Deptartment of Neurobiology and Anatomy
University of Rochester Medical Center
Rochester, NY
USA
pshr@mail.rochester.edu

MARC J. SHULMAN
VA Connecticut Healthcare System
Yale University
New Haven, CT
USA
marc.shulman@med.va.gov

DAVID M. SIBELL
Comprehensive Pain Center
Oregon Health and Science University
Portland, OR
USA
sibelld@ohsu.edu

PHILIP J. SIDDALL
Pain Management Research Institute
Royal North Shore Hospital
University of Sydney
Sydney, NSW
Australia
phils@med.usyd.edu.au

STEPHEN D. SILBERSTEIN
Jefferson Medical College
Thomas Jefferson University and
Jefferson Headache Center
Thomas Jefferson University Hospital
Philadelphia, PA
USA
stephen.silberstein@jefferson.edu

DONALD A. SIMONE
University of Minnesota
Minneapolis, MN
USA
simon003@umn.edu

DAVID G. SIMONS
Department of Rehabilitation Medicine
Emory University
Atlanta, GA
USA
loisanddavesimons@earthlink.net

DAVID SIMPSON
Clinical Neurophysiology Laboratories
Mount Sinai Medical Center
New York, NY
USA
david.simpson@mssm.edu

MARC SINDOU
Department of Neurosurgery
Hopital Neurologique
Pierre Wertheimer University of Lyon
Lyon
France
marc.sindou@chu-lyon.fr

SØREN HEIN SINDRUP
Department of Neurology
Odense University Hospital
Odense
Denmark
s.sindrup@dadlnet.dk

BENGT H. SJÖLUND
Rehabilitation and Research Centre for
Torture Victims
South Danish University
Copenhagen
Denmark
bsj@rct.dk

CARSTEN SKARKE
Institute of Clinical Pharmacology
pharmazentrum frankfurt/ZAFES
Institute of Clinical Pharmacology
Johann-Wolfgang Goethe University
Frankfurt
Germany
skarke@em.uni-frankfurt.de

KATHLEEN A. SLUKA
Physical Therapy and Rehabilitation Science
Graduate Program
University of Iowa
Iowa City, IA
USA
kathleen-sluka@uiowa.edu

INGRID SÖDERBACK
Department of Public Health and Caring Sciences
Uppsala University
Uppsala
Sweden
ingrid.soderback@pubcare.uu.se

SEYMOUR SOLOMON
Montefiore Medical Center
Albert Einstein College of Medicine
Bronx
New York, NY
USA
ssolomon@montefiore.org

CLAUDIA SOMMER
Department of Neurology
University of Würzburg
Würzburg
Germany
sommer@mail.uni-wuerzburg.de

LINDA S. SORKIN
Anesthesia Research Laboratories
University of California
San Diego, CA
USA
lsorkin@ucsd.edu

MICHAEL SPAETH
Friedrich-Baur-Institute
University of Munich
Munich
Germany
spaeth.m5@t-online.de
michael.spaeth@lrz.uni-muenchen.de

PEREGRIN O. SPIELHOLZ
SHARP Program
Washington State Department of Labor and Industries
Olympia, WA
USA
spip235@lni.wa.gov

BENJAMIN S. CARSON SR.
Department of Neurological Surgery
Johns Hopkins Hospital
Baltimore, MD
USA

PETER S. STAATS
Division of Pain Medicine
The Johns Hopkins University
Baltimore, MD
USA
pstaats@jhmi.edu

BRETT R. STACEY
Comprehensive Pain Center
Oregon Health and Science University
Portland, OR
USA

WENDY M. STEIN
San Diego Hospice and Palliative Care
UCSD
San Diego, CA
USA
wstein@sdhospice.org

CHRISTOPH STEIN
Department of Anaesthesiology and
Intensive Care Medicine
Campus Benjamin Franklin
Charité – University Medicine Berlin
Berlin
Germany
christoph.stein@charite.de

MICHAEL STEINMETZ
Department of Neurosurgery
The Cleveland Clinic Foundation
Cleveland, OH
USA

JAIR STERN
Functional Neurosurgery
Neurosurgical Clinic
University Hospital
Zürich
Switzerland

BONNIE J. STEVENS
University of Toronto and
The Hospital for Sick Children
Toronto, ON
Canada
b.stevens@utoronto.ca

CARL-OLAV STILLER
Division of Clinical Pharmacology
Department of Medicine
Karolinska University Hospital
Stockholm
Sweden
carl-olav.stiller@ki.se

JENNIFER N. STINSON
The Hospital for Sick Children and
The University of Toronto
Toronto, ON
Canada
jennifer.stinson@sickkids.ca

HENRY STOCKBRIDGE
Health and Community Medicine
University of Washington School of Public
Seattle, WA
USA
stoh235@lni.wa.gov

CHRISTIAN S. STOHLER
Baltimore College of Dental Surgery
University of Maryland
Baltimore, MD
USA
cstohler@dental.umaryland.edu

LAURA STONE
Department of Neuroscience
University of Minnesota
Minneapolis, MN
USA
stone@med.umn.edu

R. WILLIAM STONES
Princess Anne Hospital
University of Southampton
Southampton
UK
r.w.stones@soton.ac.uk

ANDREAS STRAUBE
Department of Neurology
Ludwig Maximilians University
Munich
Germany
astraube@nefo.med.uni-muenchen.de

JENNY STRONG
University of Queensland
Brisbane, QLD
Australia
j.strong@uq.edu.au

GEROLD STUCKI
Department of Physical Medicine and Rehabilitation
Ludwig-Maximilians University
Munich
Germany
gerold.stucki@med.uni-muenchen.de

CHERYL L. STUCKY
Department of Cell Biology
Neurobiology and Anatomy
Medical College of Wisconsin
Milwaukee, WI
USA
cstucky@mcw.edu

MATHIAS STURZENEGGER
Department of Neurology
University of Bern
Bern
Switzerland
matthias.sturzenegger@insel.ch

YASUO SUGIURA
Nagoya University School of Medicine
Graduate School of Medicine
Department of Functional Anatomy & Neuroscience
Nagoya
Japan
ysugiura@med.nagoya-u.ac.jp

MARK D. SULLIVAN
Psychiatry and Behavioral Sciences
University of Washington
Seattle, WA
USA
sullimar@u.washington.edu

MICHAEL J. L. SULLIVAN
Department of Psychology
University of Montreal
Montreal, QC
Canada
michael.jl.sullivan@umontreal.ca

B. SUNG
Medical Science Research Center and
Department of Physiology
Korea University College of Medicine
Seoul
Korea

RIE SUZUKI
Department of Pharmacology
University College London
London
UK
ucklrsu@ucl.ac.uk

KRISTINA B. SVENDSEN
Danish Pain Research Center
Aarhus University Hospital
Aarhus
Denmark
kristina@akhphd.au.dk

PETER SVENSSON
Department of Clinical Oral Physiology
University of Aarhus
Aarhus
Denmark
psvensson@odont.au.dk

NIGEL P. SYKES
St. Christopher's Hospice and King's College
University of London
London
UK
nigelsykes@doctors.org.uk

A. TAGHVA
Department of Neurosurgery
Johns Hopkins Hospital
Baltimore, MD
USA

KERSI TARAPOREWALLA
Royal Brisbane and Womens' Hospital
University of Queensland
Brisbane, QLD
Australia
Kersi_taraporewalla@health.qld.gov.au

RONALD R. TASKER
University of Toronto
Toronto Western Hospital
Toronto, ON
Canada

IRMGARD TEGEDER
Pharmacological Center Frankfurt
Clinical Center Johann-Wolfgang Goethe University
Frankfurt
Germany
tegeder@em.uni-frankfurt.de

ASTRID J. TERKELSEN
Danish Pain Research Center and Department of
Neurology
Aarhus University Hospital
Aarhus
Denmark
astrid@akhphd.au.dk

GREGORY W. TERMAN
Department of Anesthesiology and the
Graduate Program in Neurobiology and Behavior
University of Washington
Seattle, WA
USA
gwt@u.washington.edu

ALISON THOMAS
Lismore, NSW
Australia
alison.thomas@crsrehab.gov.au

BEVERLY E. THORN
University of Alabama
Tuscaloosa, AL
USA
bthorn@bama.ua.edu

CINDY L. THURSTON-STANFIELD
Department of Biomedical Sciences
University of South Alabama
Mobile, AL
USA
cthursto@usouthal.edu

ARNE TJØLSEN
University of Bergen
Bergen
Norway
arne.tjolsen@fys.uib.no

ANDREW J. TODD
Spinal Cord Group
Institute of Biomedical and Life Sciences
University of Glasgow
Glasgow
UK
a.todd@bio.gla.ac.uk

MAKOTO TOMINAGA
Department of Cellular and Molecular Physiology
Mie University School of Medicine
Tsu Mie
Japan
tominaga@doc.medic.mie-u.ac.jp

IRENE TRACEY
Pain Imaging Neuroscience (PaIN) Group
Department of Physiology, Anatomy and Genetics
and
Centre for Functional Magnetic Resonance
Imaging of the Brain
Oxford University
Oxford
UK
irene.tracey@anat.ox.ac.uk

TUAN DIEP TRAN
Department of Neurology
University of Michigan
and
Neurology Research Laboratory
VA Medical Center
Ann Arbor, MI
USA
and
Department of Pediatrics
University of Medicine and Pharmacy of Ho
Chi Minh City
Ho Chi Minh City
Vietnam

DIEP TUAN TRAN
Department of Integrative Physiology
National Institute for Physiological Sciences
Okazaki
Japan

ROLF-DETLEF TREEDE
Institute of Physiology and Pathophysiology
Johannes Gutenberg University
Mainz
Germany
treede@uni-mainz.de

JENNIE C. I. TSAO
Pediatric Pain Program
Department of Pediatrics
David Geffen School of Medicine at UCLA
Los Angeles, CA
USA

JEANNA TSENTER
Department of Physical Medicine and Rehabilitation
Hadassah University Hospital
Jerusalem
Israel

MAURITS VAN TULDER
Institute for Research in Extramural Medicine
Free University Amsterdam
Amsterdam
The Netherlands
mw.vantulder@vumc.nl

ELDON TUNKS
Hamilton Health Sciences Corporation
Hamilton, ON
Canada
tunks@hhsc.ca

DENNIS C. TURK
Department of Anesthesiology
University of Washington
Seattle, WA
USA
turkdc@u.washington.edu

JUDITH A. TURNER
Department of Psychiatry and Behavioral Sciences
University of Washington
Seattle, WA
USA

O. J. TWEEDIE
Royal Perth Hospital and
University of Western Australia
Crawley, WA
Australia

STEPHEN P. TYRER
Royal Victoria Infirmary
University of Newcastle upon Tyne
Newcastle-on-Tyne
UK
s.p.tyrer@ncl.ac.uk

ALEXANDER TZABAZIS
Department of Anesthesia
University of Erlangen
Erlangen
Germany
tzabazis@web.de

KENE UGOKWE
Department of Neurosurgery
The Cleveland Clinic Foundation
Cleveland, OH
USA

LINDSAY S. UMAN
Department of Psychology
Dalhousie University
Halifax, NS
Canada
luman@dal.ca

ANITA M. UNRUH
Health and Human Performance and
Occupational Therapy
Dalhousie University
Halifax, NS
Canada
aunruh@dal.ca

CHRISTIANE VAHLE-HINZ
Institute of Neurophysiology and Pathophysiology
University Hospital Hamburg-Eppendorf
Hamburg
Germany
vahle-hinz@uke.uni-hamburg.de

MUTHUKUMAR VAIDYARAMAN
Division of Pain Medicine
The Johns Hopkins University
Baltimore, MD
USA
mvaidya2@jhmi.edu

TODD W. VANDERAH
Department of Pharmacology
College of Medicine
University of Arizona
Tucson, AZ
USA
vanderah@u.arizona.edu

GUY VANDERSTRAETEN
Department of Rehabilitation Sciences and
Physiotherapy
Ghent University Hospital
Ghent
Belgium
guy.vanderstraeten@ugent.be

HORACIO VANEGAS
Instituto Venezolano de Investigaciones Cientificas
(IVIC)
Caracas
Venezuela
hvanegas@ivic.ve

JEAN-JACQUES VATINE
Outpatient and Research Division
Reuth Medical Center
Tel Aviv
Israel
vatinejj@reuth.org.il

LINDA K. VAUGHN
Department of Biomedical Sciences
Marquette University
Milwaukee, WI
USA
linda.vaughn@marquette.edu

LOUIS VERA-PORTOCARRERO
Department of Pharmacology
College of Medicine
University of Arizona
Tucson, AZ
USA
loverapo@email.arizona.edu

PAUL VERRILLS
Metropolitan Spinal Clinic
Prahran, VIC
Australia
verrills@bigpond.net.au

FÉLIX VIANA
Instituto de Neurociencias de Alicante
Universidad Miguel Hernández-CSIC
San Juan de Alicante
Spain

CHARLES J. VIERCK JR.
Department of Neuroscience and
McKnight Brain Institute
University of Florida College of Medicine
Gainesville, FL
USA
vierck@mbi.ufl.edu

LUIS VILLANUEVA
INSERM
University of Clermont-Ferrand
Clermont-Ferrand
France
luis.villanueva@u-clermont1.fr

MARCELO VILLAR
Neuroscience Laboratory
Austral University
Buenos Aires
Argentina

DAVID VIVIAN
Metro Spinal Clinic
Caulfield, VIC
Australia
dvivian@metrospinal.com.au

JOHAN W. S. VLAEYEN
Department of Medical, Clinical and Experimental
Psychology
Maastricht University
Maastricht
The Netherlands
j.vlaeyen@dep.unimaas.nl

NICOLAS VOILLEY
Institut de Pharmacologie Moleculaire et Cellulaire
Valbonne
France
voilley@ipmc.cnrs.fr

ERNEST VOLINN
Pain Research Center
University of Utah
Salt Lake City, UT
USA
epaulv@yahoo.com

LUCY VULCHANOVA
Department of Veterinary and Biomedical Sciences
University of Minnesota
St. Paul, MN
USA
lucy@med.umn.edu

PAUL W. WACNIK
Department of Pharmacology
College of Medicine
University of Minnesota
Minneapolis, MN
USA
paul.w.wacnik@medtronic.com

GORDON WADDELL
University of Glasgow
Glasgow
UK
gordon.waddell@virgin.net

GARY A. WALCO
Hackensack University Medical Center
University of Medicine and Dentistry of New Jersey
New Jersey Medical School
Hackensack, NJ
USA
gwalco@humed.com

BARBARA WALKER
Centre for Pain Management
St Vincent's Hospital
Melbourne, VIC
Australia

SUELLEN M. WALKER
University of Sydney Pain Management and
Research Centre
Royal North Shore Hospital
St. Leonards, NSW
Australia
swalker@anatomy.usyd.edu.au
suellen.walker@ucl.ac.uk

LYNN S. WALKER
Division of Adolescent Medicine and
Behavioral Sciences
Vanderbilt University Medical Center
Nashville, TN
USA
lynn.walker@vanderbilt.edu

VICTORIA C. J. WALLACE
Department of Anaesthetics
Pain Medicine and Intensive Care
Chelsea and Westminster Hospital Campus
London
UK
v.wallace@imperial.ac.uk

XIAOHONG WANG
Department of Integrative Physiology
National Institute for Physiological Sciences
Okazaki
Japan

FAY WARNOCK
Children's and Women's Hospital and
The University of British Columbia
Vancouver, BC
Canada
warnock@nursing.ubc.ca

GUNNAR WASNER
Department of Neurological Pain Research and
Therapy
Neurological Clinic
Kiel
Germany
and
Prince of Wales Medical Research Institute
University of New South Wales
Randwick, NSW
Australia
g.wasner@neurologie.uni-kiel.de

SHOKO WATANABE
Department of Integrative Physiology
National Institute for Physiological Sciences
Okazaki
Japan

LINDA R. WATKINS
Department of Psychology and
Center for Neuroscience
University of Colorado at Boulder
Boulder, CO
USA
lwatkins@psych.colorado.edu

CHRISTOPHER J. WATLING
The University of Western Ontario
London, ON
Canada
chris.watling@lhsc.on.ca

PAUL J. WATSON
University Department of Anaesthesia
University of Leicester
Leicester
UK
pjw25@le.ac.uk

PETER N. WATSON
University of Toronto
Toronto, ON
Canada
peter.watson@utoronto.ca

JAMES WATT
North Shore Hospital
Auckland
New Zealand
jameswatt@clear.net.nz

STEPHEN G. WAXMAN
Department of Neurology
Yale School of Medicine
New Haven, CT
and
VA Medical Center
West Haven, CT
USA
stephen.waxman@yale.edu

CHRISTIAN WEIDNER
Department of Physiology and Experimental
Pathophysiology
University Erlangen
Erlangen
Germany
weidner@physiologie1.uni-erlangen.de

PH. TH. M. WEIJENBORG
Department of Gynecology
Leiden University Medical Center
Leiden
The Netherlands
p.t.m.weijenborg@lumc.nl

ROBIN WEIR
Hamilton Health Sciences Corporation
Hamilton, ON
Canada

NIRIT WEISS
Departments of Neurosurgery
Johns Hopkins University
Baltimore, MD
USA

URSULA WESSELMANN
Departments of Neurology
Neurological Surgery and Biomedical Engineering
The Johns Hopkins University School of Medicine
Baltimore, MD
USA
pain@jhmi.edu

DAGMAR WESTERLING
Departments of Clinical Pharmacology
Anesthesiology and Intensive Care
Lund University Hospital
Lund
Sweden
Dagmar.westerling@skane.se

KARIN N. WESTLUND
Department of Anatomy and Neurosciences
University of Texas Medical Branch
Galveston, TX
USA
kwhigh@utmb.edu

THOMAS M. WICKIZER
Department of Rehabilitation Medicine
University of Washington
Seattle, WA
USA

EVA WIDERSTRÖM-NOGA
The Miami Project to Cure Paralysis
Department of Neurological Surgery
University of Miami
VAMC
Miami, FL
USA
ewiderstrom-noga@miami.edu

JULIE WIESELER-FRANK
Department of Psychology and Center for
Neuroscience
University of Colorado at Boulder
Boulder, CO
USA

ZSUZSANNA WIESENFELD-HALLIN
Karolinska Institute
Stockholm
Sweden
zsuzsanna.wiesenfeld-hallin@labmed.ki.se

ANN WIGHAM
McCoull Clinic
Prudhoe Hospital
Northumberland
UK
ann_wigham@hotmail.com

GEORGE L. WILCOX
Department of Neuroscience
Pharmacology and Dermatology
University of Minnesota Medical School
Minneapolis, MN
USA
george@umn.edu

OLIVER H. G. WILDER-SMITH
Pain and Nociception Research Group
Pain Centre
Department of Anaesthesiology
Radboud University Nijmegen Medical Centre
Nijmegen
The Netherlands
o.wildersmith@anes.umcn.nl

KJERSTI WILHELMSEN
Section for Physiotherapy Science
Department of Public Health and Primary Health Care
Faculty of Medicine
University of Bergen
Bergen
Norway
kjersti.wilhelmsen@isf.uib.no

VICTOR WILK
Brighton Spinal Group
Brighton, VIC
Australia
vicwilk@tpg.com.au

W. A. WILLIAMS
Royal Perth Hospital and
University of Western Australia
Perth, WA
Australia

WILLIAM D. WILLIS
Department of Neuroscience and Cell Biology
University of Texas Medical Branch
Galveston, TX
USA
wdwillis@utmb.edu

JOHN B. WINER
Department of Neurology
Birmingham Muscle and Nerve Centre
Queen Elizabeth Hospital
Birmingham
UK
j.b.winer@bham.ac.uk

CHRISTOPHER J. WINFREE
Department of Neurological Surgery
Neurological Institute
Columbia University
New York, NY
USA
cjw12@columbia.edu

JANET WINTER
Novartis Institute for Medical Science
London
UK
janet.winter@novartis.com

ALAIN WODA
Faculté de Chirurgie Dentaire
University Clermont-Ferrand
Clermont-Ferrand
France
alain.woda@u-clermont1.fr

SUNG TAE KOO WONKWANG
Korea Institute of Oriental Medicine
Korea
stkoo@klom.re.kr

LEE WOODSON
Department of Anesthesiology
University of Texas Medical Branch
and
Shriners Hospitals for Children
Shriners Burns Hospital
Galveston, TX
USA

XIAO-JUN XU
Karolinska Institute
Stockholm
Sweden

HIROSHI YAMASAKI
Department of Integrative Physiology
National Institute for Physiological Sciences
Okazaki
Japan

MICHAEL YELLAND
School of Medicine
Griffith University
Logan, QLD
Australia
myelland@bigpond.com

S. YENNURAJALINGAM
Department of Palliative Care and
Rehabilitation Medicine
The University of Texas M. D. Anderson Cancer
Center
Houston, TX
USA

DAVID C. YEOMANS
Department of Anesthesia
Stanford University
Stanford, CA
USA
dcyeomans@stanford.edu

ROBERT P. YEZIERSKI
Comprehensive Center for Pain Research and
Department of Neuroscience
McKnight Brain Institute
Gainesville, FL
USA
ryezierski@dental.ufl.edu

WAY YIN
Department of Anesthesiology
University of Washington
Seattle, WA
USA
wyin@nospinepain.com

Y. W. YOON
Medical Science Research Center and
Department of Physiology
Korea University College of Medicine
Seoul
Korea

ATSUSHI YOSHIDA
Department of Oral Anatomy and Neurobiology
Osaka University
Osaka
Japan
yoshida@dent.osaka-u.ac.jp

JOANNA M. ZAKRZEWSKA
Clinical Diagnostic and Oral Sciences
Institute of Dentistry
Barts and the London
Queen Mary's School of Medicine & Dentistry
University of London
London
UK
j.m.zakrzewska@qmul.ac.uk

HANNS ULRICH ZEILHOFER
Institute for Pharmacology and Toxicology
University of Zürich
Zürich
Switzerland
zeilhofer@pharma.unizh.ch

LONNIE K. ZELTZER
Pediatric Pain Program
Department of Pediatrics
David Geffen School of Medicine at UCLA
Los Angeles, CA
USA
lzeltzer@mednet.ucla.edu.

GIOVAMBATTISTA ZEPPETELLA
St. Clare Hospice
Hastingwood
UK
jzeppetella@stclare-hospice.co.uk

YI-HONG ZHANG
Deptartment of Anatomy and Neurobiology
University of Tennessee Health Science Center
Memphis, TN
USA
yzhang32@utmem.edu

XIJING J. ZHANG
Department of Neuroscience
University of Minnesota
Minneapolis, MN
USA
zhang036@umn.edu

MIN ZHUO
Department of Physiology
University of Toronto
Toronto, ON
Canada
min.zhuo@utoronto.ca

C. ZÖLLNER
Clinic for Anesthesiology and Operative Intensive
Medicine
Charité-University Clinical Center Berlin
Campus Benjamin Franklin
Berlin
Germany
zoellner@zop-admin.ukbf.fu-berlin.de

KRINA ZONDERVAN
Wellcome Trust Centre for Human Genetics
Oxford
UK

ZBIGNIEW ZYLICZ
St. Elizabeth Hospice
Ipswich
Suffolk
UK
zzylicz@onetel.net

Habituation

Definition

Habituation is the reverse process of sensitization, consisting of a waning response to repeated stimulation that can be rapid or gradual. It involves a reduction in excitability, and means that neurons cease to fire when stimulated. However, if the interval between stimuli is altered randomly, and the strength of the stimulus is increased, this process can be reversed.

► Infant Pain Mechanisms
► Migraine Without Aura
► Psychology of Pain, Sensitisation, Habituation and Pain

Hamstring Muscle Strain

Definition

Hamstring muscle strain produces pain in the biceps femoris muscles in the back of the thigh. Stretching the muscle can produce pain, as is found with a straight leg raising maneuver.

► Sciatica

Handicap

► Disability and Impairment Definitions

Hansen's Disease

AKI J. HIETAHARJU[1], MAIJA HAANPÄÄ;[2]
[1]Department of Neurology and Rehabilitation, Pain Clinic, Tampere University Hospital, Tampere, Finland
[2]Department of Anaesthesiology and Department of Neurosurgery, Pain Clinic, Helsinki University Hospital, Helsinki, Finland
aki.hietaharju@pshp.fi

Synonym

Leprosy

Definition

Hansen's disease is a chronic granulomatous infection of the skin and peripheral nerves caused by ► Mycobacterium leprae. It is associated with marked disabilities which result from the impairment of both sensory and motor nerve function.

Characteristics

Hansen's disease used to be widely distributed all over the world, but now the major part of the global burden of the disease is represented by resource-poor countries, in tropical and warm temperate regions. In 1985, there were an estimated 12 million people with ► leprosy worldwide, resulting in a prevalence of 12 per 10,000 (Britton and Lockwood 2004). At the beginning of 2003, the number of Hansen's disease patients receiving antimicrobial therapy was around 534,000, as reported by 110 countries. About 621,000 new cases were detected during 2002. The six top endemic countries at the start of 2003 were India, Brazil, Madagascar, Mozambique, Nepal, and Tanzania (WHO).

Mycobacterium leprae is an acid-fast gram-positive bacillus, which is supposed to be transmitted mainly by aerosol spread of nasal secretions and uptake through nasal or respiratory mucosa (Noordeen 1994). The infection is not spread by touching, because the bacterium cannot penetrate intact skin. *Mycobacterium leprae* has a peculiar ► tropism for macrophages and ► Schwann cells. After having invaded the Schwann cell, the leprosy bacilli replicate slowly over years. These bacilli show preference for growth in cooler regions of the body causing damage to superficial nerves. Peripheral nerves are affected in fibro-osseous tunnels near the surface of the skin e.g. posterior tibial nerve near the medial malleolus (Britton and Lockwood 2004).

The dynamic nature of the immune response to *Mycobacterium leprae* often leads to spontaneous fluctuations in the clinical state, which are called ► leprosy reaction's. They are divided into two types. ► Leprosy type 1 reaction or reversal reaction is caused by spontaneous increases in T-cell reactivity to mycobacterial antigens (Britton 1998). In type 1 reactions, especially borderline patients may present with reactions to nerve pain, sudden palsies, and many new skin lesions. ► Leprosy type 2 reaction or erythema nodosum leprosum, is a systemic inflammatory response to the deposition of extravascular immune complexes. It occurs only in borderline-lepromatous and lepromatous leprosy (Lockwood 1996).

Diagnosis of leprosy is clinical and based on patients having at least one of three cardinal signs, which are: (1) hypopigmented or reddish patches with definite loss of sensation, (2) thickened peripheral nerves, and (3) acid-fast bacilli on skin smears of biopsy material (WHO 1998). Leprosy is divided into five subtypes based on histologic and immunologic features: tuberculoid (▶ tuberculoid leprosy), borderline tuberculoid (▶ borderline leprosy), midborderline, borderline lepromatous and ▶ lepromatous leprosy (Ridley and Jopling 1966). These subtypes have been consolidated into two groups, paucibacillary and multibacillary, for assignment to treatment regimens. According to WHO guidelines, the former is treated with ▶ dapsone 100 mg daily and rifampicin 600 mg monthly for 6 months. In multibacillary leprosy, duration of the treatment is a minimum 2 years, and ▶ clofazimine 50 mg daily and 300 mg monthly is added to paucibacillary regimen (Britton and Lockwood 2004).

The most devastating clinical consequence of the intracutaneous nerve damage is the total sensory loss of the extremities (Brand and Fritschi 1985). Pain and temperature sensation are most strikingly decreased in early cases, and later tactile and pressure sense are also lost. Anaesthesia of the extremities predisposes the patient to chronic ulcers and severe secondary deformities, and therefore leprosy remains a significant cause of neurologic disability worldwide.

Since Hansen's disease causes severe sensory loss, it is assumed that pain is uncommon in leprosy. However, peripheral nerve pain, dysesthesias and paraesthesias may complicate leprosy, both during and after treatment. Data on consumption of analgesics by patients with neuropathic pain gives some indication of the extent of the problem. In a Malaysian study of 235 leprosy patients, neuritic pain was the main reason for consumption of analgesic preparations. In 46 patients (19.5%), an overall total intake had been more than 2 kg of analgesics. The duration of intake ranged from 2 to more than 20 years (Segasothy et al. 1986).

Acute pain in one or several nerves may be the presenting feature in Hansen's disease. Pain is a familiar symptom of reactions and neuritis, due to entrapment of the oedematous inflamed nerve in sites of predilection (Nations et al. 1998). Neuritis of cutaneous nerves may also be painful (Theuvenet et al. 1993). Peripheral nerve abscesses, which are often associated with severe acute pain, occur in all types of leprosy and a variety of nerve trunks and cutaneous nerves (Kumar et al. 1997). Leprosy related acute pain can usually be relieved by steroids or other therapeutic measures, such as anti-inflammatory drugs and immobilisation or surgical intervention.

Chronic neuropathic pain in Hansen's disease has received scant attention. Hietaharju et al. (2000) reported on moderate or severe chronic neuropathic pain in 16 patients with treated multibacillary leprosy. In 10 patients, the pain had a glove and stocking-like distribution, and in 2 patients it followed the course of a specific nerve. The quality of pain was burning in 9, biting in 3, pricking in 3, cutting in 2, and electric-shock-like in 2 patients. The occurrence of pain was continuous in 50% of the patients. In an evaluation of 303 patients from a Brazilian referral centre, 174 (57%) patients complained of neuropathic pain (Stump et al. 2002). In 84 patients (48%), pain manifested as bursts. Pain affected one or more peripheral nerve territories; ulnar nerve in 101 (58%) patients and tibial nerve course in 48 (28%). There was a polyneuropathic distribution as glove-like in 47 patients (27%), and sock-like in another 47 patients. At the time of evaluation, pain was present in 47 (27%) patients.

There is little data on the occurrence of sensory disturbances such as dysesthesias, paresthesias or allodynia in patients with leprosy. In a study by Hietaharju et al. (2000), 4 patients complained of a tingling sensation, which was considered as unpleasant and painful, i.e. they had dysesthesia. Dysesthesia followed glove and stocking-distribution in 2 patients, the course of femoral cutaneous nerve in 1 patient, and was located in both legs below mid-thigh in 1 patient. Allodynia, pain due to a stimulus that does not normally provoke pain, was noticed in 2 patients. In both of these patients, enlargement and tenderness of the nerves (cutaneous femoral, common peroneal and posterior tibial) without abscess formation was discovered in clinical examination.

The most typical sensory abnormalities in leprosy patients are severely impaired perception of tactile stimuli and mechanical and thermal pain, indicating damage of Aβ, Aδ and C fibres at the painful site (Hietaharju et al. 2000). The cases with sensory loss associated with pain suggest peripheral deafferentation, i.e. pain due to loss of sensory input into the central nervous system, as occurs with different types of lesions of peripheral nerves. However, in a considerable proportion of the patients with pain the sensory function may be quite well preserved, suggesting other pathophysiological mechanisms. Early involvement of small fibres due to mycobacterial invasion can cause dysfunction and damage leading to paresthesia and pain. Other possible explanations include the impact of previous episodes of reactions, neuritis and inflammation, which may leave the nerve fibrosed, and at risk of entrapment (Negesse 1996). Some patients may have a chronic ongoing neuritis manifesting clinically with pain (Haanpää et al. 2004). Inflammation along nerve trunks has been shown to produce ectopic activity in nerves, and therefore past or present inflammatory conditions represent a source for central sensitisation, which may manifest as chronic neuropathic pain. A delayed ▶ vasculitic neuropathy, probably precipitated by persisting mycobacterial antigen, is a rare complication of leprosy (Bowen et al. 2000). Vasculitic neuropathies, such as HIV and rheumatoid disease related neuropathies are known to be painful.

References

1. Bowen JRC, McDougall AC, Morris JH, Lucas SB, Donaghy M (2000) Vasculitic neuropathy in a patient with inactive treated lepromatous leprosy. J Neurol Neurosurg Psychiatry 68:496-500
2. Brand PW, Fritschi EP (1985) Rehabilitation in leprosy. In: Hastings RC (ed) Leprosy, 1st edn. Churchill-Livingstone, Edinburgh, pp 287-319
3. Britton WJ (1998) The management of leprosy reversal reactions. Lepr Rev 69:225-234
4. Britton WJ, Lockwood DN (2004) Leprosy. Lancet 363:1209-1219
5. Haanpaa M, Lockwood DN, Hietaharju A (2004) Neuropathic pain in leprosy. Lepr Rev 75:7-18
6. Hietaharju A, Croft R, Alam R, Birch P., Mong A., Haanpää M. (2000). The existence of chronic neuropathic pain in treated leprosy. Lancet 356:1080-1081
7. Kumar P, Saxena R, Mohan L, Thacker AK, Mukhija RD (1997) Peripheral nerve abscess in leprosy: report of twenty cases. Indian J Lepr 69:143-147
8. Lockwood DN (1996) The management of erythema nodosum leprosum: current and future options. Lepr Rev 67:253-259
9. Nations SP, Katz JS, Lyde CB, Barohn RJ (1998) Leprous neuropathy: an American perspective. Semin Neurol 18:113-124
10. Negesse Y (1996) Comment: 'silently arising clinical neuropathy' and extended indication of steroid therapy in leprosy neuropathy. Lepr Rev 67:230-231
11. Noordeen SK (1994) The epidemiology of leprosy. In: Hastings RC (ed) Leprosy, 2nd edn. Churchill-Livingstone, Edinburgh, pp 29-48
12. Ridley DS, Jopling WH (1966). Classification of leprosy according to immunity: a five-group system. Int J Lepr 54:255-273
13. Segasothy M, Muhaya HM, Musa A, Rajagopalan K, Lim KJ, Fatimah Y, Kamal A, Ahmad K.S. (1986) Analgesic use by leprosy patients. Int J Lepr Other Mycobact Dis 54:399-402
14. Stump P, Baccarelli R, Marciano L, Lauris J, Ura S, Teixeira M, Virmond M (2002) Prevalence and characteristics of neuropathic pain and consequences of the sensory loss in 303 patients with leprosy. In: Abstracts of the 10th world congress on pain, August 17-22, 2002, San Diego, California, USA. IASP Press, Seattle, p 93
15. Theuvenet WJ, Finlay K, Roche P, Soares D, Kauer JMG (1993) Neuritis of the lateral femoral cutaneous nerve in leprosy. Int J Lepr 61:592-596
16. WHO (1998) Expert Committee on Leprosy, 7th Report, pp 1-43
17. WHO. http://www.who.int/lep/ (accessed Jun 24, 2004)

Hargreaves Test

▶ Thermal Nociception Test

Head Pain

▶ Headache

Headache

NIKOLAI BOGDUK
Department of Clinical Research Royal Newcastle Hospital, University of Newcastle, Newcastle, NSW, Australia
nbogduk@mail.newcastle.edu.au

Synonyms

Head Pain; Cephalalgia

Definition

Headache is pain perceived in the head. Specifically, in order to constitute headache, the pain must be perceived in the occipital, temporal, parietal, or frontal regions of the head, or in some combination of these regions. Pain from these regions may extend to encompass the orbital region, and some forms of headache may particularly affect the orbit. Pain localized to the eye, however, is not generally regarded as headache, and is better described as eye pain. Similar, pain in the face does not conventionally constitute headache; it is regarded separately as facial pain.

Characteristics

There are many varieties of headache, with many possible causes (Headache Classification Subcommittee of the International Headache Society 2004, Olesen et al. 2000). For the most common types of headache, the actual causes are not known. Although several theories are available, they relate rather to the mechanism of pain-production, and do not explain the fundamental reason why the headache occurs. That remains unknown.

Headaches are distinguished and defined largely on the basis of their clinical features. These can be described systematically under the categories of enquiry recommended for taking a ▶ history of a pain problem (see ▶ medical history):

- Length of Illness
- Site
- Radiation
- Quality
- Intensity
- Frequency
- Duration
- Time of Onset
- Mode of Onset
- Precipitating Features
- Aggravating Features
- Relieving Features
- Associated Features

Length of Illness

This domain pertains to whether or not this is the first episode of headache that the patient has suffered.

Headache for the first time is the cardinal clue for a small set of serious headaches, such as those caused by aneurysm, subarachnoid haemorrhage, meningitis, or sudden, severe hypertension.

Site

The site in which pain is felt is of no diagnostic significance, other than to establish that the complaint is one of headache. However, whether the pain is unilateral or bilateral does bear on the diagnosis of some forms of headache. For example, tension-type headache typically affects the entire head, whereas most other forms of headache are typically, although not always, unilateral. Pain of a neuralgic quality (see below), in the distribution of the nerve affected, is diagnostic of trigeminal neuralgia, glossopharyngeal or vagal neuralgia, and C2 neuralgia.

Radiation

Noting the areas *to which* pain radiates does not help in diagnosis. Different forms of headache may have the same pattern of radiation. However, it can be helpful to recognize sites *from which* pain appears to be referred. Although the pain may be perceived in the forehead, if it appears to have spread from the occiput or neck, a possible cervical source should be considered.

Intensity

All forms of headache can be mild, moderate, or severe in intensity. So, intensity alone does not serve to discriminate different types of headache. However, certain types of headache are characterized by severe headache of sudden onset, sometimes described as "thunderclap" headache. Possible causes include subarachnoid haemorrhage, meningitis, and phaeochromocytoma.

Quality

Most headaches will be dull, aching, or throbbing in quality. These features do not help in making a diagnosis. On the other hand, a lancinating quality of pain establishes that the pain is neuralgic, and is one of the defining features of trigeminal neuralgia, glossopharyngeal or vagal neuralgia, and of C2 neuralgia. Stabbing pain, or jabs of pain, is characteristic of cluster headache, although other features more strongly define this condition.

Frequency

Of all pain problems, headache is the one condition in which frequency is a cardinal diagnostic feature. Short, repeated jabs of pain, recurring in bouts over several minutes are what characterize cluster headache. Periods of pain lasting half a day, or up to three or four days, interspersed with periods free of pain, is what characterizes migraine. Other types of headache occur in paroxysmal bouts, i.e. sustained periods of repeated jabs of intense pain that then switch off. These include chronic paroxysmal hemicrania (CPH), and SUNCT (sudden, unilateral, neuralgiform headache with conjunctival injection and tearing).

Duration

Duration of pain is often inextricably linked to frequency. In cluster headache, and its congeners, the frequency of jabs of pain is high, but the duration of each jab is short, i.e. seconds. In migraine, the headache is established and remains constant, such that its duration is measured in hours or days, but then a pain–free interval appears.

Time of Onset

This is probably an obsolete category of enquiry for diagnostic purposes. Its heritage is that early morning headache was once regarded as pathognomonic of hypertension headache, but this has been disproved. Nevertheless, sometimes the time of onset can provide clues to the cause of headache. For example, headache caused by exposure to chemicals or allergens may occur at only particular times of the day, particular days of the week, or particular seasons of the year. Synchrony with menstrual cycle strongly suggests menstrual migraine.

Mode of Onset

Severe headaches of sudden onset suggest subarachnoid haemorrhage, meningitis, or hypertension as the causes. Otherwise, most headaches come on gradually or in an unremarkable fashion. However, some forms of migraine can have a prodrome. A prodrome of neurological symptoms is virtually diagnostic of classical migraine (now known as migraine with prodrome (Headache Classification Subcommittee of the International Headache Society 2004). Some patients with migraine will suffer cravings for certain types of foods, before the onset of headache. This fits with serotonin mechanisms that on the one hand are involved with pain, and on the other hand are involved with satiety.

Precipitating Factors

Some forms of recurrent headache can be precipitated, inadvertently or consciously, by certain actions. In some patients, the pain of trigeminal neuralgia can be precipitated by touching trigger spots on the face, or in the mouth. Headache precipitated by sexual activity is referred to as "sex headache", and appears to be related to a rapid rise in blood pressure. A rare, but distinctive entity, is colloid cyst of the third ventricle, in which headache can be precipitated by extension of the head, which causes the cyst to occlude the cerebral aqueduct and precipitate a sudden rise in cerebrospinal fluid pressure. "Ice–pick headache" is the term accorded to headache precipitated by exposure to cold foods or liquids.

For headaches of recent onset, not experienced before, an antecedent event may indicate the possible or likely cause. A classical example is post-lumbar puncture headache. A vexatious issue is trauma. Patients may

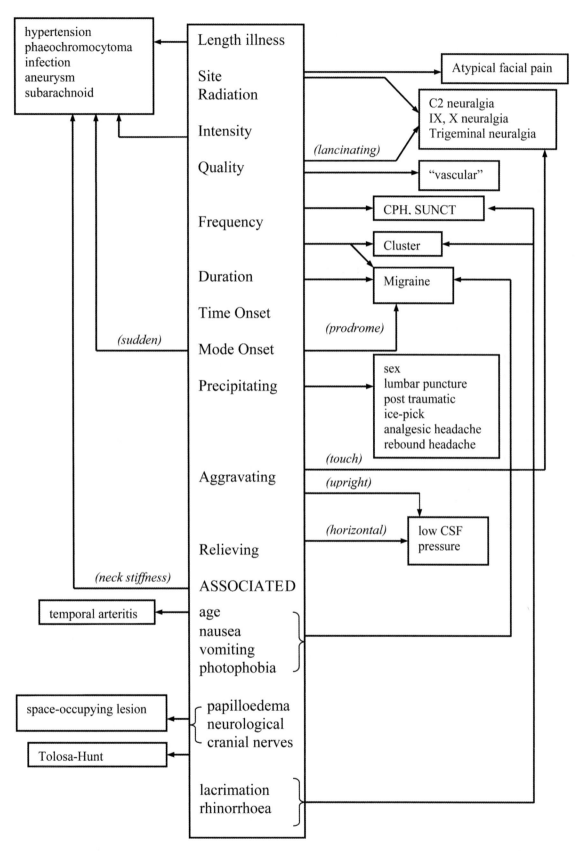

Headache, Figure 1   The differential diagnosis of headache by clinical history and examination.

report an injury that apparently caused the headache. However, a direct link between trauma and headache may be difficult to prove, and is sometimes contentious. Nevertheless, a history of trauma may be the only defining feature of some forms of headache; on which grounds the entity of "post–traumatic headache" is recognized.

Some headaches can be caused by exposure to drugs such as alcohol. Some headaches, paradoxically, can be caused by excessive consumption of analgesics. Withdrawal of analgesics can cause rebound headache.

Aggravating Factors

Few features that aggravate headache help in establishing a diagnosis, for many different forms of headache may be aggravated by activities such as turning the head, or exertion. However, certain features that appear to aggravate the pain are better classified as associated features (see below).

Relieving Factors

Many patients with headache resort to lying down. So, lying down per se is not a discriminating feature. However, when lying down promptly relieves the headache, and when resumption of the upright posture restores it, the leading diagnosis is low-pressure cerebrospinal fluid, which can be idiopathic or secondary to lumbar puncture.

Associated Features

It is in the domain of associated features that most headaches can be distinguished. Photophobia, nausea and vomiting are the cardinal diagnostic features of migraine. Lacrimation, rhinorrhoea, and conjunctival injection are reflex parasympathetic effects that occur with a family of headaches. Classically, they are the associated features of cluster headache, but they also occur in paroxysmal hemicrania and SUNCT syndrome. Papilloedema and focal neurological signs are the classic features of space occupying lesion of the cranium. Other important features are neck stiffness and Kernig's sign, which are virtually diagnostic of spread of infection or haemorrhage into the cervical subarachnoid space. Neurological signs affecting the III, IV, and VI cranial nerves are diagnostic of Tolosa–Hunt syndrome, i.e. granuloma of the cavernous sinus.

Age is an important feature. New headache in an elderly patient may be the only warning feature of temporal arteritis.

The diagnosis of acute herpes zoster can be made immediately once the eruption of vesicles occurs, but the pain may precede the eruption by up to three days.

Diagnosis

Figure 1 illustrates how taking a systematic history can allow many types of headache to be diagnosed on the basis of certain clinical features, singly or in combination. Migraine is diagnosed on the basis of periodic pain associated with photophobia, nausea, or vomiting. Cluster headache is defined by paroxysmal pain associated with lacrimation, rhinorrhoea, and conjunctival injection. Its relatives – CPH and SUNCT, only differ essentially with respect to the periodicity and duration of the headache. Intracranial lesions are diagnosed on the basis of associated neurological signs.

Certain entities, however, cannot be recognized clinically, because they do not have any distinctive features. Those entities are: benign intracranial hypertension, sphenoid sinusitis, cervicogenic headache, and tension type headache.

The first three of these entities require investigations. Benign intracranial hypertension requires a CT scan. Sphenoid sinusitis is perhaps the most "impalpable" headache. It exhibits nothing but pain, felt somewhere deep in the centre of the head. The diagnosis is established eventually by medical imaging. The diagnosis of cervicogenic headache requires the establishment of a cervical source of pain, by medical imaging or by diagnostic blocks of cervical structures or nerves.

Tension type headache is notable because there are no positive diagnostic criteria for this entity. It is a diagnosis by exclusion of other possible causes.

Other ill–defined entities include so-called "vascular headache", whose cardinal feature is throbbing pain, but which does not exhibit any of the diagnostic features of migraine.

▶ Chronic Daily Headache in Children

References

1. Headache Classification Subcommittee of the International Headache Society (2004) The International Classification of Headache Disorders, 2nd edn. Cephalalgia 24 Suppl 1:1–160
2. Olesen J, Tfelt-Hansen P, Welch KM (2000) The Headaches, 2nd edn. Lippincott Williams & Wilkins, Philadelphia

Headache, Acute Post-Traumatic

MIGUEL JA LÁINEZ-ANDRÉS[1],
ANA M PASCUAL-LOZANO[2]
[1]Department of Neurology, University of Valencia, Valencia, Spain
[2]Clinical Hospital, University of Valencia, Valencia, Spain
jlainez@meditex.es

Synonyms

Post-Traumatic Headache; PTHA

Definition

Post-traumatic headache (PTHA) is usually one of several symptoms of the "post-traumatic syndrome" and therefore may be accompanied by somatic, psychological or cognitive disturbances (Solomon 2001). A variety of pain patterns may develop after head injury and may closely resemble primary headache disorders. Common headache pathways have been described for primary and post-traumatic headaches but the pathogenesis of PTHA is still not well known (Martelli 1999).

Characteristics

Tension-type is the most common variety of PTHA (more than 80% of the patients suffered a tension-type headache after head or neck trauma), followed by cervicogenic headache. Exacerbations of migraine and cluster-like headaches also occur. Post-traumatic migraine (PTMA) represents approximately 8–10% of PTHA. This is usually a migraine without aura, often found in children, adolescents and young adults with familial history of migraine. Migraine with visual aura has been described in only a few patients (Hachinski 2000).

Mild, moderate and severe head injuries can be associated with a PTHA. Clinical quantification of traumatic brain injury patients should be based on the Glasgow Coma Scale score (GCS), duration of loss of consciousness (LOC) and presence of posttraumatic amnesia (PTA) In addition, a short practicable neuropsychological test may be useful in detecting minor memory and attentional deficits. Paradoxically, mild head injury is often accompanied by headache and additional symptoms, more frequently than moderate or severe head traumas.

To differentiate between a primary and a post-traumatic headache can be difficult in some cases. Patients who develop a new form of headache in close temporal relation to head or neck trauma should be coded as having a secondary headache. Patients in whom this type of headache was pre-existing but significantly worsened in close temporal relation to trauma, without evidence of a causal relationship between the primary headache and the other disorder, receive only the primary headache diagnosis. However, if there is both a very close temporal relation to the trauma and other good evidence that the particular kind of trauma has aggravated the primary headache, that is if trauma in scientific studies of good quality has been shown to aggravate the primary headache disorder, the patient receives the primary and the secondary headache diagnoses. In many cases of secondary headache, the diagnosis is definite only when the headache resolves or greatly improves within a specified time after effective treatment or spontaneous remission of the causative disorder. In such cases, this temporal relation is an essential part of the evidence of causation.

It is easy to establish the relationship between a headache and head or neck trauma when the headache develops immediately or in the first days after trauma has occurred. On the other hand, it is very difficult when a headache develops weeks or even months after trauma, especially when the majority of these headaches have the pattern of tension-type headache and the prevalence of this type of headache in the population is very high.

Such late onset post-traumatic headaches have been described in anecdotal reports but not in case-control studies. In accordance with new IHS Classification, that will soon be published, acute PTHA develops within 7 days after head trauma or regaining consciousness following head trauma and resolves within 3 months.

New Diagnostic Criteria for Acute Post-traumatic Headache: Acute Posttraumatic Headache with Moderate or Severe Head Injury Diagnostic Criteria

a) Headache, no typical characteristics known, fulfilling criteria C and D
b) Head trauma with at least one of the following:

1. Loss of consciousness for >30 minutes
2. Glasgow Coma Scale (GCS) <13
3. Post-traumatic amnesia for >48 h
4. Imaging demonstration of a traumatic brain lesion (cerebral hematoma, intracerebral and/or subarachnoid haemorrhage, brain contusion and/or skull fracture)

c) Headache develops within 7 days after head trauma or after regaining consciousness following head trauma
d) One or other of the following:

1. Headache resolves within 3 months after head trauma
2. Headache persist but 3 months have not yet passed since head trauma

Acute Posttraumatic Headache with Mild Head Injury

Diagnostic Criteria

a) Headache, no typical characteristics known, fulfilling criteria C and D
b) Head trauma with all the following:

1. Either no loss of consciousness, or loss of consciousness of <30 minutes duration
2. Glasgow Coma Scale (GCS) >13
3. Symptoms and/or signs diagnostic of concussion

c) Headache develops within 7 days after head trauma
d) One or other of the following:

1. Headache resolves within 3 months after head trauma
2. Headache persists but 3 months have not yet passed since head trauma.

Before new diagnosis criteria, acute-PTHA might begin less than 14 days after head or neck trauma and continue for up to 8 weeks post-injury (Headache Classification Committee of IHS 1988). Headache that develops longer than 14 days after head injury has been termed "delayed-PTHA or late-acquired headache". If such headaches persist beyond the first 3 months post-injury, they are subsequently referred to as chronic-PTHA

New Diagnostic Criteria for Chronic Post-traumatic Headache: Chronic Posttraumatic Headache with Moderate or Severe Head Injury Diagnostic Criteria

a) Headache, no typical characteristics known, fulfilling criteria C and D

b) Head trauma with at least one of the following:

1. Loss of consciousness >30 minutes
2. Glasgow Coma Scale (GCS) <13
3. Post-traumatic amnesia >48 hours
4. Imaging demonstration of a traumatic brain lesion (cerebral hematoma, intracerebral and/or sub-arachnoid haemorrhage, brain contusion and/or skull fracture)

c) Headache develops within 7 days after head trauma or after regaining consciousness following head trauma

d) Headache persists for >3 months after head trauma

Chronic Posttraumatic Headache with Mild Head Injury

Diagnostic Criteria

a) Headache, no typical characteristics known, fulfilling criteria C and D

b) Head trauma with all the following:

1. Either no loss of consciousness, or loss of consciousness of <30 minutes duration
2. Glasgow Coma Scale (GCS) >13
3. Symptoms and/or signs diagnostic of concussion

c) Headache develops within 7 days after head trauma

d) Headache persist for >3 months after head trauma

After mild head trauma, laboratory and ▶ neuroimaging investigations are not habitually needed. When the GCS score is less than 13 in the emergency room after head or neck trauma, LOC is longer than 30 min, there is PTA, neurological deficits or personality disturbances, neuroimaging studies (computer tomography scan, CT, or magnetic resonance imaging, MRI) are indicated. MRI (using at least T1 weighted, T2 weighted, proton density and gradient-echo sequence images) is much more sensitive than CT in detecting and classifying brain lesions. Within 1 week of a head injury, MRI can identify cortical contusions and lesions in the deep white matter of the cerebral hemispheres underdiagnosed by CT. MRI thus provides a sounder basis for diagnosis and treatment in patients suffering from late sequelae of cranial injuries (Voller 2001).

Complementary studies (neuroimaging, EEG, evoked potentials, CSF examination, vestibular function tests) should also be considered for patients with ongoing posttraumatic headaches. The relationship between severity of the injury and severity of the post-traumatic syndrome has not been conclusively established. Moreover, there are some controversial data. Most studies suggest that PTHA is less frequent when the head injury is more severe. Differential diagnosis may include a symptomatic headache, secondary to structural lesions and simulation. There is no evidence that an abnormality in the complementary explorations changes the ▶ prognosis or contributes to treatment. Special complementary studies should be considered on a case-by-case basis or for research purposes.

After several months, some patients developed a daily headache. In the majority of patients with episodic headaches after head injury, this condition is self-limited, but a minority of individuals may develop persistent headaches. Neurological factors have been implicated in the initial phase, psychological and legal factors (litigation and expectations for compensation) in the maintenance of them. Premorbid personality can contribute to development of chronic symptoms, affecting adjustment to injury and treatment outcome. Surprisingly, the risk of developing chronic disturbances seems to be greater for mild-moderate head injury.

Age, gender, certain mechanical factors, a low intellectual, educational and socio-economic level, previous history of headache or alcohol abuse and long duration of unconsciousness or neurological deficits after the head or neck injury, are recognized ▶ risk factors for a poor outcome. Women have higher risk of PTHA and increasing age is associated with a less rapid and less complete recovery. Mechanical impact factors, such as an abnormal position of the head (rotation or inclined) increase the risk of PTHA. Other predictor factors are presence of skull fracture, reduced value of Glasgow Scale, elevated serum protein S-100B and dizziness, headache and nausea in the emergency room (De Krujik 2002).

The role of litigation in the persistence of headache is still discussed. The relationship between legal settlements and the temporal profile of chronic-PTHA is not clearly established, but it is important to carefully assess patients who may be malingering and/or seeking enhanced compensation. In general, medico-legal issues should be solved as soon as possible.

Pathophysiology of PTHA

Pathophysiology of post-traumatic headaches is still not well understood but biological, psychological and social factors are included. In the pathogenesis, common headache pathways with primary headaches have been proposed.

During typical migraine, cerebral cortical and brain stem changes occur. The activation of the brainstem monoaminergic nuclei has been demonstrated with functional imaging studies (Bahra 2001). Disturbed neuronal calcium influx and / or hemostatic alterations have also been involved. However, these events have not been included for PTMA yet.

In recent years, several pieces of research have implicated similar neurochemical changes in both typical migraine and experimental traumatic brain injury, excessive release of excitatory amino acids, alterations in serotonin, abnormalities in catecholamines and endogenous opioids, decline in magnesium levels, abnormalities in nitric oxide formation and alterations in neuropeptides (Packard 1997). Whether these changes are determining, contributing or precipitating factors for headache in each patient is still unknown. In addition, in patients with late-PTMA a sensitization phenomenon is possible. In some patients without previous migraine and history of a recent mild head injury, trigeminal neuron sensitization could be a central cause in relation to focal lesions. Central and peripheral sensitizations have been proposed before by other authors (Malick 2000; Packard 2002).

Further researches are still necessary to clarify the relationship between chronic symptoms after mild head trauma and neuroimaging abnormalities. These abnormalities could provide a pathological basis for long-term neurological disability in patients with post-concussive syndrome. New techniques of MRI (especially diffusion tensor imaging and magnetization transfer ratio) are useful for the detection of small parenchymal brain lesions, diffuse axonal injury secondary to disruption of axonal membranes or delayed cerebral atrophy (Hofman 2002). In normal appearing white matter, magnetic resonance spectroscopy studies detect metabolic brain changes (an early reduction in N-acetyl aspartate and an increase in choline compounds), which correlate with head injury severity (Garnett 2000). Positron-emission tomography (PET), single-photon emission computed tomography (SPECT) and xenon 133 CT may provide evidence of brain perfusion abnormalities after mild head trauma and in the presence of chronic posttraumatic symptoms (Aumile 2002).

Management Strategies

Trauma-induced headaches are usually heterogeneous in nature, including both tension-type and intermittent migraine attacks. Over time, PTHA may take on a pattern of daily occurrence, although if aggressive treatment is initiated early, PTHA is less likely to become a permanent problem. Adequate treatment typically requires both "central" and "peripheral" measures. Delayed recovery from PTHA may be a result of inadequately aggressive or ineffective treatment, overuse of analgesic medications resulting in analgesia rebound phenomena or comorbid psychiatric disorders (posttraumatic stress disorder, insomnia, substance abuse, depression or anxiety) (Lane 2002).

In general, treatment strategies are based upon studies of non-traumatic headache types. Acute-PTHA may be treated with analgesics, anti-inflammatory agents and physiotherapy. PTMA may be also treated with ergotamine or triptans. Chronic-PTHA needs prophylactic medication, chronic-PTMA specific antimigraine medications. Previously amitriptyline or propranolol used alone or in combination and verapamil have been demonstrated to improve all symptoms of postconcussive syndrome, especially the migraine. Recently, Packard has published very good results with divalproex sodium as a preventive option in the treatment of PTMA (Packard 2000). Additional physical therapy, psychotherapy (bio-feedback) and appropriate educational support can be supplied, especially in patients with risk factors for poor prognosis. Explanation of the headache's nature can also improve the patient's evolution. In some cases, when a post-traumatic lesion is identified as a peripheral triggering factor for headache, specific treatment of the triggering lesion can resolve the pain. PTMA poorly treated will affect family life, recreation and employment There is no good evidence that litigation and economical expectation is associated with prolongation of headaches, however litigation should be solved as soon as is possible.

Conclusions

Trauma induced headache and headache attributed to whiplash should be treated early or associated complications will appear (daily occurrence of headache, overuse of analgesic medications and comorbid psychiatric disorders). Preventive and symptomatic treatments may be prescribed according to the clinical pattern of the headache (tension-type, migraine, cluster or cervicogenic headaches) as a primary headache. Physiotherapy, psychotherapy and resolution of litigation can be contributing factors to recovery.

References

1. Aumile EM, Sandel ME, Alavi A et al. (2002) Dynamic imaging in mild traumatic brain injury support for the theory of medial temporal vulnerability. Arch Phys Med Rehabil 83:1506–1513
2. Bahra A, Matharu MS, Buchel C et al. (2001) Brainstem activation specific to migraine headache. Lancet 357:1016–1017
3. De Kruijk JR, Leffers P, Menheere PP et al. (2002) Prediction of posttraumatic complaints after mild traumatic brain injury: early symptoms and biochemical markers. J Neurol Neurosurg Psychiatry 73:727–732
4. Garnett MR, Blamire AM, Rajagopalau B et al. (2000) Evidence for cellular damage in normal-appearing white matter correlates with injury severity in patients following traumatic brain injury: a magnetic resonance spectroscopy study. Brain 123:1043–1049
5. Hachinski W (2000) Posttraumatic headache. Arch Neurol 57:1780
6. Headache Classification Committee of the International Headache Society (1988) Classification and diagnostic criteria for headache disorders, cranial neuralgias and facial pain. Cephalalgia 8:1–96
7. Hofman PA, Verhey FR, Wilmink JT et al. (2002) Brain lesions in patients visiting a memory clinic with postconcussional sequelaes after mild to moderate brain injury. J neuropsychiatry Clin Neurosci 14:176–178
8. Lane J, Arciniegas DB (2002) Post-traumatic Headache. Curr Treat Options Neurol 4:89–104
9. Malick A, Burstein R (2000) Peripheral and central sensitization during migraine. Funct Neurol 15:28–35

10. Martelli MF, Grayson RL, Zasler ND (1999) Post-traumatic headache: neuropsychological and psychological effects and treatment implications. J Head Trauma Rehabil 14:49–69
11. Packard RC, Haw CP (1997) Pathogenesis of PTH and migraine: a common headache pathway? Headache 37:142–152
12. Packard RC (2000) Treatment of chronic daily posttraumatic headache with divalproex sodium. Headache 40:736–739
13. Packard RC (2002) The relationship of neck injury and posttraumatic headache. Curr Pain Headache Rep 6:30131–30137
14. Solomon S (2001) Post-traumatic headache. Med Clin North Am 85:987–996
15. Voller B, Auff E, Schnider P et al. (2001) To do or not to do MRI in mild traumatic brain injury? Brain Inj 15:107–115

Headache Associated with Disorders of the Cranium

▶ Headache from Cranial Bone

Headache Associated with Psychotic Disorder

▶ Headache Due to Somatoform Disorder

Headache Associated with Somatisation Disorder

▶ Headache Due to Somatoform Disorder

Headache Attributed to a Substance or its Withdrawal

STEPHEN D. SILBERSTEIN
Jefferson Medical College, Thomas Jefferson University and Jefferson Headache Center, Thomas Jefferson University Hospital, Philadelphia, PA, USA
stephen.silberstein@jefferson.edu

Synonyms

Medication-Induced Headaches; headaches associated with substances or their withdrawal

Definition

The International Headache Society (IHS) previously grouped medication-induced headaches under the rubric "headaches associated with substances or their withdrawal (Headache Classification Committee of the International Headache Society 1988)." The new IHS classification (Headache Classification Committee 2003) now calls these "headaches attributed to a substance or its withdrawal (Monteiro and Dahlof 2000)."

Food, chemical and drug ingestion or exposure can be both a cause of and a trigger for headache (Silberstein 1998). Their association is often based on reports of adverse drug reactions and anecdotal data and does not prove causality. When a new headache occurs for the first time in close temporal relation to substance exposure, it is coded as a secondary headache attributed to the substance. When a pre-existing primary headache is made worse by substance exposure, there are two possibilities. The patient can either be given only the diagnosis of the pre-existing primary headache or be given both this diagnosis and the diagnosis of headache attributed to the substance (Headache Classification Committee 2003).

Headache Attributed to Acute Substance Use or Exposure (Headache Classification Committee 2003)

Diagnostic Criteria

1. Headache fulfilling criteria 3 and 4.
2. Acute use of or other acute exposure to a substance.
3. Headache develops within 12 h of use or exposure.
4. Headache resolves within 72 h after single use or exposure.

Characteristics

Alcohol, food and food additives and chemical and drug ingestion and withdrawal have all been reported to provoke or activate migraine in susceptible individuals. Since headache is a complaint often attributed to placebo, substance-related headache may arise as a result of expectation. The association between a headache and an exposure may be coincidental (occurring just on the basis of chance) or due to a concomitant illness or a direct or indirect effect of the drug and may depend on the condition being treated. Headache can be a symptom of a systemic disease and drugs given to treat such a condition will be associated with headache. Some disorders may predispose to substance-related headache. Alone, neither the drug nor the condition would produce headache. A ▶ NSAIDs, Survey may produce headache by inducing aseptic meningitis in susceptible individuals. The possible relationships between drugs and headache are outlined below (Silberstein 1998).

Drug and Substance Related Headache

A Coincidental
B Reverse causality
C Interaction headache
D Causal

Acute: Primary effect; Secondary Effect

Acute Drug-induced Headache

Whether or not a drug triggers a headache often depends on the presence or absence of an underlying headache disorder. Headaches are usually similar to the preexisting headache. The drugs most commonly associated with acute headache can be divided into several classes (Monteiro and Dahlof 2000).

Vasodilator's

Headache is a frequent side effect of antihypertensive drugs. It has been reported with the beta-blockers, ▶ calcium channel blockers (especially nifedipine), ACE inhibitors and methyldopa. Nicotinic acid, dipyridamole and hydralazine have also been associated with headache. The headache mechanism is uncertain (Thomson Healthcare 2003).

Nitric Oxide Donor-induced Headache

Headache is well known as a side effect of therapeutic use of nitroglycerin (GTN) and other ▶ nitric oxide (NO) donors. They may cause headache by activating the trigeminal vascular pathway. There is an immediate NO donor-induced headache (GTN headache), which develops within 10 min after absorption of NO donor and resolves within 1 h after release of NO has ended. There is also a delayed NO donor-induced headache, which develops after NO is cleared from the blood and resolves within 72 h after single exposure (Ashina et al. 2000).

Phosphodiesterase Inhibitor-induced Headache

Phosphodiesterases (PDEs) are a large family of enzymes that break down cyclic ▶ nucleotide s (cGMP and cAMP). PDE-5 inhibitors include sildenafil and dipyridamole. The headache, unlike GTN-induced headache, is monophasic. In normal volunteers it has the characteristics of tension-type headache, but in migraine sufferers it has the characteristics of migraine without aura (Headache Classification Committee 2003).

Histamine-induced Headache

Histamine causes an immediate headache in non-headache sufferers and an immediate as well as a delayed headache in migraine sufferers. The mechanism is primarily mediated *via* the H_1 receptor because it is almost completely blocked by mepyramine. The immediate histamine-induced headache develops within 10 min and resolves within 1 h after absorption of histamine has ceased. The delayed histamine-induced headache develops after histamine is cleared from the blood and resolves within 72 h (Krabbe and Olesen 1980).

Nonsteroidal Anti-Inflammatory Drugs

The nonsteroidal anti-inflammatory drugs, especially indomethacin, have been associated with headache. Mechanisms include aseptic meningitis (especially with ibuprofen) and reverse causality.

Serotonin Agonists

M-chlorophenylpiperazine, a metabolite of the antidepressant trazodone, can trigger headache by activating the serotonin (5-hydroxytryptamine [HT]) 2B and 2C receptors (Brewerton et al. 1988). This may be the mechanism of headache induction during early treatment with selective serotonin reuptake inhibitors.

Foods and Natural Products (Headache Induced by Food Components and Additives)

Chocolate, alcohol, citrus fruits, cheese and dairy products are the foods that patients most commonly believe trigger their migraine, but the evidence is not persuasive.

Amino Acids

Monosodium glutamate (MSG) (Schamburg et al. 1969) and aspartame, the active ingredient of "NutraSweet," may cause headache in susceptible individuals (Schiffmann et al. 1987). Phenyl ethylamine, tyramine and aspartame have been incriminated, but their headache-inducing potential is not sufficiently validated.

Monosodium Glutamate-induced Headache (Chinese Restaurant Syndrome)

MSG can induce headache and the Chinese restaurant syndrome in susceptible individuals. The headache is typically dull or burning and non-pulsating, but may be pulsating in migraine sufferers. It is commonly associated with other symptoms, including pressure in the chest, pressure and / or tightness in the face, burning sensations in the chest, neck or shoulders, flushing of the face, dizziness and abdominal discomfort (Schamburg et al. 1969).

Aspartame

Aspartame a sugar substitute is an o-methyl ester of the dipeptide L-α-aspartyl-L-phenylalanine that blocks the increase in brain tryptophan, 5-HT and 5-hydroxyindolacetic acid normally seen after carbohydrate consumption (Schiffmann et al. 1987). It produced headache in two controlled studies but not a third (Silberstein 1998).

Tyramine

Tyramine is a biogenic amine that is present in mature cheeses. It is probably not a migraine trigger (Silberstein 1998).

Phenyl Ethylamine

Chocolate contains large amounts of β-phenyl ethylamine, a vasoactive amine that is, in part, metabolized by monoamine oxidase. The evidence to support it as a trigger is weak (Silberstein 1998).

Ethanol

Alone or in combination with ▶ congener s (wine), ethanol can induce headache in susceptible individuals. The attacks often occur within hours after ingestion. In the United Kingdom, red wine is more likely to trigger migraine than white, while in France and Italy white wine is more likely to produce headache than red. Headaches are more likely to develop in response to white wine if red coloring matter has been added.

Migraineurs who believed that red wine (but not alcohol) provoked their headaches were challenged either with red wine or with a vodka mixture of equivalent alcoholic content. The red wine provoked migraine in 9 / 11 subjects, the vodka in 0 / 11. Neither provoked headache in other migraine subjects or controls (Littlewood et al. 1988). It is not known which component of red wine triggers headache and the study may not have been blinded to oenophiles.

The susceptibility to hangover headache has not been determined. Migraineurs can suffer a migraine the next day after only modest alcoholic intake, while non-migraineurs usually need a high intake of alcoholic beverages to develop hangover headache. A few subjects develop headache due to a direct effect of alcohol or alcoholic beverages (cocktail headache). This is much rarer than delayed alcohol-induced headache (hangover headache).

Lactose Intolerance

Lactose intolerance is a common genetic disorder, occurring in over two-thirds of African-Americans, native Americans and Ashkenazi Jews and in 10% of individuals of Scandinavian ancestry. The most common symptoms are abdominal cramps and flatulence. How lactose intolerance triggers migraine is uncertain (Silberstein 1998).

Chocolate

Chocolate is the food most frequently believed to trigger headache, but the evidence supporting this belief is inconsistent (Scharff and Marcus 1999). Chocolate is probably not a migraine trigger, despite the fact that many migraineurs believe that it triggers their headache. It is the most commonly craved food in the United States. Women are more likely than men to have migraine and they crave chocolate more than men. Sweet craving is a premonitory symptom of migraine and menses are often associated with an increase in carbohydrate and chocolate craving.

Chemotherapeutic Drugs

▶ Intrathecal methotrexate and diaziquone can produce aseptic meningitis and headache. Methyldichlorophen, interferon B and interleukin 2 are all associated with headache (Boogerd 1995).

Immunomodulating Drugs

Cyclosporine, FK-506, thalidomide and antithymocyte globulin have been associated with headache (Shah and Lisak 1995).

Antimicrobial and Antimalarial Drugs

Amphotericin, griseofulvin, tetracycline and sulfonamides have been associated with headache. Chloroquine and ethionamide are also associated with headache.

Other Substances

Carbon monoxide-induced Headache (Warehouse Workers' Headache)

Typically this is a mild headache without associated symptoms with carboxyhemoglobin levels of 10–20%, a moderate pulsating headache and irritability with levels of 20–30% and a severe headache with nausea, vomiting and blurred vision with levels of 30–40%. When carboxyhemoglobin levels are higher than 40%, headache is not usually a complaint because of changes in consciousness.

Cocaine-induced Headache

Headache is common, develops immediately or within 1 h after use and is not associated with other symptoms unless there is concomitant stroke or TIA (Dhopesh et al. 1991).

Cannabis-induced Headache

Cannabis use is reported to cause headache associated with dryness of the mouth, paresthesias, feelings of warmth and suffusion of the conjunctivae (elMallakh 1987).

References

1. Ashina M, Bendtsen L, Jensen R et al. (2000) Nitric oxide-induced headache in patients with chronic tension-type headache. Brain 123:1830–1837
2. Bix KJ, Pearson DJ, Bentley SJ (1984) A psychiatric study of patients with supposed food allergy. Br J Psychiatry 145:121–126
3. Boogerd W (1995) Neurological complications of chemotherapy. In: DeWolff FA (ed) Handbook of clinical neurology. Elsevier, Amsterdam New York, pp 527
4. Brewerton TD, Murphy DL, Mueller EA et al. (1988) Induction of migraine like headaches by the serotonin agonist m-chlorophenylpiperazine. Clin Pharmacol Ther 43:605–609
5. Dhopesh V, Maany I, Herring C (1991) The relationship of cocaine to headache in polysubstance abusers. Headache 31:17–19
6. elMallakh RS (1987) Marijuana and migraine. Headache 27:442–443
7. Headache Classification Committee of the International Headache Society (1988) Classification and diagnostic criteria for headache disorders, cranial neuralgia, and facial pain. Cephalalgia 8:1–96
8. Headache Classification Committee (2003) The International Classification of Headache Disorders II. Cephalalgia (in press)
9. Krabbe AA Olesen J (1980) Headache provocation by continuous intravenous infusion of histamine, clinical results and receptor mechanisms. Pain 8:253–259
10. Littlewood JT, Glover V, Davies PT et al. (1988) Red wine as a cause of migraine. Lancet 559
11. Monteiro JM Dahlof CG (2000) Single use of substances. In: Olesen J, Tfelt-Hansen P, Welch KM (eds) The Headaches. Lippincott Williams & Wilkins, Philadelphia, pp 861–869
12. Rose FC (1997) Food and headache. Headache Quarterly 8:319–329
13. Schamburg HH, Byck R, Gerstl R et al. (1969) Monosodium L-glutamate: its pharmacology and role in the Chinese restaurant syndrome. Science 163:826–828
14. Scharff L, Marcus DA (1999) The association between chocolate and migraine: A review. Headache Quarterly 10:199–205
15. Schiffmann SS, Buckley CE, Sampson HA et al. (1987) Aspartame and susceptibility to headache. N Engl J Med 317:1181–1185

16. Shah AK Lisak R (1995) Neurological complications of immunomodulating therapy. In: DeWolff FA (ed) Handbook of clinical neurology. Elsevier, Amsterdam New York, pp 547
17. Silberstein SD (1998) Drug-induced headache. Neurol Clin N Amer 16:107–123
18. Thomson Healthcare (2003) Physicians' Desk Reference. Thomson PDR, Montvale
19. VanDenEeden SK, Koepsell TD, Longstreth WT et al. (1994) Aspartame ingestion and headaches: a randomized crossover trial. Neurology 44:1787–1793

Headache Due to Arteritis

PETER BERLIT
Department of Neurology, Alfried Krupp Hospital, Essen, Germany
peter.berlit@krupp-krankenhaus.de

Synonyms

Vasculitis; Angiitis of the CNS

Definition

Headache is the most common complaint in ▶ temporal arteritis. The major symptoms of central nervous system arteritis are multifocal neurological symptoms following ▶ stroke, in combination with headache and some degree of ▶ encephalopathy, with and without ▶ seizures. CNS-vasculitis may be part of a systemic autoimmune disease or the only manifestation of angiitis (isolated ▶ angiitis of the central nervous system – IAN).

Characteristics

Temporal Arteritis

Temporal arteritis (▶ cranial arteritis, giant cell arteritis) is an autoimmune disease of elderly people, affecting women more frequently than men (3:1). Mean age at the beginning of the disorder is 65 years or more; the disease rarely appears before the age of 50. The incidence is 18 / 100,000; there is a frequent association with HLA-DR4. The diagnosis is confirmed by the histological examination of a ▶ biopsy specimen from the temporal artery, demonstrating the arteritis with necrosis of the media and a granulomatous inflammatory exsudate containing lymphocytes, leukocytes and giant cells.

Headache is the most common complaint in temporal arteritis, associated with a markedly elevated sedimentation rate. The patient develops an increasingly intense head pain, usually unilateral, sometimes bilateral. It has a non-pulsating often sharp and stabbing character, sometimes with a temporal pronunciation. But the localization of the headache may be frontal, occipital or even nuchal (Pradalier and Le Quellec 2000). The pain increases during the night hours and persists throughout the day. Due to ischemia of the masseter muscles during mastication, ▶ jaw claudication may appear

Headache Due to Arteritis, Table 1 Frequency of signs and symptoms with temporal arteritis (adapted from Caselli and Hunder 1996)

Symptom	all (%)	initial symptom (%)
headache	72	33
polymyalgia rheumatica	58	25
malaise, weight loss	56	20
jaw claudication	40	4
fever	35	11
cough	17	8
neuropathies (mono-, or multiplex)	14	0
disorders of swallowing	11	2
amaurosis fugax	10	2
permanent loss of vision	8	3
claudication of limbs (legs)	8	0
stroke	7	0
neuro-otologic disorders	7	0
flimmer-scotoma	5	0
pain of the tongue	4	0
depression	3	0.6
diplopia	2	0
myelopathy	0.6	0

(Berlit 1997). The superficial temporal artery may be thickened and tender without pulsation –"cord-sign".

Diagnostic criteria of temporal arteritis

- age 50 years or more
- newly developed headache
- tenderness of the superficial temporal artery
- elevated sedimentation rate, at least 50 mm / h
- giant cell arteritis in a biopsy specimen from the temporal artery

Besides the headache, there may be severe pain, aching and symmetrical stiffness in proximal muscles of the limbs (polymyalgia rheumatica) in as many as 50% of patients. Many patients present the symptoms of a cryptogenic neoplasm, anorexia, loss of weight, anemia, malaise and low-grade fever.

Sudden blindness results from involvement of the posterior ciliary arteries, and blindness of one eye may be followed by the other. Other complications include the affection of intracranial or spinal vessels, necrosis of the scalp or tongue and generalization of the arteritis affecting the coronary arteries, the aorta or the intestines.

The treatment of choice at the earliest suspicion of cranial arteritis is ▶ prednisone 60–80 mg / day. If ischemic complications are present, a steroid pulse-therapy for 3 days with at least 500 mg prednisone i.v. is recommended. Patients respond quickly and often very impressively to steroids. The start of this therapy should not be delayed for the biopsy. Depending on the clinical symptoms and the sedimentation rate, steroids are gradually reduced. In the majority of patients, steroid treatment is necessary for at least 20 months; therefore a biopsy is mandatory in all cases. During the long-term course, the CRP is more helpful in the prediction of relapses than the sedimentation rate (Berlit 1997). If necessary, ▶ azathioprine or ▶ methotrexate may be used as steroid sparing agents.

Systemic Lupus Erythematosus (SLE)

▶ Systemic lupus erythematosus (SLE) is the most frequent systemic autoimmune disease, incidence 7 / 100,000 (Ruiz-Irastorza et al. 2001); the prevalence in Europe and the USA is 10 to 60 / 100,000 per year, women : men = 10 : 1. The most common age of manifestation is 15–30 years. Both migraine type headaches (see ▶ migraine) are frequent. SLE is characterized by a disturbed regulation of T- and B-cell immunity with antinuclear antibodies and autoreactivity against other autoantigens in the progressive relapsing course of the disease. The multilocular manifestations are caused by a thrombotic vasopathy or antibodies interacting with cell membrane functions; a true vasculitis is rare. Antinuclear antibodies are present in 95%, ds-DNA-antibodies in 80%. ▶ Photosensitivity of the skin with a ▶ butterfly erythema of the face are typical symptoms of SLE. Arthritis and serositis with pulmonary and cardiac manifestations are frequent. Neurological symptoms are present in about 50% of the patients, encephalopathy (60%), seizures (60%) and stroke (40%). In SLE, strokes are frequently caused by a secondary ▶ antiphospholipid syndrome (25% of all SLE patients). This diagnosis is made with the detection of lupus anticoagulant and IgG-anticardiolipin antibodies. Stroke may also be caused by cardiogenic embolism with Libmann-Sacks endocarditis or by thrombotic thrombocytopenic purpura. Some autoantibodies (ab) are associated with certain clinical manifestations, ribosomal P –psychosis, Jo 1 – polymyositis, antineuronal – epilepsy, encephalopathy. A classification of the neuropsychiatric SLE-manifestations including headache has been given by the ACR Ad Hoc Committee on Neuropsychiatric Lupus in 1999. In case-control studies, there was no difference between SLE patients and the general population regarding the prevalence and incidence of migraine or tension type headache (Fernandez-Nebro et al. 1999; Sfikakis et al. 1998). In SLE patients with tension type headache, there was an association with personality changes, emotional conflicts and depression (Omdal 2001). Most of these patients have higher disease activity scores (Amit et al. 1999). There was no association between anticardiolipin antibodies and migraine in a prospective study

(Vazquez-Cruz et al. 1990). If a SLE patient develops a new headache, a neurological examination including ▶ MRI and lumbar puncture is mandatory. The association with a ▶ pseudotumor cerebri should be excluded. Treatment of idiopathic headache syndromes in SLE is the same as in the general population. A headache as the sole neurological symptom of SLE should not alter the immunosuppressive strategy in the individual patient.

Sjögren's Syndrome

▶ Sjögren's syndrome is clinically characterized by keratoconjunctivitis sicca and symptomatic xerostomia (the sicca-syndrome) and associated with the detection of anti-Ro (SSA–97%) and anti-La (SSB–78%) autoantibodies. In addition to multifocal CNS symptoms with encephalopathy, depression or headache, a polyneuropathy and myopathy occur frequently. Whenever possible the diagnosis should be verified with a salivary gland biopsy. The incidence of migraine is higher in patients with a sicca syndrome or Raynaud phenomenon (Pal et al. 1989). ▶ Flunarizin may be helpful for prophylaxis in rheumatologic patients with migraine (Mazagri and Shuaib 1992).

Wegener's Granulomatosis (WG)

▶ Wegener's granulomatosis (WG) is a rare autoimmune disease (1 per 100,000) associated with antineutrophile cytoplasmic antibodies (c-ANCA); men are affected twice as often as women. In the limited stage of the disease, necrotizing granulomas of the nose and the paranasal sinuses may lead to compression of neighborhood structures with cranial nerve lesions, diabetes insipidus or exophthalmus. With generalization, the systemic necrotizing vasculitis involving small arteries and veins leads to affections of the lung and kidney.

In the limited stage of WG, headaches are frequent and often caused by sinusitis, non-septic meningitis or local granulomas (Lim et al. 2002). MRI may show enhancement of the basal meninges especially of the tentorium (Specks et al. 2000); the development of an occlusive or communicating hydrocephalus is possible (Scarrow et al. 1998) and must be excluded.

Prednisone and ▶ cyclophosphamide are the treatment of choice in generalized WG. In the limited stage of the disease, the combination of 2 × 800 mg sulfamethoxazole and 2 × 160 mg trimethoprim (▶ Cotrimoxazol) may be sufficient. Headaches are treated symptomatically with paracetamol or non-steroidal antiphlogistics.

Behçet's Disease

▶ Behçet's disease presents with the trias of iridocyclitis and oral and genital ulcers. The underlying systemic vasculitis of especially the veins may lead to an ▶ erythema nodosum, a thrombophlebitis, polyarthritis or ulcerative colitis. Behçet's syndrome is rare in the USA and Germany (incidence 1 / 500,000), but frequent in Turkey (300 / 100,000); men are affected twice as often as women, usually between the ages of 20 and 40. There is an association with HLA-B5. Neurological manifestations occur in approximately 30%, either as ► meningoencephalitis of the brain stem and cerebellum or as a ► sinus thrombosis, which presents often as pseudotumor cerebri (Akman-Demir et al. 1999). Headaches are the most common complaint in ► neuro-Behçet (87%). The holocephal stabbing severe pain does not usually respond to conventional analgetics, but resolves with steroid treatment. MRI and lumbar puncture are diagnostic. Steroids and immunosuppressants like azathioprine are the treatment of choice. In sinus thrombosis, anticoagulants must be given in addition.

Isolated Angiitis of the Central Nervous System – IAN (Granulomatous Arteritis of the Nervous System – GANS)

Isolated angiitis of the central nervous system – IAN (granulomatous arteritis of the nervous system – GANS) is an idiopathic medium and small vessel vasculitis affecting exclusively CNS vessels of the brain or spinal cord. About 350 cases have been documented worldwide (Schmidley 2000). The major symptoms of IAN are multifocal neurological symptoms following stroke, in combination with headache and some degree of encephalopathy, with or without seizures, cranial nerve palsies or ► myelopathy.

The encephalopathy occurs in 40–80%, subacute or chronic headaches in 40–60%, focal symptoms in 40–70% and seizures are present in 30%. An acute beginning of IAN has been described in only 11%; most patients develop the symptoms slowly and progressively. Systemic signs of inflammation (fever, ESR, CRP) are rare (10–20%). On the other hand, there are usually signs of inflammation in the CSF (pleocytosis, elevation of protein, oligoclonal banding). The specificities of cerebral ► angiography or MRI are below 30%. For definitive diagnosis of IAN, a combined leptomeningeal and parenchymal biopsy is necessary, especially in order to exclude infections or tumors (lymphoma!). Before the treatment of choice with prednisone and cyclophosphamide is established, a systemic inflammation or infection must be excluded and leptomeningeal and parenchymal biopsies must demonstrate the vascular inflammation (Moore 1989). Without histological verification of the diagnosis, blind treatment is dangerous and possibly harmful for the patient and must be strictly avoided. With immunosuppressive therapy the headaches resolve completely within a few weeks.

References

1. ACR Ad Hoc Committee on Neuropsychiatric Lupus Nomenclature (1999) The American College of Rheumatology nomenclature and case definitions for neuropsychiatric lupus. Arthritis Rheum 42:599–608
2. Akman-Demir G, Serdaroglu P, Tasci B (1999) Clinical patterns of neurological involvement in Behçet's disease: evaluation of 200 patients. The Neuro-Behçet Study Group. Brain 122:2171–2182
3. Amit M, Molad Y, Levy O et al. (1999) Headache in systemic lupus erythematosus and its relation to other disease manifestations. Clin Exp Rheumatol 17:467–470
4. Berlit P (1997) Giant Cell Arteritis. In: Lechtenberg R, Schutta HS (eds) Practice Guidelines for Neurologic Therapy. Marcel Dekker, New York
5. Caselli RJ, Hunder GG (1996) Neurologic complications of giant cell (temporal) arteritis. Sem Neurol 14:349–353
6. Fernandez-Nebro A, Palacios-Munoz R, Gordillo J et al. (1999) Chronic or recurrent headache in patients with systemic lupus erythematosus: a case control study. Lupus 8: 151–156
7. Lim IG, Spira PJ, McNeil HP (2002) Headache as the initial presentation of Wegener's granulomatosis. Ann Rheum Dis 61:571–572
8. Mazagri R, Shuaib A (1992) Flunarizine is effective in prophylaxis of headache associated with scleroderma. Headache 32:298–299
9. Moore PM (1989) Diagnosis and management of isolated angiitis of the central nervous system. Neurology 39:167–173
10. Omdal R, Waterloo K, Koldingsnes W et al. (2001) Somatic and psychological features of headache in systemic lupus erythematosus. J Rheumatol 28:772–779
11. Pal B, Gibson C, Passmore J et al. (1989) A study of headaches and migraine in Sjogren's syndrome and other rheumatic disorders. Ann Rheum Dis 48:312–316
12. Pradalier A, Le Quellec A (2000) Headache due to temporal arteritis. Pathol Biol 48:700–706
13. Ruiz-Irastorza G, Khamashta MA, Castellino G et al. (2001) Systemic lupus erythematosus. Lancet 357:1027–1032
14. Scarrow AM, Segal R, Medsger TA Jr et al. (1998) Communicating hydrocephalus secondary to diffuse meningeal spread of Wegener's granulomatosis: case report and literature review. Neurosurgery 43:1470–1473
15. Schmidley JW (2000) Central nervous system angiitis. Butterworth-Heinemann, Boston
16. Sfikakis PP, Mitsikostas DD, Manoussakis MN et al. (1998) Headache in systemic lupus erythematosus: a controlled study. Br J Rheumatol 37:300–303
17. Specks U, Moder KG, McDonald TJ (2000) Meningeal involvement in Wegener granulomatosis. Mayo Clin Proc 75:856–859
18. Vazquez-Cruz J, Traboulssi H, Rodriquez-De la Serna A et al. (1990) A prospective study of chronic or recurrent headache in systemic lupus erythematosus. Headache 30:232–235

Headache Due to Brain Metastases

Definition

Intracranial metastases are found in about 25% of all patients who have died of cancer. Some of these tumors are silent, but the majority cause the syndrome consisting of headache, nausea and vomiting, mental change, confusion, seizures and neurological deficit. Some tumors frequently produce brain secondaries (e.g. cancers of the lung and breast as well as melanoma), some only seldomly (e.g. cancer of ovary). Primary tumors, although relatively rare, can produce the same syndrome. Headache may arise from an expanding mass within the skull and distension of meninges. The treatment of choice is skull irradiation accompanied by the use of dexamethasone. The headache may get worse after morphine.

► Cancer Pain

Headache Due to Dissection

MATHIAS STURZENEGGER

Department of Neurology, University of Bern, Bern, Switzerland

matthias.sturzenegger@insel.ch

Synonyms

There are no direct synonyms for headaches resulting from dissections of cervico-cranial arteries. The location of these headaches is variable and mainly dependent on the dissected vessel segment and thus may cause differential diagnostic confusions.

Differential Diagnostic Aspects

The following three pathophysiologically poorly defined and most probably heterogeneous clinical syndromes with a diagnostic eponym may well be caused by dissection.
Sturzenegger 1995).
Carotidynia is a poorly defined syndrome with unilateral anterolateral cervical pain and tenderness. It is good advice to rule out underlying carotid dissection first, since most reports of this entity date from decades ago and the patients' carotid arteries have not been properly studied (no ultrasound, MRI, MRA or angiographic evaluation) (Biousse and Bousser 1994).
Tolosa-Hunt Syndrome (Painful Ophthalmoplegia); variable combination of periorbital pain, ipsilateral oculomotor nerve palsies, oculosympathetic palsy and trigeminal sensory loss) localize the pathological process to the region of the cavernous sinus. The causes may be traumatic, neoplastic, vascular or inflammatory. Within the inflammatory category, there is a specific subset of patients with a steroid responsive relapsing and remitting course – Tolosa-Hunt syndrome in the strict sense. The comprehensive patient evaluation is essential in establishing the correct diagnosis (Kline and Hoyt 2001).
Furthermore, the severe intensity and frequently orbital pain location of headache due to ICAD may at a first glance mimic cluster headache, but there are usually no recurrent short lasting attacks and no clustered bouts.

Definition

As already indicated by the title, the headaches are defined by their underlying pathology, i.e. dissection of the arteries. Since we are talking about headache, it is evident that we talk about dissections of cervico-cranial arteries; it is exceptional that dissection of the subclavian artery or aorta produce headache.

Pathogenesis

We have however to keep in mind that pain is usually a symptom of arterial dissections any where in the body, e.g. also of the aorta, renal or coronary arteries. The question rises why dissections are painful. Other pathologies of arterial walls may also be painful such as arteritis (e.g. giant cell arteritis) whereas atherosclerosis is usually painless.
We know that the walls of extracranial and also basal intracranial arteries are densely supplied with nociceptive, mainly trigeminal nerve fibers (Norregaard and Moskowitz 1985). These fibers are sensitive to inflammatory stimuli such as in vasculitis or to distension of the vessel wall that may take place during balloon dilatation or as a consequence of intramural hemorrhage such as in dissection. In atherosclerosis, although usually considered as an inflammatory process too, the inflammatory activity is probably simply too low to cause nociceptor discharge. It is controversial whether the irritation of the perivascular sympathetic nerve plexus, existing around the carotid as well as the vertebral arteries is another explanation or a contributing etiological factor of dissection-associated pain (De Marinis et al. 1991). In my personal experience, pain may be equally intense in dissections with definite vessel diameter extension as in those dissections without enlargement but merely vessel stenosis or occlusion. Furthermore, also from merely personal experience, pain is not more frequent in patients with Horner's syndrome compared to those without.
Dissection associated pain is usually reported with internal carotid (ICA) or vertebral artery (VA) dissections. We do not have data regarding dissection of extracranial carotid arteries and their branches or subclavian arteries and their branches, nor whether such pathologies exist and how frequently nor whether they may cause any pain. We know, that dissections may take place without causing pain. It seems to be rare, but we usually detect dissections because of their consequences such as pain or cerebral ischemia. That means that asymptomatic dissections may simply go undetected and painless dissections with other complications, such as lower cranial nerve palsy or cerebral ischemia may go unrecognized, since adequate diagnostic methods to detect dissections are not performed. In patients with "painful Horner's syndrome", many physicians have learned to think of ipsilateral internal carotid artery dissection (ICAD), but in what percentage of painless Horner's syndrome is ICAD the cause or is ICAD searched for?
The larger the affected vessel (carotid *versus* vertebral arteries) the more easily dissections are detected, i.e. can be imaged. Yet, without applying fat saturated T1 MRI sequences and, furthermore, that specific method to the appropriate vessel segment (e.g. the high cervical retromandibular ICA segment) painful ICAD without causing vessel stenosis may not be detected even when per-

forming Doppler, Duplex MRA and conventional MRI. In the VA, it is well known that for various reasons MRI, as well as Doppler / Duplex examination are much less sensitive to dissections as compared to angiography, an invasive procedure not completely without risks.

To summarize: pain may herald dissections early on, absence of pain does not exclude dissections, the frequency of painless and asymptomatic dissections is not known but they certainly exist.

Clinical Relevance

The most important aspect of headaches caused by dissections is the fact that they usually herald the onset of dissection and allow early recognition of the underlying pathology. Paying adequate attention to these warning symptoms enables the aversion of the often life-threatening sequelae of cerebral ischemia. 50–80% of patients with a dissection of the cervicocerebral arteries suffer a subsequent stroke; dissections are responsible for 20–30% of all strokes in young (<45 years) persons; warning headaches preceding stroke have been noted in 47–74% of patients with ICAD and in 33–85% of patients with VAD (Fisher 1982; Silbert et al. 1995; Sturzenegger 1994; Sturzenegger 1995).

Characteristics

Headaches caused by dissections have some typical although eventually unspecific features, which are not necessarily present in all cases. Independent of the affected vessel, these are high pain intensity, pain quality not experienced before, continuous more frequent than fluctuating pain over days, constant localization, sharp quality and tenderness of the painful head, face or neck area. Headache onset may be acute or even "thunderclap"-like suggesting subarachnoid hemorrhage, which indeed may be a complication of dissections of intracranial, especially vertebral artery, segments.

Additional characteristics are dependent on the vessel segment affected by the dissection. In the literature there are usually two broad categories, the traumatic and the spontaneous (non traumatic) dissections. This distinction is somewhat arbitrary since in many ▶ spontaneous dissections one will find some kind of so-called "trivial" trauma such as neck thrusting, a fall or certain sports or other violent physical activities with questionable significance.

From the literature one gets the impression that traumatic dissections are more frequently painless; yet this may simple be an assessment bias since in traumatic dissections there are additional injuries readily explaining pain or the health state of the patients is too serious to worry about pain or to make pain assessment possible. In the spontaneous dissection subgroup, the literature reports four major categories, extracranial carotid dissections, intracranial carotid dissections and their branches, extracranial vertebral artery dissections and intracranial vertebral artery dissections and their

branches. It may however well be that these categories are human constructions, just for educational reasons, without reflecting the reality of e.g. dissections affecting several segments of one artery or even several arteries. The vessel segments affected by dissections obviously show regional or probably ethnical variations with e.g. dissections of intracranial vertebral artery segments and their branches predominantly reported from Japan.

Spontaneous Internal Carotid Artery Dissection

The most typical clinical syndrome and the most frequent dissection is that of the extracranial segment of the internal carotid artery. Usually the most distal (high cervical, retromandibular) carotid segment just before entering the petrous canal is affected.

Spontaneous Dissection of Extracranial Internal Carotid Artery

Headache is reported in 55–95% of ICAD and was the first symptom in 47–68% (Biousse et al. 1994; Fisher 1982; Schievink 2001; Silbert et al. 1995; Sturzenegger 1995). Headache, facial or orbital pain may be the sole symptom of dissection, probably more frequently than reported so far (5%) and poses a diagnostic challenge. Local neurological manifestations (Horner's sign (35–48%), lower cranial nerve palsies (~10%) or pulsatile tinnitus (up to 30%)) are found in 30–48% of cases (Sturzenegger 1995; Sturzenegger and Huber 1993). Up to one third may complain of unilateral scalp tenderness and hair hypersensitivity. Ischemic cerebral events occur in 86% (stroke in 60% and TIA in 20%) and retinal events in 20% (Biousse et al. 1994; Schievink 2001; Sturzenegger 1995). Headache location is unilateral (79–90%), ipsilateral to the side of dissection (almost all), in the forehead (~70%), temple (~75%), eye or peri-orbital (~60%; ~10% isolated) or ear (~20%; ~10% isolated). The headache quality is steady (~75%), pulsating (25–40%), of severe intensity in 85%, thunderclap-like (14%, mimicking SAB), severe periorbital (10%, mimicking cluster headache), unique and never experienced before (65%). Headache duration is less than 1 week in 90% (range, hours to years). Anterolateral neck pain is reported by 26–60%, usually located in the upper neck behind the angle of the jaw.

Since migraine is a frequent disease, and reported in up to 40% of patients with carotid dissection and even considered a risk factor for dissection (D'Anglejean Chatillon et al. 1989), it is important not to confound migraine headaches with dissection headaches. The patient can usually distinguish these two headache types; dissection headache is a pain he never experienced before, is a continuous and not episodic pain, is not associated with general vegetative symptoms (nausea, vomiting, photophobia) and is usually constant not throbbing. Before assuming a so-called "migrainous infarct", one should exclude underlying carotid dissection as the cause of the pain and (embolic) brain ischemia. Thus, if a patient with a history of migraine, reports any change in the headache pattern (e.g. unique quality, long-lasting) or clinical characteristic, which he has not experienced before, ICAD should be considered and the appropriate investigation (ultrasound, MRI, MRA) performed soon.

The distinction from cluster headache is usually possible taking into account the duration (repetitive short attacks for cluster) and the autonomic symptoms (hyperhidrosis in cluster, anhidrosis in ICAD).

Spontaneous Dissection of the Intracranial Internal Carotid Artery

Intracranial carotid artery dissection affecting the supraclinoid portion of the ICA and or the middle and anterior cerebral arteries is very rare, especially when compared with dissections of the extracranial ICA. Whether it represents a unique entity, different from the more common extracranial variant, is unclear. Diagnosis is more difficult and usually needs angiography or high quality MRA. According to the literature, it preferentially affects very young patients (between 15 and 25 years) without any vascular risk factors. The clinical presentation comprises severe unilateral retroorbital and temporal headache followed by contralateral hemiparesis usually immediately after headache onset (Chaves et al. 2002).

Spontaneous Vertebral Artery Dissection

Dissections of the VA most frequently affect the mobile and easily distorted V3 segment. The distal extension is frequently difficult to assess and distinction between extracranial and intracranial dissection more difficult in the vertebrobasilar territory than in the carotid.

Yet it could probably be of relevance, since anticoagulation of intracranial dissections, more frequently producing aneurysms, bears a significant risk of subarachnoid hemorrhage, which may accompany intracranial VAD even without anticoagulant treatment.

Headache is reported in 69–85% and was the first symptom in 33–75% (Silbert et al. 1995; Sturzenegger 1994). Headache location is ipsilateral to the side of dissection (almost always), usually in the occiput (~ 80%). Pain always started suddenly, was of sharp quality and severe intensity, different from any previously experienced headache. Headache was steady in about 60% and pulsating in about 40%. The time course of pain was monophasic with gradual remission of a persistent headache lasting 1 to 3 weeks.

Posterior neck pain is reported by 46–80% and may be the only symptom (no associated headache). A delay between onset of head and neck pain heralding onset of dissection and neurological dysfunction is frequent (33–85%) and may be of variable duration (hours to

3 weeks). Report of this distinct type of headache should raise suspicion of an underlying dissection of a vertebral artery. Its early diagnosis and immediate anticoagulation if confined to the extracranial segments may help prevent vertebro-basilar ischemic deficits, which are frequently severe. Presenting clinical features of VAD are extremely variable and include locked-in syndrome, Wallenberg syndrome, which represents the most frequently encountered type of neurological dysfunction, cerebellar syndrome, vestibular syndrome, transient amnesia, tinnitus and hemianopia. Vertebral artery dissection may also occur silently, even without headache and is detected by chance. This seems to happen predominantly in the case of multiple dissections of cervical arteries.

Vertebral artery dissection may be caused by neck manipulation (Williams and Biller 2003). If neck pain is the sole indication for such a treatment, especially in young people who never experienced such a pain before, one should be aware that VAD may be the cause and manipulation might be fatal.

References

1. Biousse V, D'Anglejan-Chatillon J, Massiou H et al. (1994) Head pain in non-traumatic carotid artery dissection: a series of 65 patients. Cephalalgia 14:33–36
2. Biousse V, Bousser M-G (1994) The myth of carotidynia. Neurology 44:993–995
3. Chaves C, Estol C, Esnaola MM et al. (2002) Spontaneous intracranial internal carotid artery dissection. Report of 10 patients. Arch Neurol 59:977–981
4. D'Anglejean Chatillon J, Ribeiro V, Mas JL et al. (1989) Migraine –a risk factor for dissection of cervical arteries. Headache 29:560–561
5. De Marinis M, Zaccaria A, Faraglia V et al. (1991) Postendarterectomy headache and the role of the oculosympathetic system. J Neurol Neurosurg Psychiatry 54:314–317
6. Fisher CM (1982) The headache and pain of spontaneous carotid dissection. Headache 22:60–65
7. Kline LB, Hoyt WF (2001) The Tolosa-Hunt syndrome. J Neurol Neurosurg Psychiatry 71:577–582
8. Norregaard TV, Moskowitz MA (1985) Substance P and the sensory innervation of intracranial and extracranial feline cephalic arteries. Brain 108:517–533
9. Schievink WI (2001) Spontaneous dissection of the carotid and vertebral arteries. N Engl J Med 344:899–906
10. Selky AK, Pascuzzi R (1995) Raeder's paratrigeminal syndrome due to spontaneous dissection of the cervical and petrous internal carotid artery. Headache 35:432–434
11. Silbert PL, Mokri B, Schievink WI (1995) Headache and neck pain in spontaneous internal carotid and vertebral artery dissections. Neurology 45:1517–1522
12. Sturzenegger M (1994) Headache and neck pain: The warning symptoms of vertebral artery dissection. Headache 34:187–193
13. Sturzenegger M (1995) Spontaneous internal carotid artery dissection: Early diagnosis and management in 44 patients. J Neurology 242:231–238
14. Sturzenegger M, Huber P (1993) Cranial nerve palsies in spontaneous carotid artery dissection. J Neurol Neurosurg Psychiatry 56:1191–1199
15. Williams LS, Biller J (2003) Vertebrobasilar dissection and cervical spine manipulation. A complex pain in the neck. Neurology 60:1408–1409

10. LaBadie El, Glover D (1976) Physiopathogenesis of subdural hematomas. J Neurosurg 45:382–393
11. Melo TP, Pinto AN, Ferro JM (1996) Headache in intracerebral hematomas. Neurology 47:494–500
12. Rabinstein AA, Atkinson JL, Wijdicks EFM (2002) Emergency craniotomy in patients worsening due to expanded cerebral hematoma. To what purpose? Neurology 58:1367–1372
13. Weimar C, Weber C, Wagner M et al. (2003) Management patterns and health care use after intracerebral hemorrhage. A cost of illness study from a societal perspective in Germany. Cerebrovsc Dis 15:29–36

Headache Due to Low Cerebrospinal Fluid Pressure

ANDREAS R. GANTENBEIN, PETER S. SÁNDOR
Headache & Pain Unit, University Hospital Zurich, Zurich, Switzerland
peter.sandor@usz.ch

Synonyms

Spontaneous Intracranial Hypotension; Symptomatic Intracranial Hypotension; Post-Lumbar Puncture Headache; Low Intracranial Pressure Headache; Spontaneous Aliquorhea; Ventricular Collapse; Hypotension of Spinal Fluid

Definition

There are 3 types of headache attributed to low ▶ cerebrospinal fluid (CSF) pressure in the new classification of the International Headache Society (IHS, Headache Classification Committee of the International Headache Society 2004): Post-dural puncture headache (7.2.1), CSF fistula headache (7.2.2), and headache related to spontaneous low CSF pressure (7.3.3). They have in common an ▶ orthostatic component, as the headache usually begins within 15 min of standing or sitting up. The headache mainly improves in the recumbent position; however, this is a diagnostic criterion only for post- ▶ lumbar puncture in the IHS classification. The headache is associated with at least one of the following symptoms: neck stiffness, tinnitus, hypacusis, photophobia, or nausea. The aetiology is different for the 3 types. See Table 1 for compared classification criteria (Headache Classification Committee of the International Headache Society 2004).

Characteristics

In 1938, Schaltenbrand, a German neurologist, wrote about two conditions regarding cerebrospinal fluid:

a) 'Liquorrhea' involving headache and ▶ papilloedema, which later became known as pseudotumor cerebri, and
b) 'Spontaneous aliquorhea', presenting with orthostatic headaches and features of intracranial hypotension. He explained the syndrome of low CSF

pressure by three possible pathological mechanisms: decreased production, increased absorption or leakage, e.g. after a lumbar puncture (Schaltenbrand 1938).

The brain is 'swimming' in the CSF. The average weight of 1500 g is reduced to 50 g by the intracranial pressure. The remaining weight is held by the meningeal blood vessels, the outgoing cranial nerves, and microstructures. If the CSF pressure decreases, there is traction on the supporting structures of the brain. Recent MRI studies have even shown the "descending" brain (Pannullo et al. 1993). It is thought that traction on the cranial nerves (V, IX, X), on the three upper cervical nerves, and on bridging veins which are pain-sensitive structures, causes the headache and its associated features. However, there are contradictory reports to this so called 'sagging theory' (Levine and Rapalino 2001). As long as magnetic imaging cannot be performed in the erect position, it will probably be difficult to bring an end to that discussion.

Magnetic imaging of the head and spine has revolutionized the knowledge and the detection of this disorder (Fishman and Dillon 1993; Mokri 2001; Sable and Ramadan 1991). It was not until the 1990s that investigators demonstrated that the production of about 500 ml per day is relatively constant, and therefore is rarely a cause for the problems. The CSF volume is estimated to be between 150–210 ml, this means the total volume is renewed 2–3 times per day. CSF volume is smaller in women, younger, and obese persons. Most of the CSF is absorbed via the arachnoid villi into the venous sinuses and cerebral veins, and only a very small part is absorbed through simple diffusion. On this background, the most obvious and common reason for low intracranial pressure is CSF leakage. The spontaneous leaks are mostly located on the thoracic or cervical level (Sencakova et al. 2001).

Post-lumbar puncture headache happens in up to one-third of patients with lumbar puncture (Adams et al. 2002). Patients with preceding headaches, and young women with low BMI, may be at higher risk of developing headaches. Patients with postural headaches should be imaged before lumbar puncture, and if there are MRI signs of ▶ pachymeningeal enhancement, a lumbar puncture should not be performed.

Symptoms

Low CSF pressure usually causes orthostatic headaches, which develop in the upright position and improve when lying down (recumbency). The onset of the headache is usually sudden or gradual. The character of the pain is often described as severe and throbbing or dull, and it can be diffuse or focal, with a frontal or occipital localisation. The headache typically has orthostatic features in the beginning (e.g. onset within 30 min after standing up), however, these features may blur with

Headache Due to Low Cerebrospinal Fluid Pressure, Table 1 Compared diagnostic criteria of the International Headache Classification 2nd Edition regarding headache attributed to low CSF pressure

Post-dural puncture headache	CSF fistula headache	Spontaneous low CSF
Headache within 15 min of sitting or standing		
Resolving within 15 min after lying		
Associated symptoms (1 of the following):		
Neck stiffness Tinnitus Hypacusis Photophobia Nausea		
Etiology		
Dural puncture	CSF leakage: MRI evidence (pachymengial enhancement) Conventional or CT myelography, cysternography OP <60 mm CSF in sitting position	
Onset		
Within 5 days after lumbar puncture	Close relation to CSF leakage	No lumbar puncture or leakage
Resolving		
Spontaneously within 1 week or Within 48 h after treatment	Within 1 week of sealing leak	Within 72 h after blood patch

chronicity and result in a chronic daily headache which is worse when the patient is in an upright position and improves when lying down. Other exaggerating factors include movements of the head, sneezing, coughing, straining, and jugular venous compression. In general pain killers do not sufficiently improve the headache. Recumbency is often the only measure which can relieve the pain; usually within 10–15 min. Associated features can be manifold: anorexia, nausea, vomiting, vertigo, dizziness, neck stiffness, blurred vision, and even photophobia are commonly described. Tinnitus, bilateral hyp(er)acusis, unsteadiness, staggering gait, diplopia, transient visual obscuration, hiccups, and dysgeusia have been reported.

Examination

The neurological examination is typically normal. However, mild neck stiffness is frequently noted.

The CSF opening pressure is typically below 70 mm, however, it can be low normally. Fluid is typically clear and colourless, occasionally ▶ xanthochromic. The CSF protein level is usually normal, but may be high, mostly still below 100 mg/dl. Cell counts give variable results: erythrocytes and leukocytes may be normal or elevated. Cytologic and microbiologic tests are always negative, and glucose rate CSF/plasma is always between 0 and 1.

The standard diagnostic investigation for low CSF pressure and CSF leaks is MR imaging with Gadolinium. The most common abnormality is diffuse pachymeningeal enhancement (Mokri 2004). According to the Monro-Kellie doctrine (brain volume + CSF + intracranial

blood = constant) the CSF loss is compensated by venous hyperaemia. Whereas the leptomeninges have blood brain barriers, the pachymeninges (dura mater) do not and therefore accumulate the contrast medium. The enhancement is typically linear, thick and uninterrupted, and diffuse, including supra- and infratentorial meninges. Furthermore, there is commonly sinking or sagging of the brain, which can sometimes mimic Chiari I malformation, subdural fluid collections (they may be unilateral), and decrease in size of ventricles. Less common abnormalities include pituitary enlargement, engorged venous sinuses, and elongation of the brain stem. MRI of the spine can show spinal pachymeningeal enhancement, engorgement of venous plexus, and extraarachnoidal fluid, but only rarely reveal the site of the leak. The most accurate technique to find the exact site of CSF leaks is CT myelography. It is to be mentioned that different leaks and diverticles of different sizes can be found in the same patient. An exact identification of the site of the leak, however, is only necessary when surgical intervention is needed.

A CT scan of the head is usually unremarkable and therefore not very useful. Older diagnostic techniques include radioisotope cisternography with Indium-111, myelography without CT, and meningeal biopsy.

Differential-Diagnosis

Most patients present with a new onset daily headache following a lumbar puncture or another dural trauma, or, if developing spontaneously present as new daily persistent headache, which would act as a working diagnosis, unless low CSF pressure headache is diagnostically classified using imaging techniques (▶ MRI, CT myelography).

The orthostatic component is a salient feature. It is therefore hard to understand that in a recent study (Schievink 2003) spontaneous intracranial hypotension (SIH) was misdiagnosed in 94% of the reviewed cases, with a mean diagnostic delay of 13 months (median 5 weeks, range 4 days to 13 years). Sometimes associated features, such as nausea or photophobia, can mimic migraine. Especially when there is a personal or family history of headaches, the picture can be diluted. Furthermore, the orthostatic feature becomes less prominent with time. Obviously, the diagnosis of low CSF pressure headache is easier when the patient is seen at the beginning of the problem, and when there is a close temporal relationship to a lumbar puncture or another trauma affecting the spine. The differential diagnosis to the other orthostatic headache due to raised intracranial pressure should be fairly easy. Interestingly, almost all patients with low CSF pressure develop headaches, but only 30–80% of the patients with increased intracranial pressure do so (Mokri 2001).

Whereas both, low and high pressure headaches can be aggravated by coughing or straining, intracranial hypertension typically develops when lying down, especially in the morning, and is mostly present with transient visual loss or papilloedema in the neurological examination.

Management & Treatment

Fortunately, many low pressure headaches dissolve spontaneously within days. Treatments vary for the three different types of low CSF pressure headache. Conservative strategies include bed rest, fluid intake and an abdominal binder. Caffeine (250–500 mg i.v.), theophylline and to a lesser part steroids can be effective. When conservative treatments give no sufficient pain relieve within 24 h, an epidural ▶ blood patch (10–15 ml of autologous blood into the epidural space) would be indicated. Blood patches seem to have not only an immediate effect, through simple volume replacement, but also a delayed sealing of the leak. Post-lumbar puncture headaches are often relieved after the first (rarely the second) blood patch, while patients with spontaneous CSF leaks may need up to 4 or more. Instead of a second or third blood patch an epidural saline infusion could be attempted, using a catheter placed at the L2-3 level and a flow rate of 20ml/h for 72 h. If a leak is clearly located with imaging techniques and the headache is treatment refractory a surgical closure may be considered.

References

1. Adams MG, Romanowski CA, Wrench IJ (2002) Spontaneous Intracranial Hypotension – Lessons to be Learned for the Investigation of Post Dural Puncture Headache. Int J Obstet Anesth 11:65–67
2. Fishman RA, Dillon WP (1993) Dural Enhancement and Cerebral Displacement Secondary to Intracranial Hypotension. Neurology 43:609–611
3. Headache Classification Committee of the International Headache Society (2004) The International Classification of Headache Disorders, 2nd edn. Cephalalgia 24:9–160
4. Levine DN, Rapalino O (2001) The Pathophysiology of Lumbar Puncture Headache. J Neurol Sci 192:1–8
5. Mokri B (2001) Low Cerebrospinal Fluid Pressure Headache. In: Silberstein SD, Lipton RB, Dalessio DJ (eds) Wolff's Headache and Other Pain, 7th edn. Oxford University Press, New York, pp 417–433
6. Mokri B (2004) Spontaneous Low Cerebrospinal Pressure/Volume Headaches. Curr Neurol Neurosci Rep 4:117–124
7. Pannullo SC, Reich JB, Krol G et al. (1993) MRI Changes in Intracranial Hypotension. Neurology 43:919–926
8. Sable SG, Ramadan NM (1991) Meningeal Enhancement and Low CSF Pressure Headache. An MRI study. Cephalalgia 11:275–276
9. Schaltenbrand G (1938) Neuere Anschauungen zur Pathophysiologie der Liquorzirkulation. Zentralbl Neurochir 3:290–300
10. Schievink WI (2003) Misdiagnosis of Spontaneous Intracranial Hypotension. Arch Neurol 60:1713–1718
11. Sencakova D, Mokri B, McClelland RL (2001) The Efficacy of Epidural Blood Patch in Spontaneous CSF Leaks. Neurology 57:1921–1923

Headache Due to Sinus-Venous Thrombosis

VOLKER LIMMROTH, HANS-CHRISTOPH DIENER
Department of Neurology, University of Essen, Essen, Germany
volker.limmroth@uni-essen.de,
h.diener@uni-essen.de

Definition

Cerebral venous sinus thrombosis (CVST) is a rare but challenging condition and is therefore often unrecognised. Its clinical presentation may vary significantly from case to case. Headache, however, is often the very first and leading symptom. The headache is mostly described as dull holocephalic pain, of increasing intensity and can easily be mistaken for tension type headache, migraine headache or other disorders such as pseudotumor cerebri. Along with headache, additional symptoms typical to increasing intracranial pressure such as papilloedema, nausea, vomiting and cognitive decline may be present. Further symptoms are focal deficit and seizures. The headache does not typically respond to classical anti-headache drugs, which should be taken as an important sign that further evaluation is necessary. Classical patients with CVST are young females with risk factors such as oral contraceptive pill, nicotine abuse, being overweight or during pregnancy, but all age groups can be affected and CVST can evolve secondary to an adjacent infectious process; dehydration, hypercoagulable state, inflammatory disorders, malignancies or head traumas. The diagnosis can be easily confirmed by MRI with venography or modern spiral-CAT-scan.

The treatment of choice is intravenous heparin followed by oral anticoagulation for 3–6 months. The prognosis is good if treatment is initiated early but can be fatal when the condition is overlooked. Despite its low incidence, CSVT is, therefore, one of the most important differential diagnosis clinicians must bear in mind when evaluating patients with headache.

Characteristics

Pathophysiology

Venous blood drains through small cerebral veins into larger veins that empty into dural sinuses and eventually into the internal jugular veins. Pre-existing anastomoses between cortical veins allow the development of collateral circulation in the event of an occlusion. The main cerebral venous sinuses affected by CVST are the superior sagittal sinus (72%) and the lateral sinuses (70%). In about one-third of cases more than one sinus is affected, in a further 30–40% both sinuses and cerebral or cerebellar veins are involved (Ameri and Bousser 1992; Bousser and Barnett 1992; Villringer et al. 1994). In contrast to arterial thrombus, a venous thrombus evolves slowly, due good collateralisation of the venous vessels, which probably explains the usually gradual onset of symptoms, frequently over weeks and months. Sudden onset, however, may occur and may then cause predominating focal deficits rather than headache. Haemorrhagic infarction occurs in approximately 10–50% of cases, principally affecting the cortex and adjacent white matter (Bousser et al. 1985; de Bruijn et al. 1996; Buonanno et al. 1982; Provenzale et al. 1998). This is thought to be primarily due to elevated venous and capillary pressure caused by the persistence of thrombosis.

Predisposing Factors

An overview of predisposing factors is given below. In most of the cases one or more of these factors can be identified. In general, a distinction can be made between infective and non-infective causes or, as suggested by Bousser and Barnett, between local and systemic causes (Bousser and Barnett 1992). Within recent decades, infective causes have declined and are now responsible for less than 10% of cases and are mostly caused by staphylococcal infection of the face. Amongst the non-infective causes, systemic conditions such as connective tissue diseases, other granulomatous or inflammatory disorders and malignancies are the most common. Other risk factors in otherwise healthy subjects are overweight, hormonal therapy, smoking and underlying – mostly unknown – clotting disorders. In many cases several of these factors can be found.

Local causes

- penetrating head injury
- intracranial infection
- regional infection
- stroke and haemorrhage
- space occupying lesions
- neurosurgery

Systemic causes

- severe dehydration
- hormonal and endocrine causes
- cardiac disease
- red blood cell disorders
- thrombocythaemia
- coagulation disorders (acquired or hereditary)
- infusions via central venous catheter
- surgery with immobilisation
- malignancies
- inflammatory bowel disease
- connective tissue diseases
- Behcet's disease
- sarcoidosis
- nephrotic syndrome
- drugs (L-asparaginase, epsilonaminocaproic acid, ecstasy)
- sepsis and systemic infection

Clinical Presentation

Depending on the sinus involved and the extent of the venous thrombus, CVST presents with a wide spectrum of symptoms and signs. Headache is the leading symptom and present in 70–90% of cases. Other important symptoms are focal deficits such as hemiparesis and hemisensory disturbance, seizures, impairment of level of consciousness and papilloedema (Ameri and Bousser 1992; Bousser et al. 1985). The onset may also vary a great deal from acute, subacute or insidious, but most patients develop symptoms over days or weeks.

In a series of 110 cases, Ameri and Bousser (1992) found several typical clinical constellations; up to 75% of cases are characterised by a focal neurological deficit and headache, 30%–50% may present with seizures often followed by a Todd's paresis and 18–38% of cases present with a syndrome resembling benign intracranial hypertension with headache, papilloedema and visual disturbances. As indicated above, symptoms also depend on the location of the thrombus. The (isolated) thrombosis of the superior sagittal sinus (which occurs in less than 5% of the cases) presents with bilateral or alternating deficits, particularly in the lower limbs and/or seizures, the (isolated) thrombosis of the cavernous sinus (3% of the cases) with chemosis, proptosis and painful ophthalmoplegia. Patients with lateral sinus thrombosis may present with a pseudotumor cerebri-like syndrome. Recently, Farb et al. (2003), using a technique called auto-triggered elliptic-centric-ordered 3-dimensional gadolinium-enhanced MR venography, found that 27 of 29 patients with idiopathic intracranial hypertension suffered from a bilateral sinovenous stenosis which was only seen in 4 of 59 control subjects. Severe cases with the involvement of the superior sagittal sinus, the cavernous sinus and the lateral sinus, however, may present with a rapidly progressive condition including headache, nausea, pyramidal signs and deepening coma.

CVST appears to be slightly more frequent in women with a suggested female-to-male ratio of 1.29:1. Interestingly, while 61% of women with CVST were aged 20–35 years, a uniform age distribution has been suggested for men with CVST. The most likely explanation for this specific age distribution in women is the use of oral contraceptives and fact that CVST is frequently observed during pregnancies.

Diagnosis

Patients with a suspected CVST must undergo specific cranial imaging immediately. Magnetic resonance imaging (MRI) combined with magnetic resonance venography (MRV) have largely replaced invasive cerebral angiography and conventional computed tomography (CT). Modern subsecond spiral CT and multi-detector-row-CT-scanners (MDCT), however, are now able to obtain whole-brain CT venograms in less than a minute. Unlike the conventional CT scanner, MDCT scanners have sufficient speed for high resolution images of the entire brain and all dural sinuses during the peak venous enhancement (Casey et al. 1996; Wetzel et al. 1999). The technique can therefore – if available – be used as a first line diagnostic tool since the procedure is cheaper and faster than MRI/MRV. Moreover, using a CT scanner of the latest generation, a recent study has been shown that CT venography may be superior to MRV in visualising sinuses or smaller cerebral veins or cortical veins with low flow. However, it goes without saying that MRI/MRV are the imaging techniques of choice for pregnant women. Some doubtful cases may still require cerebral angiography. One of the common problems is the absence or hypoplasia of the anterior portion of the superior sagittal sinus, a normal variant that can simulate thrombosis on MRV (Provenzale et al. 1998; Wang 1996). Also, contrast enhancement along the edge of the thrombus can be mistaken for normal contrast material accumulating within a patient's sinus. Aside from confirming the diagnosis by cranial imaging, it is mandatory to search for the underlying causes including the search for local infection, head injury, malignancies, connective tissue diseases with inflammatory markers, autoantibodies and markers of coagulation disorders such as Factor V Leiden mutation if resistance to activated protein C is abnormal, activities of proteins C and S, antithrombin III, plasminogen, fibrinogen and anticardiolipin antibodies (de Bruijn et al. 1998; Deschiens et al. 1996; Kellett et al. 1998) All these investigations should probably be performed twice, i.e. before starting anticoagulation, and 6 months later after finishing since the acute status of the disease may influence the expression of these parameters.

Treatment

Only a few therapeutic trials have evaluated potential therapeutic agents in CVST. Antithrombotic treatment modalities include heparin, thrombolysis and oral anticoagulants. Einhäupl et al. (1991) in a randomised and placebo-controlled trial, demonstrated the benefits of heparin in a series of 20 patients. There was a significant difference in favour of intravenous heparin with respect to neurological recovery and mortality compared to placebo. Interestingly, in an additional retrospective analysis on 102 patients with CVST the same authors suggested heparin to be beneficial, even in those patients who had an intracranial haemorrhage prior to treatment initiation. A few years later, de Bruijn et al. (1999) compared low-molecular-weight heparin followed by warfarin, or placebo. A significant difference between the groups could not be detected in this study (de Bruijn and Stam 1999).

Several groups (Frey et al. 1999; Horowitz et al. 1995; Kim and Suh 1997; Smith et al. 1994) addressed the question of whether additional benefit could be achieved by thrombolysis via selective catheterisation of the occluded sinus. Although all studies included a small number of patients (n = between 7 and 12 patients per study), all studies suggested that the majority of patients undergoing catheterisation and thrombolysis with urokinase recovered well, and only a few patients suffered from an additional cerebral haemorrhage. Since there is no direct comparative trial between heparin and thrombolysis, the question if this approach provides an additional benefit and an acceptable benefit-to-risk ratio when compared to i.v. heparin is not answered. The disadvantage of catheterisation in patients with CVST is the significant logistic effort and expertise necessary to have this intervention always available.

There is a general agreement that oral anticoagulants should follow as treatment of the acute phase for 3–6 months. In patients with known prothrombotic conditions anticoagulation may be a life-long requirement. No agreement has been reached regarding the question whether patients who present with seizures should undergo anti-epileptic treatment after the acute phase. This decision remains to be made from case to case and under the consideration of the individual circumstances. Taken together, intravenous heparin is the first-line treatment in a dosage sufficient to increase the apTT to 2–3 times of the control value. Several authors suggest a start with a heparin bolus of 5000 U and to continue according to the apTT elevation, which mostly requires dosages between 1000 and 1600 U/h for adults. Heparin is the first-line treatment, even in the presence of haemorrhagic infarction (Bousser 1999). In case of clinical deterioration despite adequate heparinisation, selective local thrombolysis should be considered, in spite of the increased haemorrhagic risk.

H

Prognosis

Mortality in untreated cases of venous thrombosis has been reported to range from 13.8–48% (Preter et al. 1996). A recent Portuguese study suggested a morbidity of around 8% despite adequate treatment in a group of 91 prospectively analyzed consecutively admitted patients with a mean 1 year follow-up interval (Ferro et al. 2004). Interestingly, 82% of the patients recovered completely, but 59% developed thrombotic events during the follow-up, 10% had seizures and 11% complained of severe headaches. Recently Buccino et al. (2003) found a good overall outcome in a series of 34 patients with CSVT. Still, 10 patients (30%) suffered from episodic headaches, 3 patients (8.8%) from seizures, 4 patients (11.7%) from pyramidal signs and 2 (5.9%) from visual deficits and 6 patients (17.6%) from working memory deficit and depression. All these studies clearly emphasize that CSVT is a treatable condition in the majority of cases and that early diagnosis and immediate initiation of heparin treatment are the key components for a good overall outcome.

References

1. Ameri A, Bousser MG (1992) Cerebral venous thrombosis. Neurol Clin 10:87–111
2. Bousser MG (1999) Cerebral venous thrombosis: nothing, heparin, or local thrombolysis? Stroke 30:481–483
3. Bousser MG, Barnett HJM (1992) Cerebral venous thrombosis. Stroke: pathophysiology, diagnosis and management, 2nd edn. Churchill-Livingstone, New York, pp 517–537
4. Bousser MG, Chiras J, Bories J et al. (1985) Cerebral venous thrombosis –a review of 38 cases. Stroke 16:199–213
5. Buonanno FS, Moody DM, Ball TLM (1982) CT scan findings in cerebral sinus venous occlusion. Neurology 12:288–292
6. Buccino G, Scoditti U, Patteri I et al. (2003) Neurological and cognitive long-term outcome in patients with cerebral venous sinus thrombosis. Acta Neurol Scand 107:330–335
7. Casey SO, Alberico RA, Patel M et al. (1996) Cerebral CT venography. Radiology 198:163–170
8. de Bruijn SF, Stam J for the CVST Study Group (1999) Randomised, placebo-controlled trial of anticoagulant treatment with low-molecular-weight heparin for cerebral sinus thrombosis. Stroke 30:484–488
9. de Bruijn SF, Stam J, Kapelle LJ (1996) Thunderclap headache as first symptom of cerebral venous sinus thrombosis. CVST Study Group. Lancet 348:1623–1625
10. de Bruijn SF, Stam J, Koopman MM et al. (1998) Case-control study of risk of cerebral sinus thrombosis in oral contraceptive users who are cautious of hereditary prothrombotic conditions. BMJ 316:589–592
11. Deschiens MA, Conard J, Horellou MH et al. (1996) Coagulation studies, Factor V Leiden and anticardiolipin antibodies in 40 cases of cerebral venous thrombosis. Stroke 27:1724–1730
12. Einhäupl KM, Villringer A, Meister W et al. (1991) Heparin treatment in sinus venous thrombosis. Lancet 338:597–600
13. Farb RI, Scott JN, Willinsky RA et al (2003) Intracranial venous system: gadolinium-enhanced three-dimensional MR venography with auto-triggered elliptic centric-ordered sequence –initial experience. Radiology 226:203–209
14. Ferro JM, Canhao P, Stam J et al.; ISCVT Investigators (2004) Prognosis of cerebral vein and dural sinus thrombosis: results of the International Study on Cerebral Vein and Dural Sinus Thrombosis (ISCVT). Stroke 35:664–670
15. Frey JL, Muro GJ, McDougall CG et al. (1999) Cerebral venous thrombosis: combined intrathrombus rtPA and intravenous heparin. Stroke 30:489–494
16. Horowitz M, Purdy P, Unwin H et al. (1995) Treatment of dural sinus thrombosis using selective catheterisation and urokinase. Ann Neurol 38:58–67
17. Kellett MW, Martin PJ, Enevoldson TP et al. (1998) Cerebral venous sinus thrombosis connected with 20210, a mutation of the prothanbil gene. J Neurol Neurosurg Psychiatry 65:611–612
18. Kim SY, Suh JH (1997) Direct endovascular thrombolytic therapy for dural sinus thrombosis: infusion of alteplase. Am J Neuroradiol 18:639–664
19. Preter M, Tzourio C, Ameri A et al. (1996) Long-term prognosis in cerebral venous thrombosis: follow-up of 77 patients. Stroke 27:243–246
20. Provenzale JM, Joseph GJ, Barboriak DP (1998) Dural sinus thrombosis: findings on CT and MRI imaging and diagnostic pitfalls. AJR 170:777–783
21. Smith TP, Higashida RT, Barnwell SL et al. (1994) Treatment of dural sinus thrombosis by urokinase infusion. Am J Neuroradiol 15:801–807
22. Villringer A, Mehraen S, Einhäupl KM (1994) Pathophysiological aspects of cerebral sinus venous thrombosis. J Neuroradiol 21:72–80
23. Wang AM (1997) MRA of venous sinus thrombosis. Clin Neurosci 4:158–164
24. Wetzel SG, Kirsch E, Stock KW et al. (1999) Cerebral veins: comparative study of CT venography with intraarterial digital subtraction angiography. AJNR Am J Neuroradiol 20:249–255

Headache Due to Somatoform Disorder

RETO M. AGOSTI
Headache Center Hirlsanden, Zurich, Switzerland
reto.agosti@kopfwww.ch

Synonyms

Headache Associated with Somatisation Disorder; Headache Associated with Psychotic Disorder

Definition

Headaches of no typical characterisation (such as migraine or cluster headaches) with close temporal association with undifferentiated somatoform disorder (as defined by DSM IV).

Characteristics

This type of headache does not have any characteristic symptoms that are unique to these types of headaches. Any other headache type, primary (such as migraine, cluster headaches, etc) or secondary, must be excluded. By definition, there must be a close temporal relationship with the multiple symptoms of an undifferentiated somatoform disorder as defined by DSM-IV: a) A physical complaint, plus headache, that, after appropriate investigation, cannot be fully explained by a known general medical condition, or by the direct effects of a substance or medication or, when there is a related medical condition, that complaint or impairment is in excess of what would be expected from the history, examination and/or laboratory findings; and b) The physical complaint and headaches cause distress or impairment and last at least 6 months. The headache occurs exclusively during the course of the other physical complaint, and resolves after the undifferentiated somatoform disorder remits. A similar condition with clearly more stringent criteria regarding the somatoform symptoms and complaints are headaches associated with somatisation disorder, for which DSM-IV requires a minimum of eight somatoform symptoms or complaints and age of onset under 30. Both types of headaches (associated with somatoform and somatisation disorder) only entered the IHS classification of headaches in 2004, and are highly debated regarding their existence as proper diagnoses, with the persistent lack of a biological marker for primary headaches as one of the major obstacles. The diagnosis is fully based on phenomenology, and the treatment symptomatic towards treating the headaches or the underlying psychiatric disorder. A causal relationship in any direction is under debate. Association of headaches with other psychiatric disturbances such as depression, phobias etc. are classified separately. Headaches associated with somatisation disorder are rare, but headaches associated with somatoform disorder are more frequent.

References

1. American Psychiatric Association (1994) Diagnostic and Statistical Manual of Mental Disorders, 4th edn. (DSM IV) American Psychiatric Association, Washington, DC
2. Puca F, Genco S, Prudenzano MP (1999) Psychiatric Comorbidity and Psychosocial Stress in Patients with Tension-Type Headache from Headache Centers in Italy. The Italian Collaborative Group for the Study of Psychopathological Factors in Primary Headaches. Cephalalgia 19:159–164
3. Yutzy S (2003) Somatoform Disorders In: Tasman A, Kay J, Lieberman JA (eds) Psychiatry, 2nd edn. John Wiley and Sons, Chichester, pp 1419–1420

Headache, Episodic Tension Type

ANDREAS R. GANTENBEIN, PETER S. SÁNDOR
Headache & Pain Unit, University Hospital Zurich, Zurich, Switzerland
andy.gantenbein@gmx.ch, peter.sandor@usz.ch

Synonyms

Episode Tension Type Headache; Idiopathic Headache; Muscle Contraction Headache; Ordinary Headache; Psychogenic Headache; Psychomyogenic Headache; Tension Headache

Definition

The new classification of the International Headache Society (IHS) distinguishes an infrequent (less than 1 day per month) and a frequent form (at least 1 day but less than 15 days per month) of episodic tension type headache. Duration varies from minutes to days. The pain is typically bilateral, of mild to moderate intensity,

and has a ▶ pressing/tightening character. There is no worsening with routine physical activity. There is no nausea, but ▶ photophobia or ▶ phonophobia may be present. Both infrequent and frequent types can be subdivided according to the presence or absence of pericranial ▶ tenderness (jaw, scalp and neck muscles). See Table 1 for the classification criteria (Headache Classification Subcommittee of the International Headache Society 2003).

Characteristics

With a lifetime prevalence of 30–78% in general population, tension type headache is the most common primary headache and has a high socio-economic impact. The male to female ratio is 1:1.5. The prevalence in childhood ranges from 0.5–12% (Anttila et al. 2002; Rasmussen et al. 1991; Rasmussen 2001; Schwartz et al. 1998). Tension headache was first defined by the IHS classification committee in 1988. This type of headache previously had a psychological label and was thought to be caused exclusively by mental conflicts, stress, tension, or emotional overload. There was exciting little interest from research and pharmaceutical companies. However, more recently a number of studies have investigated neurobiological mechanisms. Peripheral pain mechanisms, such as myofascial tenderness, hyperalgesia and muscle hardness have been implicated in the episodic type, and dysfunction of central sensitisation in the chronic type. Overall tension-type headache appears to be a central disinhibitory phenomenon, probably with involved neurotransmitter changes, defective nociceptive control, increased sensitivity to both myofascial and vascular input, and associated personality traits (Jensen and Olesen 2000). Whether tension type headache and migraine are separate entities, as suggested by epidemiological data, or rather represent a continuum with shared pathophysiology remains controversial (Rasmussen 1996; Ulrich et al. 1996).

Symptoms

The headache can be described in simple terms as pain in the head without associated symptoms. Unlike migraine there is no sensory hypersensitivity, e.g. to sound, light, or movements. Unlike cluster headache autonomic features (tearing, redness of the eye and blocked nose) are not present. Due to the usually mild and short lasting character, patients with less frequent tension headache often view their symptoms as a nuisance and rarely seek the advice of a specialist. Accordingly, these patients often treat their headache with standard over-the-counter pain killers (often containing caffeine) or with non-pharmacological treatments, such as hot or cold packs, or massage. If the headache is more frequent it may well become distressing and interfere with daily life. This may be associated with regular intake of non-specific analgesics, and can lead to further problems, including chronification of the headache.

Headache, Episodic Tension Type, Table 1 Compared diagnostic criteria frequent episodic tension-type headache and migraine without Aura from the International Headache Classification 2nd edn

Diagnosis:	Frequent episodic tension type headache	Migraine without Aura
Number of episodes:	At least 10	At least 5
Number of days with such headache:	≥ 1 day and < 15 days per month (for at least 3 months)	< 15 days/month (untreated or unsuccessfully treated)
Duration of the headache:	30 min to 7 days	4–72 h
Pain characteristics:	At least two of the following:	At least two of the following:
	Pressing/tightening (non-pulsating) quality	Pulsating quality
	Mild or moderate intensity	Moderate or severe pain intensity
	Bilateral location	Unilateral location
	No aggravation by walking stairs or similar routine physical activity	Aggravation by or causing avoidance of routine physical activity
Accompanying Symptoms:	Both of the following:	At least one of the following:
	No nausea or vomiting (anorexia may occur).	Nausea and/or vomiting
	Photophobia or phonophobia or none	Photophobia and phonophobia

Episodic tension type headache has a high intra- and interindividual variability with respect to frequency and intensity. Additionally, the duration of each attack may range from 30 minutes to 7 days. It usually has a diffuse pressing character, often described by patients as a 'tight band around the head'. The pain is dull, persistent and often diurnal. The headache is bilateral in 80–90% of cases. Most commonly intensity is mild to moderate and may interfere with (though not usually prevent) performance of daily activities. Characteristically it is not aggravated by routine physical activity. Nausea and vomiting are absent. Patients may complain of mild intolerance to loud sound or bright light, though true photophobia or phonophobia is rare and strongly suggest migraine (certainly when both present). There is no blurred vision and no focal neurological disturbance. Patients may complain of a feeling of giddiness or light-headedness, sometimes as a consequence of hyperventilation in association with anxiety. Many patients report difficulties in concentrating and lack of interest in work and hobbies. With age, tension-type headache can increases in frequency and duration, and there tends to be more variability of localization and rarely nausea may develop (Wober-Bingol et al. 1996).

Examination

Tension type headache patients require thorough neurological examination, including inspection and palpation of ▶ pericranial muscles. Pericranial tenderness is easily recorded by small rotating movements and a firm pressure with two fingers on the frontal, temporal, masseter, pterygoid, sternocleidomastoid, splenius and trapezius muscles. A local tenderness score from 0–3 on each muscle can be summated to a total tenderness score for each individual. The use of a palpometer (pressure sensitive device) can improve validity and reproducibility. Palpation is also a useful guide for treatment strategy, and adds value and credibility to the explanations given to the patient.

Differential-Diagnosis

An accurate diagnosis is essential, and migraine, as well as secondary headache, should be excluded. Tension-type headache is sometimes difficult to distinguish from migraine in patients who have both tension headache and migraine with or without aura. It is important to educate patients in the differentiation between these headaches, as the right treatment for the right headache can be administered and medication overuse headache can be avoided. A diagnostic headache diary can be helpful to identify different patterns, since patients often describe only the characteristics of recent or the most severe attacks. In favour of tension type headache is a highly variable temporal profile and pain improvement with exercise. Unsuccessful treatment with ergotamins or triptans for acute attacks, or with beta-blockers or Flunarizin for prevention, also suggest a diagnosis of tension type headache. (Kaniecki 2002) See Table 1 for the comparison of classification criteria for migraine without aura and tension-type headache.

If headache is new (particularly over the age of 50), has a sudden onset, changes significantly in established pattern or characteristics, or does not fit a classical scheme, then secondary causes need to be excluded. Head trauma, vascular disorder, nonvascular intracranial disorder, substance abuse, noncephalic infection, metabolic disorder, and cranial structure defects can sometimes imitate tension type headache. If the neu-

Headache, Episodic Tension Type, Table 2 Acute treatment options in episodic tension-type headache

List of effective acute drugs			
Paracetamol/ Acetaminophen	1000 mg		
Aspirin	1000 mg	Steiner et al. Cephalalgia 2003	
Ibuprofen	400 mg	Packman et al. Headache 2000	
Ketoprofen	25 mg	Steiner et al. Cephalalgia 1998	
Naproxen	750 mg	Autret et al. Cephalalgia 1997	
Diclofenac	12.5–25 mg	Kubitzek et al. EurJPain 2002	
Metamizol	1000 mg	Martinez et al.	Cephalalgia 2001
Medications for children			
Ibuprofen	10 mg/KG		
Paracetamol	15 mg/KG		

rological examination is normal and the headache has no worrisome characteristics, there is no need for further investigations such as neuroimaging or lumbar puncture, and the patient can be reassured.

A number of precipitating factors have been described, including oromandibular dysfunction, non-psychological motor stress, local myofascial release of irritants, sleep deprivation, and coexisting migraine (Spierings et al. 2001). More controversial is the role of psychological factors, although the triggering of attacks by psychological stress is recognised. Up to one third of tension type headache patients show associated symptoms of depression or anxiety, though surveys of personality profiles have not demonstrated significant abnormalities (Holroyd 2002; Merikangas et al. 1994; Mitsikostas and Thomas 1999).

Management and Treatment

As yet there is no specific treatment for tension-type headache. Episodic and mild headaches are often successfully treated with non-specific analgesics, without the involvement of specialists. Drugs with evidence based benefit for acute treatment include aspirin, paracetamol and NSAIDs (Table 2). Compound analgesics should be used with caution, as repeated self-medication can yield to dependency, rebound headache and chronification. The use of drugs for more than 2–3 days per week (> 10 days per month) with associated chronic headache suggests an additional medication-overuse headache (IHS classification). The following rules apply for the acute treatment of ▶ episodic tension-type headache :

1. The analgesics should be taken at relatively high dose!
2. The intake should be as early as possible! *
3. Drugs should not be taken on more than 2 days a week!*

4. The use of compound analgesics (codeine, caffeine, etc.) should be avoided, or at least limited and carefully monitored!

*cave: balance!

As a preventative treatment for frequent tension-type headaches a typical first choice is a tricyclic antidepressant, such as Amitriptyline. High dose Magnesium may be effective. Combination with a non-pharmacological treatment, such as cognitive behavioural therapy, progressive muscle relaxation, or psychological counselling may be useful. In addition, advice may be also needed about the mechanisms of hyperventilation. Management must include elimination of exacerbating factors, such as dental pathology, sinus disease, depressive disorders, un-physiological working conditions, and disturbed sleep patterns. Physiotherapy, physical treatment (hot and cold packs), ultra-sound, electrical stimulation, posture improvement, relaxation and exercise programs are helpful in certain cases. Some patients report beneficial effects of muscle relaxants, tiger balm, and peppermint oil. (Stillman 2002)

References

1. Anttila P, Metsahonkala L, Aromaa M et al. (2002) Determinants of Tension-Type Headache in Children. Cephalalgia 22:401–408
2. Headache Classification Subcommittee of the International Headache Society (2003) International Classification of Headache Disorders, 2nd edn. Cephalalgia
3. Holroyd KA (2002) Behavioral and Psychologic Aspects of the Pathophysiology and Management of Tension-Type Headache. Curr Pain Headache Rep 6:401–407
4. Jensen R, Olesen J (2000) Tension-Type Headache: An Update on Mechanisms and Treatment. Curr Opin Neurol 13:285–289
5. Kaniecki RG (2002) Migraine and Tension-Type Headache: An Assessment of Challenges in Diagnosis. Neurology 58:15–20
6. Merikangas KR, Stevens DE, Angst J (1994) Psychopathology and Headache Syndromes in the Community. Headache 34:17–22
7. Mitsikostas DD, Thomas AM (1999) Comorbidity of Headache and Depressive Disorders. Cephalalgia 19:211–217

8. Rasmussen BK (1996) Migraine and Tension-Type Headache are Separate Disorders. Cephalalgia 16:217–220; discussion 223
9. Rasmussen BK (2001) Epidemiology of Headache. Cephalalgia 21:774–777
10. Rasmussen BK, Jensen R, Schroll M et al. (1991) Epidemiology of Headache in a General Population – A Prevalence Study. J Clin Epidemiol 44:1147–1157
11. Schwartz BS, Stewart WF, Simon D et al. (1998) Epidemiology of Tension-Type Headache. Jama 279:381–383
12. Spierings EL, Ranke AH, Honkoop PC (2001) Precipitating and Aggravating Factors of Migraine versus Tension-Type Headache. Headache 41:554–558
13. Stillman MJ (2002) Pharmacotherapy of Tension-Type Headaches. Curr Pain Headache Rep 6:408–413
14. Ulrich V, Russell MB, Jensen R et al. (1996) A Comparison of Tension-Type Headache in Migraineurs and in Non-Migraineurs: A Population-Based Study. Pain 67:501–506
15. Wober-Bingol C, Wober C, Karwautz A et al. (1996) Tension-Type Headache in Different Age Groups at Two Headache Centers. Pain 67:53–58

Headache from Cranial Bone

HARTMUT GÖBEL
Kiel Pain Center, Kiel, Germany
hg@schmerzklinik.de

Synonyms

Headache Associated with Disorders of the Cranium; Facial Pain Associated with Disorders of the Cranium

Definition

Pain in the head or face caused by a lesion within the cranial bone.

Characterisitics

Most disorders of the skull (e.g. congenital abnormalities, fractures, tumours, metastases) are not usually accompanied by headache. Exceptions of importance are osteomyelitis, multiple myeloma and Paget's disease. Headache may also be caused by lesions of the mastoid, and by petrositis. No epidemiological data are available on headaches due to lesions of the cranial bone.

The bone of the skull has limited sensitivity to pain because only a few nerve fibers enter it from the overlying periosteum. The periosteum is more pain sensitive, and skull lesions therefore produce headache, chiefly by involving it. The lesions of the skull most likely to do this are those that are rapidly expansile, aggressively osteoclastic, or have an inflammatory component.

Most skull lesions are asymptomatic and are discovered as incidental findings on roentgenograms or other imaging procedures done to investigate unrelated complaints, including fibrous dysplasia, osteomas, epidermoid cysts, metastatic cancers, hemangiomas, eosinophilic granulomas, and Paget's disease of the skull. Some of these lesions, notably hemangiomas and eosinophilic granulomas and the rare aneurysmal bone cysts, may present with a tender swelling on the calvarium but not with spontaneous headache.

Relatively few skull lesions produce headache. Multiple myeloma often presents with bone pain anywhere in the body, and skull deposits are sometimes a source of such pain. The multiplicity of the deposits, and the proclivity of the myeloma cells to produce osteoclast activating factor, are likely to account for the production of head pain by this particular bone tumor. Osteomyelitis produces spontaneous head pain because of its rapid evolution and its inflammatory component. Although most cases of Paget's disease of the skull are asymptomatic, remodeling of bone, by producing basilar invagination, may cause headache either through traction on the upper cervical nerve roots, or by the production of cerebrospinal fluid pathway distortion with hydrocephalus. Skull lesions as a cause of headache are infrequent, but usually require neurosurgical treatment. If necessary, surgical excision can serve to confirm the diagnosis and retard the progression of neurological dysfunction and head pain. Apart from specific medication, non-opioid and opioid analgesics may be used for pain relief.

References

1. Bhatoe HS (1998) Deshpande GU. Primary Cranial Ewing's Sarcoma. Br J Neurosurg 12:165–169
2. Göbel H (1997) Die Kopfschmerzen. Ursachen, Mechanismen, Diagnostik und Therapie in der Praxis. Springer Verlag, Berlin Heidelberg New York, pp 1–901
3. Göbel H, Edmeads JG (2000) Disorders of the Skull and Cervical Spine. In: Olesen J, Tfelt-Hansen P, Welch KMA (eds) The Headaches, 2nd edn. Lippincott Williams & Wilkins, Philadelphia, pp 891–898
4. Hayashi T, Kuroshima Y, Yoshida K et al. (2000) Primary Osteosarcoma of the Sphenoid Bone with Extensive Periosteal Extension – Case Report. Neurol Med Chir (Tokyo) 40:419–22
5. International Classification of Headache Disorders 2nd edn (2004) Cephalalgia 24:9–160
6. Scherer A, Engelbrecht V, Nawatny J (2001) MRI of the Cerebellopontine Angle in Patients with Cleidocranial Dysostosis. Rofo Fortschr Geb Rontgenstr Neuen Bildgeb Verfahr 173:315–318
7. Voorhies RM, Sundaresan N (1985) Tumors of the Skull. In: Wilkins RH, Rengachary SS, (eds) Neurosurgery. McGraw-Hill, New York, pp 984–1001

Headache in Aseptic Meningitis

K. RAVISHANKAR
The Headache and Migraine Clinic, Jaslok Hospital and Research Centre, Lilavati Hospital and Research Centre, Mumbai, India
dr_k_ravishankar@vsnl.com

Synonyms

Viral Meningitis; Serous Meningitis; Abacterial Meningitis; Aseptic Meningitis

Definition

▶ Aseptic Meningitis is the term applied to an acute clinical syndrome that comprises headache, fever, signs of meningeal inflammation and a predominantly lymphocytic pleocytosis with normal glucose and normal to elevated proteins in the cerebro-spinal fluid (CSF). Historically, the word 'aseptic' was introduced to denote the nonbacterial aetiology of this syndrome, and included forms of infective meningitis (viral and fungal) that were negative on routine bacteriologic stains and culture. With the introduction of polymerase chain reaction (PCR) based investigations and improved diagnostic techniques, the yield has improved, and the list of conditions that can present with a clinical picture like aseptic meningitis has expanded considerably. Although often used interchangeably, this term is therefore no longer synonymous with ► Viral Meningitis.

Characteristics

Introduction

Both infective and noninfective conditions may present with a picture that fits the definition of aseptic meningitis. Infective causes (Table 1) are mostly viral in origin and less commonly of fungal, parasitic, nonpyogenic bacterial, rickettsial or mycoplasmal origin; non-infective causes (Table 2) include tumours of the central nervous system, carcinomas, leukaemias, sarcoidosis, systemic lupus erythematosus (SLE), rheumatoid arthritis, certain drugs, vaccines, immunoglobulins, intrathecal agents and rarely some disorders of unproven aetiology like Behcets syndrome, Vogt-Koyanagi-Harada syndrome.

Aseptic meningitis is common and seen more often in children and young adults, especially during the summer months. Except in the neonatal period, the mortality and morbidity rates are low (Norris et al. 1999; Cherry 1998). Most patients with aseptic meningitis due to viral causes have a benign course and spontaneously improve, while others may run a complicated course unless specifically

Headache in Aseptic Meningitis, Table 1 Viral Conditions that may present with aseptic meningitis

Infectious Etiologies	Non-Infectious Causes
	Drugs:-
Enteroviruses, Polio, coxsackievirus, echovirus	NSAIDs
HSV types 1 and 2	Trimethoprim
Varicella-zoster virus	Azathioprine
Adenovirus	Intravenous immunoglobulin
Epstein-Barr virus	Isoniazid
LCMV	Intrathecal
HIV	Methotrexate
Influenza A and B	Vaccines
	Allopurinol

Headache in Aseptic Meningitis, Table 2 Non-Viral Conditions that may present with aseptic meningitis

Infectious Etiologies	Non-Infectious Causes
Bacteria:-	**Other Diseases:-**
M.tuberculosis	Sarcoidosis
Borrelia burgdorferi	Leptomeningeal carcinoma
Treponema pallidum	SLE
Brucella	CNS vasculitis
Mycopl.pneumoniae	Behcet disease
Fungi:-	Vogt-Koyanagi-Harada syndrome
Crypto. Neoformans	Migraine
Histo. capsulatum	
Coccidiodes immitis	
Blasto. Dermatitides	
Parasites:-	
Toxoplasma gondii	
Taenia solium	

H

treated. World-wide prevalence varies depending on geographic factors, seasonal influence, epidemiologic patterns of diseases and vaccination policies.

Clinical Features

Aseptic meningitis is characterized by abrupt onset of headache, fever and neck stiffness. Additional clinical symptomatology may vary depending on the underlying cause. Focal signs and seizures are rarely seen in aseptic meningitis, but mumps, certain arboviruses, and lymphocytic choriomeningitis virus may cause a meningoencephalitis (Rice 2001).

The headache of aseptic meningitis has no typical characteristics. It is severe, most often bilateral and may be associated with fever and vomiting. Lamonte et al. (1995), in their retrospective review of 41 patients with aseptic meningitis, noted that headache was present in all, started or worsened abruptly in 24; in 39 the headache was severe and in 6 it was the worst headache. There was no consistent pattern of location or type of pain. In all cases the headache was different from the usual headache. Systemic prodromal symptoms preceded the onset of headache in 19 patients. Nausea, vomiting, cognitive changes, back pain, blurred vision, phonophobia, photophobia and tinnitus were the associated symptoms seen in their series (Marian et al. 1995).

Migraine headache may mimic aseptic meningitis, but if a patient presents acutely with fever and headache that is bilateral, throbbing not relieved with analgesics and different from their earlier headaches, then aseptic meningitis needs ruling out. Rarely migraine itself can cause aseptic meningitis. Bartleson et al. (1981) reported a series of patients with complicated migraine and CSF pleocytosis preceded by a viral-like illness (Gomez-Aranda et al. 1997). Other causes of similar headache that may confuse include subarachnoid haemorrhage and other acute headaches.

The cell count in aseptic meningitis is usually less than 1000 per cu. mm, and there may be an early predominance of polymorphonuclear leucocytes. Repeated lumbar puncture in 8-12 hours frequently shows a change from neutrophil to lymphocyte predominance. CSF glucose levels are normal and CSF proteins may be normal or elevated. CSF culture for viruses and PCR studies help in further confirming the diagnosis.

Differential Diagnosis

Viruses are the most common causative agents, but even when all viral diagnostic facilities are available, the causal agent may be difficult to identify in a good proportion of cases. Viral pathogens may enter the CNS through the haematogenous or neural route. Neural penetration is limited to herpes viruses (HSV–1, HSV–2 and varicella zoster virus) and some enteroviruses. Exposure to mosquito or tick vectors is a risk factor for transmission (Adams and Victor 2001). Over 80% of aseptic meningitis are caused by enteroviruses (coxsackie A or B, enterovirus 68 to 71, echovirus and poliovirus), followed by the mumps virus, HSVû2, HIV, and less commonly HSV–1, varicella zoster virus (VZV), Epstein-Barr virus and cytomegalovirus (CMV). Rarely arbovirus, lymphocytic choriomeningitis virus (LCMV) and adenovirus may be responsible for similar symptoms. Influenzal and parainfluenzal illnesses can also cause aseptic meningitis. The incidence of polio and mumps in the vaccination era has decreased significantly in developed countries. In younger people, measles virus may cause aseptic meningitis that is associated with a rash (Waisman et al. 1999).

Human Immunodeficiency Virus (HIV) infection may present with aseptic meningitis, particularly at the time of seroconversion (Levy et al. 1990). Patients may present with CSF pleocytosis, elevated protein level and high intracranial pressure. Besides the usual meningeal signs, patients with HIV infection may have neurological deficits and may need imaging. Adenovirus may be a major cause of meningitis in patients with HIV infections. Varicella zoster virus can affect the immunocompromised.

Arbovirus accounts for approximately 5% of cases of aseptic meningitis in North America, and the incidence varies depending on the life cycle of arthropod vectors, animal reservoirs and their contact with humans. Some of the important viruses include Eastern and Western equine encephalitis viruses, St Louis Encephalitis virus, West Nile virus, Japanese B virus and Colorado tick fever. LCMV affects those at risk who come in contact with rodents or their excreta (Nelsen et al. 1993).

The immediate concern in practice should not be aimed at establishing a particular virus as the cause of the illness, but more importantly to exclude the few conditions with aseptic meningitis like picture, but having another underlying non-viral cause warranting specific management. In every patient with aseptic meningitis one has to look beyond viruses as the causative factor

Non-viral causes have a more complicated course but can be managed with specific treatment. Tuberculous, fungal, syphilitic, spirochaetal, rickettsial, parasitic and other mycoplasmal infections can cause aseptic meningitis, which should be suspected in the appropriate clinical setting. In the early stages, tuberculous meningitis may appear like aseptic meningitis and can be difficult to diagnose. The glucose levels are reduced only in the later stages and the organism is difficult to find. CSF features of aseptic meningitis, but without fever, may be seen with acute syphilitic meningitis. Cryptococcal infections, other fungal infections, and some rare conditions like Mycoplasma pneumonia, Brucellosis and Q fever can also present like aseptic meningitis. Brucellosis is common in specific geographic locations.

Conjuctival suffusion with transient erythema, severe leg and back pain, pulmonary infiltrates and aseptic meningitis should suggest leptospiral infection. Infection is acquired by contact with soil or water contaminated by the urine of rats, dogs, or cattle. Lyme borreliosis is a common spirochaetal cause of aseptic meningitis and meningoencephalitis. The spirochaete is tick borne, common in north eastern United States from May to July (Eppes et al. 1999).

Leukaemias in children and lymphomas in adults are common sources of meningeal reactions with aseptic meningitis like CSF picture. In these disorders, and in meningeal carcinomatosis, neoplastic cells are found throughout the leptomeninges with additional root involvement. Features of the aseptic meningitis syndrome can also be caused by brain abscess, parameningeal infections and partially treated bacterial meningitis, when it may be mistakenly diagnosed as viral aseptic meningitis. A careful history of previous antibiotic administration must therefore be obtained in all patients with meningitis.

Sarcoidosis, Behcets syndrome, vasculitis and granulomatous angiitis can present with aseptic meningitis syndrome by infiltrating the leptomeninges. These conditions, however, rarely present with a clinical picture of meningitis alone, more often they are seen with other neurological accompaniments (Gullapalli and Phillips 2002; Nelsen et al. 1993). Some chronic diseases like systemic lupus erythematosus, serum sickness and Vogt-Koyanagi-Harada syndrome, may present with aseptic meningitis (Adams and Victor 2001).

Drug induced aseptic meningitis (DIAM), either by: 1) direct irritation of the meninges with intrathecal administration, or by 2) immunological hypersensitivity to the drug, has been reported as an uncommon adverse reaction with numerous agents (Chaudhry and Cunha 1991). The major categories of causative agents are non-steroidal anti-inflammatory drugs (NSAIDs), antimicrobials, intravenous immunoglobulins, isoniazid, allopurinol and vaccines for measles, mumps and rubella. In addition to headache, there may be signs of a hypersensitivity reaction. Trimethoprim-sulphamethoxazole, azathioprine and intrathecal injections can result in the clinical findings of aseptic meningitis. The association between SLE and ibuprofen as a cause of DIAM is important to recognise. A high index of suspicion is necessary to make the diagnosis. Treatment is to withhold the drug. There are no long-term sequelae of DIAM.

Besides the typical CSF picture, it is essential to isolate the virus in CSF, stool, saliva and throat swabs using PCR and other serologic tests (Jeffery et al. 1997). It is important to enquire about a past history of infectious disease, immunisations, contact with animals, insect bites, recent respiratory or gastro-intestinal infection and recent travel. The season during which the illness occurs and the geographical location are helpful pointers.

Recurrent aseptic meningitis is also known as Mollarets meningitis and can be a diagnostic dilemma. There is spontaneous remission and no causative agent has been consistently found. It is difficult to identify the virus in the CSF. These patients need detailed investigations with repeat lumbar punctures, cytology or CSF bacterial cultures, PCR, HIV testing and MRI with contrast if necessary. Recurrence in a few cases is caused by HSV–1 and HSV–2 infections (Cohen et al. 1994).

Conclusion

Most patients with aseptic meningitis need only supportive care. It may be prudent to start antibiotics until cultures are shown to be negative, or a second examination of CSF shows a more typical picture. Most patients recover completely and rapidly when the aetiology is viral, unless there is an associated encephalitic component. Precautions should be taken when specific viruses are identified. Effective antiviral therapy is available against HSV–1, varicella and CMV. For HSV–2, acyclovir is the drug of choice. Other causes need appropriate management. Rarely, patients may have persistent headache, mild mental impairment, incoordination or weakness that lasts for months. Although aseptic meningitis is an acute illness, most patients eventually improve.

References

1. Adams RD, Victor M (2001) Viral Infections in the Nervous System. In: Adams RD, Victor M (eds) Principles of Neurology, 7th edn. McGraw-Hill, New York
2. Bartleson JD, Swanson JW, Whisnant JP (1981) A Migrainous Syndrome with Cerebrospinal Fluid Pleocytosis. Neurology 1:1257–1262
3. Chaudhry HJ, Cunha BA (1991) Drug-Induced Aseptic Meningitis: Diagnosis Leads to Quick Resolution. Postgrad Med 90:65–70
4. Cherry JD (1998) Aseptic Meningitis and Viral Meningitis. In: Feigin RD, Cherry JD (eds) Textbook of Pediatric Infectious Diseases, vol 2, 4th edn. Saunders, Philadelphia, pp 450–457
5. Cohen BA, Rowley AH, Long CM (1994) Herpes Simplex Type 2 in a Patient with Mollaret's Meningitis: Demonstration by Polymerase Chain Reaction. Ann Neurol 35:112–116
6. Eppes SC, Nelson DK, Lewis LL, Klein JD (1999) Characterization of Lyme Meningitis and Comparison with Viral Meningitis in Children. Pediatrics May 103:957–960
7. Gomez-Aranda F, Canadillas F, Marti-Masso JF et al. (1997) Pseudomigraine with Temporary Neurological Symptoms and Lymphocytic Pleocytosis. A Report of 50 Cases. Brain 120:1105–1113
8. Gullapalli D, Phillips LH (2002) Neurologic Manifestations of Sarcoidosis. Neurol Clin 20:59–83
9. Jeffery KJ, Read SJ, Petro TE et al. (1997) Diagnosis of Viral Infections of the Central Nervous System: Clinical Interpretation of PCR Results. Lancet 349:313–317
10. Levy RM, Bredesen DE, Rosenblum ML (1990) Neurologic Complications of HIV Infection. Am Fam Physician 41:517–536
11. Lamonte M, Silberstein SD, Marcelis JF (1995) Headache Associated with Aseptic Meningitis. Headache 35:520–526
12. Nelsen S, Sealy DP, Schneider EF (1993) The Aseptic Meningitis Syndrome. Am Fam Physician 48:809–815
13. Norris CM, Danis PG, Gardner TD (1999) Aseptic Meningitis in the Newborn and Young Infant. Am Fam Physician 59:2761–2770
14. Rice P (2001) Viral Meningitis and Encephalitis. Medicine 29:54–57
15. Waisman Y, Lotem Y, Hemmo M et al. (1999) Management of Children with Aseptic Meningitis in the Emergency Department. Pediatr Emerg Care 15:314–317

Health Informatics

▶ Information and Psychoeducation in the Early Management of Persistent Pain

Heart Pain

▶ Visceral Pain Model, Angina Pain

Heat Hyperalgesia

Definition

Heat hyperalgesia is increased pain produced by a normally painful heat stimulus.

▶ Neuropathic Pain Model, Partial Sciatic Nerve Ligation Model
▶ Sympathetically maintained Pain and Inflammation, Human Experimentation

Heat Lesion

▶ Radiofrequency Neurotomy, Electrophysiological Principles

Heat Sensor

▶ Capsaicin Receptor

Heightened Attention

▶ Hypervigilance and Attention to Pain

Heightened Vigilance

▶ Hypervigilance and Attention to Pain

Helical CT

▶ CT Scanning

Helicobacter Pylori

Definition

Helicobacter Pylori are bacteria that cause inflammation and ulcers in the stomach.
▶ NSAIDs, Adverse Effects

Heliotherapy

Definition

Heliotherapy is the exposure to sun rays and ultraviolet rays.
▶ Spa Treatment

Helplessness

Definition

Helplessness is a belief in one's inability to adequately manage or cope with a stressful situation and to exert any control over ones circumstances, symptoms, and life.
▶ Catastrophizing
▶ Cognitive-Behavioral Perspective of Pain

Hemianesthesia

Definition

Hemianesthesia is the sensory loss in the left or right side of the body.
▶ Central Nervous System Stimulation for Pain

Hemibody Radiation

Definition

Hemibody radiation is an external beam of radiation administered to half of the body, i.e. above or below the diaphragm, for systemic metastatic disease.
▶ Adjuvant Analgesics in Management of Cancer-Rated Bone Pain

Hemicrania Continua

LAWRENCE C. NEWMAN
Albert Einstein College of Medicine, New York, NY, USA
lnewman@chpnet.org

Definition

An under-recognized, primary headache disorder that is characterized by a constant, one-sided headache with fluctuating intensity. In general, the headache is present as a persistent background discomfort of mild to moderate intensity, but exacerbations of more severe pain, superimposed upon the baseline pain, occurs periodically. During these painful flare-ups, patients experience one or more symptoms on the side of the headache. These symptoms include, drooping of the eyelid, reddening or tearing of the eye, constriction of the pupil, and stuffiness or dripping of the nostril. Recognition of the disorder is important, because the headache responds dramatically to treatment with the anti-inflammatory medication indomethacin.

Characteristics

Hemicrania continua (HC) is an under-recognized primary headache disorder. Initially, HC was believed to be a very rare disorder, however, in headache subspecialty practices, HC is a common cause of refractory, ▶ unilateral, chronic daily headache. (Peres et al. 2001) Sjaastad and Spierings initially described the disorder in two patients with continuous headaches from onset (Sjaastad and Spierings 1984). Since that initial description, approximately 150 cases have been described in the literature.

Hemicrania continua demonstrates a marked female preponderance, with a female to male ratio of approximately 2:1. The condition most often begins during adulthood. The age of onset ranges from 5-67 years (mean 28 years) (Peres et al. 2001; Matharu et al. 2003). Most sufferers describe strictly unilateral pain, without side-shift. Rarely, bilateral pain (Pasquier et al. 1987; Iordanidis and Sjaastad 1989; Trucco et al. 1992), or pain that alternated sides, has been described (Newman et al. 1992; Newman et al. 2004). The maximal pain is experienced in the eye, temple and cheek regions. On occasion, the pain may radiate into the ▶ ipsilateral occiput, neck and retro-orbital areas.

The pain is usually described as a steady ache or throbbing pain. Superimposed upon the continuous baseline low-level discomfort, the majority of patients report exacerbations of more intense pain lasting from 20 minutes to several days. Although significantly more intense than the usual background discomfort, the painful exacerbations never reach the level experienced by ▶ cluster headache sufferers. These exacerbations may occur at any time of the day or night, and frequently awaken the patient from sleep. Migraine-like associated symptoms such as nausea, vomiting, ▶ photophobia and ▶ phonophobia often accompany these exacerbations. Rarely, painful exacerbations may be preceded by a migrainous visual aura (Peres et al. 2002). ▶ Autonomic features of cluster headache, including ipsilateral ▶ ptosis, ▶ conjunctival injection, ▶ lacrimation and nasal congestion, often accompany exacerbations of pain. When present, however, these associated features are usually much less pronounced than those seen in cluster headaches. Painful exacerbations are also associated with a sensation of ocular discomfort, often likened to a foreign body in the eye (typically reported as sand or hair). Concurrent ▶ primary stabbing headaches ("jabs and jolts") are reported by many patients, occasionally occurring only in association with the painful exacerbations. During exacerbations of pain, patients assume the pacing activity usually seen with cluster headaches. The International Headache Society (IHS) diagnostic criteria for HC are as follows:

Diagnostic Criteria

a) Headache for > 3 months fulfilling criteria B–D
b) All of the following characteristics:
  1. unilateral pain without side-shift
  2. daily and continuous, without pain-free periods
  3. moderate intensity, but with exacerbations of severe pain
c) At least one of the following autonomic features occurs during exacerbations and ipsilateral to the side of pain:
  4. conjunctival injection and/or ▶ lacrimation
  5. nasal congestion and/or ▶ rhinorrhea
  6. ptosis and/or miosis
d) Complete response to therapeutic doses of indomethacin
e) Not attributed to another disorder

Three temporal profiles of HC have been reported (Newman et al. 1994, Goadsby and Lipton 1997). A chronic form in which headaches persist unabated for years, an episodic form in which distinct headache phases are separated by periods of pain-free remissions, and an initially episodic form that over time evolves into the chronic, unremitting form. HC is chronic from onset in 53%, chronic evolved from episodic in 35%, and episodic in 12% of sufferers (Matharu et al. 2003). There are also individual case reports of atypical presentations; one patient initially experienced the chronic form that over time became episodic (Pareja 1995), another patient with the episodic form experienced headaches with a clear seasonal pattern (Peres et al. 2001).

Organic mimics of HC have been reported to occur in association with brain tumors involving the bones of the skull and skull base (Matharu et al. 2003). HC has been reported to occur in a patient diagnosed with HIV, although a causal relationship was not definitively established (Brilla et al. 1998). Rarely, the diagnosis of HC is masked by a concurrent medication rebound headache. In these instances, discontinuation of the overused analgesic is not associated with headache cessation, and the diagnosis of HC is made by exclusion (Matharu et al. 2003). In rare instances, HC followed head trauma (Lay and Newman 1999).

Hemicrania continua is often misdiagnosed. Although it is not a true cluster headache variant, HC may be mistaken for cluster if the physician focuses on the painful flare-ups with associated autonomic features. A careful history should reveal the presence of the continuous, low-level baseline discomfort in addition to the more disabling exacerbations. Additionally, the autonomic features of HC, when present, tend to be much less pronounced than those of cluster. Similarly, the associated nausea, vomiting, photophobia and phonophobia that accompany exacerbations of pain may be misdiagnosed as chronic migraine headaches. HC is distinguished from migraine by the presence of the persistent dull background discomfort.

Like all primary headache disorders, HC is diagnosed based on the patients' history, medical and neurological examinations. As it is a relatively uncommon headache disorder, and because there have been serious disorders that mimic HC, all patients with features of HC should undergo an MRI scan of the brain prior to initiating therapy.

The treatment of HC is with the medication ▶ indomethacin. In fact, the diagnosis of HC is predicated on response to treatment with indomethacin. The initial dosage is 25 mg, three times daily. If clinical response is not seen within 1–2 weeks, the dosage should be increased to 50–75 mg, three times daily. Complete response to treatment with indomethacin is prompt, usually within 1–2 days of reaching the effective dose. The typical maintenance dose ranges from 25–100 mg, daily. Skipping or delaying the dose often results in headache recurrence. An intramuscular injection of indomethacin, 50–100 mg (the "indotest") has been proposed as a diagnostic procedure for HC (Antonaci et al. 1998). Total resolution of the pain of HC was reported to occur within 2 hours of the injection. Injectable indomethacin is not available in the United States.

Patients suffering with the episodic form should be instructed to continue the medication for 1–2 weeks longer than their typical headache phase and then gradually taper the dose. For those patients with the chronic form, medication tapering should be attempted every 6 months. Patients requiring long-term indomethacin therapy should be given medications such as antacids, misoprostol, histamine H_2 blockers or proton pump inhibitors to mitigate the gastrointestinal side effects of this agent.

In patients who do not respond to treatment with adequate doses of indomethacin, another diagnosis should be considered. Other agents, which may have partial success in the treatment of HC, include naproxen and paracetamol, paracetamol in combination with caffeine, ibuprofen, piroxicam, and reficoxib (Matharu et al. 2003). Six patients who met the clinical criteria for HC, yet failed to respond to treatment with indomethacin, have been reported (Matharu et al. 2003). Nonetheless, the IHS clinical criteria for HC specify that indomethacin responsiveness is necessary for the diagnosis.

References

1. Antonaci F, Pareja JA, Caminero AB et al. (1998) Chronic Paroxysmal Hemicrania and Hemicrania Continua: Parenteral Indomethacin: The "Indotest". Headache 38:122–128
2. Brilla R, Evers S, Soros P et al. (1998) Hemicrania Continua in an HIV-Infected Outpatient. Cephalalgia 18:287–288
3. Headache Classification Subcommittee of the International Headache Society. The International Classification of Headache Disorders, 2nd edn (2004) Cephalalgia 24:1–150
4. Iordanidis T, Sjaastad O (1989) Hemicrania Continua: A Case Report. Cephalalgia 9:301–303
5. Lay C, Newman LC (1999) Posttraumatic Hemicrania Continua. Headache 39:275–279
6. Matharu MS, Boes CJ, Goadsby PJ (2003) Management of Trigeminal Autonomic Cephalgias and Hemicrania Continua. Drugs 63:1–42
7. Newman LC, Lipton RB, Russell M et al. (1992) Hemicrania Continua: Attacks May Alternate Sides. Headache 32:237–238
8. Newman LC, Lipton RB, Solomon S (1994) Hemicrania Continua: Ten New Cases and a Review of the Literature. Neurology 44:2111–2114
9. Newman LC, Spears RC, Lay CL (2004) Hemicrania Continua: A Third Case in which Attacks Alternate Sides. Headache 44:821–823
10. Pareja JA (1995) Hemicrania Continua: Remitting Stage Evolved from the Chronic Form. Headache 35:161–162
11. Pasquier F, Leys D, Petit H (1987) Hemicrania Continua: The First Bilateral Case. Cephalalgia 7:169–170
12. Peres MFP, Silberstein SD, Nahmias S et al. (2001) Hemicrania Continua is Not That Rare. Neurology 57:948–951
13. Peres MFP, Siow HC, Rozen TD (2002) Hemicrania Continua with Aura. Cephalalgia 22:246–248
14. Sjaastad S, Spierings EL (1984) Hemicrania Continua: Another Headache Absolutely Responsive to Indomethacin. Cephalalgia 4:65–70
15. Trucco M, Antonaci F, Sandrini G (1992) Hemicrania Continua: A Case Responsive to Piroxicam-beta-cyclodextrin. Headache 32:39–40

Hemicrania Continua Headache

Definition

Hemicrania continua is a continuous (always present) but fluctuating unilateral headache, moderate to severe in intensity, and accompanied by of one of the following during pain exacerbations: conjuntival injection, lacrimation, nasal congestion, rhinorrhea, ptosis, or eyelid edema. It is uniquely responsive to indomethacin.

▶ Chronic Daily Headache in Children
▶ New Daily Persistent Headache
▶ Paroxysmal Hemicrania

Hemicrania Simplex

▶ Migraine Without Aura

Hemipain

Definition

Hemipain is pain that is situated in one half of the body.

▶ Diagnosis and Assessment of Clinical Characteristics of Central Pain

Hemisection Model

▶ Spinal Cord Injury Pain Model, Hemisection Model

Hemisphere

Definition

The hemisphere is either half of the cerebrum or brain; the human brain has a left and a right hemisphere.

▶ PET and fMRI Imaging in Parietal Cortex (SI, SII, Inferior Parietal Cortex BA40)

Hemorrhagic Stroke

▶ Headache Due to Intracranial Bleeding

Hereditary Motor and Sensory Neuropathy

Definition

Hereditary motor and sensory neuropathy is an alternative name for Charcot-Marie-Tooth Disease.

▶ Hereditary Neuropathies

Hereditary Neuropathies

WILLIAM N. KELLEY, STEVEN S. SCHERER
Department of Neurology, The University of
Pennsylvania Medical School, Philadelphia, PA, USA
sscherer@mail.med.upenn.edu

Synonyms

Charcot-Marie-Tooth disease (CMT); Hereditary Motor and Sensory Neuropathy (HMSN); Dejerine-Sottas neuropathy (DSN); Congenital Hypomyelinating Neuropathy; Hereditary Neuropathy with Liability to Pressure Palsies

Definition

Hereditary neuropathies are inherited diseases that injure peripheral nerves.

Characteristics

Classification of Hereditary Neuropathies

Inherited neuropathies can be separated according to whether they are syndromic (i. e., one of a number of affected tissues), and whether they are "axonal" or "demyelinating" (whether the primary abnormality appears to affect axons/neurons or myelinating ▶ Schwann cells). Non-syndromic inherited neuropathies (Tab. 1) are usually called ▶ CMT or ▶ HMSN. Different kinds are recognized clinically, aided by electrophysiological testing of peripheral nerves (Dyck et al. 1993; Lupski and Garcia 2001; Kleopa and Scherer 2002). If the forearm motor nerve conduction velocities (NCVs) are greater or less than 38 m/s, then the ▶ neuropathy is traditionally considered to be "axonal" (CMT2/HMSN II) or "demyelinating" (CMT1/HMSN I), respectively. Some non-syndromic inherited neuropathies have been given different names because their phenotypes differ; these may be milder (e.g. HNPP) or more severe (DSN CHN). Mutations in different genes can cause a similar phenotype, and different mutations in the same gene can cause different phenotypes (Lupski and Garcia 2001; Suter and Scherer 2003; Wrabetz et al. 2004). For most of these mutations, the evidence favors the idea that the more severe phenotypes are caused by a gain of function and that (heterozygous) loss of function alleles cause milder phenotypes.

The Biology of Myelinated Axons and Neuropathies

The structure and function of myelinating Schwann cells is the basis for understanding how mutations cause inherited demyelinating neuropathies. The ▶ myelin sheath itself can be divided into two domains, compact and non-compact myelin, each of which contains a non-overlapping set of proteins (Fig. 1). Compact myelin forms the bulk of the myelin sheath. It is largely composed of lipids, mainly cholesterol and sphingolipids,

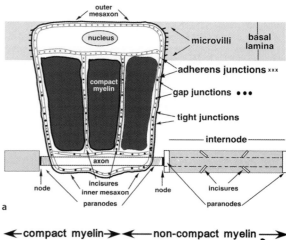

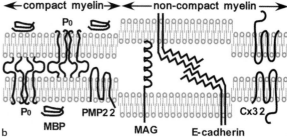

Hereditary Neuropathies, Figure 1 The architecture of the myelinated axon in the PNS. In (a) one myelinating Schwann cell has been "unrolled" to reveal the regions forming compact myelin, as well as paranodes and incisures, regions of non-compact myelin. In (b) note that P$_0$, PMP22, and MBP and are found in compact myelin, whereas Cx32, MAG and E-cadherin are localized in non-compact myelin. Modified from (Kleopa and Scherer 2002), with permission of Elsevier Science.

including galactocerebroside and sulfatide, and three proteins – MPZ/P$_0$, PMP22, and myelin basic protein (MBP). Found in the paranodes and incisures, non-compact myelin contains tight junctions, gap junctions, and adherens junctions. In most cell types, these junctions join adjacent cells, whereas in Schwann cells, they are found between adjacent layers of non-compact myelin (Scherer et al. 2004). Gap junctions formed by Cx32 may form a radial pathway, directly across the layers of the myelin sheath; this would be advantageous as it provides a much shorter pathway (up to 1000-fold) than a circumferential route.

Genetic evidence supports the long-standing doctrine that neuropathies are length-dependent, because the longest axons are the most vulnerable to defects in axonal transport (Suter and Scherer 2003). Neurofilaments and microtubules comprise the axonal cytoskeleton. Neurofilaments are composed of three subunits, termed heavy, medium, and light. Dominant mutations in the gene encoding the light subunit (*NEFL*) cause an axonal neuropathy (CMT2E, Tab. 1). Most proteins are synthesized in the cell body and transported down the axon. Microtubule-activated ATPases, known as kinesins, which are molecular motors that use microtubules as tracks, mediate axonal transport.

Hereditary Neuropathies, Table 1 Non-syndromic inherited neuropathies with a genetically identified cause The neuropathies are classified by MIM (http://www.ncbi.nlm.nih.gov/Omim/); the references for the individual mutations are compiled in the CMT mutation database (http://molgen-www.uia.ac.be/ CMTMutations/DataSource/MutByGene.cfm). Bolded diseases have pronounced affects on pain.

Disease (MIM)	Mutated gene/linkage	Clinical features
Autosomal or X-linked dominant demyelinating neuropathies		
HNPP (162500)	Usually deletion of one PMP22 allele	Episodic mononeuropathies at typical sites of compression; also mild demyelinating neuropathy
CMT1A (118220)	Usually duplication of one PMP22 allele	Onset $1^{st}-2^{nd}$ decade; weakness, atrophy, sensory loss; beginning in the feet and progressing proximally
CMT1B (118200)	MPZ	Similar to CMT1A; severity varies according to mutation (from "mild" to "severe" CTM1)
CMT1C (601098)	LITAF/SIMPLE	Similar to CMT1A; motor NCVs about 20 m/s
CMT1D (607687)	EGR2	Similar to CMT1A; severity varies according to mutation (from "mild" to "severe" CTM1)
CMT1X (302800)	GJB1	Similar to CMT1A, but distal atrophy more pronounced; men are more affected than are women
Autosomal dominant axonal neuropathies		
CMT2A (118210) CMT2A2 (609260)	KIF1Bβ MFN2	Onset of neuropathy by 10y; progresses to distal weakness and atrophy in legs; mild sensory disturbance
CMT2B (600882)	RAB7	Onset $2^{nd}-3^{rd}$ decade; severe sensory loss with distal ulcerations; also length-dependent weakness
CMT2C (606071)	12q23-24	Prominent vocal cord and diaphragmatic weakness
CMT2D (601472)	GARS	Arm more than leg weakness; onset of weakness $2^{nd}-3^{rd}$ decade; sensory axons involved
CMT2E (162280)	NEFL	Variable onset and severity; ranging from DSS-like to CMT2 phenotype; pain sensation may be diminished
CMT2-P$_0$ (118200)	MPZ	Late onset (30y or older); but progressive neuropathy; pain; hearing loss; abnormally reactive pupils
Severe demyelinating neuropathies (autosomal dominant or recessive; "CMT3 or HMSN III")		
DSS (Dejerine-Sottas Syndrome (145900)	Dominant (PMP22; MPZ; GJB1; EGR2; NEFL) and recessive (MTMR2; PRX) mutations	Delayed motor development before 3y; severe weakness and atrophy; severe sensory loss particularly of modalites subserved by large myelinated axons; motor NCVs less than 10 m/s; dysmyelination on nerve biopsies
CHN (Congenital Hypomyelinating Neuropathy; 605253)	Dominant (EGR2; PMP22; MPZ) &recessive (EGR2) mutations	Clinical picture often similar to that of Dejerine-Sottas syndrome; but hypotonic at birth
Autosomal recessive demyelinating neuropathies ("CMT4")		
CMT4A (214400)	GDAP1	Early childhood onset; progressing to wheelchair-dependency; mixed demyelinating and axonal features
CMT4B1 (601382)	MTMR2	Early childhood onset; may progress to wheelchair-dependency; focally-folded myelin sheaths
CMT4B2 (604563)	MTMR13	Childhood onset; progression to assistive devices for walking; focally-folded myelin sheaths; glaucoma
CMT4C (601596)	KIAA1985	Infantile to childhood onset; progressing to wheelchair-dependency; severe to moderate NCV slowing
CMT4D (601455)	NDRG1	Childhood onset; progression to severe disability by 50y; hearing loss and dysmorphic features
CMT4F (605260)	PRX	Childhood onset; usually progression to severe disability; prominent sensory loss
CMT4 (605253)	EGR2	Infantile onset; progressing to wheelchair-dependency

Hereditary Neuropathies, Table 1 (continued)

Disease (MIM)	Mutated gene/linkage	Clinical features
Autosomal recessive axonal neuropathies ("AR-CMT2" or "CMT 2B")		
AR-CMT2A(605588)	*LMNA* mutations	Onset of neuropathy in 2nd decade; progresses to severe weakness and atrophy in distal muscles
Hereditary Motor Neuropathies (HMN or "distal SMA")		
SMARD1 (604320)	Recessive *IGHMBP2* mutations	Distal infantile spinal muscular atrophy with diaphragm paralysis
HMN 5 (600794)	Dominant *GARS* mutations	Arm more than leg weakness; onset of weakness 2nd–3rd decade; no sensory involvement
Hereditary Sensory (and Autonomic) Neuropathies/Neuronopathies (HSN or HSAN)		
HSN-1 (162400)	Dominant *SPTLC1* mutations	Onset 2nd–3rd decade (often with phase of lacinating pain); severe sensory loss (including nociception) with distal ulcerations; also length-dependent weakness
HSN-2 (201300)	Recessive *HSN2* mutations	Childhood onset of progressive numbness in hands and feet, exacerbated by cold; reduced pain sensation; no overt autonomic dysfunction
HSN-3 (Riley-Day syndrome; 223900)	Recessive *IKBKAP* mutations	Congenital onset; dysautonomic crises; decreased pain sensation; absent fungiform papilla; overflow tears
HSN-4 (CIPA; 256800)	Recessive *NTRKA*	Dysautonomia and loss of pain sensation caused by congenital absence of sensory and sympathetic neurons
HSN-5 (608654)	Recessive *NGFB* mutations	Childhood onset; unheeded pain leads to development of Charcot joints; deceased sensation to multiple modalities
HSN with cough and gastroesophageal reflux (608088)	3p22-p24	Adult onset cough and sensory neuropathy; with sensory loss; painless injuries; and/or lacinating pains

A mutation in the gene encoding kinesin KIF1Bβ causes CMT2A1 a dominantly inherited axonal neuropathy. Mutations in the genes encoding gigaxonin and the p150 subunit of dynactin also disrupt axonal transport and cause neuropathy/neuronopathy. Defective axonal transport has been implicated in a host of other inherited neurological diseases, including the inherited spastic paraplegias, which appear to be length-dependent CNS axonopathies.

CMT and Pain

The best examples of a dominantly inherited neuropathy that is associated with pain are *MPZ* mutations, which cause a CMT2-like phenotype (CMT2-P_0), particularly the Thr124Met mutation. Several families have been found to have an adult-onset neuropathy with painful lacinations and hearing loss. Nerve biopsies from clinically affected patients show axonal loss, clusters of regenerated axons, and some thinly myelinated axons. In spite of a late onset, many patients progress relatively rapidly to the point of using a wheelchair. Neuropathic pain is not a prominent symptom in most patients with *MPZ* mutations (CMT1B).

Neuropathic pain can be a prominent feature in some CMT2 (e.g. CMT2-P_0) patients (Gemignani et al. 2004), but the genetic cause(s) of these cases is not yet known. CMT2B patients have the opposite problem –

they do not feel pain, and insensitivity to pain commonly leads to distal ulcerations in the feet, even toe amputations. CMT2B is caused by dominant mutations in *RAB7*, which encodes a member of the Rab family of Ras-related GTPases that are essential for proper intracellular membrane trafficking. RAB7 is widely expressed, including in motor and sensory neurons. A similar, ulceromutilating neuropathy has been reported in an Austrian family, which did not link to the CMT2B locus, indicating further genetic heterogeneity in this phenotype.

Hereditary Sensory (and Autonomic) Neuropathies (HSN or HSAN)

They were initially classified together for their shared characteristics - the loss of sensory (especially of small fibers) and ► autonomic fibers, resulting in severe sensory loss to the point that the hands and feet became mutilated from unheeded trauma. They proved to be genetically heterogeneous (Tab. 1). HSN-1 is an autosomal dominant trait and manifests in adolescence with small fiber sensory loss, burning pain (distal>proximal and legs>arms), pedal deformity, acromutilation, and distal weakness. It is caused by mutations in the gene encoding serine palmitoyl transferase, long-chain base subunit 1 (*SPTLC1*). The mutations that cause HSN-1 reside in a conserved region, and the corresponding mutations in the yeast enzyme act as dominants because the enzyme is part of a heterodimer.

HSN-2, HSN-3 and HSN-4 are autosomal recessive. HSN-2 begins in early childhood with similar phenotype to HSN-1. HSN-3, also known as the Riley-Day syndrome or familial dysautonomia with congenital indifference to pain, is usually caused by a mutation that leads to missplicing of IKBKAP (inhibitor of κ light polypeptide gene enhancer in B cells, kinase complex-associated protein) (Axelrod 2004). Some characteristics manifest at birth, indicating that certain populations of autonomic and sensory neurons/axons either fail to develop or are already affected, but axonal/neuronal loss progresses even after birth. Although initial deficits such as dysautonomic crises appear to stem from the loss of small fibers, large myelinated fibers are progressively affected. Loss of sensation renders patients prone to self-injury. At least two syndromic neuropathies, cold-induced sweating and Stüve-Wiedemann/ Schwartz-Jampel type 2 syndrome have features in common with HSN-3 (Tab. 2). HSN-4 is a syndromic disease, characterized by congenital insensitivity to pain with anhydrosis (hence the alternative name, CIPA syndrome), with the associated features of small fiber sensory loss, autonomic failure, mental retardation, and acromutilation. CIPA syndrome is caused by mutations in NTRKA, which encodes a receptor tyrosine kinase for nerve growth factor (Indo 2001).

Syndromic Inherited Neuropathies and Pain

Demyelinating neuropathies are part of several recessive neurological syndromes, but are typically overshadowed by other manifestations (Tab. 2). Neuropathic pain is uncommon except in metachromatic leukodystrophy. An axonal neuropathy is a part of many syndromes, and most appear to be neuron-autonomous. Discussed below are some of the inherited syndromic axonal neuropathies that have pronounced effects on pain.

Familial amyloid polyneuropathy (FAP) 1 and 2 is caused by dominant mutations in the transthyretin (*TTR*) gene – almost all are caused by a single nucleotide change that results in an amino acid substitution (Benson 2000). In the United States, the majority of mutations are found in families of European ancestry, and, in many cases, the mutations have been traced to the country of origin. Adults develop dysesthesias in the lower extremities, with or without small fiber findings such as decreased temperature sensation, and/or autonomic dysfunction-constipation and diarrhea or impotence. The progressive loss of large myelinated (sensory and motor) fibers leads to progressive sensory loss and motor impairment. Amyloidosis results from the transformation of a protein into β-structured fibrils that are deposited in various organs, causing dysfunction by their presence and magnitude. FAP 3, caused by mutations in *Apoliproprotein A1*, also causes neuropathy and neuropathic pain.

Recurrent episodes of painful brachial plexus lesions are the hallmark of hereditary neuralgic amyotrophy – a dominantly inherited disorder (Windebank 1993). Individual episodes are similar to those in idiopathic neuralgic amyotrophy; both kinds are heralded by severe pain, followed by weakness within days, and recovery over weeks to months. Episodes may be triggered by immunization and childbirth, and perivascular inflammation and Wallerian degeneration are characteristic lesions (Klein et al. 2002). Subtle dismorphic features in affected patients with the inherited form indicate that this is a syndromic disorder. Neuralgic amyotrophy is caused by mutation in *SEPT9*, but another locus is possible.

Porphyrias are caused by mutations in the genes involved in heme biosynthesis. Dominant mutations in porphobilinogen deaminase, coproporphyrinogen 3 oxidase, protoporphyrinogen oxidase, ferrochelatase may produce different syndromes (photosensitivity, psychosis, and/or liver disease), but all can cause acute attacks of abdominal pain followed by neuropathy (Windebank and Bonkovsky 1993). High levels of porphyrins are found during attacks, and may be toxic to motor axons/neurons, but why those innervating certain muscle groups are mainly affected remains to be determined. The somatic neuropathy itself is usually not painful, but it is conceivable that the abdominal pain is related to damaged visceral afferent axons. Hereditary tyrosinemia type 1 causes crises that resemble the porphyrias, including elevated urinary δ-aminolevulinic acid, except for limb pain that may be neuropathic.

Fabry disease is caused by deficiency of an X-linked lysosomal hydrolase, α-galactosidase, leading to accumulation of glycosphingolipids in many cell types, including sensory neurons. The loss of sensory axons and sensory neurons is presumed to cause neuropathic pain, which is the most common and the earliest symptom (MacDermot et al. 2001). Patients had a mean pain score of five (1–10 scale) in spite of pharmacological therapy. In addition to constant pain, patients can have severe attacks of pain, often triggered by heat, fever, alcohol, or exercise.

Concluding Thoughts

Inherited neuropathies are common, and their genetic causes are rapidly being determined. A lack of pain in certain inherited neuropathies can be related to the loss of the relevant sensory axons/neurons, particularly for HSN-1, HSN-3, and HSN-4/CIPA syndrome. Discovering the molecular causes of even rarer kinds of inherited insensibility to pain should lead to a better understanding of the neurobiology of pain. Why pain is a characteristic of some neuropathies and not others is far less clear. It seems that neuropathies that mainly affect small myelinated and unmyelinated (nociceptive and other kinds of sensory) axons are more likely to cause pain than those that chiefly affect large myelinated (mo-

Hereditary Neuropathies, Table 2   Selected syndromic inherited neuropathies For references; see the following websites: http://www.ncbi.nlm.nih.gov/Omim/; http://molgen-www.uia.ac.be/ CMTMutations/DataSource/MutByGene.cfm; and http://www.neuro.wustl.edu/neuromuscular/. Bolded diseases have pronounced affects on pain. For abbreviations; see text

Disease (MIM)	Mutated gene/linkage	Clinical features
Dominantly inherited; syndromic demyelinating neuropathies		
Wardeenburg type IV (602229)	*SOX10*	CNS and PNS dysmyelination; Hirschsprung disease
Recessively inherited; syndromic demyelinating neuropathies		
Metachromatic leuko-dystrophy (250100)	*Arylsulfatase A*	Demyelinating neuropathy; optic atrophy; mental retardation; hypotonia; phase of neuropathic pain
Globoid cell leuko-dystrophy (245200)	*Galactosylceramide β-galactosidase*	Demyelinating neuropathy; spasticity; optic atrophy; mental retardation
Dominantly inherited; syndromic axonal neuropathies		
Hereditary Neuralgic Amyotrophy (162100)	*SEPT9*	Episodes of painful neuropathies of the brachial plexus; hypotelorism; small palpebral fissures; small mouth
FAP 1 and 2 (176300)	*TTR* (Transthyretin)	Painful axonal neuropathy with prominent involvement of small axons; other organs involved; FAP 2 also has carpal tunnel syndrome
FAP 3/"Iowa" type (107680)	*Apolipoprotein A-1*	Painful axonal neuropathy; renal and hepatic disease
FAP 4/"Finnish" type (105120)	*Gelsolin* (137350)	Corneal lattice dystrophy; cranial neuropathies; peripheral neuropathy not typically painful
Acute intermittent porphyria (176000)	*Porphobilinogen deaminase*	Acute neuropathy follows crises of abdominal pain; psychosis; depression; dementia; seizures
Coproporphyria (121300)	*Coproporphyrinogen 3 oxidase*	Skin photosensitivity; psychosis; crises of acute neuropathy (and abdominal pain) are rare
Variegate porphyria(176200)	*Protoporphyrinogen oxidase*	South Africa: founder effect; symptoms similar to those in acute intermittent porphyria
Erythopoietic proto-porphyria (17000)	*Ferrochelatase*	Dermatitis; photosensitivity; liver disease; acute neuropathy rare
Fabry disease (301500)	α-*galactosidase*	X-linked; painful neuropathy even painful crises; cardiomyopathy; renal failure; angiokeratoma
Recessively inherited; syndromic axonal neuropathies		
Giant axonal neuropathy (256850)	*Gigaxonin*	Mental retardation; spasticity; kinky/curly hair
Hereditary tyrosinemia type 1 (276700)	*Fumarylacetoacetase*	Hepatic and renal disease; cardiomyopathy; crises of acute neuropathy and abdominal pain similar to those in porphyrias (but in infancy/childhood)
Tangier Disease (205400)	*ABCA1* (60046)	Atherosclerosis and/or peripheral neuropathy; syringomyelia-like loss of pain sensation can result in painless ulcerations and acromutilation
Congenital sensory and autonomic neuropathy and neurotrophic keratitis (256810)	unknown	Affects Navajo infants/children; encephalopathy; myelopathy; neuropathy resulting in painless ulcerations and acromutilation; fatal liver disease
Cold-induced sweating (272430)	*CRLF1*	Poor sucking in infancy; cold-induced sweating; diminished pain caused by cold/hot/mechanical stimuli
Stüve-Wiedemann/ Schwartz-Jampel type 2 syndrome	*LIFR*	Osteodysplasia with similar findings to HSN-3/familial dysautonomia: lack of corneal reflex, lack of fungiform papillae, tongue ulceration; also cold-induced sweating

tor and non-nociceptive sensory) axons. This reasoning does not account for why it is that neuropathic pain is more common in CMT2 than in CMT1 (Gemignani et al. 2004), and so prominent CMT2-P_0 (see above). Further, it remains to be explained why pain was much more commonly reported in a patient survey (Carter et al. 1998) than described in typical reports. Part of this discrepancy may owe to the failure to discriminate between neuropathic pain from other causes (Carter et al. 1998) as discussed by Gemignani et al. (2004).

References

1. Axelrod FB (2004) Familial Dysautonomia. Muscle Nerve 29:352–363
2. Benson MD (2000) Amyloidosis. In: Scriver CR, Beaudet AL, Sly WS, Valle D, Childs B, Kinzler KW, Vogelstein B (eds) The Metabolic and Molecular Bases of Inherited Disease, vol IV. McGraw Hill, New York, pp 5345–5378
3. Carter GT, Jensen MP, Galer BS, Kraft GH, Crabtree LD, Beardsley RM, Abresch RT, Bird TD (1998) Neuropathic Pain in Charcot-Marie-Tooth Disease. Arch Phys Med Rehabil 79:1560–1564
4. Dyck PJ, Chance P, Lebo R, Carney JA (1993) Hereditary Motor and Sensory Neuropathies. In: Dyck PJ, Thomas PK, Griffin JW, Low PA, Poduslo JF (eds) Peripheral Neuropathy. WB Saunders, Philadelphia, pp 1094–1136
5. Gemignani F, Melli G, Alfieri S, Inglese C, Marbini A (2004) Sensory Manifestations in Charcot-Marie-Tooth Disease. J Periph Nerv Syst 9:7–14
6. Indo Y (2001) Molecular Basis of Congenital Insensitivity to Pain with Anhidrosis (CIPA): Mutations and Polymorphisms in TRKA (NTRK1) Gene Encoding the Receptor Tyrosine Kinase for Nerve Growth Factor. Hum Mutat 18:462–471
7. Klein CJ, Dyck PJB, Friedenberg SM, Burns TM, Windebank AJ, Dyck PJ (2002) Inflammation and Neuropathic Attacks in Hereditary Brachial Plexus Neuropathy. J Neurol Neurosurg Psychiat 73:45–50
8. Kleopa KA, Scherer SS (2002) Inherited Neuropathies. Neurol Clin N Am 20:679–709
9. Lupski JR, Garcia CA (2001) Charcot-Marie-Tooth Peripheral Neuropathies and Related Disorders. In: Scriver CR, Beaudet AL, Sly WS, Valle D, Childs B, Kinzler KW (eds) The Metabolic Molecular Basis of Inherited Disease. McGraw-Hill, New York, pp 5759–5788
10. MacDermot KD, Holmes a, Miners AH (2001) Anderson-Fabry Disease: Clinical Manifestations and Impact of Disease in a Cohort of 98 Hemizygous Males. J Med Genet 38:750–560
11. Scherer SS, Arroyo EJ, Peles E (2004) Functional Organization of the Nodes of Ranvier. In: Lazzarini RL (ed) Myelin Biology and Disorders, vol 1. Elsevier, pp 89–116
12. Suter U, Scherer SS (2003) Disease Mechanisms in Inherited Neuropathies. Nat Neurosci Rev 4:714–726
13. Windebank T (1993) Inherited Recurrent Focal Neuropathies. In: Dyck PJ, Thomas PK, Griffin JW, Low PA, Poduslo JF (eds) Peripheral Neuropathy. W.B. Saunders, Philadelphia, pp 1137–1148
14. Windebank T, Bonkovsky HL (1993) Porphyric Neuropathy. In: Dyck PJ, Thomas PK, Griffin JW, Low PA, Poduslo JF (eds) Peripheral Neuropathy. WB Saunders, Philadelphia, pp 1161–1168
15. Wrabetz L, Feltri ML, Kleopa KA, Scherer SS (2004) Inherited Neuropathies - Clinical, Genetic, and Biological Features. In: Lazzarini RL (ed) Myelin Biology and Disorders, vol 2. Elsevier, pp 905–951

Hereditary Neuropathy with Liability to Pressure Palsies

▶ Hereditary Neuropathies

Hereditary Sensory and Autonomic Neuropathy Type IV, HSAN IV, HSAN 4

▶ Congenital Insensitivity to Pain with Anhidrosis

Hereditary Sensory Neuropathy

Definition

Hereditary Sensory Neuropathy is an inherited neuropathy that mainly affects sensory axons and/or sensory neurons.

▶ Hereditary Neuropathies

Heritability of Inflammatory Nociception

JEFFREY S. MOGIL
Department of Psychology and Centre for Research on Pain, McGill University, Montreal, QC, Canada
jeffrey.mogil@mcgill.ca

Synonyms

Inflammatory Nociception, Heritability; Inflammatory Nociception, Genotypic Influences; Inflammatory Nociception, Genetic Factors

Definition

Humans and laboratory animals display widely variable responses to inflammatory stimuli. Even when the amount of inflammation is held constant, robust individual differences in the pain accompanying that inflammation are observed. Some proportion of this variability can be attributed to inherited genetic factors, and progress is being made in identifying the relevant genes using ▶ inbred strains of mice. Genes contributing to variability in inflammatory nociception are probably distinct from genes contributing to variability in the development of inflammation itself.

Characteristics

Susceptibility to developing inflammatory pathologies like rheumatoid arthritis is considerably ▶ heritable, with one recent meta-analysis of ▶ twin studies suggesting that inherited genetic factors account for approximately 60% of the variation in disease liability (MacGregor et al. 2000). A number of animal models of autoimmune and/or inflammatory disorders have been developed, and scores of "modifier" genetic loci (i.e. non–major histocompatibility complex genes) influencing disease susceptibility or severity have been detected using ▶ quantitative trait locus (QTL) mapping (Griffiths et al. 1999). These loci show considerable overlap with the results of human genome-wide scans for ▶ genetic linkage in pedigrees of autoimmune/inflammatory disease sufferers (Becker et al. 1998). In a few cases, the precise genes and DNA variants responsible for the modified susceptibility or severity have been unambiguously identified, including ▶ single nucleotide polymorphisms (SNPs) in the human SLC22A4 gene encoding an organic cation transporter (Tokuhiro et al. 2003) and the rat *Ncf1* gene encoding a cytosolic factor in the NADPH oxidase complex (Olofsson et al. 2003).

However, the heritability of inflammatory *pain* remains poorly understood; none of the genes described above are necessarily relevant to variable pain responses given a particular degree of inflammation. A large number of ▶ transgenic knockout mice have been developed that display altered sensitivity to inflammatory nociception (see Mogil and Grisel 1998), thus providing evidence for the crucial roles of the targeted genes in the processing of inflammatory pain. Knockout mice represent a poor model to study inherited variability though, because their genetic "lesion" is far more dramatic than the subtle changes in function and expression that more generally characterize genetic variation in a population. The contrasting responses of different inbred strains of rats and mice have clearly demonstrated that assays of inflammatory nociception featuring standardized stimuli are robustly heritable. For example, recuperative licking behavior on the "tonic" or "late" phase of the ▶ formalin test – thought by many to reflect ongoing inflammatory nociception – ranges by up to 10–fold among 14 strains tested (Mogil et al. 1998) (Fig. 1). We have extensively characterized the extreme–responding strains, A/J and C57BL/6, and observed differences in formalin potency and efficacy and alterations in the timing of licking behavior in the tonic phase. However, these strains do not differ in edema produced by formalin injection, whether assessed *via* hind-paw thickness, *via* hind-paw weight, or histologically.

To provide evidence that the behavioral strain difference in licking time truly reflects a difference related to pain processing rather than non-specific factors (e.g., emotionality, locomotor activity, propensity to lick injured tissue), we conducted a study evaluating the ▶ genetic correlation between formalin-induced licking and ▶ c-fos immediate-early gene expression in the spinal cord dorsal horn. We found an extremely high correlation ($r=0.94$) between tonic-phase licking and Fos-protein immunoreactivity in the deep (laminae V/VI) but not superficial (laminae I/II) dorsal horn among eight mouse strains (Bon et al. 2002). This high correlation suggests that the strain-dependent behavioral differences are reflected in the processing of the noxious stimulus in appropriate pain–relevant ascending pathways.

As a first step to identifying the genes responsible for the robust differences between A/J and C57BL/6J mice on the formalin test, we performed a QTL mapping study in an ▶ F2 intercross of these strains (Wilson et al. 2002). Two statistically significant QTLs were identified; one of these (called *Nociq2*), on distal mouse chromosome 10, was associated with the tonic phase and accounted for 15% of the overall trait variance. In this F$_2$ population, the ≈25% of mice inheriting two copies of the A/J ▶ allele at a gene very near the end of chromosome 10 displayed 200 seconds *less* licking in the tonic phase

than mice with one or two C57BL/6J alleles. We have now provided confirmatory evidence for the existence of this formalin test-relevant gene using more advanced mapping populations (e.g. recombinant inbred strains, recombinant congenic strains) (Darvasi 1998), and have pinpointed its exact location to less than 3 cM (i.e. <3 million nucleotides; unpublished data), a genomic region containing only 14 known genes.

When genes associated with variable inflammatory pain sensitivity are identified, what will their relevance be to other pain states? Using genetic correlation analysis applied to over 22 different nociceptive assays in 12 mouse strains, we have determined that at least five fundamental 'types' of nociception exist. The defining feature of these pain types is noxious stimulus modality; that is, sensitivity to thermal stimuli is inherited similarly, but sensitivity to noxious chemical stimuli depends on a different set of genes (Lariviere et al. 2002). Generally speaking, the same mouse strains that are sensitive on the formalin test are also sensitive to injection of acetic acid, capsaicin or bee venom; such strains might not, however, be sensitive in the hot-plate test. It is interesting that the presence or absence of inflammation does *not* appear to be the defining feature, but rather the use of a noxious chemical substance producing spontaneously emitted pain behaviors. Some inflammatory mediators produce very little behavioral evidence of spontaneous pain (e.g. carrageenan), instead yielding long-lasting thermal and mechanical hypersensitivity. In these cases, what appears to be inherited in mice is not sensitivity to the mediator itself, but rather sensitivity to the evoking stimulus. That is, mouse strains sensitive to the development of thermal hypersensitivity after carrageenan injection are not the same strains that are sensitive to the development of mechanical hypersensitivity (Lariviere et al. 2002), implying the existence of modality-selective genes. Another finding from this analysis is that the same set of genes appear to be relevant to hypersensitivity states, whether they were induced by inflammation or nerve damage, possibly suggesting an important inflammatory component in the development of neuropathic pain.

The predictions described above will require the identification of many more pain variability-related genes for their evaluation. It is interesting, however, that none of the existing murine QTLs for thermal nociception (see Mogil 2004) are located on distal chromosome 10. Furthermore, an unpublished study (H.S. Hain and J.K. Belknap, personal communication) using the chemical/inflammatory acetic acid writhing test has also detected a statistically significant QTL on distal chromosome 10.

Once genes associated with variable sensitivity to inflammatory nociception are identified, the demonstration of the relevance of those genes and their common variants to humans might be important in a number

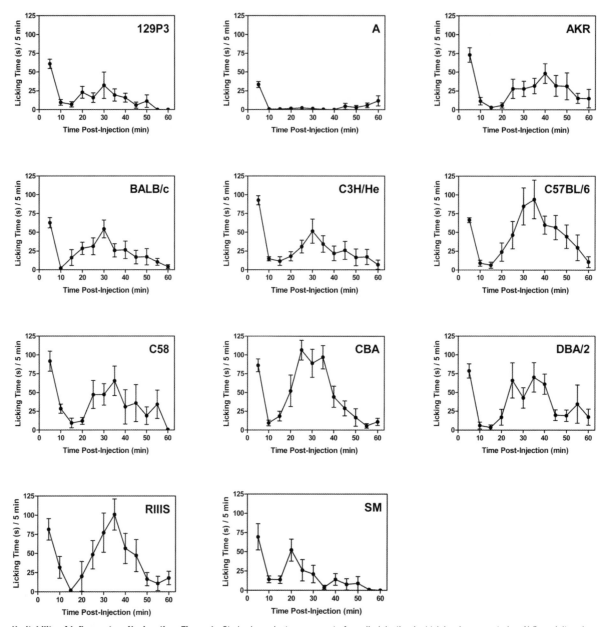

Heritability of Inflammatory Nociception, Figure 1   Strain-dependent responses to formalin injection in 11 inbred mouse strains. Naïve adult male mice were habituated to Plexiglas observation cylinders for at least 30 min. Then, 25 μl of 5% formalin was injected subcutaneously into the plantar surface of the right hind paw using a 50 μl microsyringe with a 30-gauge needle. Mice were then returned to the cylinders, and behavioral observations were begun immediately. The total time spent licking/biting the right hind paw over the next 60 min was measured with a stopwatch. Symbols represent mean ± S.E.M. time spent licking the affected hind paw in each 5-min period. These data were published in Mogil et al. (1998) in a different form.

of ways. For example, it is well appreciated that the amount of pain experienced by sufferers of osteoarthritis can not be easily predicted by the extent of their joint degeneration (e.g. Link et al. 2003). ► Genotyping of arthritis sufferers and others at relevant genes might allow better prediction and management of inflammatory pain. Finally, it should be noted that responses to analgesics used in the management of inflammatory pain are also highly variable (e.g. Walker et al. 1994) and that the ► pharmacogenetics of analgesia is also being studied (Wilson et al. 2003).

References

1. Becker KG, Simon RM, Bailey-Wilson JE et al. (1998) Clustering of non-major histocompatibility complex susceptibility candidate loci in human autoimmune diseases. Proc Natl Acad Sci USA 95:9979–9984
2. Bon K, Wilson SG, Mogil JS et al. (2002) Genetic evidence for the correlation of deep dorsal horn Fos protein immunoreactivity with tonic formalin pain behavior. J Pain 3:181–189
3. Darvasi A (1998) Experimental strategies for the genetic dissection of complex traits in animal models. Nature Genet 18:19–24
4. Griffiths MM, Encinas JA, Remmers EF et al. (1999) Mapping autoimmunity genes. Curr Opin Immunol 11:689–700

5. Lariviere WR, Wilson SG, Laughlin TM et al. (2002) Heritability of nociception. III. Genetic relationships among commonly used assays of nociception and hypersensitivity. Pain 97:75–86
6. Link TM, Steinbach LS, Ghosh S et al. (2003) MR imaging findings in different stages of disease and correlation with clinical findings. Radiology 226:373–381
7. MacGregor AJ, Snieder H, Rigby AS et al. (2000) Characterizing the quantitative genetic contribution to rheumatoid arthritis using data from twins. Arthritis Rheum 43:30–37
8. Mogil JS (2004) Complex trait genetics of pain in the laboratory mouse. In: Mogil JS (ed) The Genetics of Pain, Progress in Pain Research and Management, vol 28. IASP Press, Seattle, pp 123–149
9. Mogil JS, Grisel JE (1998) Transgenic studies of pain. Pain 77:107–128
10. Mogil JS, Lichtensteiger CA, Wilson SG (1998) The effect of genotype on sensitivity to inflammatory nociception: characterization of resistant (A/J) and sensitive (C57BL/6) inbred mouse strains. Pain 76:115–125
11. Olofsson P, Holmberg J, Tordsson J et al. (2003) Positional identification of *Ncf1* as a gene that regulates arthritis severity in rats. Nature Genet 33:25–32
12. Tokuhiro S, Yamada R, Chang X et al. (2003) An intronic SNP in a RUNX1 binding site of *SLC22A4*, encoding an organic cation transporter, is associated with rheumatoid arthritis. Nature Genet 35:341–348
13. Walker JS, Nguyen TV, Day RO (1994) Clinical response to non-steroidal anti-inflammatory drugs in urate-crystal induced inflammation: a simultaneous study of intersubject and intrasubject variability. Br J Clin Pharmac 38:341–347
14. Wilson SG, Chesler EJ, Hain HS et al. (2002) Identification of quantitative trait loci for chemical/inflammatory nociception in mice. Pain 96:385–391
15. Wilson SG, Bryant CD, Lariviere WR et al. (2003) The heritability of antinociception II: pharmacogenetic mediation of three over-the-counter analgesics in mice. J Pharmacol Exp Ther 305:755–764

Heritable

Definition

A heritable trait is one which is passed on through generations (i.e. „runs in families"), such that offspring tend to resemble their parents. The strong implication is that inherited genetic factors are responsible, although non-genomic transmission has been demonstrated. Heritability is best established in humans using *twin studies*, in which the similarity of pairs of monozygotic and dizygotic twins is compared. In animals, heritability is best established by successful selective breeding for the trait.

▶ Heritability of Inflammatory Nociception
▶ Opioid Analgesia, Strain Differences
▶ Twin Studies

Herpes Simplex Virus Vectors

Definition

Herpes simplex virus (HSV) is a human pathogen that causes the common cold sore and infections of the conjunctiva, and is a double-stranded DNA virus with a capsid and surrounding tegument and envelope. The 152 kB genome can potentially accommodate up to approximately 44 kB of foreign DNA. The propagation of replication-incompetent HSV vectors in cultured cells is accomplished using cell lines that complement essential gene products that have been removed from the vector genome. HSV vector genomes do not integrate, but remain as episomes in the nucleus of transduced cells. HSV vectors, like the parental virus, efficiently target to sensory neurons from the skin and can establish a life-long latent state in those neurons.

▶ Opioids and Gene Therapy

Herpes Virus

Definition

Herpes virus can infect nerve roots, including nerve roots of the sciatic nerve. In the case of shingles (Herpes zoster), a rash is usually present along the course of the infected nerve root.

▶ Sciatica

Herpes Zoster

Definition

Herpes zoster is an infection of the nervous system caused by the varicella zoster virus (VZV), the same virus that causes chickenpox. VZV can remain dormant in the sensory ganglia for decades after an infection. Herpes zoster results when the dormant virus in these nerves is reactivated, often as a result of decline in cellular immunity to VZV with aging or immunosuppression.

▶ Cancer Pain, Assessment in the Cognitively Impaired
▶ Postherpetic Neuralgia
▶ Postherpetic Neuralgia, Pharmacological and Non-Pharmacological Treatment Options

Herpes Zoster Pain

▶ Postherpetic Neuralgia, Etiology, Pathogenesis and Management

Heteromeric Channels

Definition

Heteromeric channels are protein complexes that form pores in the cell membrane. Typically, channels are made up of several subunits, which may be identical, result-

ing in homomeric channels, or different, resulting in heterometic channels.
- ▶ Purine Receptor Targets in the Treatment of Neuropathic Pain

Heterotopic Ossification

Definition

Heterotopic Ossification is the appearance of bony tissue elements in what are normally soft tissue structures.
- ▶ Spinal Cord Injury Pain

Heterozygosity

Definition

Heterozygosity is a state in which the maternal and paternal allele of a gene are not the same. In this common situation, the expression of that gene will depend on dominance of the alleles. In inbred strains, all heterozygosity is lost, and every gene is fixed in a homozygous state.
- ▶ Alleles
- ▶ Inbred Strains
- ▶ Opioid Analgesia, Strain Differences

Heterozygous Carriers

Definition

Heterozygous carriers refer to the state of possessing two different alleles of a particular gene, one inherited from each parent.
- ▶ NSAIDs, Pharmacogenetics

Hidden Triggers

Definition

Hidden Triggers are internal precipitating mechanisms.
- ▶ Sunct Syndrome

High Dependency or Intensive Care Units

Definition

High dependency or intensive care units are specialized wards where one or two highly trained nurses take care of each patient
- ▶ Postoperative Pain, Acute Pain Team

High Thoracic Epidural Anesthesia

Definition

High thoracic epidural anesthesia leads to a reversible cardiac sympathectomy blocking the segments T^1-T5. The epidural catheters are inserted at levels C7 -T1 or at level T^1-T2 by the median approach and with hanging drop technique.
- ▶ Postoperative Pain, Thoracic and Cardiac Surgery

High Threshold Mechanoreceptor

- ▶ Mechanonociceptors
- ▶ Nociceptors in the Orofacial Region (Skin/Mucosa)

High-Threshold Mechanosensitive Muscle Receptors

Definition

In experiments employing recordings from single muscle receptors with unmyelinated or thin myelinated afferent fibers, many units exhibit a high mechanical threshold when tested with local pressure stimuli (e.g. using a forceps with broadened tips on the exposed muscle). These receptors do not respond to passively stretching the muscle or aerobic active contractions, but require pressure stimulation of tissue-threatening and subjectively painful intensity for activation. The receptors are also typically responsive to stimulation with algesic substances. The general interpretation is that these receptors are nociceptors and induce muscle pain when activated.
- ▶ Muscle Pain Model, Ischemia-Induced and Hypertonic Saline-Induced

High Threshold Neurons

Synonym

HT neurons

Definition

HT neurons respond fairly selectively to noxious mechanical stimuli. They may have a minimal response to innocuous mechanical stimuli, but they are essentially tuned for strong stimuli. They may also respond to noxious thermal and chemical stimuli. Sometimes HT cells are referred to as nociceptive-specific neurons.
- ▶ Functional Changes in Sensory Neurons Following Spinal Cord Injury in Central Pain
- ▶ Nick Model of Cutaneous Pain and Hyperalgesia
- ▶ Spinothalamic Input, Cells of Origin (Monkey)
- ▶ Thalamus, Nociceptive Cells in VPI, Cat and Rat

High-Threshold VDCCs

▶ Calcium Channels in the Spinal Processing of Nociceptive Input

High Velocity Thrust Manipulation

▶ Spinal Manipulation, Characteristics

High-Voltage Calcium Channels

▶ Calcium Channels in the Spinal Processing of Nociceptive Input

Hindlimb Flexor Reflex

▶ Opioids and Reflexes

Hippocampal Formation or Hippocampal Region

Definition

The hippocampus (dentate gyrus and pyramidal cell fields CA1-3) and the subiculum are together referred to as the hippocampal formation, s. Hippocampus for details. Perhaps the most extensively studied structure in the brain, the hippocampal region has most often been implicated in memory processing.
▶ Hippocampus
▶ Hippocampus and Entorhinal Complex, Functional Imaging

Hippocampus

Definition

Brain structure comprising the dentate gyrus and the pyramidal cell fields of the hippocampus. There are three different pyramidal cell fields: CA1, CA2 and CA3. These subregions differ in their cellular organization and connectivity. The hippocampus is primarily organized as a unidirectional circuit. Information from the entorhinal cortex converges on the dentate gyrus, which in turn projects to field CA3, which sends projections to field CA1. The circuit is completed as CA1 projects to the subiculum, the major output region of the hippocampus. Strictly speaking, the subiculum does not form part of the hippocampus, but together the two structures make up the hippocampal formation.

▶ Hippocampus and Entorhinal Complex, Functional Imaging

Hippocampus and Entorhinal Complex, Functional Imaging

SIRI LEKNES[1, 2], IRENE TRACEY[1, 2]
[1]Pain Imaging Neuroscience (PaIN) Group, Department of Physiology, Anatomy and Genetics, Oxford University, Oxford, UK
[2]Centre for Functional Magnetic Resonance Imaging of the Brain, Oxford University, Oxford, UK
irene.tracey@anat.ox.ac.uk

H

Synonyms

Entorhinal Cortex and Hippocampus, Functional Imaging; Parahippocampal Region, Neuroimaging

Definition

The ▶ hippocampus is comprised of the dentate gyrus and the CA1, CA2 and CA3 pyramidal cell fields. The ▶ hippocampal formation consists of the hippocampus and the subiculum. The adjacent entorhinal, perirhinal, and parahippocampal cortices comprise the ▶ parahippocampal region (Fig. 1). These limbic subregions differ in their cellular organization and connectivity, but are commonly implicated in memory and emotion processing.

The hippocampus lies at the end of a cortical processing hierarchy, and the entorhinal cortex is the major source of its cortical projections. Much of the cortical input to the entorhinal cortex originates in the adjacent perirhinal and parahippocampal cortices, which in turn receive widespread projections from sensory and association areas in the frontal, temporal and parietal lobes (Squire et al. 2004).

▶ Functional imaging is a general term used to describe methodologies that allow function to be located either spatially or temporally within the brain (and other organs). The methods are generally non-invasive and used for human studies; the term neuroimaging is often used when applied specifically to brain studies. Methods include functional magnetic resonance imaging (FMRI), positron emission tomography (PET), magneto-encephalography (MEG) and electro-encephalography (EEG). Unless otherwise stated, the studies discussed in this article are FMRI or PET studies of the brain.

Characteristics

Melzack and Casey (1968) proposed that the hippocampus and associated cortices participate in mediating the aversive drives and affective characteristics of pain perception. A wide range of animal studies support the notion that pain processing is a primary function of the hip-

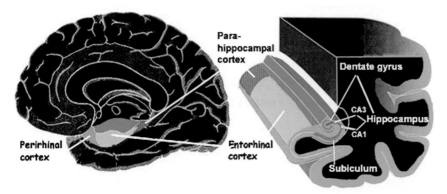

Hippocampus and Entorhinal Complex, Functional Imaging, Figure 1   (left) Medial view of the human brain outlining the perirhinal cortex (orange); parahippocampal cortex (red); and entorhinal cortex (yellow). (right) Section of the temporal lobe showing the components of the hippocampal/entorhinal complex in some detail: the dentate gyrus (pale green); the CA1 and CA3 hippocampal fields (green) that make up the hippocampus proper; the subiculum (pink); the perirhinal cortex (orange); parahippocampal cortex (red); and entorhinal cortex (yellow).

pocampal complex. Importantly, Dutar and colleagues (1985) demonstrated that septo-hippocampal neurons in rats respond directly to noxious peripheral stimulation. Similarly, functional imaging studies of pain perception have repeatedly reported a direct implication of areas within the hippocampus in the processing of nociceptive stimuli. Since nociceptive information is typically novel and of high priority, a direct role for the hippocampus in nociceptive processing is consistent with comparator theories of hippocampal function (e.g. McNaughton and Gray 2000). Comparator theory maintains that the hippocampus is involved in novelty detection and that its function is to compare actual and expected stimuli (i.e. stimuli registered in memory).

In an early PET study, Derbyshire and colleagues (1997) found hippocampal activation in response to mildly and moderately painful heat stimuli, when contrasted with warm, non-painful stimulation. Using very specific nociceptive stimuli (laser stimulation of A-δ fibers only) to subjects' left and right hands, Bingel and colleagues (2002) found bilateral activation of the amygdala and hippocampal complex. The receptive fields of hippocampal neurons are predominantly large and bilateral (Dutar et al. 1985). As other pain-related activation was lateralized, the authors suggested that the hippocampal activity reflected direct nociceptive projections to the hippocampus, perhaps revealing novelty detection (Bingel et al. 2002). Further, Ploghaus and colleagues (2001) found that pain modulation by drying stimulus temperature caused activation of a region of the hippocampus proper, consistent with a role of the hippocampus in pain intensity encoding (Fig. 2a).

Nevertheless, the large majority of human functional imaging studies of pain do not report activation of regions within the hippocampus / entorhinal complex. There are several possible explanations for this discrepancy. The first concerns the signal to noise ratio. As the complex is a relatively small structure, the spatial resolution of conventional whole-brain imaging paradigms

means that partial volume effects might occur and decrease signal to noise in this region. One caveat specific to functional imaging of this region is the implication of the hippocampus in the ▶ resting state network (Greicius and Menon 2004). PET and FMRI studies have suggested that the resting brain has a default mode of internal processing in which the hippocampus is a central component. In the neuroimaging of pain perception, nociceptive processing is commonly compared with baseline (rest) conditions. The hippocampus' involvement in resting state / baseline processing may mask out the activation of this region in such task-baseline comparisons if increased baseline activity reduces subsequent stimulation evoked responses and therefore could yield a false negative result. Another factor that may mask out activation of regions within the medial temporal lobe is the registration of individual brains onto a standard template for group comparison. Traditional techniques that optimize whole-brain alignment (e.g. aligning to the atlas of Talairach & Tournoux) do not adequately account for variations in location and shape of medial temporal lobe structures (see Squire et al. 2004 for review).

Regions within the hippocampus / parahippocampal complex have been more consistently activated in studies where pain perception has been modulated by expectation and / or anxiety. It is clear that memory (which influences expectation) modulates pain perception. While certain expectation is associated with fear, uncertain expectation is associated with anxiety. For instance, a rat experiences fear when it must enter a space where a cat is present. Anxiety, on the other hand, corresponds to the state a rat is in when it must enter a space where a cat may or may not be present. While fear facilitates rapid reactions (fight or flight) and causes distraction and analgesia from the pain, anxiety is characterized by risk assessment behavior or behavioral inhibition (the rat hesitates to enter the space where a cat might be). This behavior is associated with

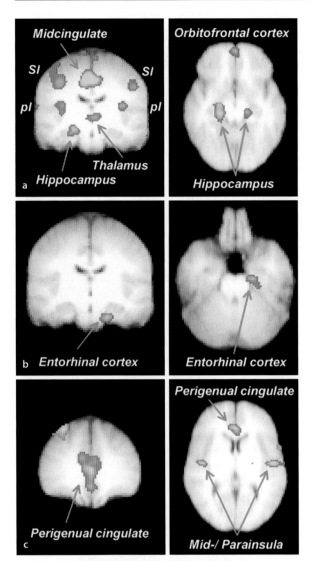

Hippocampus and Entorhinal Complex, Functional Imaging, Figure 2 (a) Temperature-related activation increases in perceived pain: Bilateral S1, dorsal margin of posterior insula, thalamus, midcingulate and right hippocampus. (b) Anxiety-related activation increases in perceived pain associated with significant activation in left entorhinal cortex. (c) Activity in the perigenual cingulated and the mid- / para insula was significantly correlated with entorhinal FMRI signal during pain modulation by anxiety. Reproduced with permission from Ploghaus et al. 2001.

and colleagues (2001) manipulated the certainty of expectation about impending nociceptive stimulation, to investigate its modulation on pain perception. This study examined the neural mechanism by which anxiety (uncertain expectation) causes increased pain perception (hyperalgesia), and contrasted it with the process by which a heightened nociceptive stimulation causes increased pain perception. The Gray-McNaughton theory proposes that the hippocampal formation responds to aversive events such as pain whenever they form part of a behavioral conflict, e.g. a conflict caused by uncertain expectation of pain. This conflict induces anxiety. Output from the comparator has two effects that underpin anxiety and behavioral inhibition. First, it tends to suppress both of the currently conflicting responses. Second, it increases the valence of the affectively negative associations of each of the conflicting goals (McNaughton and Gray 2000).

As predicted from theory, Ploghaus and colleagues reported activation of the entorhinal cortex during anxiety-driven hyperalgesia, but not during increased pain perception caused by augmented nociceptive input (Fig. 2b; Ploghaus et al. 2001). Studies of other (not anxiety-related) types of hyperalgesia typically report no significant activation of the hippocampus / parahippocampal region (e.g. Zambreanu et al. 2005). One exception is a recent FMRI study of drug modulation during pain (Borras et al. 2004). Naloxone, a predominantly μ opioid antagonist, was administered to naïve subjects in low doses. During rest (baseline) conditions where no stimulation was applied, regions in the hippocampal / entorhinal complex were activated more in the drug condition than during placebo. According to the Gray-McNaughton theory, the entorhinal cortex primes responses that are adaptive to an aversive input, such as the motor response necessary for escape from a threatening environment. Enhanced activation in this region after naloxone infusion indicates a change in basal activity, potentially lowering the threshold for activation of adaptive responses.

In line with this argument, differences between naloxone and placebo conditions during nociceptive processing were found in several areas within the hippocampus / parahippocampal region. When pain ratings were matched across conditions, an area within the posterior parahippocampal gyrus was significantly more activated in the naloxone condition. Activation of the hippocampus proper to nociceptive stimulation in the drug condition compared to the placebo condition was found only when subjects rated the pain intensity higher in the naloxone condition (nociceptive stimuli were of equal intensity across conditions). This result adds further support for the role of the hippocampus proper in pain intensity encoding. In their study of anxiety-driven hyperalgesia, Ploghaus and colleagues (2001) found that the entorhinal cortex activation was predictive of activity in the perigenual cingulate and

increased somatic and environmental attention, which can lead to anxiety-driven hyperalgesia (McNaughton and Gray 2000).

Using FMRI to investigate the effects of expectation on pain perception, Ploghaus and colleagues (2000) found that areas in the hippocampal complex were activated during mismatches between expected and actual pain. Consistent with comparator theory, the same ▶ hippocampal regions were implicated in three different types of mismatch: when no pain was expected (novelty); when the nociceptive stimulus differed from expectation; and when the painful stimulus was unexpectedly omitted. In a subsequent study, Ploghaus

Hippocampus and Entorhinal Complex, Functional Imaging, Table 1 Summary of functional imaging studies outlined here, listing stimulus type, neuroimaging technique and activations/deactivations in hippocampal/parahippocampal regions

Authors	Stimulus type		Hippocampus proper	Parahippocampal region
Derbyshire et al. 1997	Laser (heat nociception or warm)	PET	Nociceptive encoding	-
Ploghaus et al. 2000	Thermal (heat nociception or warm)	FMRI	Expectation related	Expectation related
Ploghaus et al. 2001	Thermal (heat nociception)	FMRI	Nociceptive encoding	Expectation related
Bingel et al. 2002	A-δ-specific laser	FMRI	Nociceptive encoding	-
Wilder-Smith et al. 2004	Rectal balloon distension and thermal (cold nociception)	FMRI	Patients more than controls	Patients more than controls
Borras et al. 2004	Thermal (heat nociception)	FMRI	Nociceptive encoding	May be related to shift in threshold for adaptive response
Greicius and Menon 2004	Visual (resting state examined)	FMRI	Resting state network	Resting state network
Napadow et al. 2005	Acupuncture in pain-free controls	FMRI	Deactivation	-

mid-insula (Fig. 2c). Corresponding regions of the cingulate and insular cortices were also implicated in naloxone-induced increases in pain perception (Borras et al. 2004). The authors concluded that the regions where activation by noxious heat was modulated by naloxone were the sites of action of endogenous opioid pathways involved in regulating the central nervous system response to aversive stimuli.

Some support for the involvement of the hippocampus / parahippocampal region in opioid regulation of the brain's response to nociceptive input comes from functional imaging studies of acupuncture. Several studies investigating brain responses to acupuncture in healthy, pain-free volunteers have reported ► deactivation of regions within the hippocampus / entorhinal complex (e.g. Napadow et al. 2005). A recent study examining the effects of acupuncture in chronic pain patients does not report involvement of the hippocampus or parahippocampal areas (Pariente et al. 2005), but this study did not include a contrast for deactivation of specific brain regions.

There can be little doubt that the role of the hippocampus / entorhinal complex in nociceptive processing and the generation of pain perception demands further investigation in both healthy volunteers and in clinical pain patients. So far, the functional imaging studies of pain reporting hippocampus / entorhinal complex activation have been whole-brain studies examining the effects of nociceptive stimulation on all regions of the brain. This contrasts with the neuroimaging literature on the role of the hippocampal complex in memory, where researchers have been able to focus solely on this narrow region of cortex, improving spatial resolution and avoiding registration caveats e.g. by employing partial-coverage imaging techniques (Fig. 3) (see also Squire et al. 2004). To disentangle the roles of the subregions within the hippocampus / entorhinal complex in nociceptive processing and pain perception, high-

resolution studies of this region during pain, employing similar measures, are needed. Care must also be taken to optimize study design in order to avoid the masking out of nociceptive-related hippocampal activations by processing of the resting state network.

The role of hippocampus / entorhinal complex in clinical pain is still largely unknown. A study of patients suffering from irritable bowel syndrome (IBS) has recently shown involvement of hippocampus in pain processing in patients compared to healthy controls (Wilder-Smith et al. 2004). Given the known involvement of anxiety

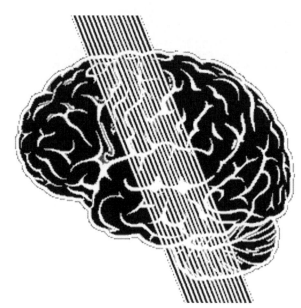

Hippocampus and Entorhinal Complex, Functional Imaging, Figure 3 Visualization of slice positioning in a high-resolution, partial-coverage study of hippocampus / entorhinal complex function. By only covering a section of the brain, resolution can be improved significantly, and it may be possible to begin disentangling the function of small subregions within the hippocampus/parahippocampal complex for nociceptive processing and pain perception.

in irritable bowel syndrome, this result lends further support to the postulated involvement of the hippocampus / entorhinal complex in anxiety-driven increases of pain perception. Further, the hippocampus may form part of a system of central involvement that drives the visceral hypersensitivity of these patients. More studies of anxiety and hippocampus / entorhinal complex function in clinical pain should shed light on the importance of centrally generated pain and hyperalgesia.

In conclusion, converging evidence from human neuroimaging and animal studies points to a direct role for the hippocampus in the processing of nociceptive information such as pain intensity encoding. Areas within the hippocampus / entorhinal complex are involved in the comparison between actual and expected nociceptive stimuli, and play a role in anxiety-driven hyperalgesia. The increases in pain perception caused by uncertain expectation may be due to a modulation of the opiate system, as hinted at by a study investigating the effects of the μ opioid antagonist naloxone (Borras et al. 2004).

References

1. Bingel U, Quante M, Knab R et al. (2002) Subcortical structures involved in pain processing: evidence from single-trial fMRI. Pain 99:313–321
2. Borras MC, Becerra L, Ploghaus A et al. (2004) fMRI measurement of CNS responses to naloxone infusion and subsequent mild noxious thermal stimuli in healthy volunteers. J Neurophysiol 91:2723–2733
3. Derbyshire SWG, Jones AKP, Gyulai F et al. (1997) Pain processing during three levels of noxious stimulation produces differential patterns of central activity. Pain 73:431–445
4. Dutar P, Lamour Y, Jobert A (1985) Activation of identified septo-hippocampal neurons by noxious peripheral stimulation. Brain Res 328:15–21
5. Greicius MD, Menon V (2004) Default-mode activity during a passive sensory task: uncoupled from deactivation but impacting activation. J Cogn Neurosci 16:1484–1492
6. McNaughton N, Gray JA (2000) Anxiolytic action on the behavioural inhibition system implies multiple types of arousal contribute to anxiety. J Affect Disord 61:161–176
7. Melzack R, Casey KL (1968) Sensory, motivational, and central control determinants of pain. In: Kenshalo DR (ed) The skin senses. Thomas, Springfield, IL, pp 423–439
8. Napadow V, Makris N, Liu J et al. (2005) Effects of electroacupuncture versus manual acupuncture on the human brain as measured by fMRI. Hum Brain Mapp 24:193–205
9. Pariente J, White P, Frackowiak RSJ et al. (2005) Expectancy and belief modulate the neuronal substrates of pain treated by acupuncture. NeuroImage 25 1161–1167
10. Ploghaus A, Narain C, Beckmann CF et al. (2001) Exacerbation of pain by anxiety is associated with activity in a hippocampal network. J Neurosci 21:9896–9903
11. Ploghaus A, Tracey I, Clare S et al. (2000) Learning about pain: The neural substrate of the prediction error for aversive events. PNAS 97:9281–9286
12. Squire LR, Stark CEL, Clark RE (2004) The Medial Temporal Lobe. Ann Rev Neurosci 27:279–306
13. Wilder-Smith CH, Schindler D, Lovblad K et al. (2004) Brain functional magnetic resonance imaging of rectal pain and activation of endogenous inhibitory mechanisms in irritable bowel syndrome patient subgroups and healthy controls. Gut 53:1595–1601
14. Zambreanu L, Wise RG, Brooks JCW et al. (2005) A role for the brainstem in central sensitisation in humans. Evidence from functional magnetic resonance imaging. Pain 114:397–407

Histamine

Definition

Histamine is a naturally occurring compound that is endogenous in mammalian tissue. It is synthesized by the decarboxylation of the amino acid histidine. It is a hydrophilic vasoactive amine and is involved in many central nervous system functions, such as arousal, the physiologic response to anxiety and stress, water retention and the suppression of eating. It has been suggested that the neuronal histamine system functions as a danger response mechanism. In skin it is intensely pruritic and painful in higher concentrations.

▶ Cancer Pain Management, Gastrointestinal Dysfunction as Opioid Side Effects
▶ Nociceptor, Categorization

Histopathological

Definition

The method of microscopical examination to derive the diagnosis from typical changes in the normal structure of tissues.

▶ Facet Joint Pain

History of Analgesics

KAY BRUNE, BURKHARD HINZ
Department of Experimental and Clinical Pharmacology and Toxicology, Friedrich Alexander University Erlangen-Nürnberg, Erlangen, Germany
brune@pharmakologie.uni-erlangen.de,
hinz@pharmakologie.uni-erlangen.de

Synonym

Analgesics, History

Definition

Attempts to relieve pain are probably as old as mankind. Dioscourides, a Greek physician, prescribed extracts of willow bark against joint pain, whilst Hildegard von Bingen and the Reverend Stone, in his famous letter to the Royal Society of Medicine in London, suggested the same therapy (Brune 1997; Rainsford 1984). Local inflammation often goes along with "general inflammation" manifested by fever and malaise. The reasons for this were recently uncovered: the release of pyrogenic cytokines such as TNFα and IL–1. Fever along with malaise was treated on the basis of the Hippocratic concept by purgation, sweating and blood-letting (Brune 1984). Such practices were continued until the 19th century (Williams 1975) – probably without success.

It was only recently that the inhibition of the cytokine effect has become feasible (Smolen et al. 2000).

Characteristics

A scientific approach to pain therapy became possible in the 19th century, with substances isolated from plants including the willow tree (salic acid esters), and then the description of the complete synthesis by Kolbe (Marburg), (Brune 1997; Rainsford 1984). To provide sufficient amounts, the first "scale up" of a synthetic process was invented and the first drug factory built (Salicylic Acid Works founded by von Heyden, 1874; 6). Salicylic acid was found to be active against fever (Buss, Switzerland) and rheumatoid arthritis (Stricker, Berlin; Mac Lagan, Dundee) (Brune 1997; Rainsford 1984; Sneader 1985).

Earlier (1806), a pharmacist in Einbeck, Sertürner, had isolated morphine, the main analgesic ingredient of the opium resin. He checked extracts from opium for sedative activity in his pack of dogs and ended up with a pure substance (morphine) (Sertürner 1806; Sneader 1985). With morphine, for the first time, a pure (crystalline) drug was available. Death due to overdose or lack of effect could now be avoided by exact dosing (Bender 1966).

New Chemicals

The next step was taken by chemists who tried to compensate for an impaired supply of opium, chinea bark (quinine) and others by chemical synthesis. It was made possible by E. Fischer's discovery of phenylhydrazine, which allowed the synthesis of nitrogen-containing ring systems. His scholar, L. Knorr, tried to synthesize quinine, but produced phenazone (Fig. 1) (Brune 1997),

which proved to be active against fever. The patent for this compound (Antipyrine[®] was bought by a dye factory in Hoechst. This was the start of the pharmaceutical company Hoechst (Brune 1997). Another chemist (F. Hoffmann) esterified salicylic acid with acetate and (re-)discovered Aspirin. This synthesis was done in another dye factory, namely Bayer (Rinsema 1999). The new science of chemistry helped to transform the dye-industry by providing both synthetic dyes and new synthetic drugs.

Pain therapy was aided by another accidental discovery. In Strasbourg, two physicians, Cahn and Hepp, attempted to eradicate intestinal worms. The worms survived, but the fever resolved (Cahn and Hepp 1886). An analysis revealed that the pharmacy had provided acetanilide rather than naphthalene. This led to the discovery of acetanilide, which was marketed by another dye factory (Kalle) under the name Antifebrin[®] (Brune 1997; Sneader 1986). Bayer further investigated acetanilide and found that a by-product of aniline dye production, namely "acetophenitidine", was equally effective. It was marketed as Phenacetin[®] (Sneader 1986). These discoveries constituted, as Tainter phrased it (Tainter 1948), "[. . .] the beginning of the famous German drug industry and ushered in Germany's forty-year dominance of the synthetic drug and chemical field." Thus, by the end of the 19th century, 4 prototype substances were available for the treatment of pain: Morphine, salicylic acid, phenazone and phenacetin.

Chemical Modifications of Analgesics

Salicylic acid, phenazone and phenacetin were widely used, and physicians soon recognized the disadvantages of these drugs. They were of low potency, and had to

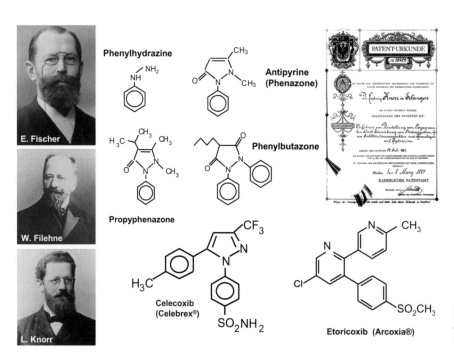

History of Analgesics,
Figure 1 Synthesis of Phenazone, the first synthetic drug ever, in Erlangen 1882.

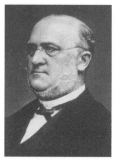
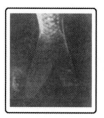
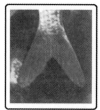
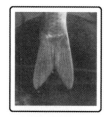

Adolf Kolbe

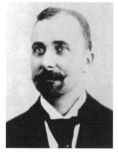
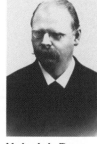
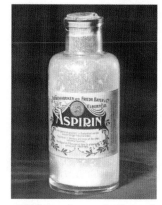

Felix Hoffmann   **Heinrich Dreser**   **1899 Implementation of Acetylsalicylic Acid (Aspirin®)**

History of Analgesics, Figure 2 Synthesis of acetylsalicyl acid in 1897.

be taken in gram quantities (spoon-wise). Sodium salicylate had an unpleasant taste. Taking several grams of phenacetin led to methaemoglobinaemia, while phenazone often caused allergic reactions. Consequently, the expanding drug industry set their chemists into action to produce improved derivatives.

F. Hoffman, a young chemist at the Bayer Company, attempted to improve the taste of salicylic acid to please his father who suffered from rheumatoid arthritis (Brune 1997; Sneader 1986). On a suggestion of v. Eichengrün (Bayer), Hoffmann produced acetylsalicylic acid, which his father preferred (Brune 1997; Sneader 1986). Acetylsalicylic acid proved difficult to handle due to its instability. Bayer, therefore, took a patent on the water-free production process invented by Hoffmann and secured the name Aspirin® (derived from acetyl and the plant spirea ulmaria). H. Dreser, the first pharmacologist at Bayer, tried to demonstrate the reduced toxicity of aspirin as compared to salicylic acid. He employed a goldfish model, believing that the "mucosa" of their fins comprised an analogue of human intestinal mucosa. Dipping the fins of goldfish into solutions of either salicylic acid or aspirin, he observed that higher concentrations of aspirin were necessary to "cloudy" the fins (Fig. 2). He concluded that this was proof of better gastrointestinal tolerability (Dreser 1899). Later, Heinrich Dreser himself recognised that he didn't measure a "gastrotoxic effect", but rather "acidity", and salicylic acid is more acidic than aspirin (Dreser 1907).

To further improve the tolerability of phenacetin, Bayer investigated a metabolite of phenacetin, acetaminophen (paracetamol). It appeared that (their) acetaminophen (due to impurities?) also caused methaemoglobinaemia. In contrast, Sterling (UK) found acetaminophen free of methaemoglobinaemia and marketed it as Panadol® (Sneader 1985).

At Hoechst, the structure of phenazone was modified. The resulting compounds amidopyrin, melubrin and dipyrone proved to be somewhat more active (Brune 1997). Roche substituted an amino group of phenazone with isopropyl. The resulting propyphenazone is still in use. It is relatively free of toxicity, i.e. it lacks kidney, GI- and bone marrow toxicity (Kaufman et al. 1991). Finally, several companies combined two active principles, e.g. by producing salts of aspirin with amidopyrine or esters between acetaminophen and salicylic acid (Benorylate®). Moreover, the three basic ingredients were mixed and supplemented, e.g. with caffeine (APC-powder); with vitamins, minerals and other partly obscure ingredients. This diversity of "drugs" pleased the consumer, but was without major medical benefit – it may rather have led to abuse and kidney toxicity (Dubach et al. 1983).

New Compounds: Pharmacology Comes into Play

In 1949, an unexpected observation once again paved the way for new analgesics. Hoping to reduce toxicity and increase effectiveness of aminophenazone, Geigy (Basel) produced an injection containing the salt of the basic aminophenazone with an acidic derivative – later named phenylbutazone (Fig. 3). This salt was found to be very active, particularly in rheumatoid pain (Brune

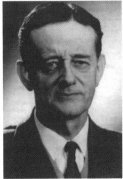

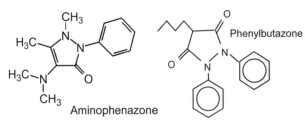

Phenylbutazone

Aminophenazone

Gerhard Wilhelmi

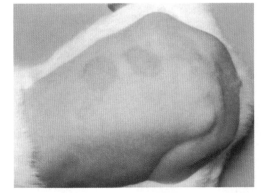

Erythema of the depilated
back of a guinea pig

History of Analgesics,
Figure 3 Synthesis of
Phemylbutazone in 1949.

1997; Sneader 1985). Burns and Brodie related this effect to phenylbutazone, which was present for much longer periods of time than aminophenazone (Domejoz 1960). The conclusion was that the "salt forming" partner of aminophenazone was the dominant active ingredient. To further investigate this clinical observation, G. Wilhelmi (Geigy) developed novel models of inflammation (Wilhelmi 1949). Phenylbutazone turned out to be particularly active in reducing the UV erythema elicited in the skin of guinea pigs (Fig. 3) (Wilhelmi 1949). It was one of the first pharmacological models of inflammation, with which several phenylbutazone analogues were found.

In the USA, C. Winter, at Merck (MSD) and later at Parke Davis, developed his models of inflammatory pain. He introduced the cotton string granuloma and the carrageenin-induced rat paw model (Shen 1984). These assays turned out to be especially useful for measuring anti-inflammatory activity (Winter et al. 1962) (Fig. 4). A similar model was employed by Randall and Selitto for detecting analgesic activity (Randall and Selitto 1957). Using these models led to the discovery of several chemical classes of analgesics. Merck identified indols (including indomethacin and sulindac, T.Y. Shen) (Shen 1984), Boots found propionic acid derivatives (ibuprofen and flurbiprofen, S. Adams; (Adams 1992), Parke Davis developed fenamates (e.g. mefenamic acid) (Shen 1984), Geigy was successful with new aryl-acetic acids, e.g. diclofenac (Shen 1984) and Rhone Poulenc with Bayer introduced ketoprofen (Shen 1984), and finally, Lombardino at Pfizer rediscovered the ketoenolic acids (phenylbutazone). The advantage of these compounds is that all pharmacokinetic parameters can be tailored by minor changes in

the molecular structure (Lombardino 1974). Pfizer's piroxicam (Otterness et al. 1982) was soon followed by tenoxicam (Roche) and meloxicam (Boehringer). All of these differ in their potency and in pharmacokinetic parameters including their metabolism and drug interactions, although their mode of action is basically the same. Most were identified using animal models before the mode of action of "aspirin-like" drugs – as these substances were formerly named – was determined. It was 70 years after the synthesis of aspirin when John

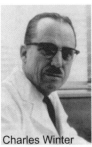

Charles Winter

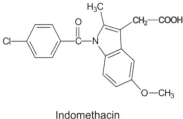

Carrageenan-induced rat paw edema

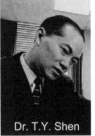

Dr. T.Y. Shen

Indomethacin

History of Analgesics, Figure 4 Carrageenin-induced rat paw model.

Vane's group could demonstrate that these compounds were inhibitors of prostaglandin synthesis (Vane 1971). This discovery, however, did not answer the question of why many of the old compounds (found by serendipity – such as phenazone, propyphenazone, phenacetin, paracetamol) were non-acidic chemicals that barely inhibited cyclooxygenases, whilst all the compounds developed in animal models of inflammation and pain were acidic and potent inhibitors (Brune 1974)? All pharmacological models inflict an acute inflammation elicited by local prostaglandin production. Consequently, drugs that work by blocking cyclooxygenases in the inflamed tissue excel in these models. Acidic compounds (comprising pKa values of around 4, ~99% protein binding and amphiphilic structures) reach long lasting high concentrations in inflamed tissue, but also relatively high concentrations in liver, kidney and the stomach wall (Brune and Lanz 1985). This skewed distribution causes complete inhibition of prostaglandin synthesis in these locations resulting in superior anti-inflammatory activity, but also liver, kidney and stomach toxicity (Brune and Lanz 1985). This distributional selectivity may have reduced some of the side-effects including CNS toxicity and increased the anti-inflammatory effects. Non-acidic compounds such as phenazone or paracetamol distribute homogeneously throughout the body. Their inhibition of prostaglandin production in inflamed tissue is small. Consequently, they are used to curb mild pain, but not inflammation. The discovery of the existence of two cyclooxygenases, COX–1 and COX–2 (Flower 2003), has changed the landscape again. It provided a new dimension of selectivity, not limited to differences of tissue distribution, but based on enzyme selectivity.

Analgesics in the Age of Molecular Pharmacology

The discovery of prostaglandins and the inhibition of prostaglandin production by aspirin-like drugs caused the investigation of the effects of anti-inflammatory steroids on prostaglandin production. Many researchers observed that steroids can reduce prostaglandin production along with anti-inflammatory activity, but do not block it completely (e.g. Brune and Wagner 1979). Only P. Needleman came up with a molecular explanation that proposed 2 different enzymes, one being regulated by steroids (Fu et al. 1990; Masferrer et al. 1990). They were soon characterized (Kujubu et al.1991). For the first time in the history of pharmacology, 2 molecular drug targets, cyclooxygenase–1 and cyclooxygenase–2 (the expression in the inflamed tissue is blocked by steroids), were identified before the biological role of the enzymes was fully known.

It was soon clear that it might be advantageous to have drugs that block only cyclooxygenase–2, because this enzyme appeared not to be involved in the production of GI-protective prostaglandins. Diclofenac and meloxicam were found to exert some, but not sufficient

selectivity to warrant GI-tolerance (Tegeder et al. 1999). This situation changed with the discovery of the highly selective sulfonomides, celecoxib and valdecoxib, and methylsulfones, rofecoxib and etoricoxib. These compounds are relatives of old compounds like phenazone (Fig. 1). They extend the paracetamol/phenazone group of non-acidic compounds which are devoid of gastrointestinal toxicity (Brune and Lanz 1985). However, these new analgesics are not free of other side effects. Inhibition of cyclooxygenase–2 affects kidney function, blood pressure and maybe more (for review, see e.g. Brune and Hinz 2004a; Hinz and Brune 2002). Another type of COX–2 selective inhibitor is Lumiracoxib. It is a relative of diclofenac and, like diclofenac, is sequestered into inflamed tissue. It combines COX–2 selectivity with selective tissue distribution (Feret 2003). The clinical success of this compound will tell us if this approach offers advantages.

Conclusion

After 120 years of development of pure analgesics, we have made some progress. Serendipity, as well as targeted research, has provided clinicians with many useful drugs that differ in many pharmacological and clinical aspects. Knowing a little of the history of their discovery and development may provide a perspective to better understand their effects and side-effects. A humble acknowledgment of the role of serendipity may change our attitude towards research and marketing claims. But then serendipity is not all, as E. Kästner, a German poet, phrased it:

Irrtümer sind ganz gut, Jedoch nur hier und da.

Nicht jeder, der nach Indien fährt, entdeckt AMERIKA.

Errors are fine, but only sometime(s).

Not everyone heading for India discovers AMERICA.

Acknowledgements

The helpful discussion with many scientists, in particular I. Otterness, A. Sallmann, T. Y. Shen (†) and G. Wilhelmi is gratefully acknowledged.

References

1. Adams SS (1992) The Propionic Acids: A Personal Perspective. J Clin Pharmacol 32:317–323
2. Bender GA (1966) Great Moments in Pharmacy. Davis & Company, Parke
3. Brune K (1974) How Aspirin Might Work: A Pharmacokinetic Approach. Agents Actions 4:230–232
4. Brune K (1984) The Concept of Inflammatory Mediators. In: Parnham MJ, Bruinvels J (eds) Discoveries in Pharmacology. Haemodynamics, Hormones and Inflammation, vol 2. Elsevier, Amsterdam, pp 487–498
5. Brune K (1997) The Early History of Non-Opioid Analgesics. Acute Pain 1:33–40
6. Brune K, Hinz B (2004a) Selective Cyclooxygenase–2 Inhibitors: Similarities and Differences. Scand J Rheumatol 33:1–6
7. Brune K, Hinz B (2004b) The Discovery and Development of Antiinflammatory Drugs. Arthritis Rheum 50:2391–2399

8. Brune K, Lanz R (1985) Pharmacokinetics of Non-Steroidal Anti-Inflammatory Drugs. In: Bonta IL, Bray MA, Parnham MJ (eds) Handbook of Inflammation, vol 5. Elsevier, Amsterdam, pp 413–449

9. Brune K, Wagner K (1979) The Effect of Protein/Nucleic Acid Synthesis Inhibitors on the Inhibition of Prostaglandin Release from Macrophages by Dexamethasone. In: Brune K, Baggiolini M (eds) Arachidonic Acid Metabolism in Inflammation and Thrombosis. Agents Actions (Suppl 4), Basel, Boston. Birkhäuser, Stuttgart pp 73–77

10. Cahn A, Hepp P (1886) Das Antifebrin, ein Neues Fiebermittel. Centralbl Klin Med 7:561–564

11. Domejoz R (1960) The Pharmacology of Phenylbutazone Analogues. Ann NY Acad Sci 1960:263

12. Dreser H (1899) Pharmacologisches über Aspirin (Acetylsalicysäure). Pflügers Arch Ges Phys 76:306–318

13. Dreser H (1907) Ueber Modifizierte Salizylsäuren. Medizinische Klinik 14:390–393

14. Dubach UC, Rosner B, Pfister E (1983) Epidemiologic Study of Analgesics Containing Phenacetin – Renal Morbidity and Mortality (1968–1979). N Engl J Med 308:357–362

15. Feret B (2003) Lumiracoxib: A Cox–2 Inhibitor for the Treatment of Arthritis and Acute Pain. Formulary 38:529–537

16. Flower RJ (2003) The Development of Cox–2 Inhibitors. Nat Rev 2:179–191

17. Fu JY, Masferrer JL, Seibert K et al. (1990) The Induction and Suppression of Prostaglandin H_2 Synthase (Cyclooxygenase) in Human Monocytes. J Biol Chem 265:16737–16740

18. Hinz B, Brune K (2002) Cyclooxygenase–2 – 10 Years Later. J Pharmacol Exp Ther 300:367–375

19. Kaufman DW, Kelly JP, Levy M et al. (1991) The Drug Etiology of Agranulocytosis and Aplastic Anemia. Oxford University Press, New York

20. Kujubu DA, Fletcher BS, Varnum BC et al. (1991) TIS10, A Phorbol Ester Tumor Promoter-Inducible mRNA from Swiss 3T3 Cells, Encodes a Novel Prostaglandin Synthase/Cyclooxygenase Homologue. J Biol Chem 266:12866–12872

21. Lombardino JG (1974) Enolic Acids with Anti-Inflammatory Activity. In: Scherrer RA, Whitehouse MW (eds) Medical Chemistry: A Series of Monographs. Academic Press, New York, pp 129–157

22. Masferrer JL, Zweifel BS, Seibert K et al. (1990) Selective Regulation of Cellular Cyclooxygenase by Dexamethasone and Endotoxin in Mice. J Clin Invest 86:1375–1379

23. Otterness IG, Larson DL, Lombardino JG (1982) An Analysis of Piroxicam in Rodent Models of Arthritis. Agents Actions 12:308–312

24. Rainsford KD (1984) Aspirin and the Salicylates. Butterworth & Co, London

25. Randall LO, Selitto JJ (1957) A Method for Measurement of Analgesic Activity on Inflamed Tissue. Arch Int Pharmacodyn 111:409–419

26. Rinsema TJ (1999) One Hundred Years of Aspirin. Medical History 43:502–507

27. Shen TY (1984) The Proliferation of Non-Steroidal Anti-Inflammatory Drugs (NSAIDS). In: Parnham MJ, Bruinvels J (eds) Discoveries in Pharmacology. Haemodynamics, Hormones and Inflammation, vol 2. Elsevier, Amsterdam, pp 523–553

28. Sertürner FW (1806) Darstellung der Reinen Mohnsäure (Opiumsäure) Nebst einer Chem. Untersuchung des Opiums. Tromsdorf J Pharm 14:47–93

29. Smolen JS, Breedveld FC, Burmester GR et al. (2000) Consensus Statement on the Initiation and Continuation of Tumour Necrosis Factor Blocking Therapies in Rheumatoid Arthritis. Ann Rheum Dis 59:504–505

30. Sneader W (1985) Drug Discovery: The Devolution of Modern Medicines. J Wiley & Sons, Chichester

31. Tainter ML (1948) Pain. Am NY Acad Sci 51:3–11

32. Tegeder I, Lotsch J, Krebs S et al. (1999) Comparison of Inhibitory Effects of Meloxicam and Diclofenac on Human Thromboxane Biosynthesis after Single Doses and at Steady State. Pharmacol Ther 65:533–544

33. Vane JR (1971) Inhibition of Prostaglandin Synthesis as a Mechanism of Action of Aspirin-Like Drugs. Nature New Biol 231:232–235

34. Wilhelmi G (1949) Guinea-Pig Ultraviolet Erythema Test. Schweiz Med Wochenschr 79:577–580

35. Williams G (1975) The Age of Agony. The Art of Healing 1700–1800. Constable, London

36. Winter CA, Risley EA, Nuss GW (1962) Carrageenin-Induced Edema in Hindpaw of the Rat as an Assay for Anti-Inflammatory Drugs. Proc Soc Exp Biol 111:544–547

Hit Rate or Sensitivity

Definition

Hit rate or sensitivity is the probability of response „A" when event A has occurred.

▶ Statistical Decision Theory Application in Pain Assessment

HIV and Pain

▶ Cancer Pain and Pain in HIV / AIDS
▶ Pain in Human Immunodeficiency Virus Infection and Acquired Immune Deficiency Syndrome

HMSN

Definition

The acronym for Hereditary Motor and Sensory Neuropathy.

▶ Hereditary Neuropathies

HNPP

▶ Hereditary Neuropathy with Liability to Pressure Palsies

Hoffman-Tinel Sign

▶ Tinel Sign

Holistic Medicine

▶ Alternative Medicine in Neuropathic Pain

Homeopathy

Definition

Homeopathy is a system of medicine developed by Samuel Hahnemann in the 19th century based on a concept of vital energy inherent in all matter, which increases in potency with repeated dilution; and on the idea that substances can be used to treat conditions that mimic their toxicity

▶ Alternative Medicine in Neuropathic Pain

Homeostasis

Definition

Homeostasis is a basic biological function associated with the maintenance of an internal environment that guarantees survival through adjusting important biological parameters (water, salt, glucose, temperature, acidity etc.).

▶ Clinical Migraine with Aura
▶ Functional Imaging of Cutaneous Pain

Homeostatic Adaptations

Definition

Physiological responses or behavioral actions which maintain or restore normal levels of biological function (e.g., maintain or restore normal body temperature).

▶ Opioids, Effects of Systemic Morphine on Evoked Pain

Homework

Definition

Activities that a patient is asked to complete or practice, usually outside of the hospital or clinic is referred to as homework.

▶ Multidisciplinary Pain Centers, Rehabilitation

Homologous Gene

Definition

An homologues gene has a similar, though often far from identical, sequence to another gene.

▶ Species Differences in Skin Nociception

Homomeric Channels

Definition

Channels are protein complexes, which form pores in the cell membrane. Typically, channels are made up of several subunits, which may be identical, resulting in homomeric channels, or different, resulting in heterometic channels.

▶ Purine Receptor Targets in the Treatment of Neuropathic Pain

Homozygous Carriers

Definition

Homozygous carriers refer to the state of possessing two identical alleles of a particular gene, one inherited from each parent.

▶ NSAIDs, Pharmacogenetics

Horsley-Clarck Apparatus or Stereotaxic Frame

Definition

Horsley-Clarck Apparatus or Stereotaxic Frame is a solid metallic frame made of two horizontal graduated bars fixed peripendicularly to a metal plate, holding a device for the fixation of the head of the animal through its upper jaw and orbits. The horizontal bars hold at mid-distance a device to fix two bars introduced into the ears (external auditory meatus).

▶ Post-Stroke Pain Model, Thalamic Pain (Lesion)

Hospice Care

Definition

Hospice care is a form of palliative or supportive care offered when the disease is at an advanced stage. The term hospice can refer to the philosophy of care, but is also used to describe the institution or site of care.

▶ Cancer Pain Management, Interface Between Cancer Pain Management and Palliative Care

Hostility

Definition

Hostility refers to "A set of negative attitudes, beliefs and appraisals concerning other". Can be inwardly directed towards oneself ("intrapunitiveness") or directed towards others ("extrapunitiveness"), Smith TW (1992).

► Chronic Gynecological Pain, Doctor-Patient Interaction

► Anger and Pain

Reference

Smith TW (1992) Hostility and Health: Current Status of a Psychosomatic Hypothesis. Health Psychology 11: 215-225.

Hot Plate Test (Assay)

Definition

Placement of the rat (or mouse) on a heated metal pad (temperature $\geq 50^\circ C$), with the time for paw licking or jumping corresponding to the latency of the test. This method is used to assess the threshold for thermonociception.

► Thalamotomy, Pain Behavior in Animals

Hot Tooth Syndrome

Definition

A tooth is sometimes described as 'hot' when it is very painful and difficult to anesthetize even with regional block anesthesia. The tooth is usually spontaneously painful, tender to touch and difficult to treat.

► Dental Pain, Etiology, Pathogenesis and Management

Household Income and Chronicity

► Pain in the Workplace, Risk Factors for Chronicity, Demographics

HPA Axis

Definition

The hypothalamus-pituitary-adrenal axis forms the basic response triad regulating endogenous glucocorticoid concentrations in the circulation.

► Fibromyalgia, Mechanisms and Treatment

HT Neurons

► High Threshold Neurons

Human Factors Engineering

► Ergonomics Essay

Human Infant Pain Neurophysiology

► Infant Pain Mechanisms

Human Models of Inflammatory Pain

LOUISE HARDING
Hospitals NHS Foundation Trust, University College London, London, UK
louise.harding@uclh.org

Synonym

Inflammatory Pain, Human Models

Definition

Research tools used to investigate the mechanisms and pharmacology of inflammatory pain and neuronal sensitisation.

Characteristics

Inflammation is a response of the body tissues to injury or irritation. Its most prominent features are pain, swelling, redness and heat. Through activation and sensitisation of nociceptors, inflammatory mediators also cause peripheral and central sensitisation of the somatosensory system, altering the way we perceive mechanical and thermal stimuli in and around inflamed skin. Studying these changes can provide information on the underlying mechanisms and, when combined with drug studies, on the pharmacology of inflammation and neuronal sensitisation. A number of experimental models have been developed for this purpose. In each model, inflammation is evoked by a different insult or injury and different models have specific characteristics. Table 1 compares the key features of the most common models which are summarised below.

The Capsaicin Model

► Capsaicin is the chemical component of chilli peppers that gives them their 'hot' quality. It directly activates ► TRPV1, a heat sensitive cationic ion channel expressed on cutaneous nociceptors, resulting in pain and inflammation. Capsaicin can either be applied topically, typically at 1 %, or injected intradermally (doses of 25–250 μg). Intradermal injection is associated with a quick hit of intense pain lasting 1–2 minutes, compared to the mild-moderate pain of topical application that develops slowly over 10–30 minutes. Both methods pro-

Human Models of Inflammatory Pain, Table 1 Comparison of somatosensory changes produced by different human models of inflammatory pain

	Capsaicin	Burn	Heat/Capsaicin	Mustard oil	Electrical	UVB	Freeze
1° heat pain[1]	yes	yes	yes	yes	yes	yes	yes
2° punctate[2]	yes	yes	yes	yes	yes	yes	yes
2° dynamic[3]	yes	yes	yes	yes	yes	no	no
dynamic duration[4]	< 1 hr	< 1 hr	4 hrs	< 1 hr	> 2 hrs	-	-
2° punctate onset[5]	< 1 hr	< 1 hr	< 1 hr	< 1 hr	< 1 hr	> 4 hrs	> 4 hrs

[1]decreased heat pain threshold in the inflamed site, [2]area of secondary punctate hyperalgesia, [3]area of secondary dynamic mechanical allodynia, [4]duration of dynamic mechanical allodynia, [5]time to onset of secondary punctate hyperalgesia. See text on individual models for data references

duce neurogenic inflammation and similar changes in somatosensory function (LaMotte et al. 1991). At the primary zone, i.e. the area of inflammation, heat pain thresholds are reduced in the capsaicin model due to sensitisation of TRPV1. Very high concentrations of capsaicin desensitise the heat responsive ion channel. This is sometimes evident following intradermal delivery, and is characterised by an increase in heat pain thresholds in a 1–3 mm area around the injection site. Surrounding the primary zone, two discrete areas of ▶ secondary hyperalgesia develop; an area of dynamic ▶ mechanical allodynia and an area of ▶ punctate hyperalgesia. These two areas differ in development time, size, pharmacological sensitivity and duration. The area of dynamic mechanical allodynia is maintained by ongoing afferent input from excited nociceptors and fades within an hour of capsaicin delivery as its concentration in the skin fades. In contrast, the area of punctate hyperalgesia, once established, appears independent of afferent input and may remain for 24 hours.

The Burn Model

In this model, heat is used to produce a first degree burn on the skin. CO_2 lasers and electronically coupled thermodes are typically used to induce the burn, by heating the skin to approximately 47°C for 7 minutes (Pedersen et al. 1998). The burn stimulus is moderately painful during its application; however, the pain quickly subsides once the heat stimulus is stopped. The injury produces a flare response similar to the capsaicin model. Evoked somatosensory changes in the primary zone are heat pain sensitisation (reduced heat pain threshold), together with a mild hypoesthesia (loss of sensation) to warming and cooling. A secondary area of punctate hyperalgesia develops around the primary zone and ▶ dynamic mechanical allodynia can also develop, but this depends on experimental conditions. Thermode size, location of skin stimulated, temperature and duration of burn stimulus shape the intensity of the burn. If the burn is very mild, insufficient afferent drive is sustained to maintain dynamic mechanical allodynia once the burn stimulus is removed.

The Heat/Capsaicin Model

This model, as it suggests, uses both heat and capsaicin to produces inflammatory pain and hyperalgesia. A heat stimulus of 45°C is applied to the skin for 5 min. followed by a 30 min. application of low dose (0.075 %) topical capsaicin (Petersen and Rowbotham 1999). This produces areas of primary and secondary hyperalgesia comparable to the capsaicin model. Like the capsaicin model, the area of dynamic mechanical allodynia starts to fade after approximately 20 minutes, but in this model the area can be rekindled by re-stimulating the treated site with a heat stimulus of 40°C for 5 minutes. This rekindling can be repeated every 20 minutes for up to four hours, providing a much longer opportunity to study the mechanisms of dynamic mechanical allodynia than the capsaicin and heat models alone.

The Mustard Oil Model

The irritant mustard oil, allyl isothiocyanate, produces characteristics of inflammation and somatosensory changes comparable to the capsaicin model, i.e. sensitisation to heat in the primary zone and secondary areas of dynamic mechanical allodynia and punctate hyperalgesia (Koltzenburg et al. 1992). Applied topically for 5 minutes, either at 100 % or diluted for a lesser effect, mustard oil produces moderate to severe pain and neurogenic inflammation. It's mechanism of action is essentially unknown. Allyl isothiocyanate has recently been shown to be an agonist of the ▶ TRPA1 receptor (previously known as ANKTM1) expressed in nociceptors (Jord et al. 2004), and this receptor may be key to its inflammatory effects. Prolonged application of mustard oil however causes blistering, which suggests the inflammation process in this model may also involve tissue damage pathways.

The Electrical Stimulation Model

As discussed, in experimental models of pain, dynamic mechanical allodynia is maintained by ongoing afferent input from excited c nociceptors. The electrical stimulation model uses continuous electrical activation of ▶ C-fibres to evoke and maintain a stable area of dynamic allodynia throughout the experimental period. Current is

H

injected at a frequency of 5 Hz and adjusted until the subject reports a pain intensity of 5/10 on a numerical pain intensity rating scale (mean current: 67 mA) (Koppert et al. 2001). This method produces an inflammatory pain response with stable dynamic allodynia for study periods of up to 2 hours. Other characteristics of this model are the reduced heat pain thresholds in the primary zone, and secondary area of punctate hyperalgesia common to most established models of inflammation.

The UVB/Sunburn Model

This model has two essential differences to those discussed so far. Firstly, there is a prolonged delay period of 6–12 hours between the inflammatory stimulus and the development of erythema and hyperalgesia. Secondly, the stimulus event used to create inflammation is not in itself painful (Bickel at al 1998). This model is particularly interesting, therefore, as the mechanisms of inflammation and hyperalgesia may differ somewhat to those evoked by direct activation of nociceptors. In this model, inflammation is produced by irradiating the skin with ultraviolet light in the UVB wavelength range (290–320 nm), typically over an area of approximately 5 cm diameter. There is considerable intersubject variability in the dose of radiation required to produce inflammation, consequently, subjects are assessed prior to the experimental period to establish the minimum dose of UVB required. For studies of ► primary and secondary hyperalgesia, three times the minimum dose required to produce ► erythema is used for experimentation. The UV model produces primary hyperalgesia to heat and secondary hyperalgesia to punctate mechanical stimuli, but not dynamic mechanical allodynia. Both primary and secondary events have a delayed onset, and are typically studied 20 hours after irradiation. This model is therefore relatively demanding, compared to other models, as subjects are required on 3 consecutive days. An advantage of this model however, is that the sensory changes are stable for 10 hours, giving a long window for detailed study.

The Freeze Lesion Model

Delayed onset hyperalgesia is also a characteristic of the freeze lesion model. Freeze lesions can be created using a 1.5 cm diameter copper rod cooled to -28°C and held perpendicularly against the skin for 10 seconds (Kilo et al. 1994). This produces mild to moderate sharp prickling pain, vasodilation of the stimulated and surrounding area and a local oedema. Pain, oedema and flushing outside the contact area subside within 2 hours; however, a discrete erythmia at the contact area remains for a number of days. No primary or secondary hyperalgesia can be detected in the first hours following the injury, but both are developed by the subsequent day. This model does not produce dynamic mechanical allodynia, and the area of punctate hyperalgesia produced by the freeze lesion

model is typically much smaller than that produced by other models.

In addition to the models described above, inflammatory pain and hyperalgesia have been reported following administration of a number of other inflammatory stimuli. This is not an exhaustive list, but for reference includes Melatin from bee venom (Sumikura et al. 2003), acidic phosphate buffered solution (Steen and Reeh 1993) complete Freunds adjuvant (Gould 2000) and bradykinin (Manning et al. 1991).

References

1. Bickel A, Dorfs S, Schmelz M et al. (1998) Effects of Antihyperalgesics on Experimentally Induced Hyperalgesia in Man. Pain 76:317–325
2. Gould HJ (2000) Complete Freund's Adjuvant-Induced Hyperalgesia: A Human Perception. Pain 85:301–303
3. Jordt SV, Bautista DM, Chuang HH et al. (2004) Mustard Oils and Cannabinoids Excite Sensory Nerve Fibres through the TRP Channel ANKTM1. Nature 427:260–265
4. Kilo S, Schmelz M, Koltzenburg M et al. (1994) Different Patterns of Hyperalgesia Induced by Experimental Inflammation in Human Skin. Brain 117:385–396
5. Koppert W, Dern SK, Sittl R et al. (2001) A New Model of Electrically Evoked Pain and Hyperalgesia in Human Skin. Anaesthesiology 95:395–402
6. Koltzenburg M, Lundberg LER, Torebjork HE (1992) Dynamic and Static Components of Mechanical Hyperalgesia in Human Hairy Skin. Pain 51:207–219
7. LaMotte RH, Shain CN, Simone DA et al. (1991) Tsai EFP. Neurogenic Hyperalgesia: Psychophysical Studies of Underlying Mechanisms. J Neurophysiol 66:190–211
8. Manning DC, Raja SN, Meyer RA, Campbell JN (1991) Pain and Hyperalgesia after Intradermal Injection of Bradykinin in Humans. Clin Pharmacol Ther 50:721–729
9. Pedersen JL, Kehlet H (1998) Hyperalgesia in a Human Model of Acute Inflammatory Pain: A Methodological Study. Pain 74:139–151
10. Petersen KL, Rowbotham MC (1999) A New Human Experimental Pain Model: The Heat/Capsaicin Sensitization Model. Neuroreport 10:1511–1516
11. Steen KH, Reeh PW (1993) Sustained Graded Pain and Hyperalgesia from Harmless Experimental Tissue Acidosis in Human Skin. Neurosci Lett 154:113–116
12. Sumikura H, Andersen OK, Drewes AM et al. (2003) A Comparison of Hyperalgesia and Neurogenic Inflammation Induced by Melittin and Capsaicin in Humans. Neurosci Lett 337:147–150

Human Thalamic Nociceptive Neurons

KAREN D. DAVIS, JONATHAN O. DOSTROVSKY
University of Toronto and the Toronto Western Research Institute, University Health Network, Toronto, ON, Canada
kdavis@uhnres.utoronto.ca, j.dostrovsky@utoronto.ca

Synonyms

Thalamic Nociceptive Neurons; Diencephalic Nociceptive Neurons in the Human; Wide dynamic range (WDR) neurons and nociceptive specific (NS) neurons in human thalamus

Definition

Central nervous system neurons whose cell bodies are located within the human thalamus (diencephalon) and that have a preferential or exclusive response to ▶ noxious stimuli.

The human thalamus, which is very similar to the monkey thalamus, includes several regions where neurons responding specifically or preferentially to nociceptive stimuli are found. However, in view of the very limited opportunities available to search for such neurons in the human and perform extensive testing on them, our knowledge concerning their properties and locations is extremely limited.

Characteristics

It is possible to directly study human thalamic nociceptive neurons during the electrophysiological mapping used by some neurosurgical teams as part of functional neurosurgical procedures for treating chronic pain, Parkinson's disease or other movement disorders (Lenz et al. 1988; Tasker and Kiss 1995). During these mapping procedures, microelectrodes are inserted into the thalamus to record the electrophysiological properties of individual thalamic neurons.

The unique opportunity afforded by functional stereotactic surgery to record and stimulate in the thalamus of awake patients, has provided some interesting findings and validation of subhuman primate studies related to thalamic function in pain. Unfortunately, the inherent limitations of these studies (time constraints, ethical considerations and lack of histological confirmation) limit the interpretation of the findings. The studies have attempted to address the following questions:

1. Where can one record nociceptive and thermoreceptive neurons?
2. What are the properties of nociceptive and thermoreceptive neurons?
3. What are the perceptual consequences of microstimulation in the regions containing nociceptive and thermoreceptive neurons?
4. Where can one evoke painful and temperature sensations by stimulating in the thalamus and what are the qualities of the sensations?
5. Are there any alterations in neuronal firing characteristics, receptive fields or stimulation-evoked sensations in chronic pain patients?

This section briefly summarizes the findings pertaining to these questions.

Nociceptive Neurons in Lateral Thalamus

The existence of nociceptive neurons in ▶ Vc (ventrocaudal nucleus often termed VP or ventroposterior nucleus) and adjacent regions has been reported by Lenz and colleagues (for review see Lenz and Dougherty 1997). The vast majority of Vc neurons are classified as non-nociceptive tactile neurons, since they respond to light touch of a distinct area of skin (i.e. the neuron's receptive field). However, there have been a few reports of some nociceptive neurons in Vc. Approximately 5–10% of Vc neurons have been classified as nociceptive, based on their responses to noxious thermal stimuli (Lenz et al. 1993a; Lenz et al. 1994). A larger proportion of Vc neurons, up to 25%, were found to respond selectively or preferentially to noxious mechanical stimuli (Lee et al. 1999; Lenz et al. 1994). These neurons were primarily located in the posterior-inferior portion of Vc. Interestingly, in the adjoining posterior-inferior area, which includes ▶ VMpo (Blomqvist et al. 2000), they identified NS neurons that responded to noxious heat, and none of the neurons in this area responded to innocuous tactile stimuli (Lenz et al. 1993a). The true proportion of thalamic nociceptive neurons may be underestimated in these studies for a variety of technical, physiological and ethical reasons. First, there are very few opportunities to test for nociceptive responses in awake human subjects, and the small body of data that has been obtained derives from patients with either movement disorders or a chronic pain condition. Second, extensive testing for nociceptive responses (both in terms of the number of neurons tested and the skin area tested) is limited due to the painful nature of the stimulus. Third, it is not clear whether there is any selection bias in the ability of microelectrodes to record from nociceptive versus tactile neurons (e.g. based on cell size, spontaneous activity, etc.).

Medial Thalamus

Much less is known regarding the role of the medial thalamus compared to the lateral thalamus in human pain, largely due to the fact that there are few opportunities to record and stimulate in this region during functional stereotactic surgery. There are some discrepancies in the incidence of medial thalamic nociceptive responses across the few published studies. One group (Ishijima et al. 1975) reported a similar proportion of mechanical- and thermally-responsive nociceptive neurons in the CM-Pf region, as compared to the findings of Lenz and colleagues in lateral thalamus. However, another group found only 2 of 318 medial thalamic neurons that responded to noxious stimuli (Jeanmonod et al. 1993). It is, however, difficult to evaluate these findings as few details were provided by the authors, and more recent studies have failed to replicate the findings (see Lenz and Dougherty 1997 for references).

Stimulation-Induced Pain

One of the unique aspects of electrophysiological studies in human patients is the ability to question the patient about sensations evoked by electrical stimulation within the brain. Electrical stimulation within Vc and adjacent regions of the thalamus usually evokes innocuous parasthesia. However, several early studies documented that stimulation in the area posterior-inferior to

Vc elicited reports of painful sensations in some patients (Halliday and Logue 1972; Hassler and Riechert 1959; Tasker 1984). Recent studies have examined the effects of stimulation in much greater detail (Davis et al. 1996; Dostrovsky et al. 2000; Lenz et al. 1993b), and these show that pain and innocuous thermal sensations can be evoked from a region at the posterior-inferior border of Vc and extending several millimeters posterior, inferior and medial. Microstimulation applied at the Vc sites of confirmed nociceptive neuronal responses rarely evokes pain, but rather produces a non-painful tingling sensation (Lee et al. 1999; Lenz et al. 1993a, b, 1994). A greater incidence of stimulation-evoked pain in Vc and the ventroposterior region has been reported in patients with a history of visceral pain, phantom pain or post-stroke pain (Davis et al. 1995; Davis et al. 1996; Davis et al. 1998; Lenz et al. 1995)

The incidence of evoked pain/thermal sensations is much higher in the posterior-inferior area than within Vc proper. Unlike the pareasthetic (tingling and 'electric shock') sensations evoked in Vc, the pain/thermal sensations are usually reported as quite natural. They are always perceived on the contralateral side of the body, and the projected fields can be quite small. The painful sensations are frequently described as burning pain. In a few cases, sensations of pain referred to deep and visceral sites have been elicited (Lenz et al. 1994; Davis et al. 1995). Lenz and colleagues have reported that microstimulation within Vc (at sites where WDR neurons responding to noxious mechanical stimuli were found) rarely results in pain, whereas at the sites in the region posterior-inferior to Vc where microstimulation evoked pain there was a high likelihood of finding nociceptive neurons (Lenz and Dougherty 1997). Histological confirmation of these stimulation and recording sites has of course not been obtained in such patients, but it seems likely that the physiologically localized region posterior-inferior to Vc corresponds anatomically to VMpo.

A few studies have reported that stimulation in the posterior aspect of medial thalamus can evoke pain (Jeanmonod et al. 1993; Sano 1979), but in most cases large tipped electrodes and high intensities were used for stimulation, so current spread is an issue. More recent studies have failed to replicate these findings.

Innocuous Cool Neurons and Sensations

Cells responding to innocuous thermal stimuli are also of great interest and highly relevant, due to the well-known association of the pain and temperature pathways. Cooling-specific neurons are only found in lamina I of the spinal and trigeminal dorsal horns, and have been shown to project to VMpo in the monkey (Dostrovsky and Craig 1996). In animal studies, cooling neurons in the thalamus have only been reported in VMpo (monkey) and medial VPM (cat). Cooling-specific neurons in human thalamus were located in

the region medial and posterior-inferior to Vc that likely corresponds to the human VMpo (Davis et al. 1999). Of particular interest was the finding that stimulation at such sites evoked cooling sensations that were graded with stimulus intensity, and that were referred to the same cutaneous region as the receptive fields of the cooling-specific neurons recorded at the site. Stimulation in this posterior-inferior region can also elicit pain (see above) and, as shown by Lenz and colleagues (1993a; 1993b), this region also contains nociceptive-specific neurons.

References

1. Blomqvist A, Zhang ET, Craig AD (2000) Cytoarchitectonic and immunohistochemical characterization of a specific pain and temperature relay, the posterior portion of the ventral medical nucleus, in the human thalamus. Brain 123:601–619
2. Davis KD, Kiss ZHT, Luo L et al. (1998) Phantom Sensations Generated by Thalamic Microstimulation. Nature 391:385–387
3. Davis KD, Tasker RR, Kiss ZHT et al. (1995) Visceral Pain Evoked by Thalamic Microstimulation in Humans. Neuroreport 6:369–374
4. Davis KD, Kiss ZHT et al. (1996) Thalamic Stimulation-Evoked Sensations in Chronic Pain Patients and in Non-Pain (Movement Disorder) Patients. J Neurophysiol 75:1026–1037
5. Davis KD, Lozano RM et al. (1999) Thalamic relay site for cold perception in humans. J Neurophysiol 81:1970–1973
6. Dostrovsky JO, Manduch M et al. (2000) Thalamic stimulation-evoked pain and temperature sites in pain and non-pain patients. In: Devor M, Rowbotham M, Wiesenfeld-Hallin Z (eds) Proceedings of the 9th World Congress on Pain. IASP Press, Seattle 7:419–425
7. Dostrovsky JO, Craig AD (1996) Cooling-specific spinothalamic neurons in the monkey. J Neurophysiol 76:3656–3665
8. Halliday AM, Logue V (1972) Painful sensations evoked by electrical stimulation in the thalamus. In: Somjen GG (ed) Neurophysiology Studied Man. Exerpta Medica, Amsterdam, pp 221–230
9. Hassler R, Riechert T (1959) Clinical and anatomical findings in stereotactic pain operations on the thalamus. Arch Psychiatr Nervenkr Z, Gesamte Neurol Psychiatr 200:93–122
10. Ishijima B, Yoshimasu N, Fukushima T et al. (1975) Nociceptive Neurons in the Human Thalamus. Confinia Neurol 37:99–106
11. Jeanmonod D, Magnin M, Morel A (1993) Thalamus and Neurogenic Pain: Physiological, Anatomical and Clinical Data. Neuroreport 4:475–478
12. Lee J, Dougherty PM, Antezana D et al. (1999) Responses of Neurons in the Region of Human Thalamic Principal Somatic Sensory Nucleus to Mechanical and Thermal Stimuli Graded into the Painful Range. J Comp Neurol 410:541–555
13. Lenz FA, Dougherty PM (1997) Pain Processing in the Human Thalamus. In: Steriade M, Jones EG, McCormick DA (eds) Thalamus, Vol II, Experimental and Clinical Aspects. Elsevier, Amsterdam, pp 617–652
14. Lenz FA, Dostrovsky JO, Kwan HC et al. (1988) Methods for Microstimulation and Recording of Single Neurons and Evoked Potentials in the Human Central Nervous System. J Neurosurg 68:630–634
15. Lenz FA, Gracely RH, Romanoski AJ et al. (1995) Stimulation in the Human Somatosensory Thalamus can Reproduce Both the Affective and Sensory Dimensions of Previously Experienced Pain. Nat Med 1:910–913
16. Lenz FA, Gracely RH, Rowland LH et al. (1994) A Population of Cells in the Human Thalamic Principal Sensory Nucleus Respond to Painful Mechanical Stimuli. Neurosci Lett 180:46–50
17. Lenz FA, Seike M, Lin YC et al. (1993a) Neurons in the Area of Human Thalamic Nucleus Ventralis Caudalis Respond to Painful Heat Stimuli. Brain Res 623:235–240

18. Lenz FA, Seike M, Richardson RT et al. (1993b) Thermal and Pain Sensations Evoked by Microstimulation in the Area of Human Ventrocaudal Nucleus. J.Neurophysiol 70:200–212
19. Tasker RR (1984) Stereotaxic surgery. In. Wall PD, Melzack R (eds) Textbook of Pain, Churchill Livingstone, pp 639–655
20. Tasker RR, Kiss ZHT (1995) The Role of the Thalamus in Functional Neurosurgery. Neurosurg Clin N Am 6:73–104

Human Thalamic Response to Experimental Pain (Neuroimaging)

ALEXANDRE F. M. DASILVA,
NOUCHINE HADJIKHANI
Martinos Center for Biomedical Imaging,
Massachusetts General Hospital, Harvard Medical
School, Charlestown, MA, USA
alexandr@nmr.mgh.harvard.edu,
nouchine@nmr.mgh.harvard.edu

Synonyms

Thalamic Response to Experimental Pain in Humans

Definition

The thalamus is the major relay structure in the forebrain for noxious and non-noxious sensory inputs. In the case of ▶ noxious stimuli, the thalamus distributes the incoming information to other specific cortical areas for proper processing of their discriminative, cognitive and affective components. Recent neuroimaging techniques can effectively detect transient thalamic neuronal activation following the application of experimental stimuli that artificially replicate painful conditions in humans.

Characteristics

Thalamic neuronal activation is frequently observed in functional neuroimaging studies following ▶ experimental pain. Through the use of neuroimaging techniques, the role of the thalamus has been gradually dissected in the nociceptive CNS network. Under those studies, experimental pain resultant of different noxious stimuli has revealed a pattern of thalamic activation that depends on the type of stimuli (e.g. thermal), area of application, and conditions inherent to the subject or patient, such as attention, or the presence of a chronic pain disorder.

Techniques

Of the neuroimaging technologies available, ▶ functional magnetic resonance imaging (fMRI) and ▶ positron emission tomography (PET) have greatly expanded our knowledge of human thalamic response to pain. Both indirectly measure the neuronal activity based on changes in the metabolism during a particular transient task (e.g. experimental pain) compared to a baseline state (e.g. no-pain state). The specific contrast for fMRI is the blood oxygenation level-dependant (BOLD) contrast, which does not require any tracer agent but relies on blood volume and blood flow, whereas radioactive labeled tracers are used to measure changes in cerebral blood flow and metabolism in PET.

Thalamic Nuclear Function

There are 14 major thalamic nuclei identified, but this number diverges depending on the histological technique applied. Some of them, or subdivisions, have specific roles in the thalamic nuclear configuration for pain processing. Activations of the ventroposterior nuclei of the ventrobasal complex (lateral), and other more medial nuclei of the thalamus, have being consistently described in neuroimaging studies. These studies confirm previous animal experiments that noxious and innocuous discriminative input from cranial and the body parts are respectively processed by the ventroposterior medial nucleus (VPM) and the ▶ ventroposterior lateral nucleus (VPL), and afterward projected to the somatosensory cortex. The lateral nuclear activation has a clear somatotopic configuration for different kinds of sensory input, while the medial thalamus, such as the ▶ dorsomedial nucleus (DM), has particular thermoreceptive functions. Noxious thermal stimulation to the facial skin of each trigeminal division in healthy human volunteers activates the contralateral VPM, while the same noxious stimulation applied to the palmar surface of the thumb activates the VPL (DaSilva et al. 2002). In both cases, during trigeminal and thumb noxious thermal stimulation, the contralateral DM nucleus of the thalamus shows activation (Fig. 1).

A specific thalamic nuclear pathway is involved in interoceptive mechanism of homeostasis: the basal part of the ventromedial nucleus (VMb) and the ▶ posterior part of the ventromedial nucleus (VMpo) play an important role in thermal nociceptive inflow through main direct projections to the insular cortex (Craig 2002). With the future improvement of the spatial resolution (2 mm for PET and <1 mm for fMRI) and signal noise rate in the neuroimaging studies, as well as the superposition of structural ▶ diffusion tensor imaging (DTI) maps to delineate nuclear architecture under the activations (Fig. 2), we will be able to precisely define the pattern of thalamic activation following painful stimulus in human (DaSilva et al. 2003; Wiegell et al. 2003).

Experimental Noxious Stimuli

Most of the noxious stimuli used in neuroimaging studies are thermal in nature, applying temperatures higher than 45C for heat pain, and usually lower than 6C for cold pain, enough to activate nociceptive fibers (C and A-delta). The noxious thermal stimuli are delivered by non-magnetic contact probes, water immersion, and laser (heat) to a particular part of the body in an alternating fashion with a non-noxious state (e.g. neutral 32C x noxious 46C). Similar noxious sensations have also been produced by interlaced application of non-noxious

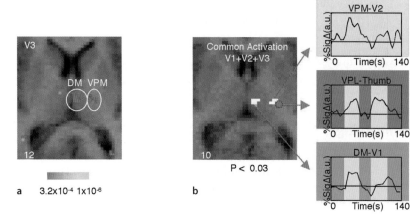

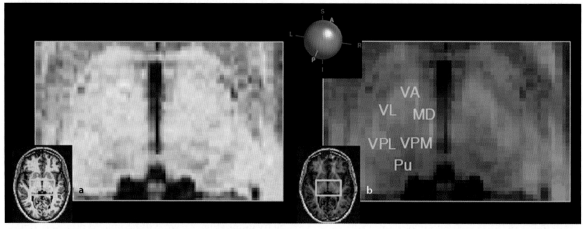

**Thalamus activation
Mandibular noxious
thermal stimulation**

**Thalamus activation
Face and Thumb noxious thermal
stimulation**

Human Thalamic Response to Experimental Pain (Neuroimaging), Figure 1   Activation in Thalamus. (a) Activation in the thalamus contralateral to a noxious thermal stimulus to the V3 (mandibular trigeminal branch) region of the face. (b) Activation in the thalamus following contralateral stimulation to the face and hand. The white areas show regions of common activation following noxious thermal stimulation to the V1 (ophtalmic), V2 (maxillary) and V3 (mandibular) distributions of the face, in regions defined as the dorsomedial (DM) and ventroposteromedial (VPM) nuclei. Activation of the thumb is mapped onto the same anatomical section (purple circle) and corresponds to the ventroposterolateral (VPL) nucleus. The regions are defined anatomically using the Talairach Atlas. Time courses of activation for each area are shown in inserts. Percent signal change is shown in arbitrary units (a.u.); numbers in bottom corners indicate the Talairach coordinate in the rostro-caudal (z) axis. (Da Silva et al. 2002).xxx

Human Thalamic Response to Experimental Pain (Neuroimaging), Figure 2   Color-coded DTI map superimposed on high-resolution anatomical image. Comparison of an axial (a) MPRAGE structural image and the corresponding (b) color-coded DTI map. The ROI is taken from the yellow box shown in the whole slice image at bottom-left. On the MPRAGE, the thalamus appears homogeneous, whereas the DTI map shows significant substructure. The thalamic nuclei have been labeled according to their anatomical position and fiber orientation. The color-coding depicts the local fiber orientation (i.e. the principal eigenvector of the diffusion tensor) with red indicating mediolateral, green anteroposterior, and blue superoinferior. The color-coding is also indicated by the red-green-blue sphere shown at top-center. Abbreviations: VA, ventral anterior; VL, ventrolateral; MD, mediodorsal; VPL, ventral posterior lateral; VPM, ventral posterior medial; Pu, pulvinar. (Da Silva et al. 2003).

warm and cold temperatures, which is known as the thermal-grill illusion of pain. Other noxious stimuli that have been used in pain studies are mechanical (e.g. tonic pressure), electrical (e.g. intramuscular electrical stimulation) and chemical (e.g. subcutaneous injection of ▶ capsaicin or ascorbic acid).

Neuroimaging studies applying experimental stimuli produce thalamic activation. Noxious and innocuous thermal stimuli (cold and heat) activate the medial and lateral thalamic nuclei, with predominant contralateral activation, while innocuous mechanical stimuli mostly activate the lateral thalamus. Noxious mechanical stimuli (tonic pressure) elicit inconsistent contralateral thalamic activation (Creac'h et al. 2000), as tonic pain (long duration) elicits less thalamic activation than phasic pain (short duration). In addition, the amount of thalamic activation observed depends on the size of the somatotopical representation of the body part being stimulated (the face has, for example, a much bigger cortical representation than the foot).

If the experimental noxious stimulus is applied to the same region but in different tissues, the thalamic activation pattern can also be distinct, as in the case of experimental skin and muscular pain (Svensson et al. 1997). Although noxious intramuscular electrical stimulation and cutaneous pain, elicited by CO_2 laser in the left brachioradialis area produce equal positive correlation between increases in regional cerebral flow (rCBF) in thalamus and anterior insula, only the cutaneous noxious stimulation shows a negative relationship in rCBF changes between thalamus and contralateral primary sensorimotor cortex, indicating a possible inhibitory mechanism between both structures.

Chemical experimental pain using capsaicin has been used in neuroimaging studies in two different ways: to induce acute and/or allodynic pain. Capsaicin is a hot pepper-derived derived substance that induces consistent ongoing pain, with a response including midline thalamic nuclei such as the DM nucleus (Iadarola et al. 1998). The cutaneous area treated with capsaicin, injected or topically applied, also develops secondary ▶ allodynia. Allodynia is a reversible state of painful sensitivity to non-noxious stimuli, such as brush and warm stimuli that replicates a clinical phenomenon common in ▶ neuropathic pain, burn lesions and ▶ migraine patients. Capsaicin-allodynia to non-noxious heat activates the medial thalamus simultaneously with the frontal cortex, orbital and dorsolateral prefrontal (DLPFC), suggesting a greater affective and cognitive response, which correlates with the higher unpleasantness rating compared to normal heat pain rating (Lorenz et al. 2003).

Conditions inherent to the subjects also affect the thalamic response to experimental pain. There is an indication that gender differences in pain perception influence thalamus function. For the same thermal noxious pain, females show a higher rating for pain intensity than males, translated into higher activation in the contralateral thalamus, as well as in the prefrontal cortex and anterior insula (Paulson et al. 1998). Male subjects demonstrate higher μ-opioid system activation than female subjects in the anterior thalamus, ventral basal ganglia and amygdala during sustained deep muscular pain (Zubieta et al. 2002). Pain perception is also altered by attention, hypnosis or pharmacologic effect through a modulation of the pain system involving mainly the thalamus and cingulated cortex. Distraction tasks presented to subjects during thermal pain correlate with decreased perception of pain, and consequently lower medial thalamic activation (Bantick et al. 2002). In a hypnotic state, the patient's reduced pain perception correlates with high functional modulation between the midcingulate cortex, the thalamus and the midbrain (Faymonville et al. 2003). Under

the influence of fentanyl, a μ-opioid receptor agonist, there is a strong attenuation of responses to noxious cold stimulation in the contralateral thalamus and primary somatosensory cortex (Casey et al. 2000).

Acute and chronic pain can alter the pattern of thalamic and cortical activation. Patients suffering acute post-dental extraction show increased response to heat pain applied to the ipsilateral hand in the somatosensory pathway, including thalamus and S1 (Derbyshire et al. 1999). This increased level of rCBF does not occur when the same noxious stimulus is applied to the hand contralateral to the dental extraction. This fact can be explained by the ongoing post-surgical inflammatory process, and its repercussions in the CNS awareness, amplifying any further sensory input from the ipsilateral areas, surrounding or distant (for safeguard) from the injury. Chronic pain disorders have shown a central distinct neuroplastic mechanism in response to the persistent pain input overflow. Instead of thalamic increase activation to painful stimulation, there is attenuation of the response and even a decrease of the rCBF in the thalamus. This is the case for ▶ fibromyalgia and neuropathic patients, where chronic thalamic activation following their persistent evoked and ongoing clinical pain, attenuates or decreases its response after time (Gracely et al. 2002; Hsieh et al. 1995; Kwiatek et al. 2000). Patients suffering from ▶ cluster headache, a primary headache disorder, also show similar results, with significantly lower rCBF changes during the headache-free period compared to control subjects in the contralateral thalamus and S1 after ipsilateral tonic cold pain stimulation (Di Piero et al. 1997).

Conclusion

Although it is clear that neuroimaging research can contribute to the understanding of the thalamic neuronal activation regarding experimental and clinical pain, its nuclear specificity is yet to be completely defined. Technical improvement of imaging tools will provide better anatomical and functional nuclear maps of the thalamus, and consequently, of its correlation with each intrinsic aspect of a noxious event.

References

1. Bantick SJ, Wise RG, Ploghaus A et al. (2002) Imaging How Attention Modulates Pain in Humans using Functional MRI. Brain 125:310–319
2. Casey KL, Svensson P, Morrow TJ et al. (2000) Selective Opiate Modulation of Nociceptive Processing in the Human Brain. J Neurophysiol 84:525–533
3. Craig AD (2002) How do you feel? Interoception: The Sense of the Physiological Condition of the Body. Nat Rev Neurosci 3:655–666
4. Creac'h C, Henry P, Caille JM et al. (2000) Functional MR Imaging Analysis of Pain-Related Brain Activation after Acute Mechanical Stimulation. AJNR Am J Neuroradiol 21:1402–1406
5. DaSilva AF, Becerra L, Makris N et al. (2002) Somatotopic Activation in the Human Trigeminal Pain Pathway. J Neurosci 22:8183–8192

6. DaSilva AF, Tuch DS, Wiegell MR et al. (2003) Diffusion Tensor Imaging – A Primer on Diffusion Tensor Imaging of Anatomical Substructure. Neurosurg Focus 15:1–4
7. Derbyshire SW, Jones AK, Collins M et al. (1999) Cerebral Responses to Pain in Patients Suffering Acute Post-Dental Extraction Pain Measured by Positron Emission Tomography (PET). Eur J Pain 3:103–113
8. Di Piero V, Fiacco F, Tombari D et al. (1997) Tonic Pain: A SPET Study in Normal Subjects and Cluster Headache Patients. Pain 70:185–191
9. Faymonville ME, Roediger L, Del Fiore G et al. (2003) Increased Cerebral Functional Connectivity Underlying the Antinociceptive Effects of Hypnosis. Brain Res Cogn Brain Res 17:255–262
10. Gracely RH, Petzke F, Wolf JM et al. (2002) Functional Magnetic Resonance Imaging Evidence of Augmented Pain Processing in Fibromyalgia. Arthritis Rheum 46:1333–1343
11. Hsieh JC, Belfrage M, Stone-Elander S et al. (1995) Central Representation of Chronic Ongoing Neuropathic Pain Studied by Positron Emission Tomography. Pain 63:225–236
12. Iadarola MJ, Berman KF, Zeffiro TA et al. (1998) Neural Activation during Acute Capsaicin-Evoked Pain and Allodynia Assessed with PET. Brain 121:931–947
13. Kwiatek R, Barnden L, Tedman R et al. (2000) Regional Cerebral Blood Flow in Fibromyalgia: Single-Photon-Emission Computed Tomography Evidence of Reduction in the Pontine Tegmentum and Thalami. Arthritis Rheum 43:2823–2833
14. Lorenz J, Minoshima S, Casey KL (2003) Keeping Pain Out of Mind: The Role of the Dorsolateral Prefrontal Cortex in Pain Modulation. Brain 126:1079–1091
15. Paulson PE, Minoshima S, Morrow TJ et al. (1998) Gender Differences in Pain Perception and Patterns of Cerebral Activation during Noxious Heat Stimulation in Humans. Pain 76:223–229
16. Svensson P, Minoshima S, Beydoun A et al. (1997) Cerebral Processing of Acute Skin and Muscle Pain in Humans. J Neurophysiol 78:450–460
17. Wiegell MR, Tuch DS, Larsson HB et al. (2003) Automatic Segmentation of Thalamic Nuclei from Diffusion Tensor Magnetic Resonance Imaging. Neuroimage 19:391–401
18. Zubieta JK, Smith YR, Bueller JA et al. (2002) mu-Opioid Receptor-Mediated Antinociceptive Responses Differ in Men and Women. J Neurosci 22:5100–5107

Hunner's Ulcer

Definition

Hunner's ulcer is a focal inflammatory lesion of the bladder wall in chronic interstitial cystitis; its surface may crack and bleed with bladder distension.

▶ Interstitial Cystitis and Chronic Pelvic Pain

HVTM

▶ High Velocity Thrust Manipulation

Hyaline Cartilage

Definition

Hyaline cartilage is translucent cartilage that is common in joints and the respiratory passages.

▶ Sacroiliac Joint Pain

Hyaluronan

BRIAN MCGUIRK
Occupational (Musculoskeletal) Medicine, Hunter Area Health Service, Newcastle, NSW, Australia
mgillam@mail.newcastle.edu.au

Synonyms

Hyaluronic acid; Viscosupplementation

Definition

Hyaluronic acid is a naturally occurring glycosaminoglycan, consisting of a repeating dimer of glucuronic acid and N-acetyl-glucosamine (Weissman and Meyer 1954). The proprietary form is known as hyaluronan. This agent is administered by intra-articular injection, as a treatment for osteoarthritis.

Characteristics

Hyaluronic acid is a widely distributed polysaccharide, which plays an important role in all mammalian connective tissues, due to its peculiar physico-chemical and biological properties. By nature of its propensity to form highly hydrated and viscous matrices, hyaluronic acid imparts stiffness, resilience and lubrication to various tissues. The unique biophysical properties of hyaluronic acid are manifested in its mechanical function in the synovial fluid, the vitreous humour of the eye, and the ability of connective tissues to resist compressive forces (Laurent 1998).

In normal human synovial fluid, hyaluronic acid has a high molecular weight and acts in a visco-elastic manner. Due to its hyaluronic acid content, joint fluid acts as a viscous lubricant during slow movement of the joint, as in walking, and as an elastic shock absorber during rapid movement, as in running.

In osteoarthritis, both the concentration and molecular weight of hyaluronic acid in the synovial fluid are reduced (Marshall 1998; George 1998), which impacts on its biophysical properties. It was this finding that gave rise to the concept of *viscosupplementation,* in which injection of exogenous hyaluronic acid into the joint space is presumed to augment the functions of endogenous hyaluronic acid.

Mechanism

The mechanism by which intra-articular hyaluronic acid works in patients with osteoarthritis remains unknown. Although restoration of the elasto-viscous properties of synovial fluid seems to be the most logical explanation, other mechanisms must exist. The actual period that the injected hyaluronic acid product stays within the joint space is in the order of hours to days, but the time of clinical efficacy is often in the order of months (Cohen 1998; Balazs and Denlinger 1993). Possible explanations include stimulation of endogenous production of hyaluronic acid; inhibition of inflammatory mediators such as cytokines and prostaglandins; stimulation of cartilage matrix synthesis as well as inhibition of cartilage degradation; and a direct protective action on nociceptive nerve endings.

Technique

Hyaluronan is injected into the joint to be treated using a strict, no-touch, aseptic technique. If an effusion is present, aspiration of the joint is recommended before the injection, in order to prevent dilution of the injectate. Excessive weight-bearing physical activity should be avoided for 1–2 days.

Applications

The US Food & Drug Administration has approved the use of hyaluronan for patients with osteoarthritis of the knee, whose joint pain has not responded to non-medicinal measures and analgesic drugs. The guidelines for osteoarthritis from the American College of Rheumatology (American College of Rheumatology Subcommittee on Osteoarthritis Guidelines 2000) state that it may be "especially advantageous in patients in whom non-selective ▶ NSAIDs and Cox-2 specific inhibitors are contra-indicated, or in whom they have been associated either with a lack of efficacy or with adverse events". Intra-articular hyaluronic acid is generally used after non-pharmacologic treatments, analgesics and a trial of several NSAIDs.

Efficacy

Since the 1970s many studies have been carried out to evaluate the efficacy of hyaluronan. Despite a number of randomised, controlled trials having been carried out, the results and their interpretation, remain conflicting. Whereas the earliest studies suggested benefits, more recent double-blind placebo-controlled trials did not show any benefit over placebo. In other studies, hyaluronan has been suggested to have an overall benefit over placebo.

An extensive review on intra-articular administration of hyaluronan, published by Brandt et al. (2000), concludes that "although several clinical trials indicate that intraarticular injection of [hyaluronan] results in relief of joint pain in patients with knee [osteoarthritis], and that this effect may last for months, similar results are seen with placebo, and it is not clear that the difference between [hyaluronan] and placebo, even if statistically significant, is clinically significant."

In response, Miller, in correspondence to the Journal of American Academy of Orthopaedic Surgeons (Miller 2001), argued that the decrease in the total number of knee replacements performed in the USA has occurred as a direct result of the use of viscosupplementation, citing a number of studies that formed the basis of the presentation to the FDA for its approval of hyaluronan as a treatment for osteoarthritis.

Side Effects

Transient localised pain and/or effusion is the most commonly reported side effect, albeit occurring in a low (0–3) percentage of patients, based on the majority of clinical trials conducted to date (Puttick et al. 1995). These resolve spontaneously within a short period. Several cases of pseudogout have been confirmed (Luzar and Altawil 1998). Long-term side-effects have not been identified.

References

1. American College of Rheumatology Subcommittee on Osteoarthritis Guidelines (2000) Recommendations for the Medical Management of Osteoarthritis of the Hip and Knee. Arthritis Rheum 43:1905–1915
2. Balazs E, Denlinger J (1993) Viscosupplementation: A New Concept in the Treatment of Osteoarthritis. J Rheumatol 20 (Suppl):3–9
3. Brandt K, Smith G, Simon L (2000) Intraarticular Injection of Hyaluronan as Treatment for Knee Osteoarthritis: What is the Evidence? Arthritis Rheum 43:1192–1203
4. Cohen M, (1998) Hyaluronic Acid Treatment (Viscosupplementation) for OA of the Knee. Bull Rheum Dis 47:4–7
5. George E (1998) Intra-Articular Hyaluronan Treatment for Osteoarthritis. Ann Rheum Dis 57:637–640
6. Laurent TC (ed) (1998) The Chemistry, Biology and Medical Applications of Hyaluronan and its Derivatives. Wenner-Gren International Series, vol 72, Portland Press, London
7. Luzar M, Altawil B (1998) Pseudogout following Intraarticular Injection of Sodium Hyaluronate Arthritis Rheum 41:939–940
8. Marshall KW (1998) Viscosupplementation for Osteoarthritis: Current Status, Unresolved Issues and Future Directions. J Rheumatol 25:2056–2058
9. Miller E (2001) Correspondence. Viscosupplementation: Therapeutic Mechanisms and Clinical Potential in Osteoarthritis of the Knee. J Am Acad Orthop Surg 9:146–147
10. Puttick M, Wade J, Chalmers A, Connell D, Rangno K (1995) Local Reactions after Intra-Articular Hylan for Osteoarthritis of the Knee. J Rheumatol 22:1311–1314
11. Weissman B, Meyer K (1954) The Structure of Hyalbiuronic Acid and of Hyaluronic Acid from Umbilical Cord. J Am Chem Soc 76:1753–1757

Hyaluronic Acid (HA)

Definition

Investigational drug for the treatment of IC; appears to temporarily replace defective mucosa.
▶ Hyaluronan
▶ Interstitial Cystitis and Chronic Pelvic Pain

Hydrodistention

Definition

Hydrodistention is the filling of bladder under anesthesia, to assess for mucosal tears, glomerulations, and bladder capacity; part of diagnostic workup as well as therapy for IC.
▶ Interstitial Cystitis and Chronic Pelvic Pain

Hydroperoxides

Definition

Hydroperoxides such as PGG_2 are required to initiate the conversion of arachidonic acid into prostaglandins.
► Cyclooxygenases in Biology and Disease

Hydrotherapy

Definition

Hydrotherapy is the external application of water, e.g. the immersion of the body in thermal water.
► Chronic Pain in Children, Physical Medicine and Rehabilitation
► Spa Treatment

Hydroxy–7.8–Dihydrocodeinone

► Oxycodone

Hypalgesia

► Hypoalgesia
► Hypoalgesia, Assessment

Hypalgia

► Hypoalgesia, Assessment

Hyperaesthesia

► Hyperalgesia

Hyperaesthesia, Assessment

KRISTINA B. SVENDSEN[1], TROELS S. JENSEN[2],
F. W. BACH[2]
[1]Danish Pain Research Center, Aarhus University Hospital, Aarhus, Denmark
[2]Danish Pain Research Center and Department of Neurology, Aarhus University Hospital, Aarhus, Denmark
kristina@akhphd.au.dk, tsj@akhphd.au.dk

Definition

Hyperaesthesia is increased sensitivity to stimulation, excluding the special senses (Merskey and Bogduk 1994). ► Allodynia and ► hyperalgesia are included in the definition.

Characteristics

Hyperaesthesia refers to both the finding of a lowered threshold to a non-noxious or a noxious stimulus, and to an increased response to suprathreshold stimuli (Merskey and Bogduk 1994). It can best be described as a leftward shift of the stimulus-response curve, which relates the response to the stimulus intensity (Fig. 1). Hyperaesthesia has to be distinguished from hyperpathia, which is a classical feature of neuropathic pain and easily demonstrated in skin territories innervated by damaged nerve fibres (Jensen et al. 2001),(Jensen and Baron 2003).

Hyperaesthesia may occur after traumatic or inflammatory injury to the skin (Treede et al. 1992) or in the undamaged skin in neuropathic pain conditions (Boivie 1999, Woolf and Mannion 1999). Hyperaesthesia may also be found in the skin area of referred muscle (Svensson et al. 1998) and visceral pain (Hardy 1950, Stawowy et al. 2002). In tissue injury, increased sensibility to stimuli may be found in both the injured area (normally called primary hyperalgesia) and in surrounding non-injured skin area (secondary hyperalgesia) (Treede and Magerl 2000).

Induction and Assessment

Hyperaesthesia may be induced by different stimulus modalities including mechanical, thermal, and chemical stimuli (Treede et al. 1992, Jensen et al. 2001, Woolf and Mannion 1999).

Hyperaesthesia can be assessed by determining ► detection thresholds for a given stimulus. In the case of noxious stimuli, pain detection and pain tolerance thresholds can be used. Assessment of hyperalgesia includes stimulus-response curves, where noxious stimuli of different intensities (e.g. thermal stimuli or

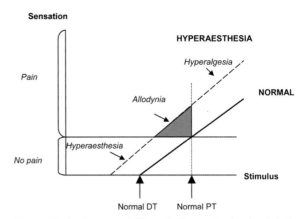

Hyperaesthesia, Assessment, Figure 1 Hyperaesthesia refers to both lowered thresholds and to increased response to suprathreshold stimuli. Decreased pain threshold is called allodynia. Increased response to normally painful stimuli is called allodynia. DT, detection threshold. PT, pain threshold.

pressure) are applied in a random order and the pain sensation/intensity is assessed for each stimulus.

Hyperaesthesia is present when the detection and/or ▶ pain threshold for a given stimulus is decreased (Fig. 1), or the response to suprathreshold stimuli is increased. In the case where pain is induced by a normally non-painful stimulus, the term allodynia is used. Increased response to normally painful stimuli, e.g. evaluated by the stimulus-response curve, is termed hyperalgesia.

Clinical Examination/Studies

Bedside sensory screening may be useful in the evaluation of the anatomical distribution and the qualitative characterisation of sensory abnormalities of the skin (Hansson and Lindblom 1992). Bedside examination includes mechanical stimuli (cotton wool, paintbrush, pressure with fingertip, pinprick), thermal stimuli (thermal rollers kept at 20° and 40°C, acetone drop) and vibration sense (tuning fork) (Table 1).

Sensory examination is normally done in the area with maximal pain and compared with the contralateral site of the body (Andersen et al. 1995, Jensen et al. 2001) or the adjacent body area not involved in disease. Hyperaesthesia is present in the case of increased sensation/pain to a non-painful (hyperaesthesia/allodynia) or a painful stimulus (hyperalgesia).

Quantitative assessment of hyperaesthesia is performed using quantitative sensory testing (QST). QST includes mechanical (▶ Von Frey hair, pressure algometry) and thermal stimuli (Thermotest) (Table 1). The results of QST from the affected site of the body are normally compared with results from an unaffected contralateral body site. However, when the contralateral site is also affected by disease, values from healthy subjects/general population may be used (Kemler et al. 2000). For standard-

ized regions such as feet, hands and face several laboratories have established normative data for thermal and mechanical stimuli. Hyperaesthesia is present in the case of lowered detection and/or pain thresholds. Pain Detection and Pain Tolerance Thresholds (see ▶ Pain Detection and Pain Tolerance Thresholds) indicates hyperalgesia.

The qualitative aspect of pain can be assessed by various questionnaires such as McGill Pain Questionnaire (Melzack 1975), verbal rating scales, visual analogue scales, numerical rating scales etc. (Turk and Melzack 1992).

Patient Example

A 54 year old man with peripheral neuropathic pain following a trauma located to the right antebrachium. The sensory function of the right hand was assessed by QST, and the results were compared with the healthy contralateral site. The patient had signs of hyperaesthesia with decreased tactile detection threshold, allodynia with decreased tactile pain threshold; decreased pressure pain threshold, decreased heat and cold pain thresholds and hyperalgesia with decreased pressure tolerance threshold (see Fig. 2). In addition he had cold allodynia evoked by acetone drop.

Experimental Studies

Human

Hyperaesthesia is found in various human pain models: Burn injury of the skin (a model of cutaneous injury) is followed by heat and mechanical allodynia in both injured and the adjacent non-injured surrounding skin (Pedersen and Kehlet 1998).

Capsaicin application of the skin produces allodynia with decreased heat pain threshold at the site of injection, and pain induced by a light normally non-painful

H

Hyperaesthesia, Assessment, Table 1 Sensory testing

	Stimulus	Method	Sensation
Bedside examination	Mechanical stimuli -Dynamic Touch -Static Touch -Punctate stimuli	Stroking the skin with a paintbrush / cotton swab Gentle pressure with fingertip Pinprick	Increased sensation/pain = hyperaesthesia
	Thermal stimuli -Cold -Warm	Metallic thermal roller kept at 20°C Acetone / menthol Metallic thermal roller kept at 40°C	
Quantitative sensory testing	Mechanical stimuli -Tactile detection threshold -Tactile pain threshold -Pressure pain threshold -Pressure pain tolerance threshold	Von Frey Hair Pressure Alogometry	Decreased threshold = hyperaesthesia
	Thermal stimuli -Cold detection threshold -Warm detection threshold -Cold pain threshold -Heat pain threshold -Heat tolerance threshold	Thermotest	

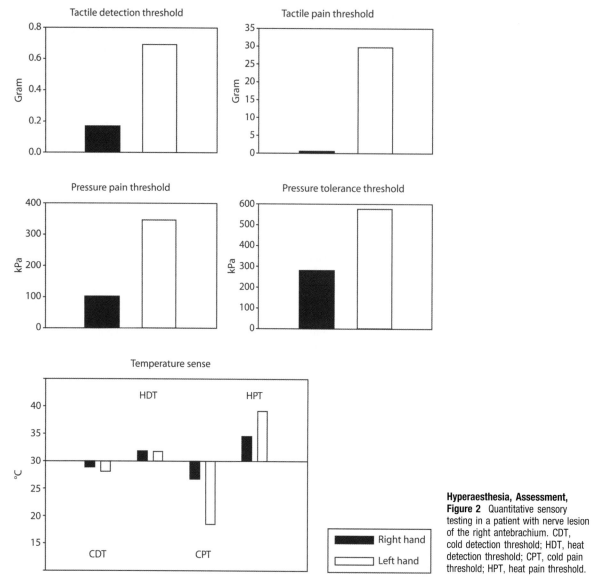

Hyperaesthesia, Assessment, Figure 2 Quantitative sensory testing in a patient with nerve lesion of the right antebrachium. CDT, cold detection threshold; HDT, heat detection threshold; CPT, cold pain threshold; HPT, heat pain threshold.

mechanical stimulus in an area surrounding the injection site (Treede et al. 1992). Burn injury has also been combined with capsaicin in a heat-capsaicin sensitisation model (Petersen et al. 2001).

Intramuscular injections of hypertonic saline, capsaicin, glutamate and other excitatory or algogenic substances have been used as a model of localised and referred muscular pain (Graven-Nielsen and Arendt-Nielsen 2003). In these muscle pain models decreased pressure pain thresholds have been found. Hypertonic saline may induce mechanical hyperaesthesia located to the overlying or adjacent skin (Svensson et al. 1998).

Animal

Strictly speaking, hyperaesthesia including allodynia and hyperalgesia with increased sensitivity to specific sensory stimulation cannot be determined in experimental animal models. Nevertheless, it is generally accepted that increased motor responses to mechanical (Von Frey hair), thermal (cold bath, hot plate, acetone, focal heat) and chemical (capsaicin) stimuli in animal models of nerve injury, inflammation or diabetes reflects a hypersensitivity of the animal to the pertinent stimulus (Scholz and Woolf 2002).

References

1. Andersen G, Vestergaard K, Ingeman-Nielsen M, Jensen TS (1995) Incidence of Central Post-Stroke Pain. Pain 61:187–193
2. Boivie J (1999). Central Pain. In: Wall PD, Melzack R (eds) Textbook of Pain. Churchill Livingstone, New York, pp 879–914
3. Graven-Nielsen T, Arendt-Nielsen L (2003) Induction and Assessment of Muscle Pain, Referred Pain, and Muscular Hyperalgesia. Curr Pain Headache Rep 7:443–451
4. Hansson P, Lindblom U (1992) Hyperalgesia Assessed with Quantitative Sensory Testing in Patients with Neurogenic Pain. In: Willis WD (ed) Hyperalgesia and Allodynia. Raven Press, New York, pp 335–343

5. Hardy JD, Wolff HG, Goodell H (1950) Experimental Evidence on the Nature of Cutaneous Hyperalgesia. J Clin Invest 29:115–140
6. Jensen TS, Baron R (2003) Translation of Symptoms and Signs into Mechanisms in Neuropathic Pain. Pain 102:–18
7. Jensen TS, Gottrup H, Sindrup SH, Bach FW (2001) The Clinical Picture of Neuropathic Pain. Eur J Pharmacol 429:1–11
8. Kemler MA, Schouten HJ, Gracely RH (2000) Diagnosing Sensory Abnormalities with either Normal Values or Values from Contralateral Skin: Comparison of Two Approaches in Complex Regional Pain Syndrome I. Anesthesiology 93:718–727
9. Melzack R (1975) The McGill Pain Questionnaire: Major Properties and Scoring Methods. Pain 1:277–299.
10. Merskey H, Bogduk N (1994) Classification of Chronic Pain: Descriptions of Chronic Pain Syndromes and Definitions of Pain Terms, Prepared by the International Association for the Study of Pain, Task Force of Taxonomy. IASP Press, Seattle
11. Pedersen JL, Kehlet H (1998) Secondary Hyperalgesia to Heat Stimuli after Burn Injury in Man. Pain 76:377–384
12. Petersen KL, Jones B, Segredo V, Dahl JB, Rowbotham MC (2001) Effect of Remifentanil on Pain and Secondary Hyperalgesia Associated with the Heat–Capsaicin Sensitization Model in Healthy Volunteers. Anesthesiology 94:15–20
13. Scholz J, Woolf CJ (2002) Can we Conquer Pain? Nat Neurosci 5 suppl: 1062–1067
14. Stawowy M, Rossel P, Bluhme C, Funch-Jensen P, Arendt-Nielsen L, Drewes AM (2002) Somatosensory Changes in the Referred Pain Area following Acute Inflammation of the Appendix. Eur J Gastroenterol Hepatol 14:1079–1084
15. Svensson P, Graven-Nielsen T, Arendt-Nielsen L (1998) Mechanical Hyperesthesia of Human Facial Skin Induced by Tonic Painful Stimulation of Jaw Muscles. Pain 74:93–100
16. Treede RD, Magerl W (2000) Multiple Mechanisms of Secondary Hyperalgesia. Prog Brain Res 129:331–41
17. Treede RD, Meyer RA, Raja SN, Campbell JN (1992) Peripheral and Central Mechanisms of Cutaneous Hyperalgesia. Prog Neurobiol 38:397–421
18. Turk DC, Melzack R (1992) Handbook of Pain Assessment. The Guilford Press, New York
19. Woolf CJ, Mannion RJ (1999) Neuropathic Pain: Aetiology, Symptoms, Mechanisms, and Management. Lancet 353:1959–1964

Hyperalgesia

ROLF-DETLEF TREEDE
Institute of Physiology and Pathophysiology, Johannes Gutenberg University, Mainz, Germany
treede@uni-mainz.de

Synonyms

Primary hyperalgesia; secondary hyperalgesia; algesia; hyperesthesia

Definition

Increased pain sensitivity. Antonym: ► hypoalgesia (decreased pain sensitivity). Increased pain sensitivity at a site of tissue damage is called primary hyperalgesia. Increased pain sensitivity in normal skin surrounding a site of tissue damage is called secondary hyperalgesia.

Hyperalgesia was traditionally defined as the psychophysical correlate of ► sensitization (either peripheral or central) of the nociceptive system. As such, it is characterized by a decreased pain threshold and increased pain to suprathreshold stimuli. The current definition by the International Association for the Study of Pain (IASP) refers only to the latter phenomenon ("increased pain to a stimulus that is normally painful"). A decreased pain threshold would operationally fulfill the IASP definition of ► allodynia ("pain induced by stimuli that are not normally painful"). This narrow definition has proved to be counterproductive for two reasons: 1) all known mechanisms of sensitization lead to changes in both threshold and suprathreshold response, 2) the extended use of the term allodynia has distracted from its initial clinical meaning and has hampered the transfer of knowledge from animal research to the clinic. Therefore, this essay uses the traditional definition of hyperalgesia as the psychophysical correlate of sensitization, which will probably be adopted by IASP in the near future.

H

Characteristics

Increased pain sensitivity (hyperalgesia) can be differentiated according to the test stimulus that is perceived as more painful, mechanical hyperalgesia, heat hyperalgesia, cold hyperalgesia, and chemical hyperalgesia (Table 1). Mechanical hyperalgesia can be further differentiated according to the size of the object contacting the skin (punctate or blunt) and the temporal dynamics of its application (static or dynamic). The underlying mechanisms are sensitization either in the periphery or in the central nervous system or both. Hyperalgesia at a site of tissue damage is called primary hyperalgesia; hyperalgesia surrounding this site is called secondary hyperalgesia. The sensory characteristics of primary and secondary hyperalgesia differ considerably (Fig. 1). Whereas primary hyperalgesia encompasses increased sensitivity to both mechanical and heat stimuli, secondary hyperalgesia is relatively specific for mechanical stimuli (Treede et al. 1992).

Primary hyperalgesia to heat stimuli is fully accounted for by ► peripheral sensitization of the terminals of primary nociceptive afferents (Raja et al. 1999). Peripheral sensitization shifts the stimulus-response function for heat stimuli to the left. This leftward shift is associated with a decreased threshold, increased responses to suprathreshold stimuli, and spontaneous activity (Fig. 2). Primary nociceptive afferents express the heat-sensitive ion channel TRPV1 (Caterina and Julius 2001). This channel can be sensitized by inflammatory mediators and the ensuing drop in heat threshold turns normal body temperature into a suprathreshold stimulus (Liang et al. 2001). Thus, primary hyperalgesia to heat can also explain ongoing pain of inflammatory origin. Secondary hyperalgesia to mechanical stimuli is not associated with any change in peripheral coding (Baumann et al. 1991), but can be explained by enhanced synaptic responses of second order neurons in the spinal cord to their normal afferent input (► central sensitization). These neurons also exhibit a drop in threshold and

Hyperalgesia, Table 1 Types of hyperalgesia and their likely mechanisms

Test stimulus	Occurrence	Afferents	Sensitization
heat	primary zone	type I &II AMH, CMH	peripheral
blunt pressure	primary zone	MIA, (type I AMH?)	peripheral
impact	primary zone	MIA, (type I AMH?)	peripheral
punctate	neuropathic secondary zone primary zone	type I AMH type I AMH type I AMH, MIA	central central peripheral/central?
stroking	neuropathic secondary zone primary zone	Aβ-LTM Aβ-LTM Aβ-LTM	central central central
cold	neuropathic pain secondary zone?	? ?	central? central?
chemical	inflammation	type II AMH, CMH, MIA ?	peripheral ?

Abbreviations: Aβ-LTM Aβ-fiber low-threshold mechanoreceptor ("touch receptor"), probably rapidly adapting subtype (Meissner corpuscle); type I AMH A-fiber nociceptor with slow high-threshold heat response (no TRPV1), probably equivalent to A-fiber high-threshold mechanoreceptor; type II AMH A-fiber nociceptor with rapid low-threshold heat response (TRPV1); CMH C-fiber mechano-heat nociceptor (TRPV1); MIA mechanically insensitive (silent) nociceptive afferent (From Treede et al. 2004).

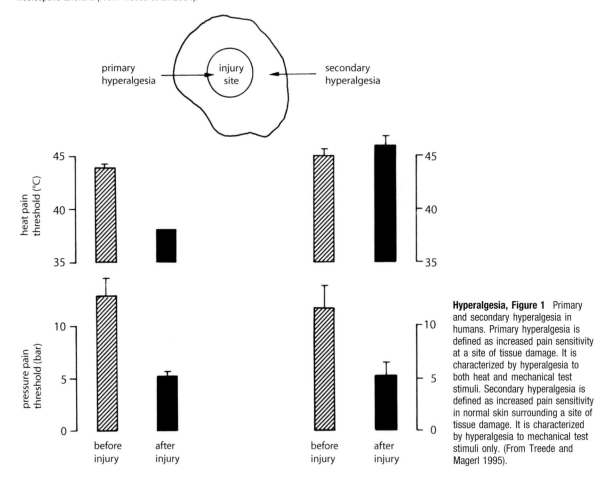

Hyperalgesia, Figure 1 Primary and secondary hyperalgesia in humans. Primary hyperalgesia is defined as increased pain sensitivity at a site of tissue damage. It is characterized by hyperalgesia to both heat and mechanical test stimuli. Secondary hyperalgesia is defined as increased pain sensitivity in normal skin surrounding a site of tissue damage. It is characterized by hyperalgesia to mechanical test stimuli only. (From Treede and Magerl 1995).

an increase in suprathreshold responses (Simone et al. 1991). In addition, expansion of the ▶ receptive field is a prominent feature of central sensitization. The molecular mechanisms of central sensitization resemble those of long-term potentiation of synaptic efficacy (LTP). LTP has been demonstrated for neurons in isolated spinal cord slices, in intact animals and on a perceptual level in human subjects (Klein 2004; Sandkühler 2000;

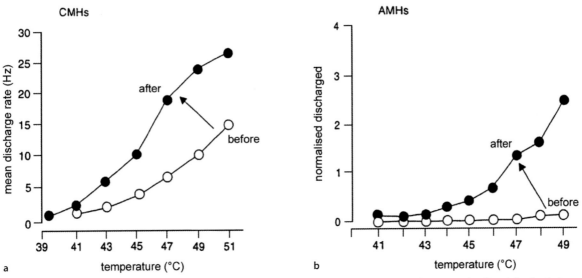

Hyperalgesia, Figure 2 Peripheral sensitization of nociceptive afferents by a burn injury in monkey. The stimulus response function relating the discharge rate of nociceptive C- (a) and A-fiber nociceptors (b) is shifted to the left following injury to the receptive field. This shift is characterized by a drop in threshold, increased responses to suprathreshold stimuli, and by spontaneous activity. Spontaneous discharges occur when the heat threshold is below body temperature. Peripheral sensitization is restricted to the injured part of the receptive field. (From Treede et al. 1992).

Treede and Magerl 1995). As a cellular correlate of learning and memory, LTP in the nociceptive system is a phylogenetically old mechanism, present even in invertebrates (Woolf and Walters 1991).

Although not characterized in as much detail, descending supraspinal mechanisms may contribute to both primary and secondary hyperalgesia, *via* reduced descending inhibition or *via* enhanced descending facilitation (Millan 2002; Porreca et al. 2002). Moreover, central sensitization may also occur at the thalamic or cortical level.

The mechanisms of cold hyperalgesia, which is a frequent finding in some ▶ neuropathic pain states, are still enigmatic (Wasner et al. 2004). Peripheral sensitization of nociceptive afferents cannot be ruled out, because the peripheral encoding of noxious cold stimuli has not been investigated sufficiently (Raja et al. 1999). Some evidence supports the concept of central disinhibition by selective loss of a sensory channel specific for non-noxious cold that exerts a tonic inhibition on nociceptive channels (Craig and Bushnell 1994). Central sensitization, similar to mechanical hyperalgesia, is another possibility.

Clinical Implications

Primary and secondary hyperalgesia occur transiently after each injury, and are hence part of the normal clinical picture of postoperative pain. Chronic inflammatory hyperalgesia resembles primary hyperalgesia. Hyperalgesia in neuropathic pain and referred hyperalgesia in visceral pain resemble secondary hyperalgesia (Treede et al. 1992). Cancer pain and musculo-skeletal pain states including low-back pain may also be accompanied by hyperalgesia. Parallel to the definition of sensi-

tization, hyperalgesia is characterized by a decrease in pain threshold, increased pain to suprathreshold stimuli and spontaneous pain.

Hyperalgesia Versus Allodynia

The current IASP taxonomy has restricted the term "hyperalgesia" to increases in pain to suprathreshold stimuli (Merskey and Bogduk 1994). But are threshold changes and suprathreshold changes two independent phenomena needing two separate terms? This question can be addressed in a clinical example, the increased pain sensitivity to punctate mechanical stimuli in patients suffering from neuropathic pain (Baumgärtner et al. 2002). Figure 3 illustrates that hyperalgesia to calibrated pinpricks in these patients is characterized by both an increase in pain to suprathreshold stimuli and a decrease in pain threshold. According to the IASP taxonomy the threshold decrease would be labeled 'allodynia', whereas the increase in pain to suprathreshold stimuli would be labeled 'hyperalgesia' (Fig. 3). Consistent use of the IASP taxonomy is obviously awkward in this case, because these observations reflect two aspects of the same phenomenon and the same data, i.e. a dramatic leftward shift of the psychometric function and upward shift of the stimulus response function of pain to the same set of test stimuli. The traditional usage of the term 'hyperalgesia' as an umbrella term for all phenomena of increased pain sensitivity describes hyperalgesia to punctate mechanical stimuli more adequately (Treede et al. 2004).

▶ Allodynia and Alloknesis
▶ Allodynia (Clinical, Experimental)
▶ Amygdala, Pain Processing and Behavior in Animals
▶ Cancer Pain

reduced threshold

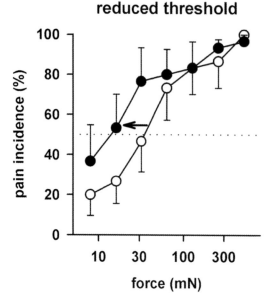

increased response

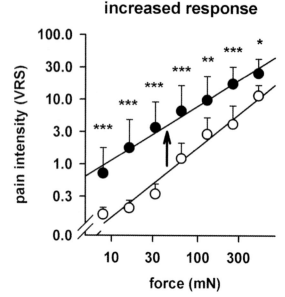

Hyperalgesia, Figure 3 Hyperalgesia to punctate mechanical stimuli in neuropathic pain. Averaged data from a group of six patients with neuropathic pain were plotted in two different ways: as incidence (left) and as intensity (right) of pain sensation in neuropathic pain skin areas (filled circles) compared to normal skin (open circles). Stimuli were graded punctate probes (diameter 0,2 mm) of seven intensities (8–512 mN). Left panel: reduced threshold (intersection with dotted line at 50%) implies pain due to a stimulus, which does not normally evoke pain ("allodynia?"). Right panel: Increased pain response to a stimulus, which is normally painful ("hyperalgesia?"). Note that both graphs are different aspects (pain incidence and pain intensity) plotted from the same data set. Arrows: leftward shift of pain incidence and upward shift of pain intensity. VRS = verbal rating scale. Mean ± SEM across subjects. Post hoc least significant differences tests: ** $p < 0.01$; *** $p < 0.001$. (From Treede et al. 2004).

▶ Cancer Pain, Animal Models
▶ Capsaicin Receptor
▶ CRPS, Evidence-Based Treatment
▶ Cytokine Modulation of Opioid Action
▶ Deafferentation Pain
▶ Diagnosis and Assessment of Clinical Characteristics of Central Pain
▶ Drugs Targeting Voltage-Gated Sodium and Calcium Channels
▶ Forebrain Modulation of the Periaqueductal Gray
▶ Freezing Model of Cutaneous Hyperalgesia
▶ Hyperaesthesia
▶ Hyperpathia
▶ Hyperpathia, Assessment
▶ Hypoesthesia, Assessment
▶ Inflammation, Modulation by Peripheral Cannabinoid Receptors
▶ Lateral Thalamic Lesions, Pain Behavior in Animals
▶ Metabotropic Glutamate Receptors in Spinal Nociceptive Processing
▶ Muscle Pain Model, Inflammatory Agents-Induced
▶ Nerve Growth Factor Overexpressing Mice as Models of Inflammatory Pain
▶ Neuropathic Pain Model, Tail Nerve Transection Model
▶ Nociceptive Circuitry in the Spinal Cord
▶ Nociceptive Processing in the Amygdala, Neurophysiology and Neuropharmacology
▶ NSAIDs, Mode of Action
▶ Opioid Receptor Trafficking in Pain States

▶ Pain Modulatory Systems, History of Discovery
▶ Percutaneous Cordotomy
▶ Polymodal Nociceptors, Heat Transduction
▶ Postherpetic Neuralgia, Etiology, Pathogenesis and Management
▶ Postherpetic Neuralgia, Pharmacological and Non-Pharmacological Treatment Options
▶ Post-Stroke Pain Model, Thalamic Pain (Lesion)
▶ Psychiatric Aspects of Visceral Pain
▶ Satellite Cells and Inflammatory Pain
▶ Spinal Cord Injury Pain Model, Contusion Injury Model
▶ Spinothalamic Tract Neurons, Central Sensitization
▶ Sympathetically Maintained Pain in CRPS II, Human Experimentation
▶ TENS, Mechanisms of Action
▶ Thalamotomy, Pain Behavior in Animals
▶ Thalamus, Clinical Pain, Human Imaging
▶ Thalamus, Dynamics of Nociception
▶ Transition from Acute to Chronic Pain
▶ Vagal Input and Descending Modulation
▶ Visceral Nociception and Pain
▶ Visceral Pain and Nociception

References

1. Baumann TK, Simone DA, Shain CN et al. (1991) Neurogenic hyperalgesia: the search for the primary cutaneous afferent fibers that contribute to capsaicin-induced pain and hyperalgesia. J Neurophysiol 66:212–227
2. Baumgärtner U, Magerl W, Klein T et al. (2002) Neurogenic hyperalgesia versus painful hypoalgesia: two distinct mechanisms of neuropathic pain. Pain 96:141–151

3. Caterina MJ, Julius D (2001) The vanilloid receptor: a molecular gateway to the pain pathway. Annu Rev Neurosci 24:487–517
4. Craig AD, Bushnell MC (1994) The thermal grill illusion: Unmasking the burn of cold pain. Science 265:252–255
5. Klein T, Magerl W, Hopf HC et al. (2004) Perceptual correlates of nociceptive long-term potentiation and long-term depression in humans. J Neurosci 24:964–971
6. Liang YF, Haake B, Reeh PT (2001) Sustained sensitization and recruitment of rat cutaneous nociceptors by bradykinin and a novel theory of its excitatory action. J Physiol 532:229–239
7. Merskey H, Bogduk N (1994) Classification of Chronic Pain. IASP Press, Seattle, p 240
8. Millan MJ (2002) Descending control of pain. Prog Neurobiol 66:355–474
9. Porreca F, Ossipov MH, Gebhart GF (2002) Chronic pain and medullary descending facilitation. TINS 25:319–325
10. Raja SN, Meyer RA, Ringkamp M et al. (1999) Peripheral neural mechanisms of nociception. In: Wall PD, Melzack R (eds) Textbook of Pain, 4th edn. Churchill Livingstone, Edinburgh, pp 11–57
11. Sandkühler J (2000) Learning and memory in pain pathways. Pain 88:113–118
12. Simone DA, Sorkin LS, Oh U et al. (1991) Neurogenic hyperalgesia: Central neural correlates in responses of spinothalamic tract neurons. J Neurophysiol 66:228–246
13. Treede RD, Magerl W (1995) Modern concepts of pain and hyperalgesia: beyond the polymodal C-nociceptor. News Physiol Sci 10:216–228
14. Treede R-D, Meyer RA, Raja SN et al. (1992) Peripheral and central mechanisms of cutaneous hyperalgesia. Prog Neurobiol 38:397–421
15. Treede R-D, Handwerker HO, Baumgärtner U et al. (2004) Hyperalgesia and allodynia: taxonomy, assessment, and mechanisms. In: Brune K, Handwerker HO (eds) Hyperalgesia: Molecular Mechanisms and Clinical Implications. IASP Press, Seattle, pp 1–15
16. Wasner G, Schattscheider J, Binder A, Baron R (2004) Topical menthol - a human model for cold pain by activation and sensitization of C nociceptors. Brain 127:1159–1171
17. Woolf CJ, Walters ET (1991) Common patterns of plasticity contributing to nociceptive sensitization in mammals and Aplysia. TINS 14:74–78

Hyperalgesia, Primary and Secondary

Definition

Primary Hyperalgesia is increased pain sensitivity at a site of tissue damage. Secondary hyperalgesia is increased pain sensitivity in normal skin surrounding a site of tissue damage. It is characterized by hyperalgesia to mechanical test stimuli.
▶ Allodynia (Clinical, Experimental)
▶ Hyperalgesia

Hyperemia

Definition

Increased blood flow or an excess of blood in a body parties known as hyperemia.
▶ Clinical Migraine with Aura

Hyperesthesia

▶ Hyperalgesia

Hyperexcitability

Definition

Large diameter sensory neurones with myelinated A-fiber axons that lie in dorsal root ganglia that project into a damaged peripheral nerve are often more easily discharged than the same type of neurone in ganglia from uninjured animals. The neurones fire from a greatly reduced current threshold. In some cases, a small depolarization produced by the local action of, e.g. a humoral substance, or by modifications in the extracellular environment (e.g. ischemia) may be enough to discharge these cells.
▶ Sympathetic and Sensory Neurons after Nerve Lesions, Structural Basis for Interactions

Hyperglycemic Neuropathy

▶ Diabetic Neuropathies

Hyperhidrosis

Definition

Hyperhidrosis means increased sweating.
▶ CRPS, Evidence-Based Treatment

Hyperknesis

Definition

Hyperknesis is the abnormal pruriceptive state in which a normally pruritic stimulus (such as a fine diameter hair which can elicit a prickle sensation followed by an itch) elicits a greater than normal duration and/or magnitude of itch.
▶ Allodynia and Alloknesis

Hyperpathia

JOHN W. SCADDING
The National Hospital for Neurology and Neurosurgery,
London, UK
jwscadding@hotmail.com

Definition

The IASP, in its Classification of Chronic Pain (1994), defines hyperpathia thus:
"Hyperpathia is a painful syndrome characterized by an abnormally painful reaction to a stimulus, as well as an increased threshold."
The following note is added:
"It may occur with ▸ allodynia, ▸ hyperesthesia, ▸ hyperalgesia, or ▸ dysesthesia. Faulty identification and localization of the stimulus, delay, radiating sensation and after-sensation may be present, and the pain is often explosive in character."

Characteristics

Introduction

Use of the term hyperpathia varies in the current scientific literature, and many avoid it. For example, in the fourth edition of The Textbook of Pain (1999), hyperpathia is mentioned by name in only 4 of 68 chapters, and possible explanations for the symptom complex are discussed in depth in only one of these. Likewise, several recent influential studies and reviews, tackling the difficult and elusive problem of linking individual symptoms and signs to underlying pathophysiological mechanisms, avoid use of the word hyperpathia altogether, or make only passing reference to it (Woolf et al. 1998; Woolf and Mannion 1999; Otto et al. 2003; Jensen and Baron 2003).
The reason is that hyperpathia describes a complex sensory experience occurring in the context of ▸ neuropathic pain. This complex can be broken down into component parts, each of which may be experienced by patients independent from the other constituent properties of hyperpathia; however, there is a tendency for the whole complex to occur in many patients suffering from neuropathic pain.

Historical Aspects

A brief historical examination reveals the variable usage of the term hyperpathia. Foerster (1927) suggested a lengthy and all-inclusive definition and description of hyperpathia, which most would agree comprehensively encapsulates the properties of stimulus-evoked painful sensations in patients suffering from neuropathic pain. He proposed the term hyperpathia be used when the following symptoms could be elicited from a regenerating area:
"a relative elevation of threshold, when the duration of the stimulus or summation of stimuli become important,

a latent period, an intensive explosive outbreak of pain of pain of abnormal unpleasant character accompanied by strong withdrawal movements, vasomotor and vegetative reactions, lack of or insufficient relationship between the strength of the stimulus and the strength of the sensation, a long after-reaction of the pain when the stimulus has ceased, irradiation, faulty localisation, and the inability to identify the nature of the stimulus which causes the pain."
Livingston (1943) equated hyperpathia with hyperalgesia:
"Any injury that directly or indirectly involves the sensory nerves may lead to the development of an abnormal sensitiveness of the skin. All sensory experiences derived from the skin may be altered in this condition, so that it is frequently called a "hyperesthesia" or a "hyperpathia". However, since the principal alteration in sensibility is an intensification of pain sensation it is more commonly referred to as a "hyperalgesia." In this state the tissues are unduly sensitive and they tend to react to the most innocuous stimuli with explosive sensations of pain accompanied by withdrawal reflexes."
Finally, Noordenbos (1959) suggests:
"Hyperpathia is present when the response to noxious or non-noxious stimuli presents the following features: delay, overshooting and after-reaction."

Definition or Description

This brief historical survey serves to emphasise two important points. The first, is the general point that a definition should include those characteristics that are the minimum necessary to categorise a condition, item or state as separate and identifiably distinct; in relation to the definition of diseases and clinical syndromes/states, a definition must have clinical relevance and usefulness. The second point, with reference specifically to the definition of hyperpathia, is that the definition is based on a collection of symptoms and signs. As is evident throughout this Encyclopaedic Reference, the last few decades have witnessed enormous progress in the basic neuroscience of pain. However, it is still not yet possible to define conditions and terms such as neuropathic pain, hyperalgesia, hyperesthesia, allodynia and hyperpathia on the basis of pathophysiological mechanisms, though there are, of course, numerous candidate mechanisms. It seems likely that each of the symptoms and signs of painful states may be produced by more than one underlying pathophysiology.
For the moment, however, we are stuck with frustratingly imprecise clinical syndromal definitions.

Symptoms and Signs Comprising Hyperpathia

It is notable that the current IASP definition of hyperpathia, quoted above, includes little detail, and it is left to the accompanying note to elaborate the symptoms. Most would agree that there are four main clinical features to hyperpathia:

1. An increased threshold to stimulation.
2. An abnormal delay in perception of a stimulus.
3. Summation, by which is meant increasingly painful sensation to a repetitive stimulus of steady intensity. Summation may take the form of an explosive, unbearable increase in pain, and it leads to brisk withdrawal from the provoking stimulus.
4. After-sensation. This is a perception by the sufferer that the stimulus evoking the pain continues after the stimulus has in fact ceased. Painful after-sensations may persist for seconds, minutes, or even hours, following brief periods of stimulation lasting only a few seconds.

Conditions in Which Hyperpathia Occurs

It is clear from numerous published accounts that hyperpathia may accompany (or, perhaps more accurately, be a part of) neuropathic pain, due to lesions at any level in the peripheral or central nervous system sensory pathways. This includes painful cutaneous scars, peripheral sensory or mixed peripheral neuropathies, brachial or lumbar plexopathies, spinal sensory radiculopathies, myelopathies, and brain stem, thalamic, sub-cortical and, very occasionally, cortical lesions. In other words, all of the many causes of neuropathic pain may be associated with hyperpathia, and multiple aetiologies are involved (Scadding 2003).

Noordenbos (1959) described in detail six patients with peripheral and central lesions, all of whom had severe hyperpathia, specifically to illustrate the occurrence of hyperpathia. Other classical accounts are to be found in Weir Mitchell et al. (1864), Riddoch (1938) and Livingston (1943).

Is Hyperpathia a Clinically Relevant and Useful Term?

Hyperpathia is very common and troublesome to patients, despite the impression one might get from perusal of the recent basic and clinical scientific literature on pain, which, as discussed above, tends to consider the component properties of hyperpathia rather than addressing hyperpathia as a whole. It is certainly highly relevant to patients. For example, a patient suffering from post-herpetic neuralgia (PHN) in a mid-thoracic dermatome, with an accompanying hyperpathic response to normally innocuous stimulation, may find the gentle rubbing of clothes on the affected area of skin quite intolerable. Indeed, for patients with PHN, it is often hyperpathia, much more than ongoing pain, which is the major component of their suffering and immobilization. Hyperpathia at other sites has the same devastating effect on the lives of numerous patients.

Although tremendous advances have been made in the measurement of pain, and particularly in the various attributes of neuropathic pain, hyperpathia is difficult to quantify, and so has tended to be underestimated in published studies (routine quantitative sensory testing does not accurately assess this).

Hyperpathia, Table 1 Possible Pathophysiological Substrates for Hyperpathia

Symptom	Mechanism
1. Increased threshold lesion	Reduced input due to sensory lesion
2. Delay in perception	Reduced large fibre input
3. Summation	Crossed after-discharge in lesionEphaptic transmission in lesion?Central sensitization
4. After-sensation	Crossed after-dischargeDRG ectopic firingCentral disinhibition

DRG, dorsal root ganglion
Woolf and Mannion (1999), Devor and Seltzer (1999), Jensen and Baron (2003)

H

Pathophysiology

Table 1 lists some possible pathophysiological substrates for the development of hyperpathia.
► Cancer Pain
► Causalgia, Assessment
► Deafferentation Pain
► Peripheral Neuropathic Pain
► Hypoesthesia, Assessment

References

1. Devor M, Seltzer Z (1999) Pathophysiology of Damaged Nerves in Relation to Chronic Pain. In: Wall PD, Melzack R (eds) Textbook of Pain, 4th edn. Churchill Livingstone, Edinburgh, ch 5, pp 129–164
2. Foerster O (1927) Die Leitungsbahnen des des Schmerzgefüls. Urban & Schwarzenberg, Wien
3. International Association for the Study of Pain (IASP) (1994) Classification of Chronic Pain. Merskey H, Bogduk N (eds) Classification of Chronic Pain: Description of Chronic Pain Syndromes and Definitions of Pain terms, 2nd edn. IASP Press, Seattle
4. Jensen TS, Baron R (2003) Translation of Symptoms and Signs into Mechanisms in Neuropathic Pain. Pain 102:1–8
5. Livingston WK (1943) Pain Mechanisms. A Physiologic Interpretation of Causalgia and its Related States. MacMillan, New York
6. Noordenbos W (1959) Pain. Problems Pertaining to the Transmission of Nerve Impulses Which Give Rise to Pain. Elsevier, Amsterdam
7. Otto M, Bak S, Bach FW, Jensen TS, Sindrup SH (2003) Pain Phenomena and Possible Mechanisms in Patients with Painful Neuropathy. Pain 101:187–192
8. Riddoch G (1938) Central Pain. Lancet 1: 1150–1156 and 1205–1209
9. Scadding JW (2003) Neuropathic Pain. Adv Clin Neurosci Rehab 3:2–5
10. Textbook of Pain (1999) Wall PD, Melzack. R (eds) 4th edition. Churchill Livingstone, Edinburgh
11. Weir Mitchell S, Morehouse GR, Keen WW (1864) Gunshot Wounds and Other Injuries of Nerves. Lippincott, Philadelphia
12. Woolf CJ, Bennett GJ, Doherty M, Dubner R, Kidd B, Koltzenburg M, Lipton R, Loeser JD, Payne R, Torebjork E (1998) Towards a Mechanism-Based Classification of Pain? Pain 77:227–229
13. Woolf CJ, Mannion RJ (1999) Neurogenic Pain: Aetiology, Symptoms, Mechanisms, and Management. Lancet 353:1959–1964

Hyperpathia, Assessment

ASTRID J. TERKELSEN, TROELS S. JENSEN
Danish Pain Research Center and Department of
Neurology, Aarhus University Hospital, Aarhus,
Denmark
astrid@akhphd.au.dk, tsj@akhphd.au.dk

Definition

Hyperpathia is a painful syndrome characterized by an abnormally painful reaction to a stimulus, especially a repetitive stimulus, as well as an increased threshold for sensory detection (Merskey and Bogduk 1994).

Characteristics

Hyperpathia includes increased ► detection threshold, steeper stimulus-response function than normal and often a time lag between stimulus and sensation, abnormal summation, after-sensations, pain radiating phenomena, faulty identification and faulty localization of the stimulus (Noordenbos 1979; Lindblom 1979; Merskey and Bogduk 1994; Bennett 1994).

Induction and assessment

Thermal-, mechanical-, and chemical- hyperpathia may exist singly or in any combination. Therefore, multiple different noxious and innocuous stimulus modalities have to be used to document or to exclude hyperpathia (Lindblom 1994) (Table 1).

Hyperpathia is assessed by performing stimulus-response curves, repetitive suprathreshold stimulation, and by asking the patient to report after-sensations, pain radiation, and coexistent phenomena.

Hyperpathia is present at increased detection threshold, decreased ► pain threshold, and ► allodynia (Fig. 1A and B, and Fig. 2B). At increased detection threshold without allodynia (Fig. 1, example 1C and 1D, and Fig. 2A), hyperpathia is present at steeper stimulus-response curve than normal (Fig. 3) or at exaggerated response (increased intensity and duration of pain) following single or repetitive suprathreshold stimulation (Table 1 and Fig. 1E).

In unilateral involvement, the contralateral mirror image area is used as control. In bilateral involvement, data should preferably be compared with normal values from sex- and age-matched controls.

Stimulus-Response

An increased sensory detection threshold (Fig. 1 and Fig. 2) characterizes hyperpathia. There can be poor localization of the stimulus and faulty identification where the patient feels pain, but not the specific modality of the stimulus (Fig. 2B) or the patient's misnaming of the stimulus modality (Fig. 3). The pain is often felt by a remarkable delay characterized by a time lag between the stimulus and the report of any sensory perception. The time lag can extend from two to three seconds to more than ten seconds .

Hyperpathia, Assessment, Table 1 Assessment of hyperpathia with Quantitative Sensory Testing (QST)

Stimuli to evoke hyperpathia	Assessment of detection threshold (DT) and pain threshold (PT)	Stimulus response function following graded innocuous and / or noxious stimuli	Repetitive suprathreshold stimulation
Thermal stimuli:			
Screening with metallic cold and heat thermorollers			
Quantitative thermal Sensory Testing with Peltier device:-Heat: -Cold:	DT, PTDT, PT	Ass. of thermal allodynia / hyperalgesia++	Repetitive heat or cold pulses++
Mechanical stimuli:			
Light touch:-Wisp of cotton:-Camel-hair brush:	–	–	Brushing with a velocity > 0.3 Hz++
Punctuate stimuli: Screening with safety pin -Von Frey hair:	DT, PT	Ass. of ► punctuate allodynia / hyperalgesia +	Multiple > 0.3 Hz pinprick stimuli +
Static stimuli: -Pressure: -Skin fold:	PTPT	Ass. of ► static allodynia / hyperalgesia++	++
Electrical stimulation:	DT, PT	+	+
Vibrametry:	DT, (PT)	+	+
Chemical stimuli:			
Topical capsaicin:	Time before detection (DT) and pain (PT)	Pain increase as a function of time	-

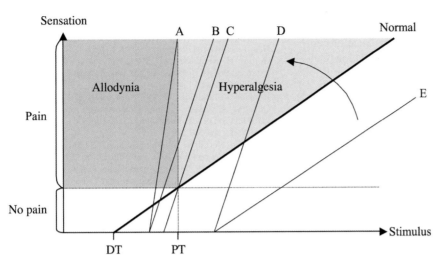

Hyperpathia, Assessment, Figure 1 Schematic description of different stimulus-response curves occurring at hyperpathia. Normal response (Normal) with normal detection threshold (DT) and normal pain threshold (PT). (A) Hyperpathia with increased DT, decreased PT, allodynia, and steeper stimulus-response curve as compared to normal. (B) Hyperpathia with increased DT, decreased PT, allodynia, hyperalgesia, and steeper stimulus-response curve as compared to normal. (C) Hyperpathia with increased DT, normal PT, hyperalgesia, and steeper stimulus-response curve. (D) Hyperpathia with increased DT, increased PT, hyperalgesia, and steeper stimulus-response curve. (E) At repetitive stimulation, pain threshold decreases and the slope of the stimulus-response curve increases thereby unmasking hyperpathia.

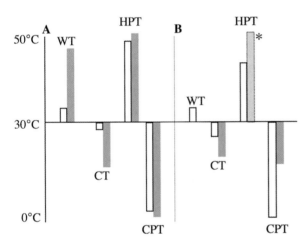

Hyperpathia, Assessment, Figure 2 Assessment of stimulus-response function of heat and cold sensation magnitude as a function of graded thermal stimulation in a 75 year old man with pain in left part of face and right leg and arm following brain stem infarct. Stimulus-response curve at right affected forearm (Affected) shows hyperpathia with steeper stimulus-response curve than at control side (Control) and faulty identification of stimulus modality with cold stimulation misnamed as heat stimulation. Control stimulus-response curve is assessed at contralateral mirror image area. Modified from Vestergaard and co-workers .

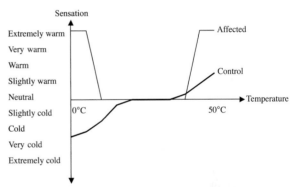

Hyperpathia, Assessment, Figure 3 Assessment of stimulus-response function of heat and cold sensation magnitude as a function of graded thermal stimulation in a 75 year old man with pain in left part of face and right leg and arm following brain stem infarct. Stimulus-response curve at right affected forearm (Affected) shows hyperpathia with steeper stimulus-response curve than at control side (Control) and faulty identification of stimulus modality with cold stimulation misnamed as heat stimulation. Control stimulus-response curve is assessed at contralateral mirror image area. Modified from Vestergaard and co-workers .

There is a steeper stimulus-response function than normal (Fig. 1 and Fig. 3) (Hansson and Lindblom 1992) with an intense, exaggerated, and explosive pain response to suprathreshold stimuli. Stimulus and response modality may be the same (► hyperalgesia) and/or different (allodynia) (Fig. 1) (Merskey and Bogduk 1994).

Temporal Summation

Hyperpathia is most likely elicited by increasing stimulus duration or by repetitive stimulation (Nordenbos 1959). Temporal summation refers to an abnormally increasing painful sensation to repetitive stimulation, although the actual stimulus remains constant and is the clinical equivalent to ► wind-up (Mendell and Wall 1965; Price et al. 1992). At repetitive stimulation above sensory detection threshold, hyperpathic subjects can report a gradual change from a faint sensation to a mildly unpleasant sensation and then a sudden exaggerated response with unbearable pain (Lourie and King 1966). During this repetitive stimulation, pain threshold decreases and the slope of the stimulus-response curve increases (Fig. 1E). This exaggerated response can be provoked by both noxious and innocuous stimuli (Table 1).

After-Sensations

After-sensations refer to abnormal persistence of pain seconds to minutes after termination of stimulation (Gottrup et al. 2003).

Pain Radiation

There may be a radiating sensation out from the point of stimulation to the cutaneous area around the stimulus or to wide adjacent areas (Bennett 1994).

Coexistent Phenomena

Hyperpathia is often accompanied by a general alerting response with strong withdrawal movements, vasomotor and vegetative reactions. It may occur with allodynia, ▶ hyperesthesia, hyperalgesia, or ▶ dysesthesia (Merskey and Bogduk 1994).

Clinical Examination/Studies

Pain history evaluates symptoms evoked by stimulation of the affected extremity like after-sensations, pain radiating phenomena, and allodynia induced by movement, non-painful cold or heat, wind touching the extremity, contact with clothing or bedlinen etc.

A bedside screening for hyperpathia is performed with heated and cold thermorollers kept at 20°C and 40°C, respectively, a wisp of cotton, and pinprick (Von Frey hair or safety pin), moving from the normal towards the painful area (Jensen et al. 2001). This screening may detect areas with possible increased sensory detection and exaggerated pain responses.

Usually the site of maximal pain reported by the patient is chosen as the test area. In this area, Quantitative Sensory Testing is performed (Fruhstorfer et al. 1976; Hansson and Lindblom 1992; Backonja and Galer 1998) to estimate detection- and pain thresholds (Table 1 and Fig. 2). At increased detection threshold, stimulus-response curves (Fig. 3) and repetitive stimulation with suprathreshold stimuli (Table 1) are performed in the test area. During examination, patient's behavioral responses are observed, such as facial expression or withdrawal from stimulus.

Experimental Studies

Hyperpathia is a clinical phenomenon and cannot be induced in human or animal experimental conditions.

▶ Allodynia (Clinical, Experimental)
▶ Amygdala, Pain Processing and Behavior in Animals
▶ Cordotomy Effects on Humans and Animal Models
▶ Nerve Growth Factor Overexpressing Mice as Models of Inflammatory Pain
▶ Opioids, Effects of Systemic Morphine on Evoked Pain

References

1. Backonja MM, Galer BS (1998) Pain Assessment and Evaluation of Patients who have Neuropathic Pain. Neurol Clin 16:775–790
2. Bennett G (1994) Neuropathic pain. In: Wall PD, Melzack R (eds) Textbook of Pain. Elsevier, Amsterdam, pp 201–224
3. Fruhstorfer H, Lindblom U, Schmidt WG (1976) Method for Quantitative Estimation of Thermal Thresholds in Patients. J Neurol Neurosurg Psychiatry 39:1071–1075
4. Gottrup H, Kristensen AD, Bach FW, Jensen TS (2003) Aftersensations in Experimental and Clinical Hypersensitivity. Pain 103:57–64
5. Hansson P, Lindblom U (1992) Hyperalgesia Assessed with Quantitative Sensory Testing in Patients with Neurogenic Pain. In: Willis WD (ed) Hyperalgesia and Allodynia. Raven Press, New York, pp 335–343
6. Jensen TS, Gottrup H, Sindrup SH, Bach FW (2001) The Clinical Picture of Neuropathic Pain. Eur J Pharmacol 19:1–11
7. Lindblom U (1979) Sensory Abnormalities in Neuralgia. In: Bonica J (ed) Advances in Pain Research and Therapy. Raven Press, New York, pp 111–120
8. Lindblom U (1994) Analysis of Abnormal Touch, Pain, and Temperature Sensation in Patients. In: Boivie J, Hansson P, Lindblom U (eds) Touch, Temperature, and Pain in Health and Disease: Mechanisms and Assessments, Progress in Pain Research and Management. IASP Press, Seattle, pp 63–84
9. Lourie H, King RB (1966) Sensory and Neurohistological Correlates of Cutaneous Hyperpathia. Arch Neurol 14:313–320
10. Mendell LM, Wall PD (1965) Responses of Single Dorsal Cord Cells to Peripheral Cutaneous Unmyelinated Fibres. Nature 206:97–99
11. Merskey H, Bogduk N (1994) Classification of Chronic Pain: Descriptions of Chronic Pain Syndromes and Definitions of Pain Terms. IASP Press, Seattle
12. Noordenbos W (1979) Sensory Findings in Painful Traumatic Nerve Lesions. In: Bonica J (ed) Advances in Pain Research and Therapy. Raven Press, New York, pp 91–101
13. Price DD, Long S, Huitt C (1992) Sensory Testing of Pathophysiological Mechanisms of Pain in Patients with Reflex Sympathetic Dystrophy. Pain 49:163–173
14. Vestergaard K, Nielsen J, Andersen G, Ingeman-Nielsen M, Arendt-Nielsen L, Jensen TS (1995) Sensory Abnormalities in Consecutive, Unselected Patients with Central Post-Stroke Pain. Pain 61:177–186

Hyperpolarization

Definition

Hyperpolarization is an increase in inside negativity of the transmembrane resting potential of an excitable cell, such as a neuron that can make a neuron less excitable and, if of sufficient magnitude, can prevent the occurrence of action potentials.

▶ Chronic Pain
▶ Descending Circuitry, Opioids
▶ Drugs with Mixed Action and Combinations, Emphasis on Tramadol
▶ Thalamic Bursting Activity

Hyperresponsiveness

Definition

Increased responsivity and improper frequency control of classes of sensory neurons in the central nervous system originated by anomalous inputs.

▶ Deafferentation Pain

Hypersensitivity

Definition

Hypersensitivity is an increased sensation of stimuli or increased scores of symptoms in response to standard stimuli.
▶ Chronic Pelvic Pain, Musculoskeletal Syndromes
▶ Deafferentation Pain
▶ Psychology of Pain, Sensitisation, Habituation and Pain
▶ Recurrent Abdominal Pain in Children
▶ Sensitization of Visceral Nociceptors

Hypersensitivity Maintained Pain

Synonyms

Central sensitization

Definition

A phenomenon developing in the central nervous system after peripheral injury by which mechanoreceptors acquire the ability to evoke pain. Clinically, it is characterized by secondary hyperalgesia, i.e. an increased painfulness of stimuli applied to a region outside the area of injury.
▶ Alpha(α) 2-Adrenergic Agonists in Pain Treatment

Hyperstimulation Analgesia

Definition

Hyperstimulation Analgesia is a short but very painful stimulation that reduces (short-term) pain.
▶ Acupuncture Mechanisms

Hypertensive Encephalopathy

Definition

Hypertensive encephalopathy is a change in the brain caused by failure of auto regulation of the cerebral circulation in the presence of severe hypertension, characterized pathologically by vasogenic cerebral edema and, sometimes, microhemorrhages and microinfarcts, and characterized clinically by headache, obtundation, seizures, visual changes, and/or focal deficits.
▶ Headache Due to Hypertension

Hypertensive Headaches

▶ Headache Due to Hypertension

Hypertonic Saline

Definition

Hypertonic saline is a solution of greater that 155 mM sodium chloride. Sodium chloride solutions of 1.0 M can be injected into muscle tissue and produce pain, presumably due to their osmotic strength.
▶ Nociceptors in the Orofacial Region (Temporomandibular Joint and Masseter Muscle)

Hypervigilance

Definition

Hypervigilance is the excessive predisposition to attend to a certain class of events, or the excessive readiness to select and respond to a certain kind of stimulus from the external or internal environment. In the context of fear of movement, hypervigilance concerns the increased attention to pain, potential signals of pain and other possible somatosensory signals. General hypervigilance is the tendency of highly anxious individuals to pay attention to other irrelevant (neutral) stimuli.
▶ Disability, Fear of Movement
▶ Dyspareunia and Vaginismus
▶ Fear and Pain
▶ Hypervigilance and Attention to Pain
▶ Muscle Pain, Fear-Avoidance Model

Hypervigilance and Attention to Pain

GEERT CROMBEZ[1], STEFAAN VAN DAMME[1], CHRISTOPHER ECCLESTON[2]
[1]Department of Experimental Clinical and Health Psychology, Ghent University, Ghent, Belgium
[2]Pain Management Unit, University of Bath, Bath, UK
geert.crombez@ugent.be,
stefaan.vandamme@ugent.be, c.eccleston@bath.ac.uk

Synonyms

Heightened Vigilance; Overalertness; Heightened Attention

Definition

▶ Hypervigilance to pain or somatic sensations is the excessive tendency to attend to pain/somatic sensations, or the excessive readiness to select pain-related information over other information from the environment. In the context of pain, hypervigilance is assumed to be initiated and maintained by its immediate threat value. ▶ Pain-related fear and ▶ Catastrophic Thinking have often been found to be strong predictors of hypervigilance to pain.

Characteristics

Chapman (1978) was one of the first to apply the construct of (hyper)vigilance to somatic sensations and pain. He referred to hypervigilance as a perceptual habit of scanning of the body for somatic sensations. Hypervigilance was thought to be an emergent property of the threat value of pain. People who appraise bodily sensations as dangerous were thought to be more likely to develop a habit of scanning the body for threatening sensations. His view is similar to the view expressed by Watson and Pennebaker (1989), who explored diverse explanations for the robust relationship between ▶ negative affectivity (NA) and somatic complaints. Indeed, an impressive number of studies has revealed that NA is strongly associated with symptom reporting and a heightened self-report of all types of physical sensations and symptoms, even in the absence of medical markers of disease. Watson and Pennebaker argued that this relationship is best explained by a hypervigilance to somatic information in persons with high levels of NA: "First, [individuals with] high NA may be more likely to notice and attend to normal body sensations and minor aches and pains. Second, because their scanning is fraught with anxiety and uncertainty, [individuals with] high NAs may interpret normal symptoms as painful or pathological" (Watson and Pennebaker 1989, p 247).

Hypervigilance has become a key theoretical and clinical construct in explaining high symptom reporting, especially in situations of medically unexplained or ambiguous sensations (Barsky and Klerman 1983; Rollman and Lautenbacher 1993). We should, however, be careful in equating high symptom reporting with hypervigilance. Hypervigilance is only one possible explanation for high symptom reporting, and other explanations using central nervous processes are often not taken into account. It is also presumptuous to conclude that a low ▶ pain threshold and a low ▶ pain tolerance are sensitive and specific indicators of hypervigilance. Hypervigilance may only be invoked as an explanatory construct when attentional processes are involved. Hypervigilance may be assessed by using self-report, psychophysiological and behavioural measures (Van Damme et al. 2004b).

In understanding hypervigilance, it is important to consider "normal" attention to pain. Eccleston and Crombez (1999) were among the first to systematically investigate the "normal" attentional processes to pain. In their cognitive-affective model of the interruptive function of pain, they argued that pain imposes an overriding priority for attentional engagement by activating a primitive defensive system that urges escape from somatic threat. Whether pain will demand attention, is the result of both pain-related characteristics (i.e. intensity, novelty, catastrophizing about pain, pain-related fear) and characteristics of other demands in the environment (monotonous environment, attention absorption in other activities). In their model, it is difficult to draw a sharp delineation between vigilance and hypervigilance. Hypervigilance to pain does not seem to result from an abnormal characteristic of the individual, such as negative affectivity. Available evidence suggests that hypervigilance to pain emerges as the working of normal attentional mechanisms in abnormal situations. Such situations are: (1) the chronic presence of high-intensity pain, (2) monotonous environments, or environments that lack external stimulation, and (3) most importantly, the high threat value of pain. Indeed, Goubert et al. (2004) found that the key mediating variable in explaining hypervigilance to pain was not an abnormally high level of negative affectivity, but the immediate threat value of pain, measured by pain-related fear and catastrophic thinking about pain (Fig. 1). Negative affectivity was best conceived as a vulnerability factor: It lowers the threshold at which pain is perceived as threatening, and at which catastrophic thoughts about pain emerge.

The idea that one is hypervigilant for threatening information is well-known in the clinical literature on fear and anxiety (Eysenck 1992; Pincus and Morley 2001). In contrast with the view of Chapman (1978), hypervigilance to threat is not restricted to one particular attentional mechanism, i.e. scanning. It is therefore reasonable to assume that hypervigilance to pain and somatic sensations may also become manifest in a variety of ways. The following example may clarify these different components: Imagine a person, afraid of back pain and (re)injury during movements, who has to resume a backstraining job after a period of pain-related work absence. The thought of going back to work will be sufficient to make him fearful. This thought may make him distracted by several irrelevant stimuli in the environment (▶ distractibility). From the moment he starts with some backstraining activities at work, he may begin to scan his body for pain or for other potential signals of bodily harm (▶ scanning). This may result in the rapid detection of any bodily sensation in his back. Attention will be drawn automatically to any change in back sensations (▶ attentional bias), and once it is detected, the person may experience difficulties disengaging attention from these somatic sensations and to re-engage attention towards his work (difficulty disengaging attention).

There are a number of promising paradigms that allow these various components of hypervigilance to pain to be disentangled (Van Damme et al. 2002; Spence et al. 2002). Studies have begun to investigate the critical role of these components in hypervigilance to pain. Results suggest that the rapid detection of pain or signals of pain is not critically dependent upon the presence of pain (attentional bias). The introduction of any somatosensory stimulus – painful or non-painful – introduces a rapid shift of attention towards that stimulus.

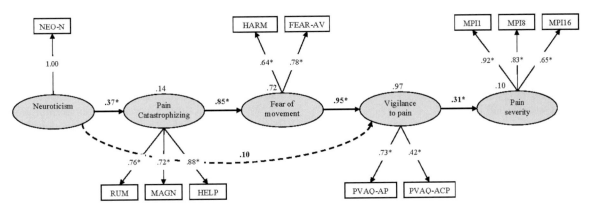

Hypervigilance and Attention to Pain, Figure 1 Psychology of Pain, hypervigilance and attention to pain.

Of more importance seems to be the effect of threat upon the difficulty disengaging from pain. Once pain or signals for pain have been detected, there is a difficulty disengaging from that threatening information. The difficulty is even more pronounced for those who catastrophize about pain (Van Damme et al. 2004a). Our understanding of hypervigilance has a number of implications. First, hypervigilance may be one mechanism by which pain-related fear may fuel avoidance. Patients with ► kinesiophobia are also hypervigilant for pain and possible signals of impending pain. Their attention dwells more on somatic sensations and will easily promote ► avoidance behaviour (Vlaeyen and Linton 2000). Second, hypervigilance to pain and somatic sensations will result in the more frequent reporting of symptoms. Third, as research shows that a high threat value of pain results in difficulty disengaging from pain and pain signals, cognitive interference will occur. Fourth, as hypervigilance seems to be mediated by the threat value of pain, distraction is probably not an effective treatment technique in patients with a high level of catastrophic thinking about pain. This was confirmed in the study by Hadjistavropoulos et al. (2000), who found that distraction was not effective in chronic pain patients with a high level of health anxiety.

References

1. Barsky AJ, Klerman GL (1983) Overview: Hypochondriasis, Bodily Complaints, and Somatic Styles. Am J Psychiatry 140:273–283
2. Chapman CR (1978) Pain: The Perception of Noxious Events. In: Sternbach RA (ed) The Psychology of Pain. Raven Press, New York, pp169–202
3. Eccleston C, Crombez G (1999) Pain Demands Attention: A Cognitive-Affective Model of Interruptive Function of Pain. Psychol Bull 3:356–366
4. Eysenck MW (1992) Anxiety: The Cognitive Perspective. Hillsdale, Lawrence Erlbaum Associates, p 195
5. Hadjistavropoulos HD, Hadjistavropoulos T, Quine A (2000) Health Anxiety Moderates the Effects of Distraction versus Attention to Pain. Behav Res Ther 38:425–438
6. Goubert L, Crombez G, Van Damme S (2004) The Role of Neuroticism, Pain Catastrophizing and Pain-Related Fear in Vigilance to Pain: A Structural Equations Approach. Pain 107:234–241
7. Pincus T, Morley S (2001) Cognitive Processing processing bias in chronic pain: A review and integration. Psychol Bull 127:599-617
8. Rollman GB, Lautenbacher S (1993) Hypervigilance Effects in Fibromyalgia: Pain Experience and Pain Perception. In: Voeroy H, Merskey H (eds) Progress in Fibromyalgia and Myofascial Pain. Elsevier Science Publishers BV, New York, pp 149–159
9. Spence C, Bentley DE, Phillips N, McGlone FP, Jones AKP (2002) Selective Attention to Pain: A Psychophysical Investigation. Exp Brain Res 145:395–402
10. Van Damme S, Crombez G, Eccleston C (2002) Retarded Disengagement from Pain Cues: The Effects of Pain Catastrophizing and Pain Expectancy. Pain 100:111–118
11. Van Damme S, Crombez G, Eccleston C (2004a). Impaired Disengagement from Pain: The Role of Catastrophic Thinking About Pain. Pain 107:70–76
12. Van Damme S, Crombez G, Eccleston C, Roelofs J (2004b) The Role of Hypervigilance in the Experience of Pain. In: Asmundson GJG, Vlaeyen J, Crombez G (eds) Understanding and Treating Fear of Pain. Oxfort University Press, pp 71–99
13. Vlaeyen JWS, Linton SJ (2000) Fear-Avoidance and its Consequences in Chronic Musculoskeletal Pain: A State of the Art. Pain 85:317–332
14. Watson D, Pennebaker JW (1989) Health Complaints, Stress, and Distress: Exploring the Central Role of Negative Affectivity. Psychol Rev 96:234–254

Hypesthesia

Definition

Hypesthesia is a decreased sensation to stimuli.
► Hypoesthesia, Assessment
► Viral Neuropathies

Hypnic Alarm Clock Headache Syndrome

► Hypnic Headache

Hypnic Headache

JAMES W. LANCE

Institute of Neurological Sciences, Prince of Wales
Hospital and University of New South Wales, Sydney,
NSW, Australia
jimlance@bigpond.com

Synonym

Hypnic Alarm Clock Headache Syndrome

Definition

Headache awakening the subject from sleep, not occurring during waking hours, usually lasting less than 180 min and not associated with autonomic features.

Characteristics

The headache is unilateral in about 40% of patients but is bilateral in the remainder. It usually develops after the age of 50 years, recurs more than fifteen times a month and is not severe but persists for more than 15 min after waking. It may be accompanied by nausea, photophobia or phonophobia, but not all three of these migrainous features. The bilateral site, mild intensity and the lack of autonomic features distinguish it from cluster headache. It usually responds to the administration of caffeine or lithium taken on retiring to bed.

Clinical Reports and Pathophysiology

Raskin (1988) first drew attention to this uncommon syndrome. He reported six patients, five of whom were male, all aged 60 years or more who were waking up consistently with generalised headaches that persisted for 30–60 min. Two volunteered that they were always woken from a dream by these headaches. Three patients reported accompanying nausea. The headaches were not alleviated by amitriptyline or propranolol but responded to lithium 300 mg or propranolol 600 mg at night. Raskin attributed the condition to a disorder of the brain's "► biological clock" in the hypothalamus, pointing out that cluster headache, cyclical migraine and manic-depression disorder were also tied to bodily rhythms and responded to lithium.

Ten of the nineteen patients described by Dodick et al. (1998) were awakened by headache at a consistent time, usually between 1.00 am and 3.00 am, giving rise to the term "alarm clock" headache. Three patients had infrequent but identical headaches during daytime naps. One described the headaches as developing during vivid dreams. Three patients mentioned infrequent nausea. It is not clear why one patient who had a severe unilateral headache with ipsilateral lacrimation and rhinorrhea was included in this series and not classified as cluster headache. An additional link with dreaming was provided by one of the three patients described by Morales-Asin at al. (1998).

In attempts to clarify this question, ► polysomnography has been carried out successfully in recording the onset of hypnic headache in six patients. Dodick (2000) found that an episode started during ► rapid eye movement (REM) sleep at a time of severe oxygen desaturation. Evers et al. (2003) reported two patients with onset during REM sleep, one of whom had periodic limb movements throughout the night. Oxygen desaturation did not exceed 85% at any time. Pinessi et al. (2003) recorded four hypnic headaches in two patients, all emerging from the REM phase of sleep without any oxygen desaturation. These authors pointed out that a patient reported by Arjona et al (2000) as being aroused by hypnic headache in stage 3 slow wave sleep, was being treated with venlafaxine, which may have altered her sleep pattern.

Cells that switch REM sleep cells off are found in the locus coeruleus and dorsal raphe nucleus and discharge regularly during waking hours, ceasing during REM sleep. Their action depends on noradrenergic and serotonergic transmission respectively. Since pathways from these areas form part of the body's endogenous pain control system their switching off could account for the onset of pain with REM sleep. (Dodick et al. 2003; Pinessi et al. 2003) The sleep-wake cycle is controlled by the suprachiasmatic nucleus of the hypothalamus and reduced ► melatonin secretion is thought to play a part in the initiation of hypnic headache.

Martins and Gouveia (2001) reported the case of a patient in remission for 10 months after lithium therapy who flew from Portugal to Brazil over three time zones. Her hypnic headaches recurred each night for 10 days while away but ceased on her return.

Summary

Evers and Goadsby (2003) have reviewed the seventy-one cases of hypnic headache reported in the literature to date. There were twenty-four men and forty-one women ranging in age from 26 to 83 years. The headache was bilateral in 61% and unilateral in 39%. It varied in frequency from one each week to six per night. It usually started 2–4 h after falling asleep, was moderate in intensity and persisted for 15 min to 3 h.

Nausea was reported by 19.4%. Mild photophobia, phonophobia or both were experienced by 6.8%. Some autonomic features such as lacrimation were recorded in six patients, two of whom developed ptosis. No relevant abnormality was found on CT, MRI, EEG or carotid Doppler ultrasound studies.

Evers and Goadsby (2003) summarised the response to treatment in reported cases. Good results were achieved by lithium in 26 / 35 patients; caffeine in 6 / 16, indomethacin in 7 / 18, flunarizine in 4 / 5, melatonin in 3 / 7 and prednisone in the only two patients in whom it had been tried (Relja et al. 2002).

References

1. Arjona JA, Jimenez-Jimenez FJ, Vela-Bueno A et al. (2000) Hypnic headache associated with stage 3 slow wave sleep. Headache 40:753–754
2. Dodick DW (2000) Polysomnography in hypnic headache syndrome. Headache 40:748–752
3. Dodick DW, Mosek AC, Campbell JK (1998) The hypnic ("alarm clock") headache syndrome. Cephalalgia 18:152–156
4. Dodick DW, Eross EJ, Parish JM (2003) Clinical, anatomical and physiologic relationship between sleep and headache. Headache 43:282–292
5. Evers S, Goadsby PJ (2003) Hypnic headache. Clinical features, pathophysiology and treatment. Neurology 60:905–909
6. Evers S, Rahmann A, Schwaag S et al. (2003) Hypnic headache –The first German cases including polysomnography. Cephalalgia 23:20–23
7. Martins IP, Gouveia RG (2001) Hypnic headache and travel across time zones: a case report. Cephalalgia 21:928–931
8. Morales-Asin F, Mauri JA, Iiguez C et al. (1998) The hypnic headache syndrome: report of three new cases. Cephalalgia 18:157–158
9. Pinessi L, Rainero I, Cicolin A et al. (2003) Hypnic headache syndrome: association of the attacks with REM sleep. Cephalalgia 23:150–154
10. Raskin NH (1998) The Hypnic headache Syndrome. Headache 28:534–536
11. Relja G, Zarzon M, Locetelli L et al. (2002) Hypnic headache: rapid and long-lasting response to predisone in two new cases. Cephalalgia 22:157–159

Hypnosis

Definition

A process of focusing attention that typically produces deep relaxation and openness to verbal suggestions; it can be performed on oneself or by others by using a combination of relaxation and intensive guided imagery techniques. The resulting altered state of consciousness is known as a trance. Hypnosis is widely used in both adults and children, and is broadly effective in the management of chronic and acute pain, especially cancer pain.

▶ Complex Chronic Pain in Children, Interdisciplinary Treatment
▶ Coping and Pain
▶ Hypnotic Analgesia
▶ Psychological Treatment in Acute Pain
▶ Relaxation in the Treatment of Pain

Hypnotherapy

▶ Therapy of Pain, Hypnosis

Hypnotic Analgesia

Donald D. Price[1], Pierre Rainville[2]
[1]Oral Surgery and Neuroscience, McKnight Brain Institute, University of Florida, Gainesville, FL, USA
[2]Department of Stomatology, University of Montreal, Montreal, QC, Canada
dprice@dental.ufl.edu, pierre.rainville@umontreal.ca

Definition

Psychological factors and interventions can sometimes powerfully modulate pain, and there is an emerging neurobiology of pain-modulatory mechanisms. Central neural mechanisms associated with such phenomena as placebo/nocebo, hypnotic suggestion (see ▶ Post-Hypnotic Suggestion), attention, distraction and even ongoing emotions are now thought to modulate pain by decreasing or increasing neural activity within many of the brain structures shown in Figure 1 (Rainville 2002). This modulation includes endogenous pain-inhibitory and pain-facilitation pathways that descend to spinal dorsal horn, the origin of ascending spinal pathways for pain as well as modulation, which takes place within cortico-limbic circuits once nociceptive information has reached cortical levels (De Pascalis 2001; Fields and Price; Hofbauer 2001; Porro et al. 2002; Rainville 2002). Hypnotically induced reduction in pain is based on changes in pain induced by suggestions and facilitated by an alteration of consciousness (Hilgard and Hilgard 1983; Price and Barrell 1990; Rainville and Price 2003). This alteration is accompanied by changes in brain activity involved in the regulation of consciousness (Rainville and Price 2003). Hypnotic changes in pain experience can consist of selective changes in the ▶ affective dimension (component) of pain, or reductions in both sensory and affective dimensions depending on the nature of the suggestions. Changes in affective and sensory components of pain are associated with corresponding changes in anterior cingulate cortical activity and somatosensory cortical activity respectively (Rainville and Price 2003; Rainville 2002). Different hypnotic analgesic approaches are clinically useful.

Characteristics

What are the Types of Hypnotic Suggestions for Analgesia

The suggestions for alteration of the experience of pain in studies of hypnotic analgesia, relate closely to the dimensions of pain and to the psychological stages of pain processing. Thus, there are suggestions that specifically target the affective-motivational dimension of pain, as distinguished from the ▶ sensory-discriminative dimension (Rainville et al. 1999). These would include suggestions for reinterpreting sensations as neutral or pleasant rather than unpleasant, as well as suggestions for reducing or eliminating the implications of threat or harm from the sensations. Then there are suggestions designed for specifically altering the quality and/or intensity of painful sensations so that they become less intense or absent altogether. There are three very different types of hypnotic suggestions for altering pain sensation in-

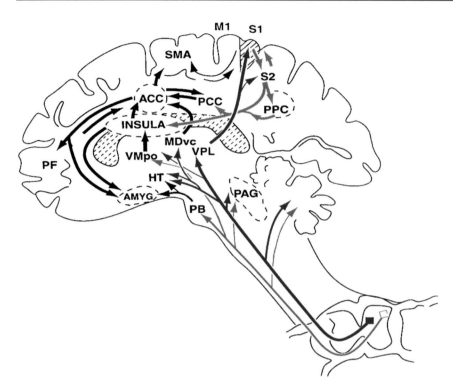

Hypnotic Analgesia, Figure 1 Schematic of ascending pathways, subcortical structures, and cerebral cortical structures involved in processing pain. PAG, periaqueductal grey; PB, parabrachial nucleus of the dorsolateral pons; VMpo, ventromedial part of the posterior nuclear complex; MDvc, ventrocaudal part of the medial dorsal nucleus; VPL, ventroposterior lateral nucleus; ACC, anterior cingulate cortex; PCC, posterior cingulate cortex; HY, hypothalamus; S-1 and S-2, first and second somatosensory cortical areas; PPC, posterior parietal complex; SMA, supplementary motor area; AMYG, amygdala; PF, prefrontal cortex (Figure from Price, Science (2001)).

tensity (De Pascalis et al. 1999; De Pascalis 2001). One type provides ▶ dissociative imagery by suggesting experiences that are disconnected from the felt sense of the body. An example would be a suggestion to imagine oneself "floating out of the body and up in the air" combined with the implicit or explicit suggestion that the pain belongs to the body and not to the one who experiences being somewhere else. Common to suggestions for dissociation, is the intention of having subjects not feel parts of their bodies that would otherwise be painful, and/or experience themselves in another location and context altogether. Another type is ▶ focused analgesia, which is intended to replace sensations of pain with others, such as numbness or warmth or with the complete absence of sensation. In complete contrast to dissociative analgesia, focused analgesia requires increased attention to the body area wherein pain is present, combined with a replaced sensation in that body area. For example, focused analgesia might include suggestions to focus on sensations in the hand, and to experience all sensations of the hand *as* if it were in a large glove. A third type of suggestion involves the reinterpretation of the meaning of the sensory experience. In this case, the significance of the experience for the integrity of the body is reduced or completely abolished, so that pain sensations are no longer associated with feelings of threat. Just as studies are needed to assess the role of hypnotic depth and individual components of hypnosis on pain, so there also need to be studies of differential effects of various types of suggestion on sensory and affective dimensions of pain experience. For example, what are the effects on

pain of suggestions exclusively designed to reinterpret the meanings of the sensations so that they are less threatening or unpleasant?

Which Types of Hypnotic Suggestions are Most Effective in Producing Analgesia

Very few hypnotic analgesia studies have directly compared effects from the different types of hypnotic suggestions described above. However, De Pascalis et al. conducted studies that compared analgesic effects produced by experimental conditions of Deep Relaxation, Dissociated Imagery, Focused Analgesia, and Placebo in comparison to a Waking Control condition (De Pascalis et al. 1999; De Pascalis 2001). They compared these conditions across groups of high, medium, and low hypnotizable participants, and utilized several dependent pain-related measures. These included pain and distress ratings, pain threshold determinations, somatosensory event-related potentials (SERP), heart rate, and skin conductance responses (SCR). The experimental stimuli consisted of non-painful and painful levels of electrical pulses delivered to the right wrist.

Of the four experimental conditions, Deep Relaxation, Dissociated Imagery, and Focused Analgesia produced statistically significant reductions on all pain-related measures among all three groups of participants (i.e. low, mid-, high). However, these analgesic effects interacted with ▶ hypnotizability, as shown in Figure 2. During Focused Analgesia, highly hypnotizable participants had larger reductions in pain ratings in comparison to low and medium hypnotizable participants. Further-

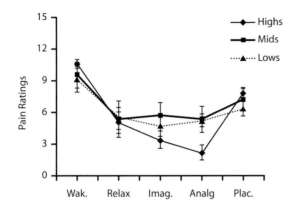

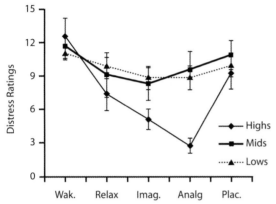

Hypnotic Analgesia, Figure 2 Pain sensory and distress ratings in response to noxious electrical stimulation delivered to the wrist in normal subjects with high (Highs), moderate (Mids), or low (Lows) hypnotic susceptibility. Both pain sensory and distress ratings decrease significantly in response to hypnotic suggestions for relaxation (Relax), dissociative imagery (Imag.), and focused analgesia (Analg), compared to the baseline wakefulness (Wak.) and placebo (Plac.) conditions. Larger pain reductions are observed in more susceptible subjects (Highs) and during focused analgesia. Also, note that there is no significant placebo analgesia observed for all three groups. (De Pascalis et al. 2001).

more, highly susceptible subjects had more pronounced reductions in distress ratings during Focused Analgesia and Dissociated Imagery, in comparison to the other two groups. Focused Analgesia produced the largest reductions in all dependent measures within highly hypnotizable participants. No significant placebo effects were obtained for any of the three groups. The combination of these results indicates several interesting features of hypnotic analgesia. First, hypnotic analgesia cannot simply be understood as a placebo effect and is more than just relaxation. Second, very different types of suggestions for analgesia are effective and are facilitated by hypnotizability. Third, hypnotic analgesia can affect physiological reflexive responses associated with pain (Hilgard and Hilgard 1983; Rainville 2002). Each of the types of hypnotic suggestion discussed so far can be given directly or indirectly. A ► direct suggestion for analgesia would be "You will notice that the pain is less intense. ..." whereas an ► indirect suggestion would be "I wonder if you will notice whether the

sensation you once experienced as painful will be experienced as just warmth or pressure or perhaps even numbness. ... " The latter is permissive, ambiguous, and refers to alternative experiences without the implication of a direct instruction. Resistance to hypnotic suggestions may be less in the case of permissive-indirect as compared to restrictive-direct suggestions, because one is not directly told what to experience. Furthermore, restrictive-direct suggestions may be perceived as unnecessarily authoritarian. One might expect that a larger proportion of people could benefit from a hypnotic approach that uses indirect suggestions and there is some, albeit limited, evidence that this is so (Price and Barber 1987; Price and Barrell 1990).

What are the Factors that Determine the Efficacy of Hypnotic Analgesia

The efficacy of hypnotic analgesia and its relationship to hypnotic susceptibility has been shown to depend on several factors (Price and Barber 1987). These include the pain dimension that is measured, baseline pain intensity, the maintained presence of the hypnotist or hypnotic suggestions, and finally hypnotic ability. Some of these factors are shown in Table 1. When suggestions were given for both reinterpreting the meaning of experimentally induced heat sensations and for experiencing them as less intense, pain sensation intensity was reduced by an average of about 50 percent, and pain unpleasantness was reduced by 87 percent in a group of sixteen subjects. Thus, pain affect was more powerfully attenuated in comparison to pain sensation. Although hypnotic suggestions exerted a more powerful reduction of pain affect than pain sensation, it was also quite apparent that both dimensions were reduced, as has been amply demonstrated in several experimental laboratories (Barber and Mayer 1977; De Pascalis et al. 1999; De Pascalis 2001; Rainville et al. 1999; Rainville 2002). Reduction in pain sensation was statistically associated with hypnotic susceptibility, albeit at modest levels (Tab. 1). Therefore, the component of the hypnotic intervention that relied on hypnotic ability and a hypnotic state was the one most influential on pain sensation intensity. Interestingly, the association became stronger with increasing levels of pain intensity (Tab. 1). It makes sense that the reduction

Hypnotic Analgesia, Table 1 Hypnotic Susceptibility and Analgesia

Stimulus Temperature	Sensory Analgesia	Affective Analgesia
	Spearman Correlation Coefficient	
44.5° C	+0.04	-0.23
47.5° C	+0.21	-0.11
49.5° C	+0.43*	-0.08
51.5° C	+0.56*	+0.10

*P<0.05

in stronger pains requires more hypnotic ability than the reduction in weaker pains. A final factor was maintained contact between the hypnotist and the subject. Statistically significant analgesia developed in one group of subjects that had maintained contact with the hypnotist during the pain testing session, and did not develop in the group that did not have maintained contact. Thus, multiple factors are involved in analgesia that results from a hypnotic intervention. These may include those that are unrelated to hypnotic susceptibility and perhaps even to a hypnotic state. Such potential multiple factors are closely related to different proposed mechanisms of hypnotic analgesia.

Rainville et al. further clarified the relationship between different types of hypnotic suggestions for analgesia, and the dimensions of pain that are modulated by these suggestions (Rainville et al. 1999). This study conducted two types of experiments, one in which hypnotic suggestions were selectively targeted toward increasing or decreasing the sensory intensity of pain, and the other in which hypnotic suggestions were targeted toward decreasing or increasing the affective dimension of pain. In both types of experiments, normal subjects who were trained in hypnosis, rated pain intensity and pain unpleasantness produced by a tonic heat pain test (^{1}-min immersion of the hand in 45.0–47.5° C water). The results of the two experiments are illustrated in Figure 3.

In the first experiment, suggestions to modulate pain sensation intensity resulted in significant changes in both pain sensation intensity ratings and pain unpleasantness ratings, that is, both dimensions were modulated in parallel. This was so, despite the fact that no suggestions were given about pain affect. In the second experiment, pain unpleasantness was significantly increased and decreased after suggestions were given for these changes, and these changes occurred without corresponding changes in pain sensation intensity. Hypnotic susceptibility (Stanford Hypnotic Susceptibility Scale Form A) was specifically associated with pain sensation intensity modulation in the first experiment (directed toward pain sensation; Spearman-r = 0.69), and with pain unpleasantness modulation in the second experiment (directed toward pain affect; Spearman-r = 0.43).

Thus, hypnotic changes in pain experience can consist of selective changes in the affective dimension of pain or reductions in both sensory and affective dimensions, depending on the nature of the suggestions. Selective changes in only affective components of pain are associated with corresponding changes in anterior cingulate cortical activity, and changes in sensory components are accompanied by corresponding changes in somatosensory cortical activity (Hofbauer 2001; Rainville 2002). Reinterpretation of meanings of pain, dissociation, and focused analgesia reflect different psychological mechanisms of hypnotic analgesia. These multiple mecha-

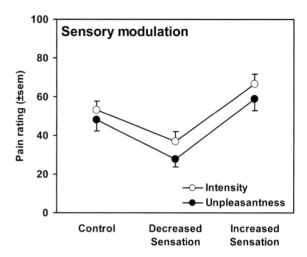

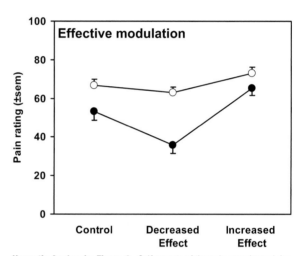

Hypnotic Analgesia, Figure 3   Self-reports of the pain experienced during the immersion of the hand in hot water following hypnotic suggestions directed at the sensory and affective dimension of pain. Suggestions directed at the sensory aspect of pain (Sensory modulation) produce parallel changes in self-reports of pain sensation intensity and unpleasantness. In contrast, suggestions for the reinterpretation of pain with decreased and increased sense of threat and discomfort (Affective modulation) produce specific changes in pain unpleasantness that largely exceed the changes in pain sensation intensity. (Rainville et al. 1999)

nisms are likely to be associated with intracortical and descending brain-to-spinal cord mechanisms, to varying extents. Although there is some evidence that hypnotic analgesia has demonstrable clinical efficacy, there is a strong need for improvements in methodologies of clinical studies. In particular, there is a need to compare the efficacy of different hypnotic approaches and provide rigorous standardized outcome measures.

It is useful to consider how results of experiments by De Pascalis et al. (De Pascalis et al. 1999; De Pascalis 2001) and Rainville et al. (Rainville et al. 1999; Rainville 2002), described above, help identify the necessary and sufficient psychological factors for hypnotic analgesia. Hypnotic analgesia cannot work only by means of distraction, because suggestions for Focused Analgesia are among the most effective, particularly among highly hypnotizable participants. Focused Analgesia requires greater not lesser attention to the body area wherein analgesia develops. Hypnotically induced changes in pain affect can occur directly through suggestions that alter the meaning of the experience of the stimulus, or indirectly through suggestions that target the pain sensation. Hypnotic changes in the latter can also occur through suggestions for dissociation or through suggestions for changes in the way the sensory qualities are experienced (e. g. numbness versus burning). Hypnotic analgesia cannot only work by means of a placebo effect, because subjects are likely to experience placebo and hypnotic suggestions differently. Moreover, there is now good evidence that ▶ placebo analgesia, but not hypnotic analgesia, requires an endogenous opioid pain-inhibitory mechanism. Placebo analgesia is naloxone reversible in studies of experimental pain, whereas several studies have shown than hypnotic analgesia is not naloxone reversible (Barber and Mayer 1977; Goldstein and Hilgard 1975). Finally, placebo analgesia, unlike hypnotic analgesia, is not significantly associated with hypnotic susceptibility (Hilgard and Hilgard 1983).

Conclusions

The combination of anatomical, psychological, and neurophysiological approaches to understanding the brain mechanisms underlying sensory and affective dimensions of pain and its modulation by psychological interventions, such as hypnotic suggestions, has led to a vastly improved ability to answer questions that only 10 years ago were relatively impenetrable. In particular, studies that combine brain imaging with psychophysical methods and sophisticated experimental designs, have led to the possibility of understanding complex mechanisms by which sensory and affective dimensions of pain are interrelated, and how these dimensions can be modulated by cognitive factors. The brain networks for these mechanisms are extensive and involve both serial and parallel circuitry, which is itself under dynamic control from several brain regions.

References

1. Barber J, Mayer D (1977) Evaluation of the Efficacy and Neural Mechanism of a Hypnoticanalgesia Procedure in Experimental and Clinical Dental Pain. Pain 4:41–48
2. De Pascalis V, Magurano MR, Bellusci A (1999) Pain Perception, Somatosensory Event-Related Potentials and Skin Conductance Responses to Painful Stimuli in High, Mid, and Low Hypnotizable Subjects: Effects of Differential Pain Reduction Strategies. Pain 83:499–508
3. De Pascalis V, Magurano MR, Bellusci A et al. (2001) Somatosensory Event-Related Potential and Autonomic Activity to Varying Pain Reduction Cognitive Strategies in Hypnosis. Clin Neurophysiol 112:1475–1485
4. Fields HL, Price D (1997): Toward a neurobiology of placebo analgesia. In: Harrington A (ed): The Placebo Effect. Harvard University Press, Cambridge, Massachusetts, pp 93-115
5. Goldstein A, Hilgard ER (1975) Lack of Influence of the Morphine Antagonist Naloxone on Hypnotic Analgesia. Proc Natl Acad Sci USA 72:2041–2043
6. Hilgard ER, Hilgard JR (1983) Hypnosis in the Relief of Pain. William Kaufmann, Los Altos, CA, pp 294
7. Hofbauer RK, Rainville P, Duncan GH et al. (2001) Cortical Representation of the Sensory Dimension of Pain. J Neurophysiol 86:402–411
8. Porro CA, Balraldi P, Pagnoni G et al. (2002) Does Anticipation of Pain Affect Cortical Nociceptive Systems? J Neurosci 22:3206–3214
9. Price DD, Barber J (1987) An Analysis of Factors that Contribute to the Efficacy of Hypnotic Analgesia. J Abnorm Psychol 96: 46–51
10. Price DD, Barrell JJ (1990) The Structure of the Hypnotic State: A Self-Directed Experiential Study. In: Barrell JJ (ed) The Experiential Method: Exploring the Human Experience. Copely Publishing Group, Massachusetts, pp 85–97
11. Rainville P, Price DD (2003). Hypnosis Phenomenology and the Neurobiology of Consciousness. Int J Clin Exp Hypn 51:105–129
12. Rainville P, Carrier B, Hofbauer RK et al. (1999) Dissociation of Sensory and Affective Dimensions of Pain using Hypnotic Modulation. Pain 82:159–171
13. Rainville P (2002) Brain Mechanisms of Pain Affect and Pain Modulation. Curr Opin Neurobiol 12:195–204

H

Hypnotic Relaxation

▶ Relaxation in the Treatment of Pain

Hypnotism

▶ Therapy of Pain, Hypnosis

Hypnotizability

Definition

Hypnotic susceptibility, hypnotic capacity or hypnotic responding delineates a variable that determines the extent to which an individual is able to respond to hypnotic suggestion. Research has shown that hypnotizability can be measured with good reliability and is a remarkably stable trait in adults. It correlates with dissociative experiences and with measures of absorption. Highly hypnotizable individuals tend to have a high imaginative capacity.

▶ Hypnotic Analgesia
▶ Therapy of Pain, Hypnosis

Hypoaesthesia

Definition

Hypoaesthesia is a decreased sensitivity to stimulation, excluding special senses.

- ▸ Hyperaesthesia
- ▸ Hypoaesthesia
- ▸ Hypoesthesia, Assessment

Hypoalgesia, Assessment

MISHA-MIROSLAV BACKONJA
Department of Neurology; University of Wisconsin-Madison, Madison, WI, USA
backonja@neurology.wisc.edu

Synonyms

Hypalgia; Assessment of Hypoalgesia

Definition

IASP Taxonomy (Merskey and Bogduk 1994) defines hypoalgesia as "decreased perception of noxious stimuli." Hypoalgesia could be in response to a wide variety of mechanical stimuli such as pinch, strong pressure or punctuate and to thermal noxious stimuli of heat and cold, basically any physical force of sufficient intensity to disrupt or threaten the integrity or homeostasis of any tissue.

In other terms, hypoalgesia is diminished experience of pain in response to a normally painful stimulus. Hypoesthesia covers the case of diminished sensitivity to stimulation that is normally not painful.

Hypoalgesia is also defined as raised threshold to painful stimuli.

Characteristics

Hypoalgesia is a ▸ negative sensory phenomenon seen exclusively in patients with neurological disease or injury, including patients with ▸ neuropathic pain (Backonja and Galer 1998; Lindblom and Ochoa 1986; Backonja 2003). Hypoalgesia indicates a decrease or loss of function that comes as a result of neurological disease or injury affecting thermonociceptive pathways, anywhere from primary afferents to cerebral cortical structures. Distinction of hypoalgesia from hypoesthesia is based primarily on the type and intensity of the stimulus applied to the thermonociceptive sensory system.

Methods of Assessment and the Interpretation

Assessment of the sensory nervous system function is most commonly done at the bedside where testing is primarily qualitative in nature, while quantitative assessment, increasingly using computerized electronic equipment, is done in a quantitative sensory laboratory (Backonja and Galer 1998; Greenspan 2001). Either should be able to detect hypoalgesia, but the way these methods arrive to the conclusion about presence and severity of hypoalgesia is distinct, and that is also reflected in the

definition. Qualitative bedside exam relies on patient report. Quantitative sensory testing arrives at its conclusion about hypoalgesia on the basis of the raised thresholds to painful stimuli.

Qualitative assessment is based on the subject's ability to compare and report quality of sensation from standard methods of stimulation, from the ▸ symptom affected areas, when it is compared to normal unaffected areas. Qualitative method is very convenient for bedside evaluations. Frequently utilized bedside methods include standard neurological examination tools such as safety pin, monofilament, and various metal objects that could be conveniently warmed or cooled in the clinical setting. A degree of quantification is possible, and requires that the subject reports whether a decrease of pain from painful stimulation is mild, moderate, severe or completely absent, when compared to a normal unaffected area. Since a qualitative method requires psychophysical interaction, this method can be used only in humans who can linguistically communicate with the examiner, and as such it cannot be used in animal models of pain studies.

Quantitative assessment of sensory deficits requires a more sophisticated approach and frequently utilizes electronically controlled devices, although a number of psychophysical methods, especially mechanical stimuli, are used and all of them place much longer time demands on patients. Traditionally this method is known as quantitative sensory testing (QST). The primary outcome of QST is determination of thresholds for specific modalities which are then compared to the established norms (Greenspan 2001; Goetz et al. 2005). Increase in threshold to painful stimuli is then interpreted as hypoalgesia. QST methods could be used not only in human studies but also in animal models.

One of the main goals of neurological evaluation is to determine the site and level of ▸ neuraxis where pathological processes that produce symptoms, including pain, originate (Dyck and O'Brien 2003). In addition to establishing the nature of ▸ neurological deficit, such as hypoalgesia to a specific modality, it is important to establish a special pattern of these abnormalities, since the pattern serves as the basis for the determination whether the lesion that is causing symptoms, including pain, involve specific peripheral nerve structures, such as peripheral nerves, plexus or the nerve root, versus central nervous system structures such as spinal cord, brainstem, subcortical or cortical structures and pathways of the brain.

Caveats and Unresolved Issues

Difficulty of assessing hypoalgesia arises from the inherent difficulty of assessing negative sensory phenomenon. For example, conceptually it is easier to illustrate ▸ positive sensory phenomenon to subjects, such as pain with instruction that 0 = none, and 10 = worst imaginable. In contrast, it is much harder conceptually to illustrate and request a rating of spontaneous loss of sensation because it is not possible to feel what one is not able to feel, in spite of the instruction that the patient is to imagine scaling between one end being a normal sensation and the other absence of sensation.

Another phenomenon that can result from painful stimulation and the one that is on the opposite end of the spectrum of sensory experience is ▶ hyperalgesia. The difficulty of assessing sensory abnormalities which are characterized by hypoalgesia to one sensory modality and hyperalgesia to another sensory modality in the same area frequently seen in patients with neuropathic pain leads to confusion not only for patients but also for inexperienced clinicians Depending on the way stimulation is conducted even when hypoalgesia is present, the outcome can be either hyperalgesia or hyperpathia. For example, in the case of partial hypoalgesia and when the stimulus is "strong enough" the outcome could be hyperalgesia, and in the case that stimulus is not "strong enough" with temporal and special summation that could result in increased pain, which would become hyperpathia. Consequently, from the pain mechanisms prospective, the relationship between hypoalgesia and hyperalgesia still far from clear. In summary, hypoalgesia is a ▶ clinical sign of neurological injury or disease, which in some patients can lead to neuropathic pain. Methods for determining the presence of hypoalgesia are qualitative, such as in bedside exam or quantitative, such as QST. Mechanisms of hypoalgesia for specific modalities, and in particular its relationship to hyperalgesia and hyperpathia, are poorly understood.

- ▶ Allodynia (Clinical, Experimental)
- ▶ Amygdala, Pain Processing and Behavior in Animals
- ▶ Cordotomy Effects on Humans and Animal Models
- ▶ Nerve Growth Factor Overexpressing Mice as Models of Inflammatory Pain
- ▶ Opioids, Effects of Systemic Morphine on Evoked Pain

References

1. Merskey H, Bogduk N (1994) Classification of Chronic Pain, vol 2. IASP Press, Seattle
2. Backonja MM, Galer BS (1998) Pain Assessment and Evaluation of Patients who have Neuropathic Pain. Neurol Clin 16:775–790
3. Lindblom U, Ochoa J (1986) Somatosensory Function and Dysfunction. In: Asbury AK, McKhann GM, McDonald WI (eds) Diseases of the Nervous System. Clinical Neurobiology. W.B. Saunders Company, Philadelphia, pp 283–298
4. Backonja M (2003) Defining Neuropathic Pain. Anesthesia Analgesia 97:785–790
5. Greenspan JD (2001) Quantitative Assessment of Neuropathic Pain. Curr Pain Headache Rep 5:107–113
6. Dyck PJ, O'Brien PC (2003) Quantitative Sensory Testing: Report of the Therapeutics and Technology Assessment Subcommittee of the American Academy of Neurology. Neurology 61:1628–1630
7. Getz KK, Cook T, Backonja MM (2005) Pain Ratings at the Thresholds are Necessary for Interpretation of Quantitative Sensory Testing. Muscle Nerve 32:179–184

Hypochondriaca

Definition

Hypochondriaca refers to a persistent conviction that one is or is likely to become ill, when a patient complains of symptoms that have no organic basis. These symptoms persist despite reassurance and medical evidence to the contrary

▶ Psychiatric Aspects of Visceral Pain

Hypochondriasis

H

Definition

Hypochondriasis is a minimum six month preoccupation with fears of having a serious disease, based on misinterpretation of bodily symptoms (e.g. a sore throat is thought to be throat cancer), which persists in spite of medical evidence that the serious disease is not present.

▶ Somatization and Pain Disorders in Children

Hypochondriasis, Somatoform Disorders and Abnormal Illness Behaviour

ISSY PILOWSKY
Emeritus Professor of Psychiatry, University of Adelaide, Adelaide, SA, Australia
issyp@med.usyd.edu.au

Synonyms

Abnormal Illness Behaviour of the Unconsciously Motivated, Somatically Focussed Type; Discordant Illness Behaviour; Dysnosognosia; somatoform disorders

Definition

In the Fourth edition of the Diagnostic and Statistical Manual of the American Psychiatric Association (1994), Hypochondriasis is defined according to the following criteria:

- Because of misinterpreting bodily symptoms, the patient becomes preoccupied with ideas or fears of having a serious illness.
- Appropriate medical investigation and reassurance do not relieve these ideas.
- These ideas are not delusional (as in Delusional Disorder) and are not restricted to concern about appearance (as in Body Dysmorphic Disorder).
- They cause distress that is clinically important or impair work, social or personal functioning.
- They have lasted 6 months or longer.

- These ideas are better explained by Generalized Anxiety Disorder, Major Depressive Episode, Obsessive-Compulsive Disorder, Panic Disorder, Separation Anxiety or a different Somatoform Disorder.

Specify when with poor insight: During most of this episode, the patient does not realize that the preoccupation is excessive or unreasonable.

It is of interest to compare this development with the earlier criteria for the diagnosis of hypochondriasis as listed in DSM–IIIR (the revised edition of DSM–III). They are as follows:

a) Preoccupation with the fear of having, or the belief that one has, a serious disease, based on the person's interpretation of physical signs or sensations as evidence of physical illness.
b) Appropriate physical evaluation does not support the diagnosis of any physical disorder that can account for the physical signs or the person's unwarranted interpretation of them, and the symptoms in 'A' are not just those of panic attacks.
c) The fear of having or belief that one has a disease persists despite medical reassurance.
d) Duration of the disturbance is at least six months.
e) The belief in A is not of delusional intensity, as in Delusional Disorder, Somatic Type (i.e. the person can acknowledge the possibility that the fear or the belief of having a serious illness is unfounded). [Comment: In which case the psychopathological phenomenon could be labelled an 'abnormal preoccupation' or an 'overvalued idea'.].

Characteristics

Hypochondriasis is regarded as one of the Somatoform Disorders in both the DSM IV, and the tenth edition of the WHO Classification of Mental and Behavioural Disorders: (ICD–10): Clinical descriptions and diagnostic guidelines.

The Somatoform disorders are defined in DSM IV as essentially the presence of physical symptoms for which there are no demonstrable organic findings or known physiological mechanisms'.

In both DSM–IV and ICD–10, a significant departure is made from the principle of classifying on the basis of phenomenological description only. Thus, in DSM–IV we find the inclusion of the statement that 'the symptoms are linked to psychological factors or conflicts'.

Illness, the Sick role, illness behaviour and abnormal illness behaviour. (Pilowsky 1969, 1978, 1997).

Illness is defined as any state of an organism which fulfils the requirements of a relevant reference group for admission to a sick role.

The Sick Role

As delineated by the sociologist Talcott Parsons (1964, 1978), the sick role is a partially and conditionally granted social role. The individual seeking this role is required to fulfil three obligations. These are: a) accept that the role is "undesirable"; one which should be relinquished a soon as possible; b) co-operate with others so as to achieve "health", and c) utilize the services of those regarded by society as competent to diagnose and treat the condition. (In technologically advanced societies, this person is usually a formally registered doctor who is granted the authority to sign 'sickness certificates')

If these obligations are met, the following privileges are granted: a) the person is regarded as not "responsible" for the condition (i.e. he cannot produce or terminate it by an act of will, and is not to be considered a malingerer); b) the person is regarded as someone requiring care, and c) is entitled to exemption from age appropriate normal obligations.

All of these definitions demonstrate how central the role of the doctor is (in Technologically advanced societies) when it comes to the allocation of healthcare resources. It also draws attention to the pressures on the Doctor-Patient relationship from without, and their inevitable interaction with interpersonal and intrapersonal forces.

Abnormal Illness Behaviour (AIB)

This is defined as: An inappropriate or maladaptive mode of experiencing, evaluating or acting in relation to one's own state of health, despite the fact that a doctor (or other recognized social agent) has offered accurate and reasonably lucid information concerning the person's health status and the appropriate course of management (if any), based on a thorough examination of all parameters of functioning (i.e. physical psychological and social) taking into account the individuals age, educational and socio-cultural background.

A detailed analysis of this definition is to be found in Pilowsky (1997).

Clinical Characteristics

Pain is a common feature of hypochondriacal disorders. Since the patient tends to reject the presence of psychological problems, such individuals are not encountered in psychiatric settings but rather in medical, surgical and, in the case of conversion disorders, in neurological clinics.

Another relevant somatoform disorder is 'conversion disorder', also known as 'Hysterical neurosis, conversion type' The difference between hypochondriasis and conversion, is that the latter is defined as manifesting 'a loss or alteration of physical functioning that suggests a physical disorder in the absence of physical signs on examination to support the presence of a physical disorder'. However 'psychological factors are judged to be aetiologically related, because of a temporal relationship between a psychosocial stressor that is apparently related to a psychological conflict or need, and initiation or exacerbation of the symptom.'

A feature often described in association with a conversion disorder is 'la belle indifference', which refers not simply to an absence of concern, but rather to a sort of positive serenity, clearly inappropriate to the apparent seriousness of the physical disability.

The condition named 'somatoform pain disorder' is described in virtually the same terms as conversion disorder, except for the statement that it is primarily characterised by: 'Pain which causes significant distress or impairment in functioning, which cannot be fully explained by a physician. It must be judged to be related to psychological factors and cannot be better explained by another disorder'.

Thus, the major difference between pain as a feature of hypochondriasis, and pain as a conversion symptom, is that in the former case there is concern and preoccupation as to what the pain may mean, in terms of specific illnesses such as cancer or heart disease; while in the latter the patient denies concern over any specific condition, but is rather troubled by the experience of pain as a cause of disability and suffering.

Management

The key to management is the establishment of an alliance with the patient. This issue is of particular salience, when the clinician is a psychologist or psychiatrist, has been discussed at length in Pilowsky (1997), because patients often consider a referral to such a person to mean that the referring doctor believes 'it is all in my mind'. By which is meant that they are being accused of malingering. Achieving an alliance is not possible unless the acceptance of the reality of the symptoms is clearly conveyed to the patient by the attention paid to the alleviation of discomfort, and prevention of further disability by appropriate supportive psychotherapeutic, physiotherapeutic and psychopharmacological (e.g. antidepressants in low doses), and if necessary by psychological methods such as cognitive-behavioural therapy. In theory, this should be easiest at the initial presentation to the first doctor who sees the patient, especially as this is usually a non-psychiatrist, and most often a family doctor who should, ideally, be well acquainted with the patient and his circumstances, as well as, hopefully, his family.

How this doctor might manage the situation has been described and researched by Goldberg et al. (1989). They have developed a methodology whereby the doctor can help the patient to reattribute the physical symptoms to psychological causes. Once this has been achieved, it is reasonable to proceed with a problem-solving approach to any of the difficulties the patient is invariably experiencing in his life (Rost and Smith 1990; Wilkinson and Mynors-Wallis 1994; Scicchitano 20000) .When a multi-modal approach is necessary, this is generally best provided by a multidisciplinary pain clinic, when it is available.

Some Pain Clinics have in-patient facilities with well trained experienced staff that are able to provide programmes for patients manifesting severe invalidism and perhaps dependence on drugs such as opiates.

References

1. American Psychiatric Association (1994) Diagnostic and Statistical Manual of Mental Disorders, 3rd edn Revised. American Psychiatric Association, Washington, DC
2. Goldberg DP, Gask L, O'Dowd T (1989) The Treatment of Somatization-Teaching Techniques of Reattribution. J Psychosom Res 33:689–696
3. Parsons T (1964) Social Structure and Personality. Collier-Macmillan, London
4. Parsons T (1978) Action Theory and the Human Condition. Free Press, New York
5. Pilowsky I (1969) Abnormal Illness Behaviour. Br J Med Psychol 42:347–351
6. Pilowsky I (1978) A General Classification of Abnormal illness Behaviours. Br J Med Psychol 51:131–137
7. Pilowsky I (1997) Abnormal Illness Behaviour. Wiley, Chichester
8. Rost KM, Smith GR Jr (1990) Improving the Effectiveness of Routine Care for Somatization. J Psychosom Res 43:463–465
9. Scicchitano JP (2000) Identification and Management of Somatisation in the Primary Care Setting in Terms of Illness Behaviour and Risk of Psychiatric Illness. PhD Thesis, University of Adelaide
10. Wilkinson P, Mynors-Wallis L (1990) Problem-Solving Therapy in the Treatment of Unexplained Physical Symptoms in Primary Care. J Psychosom Res 38:591–598
11. World Health Organisation (1992) Classification of Mental and Behavioural Disorders: Clinical descriptions and Diagnostic Guidelines. World Health Organization, Geneva

H

Hypoesthesia, Assessment

MISHA-MIROSLAV BACKONJA
Department of Neurology, University of Wisconsin-Madison, Madison, WI, USA
backonja@neurology.wisc.edu

Synonyms

Hypesthesia; hypoaesthesia

Definition

Hypoesthesia refers to decreased perception of innocuous stimuli, a condition where the body is much less sensitive than normal to stimulation that by its nature and intensity does not produce pain. Special senses are excluded (Merskey and Bogduk 1994). Hypoesthesia refers to diminished perception of a large range of mechanical stimuli such as touch, brush, pressure and vibration and thermally innocuous stimuli of warm and cold. Stimulation and locus are specified. Hypoesthesia is also defined as a raised threshold to nonpainful stimuli and this definition is used as a criterion for hypoesthesia during quantitative sensory testing (QST). There are two phenomena that are the opposite of hypoesthesia, hyperesthesia and allodynia. Hyperesthesia is increased but not painful sensation from innocuous stimulation and allodynia is pain from innocuous stimulation. If stimulation is of nature or intensity to produce tissue damage and the subject perceives it as harmless, then the phenomenon is defined as hypoalgesia.

Characteristics

Hypoesthesia is a ► negative sensory phenomenon seen primarily in patients with neurological disease or injury, including patients with ► neuropathic pain (Lindblom and Ochoa 1986; Backonja and Galer 1998; Backonja 2003). Hypoesthesia indicates decrease or loss of function that arises as a result of neurological disease or injury affecting somatic sensory and thermal pathways, anywhere from primary afferents to cerebral cortical structures. Hypoesthesia is demonstrated by means of sensory examination during which standard methods of mechanical and thermal stimulus are applied with the goal of activating specific classes of receptors. The specificity of somatic sensory pathways in conducting particular somatic sensations is significantly altered by disease and injury of the ► somatosensory nervous system and hypoesthesia is probably the most sensitive and reliable indication of such injury. In contrast, positive sensory phenomena, such as allodynia and ► hyperalgesia, are relatively frequent components of neuropathic pain; the complexity of underlying mechanisms makes them much more difficult to interpret. Understanding the relationship between injury of the somatosensory neural structures and its manifestations, such as hypoesthesia is relevant to pain mechanisms, because methods of testing and interpretations are based on the specificity of sensory modalities. Distinction of hypoesthesia from hypoalgesia is based primarily on the type and intensity of the stimulus applied to the thermonociceptive sensory system.

Methods of Assessment and Interpretation

Assessment of sensory nervous system function is most commonly done at the bedside and under these circumstances the testing is primarily qualitative in nature. Quantitative assessment increasingly utilizes computerized electronic equipment in the environment of a quantitative sensory laboratory (Backonja and Galer 1998; Greenspan 2001). Either approach should be able to detect hypoesthesia, but the ways in which these methods arrive at conclusions about the presence and severity of hypoesthesia are distinctly different and this distinction is also reflected in the definitions stated earlier. Qualitative bedside examination of the presence of hypoesthesia is based primarily on patient report that a stimulus is perceived as decreased. Quantitative sensory testing arrives at conclusions about hypoesthesia on the basis of raised thresholds to painful stimuli. Qualitative somatosensory assessment is based on the subject's ability to compare and report quality of sensation resulting from standard methods of stimulation of affected areas compared to normal unaffected areas. The qualitative method is very convenient for bedside evaluations. Frequently utilized bedside methods include standard neurological examination tools such as cotton tips, monofilaments, tuning forks for testing of vibration and various metal objects that can conveniently be warmed or cooled in the clinical setting. A degree of quantification is possible and requires that the subject report whether the decrease in perceived sensation from applied stimuli is mild, moderate, severe or completely absent when compared to a normal unaffected area. Since the qualitative method requires psychophysical interaction, this method can only be used in humans who can communicate linguistically with the examiner and hence cannot be used in infants or aphasic subjects or in animal models in somatosensory and pain research.

Quantitative assessment of sensory deficits requires a more sophisticated approach and frequently utilizes electronically controlled devices, though a number of psychophysical methods especially mechanical stimuli are used. Traditionally this method is known as quantitative sensory testing (QST). All of the quantitative methods require much longer times for completion. The primary outcome of QST is determination of thresholds for specific modalities, which are then compared, to the established norms (Greenspan 2001). Increases in the threshold to innocuous stimuli are interpreted as hypoesthesia. The QST method can be used not only in human studies but also in animal models.

A crucial step in the interpretation of QST is to obtain a pain rating at the threshold. In spite of the fact that the pain threshold is increased, the presence or absence of positive sensory phenomena, one of them being ► hyperpathia (increased threshold but even innocuous stimuli are perceived as painful) and consequently presence of a painful neuropathic disorder (Getz Kelly 2004). The advantage of testing with innocuous stimuli and detecting hypoesthesia, especially for cold detection, is that it is one of the most sensitive methods of detecting somatic sensory deficits, which characterize neurological disorders, including neuropathic pain disorders (Dyck 2000).

One of the main goals of neurological evaluation is to determine the site and level of ► neuraxis where pathological processes that produce symptoms, including pain, originate (Dyck and O'Brien 2003). In addition to establishing the nature of the ► neurological deficit, such as hypoesthesia, to a specific modality, it is important to establish the special pattern of these abnormalities, since the pattern serves as the basis for the determination as to whether the lesion that is causing symptoms including pain, involves specific peripheral nerve structures, such as peripheral nerves, plexuses or nerve roots, or central nervous system structures such as spinal cord, brainstem, subcortical or cortical structures and pathways of the brain.

Caveats and Unresolved Issues

The difficulty of assessing hypoesthesia arises from the inherent difficulty of assessing a negative sensory phenomenon. For example, it is easier conceptually to illustrate to the subjects a ▶ positive sensory phenomenon, such as pain, with instructions that 0=none and 10=worst imaginable. In contrast, it is much harder conceptually to illustrate and request a rating of spontaneous loss of sensation, because it is not possible to feel what one is not able to feel, in spite of the instruction that the patient is to imagine scaling between normal sensation and absence of sensation.

Other phenomena that can result from innocuous stimulation and are on the opposite end of the spectrum of sensory experience are hyperesthesia, allodynia or even hyperpathia. Confusion for the examiner as well as for the patient is caused by the difficulty of assessment that comes from the fact that pain disorders, most frequently neuropathic pain, are characterized by allodynia or hyperalgesia to one sensory testing modality but are also found to have evidence of hypoesthesia to another testing modality in the same area. Depending on the way stimulation is conducted, even when hypoesthesia is present, the outcome can be hyperpathia in case of repeated stimulation. For example, in the case of partial hypoesthesia when the stimulus is in the way to lead to temporal and special summation could result in increased threshold but what is perceived is painful, which is then interpreted as hyperpathia. Consequently, from the pain mechanisms perspective, the relationship of hypoesthesia and hyperpathia still far from clear.

In summary, hypoesthesia is a sensitive clinical sign of neurological injury or disease, which in some patients can lead to neuropathic pain. Methods for determining the presence of hypoesthesia are qualitative, as in bedside examination or quantitative, as with QST. Mechanisms of hypoesthesia for specific modalities and its relationship to hyperpathia are still not well understood.

References

1. Backonja M (2003) Defining neuropathic pain. Anesth Analg 97:785–790
2. Backonja MM, Galer BS (1998) Pain assessment and evaluation of patients who have neuropathic pain. Neurol Clin North Am 16:775–790
3. Dyck PJ, O'Brien PC (2003) Quantitative sensory testing: Report of the Therapeutics and Technology Assessment Subcommittee of the American Academy of Neurology. Neurology 61:1628–1630
4. Greenspan JD (2001) Quantitative assessment of neuropathic pain. Curr Pain Headache Reports 5:107–113
5. Lindblom U, Ochoa J (1986) Somatosensory function and dysfunction. In: Asbury AK, McKhann GM, McDonald WI (eds) Diseases of the Nervous System -Clinical Neurobiology. W.B. Saunders Company, Philadelphia, pp 283–298
6. Merskey H, Bogduk N (1994) Classification of Chronic Pain, vol 2. IASP Press, Seattle

Hypogastric Neurectomy

Definition

Hypogastric Neurectomy is a surgical resection of the hypogastric nerves.

▶ Visceral Pain Models, Female Reproductive Organ Pain

Hyponatremia

Definition

Hyponatremia represents less than normal levels of sodium ions, or salt, in the blood, which may result in cognitive impairment.

▶ Trigeminal Neuralgia, Diagnosis and Treatment

Hypophysectomy

Definition

Excision of the pituitary gland is known as hypophysectomy.

▶ Cancer Pain Management, Neurosurgical Interventions

Hypotension of Spinal Fluid

▶ Headache Due to Low Cerebrospinal Fluid Pressure

Hypothalamic Pituitary Axis

Definition

These organs combine with the gonads to play a critical role in the development and regulation of a number of the body's systems, such as the reproductive and immune systems.

▶ Fibromyalgia

Hypothalamus

Definition

The hypothalamus is a very prominent group of neurons located below the thalamus at the base of the brain forming the ventral-most part of the diencephalon. It is divided into three lateral levels (medial, intermediate and lateral) and five caudo-rostral levels (mammillary, posterior, intermediate, anterior, and preoptic). Its role includes the neuroendocrine regulations (arcuate, paraventricular and supraoptic nuclei), autonomic regulations (cardio-respiratory, thermoregulation, metabolic, digestive) and processing of motivational behaviors like sexual, feeding, drinking, waking/sleep state, aggressiveness and illness feeling. It is also involved in modulating nociception.

▶ Descending Circuitry, Transmitters and Receptors
▶ Parabrachial Hypothalamic and Amydaloid Projections

Hypothalamus and Nociceptive Pathways

JEAN-FRANÇOIS BERNARD
Faculté de Médecine Pitié-Salpêtrière, Institut National de la Santé et de la Recherche Médicale, INSERM U-677, Paris, France
jfbernar@ext.jussieu.fr

Definition

The hypothalamus is a complex structure that occupies the ventral half of the diencephalon below the thalamus on either side of the third ventricle. It lies just above the ▶ pituitary gland responsible for neuroendocrine secretions.

The hypothalamus includes about 40 nuclei of very different shapes and sizes. For simplification, it is generally divided into three medio-lateral zones, periventricular, medial and lateral and four caudo-rostral regions, mammillary, tuberal, anterior and preoptic. Combination of zones and regions permitted the recognition of twelve hypothalamic areas (Simerly 1995).

Neurosecretory neurons are mainly located within the periventricular zone with a particularly high density in the paraventricular nucleus. In addition, another important group of neurosecretory neurons is located in the supraoptic nucleus, a well-individualized nucleus located in the lateral region, on the lateral border of the optic chiasm. The neurosecretory system is subdivided into two parts, 1) magnocellular neurosecretory neurons (oxytocin and vasopressin), which directly innervate the posterior pituitary gland and 2) parvocellular neurosecretory neurons (corticotropin, gonadotropin, growth hormone, thyrotropin releasing hormones, somatostatin, angiotensin II and dopamine), which innervate the median eminence, the hypothalamic hormones being transported to the anterior pituitary gland *via* the hypophysial portal system (Swanson 1987).

The medial and lateral zones of the hypothalamus are chiefly devoted to the control of ▶ autonomic functions (cardiovascular, respiratory, blood fluid balance, energy metabolism, thermoregulatory and digestive) and major basic instinctive behaviors (feeding, drinking, reproductive, flight, defensive and aggressive) including the wakefulness-sleep cycles (Swanson 1987).

Characteristics

The hypothalamus is a fascinating region of the brain, which is much more than a control center for neuroendocrine secretion. Indeed, the hypothalamus is the upper center for autonomic functions and basic behaviors that assure the survival of both the individual and the species. It is easy to understand the role of the hypothalamus when it guarantees an adequate level of homeostasis for autonomic functions needed for survival. It is not so obvious to appreciate the importance of the myriad basic behaviors it generates. Thus, it is basically responsible for most of the motivations that govern our life, such as for example, hunger, the pleasures of eating and satiety, sexual desire, aggressiveness, fear, drowsiness, alertness and numerous other fundamental motivations of life. Considering these functions, it seems that the hypothalamus should play an important role in the autonomic and ▶ motivational components of pain. All the same, the precise role of hypothalamus in different components of pain remains unclear. The only clearly accepted function of the hypothalamus in pain is the neuroendocrine corticotropin response.

In humans, imagery studies indicate that the acute traumatic pain comes with a noticeable activation of the hypothalamus (Hsieh et al. 1996). However, these studies provide neither information about the activation of different hypothalamic nuclei nor data about the role of hypothalamus in pain. In fact until now, most evidence for an involvement of the hypothalamus in nociceptive processing comes from anatomical and c-fos data. Cross-checking these data with the known functions of hypothalamic nuclei, it becomes possible to make hypotheses about the involvement of the hypothalamus in pain.

Nociceptive Afferent Inputs to the Hypothalamus

The hypothalamus has three well-documented sources of nociceptive inputs, the spinal and trigeminal dorsal horn, the parabrachial area and the ventrolateral medulla (Fig. 1).

● Spinal and trigeminal inputs – a number of spinal and trigeminal neurons are labeled after a large injection of retrograde axonal tracer within the hypothalamus. Labeled neurons are located in superficial and, above all, in deep laminae of the dorsal horn i.e. in regions known to be involved in nociceptive processing. Electrophysiological studies indicate that most spino / trigemino-hypothalamic neurons respond to a variety of noxious stimuli (Burstein 1996). These data, which seem to indicate a major nociceptive input to the hypothalamus, are challenged by anterograde axonal tracing studies that show much lower spinal and trigeminal projection upon the hypothalamus (Gauriau and Bernard 2004). Comparative examination of all the studies seems to point

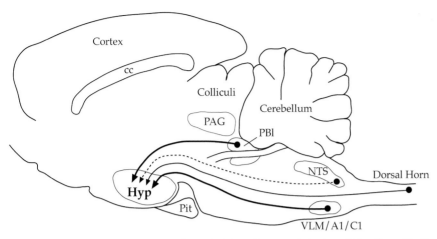

Hypothalamus and Nociceptive Pathways, Figure 1 Schematic representation, in sagittal sections, of the three main hypothalamic nociceptive inputs: the PBl, the VLM/A1/C1 region and the trigeminal and spinal dorsal horn (mainly the deep laminae). Thick line: extensive nociceptive projection; thin line: medium density nociceptive projection; dotted line: hypothetical nociceptive projection. Abbreviations: A1, A1 noradrenaline cells; C1, C1 adrenaline cells; cc, corpus callosum; Hyp, hypothalamus; NTS, nucleus tractus solitarii; PAG, periaqueductal gray matter; PBl, lateral division of the parabrachial nucleus; Pit, pituitary gland; VLM, ventrolateral medulla.

to at least a moderate but indisputable nociceptive projection, mainly to the lateral (Fig. 2) but also to the posterior and the paraventricular hypothalamic nuclei.

- Parabrachial inputs (see parabrachial hypothalamic and amygdaloid projections) –the lateral parabrachial area receives a heavy nociceptive input from spinal and trigeminal lamina I nociceptive neurons. The lateral parabrachial area projects heavily to the hypothalamic ventromedial nucleus and extensively to the retrochiasmatic, the median and the ventrolateral preoptic hypothalamus. Although less extensive, a notable projection reaches the dorsomedial, the periventricular, the paraventricular and the lateral nuclei (Fig. 2). Electrophysiological studies indicate that this strong afferent input to the hypothalamus from the parabrachial nucleus is primarily nociceptive (Bernard et al. 1996; Bester et al. 1997).
- Caudal ventrolateral medulla inputs –this reticular region includes the A1 / C1 catecholaminergic neurons and receives nociceptive inputs from both the superficial and the deep laminae of the dorsal horn. The caudal ventrolateral medulla projects extensively to the paraventricular nucleus and, to a lesser extent, to the periventricular, the supraoptic and the median preoptic hypothalamic nuclei (Fig. 2). Here again it was shown that this afferent input contains nociceptive neurons (Burstein 1996; Pan et al. 1999).

The nucleus of the solitary tract was also proposed as a nociceptive input for the hypothalamus. However, this nucleus is primarily a center for autonomic / visceral and gustatory information. The role and the importance of solitary tract neurons in conveying nociceptive messages from the spinal cord to the hypothalamus need to be confirmed.

To summarize, anatomical data indicate several hypothalamic subregions that appear to be more specifically involved in nociceptive processing:

1. The neuroendocrine group (the paraventricular nucleus and to a lesser extent the periventricular and supraoptic nuclei) that receives nociceptive messages from all the nociceptive sources described above.
2. The ventromedial nucleus, the perifornical and the retrochiasmatic areas that receive a very prominent nociceptive input from the parabrachial area.
3. The median and ventrolateral preoptic area, the dorsomedial, the lateral and the posterior hypothalamic region, which receive lower but yet substantial nociceptive inputs.

Corroborating the anatomical data closely, it was shown that various painful stimuli evoke c-fos expression in regions receiving nociceptive afferent projections. The strongest c-fos expression was observed in neuroendocrine neurons of the hypothalamus located in the paraventricular, the supraoptic and the periventricular / arcuate nuclei. A substantial c-fos expression is evoked in the posterior, the ventromedial and the dorsomedial nuclei and the retrochiasmatic, the lateral and the anterior regions of the hypothalamus (Rodella et al. 1998; Snowball et al. 2000).

Role of Hypothalamus in Visceromotor Responses to Painful Stimuli

The anatomical data indicate that both parabrachial and A1 / C1 projections to the paraventricular nucleus innervate more densely neurons containing corticotropin releasing hormone as well as ▶ magnocellular neurons (that contain vasopressin and oxytocin). Painful stimuli evoke specifically c-fos expression in neurons containing corticotropin releasing hormone, vasopressin

H

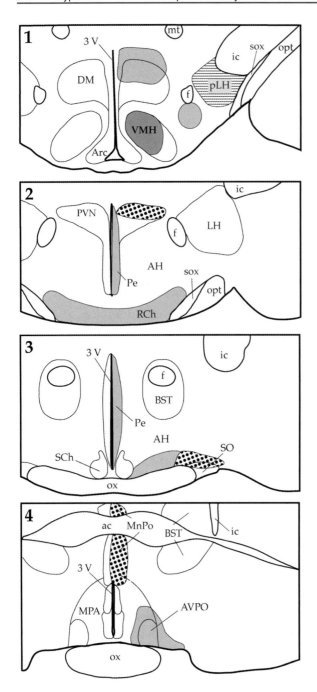

Hypothalamus and Nociceptive Pathways, Figure 2 Summary diagram illustrating, in coronal sections, the location of nociceptive projections within the hypothalamus (1–4, caudal to rostral). The parabrachial "nociceptive" area projects primarily upon the VMH (dark gray) and extensively upon the DM and the perifornical area (1), the RCh and the Pe (2), the rostral Pe and the ventral AH (3) and the AVPO (4) hypothalamic nuclei (gray). Both the parabrachial nucleus and the A1/C1 group within the ventrolateral medulla project to the PVN (2), the SO (3) and the MnPO (4) (black points). Both the parabrachial area and the spinal and trigeminal dorsal horn project to the pLH (1) (horizontal hatching). Abbreviations: 3V, third ventricle; A1/C1 A1, noradrenaline cells, C1, adrenaline cells; ac, anterior commissure; AH, anterior hypothalamic area; Arc, arcuate nucleus; AVPO, anteroventral preoptic nucleus; BST, bed nucleus of stria terminals; DM, dorsal medial nucleus; f, fornix; ic internal capsule; LH, lateral hypothalamus; MnPO, median preoptic nucleus; MPA, medial preoptic area; mt, mammillothalamic tract; opt, optic tract; ox optic chiasm; Pe, periventricular nucleus; pLH, posterior portion of lateral hypothalamus; PVN, paraventricular nucleus; RCh, retrochiasmatic area; SCh, suprachiasmatic nucleus; SO, supraoptic nucleus; sox, supraoptic decussation; VMH, ventromedial hypothalamic nucleus

and oxytocin at the levels of paraventricular, arcuate and supraoptic nuclei. This neuroendocrine response is specific for these neurohormones; it does not include gonadotropin, growth hormone, and thyrotropin releasing hormones (Pan et al. 1996).

The neuroendocrine component of pain is indisputably under hypothalamic control with well-identified pain pathways to drive it. The role of these neurohormones in pain is not completely understood. It is likely that an increase in the corticotropin hormone axis is important to cope with the dangerous or traumatic situation

that comes with pain (mobilization of metabolism and mental energy). Nonetheless, in the case of chronic pain, the stimulation of the corticotropin axis might become deleterious (anxiety, depression, decrease of immunity, neuronal loss). Vasopressin may accompany corticotropin secretion to increase or maintain blood pressure. The role and amount of oxytocin secretion in cases of acute pain remain yet poorly understood.

Importantly, psychological stress (immobilization, anxiety, and fear) acts on the corticotropin axis of the hypothalamus *via* limbic projections (bed nucleus of the stria terminalis, prefrontal cortex) different from those described for nociceptive stimuli (physical stress).

Numerous paraventricular neurons (chiefly in a dorsal position) are not neuroendocrine cells but provide descending projections to the brainstem and the spinal cord. Although the paraventricular nucleus provides the more extensive set of descending projections, other hypothalamic nuclei also receiving nociceptive messages send similar descending projections, namely the periventricular, the retrochiasmatic area, the dorsomedial, the dorsal, the perifornical and the lateral hypothalamic areas. These hypothalamic neurons project to the periaqueductal gray matter, the parabrachial area, the solitary tract, the motor vagus, the ambiguous nuclei and the ventrolateral medulla in the brainstem. In the spinal cord, they project chiefly to the sympathetic preganglionic column (Saper 1995). These hypothalamic neurons are adequately placed to drive both the sympathetic and the ▶ parasympathetic components of pain. They might, in connection with brainstem neurons, increase or decrease blood pressure and cardiac frequency and modify circulatory territory, according to the nature of the painful stimuli.

Role of Hypothalamus in Behavioral Response to Painful Stimuli

Several hypothalamic nuclei, which receive an extensive nociceptive input, play an important role in motivational components of pain.

The first group, including the ventromedial and the dorsomedial nuclei, the perifornical and the retrochiasmatic areas, is markedly involved in defensive-aggressive behavior. This group of nuclei projects extensively to the periaqueductal gray matter, each nucleus targeting a specific quadrant. The periaqueductal gray matter appears to be a major hypothalamic descending output to mediate aggressive-defensive behavior. Each nucleus of this hypothalamic group receives an extensive nociceptive input from the lateral parabrachial area, the ventromedial hypothalamic nucleus receiving the heaviest input. The ventromedial nucleus has been involved in aggressive-defensive behavior. Stimulation applied in this nucleus induces vocalization, attack, escape, piloerection, mydriasis and micturition that resemble the pseudo-affective reactions induced by noxious stimuli (Bester et al. 1997; Swanson 1987). Recently, the dorsomedial portion of the ventromedial nucleus has been shown to be responsible for the vocalization induced by painful electrical shock applied to the tail (Borszcz 2002). The ventromedial nucleus has also been involved in feeding behavior (it has long been considered as the "satiety center") and regulation of energy metabolism (Swanson 1987). Recently, the ventromedial hypothalamic nucleus has thus been proposed to be responsible for the anorexia induced by migraine (Malick et al. 2001). Pain should act on appetite *via* a parabrachio-ventromedial CCKergic link. Leptin receptors, which

are abundant in this hypothalamic nucleus, might also participate in the loss of appetite. Finally, stimulation applied within the ventromedial nuclei produces an analgesia, which is also probably mediated *via* the periaqueductal output. Thus, it appears that the medial zone of the tuberal (posterior) and the anterior hypothalamus is responsible for the defensive-aggressive and feeding motivational component of pain.

The second group, including the median and the anteroventral preoptic hypothalamic nuclei, is involved in osmotic / blood fluids balance regulation and sleep promoting / thermoregulation functions. These nuclei also receive a substantial nociceptive input from the lateral parabrachial area. The influence of nociceptive input upon the neurons of this hypothalamic region is less clear. It might alter drinking behavior, vasopressin secretion, falling asleep and the thermoregulation set point according to the nature of the nociceptive aggression (Saper et al. 2001; Swanson 1987).

The posterior portion of the lateral hypothalamus receives a diffuse but substantial nociceptive input directly from the deep laminae of the dorsal horn and indirectly *via* the internal lateral parabrachial nucleus. The role of the lateral hypothalamus in nociceptive processing remains obscure because this hypothalamic region was involved in a myriad functions, such as feeding behavior (it has long been considered to be a "feeding center"), drinking behavior and cardiovascular and visceral regulation, as well as in wakefulness and antinociceptive and rewarding mechanisms. However, the recent discovery that ▶ narcolepsy can be induced by lack of orexin / hypocretin (a peptide located in the neurons of lateral hypothalamus), indicates that the lateral hypothalamus is probably markedly involved in the wakefulness mechanism (Saper 2001). One role of nociceptive inputs upon neurons of the posterior lateral hypothalamus could be to trigger awakening.

Conclusion

Bringing together anatomical and functional data, the hypothalamus appears as a key center for most visceromotor (neuroendocrine, autonomic response) and motivational (aggressive-defensive reactions, ingestive behaviors, wakefulness, antinociception) components of pain. It yet remains to check experimentally the actual role of hypothalamic subregions and / or neuromodulators in the genesis of different components of pain. Anatomical data also indicate that hypothalamic functions are probably strongly modulated by the upper limbic structures (notably the extended amygdala and the cingulate / prefrontal cortex), which are also involved in the emotional appreciation of pain.

References

1.   Bernard JF, Bester H, Besson JM (1996) Involvement of the spino parabrachio-amygdaloid and -hypothalamic pathways in the autonomic and affective emotional aspects of pain. Prog Brain Res 107:243–255

2. Bester H, Besson JM, Bernard JF (1997) Organization of efferent projections from the parabrachial area to the hypothalamus: a Phaseolus vulgaris-leucoagglutinin study in the rat. J Comp Neurol 383:245–281
3. Borszcz GS (2002) The ventromedial hypothalamus contributes to generation of the affective dimension of pain in rats. Program N°. 653.5 2002 Abstract Viewer / Itinerary Planner. Society for Neuroscience, Washington, DC, Online
4. Burstein R (1996) Somatosensory and visceral input to the hypothalamus and limbic system. Prog Brain Res 107:257–267
5. Gauriau C, Bernard JF (2004) A comparative reappraisal of projections from the superficial laminae of the dorsal horn in the rat: the forebrain. J Comp Neurol 468:24–56
6. Hsieh JC, Stahle-Backdahl M, Hagermark O et al. (1996) Traumatic nociceptive pain activates the hypothalamus and the periaqueductal gray: a positron emission tomography study. Pain 64:303–314
7. Malick A, Jakubowski M, Elmquist JK et al. (2001) A neurohistochemical blueprint for pain-induced loss of appetite. Proc Natl Acad Sci USA. 98: 9930–9935. Erratum in: Proc Natl Acad Sci USA 98:14186
8. Pan B, Castro-Lopes JM, Coimbra A (1996) Activation of anterior lobe corticotrophs by electroacupuncture or noxious stimulation in the anaesthetized rat, as shown by colocalization of Fos protein with ACTH and beta-endorphin and increased hormone release. Brain Res Bull 40:175–182
9. Pan B, Castro-Lopes,JM, Coimbra A (1999) Central afferent pathways conveying nociceptive input to the hypothalamic paraventricular nucleus as revealed by a combination of retrograde labeling and c-fos activation. J Comp Neurol 413:129–145
10. Rodella L, Rezzani R, Gioia M et al. (1998) Expression of Fos immunoreactivity in the rat supraspinal regions following noxious visceral stimulation. Brain Res Bull 47:357–366
11. Saper CB (1995) Central autonomic system. In: Paxinos G (ed) The rat nervous system, 2nd edn. Academic Press, San Diego, pp 107–135
12. Saper C, Chou TC, Scammell TE (2001) The sleep switch: hypothalamic control of sleep and wakefulness. Trends Neurosci 24:726–731
13. Simerly RB (1995) Anatomical substrates of hypothalamic integration. In: Paxinos G (ed) The rat nervous system, 2nd edn. Academic Press, San Diego, pp 353–376
14. Snowball RK, Semenenko FM, Lumb BM (2000) Visceral inputs to neurons in the anterior hypothalamus including those that project to the periaqueductal gray: a functional anatomical and electrophysiological study. Neuroscience 99:351–361
15. Swanson LW (1987) The hypothalamus. In: Hökfelt T, Swanson LW (eds) Handbook of chemical neuroanatomy, vol 5. Integrated systems of the CNS, part I. Elsevier, Amsterdam, Oxford, pp 1–124

Hypothalamus-Anterior Pituitary-Gonadal Axis

Definition

The hypothalamus controls endocrine function by direct release of neuropeptides, or indirectly through the secretion of regulatory hormones to the anterior pituitary. These regulatory substances are secreted by the hypothalamus into the local portal plexus within the median eminence, which then drains into the blood vessels of the anterior pituitary. There are a wide number of substances released by the hypothalamus that either inhibit or stimulate the release of anterior pituitary hormones, including factors that affect the release of growth hormone, thyrotropin, and others. Related to sexual and reproductive function, the hypothalamus secretes prolactin-releasing factor (PRF), which stimulates the release of prolactin. Dopamine, also secreted by the hypothalamus, inhibits prolactin's release. Additionally, the hypothalamus secretes gonadotropin-releasing hormone (GnRH) to the pituitary gland, which triggers the secretion of luteinizing hormone (LH) from the pituitary gland. Luteinizing hormone then stimulates the Leydig cells of the testes to produce testosterone or the ovaries to produce progesterone.

▶ Cancer Pain Management, Opioid Side Effects, Endocrine Changes and Sexual Dysfunction

Hypoxia

Definition

Hypoxia is a pathological condition in which the whole organism (*generalized hypoxia*) or only a region of the organism (*tissue hypoxia*) is deprived of adequate oxygen supply.

▶ NSAIDs and Cancer

IAIABC System

► Impairment Rating, Ambiguity, IAIABC System

Iatrogenic Causes of Neuropathy

PAOLO MARCHETTINI

Pain Medicine Center, Scientific Institute San Raffaele, Milan, Italy

marchettini.paolo@hsr.it

Synonyms

Post Surgical Nerve Injury; Chronic Postoperative Pain; Chronic Post-Surgical Neuralgia

Definition

Iatros in Greek means physician, the term iatrogenic defines a pathological complication of medical care. ► Iatrogenic neuropathy is a nerve injury caused by surgical or pharmacological treatment or by its consequence.

It is estimated that iatrogenic neuropathy is a major cause of chronic pain, although the condition is still unrecognized and poorly managed. The encompassing term "► chronic post-surgical pain syndrome" which is commonly used to cluster all these not so rare outcomes of surgery, is unhelpful as it offers little insight into the pathophysiology operating in each case. For the sake of clarity, the use of the widespread terms "failed" and "syndrome" are not useful when defining post-surgical pain conditions, as they do not determine the etiology of the pain. A proper attempt to diagnose the cause of chronic post-surgical pain permits appropriate steering of the clinical management.

Characteristics

Pain and other abnormal sensory symptoms replicate the typical description of sensory aberration in mono- or poly-neuropathy (Hansson et al. 2001). Iatrogenic neuropathy however, has more psychological complications, because the recognition of nerve injury is often missed or belated. The onset of neuropathic pain can be delayed for days, weeks or, rarely, months. Doctor and patient may erroneously attribute early onset neuropathic pain to the expected "normal" post-operative pain. The operation was technically successful and there were no infections or other obvious complications. Delayed recognition may also be the consequence of immobilization by postoperative cast, bed rest, reduced activity or sedation due to anesthetic or analgesic medication. The nerve injury may selectively affect a sensory branch, hampering objective evidence of the lesion. The intensity of the pain is often unrelated to the severity of the nerve damage; indeed partial nerve injury may predispose to neuropathic pain to a greater extent than total injury. When the diagnosis is made, at times many years later, patients are frustrated by delayed treatment and by inadequate and unspecific clinical management (Horowitz 1984). The typical clinical picture of chronic pain, sensory disorder, insomnia and depression is complicated by frustration and disbelief toward physicians and other medical care providers, judged in general to be responsible for the prolonged and unnecessary suffering.

Symptoms

When a patient describes tingling (spontaneous discharges in large myelinated fibers), pins and needles (small myelinated fibers), cramps and burning (unmyelinated fibers) in the region of the surgical procedure, iatrogenic nerve injury is high on the list of differential diagnoses. The diagnosis is made based on such typical neuropathic symptoms and on the identification of sensory disorder in the anatomical territory of the injured nerve(s). It is also fundamental to search for a Tinel sign to identify the site of the injury. A condition that may hamper the diagnosis is a partial injury in continuity. Painful iatrogenic neuropathy often originates from injury confined to a sensory nerve, without evidence of muscle wasting and weakness. At times the nerve injury is rather selective, affecting small fascicular rami and may be hard to detect clinically and electrophysiologically. Command of peripheral nerve sub anatomy helps early recognition. As all neuropathic pains, iatrogenic neuralgia also can be spontaneous and evoked by stimuli to the skin or perhaps just movement. At times even minor stimuli, normally not painful, can evoke a burning and unpleasant tingling sensation or thermal sensations (dysesthesia - allodynia). Stimulus evoked pain is so distressing that patients report sensory dysfunction beyond the anatomical distribution of hypoesthesia, in territories that are wider than those supplied by the injured nerve. However, sensory dysfunction is usually confined within a territory that surrounds the cutaneous distribution of the affected plexus, root or peripheral nerve. Occasionally, the nerve injury is the consequence of progressive entrapment in the surgical scar. Such entrapment, unlike anatomical entrapment syndromes, is rarely focal, usually being more homogeneously distributed along the scar. In the early phase, ectopic neural activity may exist in the absence of nerve conduction block and neurophysiological signs may remain within normal values for a long time. The clinical equivalence is that the positive symptoms of pain, paresthesia and dysesthesia may appear without striking negative phenomena (hypo-anesthesia).

Diagnosis

In clinical practice recognizing a cutaneous nerve injury by the patient's description of tingling pins and needles and burning is relatively simple. Diagnosing an injury of nerves supplying deep structure is more demanding. In such cases the pain quality replicates the quality of a deep tissue injury, making the differential diagnosis between neuropathy and connective tissue disease not always so self-evident. Deep neuropathic pain is commonly more widespread and more difficult to localize, it is often referred at a distance from the injury site and might spread along an entire radicular territory. At times entrapment can be related to or aggravated by movement or positioning. If a nerve injury is suspected, a thorough clinical examination including sensory hyperphenomena (identification and documentation of allodynia and hyperalgesia) as well as sensory loss and motor function is required. Nerve conduction studies and quantitative sensory testing may be helpful in supporting the clinical diagnosis. When a comparison with a contralateral nerve is possible, the sensitivity of such a test is improved. The clinical assessment should also take into account that any injury to the sensory component of a motor nerve may result in pain. The motor system should be examined properly through electromyography and motor nerve conduction studies. This comprehensive sensorimotor examination allows objective identification of the neurological dysfunction. Careful evaluation means that precise follow-up can be ensured, providing a yardstick helpful in reassuring the patient that the nerve damage is not worsening and is possibly improving. Such evaluation also provides specific evidence in the event of medico-legal assessment. Assessment of the social and psychological aspects of the disease is also necessary, so that the full picture can be documented.

Epidemiology

Solid data are still much wanted. Cox et al. (1974) found a 27% incidence of neuropathic symptoms in the best-case scenario after saphenectomy. The majority of the injuries were symptomless. Only 12% of the patients, less than half of those with a clinically identifiable injury, reported subjective sensory abnormalities and only 5% of all operated patients reported pain. The most frequently injured nerves during medical interventions are 1)

brachial plexus; 2) palmar cutaneous branch of the median nerve; 3) infrapatellar cutaneous branch of the saphenous nerve, 4) ilioinguinal, iliohypogastric, genitofemoral and femoral nerves, 5) accessory and greater auricular nerves, 6) long thoracic nerve and 7) alveolar nerve. Our observation reiterates the homogeneous lists of Horowitz (1984), Dawson and Krarup (1989) and Sunderland (1991).

The surgical interventions most commonly associated with nerve injury are peripheral anesthetic nerve block, odontoiatric treatment, ENT surgery, cardiovascular surgery, orthopedic surgery and general surgery.

Odontoiatric Treatment

In endodontic surgery, nerve damage may result from direct intrusion of instruments or implants into the mandibular canal or from introducing neurotoxic substances such as paraformaldehyde close to the inferior alveolar nerve.

ENT Surgery

Nasal sinus surgery may damage the maxillary branch of the trigeminal nerve, resulting in persistent pain in the region of the eye (Neuhaus 1990).

Cardiovascular Surgery

Varicose vein striping, particularly of the saphenous vein, may result in nerve injury. After thoracotomy, a sensory disorder, in particular mechanical allodynia indicating a neuropathic component for the pain, has been found in 80 consecutive patients complaining of chronic pain after coronary artery by pass grafting (Eisenberg et al. 2001).

Orthopedic Surgery

Shoulder arthroscopy, as with all arthroscopic techniques, is becoming a more frequent cause of iatrogenesis, although reports vary widely (from 10% to one case out of 439 (Stanish and Peterson 1995).

Carpal tunnel release is a common surgical intervention that can be complicated by a lesion of the median and, more rarely, of the ulnar nerve. The reported incidence of iatrogenic nerve injury varies from five out of eighty three cases to 0.8% in a series of 3035 hands reported in a review of fourteen papers. Almost 10% of patients complaining of complications following endoscopic carpal tunnel release have neuropathic pain (Kelly et al. 1994). Breast surgery is associated with chronic pain sequels in over 20% of patients (Foley 1990). Harvesting of bone for grafting has been reported amongst the causes of injury to the lateral femoral-cutaneous nerve (Hudson et al. 1979). Incision around the knee joint has been associated with lesions of the infrapatellar branch of the saphenous nerve. In 1983, Swanson and co-workers reported a 63.2% incidence of prepatellar neuropathy in eighty-seven patients immediately after open meniscectomy, while Sherman and co-workers noted only a 0.6% incidence of reported symptoms following 2,640 arthroscopic procedures on the knee (Swanson 1983, Sherman et al. 1986). In 1995, Mochida and Kikuchi reported a 22.2% incidence of sensory disturbances in sixty-eight consecutive patients operated on between 1990 and 1991 (Mochida and Kikuchi 1995). Limb amputation is also frequently followed by chronic pain (the highest frequency reported is as high as 80% of the amputees).

General Surgery

Lymph node biopsy in the neck is sometimes associated with injury to the accessory nerve and cutaneous nerves in the neck (Murphy 1983). Ilioinguinal nerve lesion is an important complication following inguinal hernioplasty (Heise and Starling 1998). Anterior hernioplasty, which requires the dissection of spermatic cord and sensory nerves, is a more common cause of this injury. Laparoscopic repair of the hernia is increasing simultaneously with the injuries to neural structures coursing through the groin. The femoral branches of the genitofemoral nerve and the lateral cutaneous nerve of the thigh, not visible during laparoscopic inguinal hernia repair, are more vulnerable. Abdominal rectopexy has been associated with femoral nerve injury in six patients out of a series of twenty-four patients, twenty-one of whom were operated on for rectal prolapse and three for recto-rectal intussusception (Infantino et al. 1994).

Therapy

Treatment of painful iatrogenic neuropathy requires all means used in the management of any other neuropathic pain (Senegor 1991, Sindrup and Jensen 1999). In this medically provoked condition, it is even more fundamental to care for the psychological co-morbidities. These should be prevented by early recognition of the neuropathic symptoms and the identification of the injured nerve. Early recognition, besides improving pain management, avoiding psychological overlay and possibly preventing chronification, favors the reestablishment of a trustful patient doctor relationship.

References

1. Cox SJ, Wellwood JM, Martin A (1974) Saphenous nerve injury caused by stripping of the long saphenous vein. Br Med J 1:415–417
2. Dawson DM, Krarup C (1989) Perioperative nerve lesions. Arch Neurol 46:1355–1360
3. Eisenberg E, Pultorak Y, Pud D et al. (2001). Prevalence and characteristics of post coronary artery bypass graft surgery pain (PCP). Pain 92:11–17
4. Foley KM (1990) Brachial plexopathy in patients with breast cancer. In: Harris JR, Hellman S, Henderson IC et al. (eds) Breast Diseases, 2nd edn. Lippincott JB, Philadelphia, pp 722–729
5. Hansson PT, Lacerenza M, Marchettini P (2001) Aspects of clinical and experimental neuropathic pain: the clinical perspective. In: Hansson PT, Fields HL et al. (eds) Neuropathic Pain: Pathophysiology and Treatment. Progress in Pain Research and Management. IASP Press, Seattle, pp 1–18
6. Heise CP, Starling JR (1998) Mesh inguinodynia: a new clinical syndrome after inguinal herniorrhaphy? J Am Coll Surg 87:514–518
7. Horowitz SH (1984) Iatrogenic causalgia. Classification, clinical findings, and legal ramifications. Arch Neurol 41:821–824
8. Hudson AR, Hunter GA, Waddell JP (1979) Iatrogenic femoral nerve injuries. Can J Surg 22:62–66
9. Infantino A, Fardin P, Pirone E et al. (1994) Femoral nerve damage after abdominal rectopexy. Int J Colorectal Dis 9:32–4
10. Kelly CP, Pulisetti D, Jamieson AM (1994) Early experience with endoscopic carpal tunnel release. J Hand Surg (Br) 19:18–21
11. Mochida H, Kikuchi S (1995) Injury to infrapatellar branch of saphenous nerve in arthroscopic knee surgery. Clin Orthop Relat Res 320:88–94
12. Murphy TM (1983) Complications of diagnostic and therapeutic nerve blocks. In: Orkin FK, Cooperman LH (eds) Complications in anaesthesiology. Lippincott, Philadelphia
13. Neuhaus RW (1990) Orbital complications secondary to endoscopic sinus surgery. Ophthalmology 97:1512–1518
14. Senegor M (1991) Iatrogenic saphenous neuralgia: successful therapy with neuroma resection. Neurosurgery 28:295–298
15. Sherman OH, Fox JM, Snyder SJ et al. (1986) Arthroscopy-"no-problem surgery" An analysis of complications in two thousand six hundred and forty cases. JBJS 68:256–265
16. Sindrup SH, Jensen TS (1999) Efficacy of pharmacological treatments of neuropathic pain: an update and effect related to mechanism of drug action. Pain 83:389–400
17. Stanish WD, Peterson DC (1995) Shoulder arthroscopy and nerve injury: pitfalls and prevention. Arthroscopy 11:458–466
18. Sunderland S (1991) Miscellaneous causes of nerve injury. In: Sunderland S (ed) Nerve injuries and their repair. A critical appraisal. Churchill-Livingstone, Edinburgh, pp 197–199
19. Swanson AJ (1983) The incidence of prepatellar neuropathy following medial meniscectomy. Clin Orthop Relat Res 181:151–153

Iatrogenic Effect/Response

Definition

Iatrogenic effects/responses are outcomes inadvertently induced by a physician or surgeon or by medical treatment or diagnostic procedures.

▶ Acute Pain Management in Infants
▶ Cancer Pain, Assessment in Children
▶ Iatrogenic Causes of Neuropathy

Iatrogenic Neuropathy

Definition

Iatrogenic neuropathy is a nerve injury caused by surgical or pharmacological treatment, or by its consequence.

▶ Iatrogenic Causes of Neuropathy

IB4-Binding Neurons

▶ IB4-Positive Neurons, Role in Inflammatory Pain

IB4-Positive Neurons, Role in Inflammatory Pain

CHERYL L. STUCKY
Department of Cell Biology, Neurobiology and
Anatomy, Medical College of Wisconsin, Milwaukee,
WI, USA
cstucky@mcw.edu

Synonyms

IB4-Binding Neurons; GDNF-Dependent Neurons;
IB4-Positive Nociceptors

Definition

An IB4-positive neuron is a sensory neuron whose cell body lies in the dorsal root or trigeminal ganglia and whose membrane expresses surface carbohydrates (α-D galactose groups of glycol conjugates) that bind the plant lectin isolectin B4 (IB4) from *Griffonia simplicifolia* I. IB4-positive neurons have small size cell bodies and primarily give rise to unmyelinated fibers, many of which are nociceptive.

Characteristics

IB4-positive neurons comprise one of two broad classes of small diameter, C-fiber sensory neurons. The other class (IB4 negative) typically expresses neuropeptides such as substance P and calcitonin gene related peptide (CGRP) and expresses ▶ trkA receptors for ▶ nerve growth factor (NGF). IB4-positive neurons express receptors for ▶ glial cell line-derivedneurotrophic factor

(GDNF) and depend on GDNF for survival after birth (Bennett et al. 1998). IB4 positive neurons selectively express the ▶ P2X3 Receptor for ATP. IB4-positive neurons are relatively poor in expression of neuropeptides or trkA receptors (Silverman and Kruger 1990; Averill et al. 1995; Molliver et al. 1995), but some studies show overlap between IB4 binding and neuropeptide or trkA expression (Wang et al. 1994; Kashiba et al. 2001). The central terminals of IB4-positive neurons terminate predominantly in the inner ▶ lamina II of the superficial dorsal horn of the spinal cord (Gerke and Plenderleith 2004), whereas IB4-negaitve neurons terminate mainly in lamina I and outer lamina II (Fig. 1).

The neurochemical differences between IB4 positive and negative neurons suggest that the two classes of small diameter neurons may have different functional properties in conveying nociceptive information. Compared to IB4 negative neurons, IB4 positive neurons isolated from uninjured mice or rats have longer duration action potentials and higher densities of ▶ tetrodotoxin (TTX) resistant sodium channel currents (Stucky and Lewin 1999), higher densities of N-type Ca^{2+} channel currents (Wu and Pan 2004) and higher densities of voltage gated K^+ (Kv) channel currents (Vydyanathan et al. 2005). Furthermore, IB4 positive neurons from uninjured mice are significantly *less* responsive to noxious chemical stimuli, including capsaicin and protons, than IB4 negative neurons (Dirajlal et al. 2003).

Several authors have hypothesized that IB4 negative, but not IB4 positive, neurons contribute to inflammatory pain (Mantyh and Hunt 1998; Snider and McMahon 1998). To address this hypothesis, a recent study investigated whether peripheral inflammation *in vivo* alters the response properties of isolated IB4 positive or IB4 negative neurons to the noxious stimulus capsaicin, which activates the transient receptor potential vanilloid 1 (TRPV1) receptor (▶ TRPV1 receptor) (Breese et al. 2005). TRPV1 function was investigated because

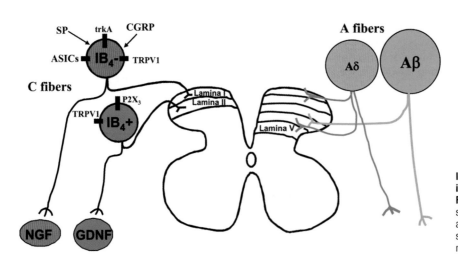

IB4-Positive Neurons, Role in Inflammatory Pain, Figure 1 Schematic of cross-section of the lumbar spinal cord and innervation by the general subclasses of primary afferent neurons.

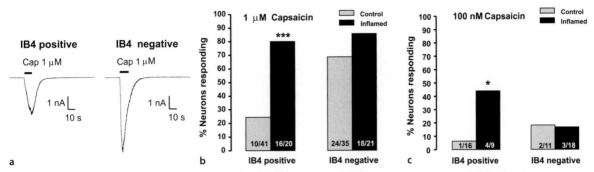

IB4-Positive Neurons, Role in Inflammatory Pain, Figure 2 Inflammation sensitizes IB4 positive neurons to capsaicin. (a) Examples of whole cell voltage clamp recordings from an IB4 positive and an IB4 negative small diameter neuron ($\leq 26 \mu$ m) that responded to 1 μ M capsaicin. (b) Percentage of IB4 positive and IB4 negative neurons from the L4/L5 DRG of control or CFA-injected mice that responded to a 10 s exposure to 1 μ M capsaicin. Capsaicin-evoked currents in all cells tested were > 40 pA.*** indicates that significantly more IB4 positive neurons from inflamed mice responded to capsaicin compared to the control IB4 positive group ($P < 0.0001$; Fisher's Exact test). (c) Percentage of IB4 positive and IB4 negative small diameter neurons isolated from the L4/L5 DRG from control or CFA-injected mice that responded to 100 nM capsaicin.* indicates that significantly more IB4 positive neurons from inflamed mice responded to capsaicin compared to control IB4 positive neurons ($P < 0.05$; Fisher's Exact test). The percentage of IB4 negative neurons that responded to 100 nM capsaicin was unaltered by inflammation. (Modified from Breese et al. 2005).

TRPV1 is a key heat transducer on nociceptors and mediates the heat hyperalgesia that accompanies peripheral inflammation (Caterina et al. 2000; Davis et al. 2000). Peripheral inflammation was induced by injection of ▶ complete Freund's adjuvant (CFA) in the hind paw of mice. Two days later, the lumbar 4–5 ganglia, which contain the cell bodies of neurons that project to the hind paw were isolated and dissociated and whole cell patch clamp recordings were performed on small diameter neurons. Fig. 2 shows that the proportion of IB4 positive neurons that respond to capsaicin with an inward current is markedly increased (3-fold) after inflammation, whereas IB4 negative neurons are unaltered. The increase in capsaicin responsiveness in IB4 positive neurons is due to increased TRPV1 function because IB4 positive neurons from ▶ TRPV1-Null Mice with CFA inflammation are unresponsive to capsaicin. Similarly, inflammation increases the proportion of IB4 positive

neurons, but not IB4 negative neurons, that respond to protons (pH 5.0) in a TRPV1-dependent manner (not shown). In parallel, CFA-induced inflammation increases by 3-fold the percentage of IB4-positive neurons that express TRPV1-immunoreactivity, but has no effect on IB4 negative neurons (Fig. 3 and Table 1).

Since the IB4 positive small diameter neurons are selectively increased in TRPV1 function and expression during peripheral inflammation, they may play an important role in inflammatory pain. Natural stimuli for TRPV1 during inflammation may be noxious heat or endogenous TRPV1 ligands including protons, N-arachidonoyl-dopamine, anandamide or eicosanoids such as leukotriene B4, 12-(S)-HPETE or 15-(S)-HPETE molecules. An increase in the number of IB4 positive neurons that respond to TRPV1 stimuli including heat or endogenous TRPV1 inflammatory ligands could increase, by ▶ spatial summation, the amount of nociceptive information transmitted to the dorsal horn of the spinal cord and ultimately contribute to inflammatory pain and hyperalgesia. The IB4-positive neurons' capacity to become sensitized highlights them as a putative target for novel therapies for inflammatory pain.

IB4-Positive Neurons, Role in Inflammatory Pain, Table 1 TRPV1-immunoreactivity in IB4 positive and IB4 negative small diameter neurons from control and CFA-injected mice

TRPV1-ir (%)	Control (%)	Inflamed (%)
% total neurons	10.7 ± 4.0	25.0 ± 3.0 *
% of IB4 positive neurons	4.5 ± 2.1	15.5 ± 3.6 †
% of IB4 negative neurons	20.9 ± 12.2	34.7 ± 8.6

m) L4/L5 DRG neurons co-stained for IB4 and TRPV1. * indicates that thepercentage of neurons that are TRPV1-mmunoreactive(TRPV1-ir) was increased in CFA-injected mice compared tocontrol mice ($P < 0.05$; two-tailed unpaired t-test). † indicates thatthe percentage of IB4 positive neurons that are TRPV1-ir wasincreased in CFA-injected mice compared to control mice ($P < 0.05$; two-tailed unpaired t-test). The percentage of TRPV1-ir IB4 negativeneurons was not significantly altered in CFA-injected mice compared to controlmice ($P > 0.3$; two-tailed unpaired t-test). n = 5 control mice (1201total neurons analyzed for TRPV1 and IB4 staining); n = 12 CFA-injected mice (1232 total neurons analyzed for TRPV1and IB4 staining) (Breese et al. 2005).

References

1. Averill S, McMahon SB, Clary DO et al. (1995) Immuno-cytochemical localization of trkA receptors in chemically identified subgroups of adult rat sensory neurons. Eur J Neurosci 7:1484–1494
2. Bennett DL, Michael GJ, Ramachandran N et al. (1998) A distinct subgroup of small DRG cells express GDNF receptor components and GDNF is protective for these neurons after nerve injury. J Neurosci 18:3059–3072
3. Breese NM, George AC, Pauers LE et al. (2005) Peripheral inflammation selectively increases TRPV1 function in IB4-positive sensory neurons from adult mouse. Pain 115:37–49
4. Caterina MJ, Leffler A, Malmberg AB et al. (2000) Impaired nociception and pain sensation in mice lacking the capsaicin receptor. Science 288:306–313

Control

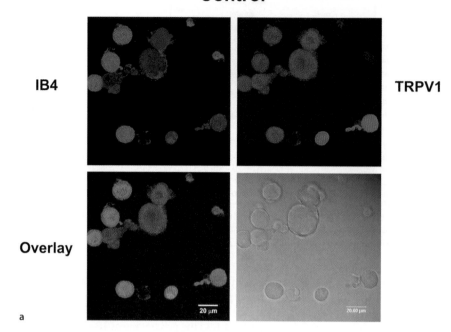

a

Inflamed

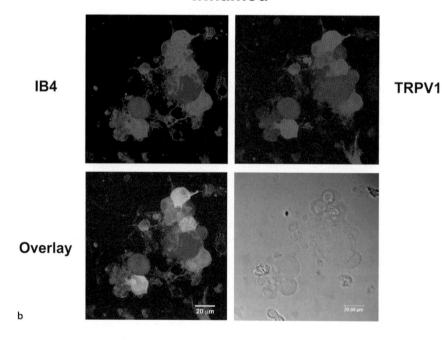

b

IB4-Positive Neurons, Role in Inflammatory Pain, Figure 3 Inflammation increases TRPV1-immunoreactivity in IB4-positive neurons. Confocal images of acutely isolated DRG neurons from control (a) and CFA-injected (b) wild-type mice that were co-stained with IB4 and a TRPV1 antibody. Lumbar 4/5 DRG neurons were isolated from control, non-injected mice or mice 22 days after CFA injection and fixed 6-9 h later for staining. Merged confocal images show that few IB4-positive neurons from control mice are TRPV1-immunoreactive, but after CFA-induced peripheral inflammation, more IB4-positive neurons are immunoreactive for TRPV1. Although neurons from control and inflamed mice were fixed at thee same time after isolation, neurons from CFA-injected mice typically exhibited more processes, less round somata and more clustering than controls.

5. Davis JB, Gray J, Gunthrope MJ et al. (2000) Vanilloid receptor-1 is essential for inflammatory thermal hyperalgesia. Nature 405:183–187
6. Dirajlal S, Pauers LE, Stucky CL (2003) Differential response properties of IB(4)-positive and -negative unmyelinated sensory neurons to protons and capsaicin. J Neurophysiol 69:1071–1081
7. Gerke MB, Plenderleith MB (2004) Ultrastructural analysis of the central terminals of primary sensory neurones labeled by trans-

ganglionic transport of Bandeiraea simplicifolia I-isolectin B4. Neuroscience 127:165–175
8. Kashiba H, Uchida Y, Senba E (2001) Difference in binding by isolectin B4 to trkA and c-ret mRNA-expressing neurons in rat sensory ganglia. Brain Res Mol Brain Res 95:18–26
9. Mantyh PW, Hunt SP (1998) Hot peppers and pain. Neuron 21:644–645
10. Molliver DC, Radeke MJ, Feinstein SC et al. (1995) Presence or absence of TrkA protein distinguishes subsets of small sensory

neurons with unique cytochemical characteristics and dorsal horn projections. J Comp Neurol 361:404–416

11. Silverman JD, Kruger L (1990) Selective neuronal glycoconjugate expression in sensory and autonomic ganglia: relation of lectin reactivity to peptide and enzyme markers. J Neurosci 23:789–801
12. Snider WD, McMahon SB (1998) Tackling pain at the source: new ideas about nociceptors. Neuron 20:629–632
13. Stucky CL, Lewin GR (1999) Isolectin B(4)-positive and -negative nociceptors are functionally distinct. J Neurosci 19:6497–6505
14. Vydyanathan A, Wu ZZ Chen SR et al. (2005) A-type voltage-gated K+ currents influence firing properties of isolectin B4-positive but not isolectin B4-negative primary sensory neurons. J Neurophysiol 93:3401–3409
15. Wang H, Rivero-Melian C, Robertson G et al. (1994) Trans-ganglionic transport and binding of the isolectin B4 from Griffonia simplicifolia I in rat primary sensory neurons. Neuroscience 62:539–551
16. Wu ZZ, Pan HL (2004) High voltage-activated $Ca^{(2+)}$ channel currents in isolectin B(4)-positive and -negative small dorsal root ganglion neurons of rats. Neurosci Lett 368:96–101

IB4-Positive Nociceptors

▶ IB4-Positive Neurons, Role in Inflammatory Pain

IBS

▶ Descending Modulation of Visceral Pain
▶ Irritable Bowel Syndrome
▶ Visceral Pain Model, Irritable Bowel Syndrome Model

IC_{50} Value

Definition

IC_{50} Value is the concentration where 50% of the inhibitory effect of a drug is reached.
▶ NSAIDs, COX-Independent Actions

Ice-Pick Pain

Definition

This describes a sharp jabbing pain in contrast to a persisting ache.
▶ Primary Stabbing Headache

Ice-Water Bucket Test

Definition

A test involving immersing an extremity into a bucket filled with ice and water, usually resulting in a temperature of 4 degrees Celsius. The test can be used as a test of pain sensitivity (e.g. by measuring how long the extremity is left immersed before pain becomes intolerable) or as a defined conditioning stimulus for testing the body's inhibitory responses to pain or nociceptive input. If the latter is intended, the extremity is left in the bucket for a defined length of time (or until a defined temperature is reached), with quantitative sensory testing (or other formal sensory testing) being performed before and after the test to quantitate the inhibitory response.
▶ Quantitative Sensory Testing

ICF

Definition

International Classification of Functioning, Disability and Health. It was developed by the World Health Organization. The ICF has addressed many of the criticisms of prior conceptual frameworks, and has been developed in a worldwide comprehensive consensus process over the few last years.
▶ Disability and Impairment Definitions

ICSI

Synonym

O'Leary-Sant Interstitial Cystitis Symptom Index

Definition

ICSI stands for O'Leary-Sant Interstitial Cystitis Symptom Index, which is utilized for quantifying the degree of symptoms associated with interstitial cystitis.
▶ Interstitial Cystitis and Chronic Pelvic Pain

IDET

Synonym

Intra Discal Electrothermal Therapy

Definition

IDET stands for Intra Discal Electrothermal Therapy – this technique is also called annuloplasty, and involves treatment of posterior annulus with heat from a thermal resistive coil in an attempt to repair, denervate and stabilize an annular tear.

▶ Discogenic Back Pain
▶ Intradiscal Electrothermal Therapy
▶ Spinal Fusion for Chronic Back Pain

Idiopathic

Definition

If a condition or disease is of unknown cause, it is described as idiopathic.

▶ Diabetic Neuropathies

Idiopathic Ataxic Neuropathy

▶ Ganglionopathies

Idiopathic Cramps

Definition

This type of cramp is the main symptom of a disease about which little is known, the cause of the cramp being obscure or speculative. Idiopathic cramps can be either sporadic or inherited, and are usually not associated with any cognitive, pyramidal, cerebellar, or sensory abnormalities.

▶ Muscular Cramps

Idiopathic Headache

▶ Headache, Episodic Tension Type

Idiopathic Myalgia

▶ Myalgia

Idiopathic Orofacial Pain

▶ Atypical Facial Pain, Etiology, Pathogenesis and Management

Idiopathic Stabbing Headache

▶ Primary Stabbing Headache

Idiopathic Vulvar Pain

▶ Vulvodynia

IEGs

▶ Immediate Early Genes

iGluRs

▶ Ionotropic Glutamate Receptors

Ignition Hypothesis

Definition

Hypothesis, proposed by Rappaport and Devor (1994), which attempts to explain paroxysmal pain in trigeminal neuralgia in terms of sustained afterdischarge and cross excitation, amplified by positive feedback among neighboring neurons in the trigeminal root and/or ganglion.

▶ Pain Paroxysms
▶ Tic and Cranial Neuralgias

IL–1beta

Definition

IL-1beta is a cytokine with many properties similar to TNF. At higher endocrine concentrations, it is associated with fever and formation of acute-phase plasma proteins in the liver.

▶ Cytokines as Targets in the Treatment of Neuropathic Pain

IL-4

Definition

Interleukin-4 is an anti-inflammatory cytokine that has also been shown to have analgesic properties.

▶ Cytokines as Targets in the Treatment of Neuropathic Pain

IL-6

Definition

IL-6 is a cytokine with mostly proinflammatory and algesic actions. It is a member of the IL-6 cytokine family that includes leukemia inhibitory factor (LIF) and ciliary neurotrophic factor (CNTF).

▶ Cytokines as Targets in the Treatment of Neuropathic Pain

IL-10

Definition

Interleukin-10 is an anti-inflammatory cytokine that has also been shown to have analgesic properties.

▶ Cytokines as Targets in the Treatment of Neuropathic Pain

Ilium

Definition

The Ilium is the upper portion of the hipbone.

▶ Sacroiliac Joint Pain

Illness Behaviour

▶ Interpersonal Pain Behaviour

Illusory Cramp

Definition

Illusory cramp is a phenomenon in which the sensation of cramping is experienced, but little or no contraction of the muscle occurs.

▶ Muscular Cramps

Imagery

Definition

Representations in the mind of visual, auditory, tactile, olfactory, gustatory or kinesthetic experiences. The subjective reality of these experiences may vary between and within individuals. Guided, directed or elicited imagery can be a potent means of changing subjective experiences of pain.

▶ Therapy of Pain, Hypnosis

IME

▶ Independent Medical Examinations

Imitation Learning

▶ Modeling, Social Learning in Pain

Immediate Early Genes

Synonym

IEGs

Definition

Immediate early genes (IEGs) are genes that are rapidly induced in the absence of de novo protein synthesis. The best characterized immediate early genes are c-jun and c-fos; both genes encode transcription factors that bind to specific regulatory sequences and activate expression of responsive genes. c-jun has a leucine zipper motif, which forms a heterodimer with a variety of proteins including c-fos. The jun-fos protein complex, also known as the activator complex (AP)-1, binds to a number of cellular promoters through a common element (5'-TGACTCA-3'). IEGs are distinct from "late response" genes, which can only be activated later following the synthesis of early response gene products. IEGs have therefore been called the "gateway to the genomic response".

▶ Amygdala, Pain Processing and Behavior in Animals
▶ NGF, Regulation during Inflammation

Immortalization

Definition

Immortalization is to confer the property of continuous division by the addition or upregulation of a gene, that when expressed in the cell, stimulates the cell to continuously divide until removed or downregulated.

▶ Cell Therapy in the Treatment of Central Pain

Immune Cell Recruitment

Definition

Inflammation induces immune cell migration from the circulation in multiple steps, including rolling, adhesion, and transmigration of immune cells through the vessel wall.

▶ Opioids and Inflammatory Pain

Immune Cells

Definition

B- and T-lymphocytes, macrophages and monocytes are immune cells patrolling through the body. They can migrate to areas with inflammation (chemotaxis).
▶ Opioid Modulation of Nociceptive Afferents in vivo

Immunocompetent Cells

Definition

Immunocompetent cells are able to respond to bacterial and viral stimuli. These cells respond by releasing classical immune mediators including proinflammatory cytokines. Within the CNS, these cells include astrocytes and microglia. Activation of these cells with immunogenic substances induces exaggerated pain.
▶ Cord Glial Activation

Immunocytochemistry

Definition

Immunocytochemistry is a method for demonstrating the localization of compounds in tissues, based on the use of antibodies.
▶ Immunocytochemistry of Nociceptors
▶ Opioid Receptors at Postsynaptic Sites

Immunocytochemistry of Nociceptors

CHERYL L. STUCKY
Department of Cell Biology, Neurobiology and Anatomy, Medical College of Wisconsin, Milwaukee, WI, USA
cstucky@mcw.edu

Synonyms

Immunohistochemistry; Immunoreactivity; Immunostaining; Neurochemistry; Neurochemical Markers; Nociceptors, Immunocytochemistry

Definition

The study of molecules or proteins (antigens) found in the cytoplasm or membrane of nociceptors by using immunologic staining methods, such as the use of fluorescent antibodies or enzymes (e.g. horseradish peroxidase). The immunocytochemistry procedure is usually performed on sections of tissue that has been fixed by a cross-linking fixative like paraformaldehyde or glutaraldehyde. Typical tissues include the dorsal root or trigeminal ganglion, peripheral nerve or target tissue such as skin. Most of these immunocytochemical markers label not only the cell bodies but also the axons and terminals of the sensory neurons.

Characteristics

Nociceptive sensory neurons express a large variety of molecules that are involved in neuronal communication and many of these molecules are present in high enough concentrations to be detected by immunocytochemical methods. For example, nociceptors contain neurotransmitters and neuropeptides which, when released from central terminals act on spinal cord neurons or when released from peripheral terminals act on other cells in the skin or target tissues. Furthermore, nociceptors express ion channels and receptors in their plasma membrane that allow them to respond to external stimuli (heat, cold, mechanical force) or internal stimuli such as molecules released by other cell types. The goal of this essay is to highlight examples of the major immunocytochemical markers that are most frequently used to characterize subpopulations of nociceptors within the ▶ dorsal root ganglion (DRG) or trigeminal ganglion. However, because DRG and trigeminal neurons are exceptionally heterogeneous with respect to their expression of peptides, enzymes and receptors, there are many molecules and subpopulations of neurons that are not described here.

Peptidergic Population: CGRP and Substance P

The most extensively characterized neuropeptides in nociceptive sensory neurons are ▶ calcitonin gene related peptide (CGRP) and ▶ substance P. The CGRP- and substance P-expressing population of small diameter neurons is frequently called the "peptidergic" population of small diameter neurons because both of these neuropeptides are found in many small diameter neurons that stain darkly with basic aniline dyes and are called "small dark cells." Small dark cells can be distinguished from large light cells, which stain clear or lightly, because they contain many neurofilaments that do not stain with the basic dyes.

Calcitonin Gene-related Peptide

CGRP is expressed by more sensory neurons than other peptides and estimates range from 20–80% of DRG or trigeminal ganglion neurons expressing CGRP. The wide range among studies is due to differences between species, the location along the cervical to sacral neuraxis, the target tissue innervated and whether or not colchicine, which blocks microtubule transport of neuropeptides, was used. Most studies agree that 35–50% of all rat lumbar DRG neurons express CGRP. Within the spinal cord, CGRP is localized exclusively in primary afferent neurons. Most CGRP-expressing sensory neurons are small or medium size in diameter (many are nociceptors), but a few are large diameter.

This is consistent with the finding that the afferent fibers of CGRP-positive neurons are primarily unmyelinated C fibers and thinly myelinated Aδ fibers and a few are large myelinated Aβ fibers (McCarthy and Lawson 1990).

Substance P

Substance P (SP) is expressed in approximately 20% of DRG neurons and most of these are small diameter neurons, although a few are medium diameter. Consistent with this, individually identified SP-expressing DRG neurons have either C fiber or Aδ fiber axons and exhibit nociceptive response properties (Lawson et al. 1997). Substance P is highly colocalized with CGRP in that nearly all SP-expressing DRG neurons also contain CGRP, although only half of the CGRP-expressing neurons also contain SP.

Other Characteristics

The peptidergic population of small dark neurons overlaps extensively with expression of ▶ trkA, the high affinity receptor for the neurotrophin ▶ nerve growth factor (NGF) and depends on NGF for survival during development (Averill et al. 1995). Because good antibodies are available for the ▶ trkA receptor, immunocytochemistry for trkA is frequently used as an alternative marker for the peptidergic population of small dark neurons. The central terminals of the peptidergic/trkA neurons are concentrated in lamina I and II outer of the superficial dorsal horn as well as in lamina V and X of the spinal cord.

CGRP-positive and SP-positive neurons innervate all types of peripheral target tissue, including skin, muscle, joint, bone and visceral organs. It is important to note that the expression pattern and levels of CGRP and SP in DRG neurons change with injury. Both CGRP and SP increase following persistent peripheral inflammation and conversely, they decrease following peripheral nerve lesion (Donnerer et al. 1992; Villar et al. 1991). This caveat must be carefully considered when using these markers to label and follow subpopulations of neurons in models of injury.

Other neuropeptides found in (typically smaller) subpopulations of mammalian DRG neurons that can be localized *via* antibody staining include somatostatin, vasoactive intestinal peptide, galanin, vasopressin, bombesin, dynorphin, enkephalin, neuropeptide Y, cholecystokinin and endothelin-1. Their distribution and characteristics will not be discussed in detail here.

Non-Peptidergic or "Peptide Poor" Population: Isolectin B4 and FRAP

The population of small dark C fiber neurons that is poor in expression of the neuropeptides CGRP or SP is typically characterized by labeling with the plant lectin, isolectin B4 (IB4). Isolectin B4 binds to surface carbohydrates, specifically the ▶ Alpha(α)-D Galactose groups of glycol conjugates (Silverman and Kruger 1990). The IB4 binding technique is most frequently used today because it is very adaptable, easy to perform, and IB4 conjugated directly to fluorescein (IB4-FITC) or other fluorescent markers can be used to label live neurons within minutes after performing physiological experiments (Stucky and Lewin 1999). However, the "peptide poor" population can also be labeled by immunoreactivity to the antibody LA4, which recognizes the α-galactose oligosaccharides (Dodd and Jessell 1985) or by the presence of the fluoride resistant acid phosphatase (FRAP) enzyme, an extra-lysosomal acid phosphatase that is resistant to fluoride ions (Silverman and Kruger 1988). The function of the α-D galactose groups is not clear, but they have been hypothesized to play a role in the cell-cell interactions during the development of connections of primary afferent neurons to the dorsal horn of the spinal cord (Dodd and Jessell 1985). The function of FRAP is not known.

Other Characteristics

The IB4 positive/FRAP positive population of small diameter neurons also expresses receptors for ▶ glial cell-line derived neurotrophic factor (GDNF) and depends on GDNF for survival during postnatal development (Molliver et al. 1997; Bennett et al. 1998). Receptors for GDNF include the ligand binding domain ▶ GFRα1 or GFRα2 and the signal transducing, tyrosine kinase domain, RET. IB4 positive neurons primarily terminate in ▶ lamina IIinner of the superficial dorsal horn of the spinal cord, a region also known as the substantia gelatinosa.

Although a number of investigations have reported a clear separation between the peptidergic/trkA and the non-peptidergic/IB4 binding populations, other reports indicate that CGRP/SP/trkA and IB4/FRAP staining overlap extensively (Wang et al. 1994; Kashiba et al. 2001). The diverse findings may be due to differences in methods used or sensitivity of detection of the labels. It is likely that there is at least a subpopulation of neurons that expresses neuropeptides and binds IB4.

Importantly, IB4 binding decreases substantially following nerve injury (Bennett et al. 1998) and therefore caution must be exercised when using this marker to label subpopulations of neurons in animal models of injury.

Neurofilament Markers: Antibodies RT97 and N52

The antibody clones RT97 and N52 both recognize the high molecular weight (200 kD) ▶ neurofilament protein NF200, which is found in sensory neurons that have myelinated axons. Both RT97 and N52 antibody labeling have been used to identify the large light population of DRG neurons. One difference between the two antibodies is that RT97 recognizes only the phosphorylated form of the 200 kD neurofilament protein whereas N52 recognizes both the phosphorylated and

I

non-phosphorylated forms of the protein. Thus, there may be some differences in the populations of neurons labeled by these two markers. An advantage of RT97 is that a cell-by-cell correlation between RT97 staining and conduction velocities has been made for rat and all A fiber (Aδ and Aβ) DRG neurons were found to be RT97-positive whereas all C fiber neurons were RT97-negative (Lawson and Waddell 1991). No such correlation between N52 and conduction velocity has yet been made.

There is almost no overlap between RT97 and IB4 staining or between N52 and IB4 staining, indicating that RT97/N52 and IB4 label distinct subpopulations of large light and small dark neurons, respectively. There is, however, significant overlap between RT97 and CGRP as approximately 30% of RT97-positive neurons contain CGRP and these are medium/large size neurons (McCarthy and Lawson 1990).

Ion Channels: TRPV1 and P2X3

Subpopulations of nociceptors can also be identified by antibodies that recognize specialized transduction molecules on the plasma membrane. Examples of these include receptors for noxious heat (TRPV1 receptor) and for ATP (P2X$_3$ receptor).

Transient Receptor Potential Vanilloid 1 (TRPV1) Receptor

The TRPV1 receptor/ion channel is the receptor for capsaicin, the potent algogen found in "hot" chili peppers (Caterina et al. 1997). Formerly known as VR1, TRPV1 is a member of the ▶ transient receptor potential family of ion channels and when activated, allows calcium and sodium to flow into the neuron, resulting in depolarization. Besides capsaicin, TRPV1 also responds to moderately noxious heat (> 43°C), acid (~pH 5.0) and a number of other endogenous ligands that may be present during inflammation or injury, including N-arachidonoyl-dopamine, anandamide or ▶ eicosanoids such as leukotriene B4, 12-(S)-HPETE or 15-(S)-HPETE molecules. Good antibodies to TRPV1 exist and TRPV1 immunoreactivity is found on many small diameter and some medium diameter sensory neurons (Caterina et al. 1997). Because capsaicin responsiveness is often used as a functional marker for nociceptors, TRPV1-immunoreactivity is frequently used as a neurochemical marker for nociceptors. Many TRPV1-immunoreactive neurons contain the neuropeptides CGRP or SP, whereas others bind IB4 (Tominaga et al. 1998). As is the case with neuropeptide immunoreactivity and IB4 binding, TRPV1 expression is also not stable after injury. The mRNA and protein for TRPV1 decreases in directly injured DRGs after ▶ axotomy or ▶ Spinal Nerve Ligation Model. Conversely, TRPV1 increases in adjacent DRGs after spinal nerve ligation and is reported to increase following peripheral inflammation (Hudson et al. 2001).

P2X$_3$ Receptor for ATP

Extracellular adenosine triphosphate (ATP) has been implicated in nociceptive signaling in normal and pathological pain conditions and ATP directly excites nociceptors. P2X$_3$ receptors are multimeric ion channels gated by ATP. They exist on native DRG neurons as either P2X$_3$ homomers or as a heteromeric combination with the P2X$_2$ receptor (P2X$_{2/3}$). Good antibodies against the P2X$_3$ receptor are available and studies document that P2X$_3$ receptors are selectively expressed on small diameter DRG neurons. Under uninjured conditions, P2X$_3$ receptors are almost exclusively localized to the IB4-binding population and only a few P2X$_3$-positive neurons contain neuropeptides (Bradbury et al., 1998). Consistent with the pattern for IB4 binding neurons, the central terminals of P2X$_3$-expressing neurons project primarily to the lamina II$_{inner}$ of the superficial dorsal horn. The expression of P2X$_3$ receptors decreases following nerve injury and this decrease can be reversed by *in vivo* administration of GDNF (Bradbury et al. 1998).

References

1. Averill S, McMahon SB, Clary DO et al. (1995) Immunocytochemical localization of trkA receptors in chemically identified subgroups of adult rat sensory neurons. Eur J Neurosci 7:1484–1494
2. Bennett DL, Michael GJ, Ramachandran N et al. 1998) A distinct subgroup of small DRG cells express GDNF receptor components and GDNF is protective for these neurons after nerve injury. J Neurosci 18:3059–3072
3. Bradbury EJ, Burnstock G, McMahon SB (1998) The expression of P2X3 purinoreceptors in sensory neurons: effects of axotomy and glial-derived neurotrophic factor. Mol Cell Neurosci 12:256–268
4. Caterina MJ, Schumacher MA, Tominaga M, Rosen TA, Levine JD, Julius D (1997) The capsaicin receptor: a heat-activated ion channel in the pain pathway. Nature 389:816–824
5. Dodd J, Jessell TM (1985) Lactoseries carbohydrates specify subsets of dorsal root ganglion neurons projecting to the superficial dorsal horn of rat spinal cord. J Neurosci 5:3278–3294
6. Donnerer J, Schuligoi R, Stein C (1992) Increased content and transport of substance P and calcitonin gene-related peptide in sensory nerves innervating inflamed tissue: evidence for a regulatory function of nerve growth factor in vivo. Neuroscience 49:693–698
7. Hudson LJ, Bevan S, Wotherspoon G et al. (2001) VR1 protein expression increases in undamaged DRG neurons after partial nerve injury. Eur J Neurosci 13:2105–2114
8. Kashiba H, Uchida Y, Senba E (2001) Difference in binding by isolectin B4 to trkA and c-ret mRNA-expressing neurons in rat sensory ganglia. Brain Res Mol Brain Res 95:18–26
9. Lawson SN, Waddell PJ (1991) Soma neurofilament immunoreactivity is related to cell size and fibre conduction velocity in rat primary sensory neurons. J Physiol 435:41–63
10. Lawson SN, Crepps BA, Perl ER (1997) Relationship of substance P to afferent characteristics of dorsal root ganglion neurones in guinea-pig. J Physiol 505:177–191
11. McCarthy PW, Lawson SN (1990) Cell type and conduction velocity of rat primary sensory neurons with calcitonin gene-related peptide-like immunoreactivity.34:623–632
12. Molliver DC, Wright DE, Leitner MJ et al. (1997) IB4-binding DRG neurons switch from NGF to GDNF dependence in early postnatal life. Neuron 19:849–861

13. Silverman JD, Kruger L (1988) Lectin and neuropeptide labeling of separate populations of dorsal root ganglion neurons and associated "nociceptor" thin axons in rat testis and cornea wholemount preparations. Somatosens Res 5:259–267
14. Silverman JD, Kruger L (1990) Selective neuronal glycoconjugate expression in sensory and autonomic ganglia: relation of lectin reactivity to peptide and enzyme markers. J Neurocytol 19:789–801
15. Stucky CL, Lewin GR (1999) Isolectin B(4)-positive and -negative nociceptors are functionally distinct. J Neurosci 19:6497–6505
16. Tominaga M, Caterina MJ, Malmberg AB et al. (1998) The cloned capsaicin receptor integrates multiple pain-producing stimuli. Neuron 21:531–543
17. Villar MJ, Wiesenfeld-Hallin Z, Xu XJ et al. (1991) Further studies on galanin-, substance P- and CGRP-like immunoreactivities in primary sensory neurons and spinal cord: effects of dorsal rhizotomies and sciatic nerve lesions. Exp Neurol 112:29–39
18. Wang H, Rivero-Melian C, Robertson G et al. (1994) Transganglionic transport and binding of the isolectin B4 from Griffonia simplicifolia I in rat primary sensory neurons. Neuroscience 62:539–551

Immunocytokines

▶ Cytokines, Effects on Nociceptors
▶ Cytokines, Regulation in Inflammation

Immunodeficient

Definition

An innate, acquired, or induced inability to develop a normal immune response.
▶ Animal Models of Inflammatory Bowel Disease

Immunoglobulin Therapy

Definition

Intravenous administration of immunoglobulin has been clinically shown to have anti-inflammatory immunomodulatory effects in GBS and CIDP. Doses required are higher than those required for immunodeficiency states.
▶ Inflammatory Neuritis

Immunohistochemistry

Definition

Immunohistochemistry is a staining method using the principle of antigen-antibody interactions to demonstrate a defined protein in tissue sections.
▶ Immunocytochemistry of Nociceptors
▶ Toxic Neuropathies

Immuno-Inflammatory Muscle Pain

▶ Muscle Pain in Systemic Inflammation (Polymyalgia Rheumatica, Giant Cell Arteritis, Rheumatoid Arthritis)

Immunoisolation

Definition

When supplying donor grafted tissue or cells, immunoisolation allows the separation of that tissue from the host, for example in an inert device that cannot be detected by the host immune system. Such a procedure is more likely to lead to long-term survival of donor tissue or cells.
▶ Cell Therapy in the Treatment of Central Pain

Immunoreactivity

▶ Immunocytochemistry of Nociceptors

Immunostaining

▶ Immunocytochemistry of Nociceptors

Immunosuppression

Definition

Inhibiting the activation and function of immune cells either by disease, or by drugs.
▶ Proinflammatory Cytokines
▶ Vascular Neuropathies

Impact of Familial Factors on Children's Chronic Pain

LINDSAY S. UMAN[1], CHRISTINE T. CHAMBERS[2]
[1]Department of Psychology, Dalhousie University, Halifax, NS, Canada
[2]Departments of Pediatrics and Psychology, Dalhousie University and IWK Health Centre, Halifax, NS, Canada
luman@dal.ca, christine.chambers@dal.ca

Synonyms

Psychosocial factors; Familial Factors; Parental Response; Family Environment

Definition

Of the many psychosocial variables known to affect chronic pain in children, the family has emerged as one of the more prominent. Families are involved in all aspects of their children's pain, including assessment and management. It is now generally accepted that parents play an important role in influencing how their children learn to respond to pain. Having a child with chronic pain can also place a significant emotional and financeial burden on families. This review will provide a brief description of the major research areas examining the impact of familial factors on children's chronic pain. Several more comprehensive reviews of family factors and pain are also available elsewhere (e.g. Chambers 2003; Palermo 2000).

Characteristics

It has long been observed that ▶ chronic pain tends to run in families, whereby children who report pain are likely to have parents who report pain and *vice versa*. The majority of the studies examining aggregation of pain in families have been retrospective; however, a large-scale prospective study found considerable support for the association between pain and pain-related disability among children and their parents (Goodman et al. 1997). Although genetic predisposition and shared environment may account in part for the tendency for pain to run in families, psychological processes, particularly ▶ social learning theory and ▶ operant conditioning, have emerged as important in understanding how children acquire information about how to respond to pain. These theories indicate that children can learn how to cope with pain from their parents through various pathways. For example, children may learn through direct parental instruction or reprimands (i.e. being told to respond or not respond in a certain way to pain) as well as through observational or vicarious learning (i.e. by watching how the parent responds to his / her own pain) (Craig 1986). Parents may also indirectly teach their children about how to express pain by how they react to their children's expressions of pain (e.g. by providing special time or exemptions when the child has pain). These childhood learning experiences may, in turn, provide the foundation for the development of pain-related behaviours and coping styles later in life. Fortunately, there is evidence that parental behaviour and responses to pain can be modified successfully in order to produce improvements in pain and coping in children.

In addition to what can be explained by various learning theories, there is some evidence for the role of general parenting style and other familial characteristics in childhood pain. Although certain parenting styles such as over-protectiveness, discouragement of adaptive strategies, and encouragement of maladaptive strategies have been associated with poorer functioning in children with chronic pain, the evidence regarding the importance of these characteristics has been inconsistent at best (Chambers 2003). A recent study found that parent-child interactions during an exercise task were not related to children's general pain coping strategies nor their level of pain-related disability (Reid et al. 2005). However, parents' discouragement of coping in response to their children's negative statements about pain made it more difficult for the children to maintain task activity.

Parental Responses to Chronic Pain

The ways in which parents choose to respond to their children's pain complaints can have significant consequences for how children learn to express them (Walker and Zeman 1992). Principles of both positive and negative reinforcement can influence pain expression in children. ▶ Positive reinforcement may include providing tangible treats such as presents or favourite foods, as well as non-tangible rewards such as special privileges, sympathy and increased attention for pain behaviours. ▶ Negative reinforcement may include allowing the child to stay home from school, as well as exemption from chores and other unpleasant or anxiety-provoking activities (e.g. music lessons, sport practices). Both positive and negative reinforcement may inadvertently reward pain behaviours and encourage their display, while simultaneously discouraging adaptive coping in the face of pain.

This combination of reinforcement can lead to problematic consequences, as children may learn to adopt a ▶ sick role. Children may be motivated to adopt the sick role because it provides an acceptable excuse for exemption from responsibilities as well as less than desirable performance or behaviour (Walker and Zeman 1992). There is evidence that parents are more likely to excuse the misbehaviour of children with physical illnesses when there is a medical explanation or known organic aetiology for the pain compared to children with medically unexplained pain (Walker et al. 1995). The Illness Behavior Encouragement Scale (IBES) was developed by Walker and Zeman (1992) in order to assess and quantify parental responses to child illness and pain behaviours. The IBES is a 12-item scale with questions related to how parents respond when their child is ill or experiencing pain (e.g. "How often do you let your child stay home from school when he / she has pain?"). The questions are designed to provide information about the extent to which parents reinforce or provide encouragement for sick role behaviours. Research using the IBES has shown that mothers tend to encourage the sick role more than fathers, and that girls perceive their parents as more encouraging of illness behaviour than do boys. The IBES is a useful tool for elucidating and targeting maladaptive parental behaviours (for research and in clinical practice) that could be altered in order to promote better child health and pain management.

Family Involvement in Interventions for Chronic Pain

Psychological interventions for chronic pain are typically cognitive-behavioural (▶ cognitive-behavioural therapy) in nature and frequently involve training parents to encourage positive coping behaviours and take attention away from maladaptive behaviours in their children. Interventions that involve parents have been shown to be more effective than those targeting the child alone and are also more likely to result in maintained gains over time. For example, in a study examining the role of parent-mediated management of childhood migraines, it was found that the children undergoing ▶ biofeedback treatment whose parents also received pain management guidelines displayed significantly greater reductions in headache frequency and were more likely to be headache-free than children whose parents did not receive these guidelines (Allen and Shriver 1998). Parents were taught how their own behaviour can influence the pain behaviour of their children, and they were also trained to encourage adaptive coping while discouraging maladaptive pain behaviours.

Several studies have also examined the role of short-term cognitive-behavioural family interventions for paediatric recurrent abdominal pain (Sanders et al. 1989; Sanders et al. 1994). A recent study by Robins and colleagues (2005), in which parents were taught to be active partners in their children's pain management intervention (e.g. by involving the parent as a "coach" and restricting the extent to which secondary gains from sick behaviours were provided), found that children whose families had been involved in their treatment reported significantly less abdominal pain and had fewer school absences as compared to children who received standard medical care.

The research to date suggests that involving the family in the management of chronic pain in children is advantageous. Most of the interventions involving parents have been based on behavioural principles. Future research is needed to examine the value of ▶ family systems oriented approaches in pain management in children.

Impact of Pain on the Family

While it is generally understood that families can significantly impact their children's pain, only recently has the reciprocal impact of pain on the family been acknowledged. Parenting a child with chronic pain typically involves extensive financial and emotional costs to the family, in the form of multiple medical appointments, missed time from work or school and increased stress. In a study examining the effect of chronic pain on the quality of life in adolescents and their families, it was found that more intense and frequent chronic pain in adolescents was associated with decreased self-reports of quality of life related to psychological functioning as well as physical and functional status (Hunfeld et al. 2001). Many children with chronic pain do not have an identified organic disease or underlying biological explanation for the pain, which can be an additional source of frustration for families who desire a definitive diagnosis with a time-limited treatment plan (Hunfeld et al. 2002). Treatment of a child with chronic pain is typically an ongoing long-term process, involving a multi-disciplinary team of health-care professionals. Given the numerous family resources (e.g. parental attention) devoted to caring for a child with chronic pain, it is possible that non-ill family members (e.g. siblings) may inadvertently feel neglected and resentful. Thus, caring for a child with chronic pain is a process that affects all members of the family in some capacity. Additional research is needed to further delineate the complex ways that pain can influence the health and well-being of children and their families.

Conclusion

It should be clear that familial factors are important to consider when evaluating a child with chronic pain. These family influences are multi-faceted and dynamic and can interact with various other biological, psychological and social factors over time. Children learn how to cope with and express their pain from their parents. Parental responses to child pain including positive and negative reinforcement, may foster and encourage sick role behaviours. Involving parents in interventions for chronic pain in children appears beneficial, and the financial and emotional burden related to caring for a child with chronic pain should also be considered.

References

1. Allen JD, Shriver MD (1998) Role of parent-mediated pain behavior management strategies in biofeedback treatment of childhood migraines. Behav Ther 29:477–490
2. Chambers CT (2003) The role of family factors in pediatric pain. In: McGrath PJ, Finley GA (eds) Pediatric Pain: Biological and Social Context, Progress in Pain Research and Management, vol 26. IASP Press, Seattle, pp 99–130
3. Craig KD (1986) Social modeling influences: Pain in context. In: Sternbach RA (ed) The Psychology of Pain, 2nd edn. Raven Press, New York, pp 67–95
4. Goodman, JE, McGrath PJ, Forward SP (1997) Aggregation of pain complaints and pain-related disability and handicap in a community sample of families. In: Jensen TS, Turner JA, Wiesenfeld-Hallin Z (eds) Proceedings of the 8th World Congress on Pain, Progress in Pain Research and Management, vol 8. IASP Press, Seattle, pp 673–682
5. Hunfeld JAM, Perquin CW, Duivenvoorden HJ et al. (2001) Chronic pain and its impact on quality of life in adolescents and their families. J Pediatr Psychol 26:145–153
6. Hunfeld JAM, Perquin CW, Hazebroek-Kampschreur AAJM et al. (2002) Physically unexplained chronic pain and its impact on children and their families: The mother's perception. Psychol Psychother 75:251–260
7. Palermo T (2000) Impact of recurrent and chronic pain on child and family daily functioning: A critical review of the literature. Dev Behav Pediatr 21:58–69

8. Reid GJ, McGrath PJ, Lang BA (2005) Parent-child interactions among children with juvenile fibromyalgia, arthritis, and healthy controls. Pain 113:201–210
9. Robins PM, Smith SM, Glutting JJ et al. (2005) A randomized controlled trial of a cognitive-behavioral family intervention for pediatric recurrent abdominal pain. J Pediatr Psychol 30:397–408
10. Sanders MR, Rebgetz M, Morrison M et al. (1989) Cognitive-behavioral treatment of recurrent nonspecific abdominal pain in children: An analysis of generalization, maintenance, and side effects. J Consult Clin Psychol 57:294–300
11. Sanders MR, Shepherd RW, Cleghorn G et al. (1994) The treatment of recurrent abdominal pain in children: A controlled comparison of cognitive-behavioral family intervention and standard pediatric care. J Consult Clin Psychol 62:306–314
12. Walker LS, Zeman JL (1992) Parental response to child illness behaviour. J Pediatr Psychol 20:329–345
13. Walker LS, Garber J, Van Slyke DA (1995) Do parents excuse the misbehavior of children with physical or emotional symptoms? An investigation of the pediatric sick role. J Pediatr Psychol 20:329–345

Impact on Activities of Daily Living

▶ Rating Impairment Due to Pain in a Workers' Compensation System

Impairment

Definition

Impairment is a loss, loss of use, or derangement of any body part, organ system, or organ function as a direct consequence of illness.
▶ Disability and Impairment Definitions
▶ Disability, Upper Extremity
▶ Pain as a Cause of Psychiatric Illness
▶ Physical Medicine and Rehabilitation, Team-Oriented Approach

Impairment Due to Pain

▶ Rating Impairment Due to Pain in a Workers' Compensation System

Impairment Evaluation

Definition

Evaluations performed by a physician to determine the presence and/or severity of a claimant's impairment. The evaluations are often commissioned by insurance companies or disability agencies.
▶ Impairment, Pain-Related

Impairment, Functions Loss

▶ Disability, Upper Extremity

Impairment, Pain-Related

JAMES P. ROBINSON
University of Washington Pain Center, University of Washington, Seattle, WA, USA
jimrob@u.washington.edu

Synonyms

Organ or Body Part Dysfunction; activity limitation; disability; Pain-Related Impairment

Definition

"Impairment" does not have a unique definition. The American Medical Association (AMA) defines it as: "A loss, loss of use, or derangement of any body part, organ system, or organ function" (p. 2) (Cocchiarella and Andersson 2001). The World Health Organization gives the following definition: "Impairments are problems in body function or structure as a significant deviation or loss" (p. 226) (World Health Organization (2001). The United States Social Security Administration defines impairments as "anatomical, physiological, or psychological abnormalities that can be shown by medically acceptable clinical and laboratory diagnostic techniques" (p. 3) (US Government Printing Office 1994). The present essay focuses on impairment as conceptualized by the AMA in Guides to the evaluation of permanent impairment, 5th edition (Cocchiarella and Andersson 2001).

Characteristics

Although the above definitions of impairment differ somewhat, they all emphasize that impairments are biomedical abnormalities that can be analyzed at the level of organs or body parts. In fact, a critical distinction between impairment and disability is that they address limitations at different levels of analysis – impairment refers to a limitation in the function or structure of an organ or body part, whereas disability refers to a limitation in the behavior of a person. This distinction is reflected in the syntax used to describe impairments and disabilities. For example, one would say "Ms. Smith's right leg is weak because of her polio" to describe her impairment, and "Ms. Smith is unable to walk up stairs" to describe her consequent disability.

Since impairment refers to the function or structure of organs or body parts rather than to the behavior of people, observers often assume that physicians can perform impairment evaluations objectively and relatively independently of the persons to whom the organs/body parts belong. For example, a physician could assess renal impairment on the basis of creatinine clearance or cardiac impairment on the basis of ejection fraction. Thus, ▶ impairment evaluations are thought to bypass the complications that arise when examiners try to understand claimants at the "whole person" level, or to perform analyses that rely on claimants' self-reports and voluntary behavior.

The Significance of Impairment Evaluations

Agencies that administer disability programs need a method to determine whether people who seek benefits are actually disabled – i.e. whether they have medical conditions that significantly limit their ability to carry out certain activities. Among individuals who allege disability, ones who are truly disabled need to be distinguished from ones who cannot perform activities because of non-medical circumstances (e.g. inability to find work due to an economic depression), and from ones who will not perform activities, even though they are capable of doing so. Physicians are often enlisted to make the above distinctions by objectively evaluating medical factors that may underlie a claimant's allegations of incapacitation. For at least the past 45 years, the AMA has persuasively argued that physicians can evaluate these medical factors by performing impairment evaluations. In fact, most physicians and disability adjudicators think of impairment evaluations as being synonymous with evaluations of medical factors that contribute to disability.

In practice, agencies that administer work disability programs often combine impairment data with non-medical data (e.g. educational background and prior work history) to determine whether an individual is actually disabled from work. The logic of this approach can be summarized as follows:

1. Work disability results from a combination of medical and non-medical factors.
2. Impairment evaluations measure the medical component of disability – i.e. the severity of medical factors that contribute to work disability, therefore,
3. Work disability awards should be based on impairment evaluations supplemented by non-medical data.

The Problem of Subjective Factors

However elegant the above syllogism appears to be, it leaves out an important category of information – the self-reports that disability applicants provide about their experiences as they try to engage in activities (Robinson et al. 2004). These reports provide a first-person perspective that, in principle, might be very important to the assessment of an applicants' disability.

In particular, applicants can provide subjective data regarding a variety of aversive experiences – such as anxiety, pain, fatigue, or subjective weakness – that make it difficult for them to engage in normal activities. Pain is the most common of the aversive experiences reported by applicants for work disability benefits.

The potential importance of subjective experiences is highlighted by Osterweis et al. in an Institute of Medicine monograph on the role of pain in disability awards by the Social Security Administration:

The notion that all impairments should be verifiable by objective evidence is administratively necessary for an entitlement program. Yet this notion is fundamentally at odds with a realistic understanding of how disease and injury operate to incapacitate people. Except for a very few conditions, such as the loss of a limb, blindness, deafness, paralysis, or coma, most diseases and injuries do not prevent people from working by mechanical failure. Rather, people are incapacitated by a variety of unbearable sensations when they try to work (p. 28) (Osterweis et al. 1987).

Pain and other unbearable sensations cannot be incorporated into impairment evaluations, as conceptualized in the AMA system, for two reasons. First, since pain is inherently subjective, the methods used to assess it violate the tenet that impairment evaluations should be based on objective indices of the function of organs or body parts. Secondly, pain and its effects need to be analyzed at the level of the whole person, rather than at the level of a specific organ or body part. People with chronic pain typically attribute their pain and activity limitations to dysfunction of an organ or body part. However, these subjective reports are difficult to assess precisely because examination of the involved organ or body part often does not identify abnormalities that make the pain reports inevitable. It often appears to an observer that the affected organ or body part is capable of functioning, but that the claimant does not use it normally because of pain. The observer must consider the person as a whole in order to make sense of the situation. Thus, the assessment of incapacitation secondary to pain violates the tenet that impairment evaluations should assess the functioning of organs or body parts, rather than the functioning of an individual as a whole.

Attempts to Solve the Conundrum

At one level, the question of whether pain-related activity limitations can be construed as impairments is a simple one of semantics. In principle, it can be resolved in at least two ways. One is to expand the definition of "impairment", so that the concept includes limitations secondary to pain. A second strategy is to retain the interpretation of impairment as a problem at the level of organs or body parts, but to stipulate that in the medical assessment of a disability applicant, a physician should evaluate both impairment and subjective factors – such as pain – that contribute to the applicant's activity limitations.

Regardless of the semantic issue of whether or not pain is construed as a type of impairment, disability systems face a dilemma regarding the weight they place on pain and other subjective factors (such as fatigue or perceived weakness) during disability determinations. If a system equates impairment with the medical component of disability, it will ignore the subjective factors that often play a dominant role in preventing people from working. Such a system would be objective, but might also be somewhat irrelevant, since it would systematically exclude important factors that bear on the ability of an individual to work. Conversely, a system that gives undue weight to the subjective reports of claimants may inappropriately reward ▶ symptom magnifier s and ▶ malingerer s. The challenge is to develop a disability assessment system that strikes a reasonable balance between the weight given to ▶ objective factors (such as amputations) and ▶ subjective factors (especially pain). No disability system has been able to resolve this challenge in a completely satisfactory way.

References

1. Cocchiarella L, Andersson GBJ (2001) Guides to the Evaluation of Permanent Impairment, 5th edn. AMA Press, Chicago, Illinois
2. Osterweis M, Kleinman A, Mechanic D (1987) Pain and Disability. National Academy Press, Washington, DC
3. Robinson JP, Turk DC, Loeser JD (2004) Pain, Impairment, and Disability in the AMA Guides. J Law Med Ethics 32:315–326
4. US Government Printing Office (1994) Disability Evaluation under Social Security (SSA Publication No. 64-039). Washington, DC
5. World Health Organization (2001) International Classification of Functioning, Disability and Health. World Health Organization, Geneva

Impairment Rating

▶ Impairment Rating, Ambiguity
▶ Impairment Rating, Ambiguity, IAIABC System
▶ Rating Impairment Due to Pain in a Workers' Compensation System

Impairment Rating, Ambiguity

ALAN L. COLLEDGE, GREGORY KROH
Utah Labor Commission, International Association of Industrial Accident Boards and Commissions, Salt Lake City, UT, USA
farmboyac@msn.com

Synonyms

Workers' compensation; Permanent Partial Impairment; Permanent Partial Disability; Ambiguity

Definitions

Permanent partial impairment – a permanent loss of or abnormality of psychological, physiological, or anatomical structure or function permanent.

Permanent partial disability – a permanently reduced ability to engage in substantial gainful employment by reason of any physical or mental impairment.

Characteristics

Permanent injury compensation is a large and growing component of workers' compensation system cost. In the US, it represents about two thirds of all indemnity benefits (Berkowitz and Burton 1987). Moreover, the frequency and cost of permanent injury is increasing as a share of all workers' compensation claims. Citing data from the National Council on Compensation Insurance, David Durbin states, "During the six-year period from 1988 to 1994, average PPD [permanent partial disability] costs increased 25%, an increase of approximately 4% per year, while the frequency increased almost 29% or 4.4% annually. These increasing average costs and frequencies have resulted in an increase in the permanent partial cost per worker of approximately 52% (over 7% annually) over the same six year period" (Durbin and Kish 1998).

Numerous wage-loss studies document that in virtually every state, and every classification of claimants, compensation awards are smaller than the actual or predicted wage losses that workers incur after an injury. Moreover, the correlation between impairment ratings and actual economic losses following injury are poor. For example, the statistical work by Durbin and Kish tries to measure the consistency of initial physician impairment ratings, disability ratings awarded, and final compensation given to injured workers across various US jurisdictions. They concluded that:

The results show that impairment ratings are only one of a variety of factors that systematically influence the size of a final disability award. Specifically, even for cases with benefits awarded for non-economic loss, in addition to the treating physician's determination of physical impairment, the determination of the degree of permanent disability appears to take into account factors such as age, sex, pre-injury wage, weekly temporary total benefits, and whether an attorney is involved in the case. Moreover, even after these other factors are considered, a less than one-to-one relationship exists between impairment and final disability ratings, which might be expected.

Similar results were found by Park and Butler (2000). They found that degrees of permanent impairment assigned by physicians, even under Minnesota's relatively well administered guidelines, were not statistically related to the reduction in pre-injury wages after the injury. Even after adjusting permanent injury awards for age, occupation, and other economic factors, they found that the impairment ratings had a very poor statistical relation to the actual wage loss. This finding is consistent with mainstream belief by medical and non-medical researchers in workers' compensation.

Several factors account for this lack of correlation between permanent disability compensation and wage loss. First, most jurisdictions do not consciously or deliberately set out to provide benefit levels that match the future loss of earnings. The statutes and rules that establish permanent injury compensation do not equate impairment with disability, nor do they explicitly state what the PPD award is intended to compensate. Rather, benefit levels are set in a political arena. The employer's cost of workers' compensation, and how that affects the competitive position of one jurisdiction relative to its competitors, is a far more common metric in the political debate than statistical measures of wage loss from permanent injuries.

Second, differences across workers cause the permanent disability formulae to be relatively more generous to some injured workers and relatively prone to under compensate others. Especially in pure impairment states, the rules for scheduled injury benefits impose uniform awards for each degree of physical loss, e.g. a 5% loss of the wrist is the same for a concert violinist and cement finisher. These uniform awards do not address the fact that relatively minor impairments often cause severe job limitations for construction workers, but minimal or no job limitations for office workers. In addition, younger workers tend to be under compensated for permanent injury relative to workers nearing retirement.

The focus of this paper is on the third reason for lack of predictability of impairment ratings: the physical measurements of bodily loss are not reliably and consistently measured by doctors. Doctors do not set benefit levels for specific injuries, but the measurement of physical loss they provide translates directly into dollar benefits. This lack of consistency among rating physicians is widely observed (for a review see Colledge 1994).

Much anecdotal evidence and a few formal studies suggest that a major problem with the system revolves around the consistency and defensibility of permanent impairment ratings made by physicians. Complaints in this area are routinely reported in the trade press. From the anecdotal evidence, the problem seems to exist in many jurisdictions.

Inconsistencies have been demonstrated when similar injury cases have been presented to multiple practitioners, and when the same practitioner has evaluated similar cases through time.

For example, in a 1999 study by the State of Texas, a significant number of the cases with multiple impairment ratings for the same injury showed disparities of 5% or greater: Specifically, the study found that 24% of injured workers with multiple impairment ratings had no difference between the first and last ratings, 29% had a difference of 5–10 percentage points, and 14% had a difference of 10 percentage points or more. One of the authors has documented similar inconsistencies in the State of

Utah prior to that state's recodification of impairment rating guides (Colledge 2001).

Multiple factors contribute to these inconsistencies. A major source of the problem is that state laws and regulations related to impairment and disability evaluation are often poorly crafted and are inconsistent in awarding payment, how benefit levels are set, and the formulas and procedures for guiding physician impairment ratings. Victor and Boden (1991) contend that the clarity of law on evaluating permanent injury helps control disputes. Even if laws and regulations are consistent within states, there are often inconsistencies in methods and expectations across states. This is problematic for doctors who have multi-state practices or attempt to deal with these issues from a national perspective. Another challenge for doctors is that state laws, regulations, and administrative law judges are sometimes out of step with the best available medical evidence.

Finally, injuries differ greatly in the ease with which they can be rated. A wide variety of common injuries are amenable to reasonably concrete and precise formulae, which convert measured losses to percentages of loss of use of a limb or the whole body. This type of injury is often classified as a scheduled injury. The rating of many scheduled injuries is not particularly difficult or ambiguous for a reasonably trained practitioner. For example, amputations or total loss of use of extremities are not a major source of error or inconsistency. They are objective and relatively easy to measure.

Problems can arise, though, in the evaluation of partial loss to an extremity. At what point does nerve, tendon, joint, or muscle damage render an arm or hand functionally useless? The rules on rating such partial disabilities are variable from jurisdiction to jurisdiction. A much greater problem arises in rating injuries to the spine, which are governed by much more general and subjective guidelines.

Psychological or mental injury and all the related behavioral and motivational consequences are another intractable problem. Psychological injury is real, but it is very difficult to differentiate from pre-existing psychological illness not related to the workplace and it is difficult to rate or measure. For these reasons psychological injury is a lightning rod where it is being compensated by workers' compensation. New South Wales is one recent example: "...the rights of the people of NSW have been gravely compromised by the Government's subsequent decision to use the very flawed and unfair Psychiatric Impairment Rating Scale (PIRS) to measure such impairments, and by excluding psychologists from assessment of psychological and psychiatric impairment. Apparently the Government is attempting to save on compensation payouts at the expense of psychologically impaired workers. This is a dangerous election ploy. (Lynette Shumack, NSW Executive, The Australian Psychological Society, April 5, 2002)

Rating pain is the greatest problem of all. Some jurisdictions take the position that pain is not compensable in workers' compensation. Others hold that the pain must be directly linked to the loss of use of body part, e.g. acute pain limiting the range of motion on a limb. Policy makers in such jurisdictions apparently hold the belief that workers' compensation is a no fault system that tries to get away from the problems of measuring pain and suffering that are so difficult to assign values to in civil tort cases. Other jurisdictions make some allowance for pain, if only in an indirect or implicit way. For example, some jurisdictions assign minimum impairment ratings for surgery even if the outcome was rated as 100% successful in restoring function. This might implicitly be regarded as a reward to the injured worker for the uncertainty and trauma of the surgical procedure.

In the ideal situation, a skilled practitioner using a well-defined set of criteria might be able to fairly rate the intangibles of an injury, most importantly pain. However, there is ample evidence to suggest that pain is difficult to evaluate and subject to a host of psycho-social overlays that have nothing to do with the injury itself.

Inconsistencies develop not only over the severity of impairment associated with an injury, but also over causation of the impairment. Disagreements regarding causation are particularly likely to occur when workers sustain covert injuries (such as repetitive strain injuries of the upper extremity) rather than overt ones (such as an upper extremity fracture), when an injury is superimposed on a chronic musculoskeletal condition, workers present with symptoms that do not have a clear cause or etiology, e.g. sick building syndrome or stress claims.

The consequences of the Inconsistencies described above are substantial. They tend to lead to "deuling doctors" (that is, differences of opinion between the treating physician and an expert hired by the payer of the claim), delays, and high cost litigation. In general, disputes over medical evidence are very expensive. The personnel and the support system needed for hearings tend to be among the most expensive parts of a workers' compensation agency budget. State agencies are continually experimenting with techniques to reduce case backlogs and speed decisions. Delays and other inefficiencies stimulate legislative inquiries, and as constituent frustration levels rise, lawmakers are inclined to "reform" the system. Some states go through a cycle of reform-dissatisfaction-reform

For these reasons it is vital that permanent injury benefits be managed better in most states. The keys to success:

- Fixed conditions under which permanent injury benefits can be awarded.
- A clear trigger for when permanent injury can be evaluated.
- Well defined responsibilities for the physician who is to make the legally required medical determinations.
- Uniform procedures for the measurement and evaluation of the parameters of permanent impairment to the body.
- An objective way to express the basis for the impairment rating.

Whenever any one of these is lacking, doubt and mistrust by workers or their employers enters into the benefit award. Also, opportunists find ways to exploit the ambiguity to maximize gains by "gaming" the system. Gaming the system or adversarial disputes are signs of system failure in workers' compensation.

The State of Wisconsin presents an example of a very smoothly functioning impairment system for scheduled injuries. Wisconsin Administrative Rule 80.20 specifies quite clearly how impairments from scheduled injuries translate into percentages of body part loss. Loss of motion of fingers is a good example: the physician need only measure the loss of flexion and extension at each joint of the injured finger(s) to produce a precise measure of impairment under Wisconsin law. Even more serious/complex injuries to the knee have explicit standards. Finger and knee impairment ratings by treating physicians are almost never challenged by claims adjusters and virtually never litigated.

The role of physician or administrative judgment has been circumscribed by many jurisdictions. They have reacted to ambiguity in various ways: 1) eliminating the compensability of a class of injuries, 2) constraining the range of judgment about certain injuries, or 3) assigning a narrow range of estimates. These understandable responses to uncertainty have the undesirable consequence of introducing inequity. Some workers are simply not compensated as much as they should be relative to other workers with more tangible and specific injuries. This is a political, not medical, issue. Clearly, simple and direct rules work. They mete out compensation with efficiency and speed. Of course, some would object that "cookie cutter" justice is unfair. Yet, the very basis of workers' compensation is accepting administrative simplicity in benefit delivery for the individualistic tort based approach to equitable benefit determination.

In a companion essay (Impairment – Ambiguity, Part 2 – the IAIABC System), the work of the International Association of Industrial Accident Boards and Commissions (IAIABC) to improve the process of rating injuries is described.

References

1. Berkowitz, Monroe, Burton J (1987) Permanent Disability Benefits in Workers' Compensation. W.E. Upjohn Institute for Employment Research, Kalamazoo, Mich
2. Colledge A (1994) Impairment Ratings. Occupational Health and Safety, July 1994
3. Colledge A, Sewell J, Hollbrook B (2001) Impairment Ratings in Utah, Reduction of Variability and Litigation within Workers' Compensation. Disability Medicine, ABIME 1

4. Durbin D, Kish J (1998) Factors Affecting Permanent Partial Disability Ratings in Workers' Compensation. J Risk Insur Mt. Vernon; Mar 1998
5. Park Y-S, Butler R (2000) Permanent Partial Disability Awards and Wage Loss. J Risk Insur 67:331–350
6. Shumack L (2002) NSW Executive. The Australian Psychological Society, April 5
7. Victor R, Boden L (1991) Model States Show Lawsuits Can Be Prevented. National Underwriter, Chicago

Impairment Rating, Ambiguity, IAIABC System

ALAN L. COLLEDGE, GREGORY KROH
Utah Labor Commission, International Association of Industrial Accident Boards and Commissions, Salt Lake City, UT, USA
farmboyac@msn.com

Synonyms

Workers' compensation; Permanent Partial Impairment; Permanent Partial Disability; Ambiguity; IAIABC system

Definitions

Permanent partial impairment is defined as a permanent loss of or abnormality of psychological, physiological, or anatomical structure or function permanent.

Permanent partial disability is defined as a permanently reduced ability to engage in substantial gainful employment by reason of any physical or mental impairment.

Characteristics

In the past, many jurisdictions, especially in North America, have deferred to the American Medical Association (AMA) Guides for rating occupational injuries. These guides have gone through years of evolution and are now in their 5th edition. The evolution has not mitigated disputes over the clarity and consistency of the guides. Spieler et al. (2000) best catalogued the shortcomings of the AMA Guides in the Journal of the American Medical Association. A survey done by the International Association of Industrial Accident Boards and Commissions (IAIABC) of workers' compensation agencies showed a high degree of dissatisfaction with the AMA 5th Edition.

Unfortunately, because of the lack of sensitivity and specificity of the Guides for evaluating impairment in injured workers, some jurisdictions have set out their own standards. As an example, the background section to the 1996 Florida Uniform Impairment Rating Schedule states:

In the past, much confusion has resulted from inadequate understanding by physicians and others of the scope of medical responsibility in the evaluation of permanent disability, and the difference between "permanent disability" and "permanent impairment." It is vitally important for every physician to be aware of his or her proper role in the evaluation of permanent disability under any private or public program for the disabled. It is equally important that physicians have the necessary authoritative material to assist them in competently fulfilling their particular responsibility – the evaluation of permanent impairment (Section 440.1 3, Florida Statutes).

Wisconsin, Florida and at least seven other jurisdictions in the US have developed their own guides for impairment rating. To date, there has been little sharing of information among the states on "best practices."

During the Fall of 2001, the International Association of Industrial Accident Boards and Commissions (IAIABC) began to study the feasibility of a way to assist physicians in rating permanent occupational injuries. A special committee of 16 doctors and other medical experts was formed to develop a supplemental guide to the AMA Guides. Its focus was on occupational impairment rating and injury types that are most difficult to rate.

These supplemental guides contain:

- An introduction to practitioners on the nature of occupational impairment rating.
- Definitions of key terms and concepts, such as maximum medical improvement.
- Discussion of general issues, especially the measurement of pain.
- Guides to rating surgical and non-surgical injuries of the back.
- Guides for rating the upper and lower extremities.
- Standardized reporting worksheets.

An introduction to impairment rating is critical because many physicians who do ratings are unsure of their role, or have misunderstandings about the rating procedure in a given jurisdiction. This is particularly true of those who only do ratings on an occasional or infrequent basis, or who are confronted with a rating scheme from a jurisdiction outside their normal practice.

Methodology

The Impairment Rating Committee embraced some guiding principles in their development of the supplemental guides:

- They should be based on the best available empirical evidence on the reliability of tests, measurements, and correlations of measurements to biomechanical limits on the normal use and functioning of the body.
- They should be practical in their administration by physicians.
- They should be clearly explainable to practitioners.

These principles are challenging to implement. They involve tradeoffs. For example, sophisticated measures that might be arguably more precise might be impractical and costly for a non-specialist physician. Also, the goals of objectivity and practicality often fly in the face of individual equity. The participants in the preparation of the draft IAIABC guides have elected to err on the side of simple consistent rules based on objective medical evidence.

Pain is a particularly controversial issue. It is a real consequence of injury and surely affects post injury reintegration into work and non-work activities of daily living. Having said this, the committee could not find many reliable and practical tools for rating most injuries for residual pain. Some psychological tools may be able to consistently differentiate between simulated pain and "really experienced" pain. Further, such tools may be able to gauge the approximate degree of experienced pain. However, the tools available to the drafters appeared to fall short of being easily learned and applied by treating physicians who do not specialize in occupational injury.

Results

To date, provisional Supplemental Guides have been produced. They provide specific guidance on issues not fully or clearly addressed in the AMA Guides.

Part 1 of the Supplemental Guides provides general background on the workers' compensation system and the role of the physician in awarding benefits for permanent work injuries. Much of this educational material is common knowledge for jurisdictional administrators, workers' compensation managers, and claims adjustors. Yet, it is surprising how few physicians who do not practice occupational medicine understand these fundamental concepts. The physician-rater must have an appreciation of their role in the benefit process for the system to work in accordance with the law.

This first part also reviews some of the generic concepts of impairment rating, such as maximum medical improvement and apportionment of injury. The highly controversial subject of pain is also addressed.

Part 2 of the Supplemental Guides addresses issues and problems associated with injuries to the back.

Part 3 is for rating upper and lower extremities to the draft guides.

The review process of the exposure draft of the Supplemental Guides continues. The current status of the Supplemental Guides can be viewed at http://www.iaiabc. org/Impairment/Impairment_index.htm

Impairment Ratings for Pain

The IAIABC system stresses the importance of simplicity, consistency and objective medical evidence in the assessment of impairment. Impairment ratings based on these principles are possible for many common injury types, but objective, consistent methods have not yet been developed for subjective conditions such as pain and psychological injury. Therefore, the IAIABC supplemental guides do not offer a comprehensive method for rating these conditions, although they do provide methods for rating selected conditions such as phantom pain from amputation. Of course this does not mean that subjective injury is not real. Evaluating and compensating it pose great practical problems – in particular increases in disputes, challenges, and litigation, which many jurisdictions want to avoid. In effect, the Supplemental Guides subordinate the quest for better individual equity on claims to overall system savings. Thus, purely subjective conditions, if they are to be compensated, should be addressed by explicit norms and rules outside the purview of medical examiners and raters.

Uses to Date

To date, the best practical application of the Supplemental Guides is in the State of Utah. In many respects the guides resemble administrative rules adopted by that state for the rating of permanent injuries.

The use of the Utah guides has had a dramatic reduction on litigation over impairment disputes. Less than one percent of claims with permanent disability are litigated since the revised impairment guides were adopted in 1997. This produced a dramatic cost savings to the Utah Labor Commission, since the direct cost to the agency is estimated to be $5,200 per case litigated. The chief administrator of the Utah Commission reports that the 1997 guides have been well received by attorneys, insurers, and worker representatives.

The IAIABC supplemental guides will not displace the need for the AMA guides. Rather, they provide support, clarification, and extension of the AMA guides. Individual states may wish to adopt portions of the IAIABC guides for specific issues or classes of claims.

Conclusions

Ambiguity and uncertainty over rating permanent injury produce higher administrative costs for workers' compensation systems, because: (1) Multiple examinations caused by disputed ratings are expensive, and (2) litigation over large discrepancies in ratings causes delay in benefits and further administrative cost.

One cure for the above problems of compensating for permanent injury is to establish clear and simple rules for awarding benefits. The downside to simplicity is a loss of individual equity and fairness among injured workers, i.e. some are relatively better off, and some are disadvantaged by rules that do not take into consideration how their physical loss has affected their earnings potential. This paper has argued for rating systems that stress objective medical evidence and consistent guidelines. These emphases are possible for many common injury types, but objective, consistent methods have not yet been developed for subjective conditions such as pain and psychological injury. Therefore, the IAIABC supplemental guides do not offer a comprehensive method for rating these conditions, although it does

sory connectivity in the brain could be examined. They are most suitable for infants as they are non-invasive and can be repeated without risk.

Indeed, NIRS has been used already in a preliminary investigation of the maturation of the response within the cerebral cortex to noxious stimulation caused by heel lance (Slater et al. 2005). The responses were studied using double channel NIR spectrophotometry and demonstrated that infants over a wide range of PMA from 29 to 42 weeks show a large response, localised to the somatosensory areas of the cerebral cortex, resulting from noxious stimulation.

Somatosensory evoked potentials (SEPs) can be reliably elicited from 27 weeks PMA and the appearance of the SEP waveform does not alter from that time until 40 weeks PMA (Pike et al. 1997). SEPs have been used to investigate the integrity of somatosensory pathways during the newborn period and in infancy, and as prognostic indicators of neurological impairment in high-risk infants (Pierrat et al. 1993). However, they have not yet been used to investigate the development of sensory processing in infants and young children, and it would be very interesting to observe the development of sensory connections within the brain in these age groups using this method.

Conclusions

It is evident that the study of neurophysiological phenomena can provide direct and quantitative information concerning processing of sensory information in the developing nervous system. It is also true that there are structural and functional features of this immature system that have a profound influence on pain processing in the newborn and infant. Furthermore, laboratory and clinical investigation of both mechanisms and behaviour have provided information about pain processing at the spinal cord level, but the challenge is to unravel the mystery of how much of a noxious stimulus reaches and is processed in the brain of the newborn and infant, and how this can be investigated. In the mean time, the information that we already have is sufficient to tell us that the management of pain in infancy requires not only the limitation of procedures as far as possible, but also careful and creative management of analgesia.

References

1. Andrews KA (2003) The human developmental neurophysiology of pain. In: Schechter NL, Berde CB, Yaster M (eds) Pain in Infants, Children, and Adolescents, 2nd edn. Lippincott Williams & Wilkins, Philadelphia
2. Andrews KA, Fitzgerald M (1994) The cutaneous withdrawal reflex in human neonates: sensitization, receptive fields, and the effects of contralateral stimulation. Pain 56:95–101
3. Andrews KA, Fitzgerald M (1999) The cutaneous flexion reflex in human neonates: a quantitative study of threshold and stimulus / response characteristics, following single and repeated stimuli. Dev Med Child Neurol 41:696–703
4. Andrews KA, Fitzgerald M (2000) Mapping of the area of secondary hypersensitivity around a surgical wound in human in-
fants using the abdominal skin reflex threshold. Eur J Neurosci 12 (Suppl. 11):71
5. Andrews KA, Fitzgerald M (2002) Wound sensitivity as a measure of analgesic effects following surgery in human neonates and infants. Pain 99:185–195
6. Andrews KA, Desai D, Dhillon HK et al. (2002) Abdominal sensitivity in the first year of life: comparison of infants with and without unilateral hydronephrosis. Pain 100:35–46
7. Cummings EA, Reid GJ, Finley GA et al. (1996) Prevalence and source of pain in pediatric inpatients. Pain 68:25–31
8. Dubner R (1992) Hyperalgesia and expanded receptive fields, editorial comment. Pain 48:3–4
9. Fitzgerald M, Koltzenburg M (1986) The functional development of descending inhibitory pathways in the dorsolateral funiculus of the newborn rat spinal cord. Dev Brain Res 24:261–270
10. Fitzgerald M, Millard C, MacIntosh N (1989) Cutaneous hypersensitivity following peripheral tissue damage in newborn infants and its reversal with topical anaesthesia. Pain 39:31–36
11. Fitzgerald M, Jennings E (1999) The postnatal development of spinal sensory processing. Proc Natl Acad Sci USA 96:7719–7722
12. Giamberardino MA (2000) Visceral hyperalgesia. In: Devor M, Rowbotham MC, Wiesenfeld-Hallin Z (eds) Proceedings of the 9th World Congress on Pain. IASP Press, Seattle, pp 523–550
13. Jain A, Rutter N (2000) Local anaesthetic effect of topical amethocaine gel in neonates: randomised controlled trial. Arch Dis Child Fetal Neonatal Ed 82:42–45
14. Pierrat V, Eken P, Duquennoy C et al. (1993). Prognostic value of early somatosensory evoked potentials in neonates with cystic leukomalacia. Dev Med Child Neurol 35:683–690
15. Pike AA, Marlow N, Dawson C (1997) Posterior tibial somatosensory evoked potentials in very preterm infants, Early Human Dev 47:71–84
16. Slater R, Gallella S, Boyd SG et al. (2005) Noxious stimulation causes functional activation of the somatosensory cortex in newborn infants. Early Human Dev
17. Taylor M J (2003) Where and when in the developing brain: neurophysiology of cognition in infants and children. Int J Psychophysiol 51:1–3

Infant Pain Reduction/Therapy/Treatment

▶ Acute Pain Management in Infants

Inflammation

Definition

Inflammation is a complex response to areas affected by injury or disease, which is meant to protect tissues, but is often a major source of damage. It involves the recruitment and activation of various cells (leukocytes and macrophages) and extracellular proteins, and is induced and maintained by numerous mediators like cytokines, histamine, plasma proteases, arachidonic acid metabolites (prostaglandins, leukotriens), growth factors and ions (potassium, protons).The main signs of inflammation are dolor, rubor, calor and tumor. Dolor, or pain, occurs due to activation of nociceptors that become sensitized with a lower threshold for activation. Rubor, or redness, is due to local vasodilatation with increased blood flow in the affected area. Calor, or heat, is due to a combination of increased local blood flow and an increase in cellular metabolic activity. Tumor or swelling occurs due to an increase in capillary permeability with plasma extravasation and localized edema. This may be exacerbated by restricted function in the affected area.

- ▶ Acid-Sensing Ion Channels
- ▶ COX–2 Inhibitors
- ▶ Lower Back Pain, Physical Examination
- ▶ Opioids in the Periphery and Analgesia
- ▶ Pain Modulatory Systems, History of Discovery
- ▶ Postoperative Pain, COX-2 Inhibitors

Inflammation, Modulation by Peripheral Cannabinoid Receptors

ISOBEL LEVER
Neural Plasticity Unit, Institute of Child Health,
University College London, London, UK
i.lever@ich.ucl.ac.uk

Definition

Cannabinoids are chemical compounds derived from the *cannabis sativa* plant and their synthetic analog. Pain responses resulting from inflammation can be reduced by cannabinoids, applied locally to peripheral tissues at systemically inactive doses. This analgesic mechanism involves the activation of peripheral cannabinoid receptors outside the CNS, making it distinct from the analgesic action of cannabinoids operating at receptors in the spinal cord and brain.

Characteristics

Two G-protein coupled receptors that respond to cannabinoids (CBs) have been identified so far and named CB_1 and CB_2. There is also evidence for additional cannabinoid receptor sub-types, which have yet to be characterised (Howlett et al. 2002). CB_1 receptors are found primarily in CNS neurones, and the majority of CB_2 receptors are expressed peripherally by cells with inflammatory and immune response functions. Both CB receptor sub-types have been detected in peripheral tissues from rat, mouse and human (Howlett et al. 2002), with evidence for CB_1 expression in peripheral neurones and glia, as well as on immune cells (although expression levels are lower than for CB_2 receptors) (Howlett et al. 2002, Walter and Stella 2004). Richardson et al. (1998) first demonstrated modulation of inflammatory pain states by the activation of peripheral cannabinoid receptors in an animal model of inflammatory pain. Injection of the inflammatory agent carrageenan into rat hind paw skin was used to induce a localised inflammatory response (measured by paw oedema due to ▶ plasma extravasation caused by increased microvasculature permeability) and

▶ hyperalgesia (measured by increased behavioural responses to noxious stimuli). After inflammatory injury, both the effects of paw oedema and thermal hyperalgesia were attenuated by a local injection of a small dose of the cannabinoid anandamide (AEA) to the paw skin, but not when the same dose of AEA was applied systemically. Co-administration of a selective antagonist to the CB_1 receptor (SR141716), to the paw skin, reversed the effect of AEA on thermal hypersensitivity. It also attenuated the cannabinoid-mediated reduction of plasma extravasation (stimulated by a ▶ capsaicin -induced ▶ neurogenic inflammation), thus demonstrating both an anti-hyperalgesic as well as an anti-inflammatory action of cannabinoids operating via peripheral CB_1 type cannabinoid receptors.

Local application of other cannabinoids: WIN55, 212-2, HU-210, methanandamide as well as AEA, in the formalin model of the rat hind paw skin inflammation, confirmed a reduction in pain behaviour via the activation of peripheral CB_1 receptors (Calignano et al. 1998). The ▶ endocannabinoid ligand AEA was similarly effective in this model and could be detected in paw tissue, along with a related endogenous compound Palmitoylethanolamide (PEA), which does not bind to any known cannabinoid receptor but the actions of which are reversed by the CB_2 receptor antagonist SR144528 (Howlett et al. 2002). Interestingly, when both of these compounds were injected into the paw together they produced a synergistic reduction of pain behaviour (Calignano et al. 1998). However, the anti-hyperalgesic effects of PEA were attenuated by local blockade of CB_2 but not CB_1 receptors in paw skin tissue. The contribution of CB_2 receptor signalling to the peripheral action of cannabinoids indicated by this study has since been confirmed, by using newly developed ligands that are selective for the CB_2 cannabinoid receptor sub-type (Malan et al. 2003). Application of the selective CB_2 receptor agonist AM1241 to inflamed rat paw skin tissue can reduce both mechanical and thermal hyperalgesic responses, an action which can also be locally reversed by CB_2 receptor antagonists (Quartilho et al. 2003, Hohmann et al. 2004). Other CB_2 receptor agonists have also been shown to be effective against paw tissue oedema when they were administered systemically (Clayton et al. 2002; Malan et al. 2003). Thus, cannabiniods have a dual anti-inflammatory and anti-hyperalgesic action mediated by both CB_1 and CB_2 peripheral cannabinoid receptor sub-types.

The Anti-Hyperalgesic Action of Peripheral CB Receptors

Behavioural studies report that cannabinoid receptors can be exogenously activated in inflamed hind paw skin, to produce a reduction in pain responses to noxious stimuli. Also, AEA and PEA (compounds that endogenously activate cannabinoid receptor signalling pathways) can be detected in this tissue (Calignano et al. 1998). It is therefore possible that these compounds interact with cannabinoid receptors on the peripheral endings of cutaneous ▶ nociceptive sensory neurones, in order to directly modulate the transmission of nociceptive signals to the CNS. As evidence of this mechanism, the local application of CB_1 and CB_2 receptor agonists to carrageenan-inflamed skin can reduce the responses of spinal cord cells receiving noxious mechanical inputs from this area (Kelly et al. 2003; Sokal et al. 2003). CB_1 receptors can also inhibit ▶ neurosecretion of the vasodilatory peptide CGRP from peripheral terminals of capsaicin-sensitive neurones in isolated paw skin (Richardson et al. 1998). This also suggests that cannabinoids might have a direct modulatory action on the signalling functions of nociceptive sensory neurones. In support of this mechanism, CB_1 mRNA and protein has been detected in the cell bodies of hind limb sensory nerves contained within dorsal root ganglia (DRG) (Bridges et al. 2003). However, the distribution of these receptors among the small, peptide-containing soma that are typical of nociceptive nerve fibres, was found to be limited in favour of intermediate to large-sized cells, which predominately have non-nociceptive sensory functions. It should be noted, however, that there is currently a discrepancy between the CB_1 receptor distribution reported in DRG tissue versus cultured DRG neurones (Bridges et al. 2003). CB_2 receptors have not been found on adult DRG neurones, although, as with CB_1, the presence of these receptors in functionally significant but as yet undetectable amounts *in vivo*, cannot be entirely ruled out. Functional CB_1 receptors have been demonstrated on cultured sensory neurones, where they are reported to signal via inhibitory $G_{i/o}$ proteins, to inhibit N-type voltage-activated calcium currents. Crucially, the activity of these receptors has not been demonstrated on small-sized CGRP-containing sensory neurones *in vitro* (Khasabova et al. 2004).

The Anti-Inflammatory Action of Peripheral CB Receptors

An alternative mechanism to explain the anti-hyperalgesic action of cannabinoids is linked to anti-inflammatory effects of these compounds in peripheral tissues. CB agonists may indirectly inhibit transmission in nociceptive afferents by reducing the release of by-products of inflammatory and excitotoxic processes, which serve to sensitise peripheral nociceptive fibres to mechanical and thermal stimuli. Cannabinoid receptors are present on cells that are functionally involved in immune responses to tissue injury, including B and T cells, natural killer cells, neutrophils, macrophages and mast cells (Howlett et al. 2002; Samson et al. 2003; Walter and Stella 2004). Furthermore, mitogen activation of some immune cells, such as human lymphocytes, has been shown to stimulate an up-regulation of cannabinoid receptors and also trigger the production of endocannabinoids (Howlett et al. 2002; Walter and Stella 2004). Taken together, this evidence suggests

that cannabinoids are endogenous immuno-modulators. Suppression of the pro-inflammatory functions of glial and immune cells (Walter and Stella 2004) is believed to mediate the inhibitory effects of cannabinoids on oedema and plasma extravasation. However, much of the evidence for cell-specific regulatory actions of cannabinoids has been derived from studies with isolated cell lines.

Cannabinoids are reported to reduce the production and release of pro-inflammatory signalling molecules, including tumour necrosis factor, nitric oxide and interleukin, and to enhance the release of anti-inflammatory cytokines like the IL-1 receptor antagonist, IL-4 and IL-10 (Molina-Holgado et al. 2003; Howlett et al. 2002; Walter and Stella 2004). Nerve growth factor (NGF) is an important mediator of inflammatory responses due to its ability to recruit and activate mast cells, and also to directly sensitise the receptors involved in transducing noxious stimuli on sensory neurones. Intradermal injections of NGF are used to artificially produce inflammation and hyperalgesia, and AEA and PEA compounds can be used to alleviate both effects, operating via CB_1 and CB_2 receptors, respectively (Farquhar-Smith et al. 2003). The action of NGF in tissues is amplified by mast cell function, as these cells produce and release NGF locally, as well as being activated by it. They also synthesise and release other inflammatory mediators that increase local vascular permeability and others, like serotonin, which can sensitise nociceptors. The ability of CB_1 and CB_2 receptor signalling to reduce inflammatory responses has been linked to their regulation of mast cell function (Samson et al. 2003). CB_1 receptor activation on mast cell lines is linked to the suppression of serotonin secretory responses, whereas co-expressed CB_2 receptors regulate the activation of signalling pathways that regulate gene expression. Mast cells have also been reported to produce endocannabinoids and PEA, suggesting the existence of an autocrine regulatory signalling pathway involving cannabinoids in these cells (Samson et al. 2003). Cannabinoids are also reported to suppress immune cell proliferation and chemotactic processes, which contribute to the establishment of inflammatory sites in tissues (Howlett et al. 2002; Walter and Stella 2004). Specifically, PEA has been shown to reduce neutrophil accumulation in hind paw skin inflamed by NGF injections (Farquhar-Smith et al. 2003). This is speculated to involve peripheral CB_2 receptor signalling pathways, which act to reduce the production and/or release of mast cell-derived neutrophil chemotactic factors, such as Leukotriene B4 or even NGF itself.

PEA and endocannabinoids like AEA are likely by-products of the inflammatory and excitotoxic processes occurring after tissue injury, providing endogenous signalling molecules to activate CB_1 and CB_2 receptor pathways. There is evidence that CB receptors are endogenously activated in inflamed skin tissue, as administration of CB_2 receptor antagonists alone to non-inflamed paw tissue increased the mechanical hypersensitivity and tissue oedema caused by a subsequent carrageenan inflammation (Clayton et al. 2002). Also, the injection of both CB_1 and CB_2 receptor antagonists to hind paws before inflammation by formalin, led to an enhancement of pain responses. This result similarly indicates that cannabinoid receptors are tonically activated in peripheral tissue (Calignano et al. 1998).

In summary, cannabinoids can act at CB_1 and CB_2 receptors in peripheral tissue to modulate immune and nociceptor functions: They suppress the pro-inflammatory actions of immune and glial cells leading to the reduction of tissue inflammation, and reduce the hypersensitivity of sensory nerves responding to mechanical and thermal pain stimuli. These are two ways in which the action of cannabinoids at local receptors in peripheral tissue could be effective in altering pain responses to inflammatory injury. This peripheral action is of potential therapeutic importance because it presents a way of delivering the analgesic benefit of cannabinoid compounds, whilst circumventing their centrally mediated psychoactive side effects.

References

1. Bridges D, Rice ASC, Egertova M, Elphick MR, Winter J, Michael GJ (2003) Localisation of Cannabinoid Receptor 1 in Rat Dorsal Root Ganglion Using *In Situ* Hybridisation and Immunohistochemistry. Neurosci 119:803–812
2. Calignano A, La Rana G, Giuffrida A, Peiomelli D (1998) Control of Pain Initiation by Endogenous Cannabinoids. Nature 394:277–280
3. Clayton N, Marshall FH, Bountra C, O'Shaughnessy CT (2002) CB1 and CB2 Cannabinoid Receptors are Implicated in Inflammatory Pain. Pain 96:253–260
4. Farquhar-Smith WP, Rice ASC (2003) A Novel Neuroimmune Mechanism in Cannabinoid-Mediated Attenuation of Nerve Growth Factor-Induced Hyperalgesia. Anesthesiology 99:1391–1401
5. Hohmann AG, Farthing JN, Zvonok AM, Makriyannis A (2004) Selective Activation of Cannabinoid CB2 Receptors Suppresses Hyperalgesia Evoked by Intradermal Capsaicin. J Pharmacol Exp Ther 308:446–453
6. Howlett AC, Barth F, Bonner TI, Cabral G, Casellas P, Devane WA, Felder CC, Herkenham M, Mackie K, Martin BR, Mechoulam R, Pertwee RG (2002) International Union of Pharmacology. XXVII. Classification of Cannabinoid Receptors. Pharmacol Rev 54:161–202
7. Kelly S, Jhaveri DM, Sagar DR, Kendall DA, Chapman V (2003) Activation of Peripheral Cannabinoid CB1 Receptors Inhibits Mechanically Evoked Responses of Spinal Neurons in Non-Inflamed Rats and Rats with Hind Paw Inflammation. Eur J Neurosci 18:2239–2243
8. Khasabova IA, Harding-Rose C, Simone DA, Seybold VS (2004) Differential Effects of CB1 and Opioid Agonists on Two Populations of Adult Rat Dorsal Root Ganglion Neurons. J Neurosci 24:1744–1753
9. Malan TP, Ibrahim MM, Lai J, Vanderah TW, Makriyannis A, Porreca F (2003) CB2 cannabinoid Receptor Agonists: Pain Relief Without Psychoactive Effects? Curr Opin Pharmacol 3:62–67
10. Molina-Holgado F, Pinteaux E, Moore JD, Molina-Holgado E, Guaza C, Gibson RM, Rothwell NJ (2003) Endogenous Interleukin-1 Receptor Antagonist Mediates Anti-Inflammatory and Neuroprotective Actions of Cannabinoids in Neurons and Glia. J Neurosci 23:6470–6474
11. Quartilho A, Mata HP, Ibrahim MM, Vanderah TW, Porreca F, Makriyannis A, Malan TP (2003) Inhibition of Inflammatory Hyperalgesia by Activation of Peripheral CB2 Cannabinoid Receptors. Anesthesiol 99:955–960
12. Richardson JD, Kilo S, Hargreaves KM (1998) Cannabinoids Reduce Hyperalgesia and Inflammation via Interaction with Peripheral CB1 Receptors. Pain 75: 111–119
13. Walter L, Stella N (2004) Cannabinoids and neuroinflammation. Brit J Pharmacol 141:775–785
14. Samson MT, Small-Howard A, Shimoda LMN, Koblan-Huberson M, Stokes AJ, Turner H (2003) Differential Roles of CB1 and CB2 Cannabinoid Receptors in Mast Cells. J Immunol 170:4953–4962
15. Sokal DM, Elmes SJR, Kendall DA, Chapman V (2003) Intraplantar Injection of Anandamide Inhibits Mechanically-Evoked Responses of Spinal Neurones via Activation of CB2 Receptors in Anaesthetised Rats. Neuropharmacol 45:404–411

Inflammation, Neuropeptide Release

▶ Neuropeptide Release in Inflammation

Inflammation, Role of Peripheral Glutamate Receptors

SUSAN M. CARLTON
University of Texas Medical Branch, Galveston, TX, USA
smcarlto@utmb.edu

Synonyms

Peripheral Glutamate Receptors, Role in Inflammation

Definition

Inflammation and its accompanying pain is a complicated process. Recently it has been reported that peripheral glutamate and peripheral glutamate receptors contribute to inflammatory pain and these data are summarized here.

Characteristics

There are several lines of evidence that glutamate receptors in the skin contribute to inflammatory pain. The data are derived from anatomical, behavioral and physiological experiments.

Anatomical studies in the ▶ dorsal root ganglia (DRG) indicate that ▶ ionotropic glutamate receptors (iGluR) are expressed by significant populations of sensory neurons. N-methyl-D-aspartate receptor 1 (NMDAR1) receptors are localized in virtually all DRG cells, however, only subpopulations of DRG neurons express kainate and α-amino-3-hydroxy-5-methyl-4-isoxazole propionic acid (AMPA) receptors (Sato et al. 1993). Immunohistochemistry at the electron microscopic level demonstrates that $48 \pm 18\%$ of unmyelinated axons in the rat digital nerve are positively labeled for the NMDAR1 subunit, while $27 \pm 3\%$ and $23 \pm$

8% are labeled for subunits of the kainate and AMPA receptor (Coggeshall and Carlton 1998). Forty-eight hours after intraplantar injection of complete Freund's adjuvant (CFA), there is a significant increase in the number of digital axons expressing the iGluRs (Carlton and Coggeshall 1999). The percentage of NMDAR1-labeled fibers increases from 48% to 61%, for kainate the increase is from 27% to 47% and for AMPA it is from 23% to 43%. These results suggest that there is an increased potential for activation of glutamate receptors in the inflamed state. ► Metabotropic glutamate receptors (mGluRs) have also been localized in primary sensory neurons (Bhave et al. 2001; Carlton et al. 2001). At this time it is unknown whether their expression changes during inflammation.

In behavioral studies, activation of these peripheral receptors following intraplantar injection of glutamate (Carlton et al. 1995) or injection of more selective iGluR or mGluR agonists in normal skin results in increased mechanical sensitivity as well as thermal sensitivity (Zhou et al. 1996; Carlton et al. 1998; Bhave 2001; Zhou et al. 2001). Intraplantar injection of 1 mM NMDA in normal animals produces a change in mechanical sensitivity equivalent to that seen 48 h post-CFA injection. Furthermore, concentrations of NMDA that have no effect in normal animals produce a significant reduction in mechanical thresholds in the inflamed hind paw (Du et al. 2003). This data suggests that subthreshold concentrations of glutamate may result in activation of glutamate receptors in the inflamed hind paw. Locally applied iGluR or Group I mGluR antagonists and Group II mGluR agonists can reduce nociceptive behaviors in several models of inflammation including those due to formalin, carrageenan, CFA and mustard oil (Carlton 2001; Neugebauer and Carlton 2002).

Recording from identified nociceptors using an *in vitro* skin-nerve preparation demonstrates that normal nociceptors are excited and sensitized by application of glutamate (Du et al. 2001) or NMDA (Du et al. 2003). Both Aδ and C nociceptors show a significant increase in activity compared to background when their receptive fields are exposed to 300 μM glutamate. Surprisingly, 1 mM glutamate results in lesser activity, however, it is possible that a desensitization of receptors occurs at this higher concentration. Furthermore, a 2 min exposure to 300 μM glutamate will increase unit responses to heat. This heat sensitization can occur whether the unit is excited by glutamate or not (Du et al. 1001). In 48 h CFA-inflamed skin, there is a slight shift to the left in the dose-response curve for NMDA-induced activation of nociceptors compared to normal skin, indicating that the amount of NMDA required to induce nociceptor activation is reduced 10-fold in inflamed skin. Furthermore, the percentage of NMDA-activated nociceptors and NMDA-induced discharge rates in these nociceptors is significantly increased in inflamed compared to normal skin and this activity can be blocked by co-application of the NMDA antagonist MK-801 (Du et al. 2003). Thus, it is clear that responses of nociceptors to glutamate stimulation change in the inflamed state.

A major source of ligand for activation of these peripheral receptors in normal and inflamed skin is the primary afferent terminals themselves since over 90% of DRG cells contain glutamate at concentrations considered to be higher than that representing metabolic stores. Stimulation of primary afferent fibers in the non-noxious or noxious range results in release of glutamate from peripheral primary afferent terminals (deGroot et al. 2000). The endogenous glutamate could then initiate or enhance the activity of nociceptors in the microenvironment through paracrine or autocrine stimulation (Fig. 1). There are several lines of evidence that glutamate content increases in inflamed tissue in both animal and human studies. Nerves innervating inflamed knee joints show an increase in glutamate immunoreactivity suggesting enhanced glutamate content (Westlund et al. 1992). There is increased glutamate content in inflamed hind paws as measured by microdialysis (Omote et al. 1998). The macrophages and serum that infiltrate inflamed regions will also contribute to the glutamate content (Piani et al. 1991; McAdoo et al. 1997). In human studies glutamate content increases in the synovial fluid of arthritic patients (McNearney et al. 2000). There is a ready source of ligand for glutamate receptors in inflamed regions (Fig. 2).

That glutamate receptors and ligand contribute to nociception and that both receptors and ligand increase during inflammation have clinical relevance. It has been demonstrated that iGluRs are present on unmyelinated axons in human skin (Kinkelin et al. 2000). Also, local treatment of the skin with ketamine, an NMDAR antagonist reduces hyperalgesia associated with experimental burn injuries (Warncke et al. 1997). Formulation of glutamate receptor antagonists that do not cross the blood brain barrier could be useful in reducing peripheral nociceptor activity while avoiding central side effects. Glutamate antagonists could be used in the periphery in combination with drugs that target the central nervous system to reduce both peripheral and central sensitization. These glutamate receptor antagonists would offer a non-opiate method for control of inflammatory pain.

References

1. Bhave G, Karim F, Carlton SM et al. (2001) Peripheral group I metabotropic glutamate receptors modulate nociception in mice. Nat Neurosci 4:417–423
2. Carlton SM (2001) Peripheral excitatory amino acids. Curr Opin Pharm 1:52–56
3. Carlton SM, Hargett GL, Coggeshall RE (1995) Localization and activation of glutamate receptors in unmyelinated axons of rat glabrous skin. Neurosci Lett 197:25–28
4. Carlton SM, Zhou S, Coggeshall RE (1998) Evidence for the interaction of glutamate and NK1 receptors in the periphery. Brain Res 790:160–169
5. Carlton SM, Coggeshall RE (1999) Inflammation-induced changes in peripheral glutamate receptor populations. Brain Res 820:63–70

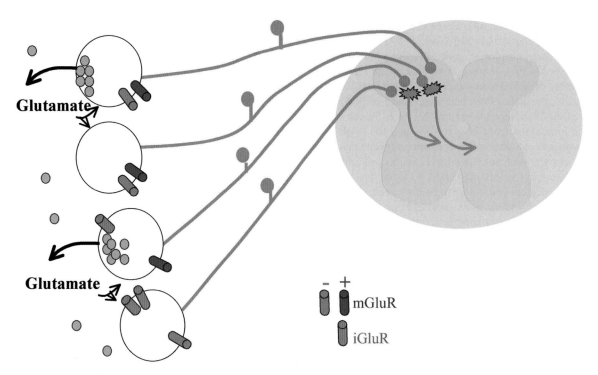

Inflammation, Role of Peripheral Glutamate Receptors, Figure 1   Glutamate-evoked activity in normal nociceptors. This schematic drawing depicts nociceptors terminating in the skin. In the normal state, many of the terminals contain glutamate in vesicles that are released upon stimulation. Through autocrine and/or paracrine routes, glutamate receptors (iGluRs, mGluRs) on nociceptors can be activated, modulating nociceptive transmission to the spinal cord.

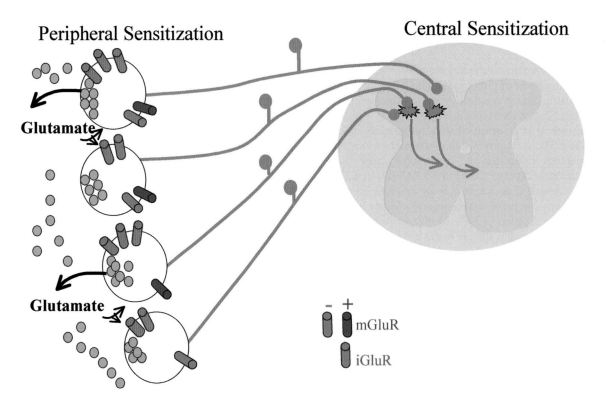

Inflammation, Role of Peripheral Glutamate Receptors, Figure 2   Glutamate-enhanced nociception in inflammation. In the inflamed state, there is an increase in glutamate content in terminals innervating the inflamed region, an increase in the number of glutamate receptor (GluR)-containing axons and thus an increased probability of GluR activation. In the inflamed region, other elements may contribute to an increase in glutamate content in the vicinity including mast cells and serum from leaky blood vessels. All of these factors will lead to enhanced nociceptive transmission.

6. Carlton SM, Hargett GL, Coggeshall RE (2001) Localization of metabotropic glutamate receptors 2/3 on primary afferent axons in the rat. Neuroscience 105:957–969
7. Coggeshall RE, Carlton SM (1998) Ultrastructural analysis of NMDA, AMPA and kainate receptors on unmyelinated and myelinated axons in the periphery. J Comp Neurol 391:78–86
8. deGroot JF, Zhou S, Carlton SM (2000) Peripheral glutamate release in the hindpaw following low and high intensity sciatic stimulation. NeuroReport 11:497–502
9. Du J, Koltzenburg M, Carlton SM (2001) Glutamate-induced excitation and sensitization of nociceptors in rat glabrous skin. Pain 89:187–198
10. Du J, Zhou S, Coggeshall RE et al. (2003) N-methyl-D-aspartate-induced excitation and sensitization of normal and inflamed nociceptors. Neuroscience 118:547–562
11. Kinkelin I, Brocker E.-B, Koltzenburg M et al. (2000) Localization of ionotropic glutamate receptors in peripheral axons of human skin. Neurosci Lett 283:149–152
12. McAdoo DJ, Hughes M, Xu G.-Y et al. (1997) Microdialysis studies of the role of chemical agents in secondary damage upon spinal cord injury. J Neurotrauma 14:507–515
13. McNearney, T, Speegle, D, Lawand NB et al. (2000) Excitatory amino acid profiles of synovial fluid from patients with arthritis. J Rheumatol 27:739–745
14. Neugebauer E, Carlton SM (2002) Peripheral metabotropic glutamate receptors as drug targets for pain relief. Expert Opin Ther Targets 6:349-361
15. Omote, K, Kawamata T, Kawamata M et al. (1998) Formalin-induced release of excitatory amino acids in the skin of the rat hindpaw. Brain Res 787:161–164
16. Piani D, Frei K, Do KQ et al.(1991) Murine brain macrophages induce NMDA receptor mediated neurotoxicity *in vitro* by secreting glutamate. Neurosci Lett 133:159–162
17. Sato K, Kiyama H, Park HT et al. (1993) AMPA, KA and NMDA receptors are expressed in the rat DRG neurones. NeuroReport 4:1263–1265
18. Warncke T, Jorum E, Stubhaug A (1997) Local treatment with the N-methyl-D-aspartate receptor antagonist ketamine, inhibits development of secondary hyperalgesia in man by a peripheral action. Neurosci Lett 227:1–4
19. Westlund KN, Sun YC, Sluka KA et al. (1992) Neural changes in acute arthritis in monkeys. II. Increased glutamate immunoreactivity in the medial articular nerve. Brain Res Rev 17:15–27
20. Zhou S, Komak S, Du J et al. (2001) Metabotropic glutamate 1α receptors on peripheral primary afferent fibers: their role in nociception. Brain Res 913:18–26
21. Zhou Z, Bonasera L, Carlton SM (1996) Peripheral adminsitration of NMDA, AMPA or KA results in pain behaviors in rats. NeuroReport 7:1–6

Inflammatory

Definition

Pertaining to the local response to an injury (usually including redness, warmth and pain).
▶ Pain Modulatory Systems, History of Discovery

Inflammatory Bowel Disease, n Animal Models

▶ Animal Models of Inflammatory Bowel Disease

Inflammatory Hyperalgesia by Skin Freezing

▶ Freezing Model of Cutaneous Hyperalgesia

Inflammatory Mediators

Definition

Inflammatory mediators comprise of a variety of endogenous substances including bradykinin, serotonin, histamine, prostaglandins, leukotrienes, amines, purines, cytokines and chemokines that are released in inflammation. They act on primary afferent nociceptors to cause pain by either inducing activity in nociceptors (activation/ excitation), or increasing nociceptor responses evoked by other stimuli (sensitization). In addition, inflammatory mediators cause the local release of other mediators from leucocytes and phagocytotic cells and attract leucocytes to the site of inflammation. Inflammatory mediators are involved in the process of removal of injured tissue and repair of the injured site. The role of inflammatory pain in this protective process is to prevent further trauma to the already injured tissue.
▶ Neuropeptide Release in Inflammation
▶ Perireceptor Elements
▶ Quantitative Thermal Sensory Testing of Inflamed Skin

Inflammatory Myopathies

▶ Myositis

Inflammatory Neuritis

LINDA S. SORKIN
Anesthesia Research Laboratories, University of California, San Diego, CA, USA
lsorkin@ucsd.edu

Synonyms

Nerve Inflammation; Neuritis; Inflammatory Neuropathy

Definition

Inflammation of a nerve or nerves. Note: Not to be used unless inflammation is thought to be present (Linblom et al. 1986), however this should include presence of neuroimmune reactions.

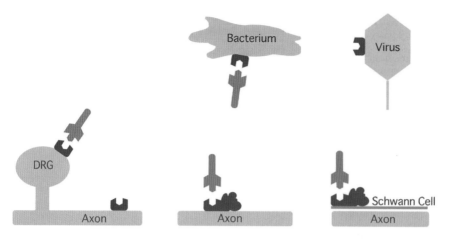

**Inflammatory Neuritis,
Figure 1** This schematic illustrates the principle of molecular mimicry. If bacteria/ viruses and Schwann cells/axons contain similar surface epitopes, antibodies generated as part of a normal immune response can cross-react with the neural elements and trigger a local immune cascade around the nerve. The epitope can be part of a more complex antigen as long as it is exposed. Exogenously administered antibody can trigger similar immune responses.

Characteristics

Inflammation of sensory nerves leading to pain is a common clinical occurrence. The etiology can range from responses to a local infection to neuroimmune reactions. In the latter case, antibodies generated in response to bacteria or viruses attack an axon or cell body of a sensory nerve or elements of local Schwann cells (usually myelin) because these structures share the epitope to which the antibody was originally directed. The autoimmune reaction resulting from this shared identity is termed molecular mimicry (Fig. 1). Alternatively, exogenous antibodies administered as part of a therapeutic regime can elicit similar responses resulting in an iatrogenic neuritis. In all cases, local immune reactions alter the microenvironments of the affected nerves. Under some conditions, the response seems to involve ▶ complement activation, in others activation of T and/or B cells is implicated. Frank infiltration of T cells, macrophages and neutrophils can occur, but perhaps due to the non-linearity of the inflammation, are not always seen in biopsy or autopsy specimens. Generation of prostaglandins, pro-inflammatory ▶ cytokines, oxygen free radicals and nitric oxide may all play a role in the immune cascade and help to break down the blood-nerve barrier. Antibody attack and/or the presence of pro-inflammatory agents within the local milieu can alter the activity of and/or destroy nerve fibers depending on the duration and severity of the response. When this includes A-delta and C nociceptive fibers, the disease is often characterized by painful dysesthesias during at least part of its course. Observed pathology can range from edema and axonal irritation, through localized demyelination with a resultant conduction slowing to irreversible axonal loss. Pain is frequently a prominent symptom of several stages of neuritis, but is not necessarily present throughout the full course of the disease.

Animal Models

Current animal models of neuritis with documented pain behavior involve placement of pro-inflammatory sub-

stances on or around the mid sciatic nerve (Eliav et al. 1999; Sorkin and Doom 2000; Gazda et al. 2001). These tend to model the less severe end of the nerve damage continuum with the most prominent change in pathology being a reversible edema of the affected nerve. Resident peri-sciatic immune cells may increase local release of interleukins, tumor necrosis factor (▶ TNF) and oxygen free radicals in the absence of prominent changes in the number of infiltrating immune cells (Gazda et al. 2001). However, application of complete Freund's adjuvant (CFA) to the nerve results in increases in both CD4 and CD8 staining T-lymphocytes (Eliav et al. 1999). Increases in endogenous pro-inflammatory substances in these models are local and are not observed in plasma. Epineural application of pro-inflammatory agents uniformly results in a profound mechanical ▶ allodynia in the ipsilateral hind paw of the affected nerve. Increasing the severity of the insult (dose of the inflammatory agent) serves to make the allodynic portions of the skin bilateral (mirror image pain). The pain behavior is reversed by spinal administration of glial inhibitors, p38 MAP kinase antagonists, antagonists to pro-inflammatory cytokines, N-methyl D-aspartate receptor antagonists and κ-opioids, but not by morphine (Eliav et al. 1999; Milligan et al. 2003).

Interestingly, epineural TNF or CFA elicits bursting activity in unmyelinated C nociceptive fibers and to a lesser extent in the finely myelinated A-delta fibers (Sorkin et al. 1997), (Eliav et al. 2001). The TNF-induced axonal firing is enhanced in conditions of inflammation and/or nerve damage. Systemic or intrathecal administration of exogenous antibody to a ganglioside found in peripheral nerve (GD_2 ganglioside) also produces mechanical allodynia in the absence of detectable thermal hyperalgesia. Like TNF administration, GD_2 ganglioside results in bursting activity in peripheral C fibers at a higher frequency than in A-delta afferent fibers within the sural nerve (Xiao et al. 1997). Low dose intravenous lidocaine (1–2 μg/ml plasma levels) temporarily turns off the ectopic activity, indicating that sodium channel stabilizing agents may be an effective treatment for the symptomatology, but not the origins, of the neuritis-associated pain.

While animal models for multiple sclerosis (experimental autoimmune encephalomyelitis) are used and might model more severe inflammatory neuritis, these models are not routinely examined for pain behavior.

Clinical Syndromes

Neuritis resulting from probable autoimmune pathogenesis has several common characteristics. There is a known or presumed antibody response against an epitope found within the peripheral nerve. The most common epitopes involved in molecular mimicry resulting in neuritis are the gangliosides and myelin-associated proteins (MAG) found in cell surface membranes. Neural membranes are enriched with sialic acid containing sphingolipids, including gangliosides. Detectable plasma levels of antibodies to several disialosyl gangliosides are associated with sensory ataxic neuropathy, Miller-Fisher syndrome and many variants of ▶ Guillain-Barré syndrome (GBS) (Quarles and Weiss 1999). In the first month of the disease, 70%–90% of GBS patients complain of severe pain (Moulin et al. 1997). Acute GBS has been reported secondary to *Campylobacter jejuni*, Epstein-Barr virus and cytomegalovirus. More rarely it has occurred following therapeutic administration of ganglioside mixtures (Illa et al. 1995). Interestingly, systemic administration of GD_2 ganglioside as an immunotherapy results in a whole body allodynia; nerve biopsy in adult patients (who have more severe symptoms than pediatric patients) indicated demyelination and mononuclear infiltrates in both the endoneurial and perivascular spaces (Saleh et al. 1992). Thus, exogenous antibodies to nerve gangliosides can initiate a prominent neuritis. High plasma levels of IgM antibodies to MAG are also associated with neuropathic syndromes with a strong sensory deficit. Various circulating antibodies against neural tissue, including GD_{1a} and GD_{1b} gangliosides, have been found in patients with ▶ chronic inflammatory demyelinating polyneuropathy (CIDP). However, much evidence points to T cell and macrophage initiated involvement (van der Meche and van Doorn 1995). Pain is less frequently reported overall in CIPD (about 20%), however, when the population is restricted to patients with sensory variants, it approaches that of GBS. Infiltration of inflammatory cells into the endoneurium is less common in CIPD than in GBS. If perivascular infiltrates occur, they are found primarily in the epineurium. Disease pathology including demyelination and decreases in nerve conduction velocity can be reproduced in experimental animals by injection of plasma from patients (Dalakas 1995).

In both GBS and CIPD timely removal of antibodies using plasma exchange or suppression of their synthesis by ▶ immunoglobulin therapy remains the most effective treatment. An early study of diabetic patients with polyneuropathy that meets the electrophysiological criteria for CIPD suggests that immunoglobulin therapy may elicit clinical improvement in this population indicating similar etiologies for both diseases (Sharma et al. 2002).

References

1. Dalakas M C (1995) Basic aspects of neuroimmunology as they relate to immunotherapeutic targets: present and future prospects. Ann Neurol 37 Suppl 1:S2–13
2. Eliav E, Herzberg U, Caudle RM (1999) Neuropathic pain from an experimental neuritis of the rat sciatic nerve. Pain 83:169–182
3. Eliav E, Benoliel R, Tal M (2001) Inflammation with no axonal damage of the rat saphenous nerve trunk induces ectopic discharge and mechanosensitivity in myelinated axons. Neurosci Lett 311:49–52
4. Gazda L S, Milligan ED, Hansen MK et al. (2001) Sciatic inflammatory neuritis (SIN): behavioral allodynia is paralleled by peri-sciatic proinflammatory cytokine and superoxide production. J Peripher Nerv Syst 6:111–129
5. Illa I, Ortiz N, Gallard E et al. (1995) Acute axonal Guillain-Barré syndrome with IgG antibodies against motor axons following parenteral gangliosides. Annals of Neurology 38:218–224
6. Linblom U, Mersky H, Mumford JM et al. (1986) Pain terms: a current list with definitions and usage. Pain Suppl. 3:S215–S221
7. Milligan E D, Twining C, Chacur M et al. (2003) Spinal glia and proinflammatory cytokines mediate mirror-image neuropathic pain in rats. J Neurosci 23:1026–1040
8. Moulin D E, Hagen N, Feasby TE et al. (1997) Pain in Guillain-Barré syndrome. Neurology 48:328–331
9. Quarles R H, Weiss MD (1999) Autoantibodies associated with peripheral neuropathy. Muscle Nerve 22:800–822
10. Saleh MN, Khazaeli MB, Wheeler RH et al (1992) Phase I trial of the chimeric anti-GD2 monoclonal antibody ch14.18 in patients with malignant melanoma. Human Antibodies and Hybridomas 3:19–24
11. Sharma KR, Cross J, Ayyar DR et al (2002) Diabetic demyelinating polyneuropathy responsive to intravenous immunoglobulin therapy. Arch Neurol 59:751–757
12. Sorkin LS, Doom C (2000) Epineurial application of TNF elicits an acute mechanical hyperalgesia in the awake rat. J Peripheral Nervous Sys 5: 96–100
13. Sorkin L S, Xiao WH, Wagner R et al (1997) Tumour necrosis factor-alpha induces ectopic activity in nociceptive primary afferent fibres. Neuroscience 81:255–262
14. van der Meche FGP, van Doorn A (1995) Guillain-Barre syndrome and chronic inflammatory demyelinating polyneuropathy: immune mechanisms and update on current therapies. Ann Neurol 37 Suppl 1:S14–31
15. Xiao W H, Yu AL, Sorkin LS (1997) Electrophysiological characteristics of primary afferent fibers after systemic administration of anti-GD2 ganglioside antibody. Pain 69:145–151

Inflammatory Neuropathy

▶ Inflammatory Neuritis

Inflammatory Nociception, Genetic Factors

▶ Heritability of Inflammatory Nociception

Inflammatory Nociception, Heritability

▶ Heritability of Inflammatory Nociception

Inflammatory Nociceptor Sensitisation, Prostaglandins and Leukotrienes

BLAIR D. GRUBB
Department of Cell Physiology and Pharmacology,
University of Leicester, Leicester, UK
bdg1@leicester.ac.uk

Synonyms

Prostaglandins in Inflammatory Nociceptor Sensitisation; Leukotrienes in Inflammatory Nociceptor Sensitisation

Definition

The term prostaglandins (PG) describes a group of oxygenated polyunsaturated fatty acids containing a cyclopentane ring and two alkyl side chains that are derived from arachidonic acid by the action of cyclooxygenase (cox) enzymes. The alphanumeric nomenclature (e.g. E_2, I_2, D_2, $F_{2\alpha}$) describes the nature and position of side groups and double bonds on the cyclopentane ring and of double bonds on the alkyl side groups. The leukotrienes (e.g. LTB_4, LTC_4, LTD_4) are a related group of conjugated trienes synthesised from arachidonic acid by the enzyme 5-lipoxygenase (Benedetto et al. 1987).

Characteristics

The link between PG synthesis and nociceptors' sensitisation was established over 30 years ago when it was discovered that non-steroidal anti-inflammatory drugs (NSAIDs) produced analgesia by inhibiting PG synthesis (Vane 1971; Ferreira, 1972). PGs elicit nociceptor sensitisation by lowering mechanical and thermal activation thresholds in nociceptive nerve endings thus reducing the stimulus intensity required to elicit action potential firing in the afferent axon.

PGs are synthesised by cyclooxygenase (cox) enzymes from their natural precursor arachidonic acid (Fig. 1). Three cox isoforms have been cloned in mammalian species, cox-1, -2 and -3. Cox-1 is a constitutively expressed isoform present in most tissues and is responsible for PG synthesis associated with normal physiological processes. Cox-2 is constitutively expressed in some tissues, e.g. brain, spinal cord and kidney, but in most tissues expression levels are low unless the tissues are damaged. Cox-2 gene expression is up-regulated in somatic and neural tissues 3–12 hours after tissue damage as part of the normal immune response. Since PGs are lipids and cannot be stored inside cells, tissue damage results in an increase in extracellular levels of PGs, which can contribute to the sensitisation of nociceptors. Cox-3 was identified only recently and is a splice variant of cox-1 that is present in dog and appears to be the molecular target for acetaminophen (paracetamol) in this species. In humans, however, cox-3 protein is probably not expressed due to a frame-shift mutation that results in an incomplete gene product.

Although several different PG species exist, only PGE_2 and PGI_2 (prostacyclin) produce pronounced nociceptors' sensitisation to mechanical and thermal stimuli (Schaible and Grubb 1993; Bley et al. 1998). It should be noted, however, that PGs can also directly excite some nociceptive nerve terminals suggesting that they might have more than one mode of action (Birrell et al. 1991; Shepelmann et al. 1992; Schmelz et al. 2003). There are many examples of PG sensitisation of nociceptors skin, muscle and joint *in vivo*. The sensitisation of joint afferents has been studied extensively in studies where these compounds or their analogues have been applied by close arterial injections. PGE_2 primarily elicits sensitising responses to mechanical stimuli whilst PGI_2 and analogues produce both sensitisation and excitation. Interestingly, PGs do not act independently to produce nociceptor sensitisation but act in concert with other inflammatory mediators. A good example of this is PGE_2-mediated enhancement of bradykinin responses in articular nociceptors. Bradykinin alone is a potent algogen and electrophysiological recordings from naïve primary afferents show that it directly activates a proportion of nociceptors and also enhances responses to mechanical stimuli. In the presence of PGs however, these actions are significantly enhanced (Schaible and Schmidt 1988; Birrell et al. 1993). Interestingly, bradykinin-induced sensitisation of nociceptors to some stimuli can be attenuated by NSAIDs suggesting that a component of the bradykinin effect itself involves synthesis of PGs (Pethö et al. 2001)

PGs elicit nociceptor sensitisation by binding to G-protein coupled PG receptors on nerve terminals and inducing changes in membrane excitability. PG receptors are named after the PG species that is the endogenous ligand (EP, IP, DP and FP). There are four EP receptor subtypes, EP_{1-4}, and two of these, EP_1 and EP_3, can express varying numbers of splice variants in different species. The EP_3 receptor is most prolific in this respect having up 9 splice variants dependent on species. By contrast there are only single IP, DP and FP receptor subtypes. This diversity of receptors and receptor subtypes mean that a number of signalling cascades are activated by PGs depending on the receptor subtype that is expressed in each tissue. In sensory neurones, mRNA for all EP receptors and for IP receptors has been identified (Oida H 1995; Donaldson et al. 2001) (Fig. 1). However, a lack of suitable antibodies

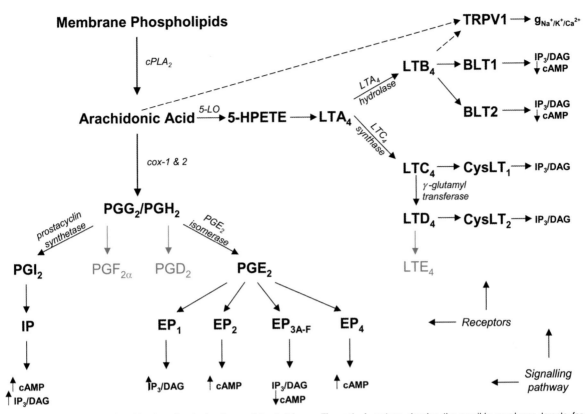

Inflammatory Nociceptor Sensitisation, Prostaglandins and Leukotrienes, Figure 1 A cartoon showing the possible membrane targets for prostaglandins and leukotrienes in nociceptors' peripheral terminals. Prostaglandins seem to mediate their effects through GPCRs located on the cell membrane whilst leukotrienes can elicit either direct or indirect effects. Solid lines indicate pathways for which there is solid evidence whilst dotted lines show possible pathways.

has precluded an objective assessment of PG receptor distribution in sensory ganglia and there is little known about the co-expression of individual prostaglandin receptors/subtypes with phenotypic markers of different class of primary afferent neurones, e.g. peptidergic nociceptors (CGRP expressing), non-peptidergic (labelled by isolectin B4) and non-nociceptive fibres (labelled by microfilament protein antibody, RT-97).

EP_1 receptors couple primarily to the $G_{q/11}$ family of G-proteins and their activation results in an activation of protein kinase C (PKC) and elevated levels of inositol 1,4,5 trisphosphate (IP_3) and diacylglycerol. This results in an increase in intracellular calcium and activation of protein kinase C, which may underlie the regulation of ion channel conductances or mechanical or thermal transducer proteins. EP_2 and EP_4 receptors couple to the G_s family of g-proteins and ligand binding results in activation of adenylyl cyclase and an increase in intracellular concentrations of cAMP and protein kinase A (PKA). Like PKC, PKA can phosphorylate and regulate a number of different ion channels to change membrane excitability. The G-protein coupling of EP_3 receptors is less well understood since there is a multitude of similar but subtly different splice variants in different species. It is clear, however, that depending on the spice variant

concerned, $G_{q/11}$, $G_{i/o}$ (or even G_s) proteins could be activated following ligand binding to EP_3 receptors. IP receptor coupling is primarily G_s linked, although some studies have suggested that there is a $G_{q/11}$-mediated activation of phosphoinositide turnover (Bley et al. 1998) (Fig. 1).

Primary afferent nociceptors are phenotypically distinct, expressing a number of ion channels that can be modulated by PGs. PGE_2 can regulate the mechanical and thermal transduction processes by modulating capsaicin/heat-sensitive TRPV1 currents and mechanosensitive currents in sensory neurones through PKA-dependent pathways (Lopshire and Nicol 1998; Cho et al. 2002). In addition to transducer channels, PGE_2 can modulate the activity of a number of channels that regulate action potential threshold and firing frequency (Fig. 2). In dorsal root ganglion neurons, for example, the activation kinetics (firing threshold) of the tetrodotoxin-resistant sodium current is altered by PGE_2 (England et al. 1996) through cAMP/PKA-dependent phosphorylation of $Na_{V1.8}$ (Fitzgerald et al. 1999) and PKC-dependent mechanisms (Gold et al. 1998).

Potassium channels that control action potential repolarisation are also targets for PGs. PGE_2 and PGI_2 inhibit

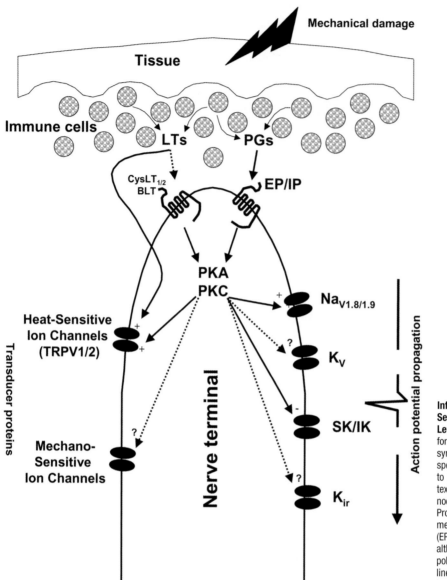

Inflammatory Nociceptor Sensitisation, Prostaglandins and Leukotrienes, Figure 2 Pathways for prostaglandin and leukotriene synthesis showing the chemical species that have been shown to sensitise nociceptors in bold text. Those not implicated in nociceptors sensitisation are in grey. Prostaglandins and leukotrienes mediate their actions through GPCRs (EP$_{1-4}$, IP, BLT1 & 2, CysLT$_{1/2}$) although leukotrienes and related polyunsaturated fatty acids (dashed lines) can directly gate the TRPV1 ion channel.

delayed rectifier potassium currents to increase cell excitability and action potential firing (Nicol et al. 1997; Jiang et al. 2003). In addition, calcium-activated potassium channels present in nociceptors are modulated by PGE$_2$ resulting in a decrease in spike frequency adaptation and an increase in action potential firing frequency (Weinreich and Wonderlin 1987).

In comparison to PGs, the role of leukotrienes and their receptors in nociceptors sensitisation has been neglected. There is good evidence showing that leukotrienes are present in inflammatory exudates but a limited number of studies where leukotrienes have been implicated in nociceptor sensitisation (Martin et al. 1987; Madison et al. 1990). Furthermore, it is not yet known whether leukotriene receptors are present on nociceptors terminals nor if they mediate the sensitising actions of leukotrienes (Figs. 1 and 2). Indeed there is much better evidence that leukotrienes can influence nociceptor sensitisation through direct interactions with ion channel proteins. This has been demonstrated for LTB$_4$, which is structurally related to capsaicin and activates TRPV1, the heat sensitive ion channel, by binding to the cytoplasmic domain of this protein (Hwang et al. 2000). Furthermore a number of other ion channels are known to be modulated by leukotrienes in different tissues, although it is not yet known whether this occurs in nociceptors.

References

1. Benedetto C, McDonald-Gibson RG, Nigam S et al. (1987) Prostaglandins and related substances: a practical approach. IRL Press Ltd, Oxford, Washington

2. Birrell GJ, McQueen DS, Iggo A et al. (1991) PGI2-induced sensitisation of articular mechanonociceptors. Neurosci Lett 124:5–8
3. Birrell GJ, McQueen DS, Iggo A et al. (1993) Prostanoid-induced potentiation of the excitatory and sensitising effects of bradykinin on articular mechanonociceptors in the rat ankle joint. Neuroscience 54:537–544
4. Bley KR, Hunter JC, Eglen RM et al. (1998) The role of IP prostanoid receptors in inflammatory pain. Trends Pharmacol Sci 19:141–147
5. Cho H, Shin J, Shin CY et al (2002) Mechanosensitive ion channels in cultured sensory neurons of rats. J Neurosci 22:1238–1247
6. Donaldson LF, Humphrey PS, Oldfield S et al. (2001) Expression and regulation of prostaglandin E receptor subtype mRNAs in rat sensory ganglia and spinal cord in response to peripheral inflammation. Prostaglandins Other Lipid Mediat 63:109–122
7. England S, Bevan S, Docherty RJ (1996) PGE$_2$ modulates the tetrodotoxin-resistant sodium current in neonatal rat dorsal root ganglion neurones via the cyclic AMP-protein kinase A cascade. J Physiol 495:429–440
8. Ferreira SH (1972) Prostaglandins, aspirin-like drugs and analgesia. Nat New Biol 240:200–203
9. Fitzgerald EM (1999) cAMP-dependent phosphorylation of the tetrodotoxin-resistant voltage-dependent sodium channel SNS. J Physiol 516:433–466
10. Gold MS, Levine JD, Correa AM (1998) Modulation of TTX-R I_{Na} by PKC and PKA and their role in PGE$_2$-induced sensitisation of rat sensory neurones *in vitro*. J Neurosci 18:10345–10355
11. Hwang SW, Cho H, Kwak J et al. (2000) Direct activation of capsaicin receptors by products of lipoxygenases: Endogenous capsaicin-like substances. PNAS 97:6155–6160
12. Jiang X, Zhang YH, Clark JD et al. (2003) Prostaglandin E2 inhibits the potassium current in sensory neurones from hyperalgesic Kv1.1 knockout mice. Neuroscience 119:65–72
13. Lopshire JC, Nicol GD (1998) The cAMP transduction cascade mediates the prostaglandin E2 enhancement of the capsaicin-elicited current in rat sensory neurons: whole cell and single channel studies. J Neurosci 18:6081–6092
14. Madison S, Whilsel EA, Suarez-Roca H et al. (1990) Sensitising effects of leukotriene B4 on intradental primary afferents. Pain 49:99–104
15. Martin HA, Basbaum AI, Kwiat GC et al. (1987) Leukotriene and prostaglandin sensitisation of cutaneous high threshold C- and A-delta mechanonociceptors in the hairy skin of the rat hindlimbs. Neuroscience 22:651–659
16. Nicol GD, Vasko MR, Evans AR (1997) Prostaglandins suppress an outward potassium current in embryonic rat sensory neurones J Physiol 77:167–176
17. Oida H, Namba T, Sugimoto Y et al (1995) *In situ* hybridization studies of prostacyclin receptor mRNA expression in various mouse organs Br J Pharmacol 116:2828–2837
18. Pethö G, Derow A, Reeh PW (2001) Bradykinin-induced nociceptor sensitisation to heat is mediated by cyclooxygenase products in isolated rat skin. Eur J Neurosci 14:210–218
19. Schaible H-G, Grubb (1993) Afferent and spinal mechanisms of joint pain. Pain 55:5–54.
20. Schaible H-G, Schmidt RF (1988) Excitation and sensitisation of fine articular afferents from cat's knee joint by prostaglandin E$_2$. J Physiol 403:91–104
21. Schepelmann K, Meßlonger K, Schaible H-G et al. (1992) Inflammatory mediators and nociception in the joint: Excitation and sensitization of slowly conducting afferent fibres of the cat's knee by prostaglandin I$_2$. Neuroscience 50:237–247
22. Schmelz M, Schmidt R, Weidner C et al. (2003) Chemical response pattern of different classes of c-nociceptors to pruritogens and algogens. J Neurophysiol 89:2441–2448
23. Vane JR (1971) Inhibition of prostaglandin synthesis as a mechanism of action for aspirin-like drugs. Nat New Biol 231:232–235
24. Weinreich D and Wonderlin WF (1987) Inhibition of calcium-dependent spike after-hyperpolarisation increases excitability of rabbit visceral sensory neurones. J Physiol 294:415–427

Inflammatory Pain

Definition

Inflammatory pain is that which is associated with chronic inflammation (e.g. present in arthritis, back pain or tempomandibular joint disorders).

▶ NSAIDs, Mode of Action

Inflammatory Pain and NGF

DAVID BENNETT

Department of Neurology, King's College Hospital, London, UK

dlhbennett@talk21.com

Definition

Inflammation is the body's reaction to injury in which part of the body becomes hot, red, swollen and painful. At the cellular level initially neutrophils and subsequently macrophages infiltrate the affected area. Many chemical mediators are involved in this process one of which is nerve growth factor (NGF). NGF is a secreted protein of molecular mass of 13 kD which exists as a homodimer. It is a member of the neurotrophin family, which also includes brain derived neurotrophic factor (BDNF), neurotrophin-3 (NT3) and neurotrophin-4/5 (NT4/5). NGF binds to both a high affinity tyrosine kinase receptor trkA and a low affinity receptor p75.

Characteristics

NGF is the archetypal 'target derived neurotrophic factor' and was initially characterised for its neurodevelopmental effects. During the period of naturally occurring cell death, the survival of post-ganglionic sympathetic neurons and small diameter nociceptive sensory neurons is critically dependent on limiting amounts of NGF produced in their target fields. This role of NGF is shown in people who have a mutation in the trkA NGF receptor resulting in congenital insensitivity to pain and anhidrosis in which nociceptive neurons and sympathetic neurons fail to develop (Indo 2002). During development, virtually all small diameter nociceptive neurons express trkA and are NGF dependent; however this receptor is down-regulated during the postnatal period (Bennett et al. 1996). In the adult trkA expression is restricted to those small diameter DRG cells which express the neuropeptides substance P (SP) and calcitonin gene related peptide (CGRP) (Fig. 1). There is a second group of small diameter DRG cells which do not express neuropeptides but possess cell surface glycoconjugates that bind the lectin isolectin B4 (IB4). These cells do not possess trkA receptors but express receptors for and are sensitive to another trophic factor glial cell line-derived neurotrophic factor.

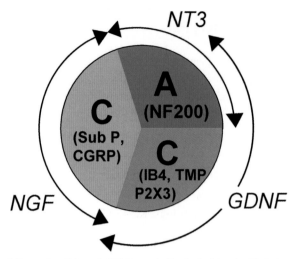

Inflammatory Pain and NGF, Figure 1 Pie chart relating trophic factor sensitivity to the different neurochemically defined classes of DRG cells. Large diameter DRG cells (A-fibres) have myelinated axons and express the neurofilament NF200. These cells are responsive principally to the trophic factors NT-3 and GDNF. Small diameter DRG cells (C-fibres) have unmyelinated axons and can be broadly divided into two groups. The first group express the neuropeptides SP and CGRP and are NGF sensitive. The second group are non-peptidergic and bind the lectin IB4, these cells are GDNF sensitive.

NGF expression is required for the maintenance of a healthy neuronal phenotype in adult peptidergic DRG cells. NGF deprivation *in vivo* results in reduced thermal and chemical sensitivity in these neurons which is accompanied by a withdrawal of their terminals from their target fields (McMahon et al. 1995).

There is now strong evidence that NGF is an important mediator of inflammatory pain hypersensitivity: NGF levels increase following inflammation, NGF has been shown to sensitise nociceptive systems and most importantly blocking NGF bioactivity reduces inflammatory pain. The expression of NGF increases rapidly following an inflammatory stimulus and such increased levels have been shown in animals after inflammation induced by skin wounding, skin blistering, ultraviolet light, complete Freund's adjuvant, carrageenan and in a model of cystitis. Increased NGF levels have also been demonstrated in the bladder of patients with cystitis and in the synovial fluid of patients with arthritis. Studies in cell culture indicate that many growth factors and cytokines can increase NGF mRNA levels and NGF secretion these include: interleukin-1 (Il-1), Il-4, Il-5, tumour necrosis factor α (TNFα), transforming growth factor β (TGF β), platelet-derived growth factor (PDGF), acid and basic fibroblast growth factors (FGF-1, FGF-2) and epidermal growth factor (EGF). Both IL1 and TNFα have been shown to be important in increasing NGF levels *in vivo* (Safieh-Garabedian et al. 1995; Woolf et al. 1997). Some agents have been shown to consistently reduce NGF mRNA levels and secretion; these include glucocorticoids and the interferons.

The administration of small doses of NGF to adult animals and man can produce pain and hyperalgesia. In rodents a thermal hyperalgesia develops within 30 minutes of systemic NGF administration and both a thermal and a mechanical hyperalgesia is present after a couple of hours (Lewin et al. 1993). Subcutaneous NGF produces a thermal and mechanical hyperalgesia at the injection site (Andreev et al. 1995). In humans intravenous injections of very low doses of NGF produce widespread myalgia and hyperalgesia at the injection site. Injection site hyperalgesia was a prominent side effect in trials of the use of NGF in the treatment of diabetic neuropathy (Apfel et al. 2000).

The critical test of the hypothesis that NGF has a role in mediating inflammatory pain was to show that blocking NGF bioactivity could reduce the hyperalgesia induced by inflammation and this has now been demonstrated by multiple groups using different model systems. We have used a fusion protein of the ligand binding domain of the trkA receptor and Fc region of human IgG (McMahon et al. 1995). This binds to and therefore blocks the activity of endogenous NGF. Application of trkA-IgG either locally or systemically could significantly reduce the thermal hyperalgesia resulting from intra-plantar administration of carrageenan in the rodent (Fig. 2). This molecule also prevents the development of thermal hyperalgesia following skin incision and detrusor hyperexcitability in a rodent model of cystitis. Similar findings have been shown using function blocking antibodies to NGF in inflammation evoked by complete Freund's adjuvant (Woolf et al. 1994; Safieh-Garabedian et al. 1995). Blocking NGF reduces thermal hyperalgesia and in some studies mechanical hyperalgesia, without altering many of the other aspects of the inflammatory process such as the degree of oedema. There is now in-

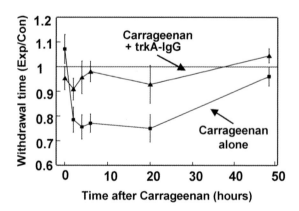

Inflammatory Pain and NGF, Figure 2 An NGF sequestering molecule trkA-IgG was used to investigate the role of NGF in inflammation. Thermal hyperalgesia develops in rats within hours following intraplantar injection of carrageenan. Animals which are inflamed and concurrently treated with trkA-IgG fail to develop most of the thermal hyperalgesia. Adapted from McMahon et al. 1995.

creasing understanding of how NGF contributes to inflammatory pain.

NGF administration causes a sensitisation of nociceptors to both thermal and chemical stimuli. These effects are probably mediated by a combination of acute changes in second messenger pathways within the nociceptor terminal itself as well as more chronic changes in gene expression within nociceptive neurons. The mechanisms by which NGF produces nociceptor sensitisation are the subject of a separate chapter, NGF sensitization of nociceptors. The algesic actions of NGF are not only limited to peripheral actions but in addition it has secondary effects on the spinal processing of nociceptive information. Firstly, the activation and sensitization of primary afferent nociceptors may lead to sufficient afferent activity to trigger central changes. Peripheral NGF administration to some visceral structures results in somatotopically appropriate induction of *c-fos* in the dorsal horn. Secondly NGF can modulate the expression of a number of neuropeptides and neuromodulators expressed within nociceptive neurons. NGF administration has been shown to increase the expression of SP and CGRP within nociceptive neurons both *in vitro* and *in vivo*. Following NGF treatment the release of SP within the dorsal horn is increased. The release of sensory neuropeptides is a well-known trigger for the induction of central sensitisation. Several hours after systemic NGF treatment, C-fibre stimulation produces greater than normal amounts of central sensitisation seen as wind-up of ventral root reflexes (Thompson et al. 1995). A-fibres also develop the novel ability to produce wind-up during inflammation and this may be secondary to novel SP expression within A-fibres (Thompson et al. 1995; Neumann et al. 1996). NGF can also modulate the central processing of nociceptive information through a novel mechanism-by increasing the expression and release of a second neurotrophic factor BDNF. BDNF is normally expressed within the NGF sensitive population of small diameter DRG cells and is anterogradely transported to their terminals within the superficial laminae of the dorsal horn where it is present within dense core vesicles (Michael et al. 1997). NGF and inflammation increase the expression of BDNF within these cells. The elevated expression of BDNF is accompanied by increased release of this factor following C-fibre stimulation. Exogenous BDNF results in facilitation of the flexor reflex (Kerr et al. 1999). This facilitation is mediated through activation of ERK MAP kinase in dorsal horn neurons, phosphorylation of the NMDA receptor subunit 1 and facilitation of NMDA receptor mediated responses (Lever et al. 2003). A trkB-IgG fusion protein has been used to sequester endogenous BDNF released within the dorsal horn and has demonstrated that BDNF has a role in the generation of hyperalgesia produced by inflammation or NGF administration (Kerr et al. 1999; Mannion et al. 1999).

In summary inflammation leads to a rapid induction of NGF expression and this can lead to a sensitisation of pain signalling systems via both peripheral and central mechanisms. There is now strong evidence that blocking NGF bioactivity reduces inflammatory hyperalgesia. NGF therefore provides a novel analgesic target and indeed clinical trials of the use of function blocking molecules in the treatment of inflammatory pain are under way.

References

1. Andreev NY, Dimitrieva N, Koltzenburg M et al. (1995) Peripheral administration of nerve growth factor in the adult rat produces a thermal hyperalgesia that requires the presence of sympathetic post-ganglionic neurones. Pain 63:109–115
2. Apfel SC, Schwartz S, Adornato BT et al. (2000) Efficacy and safety of recombinant human nerve growth factor in patients with diabetic polyneuropathy: A randomized controlled trial. rhNGF Clinical Investigator Group. JAMA 284:2215–2221
3. Bennett DL, Averill S, Clary DO et al. (1996) Postnatal changes in the expression of the trkA high-affinity NGF receptor in primary sensory neurons. Eur J Neurosci 8:2204–2208
4. Indo Y (2002) Genetics of congenital insensitivity to pain with anhidrosis (CIPA) or hereditary sensory and autonomic neuropathy type IV. Clinical, biological and molecular aspects of mutations in TRKA(NTRK1) gene encoding the receptor tyrosine kinase for nerve growth factor. Clin Auton Res 12 Suppl 1:120–132
5. Kerr BJ, Bradbury EJ, Bennett DL et al. (1999) Brain-derived neurotrophic factor modulates nociceptive sensory inputs and NMDA-evoked responses in the rat spinal cord. J Neurosci 19:5138–5148
6. Lever IJ, Pezet S, McMahon SB et al. (2003) The signaling components of sensory fiber transmission involved in the activation of ERK MAP kinase in the mouse dorsal horn. Mol Cell Neurosci 24:259–270
7. Lewin GR, Ritter AM, Mendell LM (1993) Nerve growth factor-induced hyperalgesia in the neonatal and adult rat. J Neurosci 13:2136–2148
8. Mannion RJ, Costigan M, Decosterd I et al. (1999) Neurotrophins: peripherally and centrally acting modulators of tactile stimulus-induced inflammatory pain hypersensitivity. Proc Natl Acad Sci USA 96:9385–9390
9. McMahon SB, Bennett DL, Priestley JV et al. (1995) The biological effects of endogenous nerve growth factor on adult sensory neurons revealed by a trkA-IgG fusion molecule. Nat Med 1:774–780
10. Michael GJ, Averill S, Nitkunan A et al. (1997) Nerve growth factor treatment increases brain-derived neurotrophic factor selectively in TrkA-expressing dorsal root ganglion cells and in their central terminations within the spinal cord. J Neurosci 17:8476–8490
11. Neumann S, Doubell TP, Leslie T et al. (1996) Inflammatory pain hypersensitivity mediated by phenotypic switch in myelinated primary sensory neurons. Nature 384:360–364
12. Safieh-Garabedian B, Poole S, Allchorne A et al. (1995) Contribution of interleukin-1 beta to the inflammation-induced increase in nerve growth factor levels and inflammatory hyperalgesia. Br J Pharmacol 115:1265–1275
13. Thompson SW, Dray A, McCarson KE et al. (1995) Nerve growth factor induces mechanical allodynia associated with novel A fibre-evoked spinal reflex activity and enhanced neurokinin-1 receptor activation in the rat. Pain 62:219–231
14. Woolf CJ, Safieh-Garabedian B, Ma QP et al. (1994) Nerve growth factor contributes to the generation of inflammatory sensory hypersensitivity. Neuroscience 62:327–331
15. Woolf CJ, Allchorne A, Safieh-Garabedian B et al. (1997) Cytokines, nerve growth factor and inflammatory hyperalgesia: the contribution of tumour necrosis factor alpha. Br J Pharmacol 121:417–424

Inflammatory Pain and Opioids

▶ Opioids and Inflammatory Pain

Inflammatory Pain, Human Models

▶ Human Models of Inflammatory Pain

Inflammatory Pain Models

Definition

The inflammatory process can be classified in three distinct phases: an acute and subacute phase, characterized by local vasodilatation, increased capillary permeability and infiltration of phagocytotic cells, and a chronic proliferative phase, in which tissue degeneration and fibrosis occur. According to these phases, *in vivo* animal models of inflammation/inflammatory pain have been developed. Models for testing acute and subacute inflammation are, for example, UV-induced erythema in guinea-pigs, and oxazolone- or croton-oil-induced ear edema in mice. A well-established model of chronic inflammation is adjuvant-induced arthritis in rats produced by intradermally inoculating a suspension of Mycobacterium butyricum into both hindpaws. To study visceral inflammation, experimental colitis is caused by rectal instillation of trinitrobenzene sulfonic acid. Local inflammation to measure inflammatory pain in animals is induced by intraarticular or intraplantar injection of carrageenan or formalin.

▶ Neuropeptide Release in Inflammation

Inflammatory Syndrome

▶ Lower Back Pain, Physical Examination

Infliximab

Definition

Monoclonal antibodies to TNFα that serve as a TNFα inhibitor in human autoimmune disorders.

▶ Cytokines as Targets in the Treatment of Neuropathic Pain

Inflow Artefacts

Definition

Susceptibility artifacts. In MRI, susceptibility artifacts are caused, for example, by medical devices in or near the magnetic field or by implants of the patient. These materials with magnetic susceptibility distort the linear magnetic field gradients, which results in bright areas (misregistered signals) and dark areas (no signal) nearby the magnetic material.

▶ Amygdala, Functional Imaging

Information and Psychoeducation in the Early Management of Persistent Pain

STEVEN J. LINTON
Department of Occupational and Environmental Medicine, Department of Behavioral, Social and Legal Sciences, Örebro University Hospital, Örebro, Sweden
steven.linton@orebroll.se

Synonyms

Education; Back Schools; Pain Schools; Patient Information; Health Informatics; Psychoeducation

Definition

Educational and informational approaches are concerned with providing patients with knowledge about their painful illness that will help them to cope better with the problem. Psychoeducation refers to approaches that in particular utilize psychological knowledge and advice, often provided in a "study group" format. In part, the aim is to provide basic knowledge about pain and how it operates, in order to increase knowledge and decrease distress and uncertainty about the pain problem. Moreover, informational activities almost always strive to change the patient's behavior to enhance coping.

Characteristics

Modern approaches to back and neck pain stress self-management. In order to achieve this, patients need to understand their problem and how they can manage it and consequently change their behavior in accordance. For example, a patient may need to understand that the pain itself is not harmful and that activity will enhance recovery. Further, the patient may be asked to engage in exercises, to take pain relievers on a specific time basis in order to remain active and to practice relaxation.

A lack of information or knowledge may therefore have grave consequences in the treatment of musculoskeletal pain for three reasons. First, lack of a correct explanation of the illness, its cause, course and treatment may well lead to uncertainty and an increase in anxiety and psychological distress. In other words, patients may worry and suffer needlessly. Second, when not properly informed, patients may not feel engaged in the process. Decisions about assessment and treatment may be perceived as over the head of the patient, thus pre-empting active participation. Third, self-care by the patient may be limited if the patient does not understand its importance. For example, patients may be unclear as to what they should do to enhance recovery. Moreover, if instead the patient feels she is being "taken care of", this may reduce motivation to engage in self-care activities. This is particularly salient because many of the self-care activities such as exercise involve considerable time and effort. Thus, there is good reason to believe that educational interventions may serve an important purpose.

Since communication problems in medicine are common, several attempts have been made to provide patients with clear information. In the rehabilitation clinic, patient information is sometimes used as a basic building block in multidimensional treatments for chronic pain that include many components. It is difficult to ascertain the extent of the effect of such information in relation to the effects of the other components. However, including such information is probably not particularly effective because the information is often limited in scope and provided to patients with difficult problems. At best, the information may be necessary but not sufficient to produce significant improvements (Burton and Waddell 2002).

Another approach has been to provide general health information. Some health authorities for example, have provided booklets designed to help patients self-manage minor illnesses such as colds, flu and cuts. However, controlled scientific tests of their effectiveness have been quite disappointing, as these booklets have little or no effect in reducing the number of clinical consultations e.g. (Heaney et al. 2001).

Written Materials

To be effective, written information needs to be read, understood, believed relevant and acted upon. A review of these premises however, shows that it is far from the usual case (Ley 1997). Indeed, written information as the only intervention appears to have small effect in changing behaviors. However, it might be incorporated into practices to enhance communication.

In the musculoskeletal pain area, several attempts have been made to provide patients with concrete educational materials in the form of pamphlets, books, videos or Internet services. These materials reflect different approaches primarily to back pain. Historically, written material was based on an ergonomic approach to back pain, where patients were provided with information about the structure of the spine and how injuries may occur. The message was focused on avoiding movements that are not ergonomic. In addition, these booklets

usually advised patients to contact their doctor if any of a host of pain situations occurred. Not surprisingly this type of information has not proved to be effective in lowering distress, absenteeism or consultation (Burton and Waddell 2002).

There is now rather extensive theoretical and scientific knowledge on which to base potent patient information. As a result, the current trend is to combine the growing evidence about the role of psychosocial factors and the emergence of guidelines. It has become evident that psychosocial factors may create barriers for recovery and return to work. This idea is based on recent knowledge that psychological factors are strongly associated with the transition from acute to chronic pain (Linton 2000). At the same time, several authorities have developed guidelines for the treatment of back pain that are derived from the scientific literature. Although the guidelines vary (Koes et al. 2001), there are a number of key recommendations included in most. These include prescribing activity rather than rest and providing reassurance to reduce anxiety and fear. Written materials have been developed to provide patients with the key messages. Consequently, these pamphlets often provide clear messages aimed at reducing fear, avoidance of activities and distress, e.g. (Symonds et al. 1995).

A review of the studies employing written materials indicates that under certain conditions they can be effective (Burton and Waddell 2002). While written information remains a rather weak intervention, a coordinated effort where the information is employed to enhance the messages and advice provided by clinicians, may be of value. Carefully selected and presented information presented in an uncompromising style that is in line with current management guidelines can have a positive effect on the beliefs patients have, as well as on clinical outcomes.

Schools

A number of educational efforts have been initiated in the form of a "school" or study group; these include back schools, neck schools and pain management schools. They assume that an important reason why people develop problems is a lack of knowledge. Back schools, for example, may include a wide range of topics, but typically focus on body mechanics and ergonomics. Other topics normally included are exercise, lifting and stress. A trained professional such as a physical therapist almost always provides these educational efforts in groups. However, there is great variation in the content, number and length of sessions.

Unfortunately, the school concept has demonstrated limited effects. In a review of the effects as an early, preventive intervention, it was concluded that neck and back schools were not effective (Linton and van Tulder 2001). While other reviews find some effects on knowledge and correct back posture, there is considerable agreement that back schools, at best, have only slight effects on variables such as health care utilization or absenteeism and virtually no effects on clinical variables such as pain intensity (Maier-Riehle and Harter 2001).

Psychoeducation: CBT Groups as an Early Intervention

These learning experiences focus on psychological aspects of pain, such as developing effective coping strategies, altering dysfunctional attitudes or alleviating fears about the problem. These interventions are almost always provided in groups and are a method of providing a psychologically oriented therapy in an effective and inexpensive way. A key concept is promoting self-help. A psychoeducational group program, based on cognitive behavioral therapy, was developed for patients with arthritis and then modified to be applicable for musculoskeletal pain problems (Lorig et al. 1993). In one study, chronic pain patients were randomly assigned to either the psychoeducation program or to a waiting list control (LeFort et al. 1998). The course offered six 2 h sessions designed to maximize group problem solving and self-management skills. Results indicated that the educational intervention group made significant improvements in pain, vitality, functioning, satisfaction and self-efficacy in comparison to the control group.

More recently, programs have also been adapted for early intervention aimed at preventing the development of chronic back or neck pain (Linton 2002). Although neck and back pain are very common, only a relatively small number of patients develop persistent problems restricting work capacity and requiring health care. However, these small numbers consume the majority of the resources. Consequently, identification and providing early, preventive interventions could be an effective strategy to reduce the problem. Psychological factors have been found to be an important link in the transition from acute to persistent back pain, and therefore psychologically oriented interventions seem to be needed to address the problem properly (Linton 2000). This is a particularly relevant idea because early interventions focus on changing the participant's behavior and lifestyle.

The effects of providing an early, cognitive behavioral group intervention were tested in a randomized study of 255 primary care back pain patients (Von Korff et al. 1998). The cognitive behavioral intervention consisted of four sessions focusing on problem solving skills, activity management and educational videos. Relative to the control group, those receiving the cognitive behavioral group intervention significantly reduced their worry and disability and increased their self-help skills. Similar results have been reported in other studies (Moore et al. 2000; Saunders et al. 1999).

A cognitive behavioral intervention was specifically developed for primary care patients found to be at risk on psychosocial variables. In this program patients meet six times in groups of about 8 people for 2 h once a week. The course is led by a professional and is based on helping participants to change their beliefs and behaviors. Several steps are taken to enhance engagement, such as prompting discussion, homework and "hands on" skills training. Each session contains a review of homework, a short presentation of educational material, problem solving, coping skills acquirement and individualized homework assignments. The end product for participants is a personalized coping program that they design themselves. The utility of this approach has been tested in four separate randomized controlled trials (Linton and Andersson 2000; Linton et al. 2001; Linton et al. 2006). All of these studies have demonstrated that this intervention has a clear preventive effect on future sick absenteeism and function. Thus, there is support for the contention that a psychoeducational intervention designed to match the psychological needs of the participants may help prevent the development of persistent musculoskeletal pain.

References

1. Burton AK, Waddell G (2002) Educational and informational approaches. In: Linton SJ (ed), New avenues for the prevention of chronic musculoskeletal pain and disability. Elsevier, Amsterdam, pp 245–258
2. Heaney D, Wyke S, Wilson P et al. (2001) Assessment of impact of information booklets on use of healthcare services: Randomized controlled trial. BMJ 322:1218
3. Koes BW, van Tulder MW, Ostelo R et al. (2001) Clinical guidelines for the management of low back pain in primary care. Spine 26:2504–2514
4. LeFort SM, Gray-Donald K, Rowat KM et al. (1998) Randomized controlled trial of a community-based psychoeducation program for the self-management of chronic pain. Pain 74:297–306
5. Ley P (1997) Written communication. In: Baum A, Newman S, Weinman J et al. (eds) Cambridge handbook of psychology, health, and medicine. Cambridge University Press, Cambridge, pp 331–334
6. Linton SJ (2000) A review of psychological risk factors in back and neck pain. Spine 25:1148–1156
7. Linton SJ (ed) (2002) New avenues for the prevention of chronic musculoskeletal pain and disability, vol 1. Elsevier Science, Amsterdam
8. Linton SJ, Andersson T (2000) Can chronic disability be prevented? A randomized trial of a cognitive-behavior intervention and two forms of information for patients with spinal pain. Spine 25:2825–2831
9. Linton SJ, Ryberg M (2001) A cognitive-behavioral group intervention as prevention for persistent neck and back pain in a non-patient population: A randomized controlled trial. Pain 90:83–90
10. Linton SJ, van Tulder MW (2001) Preventive interventions for back and neck pain: What is the evidence? Spine 26:778–787
11. Linton SJ, Boersma K, Jansson M et al. (2006) The effects of cognitive-behavioral and physical therapy preventive interventions on pain related sick leave: A randomized controlled trial. Clin J Pain (in press)
12. Lorig K, Mazonson PD, Holman HR (1993) Evidence suggesting that health education for self-management in patients with chronic arthritis has sustained health benefits while reducing health care costs. Arthritis Rheum 36:439–446
13. Maier-Riehle B, Harter M (2001) The effects of back schools: A meta-analysis. Int J Rehab Med 24:199–206
14. Marhold C, Linton SJ, Melin L (2001) Cognitive behavioral return-to-work program: effects on pain patients with a history of long-term versus short-term sick leave. Pain 91:155–163
15. Moore J, Von Korff M, Cherkin D et al. (2000). A randomized trial of a cognitive-behavioral program for enhancing back pain self care in a primary care setting. Pain 88:145–153

Intensity of Pain

Definition

Intensity of pain is scored on a verbal points scale. 0 no pain; 1 mild pain, does not interfere with activities; 2 moderate pain, inhibits, but does not prohibit activities; 3 severe pain, prohibits activities. It may alternatively, be measured in a visual analogue scale (VAS).
► Sunct Syndrome

Intensity of Ultrasound

Definition

The intensity is power per unit area.
► Ultrasound Therapy of Pain from the Musculoskeletal System

Intentionality

Definition

A complex adaptive system has intentionality when it exhibits directedness toward some future state or goal. Intent comprises of the endogenous initiation, construction and direction of perception, action and goal-directed behavior.
► Consciousness and Pain

Intercostal Space

Definition

A potential space at the inferior margin of each rib through which the intercostal nerve, vein, and artery travel for each rib. The intercostal nerve provides sensory and motor function to the superficial chest and abdominal wall.
► Postoperative Pain, Regional Blocks

Interdisciplinary

Definition

Interdisciplinary refers to a team or collaborative process where members of different disciplines assess and treat patients jointly.
► Complex Chronic Pain in Children, Interdisciplinary Treatment
► Physical Medicine and Rehabilitation, Team-Oriented Approach

Interdisciplinary Pain Management Programs

► Interdisciplinary Pain Rehabilitation

Interdisciplinary Pain Rehabilitation

CHRIS J. MAIN
University of Manchester, Manchester, UK
cmain@fs1.ho.man.ac.uk

Synonyms

Interdisciplinary Pain Management Programs; Cognitive-Behavioral Programs

Definition

Interdisciplinary pain management (IPM) does not offer cures for pain but comprises an integrated biopsychosocial approach to pain management from a team of health care professionals with the aim of maximizing the patient's own ability to manage their pain and pain associated dysfunction. A range of cognitive and behavioural strategies focused on re-activation and minimisation of unnecessary physical and psychosocial dysfunction are used. Perhaps most important of all as a defining characteristic of IPM is the promulgation of self-help and personal responsibility. This is evident particularly in the emphasis on active rather than passive approaches to treatment.

Characteristics

The University of Washington in Seattle pioneered multidimensional treatment, research, education and interdisciplinary working in the field of pain. From the perspective of interdisciplinary pain management, its 5th mission statement was critically important: "To enhance interaction and communication among all pain investigators at the University of Washington and to encourage cross-fertilization of ideas on pain research and therapy" (Bonica 1990). The "Seattle model" became not only an example of a practical implementation of a biopsychosocial model of pain, but also an illustration of the mutual inter-dependence of clinical practice, teaching, training and research.

More specifically, in the early days, the Seattle group promoted a view of illness that incorporated both physical and behavioural aspects. Although most pain management programs now would define themselves as cognitive behavioural in their orientation, the power and incisiveness of the behavioural component (Fordyce 1976) in the original Seattle model was critical to the development of modern inter-disciplinary pain management. During the last 30 years, variants of the Seattle model have appeared all over the world.

Modern pain management programs (PMPs) contain a number of discrete elements blended into a package of care. Each of these elements has its own pedigree as an approach to treatment and each element has its origins in a particular perspective on the nature of pain. Typically these will include rationalisation of medication use, development of individually tailored re-activation programs, training in problem solving techniques and enhancement of adaptive pain coping strategies including goal setting and pacing, with the objective of maximising positive adaptation. Programs differ in the extent to which they have a specific work focus.

An appropriate educational component is a major ingredient of all PMPs, but it seems that education, although necessary, is not sufficient for established pain programs. It seems that unless increased understanding leads to significant behavioural change, it is of little value.

Specific therapeutic objectives usually include decreasing stiffness and immobility, recovery of fitness, development of strength and the reversal of the "disuse syndrome", treatment of distress (including depression) and the modification of pain behaviour. They differ from the "sports medicine approach", typified in functional restoration programs (Mayer and Gatchell 1988), in that they usually place less emphasis specifically on strength and mobility and have traditionally focused on clinical rather than on occupational outcomes.

It is not possible to overstress the importance of the behavioural perspective as an alternative to the disease / pathology model in offering a new and alternative understanding of pain. It has led to the focus on pain management as an alternative to cure, which is not available for many pain conditions. More recently incorporation of the cognitive perspective (Turk and Okifuji 2003; Turk et al. 1983) has produced a psychologically oriented approach which, with a focus on re-activation and self-management, is frequently described as a cognitive behavioural program and has become the treatment of choice for the dysfunctional chronic pain patient, with clear scientific evidence of its efficacy (Morley et al. 1999) over more narrowly focused traditional approaches.

Desirable Characteristics of PMPs

The British and Irish chapter of the International Association for the Study of Pain, therefore, inspired by the IASP report (IASP 1990) and by Sanders (1994) recently produced a set of "desirable characteristics" for PMPs (Pain Society 1997). The key features are:

- Behavioural rather than a disease perspective
- Focus on pain management rather than cure
- Blend of ingredients
- Interdisciplinary skill-mix
- Incorporation of group therapy

- Emphasis on active rather than passive approaches to treatment
- Promulgation of self-help and patient responsibility

The Context of Pain Management

There is a gradient of complexity in pain management, ranging from specific types of individualized intervention such as medication adjustment, spinal manipulation or provision of educational material to "packages of care" involving not only multifaceted treatment but also intervention by a range of professionals using a team approach. Multidisciplinary treatment undoubtedly offers a much wider range of potential therapeutic options that can be offered by a single-handed practitioner, but there are also inherent dangers of iatrogenic confusion or distress if the patient is given inconsistent information or offered a package of care that is poorly integrated or even contradictory. Integrated care has become known as interdisciplinary pain management. The potential limitations of a multidisciplinary approach (in contrast to an interdisciplinary approach) are:

- Poor communication leading to a lack of awareness of problem areas. (For example, the physiotherapist may be unaware that a patient has an alcohol problem).
- Fragmentation of the approach to treatment and assessment in which the patient's problems are tackled sequentially rather than in an integrated fashion. The patient then comes to view the different professionals as having over-prescribed roles, making it difficult tackle inter-dependent problems.
- There may be unnecessary duplication of certain parts of the assessment procedure. This in not only inefficient but can be irritating to patients.
- Different management strategies may be employed in dealing with the same problem.
- Patients and their relatives may receive conflicting information from different disciplines leading to confusion on their part about which approach should be adopted.
- In certain cases manipulative patients can "play off" one team member against other members.
- Restricted communication within the multidisciplinary team may lead to a sense of isolation and lack of support among individual team members

General Advantages of the Interdisciplinary Approach

In interdisciplinary pain management, a special effort is made to offer a consistent and coherent approach to both assessment and management. The structuring and delivery of IPM is dealt with in detail elsewhere (Main and Spanswick 2000), but for present purposes a number of strategies merit consideration. In the interdisciplinary team, according to Melvin (1980) "...individuals not only require the skills of their own disciplines, but also have the added responsibility of the group effort on behalf of the activity or client involved. ...The group activity of an interdisciplinary team is synergistic, producing more than each individually and separately could accomplish" (p 379).

Two differing patterns of co-operation within the interdisciplinary team have been described (Finset et al. 1995). In the co-ordinated interdisciplinary team, mutual goals are set and the individuals from each discipline attempt to work on these goals in their individual sessions. In the integrated interdisciplinary team, mutual goals are worked on in joint treatment sessions with members of different disciplines participating in the sessions. The treatment could not be carried out by individual members of the team alone.

The key features of an interdisciplinary team are as follows:

- The team members share common assessment and treatment goals.
- The main task of all members of the team is to deliver treatments that are dependent on the patient's needs, not on the constraints of the individual disciplines involved.
- Unlike multidisciplinary teams, interdisciplinary teams are not necessarily led by a member of the medical profession. They are most likely to be led by an experienced clinician who has knowledge not only of working with patients with chronic pain but also a knowledge of working in a team.
- There are core areas of speciality unique to each discipline, but these are secondary to the goals of the team as a whole.
- Team members will have explicit knowledge of the skills of other disciplines involved in the team.
- Effective communication occurs between all team members
- All team members have equal status within the team
- Decisions are arrived at after considering input from all team members

Recommendations for the development, establishment and maintenance of the interdisciplinary team include:

- The philosophy of the team should be made articulate in an agreed policy document and made explicit to all members. This should be re-appraised at regular intervals and modified if necessary.
- There must be a system for staff induction and training, with a focus particularly on processes within groups, the development of core team skills required and education regarding the work of other disciplines.
- Communication is vital to the effective running of the team and a considerable amount of time should be spent on this area, both formally and informally, including regular team meetings. However, team meetings are expensive, therefore it is of importance that they are conducted efficiently and effectively.

- Meetings should have a clear agenda, with effective firm leadership to ensure focus, concluding with action points within a spirit of group cohesiveness.
- Rules of confidentiality concerning both staff and patients must be made explicit.

Team Maintenance

When different disciplines set up and work as an interdisciplinary team, this can give rise to problems in managerial, organisational and inter-personal areas. Strategies to assist integration of external hospital managers might include involving management during the early stages of planning and development of the team, discussion with management of the policy document and associated specific working practices required and developing specific and relevant outcome measures.

Ensure effective and efficient time management not only in patient assessment and treatment delivery, but also in decision-making and audit. Clinic structuring and minimisation of inappropriate referrals and failure to attend appointments lessen the dangers of fragmentation of the team and formation of "splinter groups" within the team. Ensure that good communication occurs between all team members by controlling the size of the team and encouraging cohesiveness by using team-building techniques. Any communication or interpersonal problems between team members need to be dealt with as early as possible. There should be time set aside specifically for team development and team building; this is particularly important in the early stages of forming an interdisciplinary team. Pay particular attention to the integration of new members to the team. A 'probationary period' may be extremely useful. Ensure the availability of support systems to help team members cope with the emotional pressures that can occur when working with such a demanding group of patients.

Conclusion

The interdisciplinary clinic would seem to have a number of specific advantages over uni-professional or multi-disciplinary clinics. The principal advantages include:

1. Greater range of professional expertise, permitting a wider range of treatment options
2. Decreased likelihood of inappropriate interventions as a consequence of failure to recognise (or take adequately into account) important obstacles to recovery
3. Minimising the likelihood of producing further iatrogenic distress and confusion
4. Coherent and integrated treatment approach, with clear identification of goals and responsibilities

It could, I think, reasonably be argued that the framework, with its range of options and integration of perspectives, offers the potential for optimal clinical care. Clinicians who have genuinely embraced the inter-disciplinary perspective seem to find it a professionally stimulating and satisfying approach to clinical management.

There are however potential difficulties with the approach. Some of the more frequent difficulties include patient and staff scheduling, negotiating adequate time for initial assessment and failure amongst the staff to arrive at an agreed clinical formulation and treatment plan. Indeed over the last decade, there have been increasing difficulties in obtaining and securing funding for such clinics, particularly those run on an in-patient basis. Nonetheless, as a way of managing patients, the inter-disciplinary approach as developed in the early pain management programs has offered a powerful new way of managing patients and the philosophy and practice have had a powerful influence on the design and establishment of modern pain management, not only in tertiary health care, but also in secondary prevention and in occupational settings.

References

1. Bonica JJ (1990) Multidisciplinary / interdisciplinary pain programs. In: Bonica JJ (ed) The management of pain, 2nd edn. Lea & Febiger, Philadelphia, pp 197–208
2. Finset A, Krogstad JM, Hansen H et al. (1995) Team development and memory training in traumatic brain jury rehabilitation: two birds with one stone. Brain Inj 9:495–507
3. Fordyce WE (1976) Behavioral methods for chronic pain and illness. C.V. Mosby, St. Louis
4. IASP (1990) Desirable characteristics for pain treatment facilities (Report of Task Force on Guidelines for Desirable Characteristics for Pain treatment Facilities). IASP, Seattle
5. Loeser JD (1990) Interdisciplinary, multimodal management of chronic pain In: Bonica JJ (ed) The management of pain, 2nd edn. Lea & Febiger, Philadelphia, pp 2107–2120
6. Main CJ, Spanswick CC (2000) Pain management: an interdisciplinary approach. Churchill-Livingstone, Edinburgh
7. Mayer TG, Gatchel R (1988) Functional Restoration for spinal disorders. The sports medicine approach. Lea & Febiger, Philadelphia
8. Melvin JL (1980) Interdisciplinary and Multidisciplinary Activities and the ACRM. Arch Phys Med Rehab61:379–380
9. Morley S, Eccleston C, Williams A (1999) A Systematic review and meta-analysis of randomised controlled trials of cognitive behaviour therapy and behaviour therapy for chronic pain in adults, excluding headache. Pain 80:1–13
10. Pain Society (1997) Desirable characteristics for pain management programmes: Report of a Working Party of the Pain Society of Great Britain and Ireland (The British and Irish Chapter of the International Association for the Study of Pain). The Pain Society, London
11. Sanders SH (1994) An image problem for pain centers: relevant factors and possible solutions. APS Bull Jan / Feb:17–18
12. Turk DC, Okifuli A (2003) In: Melzack R, Wall PD (eds) Handbook of pain management: a clinical companion to Wall and Melzack's textbook of pain. Churchill-Livingstone, Edinburgh, pp 533–541
13. Turk DC, Meichenbaum DH, Genest M (1983) Pain and behavioural medicine. A cognitive-behavioural perspective. The Guilford Press, New York & London

Interlaminar Epidural Steroid Injection

▶ Epidural Steroid Injections for Chronic Back Pain

Interleukin(s) (IL)

Definition

A group of molecules within the cytokine family involved in signaling between cells participating in immune and inflammatory events; distinct interleukins are defined by different numbers and letters (e.g. IL–1α, IL–1β and IL-6).

▶ Cytokines as Targets in the Treatment of Neuropathic Pain
▶ Wallerian Degeneration

Intermittent Claudication

Definition

Intermittent claudication is a condition that is characterized by pain and lameness during muscular exercise or – in the leg – during walking. The most frequent cause is narrowing of arteries in the lower leg and foot by arteriosclerosis.

▶ Muscle Pain Model, Ischemia-Induced and Hypertonic Saline-Induced

Internal Capsule

Definition

White matter pathway carrying fibers afferent to the cortex from the thalamus and efferent from the cortex to nuclei of the brain and to the spinal cord.

▶ Deep Brain Stimulation

Internal Disc Disruption

Definition

Ruptured vertebral disc at the center of the nucleus pulposis.

▶ Chronic Low Back Pain, Definitions and Diagnosis

Internal Neurolysis

Definition

Scarring related to a peripheral nerve can be external, causing adherence of the entire nerve to an adjacent structure, such as the roof of the carpal tunnel for the median nerve. When sufficient chronic compression or direct trauma create scarring between the fascicles of the peripheral nerve, there is internal scarring. The microsurgical release of this interfascicular scarring is termed an „internal neurolysis".

▶ Carpal Tunnel Syndrome

Internal Validity

Definition

The treatment and comparison groups are selected and compared in such a manner that the observed differences between them on the dependent variables under study, may only be attributed to the hypothesized intervention under investigation.

▶ Lumbar Traction

Internalization

Definition

Endocytosis; movement of proteins from the plasma membrane of a cell to intracellular compartments.

▶ Opioid Receptor Trafficking in Pain States

Internalization of Receptors

Definition

Endocytosis of surface membrane receptors after they bind a ligand. The receptors may later be recycled and reinserted into the membrane. When internalization occurs, it can be assumed that the ligand has been released in response to a stimulus. For example, when neurokinin-1 receptors are internalized, it is presumed that substance P (or a related neurokinin) has been released from nearby presynaptic terminals. Observation of this phenomenon is an indirect way of demonstrating the release of certain neurotransmitters.

▶ Visceral Pain Model, Lower Gastrointestinal Tract Pain

International Narcotics Control Board

Synonyms

INCB

Definition

An element of the United Nations drug control program. It is charged with prevention of illegal growth, manu-facture, and distribution of narcotic and other controlled medications for non-medical or non-scientific use. Its activities are set forth by the Single Convention on Narcotic Drugs and the Convention on Psychotropic substances. It has recommended that governments facilitate the availability for the treatment of chronic pain including cancer pain. It collaborates closely with the World Health Organization.

▶ Cancer Pain Management, Undertreatment and Clinician-Related Barriers

Interneuron

Definition

An interneuron is a neuron that communicates only to other neurons; they are often inhibitory.

▶ Nociceptive Circuitry in the Spinal Cord
▶ Somatic Pain
▶ Thalamocortical Loops and Information Processing
▶ Visceral Nociception and Pain

Interoception

Definition

The term interoception is often used to define perceptual experiences that are not determined by "outside" stimuli. It refers to the sense of the physiological condition of the body and links sensations such as thirst, hunger, cold and warmth and pain with emotional experience (feelings) and motivation, as it drives the individual towards adaptive behavior in order to establish homeostasis (e.g. by drinking, eating and protection against environmental challenges).

▶ Angina Pectoris, Neurophysiology and Psychophysics
▶ Functional Imaging of Cutaneous Pain
▶ Spinothalamic Tract Neurons, in Deep Dorsal Horn
▶ Thalamus, Visceral Representation
▶ Trigeminal Brainstem Nuclear Complex, Anatomy

Interpersonal Pain Behaviour

PAUL J. WATSON
University Department of Anaesthesia, University of Leicester, Leicester, UK
pjw25@le.ac.uk

Synonyms

Pain behaviour; non-organic signs; Illness Behaviour

Definition

Pain behaviour has been defined by Loeser and Fordyce (1983) as "all outputs that a reasonable observer would characterise as suggesting pain". These include posture, facial expression, verbalization, lying down, taking medicines, seeking medical assistance and receiving compensation.

Characteristics

Pain behaviours can be subdivided by how they are assessed, self report behaviours include pain reporting and self-reported responses to pain; externally validated behaviours, include consultation rates, work absence and receipt of wage compensation; and overt pain behaviours that are observable such as changes in posture, mobilisation and vocalisation associated with pain.

Pain behaviour is the product of both respondent and operant conditioning. Movement, for example bending in the case of a person with back pain, which causes pain, may lead to the modification of movement or avoidance of that activity, at least until the symptoms resolve (respondent conditioning). In this case, the restriction of movement or guarding is in response to the expectation of pain on movement, rather than in direct response to the pain itself (classical conditioning).

If the person with back pain is observed restricting their movement, or if they also moan or groan when moving, this might action sympathetic attention from others. If this attention is valued, a pattern might develop where the behaviour is expressed in order to elicit sympathetic attention (operant conditioning). The adoption of pain behaviours may also allow the patient to avoid an aversive experience, such as a stressful workplace. If the pattern of behaviour is regularly reinforced, through regular favourable attention and avoidance of difficult situations, it may become very difficult to extinguish.

The demonstration of pain behaviour is a form of social communication and it is normal to express such behaviours when in pain. The behavioural expression of pain is a function of social learning and as such is highly influenced by life experiences, culture and the social environment. Behavioural theorists, such as Fordyce (1976), suggested that pain behaviour, as well as being a communication of pain, may serve a purpose as an adaptive response to acute pain to provide a period of reduced activity in response to pain to allow repair. However, such behaviours become inappropriate and maladaptive if they persist. In this regard, behavioural theorists maintain that persistent, and persistently reinforced, pain behaviours result in high levels of physical and psychological disability (Keefe and Lefebvre 1994; Keefe and Smith 2002). Romano et al. (1995) demonstrated a relationship between spouse solicitousness and pain behaviour. In a group of patients who reported high levels of pain, patients who had solicitous spouses had higher levels of pain behaviour and higher levels of disability than patients with non-solicitous spouses. In an earlier experiment, Romano et al. (1992) found that spouse behaviours not only followed patient demonstrations of pain behaviours but they also preceded patient behaviours, for example, as the patient started a task which normally produced pain behaviour. The authors contended that this demonstrated the behaviours had been rehearsed and reinforced over time.

Hadjistavropoulos and Craig (2002) have argued that pain behaviours can operate at a subtle, automatic level. Although they recognise that overt behaviours can be exaggerated, they contend that such conscious exaggeration can be, in part, identified. They further argue that observed pain behaviours, if assessed appropriately, can give a better representation of pain than self-report. In their interpretation, self-report always involves higher mental processes, requires attention to the task and focuses attention towards the pain, which might compromise coping and thus influence the report, whereas the automaticity of facial expression and body movement is less compromised. They argue for a combination of measures encompassing self-report and behavioural observation.

Assessment of Pain Behaviours

Pain behaviour can be reliably assessed by patient self-report, through observation or third party validation.

Simple self-report diaries have been used extensively in research and clinical practice. Patients are required to report medication usage, pain report and "uptime" – the length of time spent out of a reclining position (Follick et al. 1984; Keefe and Lefebvre 1994). Structured format questionnaires have been developed asking the patient to identify the types of pain behaviour they engage in and the frequency. Some questionnaires also assess the responses of the patient's spouse or significant other to their pain behaviour (Kerns et al. 1985).

Assessments of overt pain behaviours require the patient to be observed over a period of time. Such measures can be used in the inpatient setting or outpatient setting using standardised structured assessments (Richards et al. 1982; Vlaeyen at al. 1987), behaviour is recorded by trained personnel on standard assessment sheets. The advantage of these is that they allow observation over a long period of time. The disadvantage is that the patient may avoid all pain provoking activities during the period of assessment. The sample of behaviour must include observation of the patient performing activities which would elicit pain behaviours, for example sitting, walking and performing everyday tasks.

Keefe and Block (1982) defined a list of observed pain behaviours in subjects with chronic pain that has been successfully used in a number of other painful conditions. Subjects are required to perform a number of tasks; sitting, walking, getting into and out of a chair and onto and up from a bed. Standardised video taping procedures are used and the occurrence of key behaviours of limping, facial grimacing, stopping and resting, touching or holding the affected area, guarding and bracing the affected part and verbalisation, such as reporting pain and sighing or groaning, are recorded. Such a system demonstrated high inter-rater reliability, test/re-test reliability and good internal consistency. Behaviours have also been observed to reduce after pain management or pain relieving interventions.

In response to criticism that the videotape procedure was not sufficiently exacting to allow expression of pain behaviours, Keefe and Dunsmore (1992) and Koho et al. (2001) developed a video-based assessment during functional task performance using a similar list of behaviours, and demonstrated a similar level of reliability.

A very subtle approach to assessment is offered by Craig et al. (1992); the Facial Coding System relies on change in facial expression. It has been well validated in groups from new born to adults, and has evidence to suggest that it can separate genuine from faked expressions of pain (Craig et al. 1991). Hadjistavropolous and Craig (2002) argue that it is a better reflection of automaticity in pain expression, and less influenced by volitional control than other assessments of overt behaviour.

Videotaping and rating assessments is time consuming and requires training. A number of assessments of pain behaviour in real time have been developed for use during clinical examination. Waddell and colleagues developed a list of self-reported symptoms and responses to examination that were unlikely to be associated with underlying pathology in groups of low back pain patients (Waddell et al. 1980; Waddell et al. 1984). The assessment can be performed relatively quickly by a single clinician, but it has not been used to formally assess pain behaviour or responses to treatment, the focus has mainly been in identifying people who are unlikely to respond well to treatments. A more recent and comprehensive assessment has been developed by Prkachin et al. (2002). This requires an independent observer to be present at a standardised back pain assessment to record pain behaviours. The advantages of such "real time" assessments is they give the clinician instant feedback of the results.

Purpose of Assessing Pain Behaviours

Reducing pain behaviour is a focus of behavioural pain management programmes, and is often a declared aim of multidisciplinary cognitive behavioural pain management programmes (Turk and Flor 1987; Watson 2003). Significant reductions in pain behaviour scores following interventions have been reported.

Misinterpretation of Pain Behaviours

Pain behaviour is the consequence of an individual's experience of an internal state, which is then encoded into an expressive behaviour that then allows the observer to make a judgement about that experience. In this, it is a normal communication of suffering from one individual to another. However, pain behaviour is sometimes interpreted as "exaggerated" illness presentation. It is important to bear in mind that even some gross pain behaviours are rarely a conscious attempt to mislead, and alone are not evidence of malingering (Main and Waddell 1998). Clinicians are trained to "match" the observed pain behaviours to the report of pain and the extent and severity of the pathology, but interpreting behaviour purely in such terms might lead to misinterpretation on the part of the clinician. Such responses cannot be taken out of the context of the patient's expectations of the assessment, his/her previous experience of assessment and their psychological distress at the time of the assessment. A desire to access treatment may result in the patient trying to convince the clinician of the veracity of their condition through their overt behaviour, obvious scepticism by the clinician may enhance this. The observer should also be aware of his or her own bias in interpreting pain behaviour. For example, clinicians have been shown to underestimate pain reported by men but give higher estimates of pain intensity in women. The physical attractiveness of the patient also influences the clinician, with less attractive patients being rated as having more pain (Hadjistavropoulos et al. 1996).

Special Groups

The traditional reliance on pen and paper self-report requires higher cognitive function and adequate language skills and vocabulary. Some people suffering pain are unable to express themselves adequately due to cognitive impairment, impaired consciousness, speech deficits or because they and the observer do not share a common language. Self-report measures are also inappropriate for neonates and infants. It is not the purpose of this essay to discuss these groups in detail but it is when working with such groups that pain behaviour assessments are particularly useful. Although a number of assessments have been developed for specific groups, much more work is required to develop instruments for use in those with severe physical disabilities and in elderly patients with profound cognitive impairment.

Pain is a multidimensional phenomenon, although many have suggested that is an intensely private experience and can only be assessed through the report of the person suffering it. In truth, pain is rarely entirely private, people also communicate through characteristic behaviours which can be reliably measured. Observing

I

pain behaviours can offer additional information to give a multidimensional perspective on the personal pain experience.

References

1. Craig KD, Hyde SA, Patrick CJ (1991) Genuine, Suppressed and Faked Facial Behavior during Exacerbation of Chronic Low Back Pain. Pain 46:161–172
2. Craig KD, Prkachin KM, Grunau RVE (1992) The Facial Expression of Pain. In Turk DC and Melzack R (eds) Handbook of Pain Assessment. Guildford, New York, pp 255–274
3. Follick MJ, Ahern DK, Laser-Wolston (1984) Evaluation of Daily Activity Diary for Chronic Pain Patients. Pain 19:373–382
4. Fordyce WE (1976) Behavioural Methods for Chronic Pain and Illness. Mosby, St. Louis
5. Hadjistavropoulos T, Craig KD (2002) A Theoretical Framework for Understanding Self-Report and Observational Measures of Pain: A Communications Model. Behav Res Ther 40:551–570
6. Hadjistavropoulos T, McMurtry B, Craig KD (1996) Beautiful Faces in Pain: Biases and Accuracy in the Perception of Pain. Psychol Health 11:411–420
7. Keefe FJ, Block AR (1982) Development of an Observational Method for Assessing Pain Behaviour in Chronic Low Back Pain Patients. Behav Ther 13: 363–375
8. Keefe FJ, Dunsmore J (1992) Pain Behaviour Concepts and Controversies. Am Pain Soc J 2:92–100
9. Keefe FJ, Lefebvre (1994) Pain Behaviour Concept. Controversies, Current Status and Future Directions. In: Gebhart G, Hammond DL, Jensen TS (eds) Proceedings of the VIIth World Congress on Pain. Elsevier, New York
10. Keefe FJ, Smith S (2002) The Assessment of Pain Behaviour: Implications for Applied Psychology and Future Research Directions. Appl Psychophysio Biofeedback. 27:117–127
11. Kerns RD, Turk DC, Rudy TE (1985) The West Haven-Yale Multidimensional Pain Inventory (WHYMPI) Pain 23:345–356
12. Koho P, Aho S, Watson P et al. (2001) Assessment of Chronic Pain Behaviour: Reliability of the Method and its Relationship with Perceived Disability, Physical Impairment and Function. J Rehabil Med 33:128–132
13. Loeser JD, Fordyce WE (1983) Chronic pain. In: Carr JE, Dengerik HA (eds) Behavioural Science in the Practice of Medicine. Elsevier, Amsterdam
14. Main CJ, Waddell G (1998) Behavioral Responses to Examination. A Reappraisal of the Interpretation of "Non-Organic Signs" Spine 23:2367–2371
15. Prkachin KM, Hughes E, Schultz I et al. (2002). Real-Time Assessment of Pain Behavior during Clinical Assessment of Low Back Pain Patients. Pain 95:23–30
16. Richards AH, Nepomuceno C, Riles M, Suer Z (1982) Assessing Pain Behaviors: The UAB Pain Behavior Scale. Pain 12:393–398
17. Romano JM, Turner JA, Jensen MP et al. (1992) Sequential Analysis of Chronic Pain Behaviors and Spouse Responses. J Consult Clin Psychol 60:777–782
18. Romano JM, Turner JA, Jensen MP et al. (1995) Chronic Pain Patient-Spouse Interactions Predict Pain Disability. Pain 15:300–306
19. Turk DC, Flor H (1987) Pain greater than Pain Behaviours: The Utility and Limitations of the Pain Behaviour Construct. Pain 31:277–295
20. Vlaeyen JWS, Van Eek HV, Groenman NH et al. (1987) Dimensions and Components of Observed Chronic Pain Behaviour. Pain 31:65–75
21. Waddell G, McCulloch JA, Kummel E et al. (1980) Non-Organic Signs in Low Back Pain. Spine 5:117–125
22. Waddell G, Main CJ, Morris EW et al. (1984) Chronic Low Back Pain, Psychologic Distress and Illness Behavior. Spine 9:209–213
23. Watson PJ (2003) Interdisciplinary Pain Management in Fibromyalgia. In: Chaitow L (ed) Fibromyalgia: A Practitioners Guide to Treatment. 2nd Edition. Harcourt Brace, Edinburgh

Interprofessional Approach

Definition

Healthcare professionals co-working in an integrated process.
▶ Physical Medicine and Rehabilitation, Team-Oriented Approach

Interscalene

Definition

Pertaining to the potential fascial space between the anterior and meddle scalene muscles in the neck through which the brachial plexus traverses.
▶ Postoperative Pain, Regional Blocks

Interscalene Block

Definition

Injection via a needle or catheter of local anesthetic at the interscalene groove to block sensory and/or motor innervation of the brachial plexus.
▶ Acute Pain in Children, Post-Operative

Interspike Interval

Synonyms

ISI

Definition

Interspike interval is the time interval (usually measured in milliseconds) between action potentials discharged by a neuron.
▶ Central Pain, Human Studies of Physiology
▶ Chronic Pain
▶ Thalamic Bursting Activity

Interstitial Cystitis and Chronic Pelvic Pain

ELLIOT M. PAUL, EVAN R. EISENBERG, ROBERT M. MOLDWIN
Department of Urology, Long Island Jewish Medical Center, New York, NY, USA
eliepaul@yahoo.com

Synonyms

Interstitial Cystitis; Pelvic Pain Syndrome of Bladder Origin; Chronic Pelvic Pain, Interstitial Cystis

Definition

Interstitial Cystitis (IC) is a chronic pelvic pain syndrome largely defined by its symptoms, which include urinary urgency, frequency, and pelvic pain-all in the absence of well-defined pathologies such as urinary tract infection or bladder cancer. The "classic" form of interstitial cystitis is that marked by gross erythematous changes of the bladder wall, representing panmural inflammation, fibrosis and granulation tissue. These so called "Hunner's" patches or ulcers, originally described by Guy Hunner, are identified in only 5–10% of IC patients (Hunner 1915). The remaining "non-classic" IC patients have a normal cystoscopic appearance. The prevalence of IC is 10–55 cases/100,000 population in the United States, and affects women 10 times as frequently as men. Recent literature has highlighted the similarities between this condition and non-bacterial prostatitis and prostatodynia (reclassified as category III A and B chronic pelvic pain syndrome, respectively). The quality of life for patients with IC is typically poor, with 50% reporting the inability to work fulltime and 60% complaining of dyspareunia (Ratner et al 1994). There is no known cure for IC, and no single therapy has been shown to alleviate the symptoms in all afflicted patients.

Characteristics

Interstitial cystitis is a chronic pelvic pain syndrome presenting at any age, but most commonly in the 3rd through to 5th decades of life. The syndrome is characterized by irritative voiding symptoms and pelvic discomfort, in the absence of a urinary tract infection or any other definable pelvic pathology that might give rise to such symptoms. Pain associated with bladder filling is common. In fact, urinary frequency, both during the day and at nighttime, is usually a product of the patient's desire to maintain the lowest pain level possible.

A wide spectrum of symptom severity is common amongst IC patients. For example, many patients with mild symptoms may complain of pelvic pressure worsening with bladder filling and void 2–3 times per evening. Severe patients may be incapacitated by pelvic pain and void every 5–10 minutes throughout the day and night. Urinary hesitancy is a frequent complaint. The National IC Database Study noted this symptom in 78% of patients (Kirkemo et al 1997). A retrospective review of 100 consecutive IC patients in our facility revealed a decrease in the force of the urinary stream (75%), urinary hesitancy (73%), the need to strain with urination (70%), and dyspareunia (45%).

Misdiagnosis of patients with either bacterial cystitis or bladder motor overactivity is common. Hence, many patients have been treated empirically with antibiotics and/or anticholinergic agents without success. Likewise, the symptoms of interstitial cystitis may vary with the menstrual cycle, often leading to a misdiagnosis of endometriosis. Unlike endometriosis, menstrual amelioration of symptoms is common in the IC patient. One study found that 38% of chronic pelvic pain patients presenting for laparoscopic evaluation (presumably to diagnose endometriosis) were ultimately diagnosed with interstitial cystitis (Clemons et al 2002).

Pathophysiology

Many theories to explain the pathogenesis of IC have been proposed, yet its true etiology remains elusive. Some suggest the presence of an unknown infectious etiology (Duncan and Schaeffer 1997), while others postulate that the urothelial surface and its protective bladder surface mucin are dysfunctional, thus allowing noxious solutes in the urine to gain access to underlying tissue (Parsons et al 1991). Alternative hypotheses include a neurogenic component (Pang et al 1995), excessive mast cell activation (Theoharides et al 2001), an autoimmune process (Anderson et al 1989), or a combination of some or all of these factors, as depicted in Figure 1.

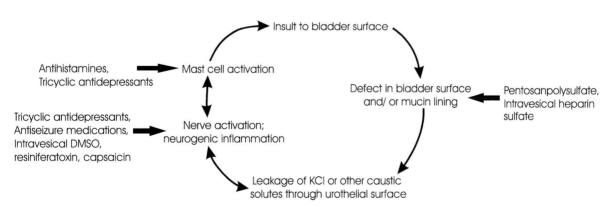

Interstitial Cystitis and Chronic Pelvic Pain, Figure 1   Schematic of several pathologies seen in interstitial cystitis and theoretical interaction between them. Note therapies available that address the various described pathologies.

Interstitial Cystitis and Chronic Pelvic Pain, Table 1

Differential Diagnosis
Bladder Calculi
Cystitis (infectious, radiation-induced, iatrogenic)
Neurological
Prostatitis
Sexually Transmitted Disease
Urethrocele, Cystocele
Urethral Diverticulum
Pelvic Floor Dysfunction
Gynecological Disorders (i. e. Endometriosis, PID)
Bladder Cancer/Carcinoma in situ

Diagnosis

Unfortunately, the diagnosis of IC remains one of exclusion (Table 1).

The National Institute of Diabetes, Digestive and Kidney Diseases established a set of diagnostic criteria for IC (Table 2), however, many physicians consider these criteria to be too restrictive and useful only for research purposes. In fact, it has been stated that as many as 60% of IC patients would be missed if these criteria were employed (Hanno et al 1999).

In clinical practice, the diagnosis is generally made by history, physical exam, urine analysis and culture, urine cytology, and cystoscopy, with or without bladder ▶ hydrodistention, under general anesthesia. Standard office cystoscopy demonstrates a normal bladder surface in 90–95% of patients. 5–10% of patients will have gross inflammatory changes of the bladder wall, termed Hunner's patches. Hydrodistention, filling the bladder to a relatively high pressure (80–100 cm H_2O) under anesthesia, has been employed to aid in the diagnosis of interstitial cystitis. Frequent findings with hydrodistention include the development of ▶ glomerulations (punctuate hemorrhages found in all regions of the bladder surface), mucosal tears, and a decreased bladder capacity. Other tests often employed during the evaluation of IC include ▶ potassium sensitivity testing (intravesical infusion of a potassium solution which often elicits pain in these patients), and urodynamics. Radiographic imaging may be used to exclude other pelvic pathology.

Various questionnaires have been created in order to assist in the diagnosis and as a measure of treatment responsiveness for patients with interstitial cystitis. The Pelvic Pain, Urgency, and Frequency (▶ PUF) Patient Symptom Scale and the O'Leary-Sant Intersitial Cystitis Symptom Index (▶ ICSI) are the most commonly used questionnaires for these purposes.

Treatment

The absence of a standardized treatment protocol for IC continues to frustrate patients as well as physicians. Regimens include dietary changes, oral agents, intravesical therapies, and surgical intervention. In most instances, a combination of therapies may be used in any given patient, many of which have an impact on pathologies identified in IC patients.

Dietary changes: Although no formal clinical trials have been carried out, many interstitial cystitis patients appear to have symptom exacerbation with the intake of various foods and beverages including: citrus fruits, carbonated beverages, alcoholic beverages, spicy foods, foods with high potassium content, caffeinated items, and artificial sweeteners (Table 3).

Not every IC patient is sensitive to each of these products, and patients are therefore encouraged to start with a bland diet and slowly add potentially irritating items. As a response to urinary frequency, many IC patients will decrease their fluid consumption, ultimately resulting in concentrated urine and as a consequence more bladder-based pain. An increase in fluid intake may therefore be helpful. Smoking may also worsen symptoms and should similarly be discouraged.

Behavioral Therapies

Bladder training, to gradually increase intervals between voids, may aid a minority of patients with IC, mostly those with more benign symptomatology. Similar behavioral therapy, using relaxation and distraction techniques, in order to assist the bladder training process, may be useful in some instances. Pelvic floor relaxation exercises and gentle stretching may be similarly beneficial in a small subset of patients with IC.

Other options include bladder retraining protocols (teaching patients to progressively increase intervals between voids, after their pain is controlled) and the use of support services, such as the Interstitial Cystitis Association (website: www.ichelp.org; telephone support: 1-800-help-ICA).

Oral Therapies: Pentosan Polysulfate Sodium (PPS) (▶ Elmiron) is often used as first-line therapy for the treatment of IC, and remains the only FDA approved oral medication for the treatment for IC. PPS is a synthetic glycosaminoglycan, very similar in molecular structure to the constituents of bladder surface mucin. One theory of IC pathogenesis is a defect in this layer that allows noxious urine solutes access to underlying tissue, thus beginning a cascade of nerve sensitization and/or inflammation. PPS's presumed mechanism of action is that it "augments" this layer and thus provides a slow improvement in symptoms. In one study, 38% of those treated with Pentosan Polysulfate Sodium experienced >50% improvement in pain compared to 18% in a placebo group (Parsons et al 1993). It is a well-tolerated

Interstitial Cystitis and Chronic Pelvic Pain, Table 2 NIDDK Criteria for the Diagnosis of I.C.

Required Findings	Automatic Exclusions
Hunner's Ulcers or diffuse glomerulations after hydrodistention *and* Pain associated with the bladder or urinary urgency	Less than 18 years of age
	Duration of symptoms less than 9 months
	Urinary frequency of less than 8 times per day
	Absence of nocturia
	Presence of bladder tumors
	Radiation cystitis
	Tuberculous cystitis
	Bacterial cystitis or prostatitis
	Vaginitis
	Cyclophosphamide cystitis
	Urethral diverticulum
	Uterine, cervical, vaginal, or urethral cancer
	Active herpes
	Bladder or lower ureteral calculi
	Symptoms relieved by antibiotics, urinary antiseptics, analgesics, anticholinergics, antispasmotics
	Involuntary bladder contractions
	Bladder capacity less than 350 cc while awake

Interstitial Cystitis and Chronic Pelvic Pain, Table 3 Foods that may Worsen Symptoms of Interstitial Cystititis

Aged cheeses	Cranberries	Nuts (except cashews, pine nuts)	Vinegar
Sour cream	Grapes	Alcoholic beverages	Citric acid
Yogurt	Nectarines	Carbonated beverages	Benzol alcohol
Chocolate	Peaches	Coffee	Monosodium glutamate (MSG)
Fava beans	Pineapples	Tea	Artificial sweeteners
Lima beans	Plums	Fruit juices	Saccharine
Pickles	Pomegranates	Mayonnaise	Preservatives
Sauerkraut	Rhubarb	Ketchup	Artificial ingredients
Onions	Strawberries	Mustard	Artificial colors
Tofu	Rye bread	Salsa	Tobacco
Soy beans	Sourdough bread	Spicy foods	Caffeine
Tomatoes	Smoked meats	Soy sauce	Diet pills
Apples	Smoked fish	Miso	Junk foods
Apricots	Anchovies	Salad dressing	Recreational drugs
Avocados	Caviar		Cold medications
Bananas	Chicken livers		Allergy medications
Cantaloupes	Salad dressing		
Citrus fruits			

agent with few side effects. Standard dosing is 100 mg, three times daily.

Various analgesic agents have been prescribed for patients with IC. NSAIDS may have some theoretical benefit in reducing the associated inflammation, however, there is the potential to paradoxically worsen the symptoms of IC due to the release of histamines. Short-term narcotic therapy is frequently used for symptom flares, and chronic narcotic therapy may be indicated in selected patients.

The inhibition of histamine release from mast cells can be accomplished with the use of antihistamines, such as hydroxyzine or tricyclic antidepressants (TCAs), such as amitriptyline. Amitriptyline and other TCAs have many other effects that are useful in the treatment of IC. Apart from their analgesic activity, their anticholinergic effect may be helpful in patients with concomitant bladder over activity (~15%). Many patients with IC may have poor urinary flow rates secondary to pelvic floor spasm. TCAs should be avoided or low doses used in IC patients, for fear of reducing flow further or promoting acute urinary retention. These agents may cause fatigue and are therefore taken in the evening to promote better sleep and decrease nocturia. Pain, nocturia, and urinary frequency are the symptoms most typically reduced by these agents.

Lastly, the use of antispasmodics and antiseizures medications have been described to aid in the relief of the debilitating symptoms associated with IC.

Intravesical Therapies

50% Dimethyl sulfoxide (DMSO) (Rimso-50®) is the only FDA-approved intravesical therapeutic agent for interstitial cystitis. Its precise method of action is unknown, however, it possesses anti-inflammatory, analgesic, and muscle-relaxing properties and appears to increase bladder capacity in many patients. DMSO may provide symptomatic relief in the majority of patients, however, repeated treatments are often necessary. Furthermore, the first several treatments may cause symptoms to flare.

Heparin sulfate (10,000 units in 10 ml sterile water) has also been used as an intravesical agent for the treatment of IC. Heparin sulfate is a normal component of the bladder's protective mucus layer. Like PPS, heparin's theoretical mechanism of action is an augmentation of the bladder's normal protective coating, thus preventing noxious bladder solutes from stimulating the bladder surface. One study reported clinical improvement in 56% of patients treated with intravesical heparin 3 times per week for 3 months, and continued remission for nearly all patients treated for six to twelve months (Parsons et al 1994). Others demonstrated the enhanced effects of a combination of DMSO and heparin compared with either agent alone (Perez-Marrero et al 1993). Relapse rates were reduced and duration of remissions were extended with this protocol. At our institution, we use a cocktail comprised of 20,000 units of heparin sulfate, 40 mg triamcinolone, and 30 ml of 1:1 0.5% bupivicaine and 2% viscous lidocaine, which has resulted in a >50% decrease in pain (visual analogue scores) in 71% of IC patients, often for many weeks.

Outside of the United States, ▶ hyaluronic acid (HA) and ▶ resiniferatoxin (RTX) are being investigated for their potential to improve the symptoms associated with IC. RTX appears to desensitize bladder nerve fibers, while HA, like heparin sulfate, theoretically augments bladder surface mucin. These agents may ultimately prove to have clinically significant benefits, and may add to our intravesical armamentarium against the symptoms of IC.

Surgery

As a last resort, surgery has been employed in a desperate attempt at providing relief for those with the most debilitating symptoms. ▶ Hunner's ulcer fulguration, transurethral excision of ulcers, subtotal cystectomy with bladder augmentation, and even total cystectomy are all options. Fulgurations and excisions of well-defined lesions, although not major surgeries can result in clinical remissions, however, long-term symptom relief is rarely achieved. Subtotal cystectomy with bladder augmentation (using a portion of detubularized bowel) is best performed in patients with severely diminished bladder capacities and unrelenting symptoms. Although the benefit of this procedure is that the urethra and bladder trigone are left intact, morbidity includes the potential for postoperative urinary retention (and the subsequent need to perform life-long intermittent catheterization) and persistence of pain. Total cystectomy may also be considered in patients refractory to other conservative modalities.

Conclusion

The diagnosis of interstitial cystitis remains one largely based upon presenting symptoms consistent with an irritative/painful bladder-based syndrome. Primary evaluation is dedicated to eliminating well-defined pathologies that might account for similar complaints. Further confirmatory testing, such as bladder hydrodistention under anesthesia or intravesical potassium chloride challenge, may be helpful at defining the bladder as the source of symptoms. Treatment options run the gambit from dietary changes to oral medications to cystectomy. Although no cure is at hand, a combination of conservative modalities may afford significant symptom relief to the majority of IC patients.

▶ Dyspareunia and Vaginismus

▶ Opioids and Bladder Pain/Function

References

1. Anderson JB, Parivar F, Lee G, Wallington TB, MacIver AG, Bradbrook RA, et al (1989) The Enigma of Interstitial Cystitis: An Autoimmune Disease? Br J Urol 63:58–63
2. Clemons JL, Arya LA, Myers DL (2002) Diagnosing Interstitial Cystitis in Women with Chronic Pelvic Pain. Obstet Gynecol 100:337–341
3. Duncan JL, Schaeffer AJ (1997) Do Infectious Agents Cause Interstitial Cystitis? Urology 49(Suppl 5A):48–51
4. Hanno PM, Landis JR, Matthews-Cook Y, Kusek J, Nyberg L Jr (1999) The Diagnosis of Interstitial Cystitis Revisited: Lessons Learned from the National Institutes of Health Interstitial Cystitis Database Study. J Urol 161:553–557
5. Hunner G L (1915) A Rare Type of Bladder Ulcer in Women: Report of Cases. Boston Med Surg J 172:660–665
6. Kirkemo A, Peabody M, Diokono AC, Afanasyev A, Nyberg LM, Landis JR, et al (1997) Associations Among Urodynamic Findings and Symptoms in Women Enrolled in the Interstitial Cystitis Database (ICDB) Study. Urology 49(Suppl 5A):76–80
7. Parsons CL, Lilly JD, Stein P (1991) Epithelial Dysfunction in Nonbacterial Cystitis (Interstitial Cystitis). J Urol 145: 732–735
8. Pang X, Marchand J, Sant GR, Kream RM, Theoharides TC (1995) Increased Number of Substance P Positive Fibers in Interstitial Cystitis. Br J Urol 75:744–750

9. Ratner V, Slade D, Greene G (1994) Interstitial Cystitis. A Patient's Perspective. Urol Clin NA 21: 1–5
10. Theoharides T, Duraisamy K, Sant G (2001) Mast Cell Involvement in Interstitial Cystitis: A Review of Human and Experimental Evidence. Urology 57(Suppl 6A):47–55
11. Parsons CL, Benson G, Childs S, Hanno P, Sant GR Webster G (1993) A Quantitatively Controlled Method to Study Prospectively Interstitial Cystitis and Demonstrate the Efficacy of Pentosanpolysulfate. J Urol 150:845–848
12. Parsons CL, Housley T, Schmidt JD, Lebow D (1994) Treatment of Interstitial Cystitis with Intravesical Heparin. Br J Urol 73:504–507
13. Perez-Marrero R, Emerson LE, Maharajh DO, Juma S (1993) Prolongation of Response to DMSO by Heparin Maintanance. Urol 41(1 Suppl):64–66

Interventional Therapies

Definition

In relation to low back pain, these typically encompass spinal surgery and a variety of injection therapies such as epidural steroid injections.

▶ Disability, Effect of Physician Communication

Intervertebral Disc

Definition

The portion between each vertebral body, composed of the annulus fibrosis and the nucleus pulposis.

▶ Chronic Low Back Pain, Definitions and Diagnosis

Intervertebral Foramen, Cervical

Definition

The cervical intervertebral foramen lies between adjacent cervical vertebrae and serves as the bony conduit through which the spinal nerve root exits the bony spinal canal. Its roof and floor are formed by the pedicles of consecutive vertebrae. Its posterolateral wall is formed largely by the superior articular process of the lower vertebra, and in part by the inferior articular process of the upper vertebra and the capsule of the zygoapophysial joint. The lower end of the upper vertebral body, the uncinate process of the lower vertebra, and the posterolateral corner of the intervertebral disc form the anteromedial wall.

▶ Cervical Transforaminal Injection of Steroids

Intra-Articular Blocks and Thoracic Medial Branch Blocks

▶ Thoracic Medial Branch Blocks and Intra-Articular Blocks

Intra-Articular Injections of Steroids

Nikolai Bogduk
Department of Clinical Research, Royal Newcastle Hospital Newcastle, University of Newcastle, Newcastle, NSW, Australia
nik.bogduk@newcastle.edu.au

Synonyms

Intra-Articular Steroid Injections; intra-articular corticosteroids; Intra-Articular Steroid Injections

Definition

Intra-articular injections of corticosteroids are a treatment for pain, ostensibly stemming from a synovial joint, in which a corticosteroid preparation is injected into the cavity of the painful joint. The injections may be blind or fluoroscopically guided.

Characteristics

Intra-articular injections of steroids were originally used as a treatment for overtly inflammatory joint diseases, such as rheumatoid arthritis. Their use for rheumatoid arthritis is not questioned. For that condition, intra-articular injections of steroids are held to be a useful adjunct to other therapy. They are not portrayed as a singular or curative treatment. They are used to suppress joint inflammation rapidly, while drug therapy is used to modify the disease process, long-term.

The success of intra-articular injections of steroids for rheumatoid arthritis inspired their use for other painful conditions of joints, notably and most commonly osteoarthritis. In practice, any painful joint can be treated, and most joints of the body have attracted this form of treatment. The treatment has become very popular, and is used not just by rheumatologists but also by orthopaedic surgeons, anaesthetists, physiatrists, and pain specialists. The literature on its efficacy, however, is sobering.

Rationale

The implicit rationale for the injection of steroids is that they relieve pain by suppressing inflammation. However, whereas this rationale is applicable to overtly inflammatory joint diseases, it is harder to sustain for osteoarthritis or undiagnosed joint pain. The evidence is weak or lacking that these latter conditions involve significant inflammation, if at all.

Rarely recognized in the literature is the fact that corticosteroids have a long-term local anaesthetic effect (Johansson et al. 1990). This effect, rather than any anti-inflammatory action, may be the basis for the observed relief of pain following intra-articular injection.

Technique

The technique for intra-articular injection differs according to the joint targeted. Common to all techniques is the need to place a needle in the cavity of the target joint. Large joints, such as the knee are readily accessed, using palpation as a guide. The smaller the joint, and the deeper in the body that it lies, the more difficult it is to enter the joint accurately with a needle. Smaller and deeper joints can be accessed under fluoroscopic guidance.

Any of a number of corticosteroid preparations can be used. Those most commonly used contain betamethasone, dexamethasone, triamcinolone, or methylprednisolone. Often these corticosteroids are provided in a depot preparation which allows for sustained, slow release of the active agent.

Application

Although any joint can be targeted, the literature describes the use of intra-articular steroids for the larger joints of the body, and some small ones. Most of the literature is anecdotal in nature, but there have been some controlled trials and systematic reviews.

Shoulder Joints

A systematic review (Buchbinder et al. 2003) assessed the literature on steroid injections for two common conditions of the shoulder. For rotator cuff disease, it found that subacromial steroid injection had a small benefit over placebo in some trials, but no benefit over NSAIDs was demonstrated. For adhesive capsulitis, two trials suggested a possible early benefit of intraarticular steroid injection over placebo; and one trial suggested short-term benefit of intra-articular corticosteroid injection over physiotherapy in the short-term. Subsequent studies have shown that subacromial injections of steroids are no more effective than placebo for post-traumatic impingement of the shoulder (McInerney et al. 2003), and injection therapy is no more effective than physiotherapy for stiff shoulder (Hay et al. 2003). For adhesive capsulitis, fluoroscopically guided injections followed by exercises are more effective than injections alone or physiotherapy alone (Carette et al. 2003). For frozen shoulder, distension of the glenohumeral joint with steroids is more effective than sham treatment for three weeks, but thereafter the differences attenuate (Buchbinder et al. 2004).

Acromioclavicular Joint

Few studies have addressed treatment of pain stemming from the acromioclavicular joint. The one controlled study found intra-articular steroids to be no more effective than placebo (Jacob and Sallay 1997).

Knee Joint

Reviews have concluded that intra-articular steroids for osteoarthritis of the knee are more effective than placebo, but they only have a short-term effect (3 weeks) (Arroll and Goodyear-Smith 2004; Creamer 1999; Raynauld et al. 2003; Towheed and Hochberg 1997). Steroid injec-

tions confer no long-term benefit for osteoarthritis of the knee (Creamer 1999).

Hip Joint

Although the hip joint has been less studied than the knee, the efficacy of intra-articular steroids seems to be the same. Injection of steroids is more effective than injection of local anaesthetic alone, but only for about 3 weeks (Kullenberg et al 2004).

Thumb

The carpometacarpal joint of the thumb is another site affected by painful osteoarthritis, and which attracts treatment with intra-articular injection of steroids. A controlled trial, however, found no ► Attributable Effect for this treatment (Meenagh et al 2004).

Neck Pain

Injections of steroids into the cervical zygapophysial joints have been used to treat chronic neck pain. A controlled study, however, found that injection of steroids was no more effective than injection of local anaesthetic alone, and that the beneficial effects of both agents rapidly disappeared in about 2 weeks (Barnsley et al. 1994).

Back Pain

Injection of steroids into the lumbar zygapophysial joints has been a popular treatment for low back pain. A review of the observational studies and the controlled studies available, found that injection of steroids is no more effective than sham therapy (Bogduk 2005).

Interpretation

The popularity of intra-articular injections of steroids for joint pain is not matched by the literature concerning their efficacy. For all joints that have been studied, the pattern is the same. Either the injections are not more effective than placebo or sham therapy, or any pain-relieving effects last for only a matter of a few weeks.

References

1. Arroll B, Goodyear-Smith F (2004) Corticosteroid Injections for Osteoarthritis of the Knee: Meta-Analysis. BMJ 328:869
2. Barnsley L, Lord SM, Wallis BJ et al. (1994) Lack of Effect of Intraarticular Corticosteroids for Chronic Pain in the Cervical Zygapophyseal Joints. N Engl J Med 330:1047–1050
3. Bogduk N (2005) A Narrative Review of Intra-Articular Corticosteroid Injections for Low Back Pain. Pain Medicine 6:297–298
4. Buchbinder R, Green S, Youd JM (2003) Corticosteroid Injections for Shoulder Pain. Cochrane Database Syst Rev CD004016
5. Buchbinder R, Green S, Forbes A et al. (2004) Arthrographic Joint Distension with Saline and Steroid Improves Function and Reduces Pain in Patients with Painful Stiff Shoulder: Results of a Randomised, Double Blind, Placebo Controlled Trial. Ann Rheum Dis 63:302–309
6. Carette S, Moffet H, Tardif J et al. (2003) Intraarticular Corticosteroids, Supervised Physiotherapy, or a Combination of the Two in the Treatment of Adhesive Capsulitis of the Shoulder: A Placebo-Controlled Trial. Arthritis Rheum 48:829–838

7. Creamer P (1999) Intra-Articular Corticosteroid Treatment in Osteoarthritis. Curr Opin Rheumatol 11:417–421
8. Hay EM, Thomas E, Paterson SM et al. (2003) A Pragmatic Randomised Controlled Trial of Local Corticosteroid Injection and Physiotherapy for the Treatment of New Episodes of Unilateral Shoulder Pain in Primary Care. Ann Rheum Dis 62:394–399
9. Jacob AK, Sallay PI (1997) Therapeutic Efficacy of Corticosteroid Injections in the Acromioclavicular Joint. Miomed Sci Instrum 34:380–385
10. Johansson A, Hao J, Sjolund B (1990) Local Corticosteroid Application Blocks Transmission in Normal Nociceptive C-Fibres. Acta Anaesthesiol Scand 34:335–338
11. Kullenberg B, Runesson R, Tuvhag R et al. (2004) Intraarticular Corticosteroid Injection: Pain Relief in Osteoarthritis of the Hip? J Rheumatol 31:2265–2268
12. McInerney JJ, Dias J, Durham S et al. (2003) Randomised Controlled Trial of Single, Subacromial Injection of Methylprednisolone in Patients with Persistent, Post-Traumatic Impingement of the Shoulder. Emerg Med J 20:218–221
13. Meenagh GK, Patton J, Kynes C et al. (2004) A Randomised Controlled Trial of Intra-Articular Corticosteroid Injection of the Carpometacarpal Joint of the Thumb in Osteoarthritis. Ann Rheum Dis 63:1260–1263
14. Raynauld JP, Buckland-Wright C, Ward R et al. (2003) Safety and Efficacy of Long-Term Intraarticular Steroid Injections in Osteoarthritis of the Knee: A Randomized, Double-Blind, Placebo-Controlled Trial. Arthritis Rheum 48:370–377
15. Towheed TE, Hochberg MC (1997) A Systematic Review of Randomized Controlled Trials of Pharmacological Therapy in Osteoarthritis of the Knee, with an Emphasis on Trial Methodology. Semin Arthritis Rheum 26:755–770

Intra-Articular Morphine

Definition

Local application of morphine in patients undergoing arthroscopic knee surgery, which induces significant postoperative pain reduction lasting up to 24 hours.
▶ Opioids and Inflammatory Pain

Intra-Articular Sacroiliac Joint Block

▶ Sacroiliac Joint Blocks

Intra-Articular Steroid Injections

▶ Intra-Articular Injections of Steroids

Intra Discal Electrothermal Therapy

▶ IDET

Intracellular Labeling

Definition

Intracellular labeling is a technique that stains a single neuron by injecting a neural tracer intracellulary through a glass microelectrode containing the tracer.
▶ Trigeminal Brainstem Nuclear Complex, Anatomy

Intracerebral Hematoma Apoplexy

▶ Headache Due to Intracranial Bleeding

Intracerebroventricular Drug Pumps

▶ Pain Treatment, Implantable Pumps for Drug Delivery

Intracerebroventricular, Intracerebral and Intrathecal

Definition

Drugs are frequently administered directly into the brain of experimental animals because such drugs may not penetrate the blood-brain barrier, or systemic administration of such drugs is prohibited by cost. Intracerebroventricular (i.c.v.) injections are made into the cerebral ventricle of the brain. Intracerebral (i.c.) injections are made into brain tissue and generally require stereotaxic implantation of microinjection guide sleeves in order to deliver the drug to a specific locus in the brain. Intrathecal (i.t.) injections are made into the cerebrospinal fluid that bathes the spinal cord.
▶ Nitrous Oxide Antinociception and Opioid Receptors
▶ Proinflammatory Cytokines

Intracranial

Definition

Structures located within the skull.
▶ Pain Treatment, Intracranial Ablative Procedures

Intracranial Ablative Procedures

▶ Pain Treatment, Intracranial Ablative Procedures

Intracranial Nociceptors

► Nociceptors in the Orofacial Region (Meningeal/ Cerebrovascular)

Intractable

Definition

Persistence of an abnormal or harmful function despite usual treatment. For instance, intractable pain that persists after the etiology is treated and defies usual pain treatments.
► Pain Treatment, Intracranial Ablative Procedures

Intracutaneous Injection Pain

► Autologous Thrombocyte Injection as a Model of Cutaneous Pain

Intradental Nociceptors

► Nociceptors in the Dental Pulp

Intradermal

Definition

Intradermal relates to areas between the layers of the dermis (skin).
► PET and fMRI Imaging in Parietal Cortex (SI, SII, Inferior Parietal Cortex BA40)

Intradiscal Electrothermal Anuloplasty

► Intradiscal Electrothermal Therapy

Intradiscal Electrothermal Therapy

Kevin Pauza, Nikolai Bogduk
Tyler Spine and Joint Hospital, Tyler, TX, USA
kevinpauza@tyler.net, nik.bogduk@newcastle.edu.au

Synonyms

IDET; intradiscal eletrothermal anuloplasty

Definition

Intradiscal Electrothermal Therapy (IDET) is a treatment devised to relieve the pain of internal disc disruption. It involves threading into the painful disc a flexible, wire electrode, which is used to heat the tissues of the posterior anulus fibrosus in an effort to relieve the pain.

Characteristics

IDET was born of the desire and need for a procedure for the treatment of discogenic low back pain, other than major surgical procedures such as fusion and disc replacement. Since its introduction into clinical practice, it has met with variable acceptance and considerable criticism. Much of the resistance, however, has been financial and social in nature, with insurers concerned about the costs of a new and potentially popular procedure, and some critics expressing concerns that much of the literature on the efficacy of the procedure is being published by its inventors.

Indications

The procedure is expressly indicated for low back pain caused by internal disc disruption. Practitioners, however, differ in how rigorously they make this diagnosis. Some rely only on the results of lumbar discography. Others insist on more rigorous criteria (Karasek and Bogduk 2001) that include demonstration of a radial fissure on post-discography CT (See: CT scan.). Nevertheless, discography is common to both approaches and is essential for the diagnosis of discogenic pain.

Eligibility criteria for IDET (Karasek and Bogduk 2001):

• Chronic, intrusive low back pain for greater than 3 months
• Failure to achieve adequate improvement with comprehensive nonoperative treatment
• No red flag condition
• No medical contraindications
• No neurologic deficit
• Normal straight-leg raise
• Nondiagnostic MRI scan
• No evidence for segmental instability, spondylolisthesis at target level
• No irreversible psychological barriers to recovery
• Motivated patient with realistic expectations of outcome
• No greater than 25% loss of disc height
• Criteria for IDD satisfied, viz.

 – Disc stimulation is positive at low pressures (< 50 psi)
 – Disc stimulation reproduces pain of intensity > 6/10
 – Disc stimulation reproduces concordant pain

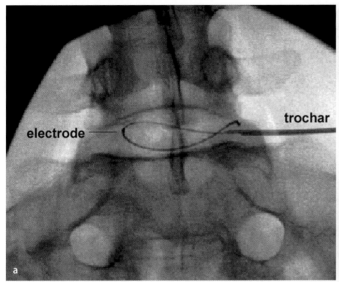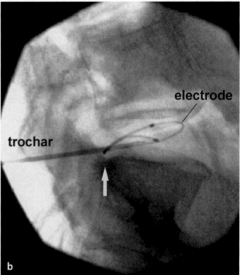

Intradiscal Electrothermal Therapy, Figure 1   Radiographs of an IDET procedure on an L5-S1 disc. (a) Postero-anterior view. The electrode has been threaded through a trochar, into and around the disc. (b) Lateral view. The electrode has passed through the outer, posterior annulus (arrow). Adapted from the Practice Guidelines for Spinal Diagnostic and Treatment Procedures of the International Spinal Intervention Society (Bogduk 2003).

- CT discography reveals a Grade 3 or greater anular tear
- Control disc stimulation is negative at one and preferably two, adjacent levels

Rationale

The professed rationale of IDET varies between proponents. None has been tested, and none has been validated. Amongst the conjectures is that heating the posterior anulus: stiffens the collagen of the disc (Saal and Saal 2000a); denatures chemical exudates in radial and circumferential fissures; seals fissures; and destroys nociceptive nerve endings (Karasek and Bogduk 2001).

Technique

Practitioners differ in the manner in which they execute IDET. Indeed, the procedure has undergone various modifications since its original description.

Common to all variants is the introduction of a flexible electrode into the disc. A trochar is passed into the disc along a posterolateral trajectory, such that its tip reaches the inner boundary of the anulus fibrosus. Through the trochar, a wire electrode is threaded and then navigated within the disc to assume a circumferential disposition, parallel to the lamina of the anulus. The objective is to place the 50 length of the active tip of the electrode across the radial fissure in the disc (Fig. 1).

The original description of the procedure required that the electrode be placed across the junction of the outer nucleus pulposus and the inner anulus fibrosus (Saal and Saal 2000a) (Fig. 2a). Subsequent variations have included: placing the electrode as far peripherally as possible in the outer anulus; attempting multiple placements

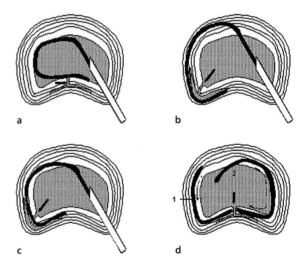

Intradiscal Electrothermal Therapy, Figure 2   Variants of intradiscal electrothermal therapy. (a) The original description, in which the electrode is placed across the base of the radial fissure (arrowed) in the plane of the junction of the outer nucleus and inner anulus. (b) A variant in which the electrode is placed in the outermost annulus, parallel and external to the circumferential extension of the radial fissure (arrowed). (c) A variant in which the electrode is placed around the inner annulus, through the radial fissure (arrowed), but internal to its circumferential extension. (d) A variant in which the radial and circumferential fissures are attacked with two electrodes (1 and 2), introduced from opposites sides of the disc. Adapted from the Practice Guidelines for Spinal Diagnostic and Treatment Procedures of the International Spinal Intervention Society (Bogduk 2003).

but at different heights within the anulus; and approaching the target fissure from both sides, and at different heights (Figs. 2b, 2c, 2d).

Efficacy

In observational studies, practitioners of IDET have reported outcomes of various magnitudes for different du-

Intradiscal Electrothermal Therapy, Table 1 Outcomes of IDET based on observational studies: a: Visual analog pain scale (0–100). b: Physical Functioning on the SF36 (0–100). c: Change in visual analog pain scale (0–100). d: Roland-Morris Disability Questionnaire (0–30). e: Bodily Pain on the SF36. f: Oswestry Disability Inventory (0–100). g. Reported as 8–24 months

Study	N	Outcome Measures	Baseline	6 M	12 M	24 M
Saal and Saal (2000b, 2002)	58	VAS[a] Mean	66		35	34
		Sd	19		23	20
		SF36:PF[b] Mean	40		60	72
		Sd	25		22	23
Lutz and Lutz (2003)	33	VAS[a] Mean	75		39[g]	
		Sd	24		30	
		RMDQ[d] Mean	14		7[g]	
		Sd	5.9		7.2	
Lee et al. (2003)	62	VAS[a] Mean	79			47
		Sd	13			30
		RMDQ[d] Mean	15			8.8
		Sd	5.3			7.5
Cohen et al. (2003)	79	> 50% relief		0.48		
		VAS[a] mean	59	21		
		Sd	18	13		
		> 90% relief		0.10		
Gerszten et al. (2002)	27	SF36: BP[e]	27		38	
		SF36: PF[b]	32		47	
		ODI[f]	34		30	

rations of follow-up (Table 1). Most of these studies have reported clinically significant reductions in pain. Some have reported sustained relief for up to two years and beyond.

Others, however, have reported less than impressive outcomes. One retrospective audit found that 50% of patients were dissatisfied with their outcome one year after treatment; and only 39% had less pain (Davis et al. 2004). The other reported that 55% of patients still required treatment after IDET; but 39% resumed or remained at work (Webster et al. 2004).

Another study found that it was unable to achieve good outcomes in the same proportion of patients as reported in the more favourable outcome studies (Freedman et al. 2003). Nevertheless, it found some patients who had satisfying relief. The authors concluded that, although IDET was not a substitute for fusion, it nevertheless could be entertained as an option prior to undertaking fusion as a treatment.

Two controlled trials have produced favourable results (Table 2). In one (Bogduk and Karasek 2002), IDET was compared with the efficacy of a rehabilitation program. A significantly greater proportion of patients treated with IDET achieved relief of pain, which endured for up to two years. In particular, 20% achieved complete relief of pain, and 57% achieved greater than 50% relief of pain. In the other study (Pauza et al. 2004), IDET was found to achieve a significantly greater reduction in pain than did sham treatment.

Another controlled study failed to find any difference in outcome between patients treated with IDET or sham therapy (Freeman et al. 2003). In that study, however, no patients benefited from either therapy. No placebo effect was encountered in either group.

Definition

Irritable bowel syndrome (IBS) is the most commonly reported functional gastrointestinal disorder effecting the large bowel and rectum. It is a syndrome characterized by abdominal pain or discomfort and altered defecation (such as diarrhea or constipation, other common symptoms are bloating, passing mucus in the stools, or a sense that the bowels were not completely emptied) without abnormalities on conventional medical tests. It is one of the most commonly seen conditions by gastroenterologists in clinical practice. IBS is not an inflammatory bowel disease, and should be diagnosed using the consensus 'Rome' clinical criteria. These are:
1. Three months of continuous or recurring symptoms of abdominal pain or irritation that may be relieved with a bowel movement, may be coupled with a change in frequency, or may be related to a change in the consistency of stools;
2. Two or more of the following are present at least 25 percent of the time: a change in stool frequency, noticeable difference in stool form, passage of mucus, bloating or altered stool passage including sensations of incomplete evacuation, straining, or urgency.
► Amygdala, Functional Imaging
► Amygdala, Pain Processing and Behavior in Animals
► Chronic Gynaecological Pain, Doctor-Patient Interaction
► Descending Modulation of Visceral Pain
► Postsynaptic Dorsal Column Neurons, Responses to Visceral Input
► Psychological Aspects of Pain in Women
► Thalamus
► Thalamus and Visceral Pain Processing (Human Imaging)
► Thalamus, Clinical Visceral Pain, Human Imaging
► Visceral Pain Model, Irritable Bowel Syndrome Model

Irritable Bowel Syndrome Model

► Visceral Pain Model, Irritable Bowel Syndrome Model

Irritant

Definition

An irritant is a chemical used in prolotherapy solutions which acts by damaging cells directly or rendering them antigenic. They include phenol, guaiacol and tannic acid.
► Prolotherapy

Ischemia

Definition

Insufficient or suppressed blood supply to an organ caused by blockage of a blood vessel (blood clot, atherosclerosis plaque, contractions, artery spasms). It prevents the tissue from receiving nutrients and oxygen and leads to accumulation of metabolic wastes like carbon dioxide and metabolic acids, and thus induces local acidosis.
► Acid-Sensing Ion Channels
► TRPV1, Regulation by Protons

Ischemia Model

► Spinal Cord Injury Pain Model, Ischemia Model

Ischemic Heart Disease

Definition

Is a condition in which blood flow (and thus oxygen and nutrients) is reduced in areas of the heart where the diameters of the coronary arteries are significantly narrowed.
► Visceral Pain Model, Angina Pain

Ischemic Neuropathies

► Vascular Neuropathies

Ischemic Pain/Test

Definition

Experimental ischemic pain from skeletal muscles can be easily produced by exercising a limb or an arm during a temporary block of the arterial blood supply.
► Tourniquet Test

ISH

► Idiopathic Stabbing Headache

ISI

► Interspike Interval

Island of Reil

▶ Insular Cortex, Neurophysiology and Functional Imaging of Nociceptive Processing

Isolectin B4

Definition

The isolectin B4 of the plant lectin Griffonia simplicifolia recognizes a sugar moiety found selectively on the surface of small myelinated and unmyelinated nerve fibers, and is a useful marker for nociceptive neurons.
▶ Nociceptor, Categorization
▶ Trigeminal Brainstem Nuclear Complex, Immunohistochemistry and Neurochemistry

Itch/Itch Fibers

MARTIN SCHMELZ
Institute for Anesthesiology and Operative Intensive Medicine, Fakulty for Clinical Medicine Mannheim, University Heidelberg, Mannheim, Germany
martin.schmelz@anaes.ma.uni-heidelberg.de

Synonyms

Pruritus

Definition

Itch (Latin: *pruritus*) obviously serves nociceptive functions, but it is clearly distinct from pain sensation. It is restricted to the skin and some adjoining mucosae. Whereas painful stimuli inflicted on the skin provoke withdrawal reflexes, itching stimuli provoke the very characteristic scratching reflex. This reflex pattern indicates that the neuronal apparatus for itch has developed as a nocifensive system for removal of irritating objects and agents affecting the skin. One might also describe scratching as a reflex pattern that is used in situations in which the noxious stimulus has already invaded the skin. In this situation withdrawal would be useless; instead localizing the injured site by scratching and a close inspection appears to be more adequate.

Characteristics

C-fibers, responding to histamine application in parallel to the itch ratings of subjects have been discovered among the group of mechano-insensitive C-afferents (Schmelz et al. 1997) suggesting that there is a specific pathway for itch (Fig. 1). In contrast, the most common type of C-fibers, mechano-heat nociceptors (CMH or polymodal nociceptors) are either insensitive to histamine or only weakly activated by it (Schmelz et al. 2003b). This fiber type cannot account for the prolonged itch induced by the intradermal application of histamine.

The histamine-sensitive or 'itch' fibers or pruriceptors are characterized by a particular low conduction velocity, large innervation territories, mechanical unresponsiveness and high transcutaneous electrical thresholds (Schmelz et al. 2003b). In line with the large innervation territories of these fibers, two-point discrimination for histamine-induced itch is poor (15 cm in the upper arm).

The relative prevalence of the different C-fiber types has been estimated from recordings in the superficial peroneal nerve. About 80% are polymodal nociceptors, which respond to mechanical, heat and chemical stimuli. The remaining 20% do not respond to mechanical stimulation. These fibers are mainly "mechano-insensitive nociceptors" (Schmidt et al. 1995), which are activated by chemical stimuli (Schmelz et al. 2000), and can be sensitized to mechanical stimulation in the presence of inflammation (Schmelz et al. 2000; Schmidt et al. 1995). Among the mechano-insensitive afferent C-fibers, there is a subset of units that have a strong and sustained response to histamine. They comprise about 20% of the mechano-heat-insensitive class of C-fibers, i.e. about 5% of all C-fibers in the superficial peroneal nerve.

Specific Spinal Pruriceptive Neurons

The concept of dedicated pruriceptive neurons has now been complemented and extended by recordings from the cat spinal cord. A specific class of dorsal horn neurons projecting to the thalamus has been demonstrated, which respond strongly to histamine administered to the skin by iontophoresis (Andrew and Craig 2001). The time course of these responses was similar to that of itch in humans and matched the responses of the peripheral C-itch fibers (Fig. 1). These units were also unresponsive to mechanical stimulation and differed from the histamine insensitive nociceptive units in lamina I of the spinal cord. In addition, their axons had a lower conduction velocity and anatomically distinct projections to the thalamus. Thus, the combination of dedicated peripheral and central neurons with a unique response pattern to pruritugenic mediators and anatomically distinct projections to the thalamus, provide the basis for a specific neuronal pathway for itch.

Peripheral Sensitization

Increased intradermal nerve fiber density has been found in patients with chronic pruritus. In addition, increased epidermal levels of neurotrophin 4 (NT4) have been found in patients with atopic dermatitis and massively increased serum levels of NGF and SP have been found to correlate with the severity of the disease in such patients (Toyoda et al. 2002). Increased fiber density and higher local NGF concentrations were also found in patients with contact dermatitis. It is known

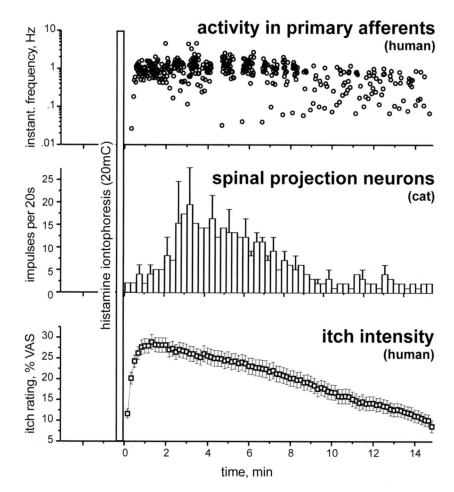

Itch/Itch Fibers, Figure 1 In the upper panel instantaneous discharge frequency of a mechano- and heat insensitive C-fiber (CMiHi) in the superficial peroneal nerve following histamine iontophoresis (20 mC; marked as open box in the diagram) is shown. In the central panel activation of a spinal projection neuron following histamine iontophoresis is depicted. The lower panel shows average itch magnitude ratings of a group of 21 healthy volunteers after an identical histamine stimulus. Ratings at 10 s intervals on a visual analogue scale with the end points "no itch" - "unbearable itch" Bars: standard error of means (modified from Schmelz et al. 1997 and Andrew et al. 2001).

that NGF and NT4 can sensitize nociceptors. These similarities between localized painful and pruritic lesions might suggest that similar mechanisms of nociceptor sprouting and sensitization exist on a peripheral level.

Central Sensitization

There is a remarkable similarity between the phenomena associated with central sensitization to pain and itch. Activity in chemo-nociceptors leads not only to acute pain but, in addition, can sensitize second order neurons in the dorsal horn, thereby leading to increased sensitivity to pain (hyperalgesia).

In itch processing, similar phenomena have been described; touch or brush-evoked pruritus around an itching site has been termed 'itchy skin' (Bickford 1938). Like allodynia, it requires ongoing activity in primary afferents and is most probably elicited by low threshold mechanoreceptors (A-β fibers). Also more intense prick-induced itch sensations in the surroundings, 'hyperknesis', have been reported following histamine iontophoresis in healthy volunteers (Atanassoff et al. 1999).

The exact mechanisms and roles of central sensitization for itch in clinical conditions have still to be explored, whereas a major role for central sensitization in patients with chronic pain is generally accepted. It should be noted that there is also emerging evidence for corresponding phenomena in patients with chronic pain and chronic itch. In patients with neuropathic pain, it has recently been reported that histamine iontophoresis resulted in burning pain instead of pure itch, which would be induced by this procedure in healthy volunteers (Birklein et al. 1997; Baron et al. 2001). This phenomenon is of special interest as it demonstrates spinal hypersensitivity to C-fiber input. Conversely, normally painful electrical, chemical, mechanical and thermal stimulation is perceived as itching when applied in or close to lesional skin of atopic dermatitis patients (Ikoma et al. 2003).

Long lasting activation of pruriceptors by histamine has been shown experimentally to induce central sensitization for itch in healthy volunteers (Ikoma et al. 2003); following the application of histamine *via* dermal microdialysis fibers, low pH stimulation of the skin close to the histamine site was perceived as itch instead of pain. Ongoing activity of pruriceptors, which might underlie the development of central sensitization for itch, has already been confirmed microneurographically in a patient with chronic pruritus (Schmelz et al. 2003a).

While there is obviously an antagonistic interaction between pain and itch under normal conditions, the patterns of spinal sensitization phenomena are surprisingly similar. It remains to be established whether this similarity will also include the underlying mechanism, which would also imply similar therapeutic approaches, such as gabapentin or clonidine, for the treatment of neuropathic itch.

References

1. Andrew D, Craig AD (2001) Spinothalamic lamina 1 neurons selectively sensitive to histamine: a central neural pathway for itch. Nat Neurosci 4:72–77
2. Atanassoff PG, Brull SJ, Zhang J et al. (1999) Enhancement of experimental pruritus and mechanically evoked dysesthesiae with local anesthesia. Somatosens Mot Res 16:291–298
3. Baron R, Schwarz K, Kleinert A et al. (2001) Histamine-induced itch converts into pain in neuropathic hyperalgesia. Neuroreport 12:3475–3478
4. Bickford RGL (1938) Experiments relating to itch sensation, its peripheral mechanism and central pathways. Clin Sci 3:377–386
5. Birklein F, Claus D, Riedl B et al. (1997) Effects of cutaneous histamine application in patients with sympathetic reflex dystrophy. Muscle Nerve 20:1389–1395
6. Ikoma A, Rukwied R, Stander S et al. (2003) Neuronal sensitization for histamine-induced itch in lesional skin of patients with atopic dermatitis. Arch Dermatol 139:1455–1458
7. Schmelz M, Schmidt R, Bickel A et al. (1997) Specific C-receptors for itch in human skin. J.Neurosci 17:8003–8008
8. Schmelz M, Schmidt R, Handwerker HO et al. (2000) Encoding of burning pain from capsaicin-treated human skin in two categories of unmyelinated nerve fibres. Brain 123:560-571
9. Schmelz M, Hilliges M, Schmidt R et al. (2003a) Active "itch fibers" in chronic pruritus. Neurology 61:564–566
10. Schmelz M, Schmidt R, Weidner C et al. (2003b) Chemical response pattern of different classes of C-nociceptors to pruritogens and algogens. J Neurophysiol 89:2441–2448
11. Schmidt R, Schmelz M, Forster C et al. (1995) Novel classes of responsive and unresponsive C nociceptors in human skin. J Neurosci 15:333–341
12. Toyoda M, Nakamura M, Makino T et al. (2002) Nerve growth factor and substance P are useful plasma markers of disease activity in atopic dermatitis. Br J Dermatol 147:71–79

ITCH MAN

Definition

A scale to quantify the severity of itching on a 10 point scale. It was developed and copyrighted by P. Blakeney and J. Marvin, Shriners Hospitals for Children, Galveston, Texas

▶ Pain Control in Children with Burns

Itchy Skin

Definition

The cutaneous areas of abnormally enhanced itch that are characterized by a greater than normal sensation of itch in response to a normally itchy stimulus (*hyperknesis*), and/or a sensation of itch evoked by stimuli that normally do not elicit itch (*alloknesis*). These states are sometimes accompanied by mild hyperalgesia in which a normally painful stimulus can evoke a greater than normal magnitude and duration of pain.

▶ Allodynia and Alloknesis

IUPHAR

Definition

The IUPHAR recommend that the opioid receptors should be called MOP (μ or mu receptor), DOP (δ or delta receptor), KOP (kappa receptor) or NOP (orphan receptor).

▶ Postoperative Pain, Opioids

Jab-Like and Jolt-Like Headache

Definition

Jab-Like and Jolt-Like Headache refers to a benign stabbing headache.
▶ Primary Exertional Headache

Jabs and Jolts Syndrome

▶ Primary Stabbing Headache

Japanese Meridian Therapy

▶ Acupuncture

Jaw Claudication

Definition

Pain during mastication due to ischemia of the masseter muscles in temporal arteritis.
▶ Headache Due to Arteritis

Jaw-Muscle Silent Periods (Exteroceptive Suppression)

GIORGIO CRUCCU
Department of Neurological Sciences, La Sapienza University, Rome, Italy
Cruccu@uniroma1.it

Synonyms

Masseter inhibitory reflex; Masseter Silent Periods; Exteroceptive Suppression

Definition

The jaw-muscle silent periods are trigemino-trigeminal inhibitory reflexes elicited by electrical, mechanical, or radiant heat stimuli delivered to the oral region (in the territory of the maxillary and mandibular trigeminal divisions); on electromyographic recordings from contracted jaw-closers, this reflex inhibition appears as an early and a late phase of suppression, also called ES1 and ES2 exteroceptive suppressions or SP1 and SP2 silent periods.

Characteristics

Whereas in the reflex control of jaw movement in lower mammals, the jaw-opening and jaw-closing muscles act in equilibrium, in humans the jaw-openers (digastric and suprahyoid muscles) play a marginal role. The jaw-closers (masseter, temporalis and pterygoid muscles) serve both functions, for reflex jaw closing under normal circumstances (excitation) and for reflex jaw opening when they undergo inhibition. The jaw-closers are excited by way of the Aα muscle spindle input and strongly inhibited by way of Aβ capsulated mechanoreceptors and Aδ free nerve endings. The powerful inhibition exerted by cutaneous and intraoral mechanoreceptors probably compensates for the unusual organization of the jaw-closing motoneurons, which undergo inhibitory control neither by reciprocal nor by recurrent inhibition. Electrical or mechanical stimuli delivered to the oral region evoke a reflex inhibition of the jaw-closing muscles, the ▶ masseter inhibitory reflex (Fig. 1). On EMG recordings from contracted jaw-closers, this reflex inhibition appears as an early and a late phase of suppression, also called ▶ ES1 and ES2 exteroceptive suppressions (Godaux and Desmedt 1975), or ▶ SP1 and SP2 silent periods (Cruccu and Deuschl 2000). Probably because electrical stimuli yield a mixed – nociceptive and non-nociceptive – input, whether the first or the second or both components are ▶ nociceptive reflexes remains controversial (Miles and Turker 1987). Innocuous mechanical stimuli will elicit both components, however, and indirect evidence supports the view that the afferents belong to the intermediately myelinated Aβ group. Afferent impulses reach the pons *via* the sensory mandibular or maxillary root of the trigeminal nerve. The first inhibitory

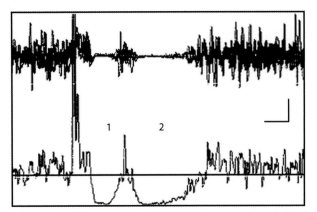
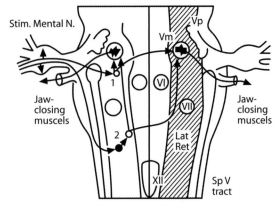

Jaw-Muscle Silent Periods (Exteroceptive Suppression), Figure 1 Masseter inhibitory reflex and brainstem circuits. Left: first (1) and second (2) inhibitory periods. Recording from the right masseter muscle. Stimulation of the right mental nerve. Upper traces: 8 trials are superimposed. Lower trace: rectified and averaged signal. The horizontal line indicates 80% of the background EMG level. Calibration 20 ms / 200 μV. Right: schematic drawing of the reflex circuits. Afferents for the first inhibitory period connect with an inhibitory interneuron (1) located close to the ipsilateral trigeminal motor nucleus. The afferents for the second inhibitory period descend along the spinal trigeminal tract and connect with a multisynaptic chain of excitatory interneurons. The last interneuron is inhibitory (2) and projects bilaterally onto the jaw-closing motoneurons. Vm, trigeminal motor nucleus; Vp, trigeminal principal sensory nucleus; Sp V tract, spinal trigeminal tract; VI, abducens nucleus; VII, facial nucleus; XII, hypoglossal nucleus; Lat Ret, lateral reticular formation. (From Cruccu and Deuschl 2000).

period (10–13 ms latency) is probably mediated by one inhibitory interneuron, located close to the ipsilateral ► trigeminal motor nucleus. This interneuron projects onto jaw-closing motoneurons bilaterally. The whole circuit lies in the mid-pons. The afferents for the second inhibitory period (40–50 ms latency) descend in the ► spinal trigeminal complex and connect to a polysynaptic chain of excitatory interneurons, probably located in the ► medullary lateral reticular formation. The last interneuron of the chain is inhibitory and gives rise to ipsilateral and contralateral collaterals that ascend medially to the right and left spinal trigeminal complexes, to reach the trigeminal motoneurons (Cruccu et al. 2005; Ongerboer de Visser et al. 1990).

As shown by experiments with noxious, high-intensity laser stimuli directed to the perioral region, selective activation of Aδ afferents elicits a single, late (70 ms latency) silent period in jaw-closing muscles (Ellrich et al. 1997; Romaniello et al. 2002). This nociceptive reflex (► laser silent period, LSP) is supposedly mediated by the spinal trigeminal nucleus, pars caudalis.

Technical Requirements and Normal Values

The masseter inhibitory reflex is usually evoked by transcutaneous electrical stimulation of the mentalis territory (to test the mandibular division) or of the infraorbital territory (to test the maxillary division), by placing the cathode on the skin overlying the mental or the infraorbital foramen and the anode 2 cm laterally. A stimulus lasting 0.1 ms delivered at an intensity of about 3 × the sensory threshold allows best visualization of the first and second inhibitory periods without causing excessive discomfort. The patient clenches the teeth at maximum strength, receives the stimulus and is then allowed

a few seconds' rest. At least 8 trials, but preferably 16, are repeated and superimposed. Quantitative studies of the excitability of the brainstem inhibitory interneurons require measurement of the size of responses (e.g. area of suppression); the level of background EMG activity must be kept constant and the signal is full-wave rectified and averaged (Fig. 1).

The onset latency should correspond to the beginning of the EMG suppression. This is usually taken at the intersection between the inhibitory shift and a line corresponding to 80% of the mean background EMG activity. The size of the response can be evaluated by measuring the area of suppression or the duration, taking the end-latency at the point when EMG returns to 80%. The onset latency is the most reliable measure for clinical applications (Table 1 shows normal values). The latency of the first inhibitory period (though not the second) has a rel-

Jaw-Muscle Silent Periods (Exteroceptive Suppression), Table 1 Masseter Inhibitory Reflex in 100 normal subjects aged 15–80 years

Latency (ms)	First inhibitory period (SP1 or ES1)	Second inhibitory period (SP2 or ES2)
Median	12	45
Mean	11.8	45.1
SD	0.8	5.2
Range	10–13.6	38–60
20-year old subjects*	11.1	42
70-year old subjects*	12.3	48

*standard curve calculations for age-latency (from Cruccu and Deuschl 2000)

atively narrow range of variability, thus allowing comparisons between subjects. The intraindividual latency difference between sides is small (range 0–1.2 ms, mean 0.3 ms ± [SD] 0.37 ms in 100 normal subjects). A latency difference between sides larger than 1.2 ms is abnormal. The second inhibitory period is considered abnormal if it is absent unilaterally or the latency difference between sides exceeds 8 ms. The second inhibitory period may be absent bilaterally in elderly patients or in patients with malocclusion (Cruccu et al. 1997).

Clinical Applications

Brainstem inhibitory reflexes cannot be tested by clinical procedures alone. In some patients, clinical examination discloses no signs of trigeminal impairment, yet testing the masseter inhibitory reflex reveals trigeminal or brainstem dysfunction. As in ► blink reflex studies, the pattern of abnormality (afferent, mixed or efferent) provides information on the site of the lesion (Cruccu et al. 2005; Ongerboer de Visser et al. 1990). Nevertheless, except in rare conditions such as a purely motor trigeminal neuropathy and hemimasticatory spasm, the "efferent" type of abnormality (abnormal responses confined to the muscle on one side, regardless of the side of stimulation) is extremely uncommon.

The two inhibitory periods of the masseter inhibitory reflex have distinct EMG features and clinical applications. The first inhibitory period appears to be insensitive to peripheral conditioning and suprasegmental modulation, its latency varies little and it is probably mediated by a small number of afferents. For these reasons it is the best available response for assessing function of the maxillary and mandibular afferents in focal and in generalized diseases. In patients with symptomatic ► trigeminal neuralgia or focal lesions within the pons, it has a diagnostic sensitivity similar to that of the R1 blink reflex (Cruccu and Deuschl 2000; Cruccu et al. 2005). The second inhibitory period is far less sensitive than the first to lesions along the reflex arc. Being mediated by a multisynaptic chain of interneurons of the lateral reticular formation however, it is modulated by suprasegmental influences. Like the R2 blink reflex, the second inhibitory period shows a strongly enhanced recovery cycle in patients with extrapyramidal disorders and an increased habituation in hemiplegia (Cruccu and Deuschl 2000). The second inhibitory period (recorded from the temporalis muscle and called ES2) is a focus of research in several centers for patients with headache. Although the findings are still controversial, some data suggest that this response might help in differentiating tension-type headache from vasomotor headaches (Schoenen et al. 1987).

Unlike the electrically elicited masseter inhibitory reflex (Cruccu et al. 1997), the laser silent period, a purely nociceptive reflex, has been demonstrated to undergo modulation by experimental pain and found to be absent in patients with ► temporo-mandibular pain (Romaniello et al. 2002, 2003).

References

1. Cruccu G, Deuschl G (2000) The clinical use of brainstem reflexes and hand-muscle reflexes. Clin Neurophysiol 111:371–387
2. Cruccu G, Frisardi G, Pauletti G et al. (1997) Excitability of the central masticatory pathways in patients with painful temporomandibular disorders. Pain 73:447–454
3. Cruccu G, Iannetti GD, Marx JJ et al. (2005) Brainstem reflex circuits revisited. Brain 128:386–394
4. Ellrich J, Hopf HC, Treede RD (1997) Nociceptive masseter inhibitory reflexes evoked by laser radiant heat and electrical stimuli. Brain Res 764:214–220
5. Godaux E, Desmedt JE (1975) Exteroceptive suppression and motor control of the masseter and temporalis muscles in normal man. Brain Res 85: 447–458
6. Miles TS, Turker KS (1987) Reflex responses of motor units in human masseter muscle to electrical stimulation of the lip. Exp Brain Res 65: 331–336
7. Ongerboer de Visser BW, Cruccu G, Manfredi M et al. (1990) Effects of brainstem lesions on the masseter inhibitory reflex. Functional mechanisms of reflex pathways. Brain 113:781–792
8. Romaniello A, Arendt-Nielsen L, Cruccu G et al. (2002) Modulation of trigeminal laser evoked potentials and laser silent periods by homotopical experimental pain. Pain 98:217–228
9. Romaniello A, Cruccu G, Frisardi G et al. (2003) Assessment of nociceptive trigeminal pathways by laser-evoked potentials and laser silent periods in patients with painful temporomandibular disorders. Pain 103:31–39
10. Schoenen J, Jamart B, Gerard P et al. (1987) Exteroceptive suppression of temporalis muscle activity in chronic headache. Neurology 37:1834–1836

J

Job Analysis

Definition

Job analysis includes description of work tasks; methods, techniques or processes involved and the work devices used, results; worker (skills, knowledge, adaptations needed). Job analysis may expose environmental and organizational factors needed to accomplish the work tasks. The Revised Handbook of Analyzing Jobs (RHAJ) explores the procedures and techniques used to analyze jobs and to record the analyses. Such analyses underlie, and are congruent with, the occupational definitions of the Dictionary of Occupational Titles (DOT. A job analysis according to R/HAJ) addresses the worker's relationship to data, people, and things (i.e. Worker Functions), the methodologies and techniques employed (i.e. Work Fields), the machines, tools, equipment, and work aids used (MTEWA), the material, procedures, subject matter, or services (MPSMS), and what worker attributes contribute to successful job performance (Worker Characteristics).

► Vocational Counselling

Job Capacity Evaluation

► Disability, Functional Capacity Evaluations

Job Demands

Definition

Job demands are the mental and physical requirements necessary to fulfill requirements associated with specific jobs.

▶ Pain in the Workplace, Risk Factors for Chronicity, Workplace Factors

Job Requirements

Definition

Job requirements are the demands an occupation or job tasks place on a worker for expected quality and quantity standard. The Dictionary of Occupational Titles (DOT) defines more than 20 000 occupations in the Labor Market in standards of Worker Functions; Work Fields, MPSMS, and Worker Characteristics.

▶ Vocational Counselling

Job Satisfaction

Definition

A measure of how happy or pleased someone is with different aspects of the work environment or the occupation as a whole.

▶ Pain in the Workplace, Risk factors for Chronicity, Job Demands

Job Site Evaluation

▶ Situational Assessment

Joint Deformities

Definition

Joint deformities are changes from the typical size or shape of a particular joint.

▶ Chronic Pain in Children, Physical Medicine and Rehabilitation

Joint Nociceptors

▶ Articular Nociceptors

JRA

▶ Juvenile Rheumatoid Arthritis

Junctional DREZ Coagulation

▶ DREZ Procedures

Just-Noticeable-Difference

Definition

On a stimulus continuum a, what is the smallest increment? (a) such that a+?(a) just noticeably exceeds a? This minimum increment of stimulus intensity is usually called the 'just-noticeable-difference' (JND or 'difference threshold' or 'difference limen').

▶ Pain Evaluation, Psychophysical Methods

Juvenile Rheumatoid Arthritis

Synonyms

JRA

Definition

Is a condition characterized by joint inflammation and stiffness for more than 6 weeks in children 16 years or younger. The inflammation causes redness, swelling, warmth, and soreness in the joints. Any joint can be affected and inflammation may limit the mobility of affected joints. JRA is a disease of the immune system. In JRA, the immune system attacks the body's own healthy cells, which causes inflammation in the lining and connective tissues of the joints.

▶ Experimental Pain in Children

Juxtaglomerular Apparatus

Definition

The functional entity in the kidney that consists of juxtaglomerular cells (epithelioid cells in the media of the afferent arterioles) and the macula densa (tubular epithelium at the region of afferent arteriole and efferent arteriole to the glomerulus), and is involved in the regulation of salt and water excretion and renal blood flow.

▶ NSAIDs, Adverse Effects

K/C Arthritis

▶ Arthritis Model, Kaolin-Carrageenan Induced Arthritis (Knee)

K⁺ Channel

Definition

K⁺ channel is a voltage-dependent permeation pathway for potassium ions.
▶ Ion Channel
▶ Ionotropic Receptor
▶ Trafficking and Localization of Ion Channels

Kainate-Induced Lesion

Definition

Neuronal death due to injection of the excitotoxin Kainate.
▶ Lateral Thalamic Lesions, Pain Behavior in Animals

Kainate Receptor

Definition

A type of ionotropic glutamate receptor that is activated by the agonist kainate. However, it should be noted that kainate will also activate other glutamate receptors, and thus should not be regarded as a specific agonist. Kainate receptors comprise of several subunits (GluR5, GluR6, GluR7, KA1, KA2) that form a heteromeric receptor-ion-channel complex.
▶ Nociceptive Neurotransmission in the Thalamus

Kaolin

Definition

Hydrated aluminium silicate.
▶ Amygdala, Pain Processing and Behavior in Animals
▶ Arthritis Model, Kaolin-Carrageenan Induced Arthritis (Knee)

Kaolin-Carrageenan Induced Arthritis

Definition

Animal model of inflammatory pain arising from the knee joint, mimicking osteoarthritis in humans.
▶ Arthritis Model, Kaolin-Carrageenan Induced Arthritis (Knee)
▶ Nociceptive Processing in the Amygdala, Neurophysiology and Neuropharmacology

Kapanoll

Definition

Kapanol is a formulation of morphine prepared as polymer coated sustained release pellets contained in a capsule.
▶ Post-Operative Pain, Morphine

Kappa(κ) Opiate/Opioid Receptors

Synonyms

KOP

Definition

One of three major opiate receptors that have been cloned (delta and mu receptors are the other two). The predominant kappa receptor is kappa₁, which has dynorphin A as the endogenous ligand. Several other kappa receptor classes have been defined. Also known as OP2 receptors, they are found in cerebral cortex,

amygdala, hippocampus, thalamus, hypothalamus, mesencephalon, pons, medulla and spinal cord. They are associated with analgesia, sedation, dysphoria and miosis.
▶ Opiates During Development
▶ Opioids, Kappa Receptors and Visceral Pain
▶ Opioid Receptors
▶ Pain Modulatory Systems, History of Discovery
▶ Postoperative Pain, Transition from Parenteral to Oral

Keratinocytes

Definition

Keratinocytes are cells in skin that secrete keratin as well as neurotrophins. Basal keratinocytes release NGF, whereas suprabasal keratinocytes release NT-3.
▶ Nerve Growth Factor, Sensitizing Action on Nociceptors

Ketalar

▶ Postoperative Pain, Ketamine

Ketamine

▶ Postoperative Pain, Ketamine

Kidney Stone Pain

▶ Visceral Pain Model, Kidney Stone Pain

Kinesiophobia

Definition

Kinesiophobia is an excessive, irrational, and debilitating fear of physical movement and activity resulting from a feeling of vulnerability to painful injury or (re)injury.
▶ Disability, Fear of Movement
▶ Fear and Pain
▶ Hypervigilance and Attention to Pain
▶ Muscle Pain, Fear-Avoidance Model

Kinesthesia

Definition

Conscious information about body position and movement.
▶ Postsynaptic Dorsal Column Neurons, Responses to Visceral Input

Knee Joint Nociceptors

▶ Nociceptor Generator Potential

Knockout Mice

Definition

Mice in which a portion of a specified gene is disrupted or removed, eliminating the corresponding protein.
▶ Opioid Receptors

KOP Receptor

Definition

The term κ-opioid peptide receptor represents the G-protein coupled receptor that responds selectively to a group of largely experimental opioid drugs. It is expressed in areas of the nervous system that moderately mediate analgesia, with a side-effect profile distinct from μ-opioids. The KOP receptor protein is produced by a single gene. When activated, the KOP receptor predominantly transduces cellular actions via inhibitory G-proteins. The electrophysiological consequences of KOP receptor activation are usually inhibitory.
▶ Kappa(κ) Opiate/Opioid Receptors
▶ Opioid Electrophysiology in PAG

KOR–1

Definition

KOR–1is a clone encoding a kappa$_1$ opioid receptor.
▶ Opioid Receptors

Kyphotic

Definition

Characteristic of or suffering from kyphosis, an abnormality of the vertebral column.
▶ Lower Back Pain, Physical Examination

La Belle Indifference

Definition

Individuals with a health condition or pain problem who seem to appear unconcerned about the nature or implications of their condition. For children with certain complex pain conditions, either children or their parents may exhibit „la belle indifference". In some cases, children may be unable to walk during the physical examination but parents are totally unaffected.

▶ Chronic Daily Headache in Children

Labor Pain

▶ Gynecological Pain, Neural Mechanisms
▶ Obstetric Pain

Labor Pain Model

▶ Visceral Pain Models, Female Reproductive Organ Pain

Laboratory Findings

Definition

Anatomical, physiological, or psychological phenomena that can be shown by the use of medically acceptable laboratory diagnostic techniques. Some of these diagnostic techniques include chemical tests, electrophysiological studies (electrocardiogram, electroencephalogram, etc.), medically acceptable imaging tests (X-rays, CAT scans, etc.), and psychological tests.

▶ Disability Evaluation in the Social Security Administration

Laboratory Pain

▶ Experimental Pain in Children

Lacrimation

Definition

Lacrimation is the tearing of an eye. During acute bouts of cluster headache and during exacerbations of hemicrania continua, the eye on the side of the pain often tears.

▶ Hemicrania Continua

Laminae I and V Neurones

Definition

Lamina I and V Neurones are neurones located in the superficial dorsal horn and deeper layers, respectively. Also known as the marginal layer of Waldeyer, Lamina 1 is the most superficial lamina of the dorsal horn in Rexed's classification. It is a very thin layer of small neurons that often send long distance ascending projections to the brain. Numerous are nociceptive (often nociceptive specific), with a smaller number being thermoreceptive or sensitive to itch inducing stimuli.

▶ Nociceptor, Categorization
▶ Opioids in the Spinal Cord and Central Sensitization
▶ Parabrachial Hypothalamic and Amydaloid Projections
▶ Spinomesencephalic Tract
▶ Spinothalamocortical Projections from SM
▶ Thalamic Nuclei Involved in Pain, Cat and Rat

Laminae II$_{outer}$ and Lamina II$_{inner}$

Definition

The spinal cord in cross section has been divided into areas based on morphological characteristics (Rexed 1952). Laminae I and II comprise of the most superficial aspect of the dorsal horn of the gray matter, and are known to receive the central terminal projections of many unmyelinated (C-fiber) and thinly-myelinated (Aδ-fiber) nociceptors. Lamina II is also known as the "substantia gelatinosa." The inner aspect of Lamina II receives the projections of many IB4-positive unmyelinated neurons. The outer aspect of Lamina II and Lamina I receive the terminals of many peptidergic unmyelinated neurons.

▶ IB4-Positive Neurons, Role in Inflammatory Pain
▶ Immunocytochemistry of Nociceptors
▶ Morphology, Intraspinal Organization of Visceral Afferents
▶ Nociceptor, Categorization

References

1. Rexed B (1952) The Cytoarchitectonic Organization of the Spinal Cord in the Rat. J. Comp. Neurol. 96: 415-466

Lamina Propria

Definition

A thin vascular layer of connective tissue beneath the epithelium of an organ.

▶ Animal Models of Inflammatory Bowel Disease

Laminae I/II Inputs to the Thalamus

▶ Spinothalamic Terminations, Core and Matrix

Laminae IV-IV, X

Definition

The basal parts of the dorsal horn and the area around the central canal of the spinal cord, respectively. These areas correspond with the nucleus proprius and central gray of the spinal cord.

▶ Morphology, Intraspinal Organization of Visceral Afferents

Laminectomy

Definition

Laminectomy is the excision of the posterior arch of a vertebra.

▶ Chronic Back Pain and Spinal Instability

Lancinating Pain

▶ Pain Paroxysms

Langerhans Cells

Definition

Langerhans cells are dendritic cells in the epidermis. They have phagocytic properties and are responsible for antigen presentation in a variety of CD4-dependent immune responses. They are involved in the early stages of contact dermatitis, skin graft rejection or HIV–1 infection.

▶ Neuropeptide Release in the Skin

Laparoscopic Pain Mapping

▶ Chronic Pelvic Pain, Laparoscopic Pain Mapping

Laparoscopy

Definition

Laparoscopy is a diagnostic tool designed to visualize the peritoneal cavity and the structures within by means of a laparoscope, which is a miniature telescope.

▶ Dyspareunia and Vaginismus

Laparoscopy (for Pain) under Local Anesthesia

▶ Chronic Pelvic Pain, Laparoscopic Pain Mapping

Large Fibers

Definition

Large fibers is a collective term for large myelinated nerves, including motor nerves and the proprioceptive type of sensory nerves, also large-diameter nerves.

▶ Toxic Neuropathies

Large Fiber Neuropathy

Definition

Peripheral nerve disorders mainly affecting large myelinated nerves (large fibers).

▶ Toxic Neuropathies
▶ Ulceration, Prevention by Nerve Decompression

Location of cannula tips

Vehicle injection

Kainate injection

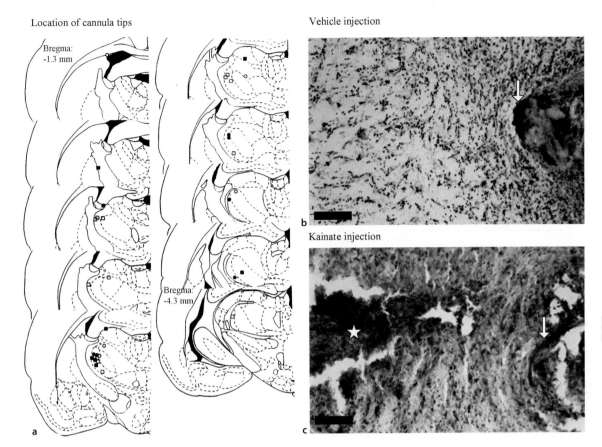

Lateral Thalamic Lesions, Pain Behavior in Animals, Figure 1 (a) Schematic representation of cannula tip locations for the Surgery (■), Vehicle injection (□), Kainate Miss (○) and Kainate Hit (·) groups based on plates from Paxinos and Watson (1986). (b) Photomicrograph of a subject that received vehicle injection within the region of the VPL. The arrow indicates the boundary of the cannula tip (dorsal aspect is right). (c) Photomicrograph of a subject that received kainate injection within the region of the VPL. The arrow indicates the boundary of the cannula tip and the star indicates the area of pronounced glial proliferation (dorsal aspect is right). All subjects included in the Kainate Hit group had cannula tip locations on target with the VPL and pronounced glial proliferation. Scale bar = 250 μM

the thalamotomy findings. First, the lateral thalamus is traditionally considered as a relay station, transmitting sensory input to the primary somatosensory cortex. Consequently, the initial expectation would be that a lesion of the VPL would result in contralateral loss of processing of somatosensory input, possibly reflected as a decrease in nociceptive threshold (► analgesia). However, the observation of pain behavior following thalamotomy in rats is an outcome that is opposite to the expectations provided by the traditional concept of the thalamus. This outcome highlights the complex nature of the somatosensory pathways responsible for transmitting nociceptive signals. Second, the experimental results following thalamotomy in rats have not addressed specific hypotheses that have been proposed for ► central pain syndrome. It remains to be determined if thalamotomy pain behavior in animals is based on: 1) irritable focus created at the site of injury, 2) sympathetic dysfunction, 3) hypothalamic dysfunction, 4) deafferentated central sensory nuclei, 5) hyperactivity

of deafferentated nonspecific reticulothalamic pathways, and 6) deafferentation of cortical nociceptive pathways.

Thalamic stimulation has been used to relieve clinical pain syndromes (Duncan et al. 1998; Marchand et al. 2003; Mazars et al. 1975). Paradoxically, thalamic stimulation has also been reported to induce pain (Lenz et al. 1995), an effect that is most likely due to the location of the stimulating electrode. Moderate increases in the function of the VPL, such as that produced by electrical stimulation or by microinjection of physiological concentrations of excitatory neurotransmitters or reuptake inhibitors, may be a suitable means of treatment for ► central pain syndrome.

References

1. Dejerine J, Egger M (1903) Le Syndrome Douloureauz Thalamique. Rev Neurol 14:521–532
2. Duncan G, Kupers R, Marchand S et al . (1998) Stimulation of Human Thalamus for Pain Relief. J Neurophysiol 80:3326–3330

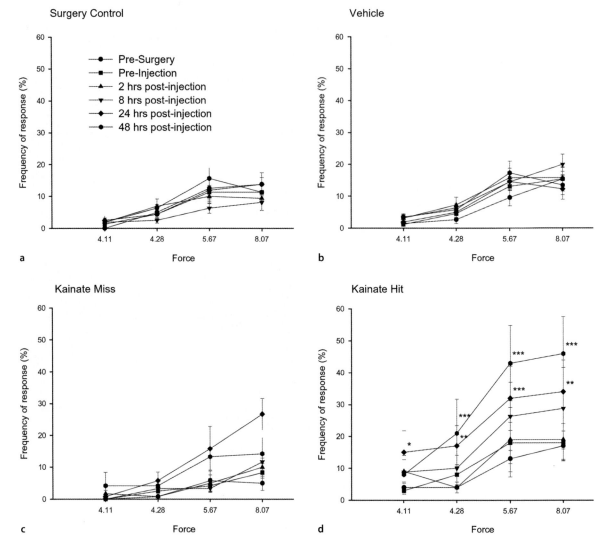

Lateral Thalamic Lesions, Pain Behavior in Animals, Figure 2   The symbol and line plots summarizes the effects of surgery alone (a), vehicle injection (b), injection of kainate confined to nuclei outside of the VPL (c) and injection of kainate localized to the VPL (d) on the mean percent of paw withdrawal response (± SEM) to punctate stimulation of the hindpaw. The responses to four intensities of punctate stimuli are shown at several time points including pre-surgery, pre-injection, 2, 8, 24 and 48 h post-injection. * = p < 0.05, ** = p < 0.01, *** = p < 0.001 compared to pre-surgery baseline

3. Fuchs PN, Lee JI, Lenz FA (2001) Central Pain Secondary to Intracranial Lesions. In: Burchiel KJ (ed) Pain Surgery. Thieme, New York
4. LaBuda CJ, Cutler TD, Dougherty PM et al. (2000) Mechanical and Thermal Hypersensitivity Develops following Kainite Lesion of the Ventral Posterior Lateral Thalamus in Rats. Neurosci Lett 290:79–83
5. Lenz FA, Gracely RH, Romanoski AJ et al. (1995) Stimulation in the Human Somatosensory Thalamus can Reproduce Both the Affective and Sensory Dimensions of Previously Experienced pain. Nature Med 1:910–913
6. Marchand S, Kupers RC, Bushnell MC et al. (2003) Analgesic and Placebo Effects of Thalamic Stimulation. Pain 105:481–488
7. Mazars GJ (1975) Intermittent Stimulation of Nucleus Ventralis Posterolateralis for Intractable Pain. Surg Neurol 4:93–95
8. Pagni CA (1976) Central Pain and Painful Anesthesia. Prog Neurol Surg 8:132– 257
9. Paxinos G, Watson C (1986) The Rat Brain in Stereotaxic Coordinates. Academic Press, New York
10. Saadé NE, Kafrouni AI, Saab CY et al. (1999) Chronic Thalamotomy Increases Pain-Related Behavior in Rats. Pain 83:401–409

Lateral Thalamic Nuclei

Definition

The lateral thalamic nuclei includes VPL, VPM and other secondary nuclei. Activation of these neurons by the spinothalamic tract is important for sensory discrimination.

▶ Lateral Thalamic Lesions, Pain Behavior in Animals
▶ Parafascicular Nucleus, Pain Modulation
▶ Spinothalamic Tract Neurons, Visceral Input

Lateral Thalamic Pain-Related Cells in Humans

ANDRES FERNANDEZ, SHINJI OHARA,
NIRIT WEISS, STAN ANDERSON, FRED A. LENZ
Departments of Neurosurgery, Johns Hopkins
University, Baltimore, MD, USA
Flenz1@jhmi.edu

Synonyms

Pain System; ventral posterior nucleus of thalamus; posterior nucleus; Thermoreception; mechanoreception

Definition

Neurons located in the human ▶ thalamus that respond selectively or differentially to painful stimuli.

Characteristics

Studies of patients at autopsy after lesions of the ▶ STT show that the human STT ascends to the thalamus medial to the medial geniculate (Mehler 1966) before terminating in the magnocellular medial geniculate, limitans and Vc portae nuclei, posterior to Vc (Mehler 1966). More anteriorly, the STT makes its most dense termination as irregular clusters in Vc (Mehler 1966). The STT terminations are concentrated in posterior inferior Vc and in dorsal Vc parvocellularis (Mehler 1966). Similarly, in monkeys, STT terminals occur as dense clusters in VPL (Boivie 1979; Apkarian and Hodge 1989). A more uniform, less dense termination is found in ventral posterior inferior - VPI (Apkarian and Hodge 1989), in the posterior nuclear group including posterior nucleus (Boivie 1979), pulvinar oralis, limitans, magnocellular medial geniculate, suprageniculate nuclei (Apkarian and Hodge 1989) and in the posterior division of the ventral medial nucleus (Blomqvist et al. 2000). Anatomic studies in patients following cordotomy demonstrate that nuclei where the STT terminates in humans are similar to those in monkeys (Mehler 1966). Finally, an area posterior, inferior and medial to monkey ventral posterior (▶ VP), corresponding to human Vc, is a proposed pain-related nucleus (ventral medial pars posterior - VMpo) (Blomqvist et al. 2000). Thus there is ample evidence of inputs from the STT to the region of Vc that could explain the occurrence of cellular responses to noxious and thermal stimuli.

Our physiological studies have demonstrated that cells in and posterior inferior to the human principal somatic sensory nucleus (ventral caudal – Vc) respond to painful mechanical stimuli (Lenz et al. 1994), painful heat stimuli (Lenz et al. 1993) and innocuous cool stimuli (Lenz and Dougherty 1998). The degree of convergence of thermal and mechanical modalities graded into the painful range has not previously been studied. Cells responding to both types of stimuli may explain both

the sensation of pain, i.e. hyperalgesia and allodynia, evoked by normally nonpainful stimuli (Fruhstorfer and Lindblom 1984) and the alleviation of pain by thermal stimuli. The responses of human thalamic cells to painful and nonpainful thermal and mechanical stimuli in patients undergoing thalamic procedures for the treatment of movement disorders were examined.

The largest study of human cells responding to both thermal and mechanical stimuli graded into the painful range explored these neuronal responses in the region of Vc of 24 patients undergoing surgery for treatment of movement disorders (Lee et al. 1999). Preoperative somatic sensory testing was carried out with a series of thermal and somatic stimuli into the painful range on all patients. Intraoperative testing was carried out on 57 cells in the region where cells responded to innocuous cutaneous somatic sensory stimuli. Thermal stimuli consisted of contact cold or heat from 6 to 51°C. The somatic series included stimulation with a camel hair brush and large, medium and small arterial clips. Preoperative somatic sensory testing established that both the mechanical and thermal series of stimuli spanned intensities extending into the painful range.

Of 57 cells tested, 15 had a graded response to mechanical stimuli extending into the painful range and thus were classified in the ▶ wide dynamic range (WDR) category. The mean stimulus-response function of cells in the WDR class, normalized to baseline, showed a four-fold mean increase in firing rate above baseline across the mechanical series of stimuli. Seven of these cells also responded to heat stimuli extending into the painful range (WDR-H) and 2 responded to cold stimuli (WDR-C). Twenty-five cells were in a class (multiple receptive – MR) that showed a response to both brush and compressive stimuli, although the responses were not graded into the painful range. Three of these cells (MR-H) had a response to heat stimuli and 5 cells responded to cold stimuli (MR-C). Nine cells responded to brushing without a response to the compressive stimuli (low threshold – LT). Although we have no direct anatomic evidence to confirm electrode location, the present results are consistent with monkey studies and suggest that cells differentially responsive to mechanical stimuli are located in Vc, Vcpc, Vcpor and anterior Po.

Brief stimuli spanning the range of the VAS (0–10) were used with preoperative training and intraoperative testing in the present study. This is unlike studies of awake monkeys where intense noxious stimuli were not used (Bushnell et al. 1993; Bushnell and Duncan 1987). The intense stimuli used in the present study may explain the large proportion of WDR cells in the region of Vc in this study. Another human study did not demonstrate WDR cells in the region of Vc (Tasker et al. 1997). The lack of such cells may be due to the stimuli used, although details of the methods have not been published for that study.

L

Microstimulation studies suggest that there is partitioning of thermal/pain sensations at different locations in the region of Vc. Stimulation sites where thermal/pain sensations are evoked are located near the posterior border of the core and within the posterior inferior region (Lenz et al. 1993). Microstimulation in the postero-inferior region evokes thermal sensations or pain often referred to large RFs and subcutaneous structures. Other reports identify sites where pain but not thermal sensations are evoked posterior and inferior to the core (Dostrovsky et al. 1991).

The largest study of micro-stimulation-evoked sensations in Vc reports explorations during stereotactic procedures for the treatment of tremor in 124 thalami and 116 patients. Core was defined as the area above the most inferior cell with a response to nonpainful cutaneous stimulation and anterior to the most posterior cell of this type. Warm sensations were evoked more frequently in the posterior region than in the core. The proportion of sites where microstimulation evoked cool and pain sensations did not differ between the core and the posterior region. In the posterior region, however, warm sensations were evoked more frequently in the lateral plane (10.8%) than in the medial planes (3.9%). No mediolateral difference was found for sites where pain and cool sensations were evoked. The presence of sites where stimulation evoked taste or where RFs and PFs were located on the pharynx were used as landmarks of a plane located as medial as VMpo. Microstimulation in this plane evoked cool, warm, and pain sensations. The results suggest that thermal and pain sensations are processed in the region of Vc as far medial as VMpo. Therefore, thermal and pain sensations seem to be mediated by neural elements in a region probably including the core of Vc, VMpo and other nuclei posterior and inferior to Vc.

Nociceptive neurons (see ▶ Human Thalamic Nociceptive Neurons) have been identified in the human medial thalamus. Ishijima et al found that one quarter (20/80) of the cells they recorded from the central medial/parafascicularis complex of man responded to noxious pinprick (Ishijima et al. 1975). None of these cells responded to non-noxious cutaneous stimuli. One group of cells responded to painful stimuli with long latency and showed prolonged after-discharges while others had a time course similar to the stimulus. Another study (Tsubokawa and Moriyasu 1975) also found a relatively large number of nociceptive neurons which they localized to the central medial nucleus. Neither of these reports has been confirmed by more recent studies of patients with neuropathic pain (Rinaldi et al. 1991). Instead cells with very high rates of spontaneous bursting discharge activity were reported in the more recent studies.

Studies of nociceptive responsive cells in humans are consistent with the results reported in awake and anesthetized monkeys. In a study of responses of cells in VPM of awake monkeys to graded mechanical stimuli (Bushnell and Duncan 1987), 10% of cells (9/89) are classified as WDR. These cells were clustered in ventral VPM. Another study reports 22 thermal responsive cells from a population of hundreds recorded in alert, trained, *Cynomologous* monkeys (Bushnell et al. 1993). Eighteen percent (4/22) of these cells responded to noxious heat only. No such cells were found in the present analysis, perhaps because of the search stimuli used. Among cells with a WDR mechanical response pattern, those that also responded to heat stimuli graded into the noxious range comprised 27% of cells (6/22) in that series.

Cells in VP, VPI and Po of anesthetized monkeys can respond to innocuous stimuli (Apkarian and Shi 1994). In a recent study forty cells responded to noxious mechanical stimuli; of these 23 cells also responded to noxious heat and 9 responded to noxious cold. These cells were located in VPI and Po more commonly than in VP. Studies in awake squirrel monkeys have found that 8% (3/36) to 12% (9/76) of cells in VP responded to noxious mechanical stimuli (Casey and Morrow, 1983). These cells were widely distributed throughout VP. In another study, a smaller number of WDR and HT cells were found throughout VP in anesthetized rhesus monkeys (73 cells/thousands of cells) (Chandler et al. 1992). Overall, monkey studies suggest that cells responsive to innocuous and noxious inputs are located in VP, VPI and Po. Cells responding to cold stimuli have tentatively been located in the region proposed to correspond to human VMpo (Davis et al. 1999). Although we have no direct anatomic evidence, the present results are consistent with monkey studies and suggest that cells responsive to painful mechanical stimuli are located in Vc, Vcpc, Vcpor and Po.

Blockade of the activity of these cells by thalamic injection of local anesthetic significantly interferes with the monkey's ability to discriminate temperature in both the innocuous and noxious range (Duncan et al. 1993). These studies establish that cells in the region of the monkey principal somatic sensory nucleus are involved in pathways signaling cutaneous thermal sensations into the noxious range. Therefore, the region of Vc is a pain-signaling pathway, as demonstrated by the presence of afferent connections from the STT, of cells responding to noxious stimuli, of sites where stimulation evokes pain and of sites where lesions relieve pain (Duncan et al. 1993). This is strong evidence for a role of Vc and adjacent nuclei in the human pain system.

References

1. Apkarian AV, Hodge CJ (1989) Primate spinothalamic pathways: III. Thalamic terminations of the dorsolateral and ventral spinothalamic pathways. J Comp Neurol 288:493–511
2. Apkarian AV, Shi T (1994) Squirrel monkey lateral thalamus. I. Somatic nociresponsive neurons and their relation to spinothalamic terminals. J Neurosci 14:6779–6795

3. Blomqvist A, Zhang ET, Craig AD (2000) Cytoarchitectonic and immunohistochemical characterization of a specific pain and temperature relay, the posterior portion of the ventral medial nucleus, in the human thalamus. Brain 123:601–619
4. Boivie J (1979) An anatomic reinvestigation of the termination of the spinothalamic tract in the monkey. J Comp Neurol 186:343–369
5. Bushnell MC, Duncan GH (1987) Mechanical response properties of ventroposterior medial thalamic neurons in the alert monkey. Exp Brain Res 67:603–614
6. Bushnell MC, Duncan GH, Tremblay N (1993) Thalamic VPM nucleus in the behaving monkey. I. Multimodal and discriminative properties of thermosensitive neurons. J Neurophysiol 69:739–752
7. Casey KL, Morrow TJ (1983) Ventral posterior thalamic neurons differentially responsive to noxious stimulation of the awake monkey. Science 221:675–677
8. Chandler MJ, Hobbs SF, Fu Q-G et al. (1992) Responses of neurons in ventroposterolateral nucleus of primate thalamus to urinary bladder distension. Brain Res 571:26–34
9. Davis KD, Lozano AM, Manduch M et al (1999) Thalamic relay site for cold perception in humans. J Neurophysiol 81:1970–1973
10. Dostrovsky JO, Wells FEB, Tasker RR (1991) Pain evoked by stimulation in human thalamus. In: Sjigenaga Y (ed) International symposium on processing nociceptive information. Elsevier, Amsterdam, pp 115–120
11. Duncan GH, Bushnell MC, Oliveras JL et al. (1993) Thalamic VPM nucleus in the behaving monkey. III. Effects of reversible inactivation by lidocaine on thermal and mechanical discrimination. J Neurophysiol. 70:2086–2096
12. Fruhstorfer H, Lindblom U (1984) Sensibility abnormalities in neuralgic patients studied by thermal and tactile pulse stimulation. In: von Euler C (ed) Somatosensory mechanisms. MacMillian, London, pp 353–361
13. Ishijima B, Yoshimasu N, Fukushima T et al. (1975) Nociceptive neurons in the human thalamus. Confin Neurol 37:99–106
14. Lee J-I, Antezanna D, Dougherty PM et al. (1999) Responses of neurons in the region of the thalamic somatosensory nucleus to mechanical and thermal stimuli graded into the painful range. J Comp Neurol 410:541–555
15. Lenz FA, Dougherty PM (1998) Cells in the human principal thalamic sensory nucleus (Ventralis Caudalis -Vc) respond to innocuous mechanical and cool stimuli. J Neurophysiol 79:2227–2230
16. Lenz FA, Gracely RH, Rowland LH et al. (1994) A population of cells in the human thalamic principal sensory nucleus respond to painful mechanical stimuli. Neurosci Lett 180:46–50
17. Lenz FA, Seike M, Richardson RT et al. (1993) Thermal and pain sensations evoked by microstimulation in the area of human ventrocaudal nucleus. J Neurophysiol 70:200–212
18. Mehler WR (1966) The Posterior Thalamic Region in Man. Confin Neurol 27:18–29
19. Rinaldi PC, Young RF, Albe-Fessard DG et al. (1991) Spontaneous neuronal hyperactivity in the medial and intralaminar thalamic nuclei in patients with deafferentation pain. J Neurosurg 74:415–421
20. Tasker RR, Davis KD, Hutchinson WD et al. (1997) Subcortical and thalamic mapping in functional neurosurgery. In: Gildenberg PL, Tasker RR (eds) Stereotactic and Functional Neurosurgery. McGraw-Hill, New York, pp 883–923
21. Tsubokawa T, Moriyasu N (1975) Follow-up results of centre median thalamotomy for relief of intractable pain. A method of evaluating the effectiveness during operation. Confin Neurol 37:280–284

Laughing Gas

▶ Nitrous Oxide Antinociception and Opioid Receptors

Law of Bell and Magendie

Definition

The ventral root contains motor fibers and the dorsal root contains sensory fibers.

▶ Dorsal Root Ganglionectomy and Dorsal Rhizotomy

LCN

▶ Lateral Cervical Nucleus

Learned Helplessness

Definition

Experimental paradigm where animals learn to stop attempting to escape inescapable shock.

▶ Pain Modulatory Systems, History of Discovery

LEF

▶ Laser Evoked Field

Lemington 5 Element Acupuncture

▶ Acupuncture

Lemnicus Trigeminalis

▶ Trigeminothalamic Tract Projections

Lemniscal Fibers

Definition

A band or bundle of ascending fibers from the secondary sensory nuclei to the ventral posterior part of the opposite thalamus. Lemniscal fibers conveying sensory discriminative component of pain information.

▶ Trigeminothalamic Tract Projections

LEP

▶ Laser-Evoked Potential

Lepromatous Leprosy

Definition

Lepromatous leprosy is the most malignant and infectious type of leprosy. It is characterized by widespread dissemination of leprosy bacilli in the tissues due to poor immune response to infection. Clinical features include widespread, symmetrical and innumerable macules, which may progress to form nodules and infiltrations. The manifestations of nerve damage appear slowly.
▶ Hansen's Disease

Leprosy

Definition

Also called Hansen's disease. It is a slowly progressive, chronic infectious disease caused by *Mycobacterium leprae*. It is characterized by granulomatous or neurotrophic lesions in the skin, nerves and viscera.
▶ Hansen's Disease

Leprosy Reaction

Definition

An acute or subacute hypersensitivity state occurring during the course of anti-leprosy treatment or in untreated leprosy. They are divided into two types: type 1 reaction and type 2 reaction.
▶ Hansen's Disease

Leptomeninges

Definition

A collective name for the arachnoid and pia mater membranes, the two innermost layers of the meninges, and between which the cerebrospinal fluid circulates.
▶ Diencephalic Mast Cells

Leptomeningitis

Definition

Inflammation of the leptomeninges (pia mater and arachnoid).
▶ Viral Neuropathies

Lesion

Definition

Selective controlled destruction of a structure within the brain.
▶ Pain Treatment, Intracranial Ablative Procedures

Leucoencephalopathy

Definition

Reversible posterior leucoencephalopathy is an MRI appearance seen in hypertensive encephalopathy, and consists of T2-weighted and FLAIR changes in the cerebral and brainstem white matter, most prominent in the distribution of the vertebrobasilar circulation.
▶ Headache Due to Hypertension

Leukocytes

Definition

White blood cells that are important in the induction of the immune response and host defense.
▶ Cytokines, Effects on Nociceptors

Leukotrienes

Definition

Leukotrienes are hormone-like, lipid-soluble regulatory molecules constructed from arachidonic acid by lipoxygenases. They participate in the regulation of diverse body functions such as bronchial constriction and allergic reactions.
▶ NSAIDs, Adverse Effects

Leukotrienes in Inflammatory Nociceptor Sensitisation

▶ Inflammatory Nociceptor Sensitisation, Prostaglandins and Leukotrienes

Levator Ani Syndrome

Definition

A myofascial pain syndrome with painful, more or less permanent, spasms of the puborectal and levator ani muscles.
▶ Pudendal Neuralgia in Women

Level of the Measurement Scale

Definition

Nominal scale: An arrangement of values of a categorical variable that has no meaningful order (such as hair color or occupation).
Ordinal scale: An order that can be imposed on the values of a variable in a subject, where the order ranges from the highest value (such as "very interested") to the lowest value (such as "not at all interested").
Interval scale: An interval scale allows for the classification and labeling of elements or objects into categories based on defined features that are numerically ranked or otherwise ordered with respect to one another. In addition, equal differences between numbers reflect equal magnitude differences between the corresponding categories. Thus, this scale has nominal and ordinal properties and in addition it incorporates a zero, but this zero value is not absolute (lacks true meaning). The lack of an absolute zero means that this scale cannot be used to calculate the ratio of two values (cannot say – one level is twice as „painful" as another level). A common example of an interval scale is the (continuous) scale of a thermometer.
Ratio scale: The ordering of numeric values when zero is meaningful (such as money or weight). Ratio scales incorporate the properties of the 3 other scales; and because they make use of a meaningful 0, their values can be interpreted to mean a true difference between numbers, and the numbers reflect true ratios of magnitude.
▶ Pain Assessment in Neonates
▶ Pain Measurement by Questionnaires, Psychophysical Procedures and Multivariate Analysis

LFP

▶ Local Field Potential

Liberation

Definition

The liberation of a drug describes its release from the pharmaceutical product.
▶ NSAIDs, Pharmacokinetics

Libido

Definition

Libido, the desire for sexual intimacy, may be altered by emotional, metabolic, and physiologic phenomenon, as well as by many medications.

▶ Cancer Pain Management, Opioid Side Effects, Endocrine Changes and Sexual Dysfunction

Lichen Sclerosis

Definition

Lichen sclerosis is a painful skin condition generally affecting the vulva (or penis) and anus. It is characterized by thinning and white patches of skin, itching and/or burning, painful sexual intercourse, and sores or lesions resulting from scratching. If left untreated, it can result in fusing of the skin, atrophy, and narrowing of the vagina.
▶ Clitoral Pain
▶ Dyspareunia and Vaginismus

Lidocaine

▶ Postoperative Pain, Lignocaine

Lifetime Prevalence

Definition

Lifetime prevalence is the total number of persons known to have had the disease or attribute for at least part of their life
▶ Prevalence of Chronic Pain Disorders in Children

Ligands

Definition

Chemicals that have an affinity for a receptor.
▶ Alternative Medicine in Neuropathic Pain

Lightning Pain

▶ Pain Paroxysms

Lignocaine

▶ Post-Operative Pain, Lignocaine

Likert Scale

Definition

A Likert scale presents a set of attitude statements and asks respondents to express agreement or disagreement on a numerical scale. Each degree of agreement is given a numerical value. Thus, a total numerical value can be calculated from all the responses.

▶ Pain Inventories

Limb Amputation

Definition

Limb amputation (removal of a limb) may be caused by surgery or trauma. In Western countries, limb amputation is most often performed because of medical disease. Many amputees experience phenomena as phantom pain, phantom sensation and stump pain.

▶ Postoperative Pain, Postamputation Pain, Treatment and Prevention

Limbic Forebrain Matrix

▶ Thalamo-Amygdala Interactions and Pain

Limbic Forebrain/System

Definition

The Limbic Forebrain/System is a set of structures deep in the brain, including the amygdala, hypothalamus and the parahippocampal and cingulate gyri, which are commonly grouped together as the limbic system. At the cortical level, it also includes the insular cortex and the cingulate cortex. These areas are phylogenetically older than the surrounding neocortex. The amygdala and the hippocampus form the central axis of the limbic system. The limbic structures are involved in the processing of emotion and motivation and are critical for normal human functioning.

▶ Amygdala, Functional Imaging
▶ Arthritis Model, Kaolin-Carrageenan Induced Arthritis (Knee)
▶ Cingulate Cortex, Functional Imaging
▶ Hippocampus and Entorhinal Complex, Functional Imaging
▶ Nociceptive Processing in the Cingulate Cortex, Behavioral Studies in Humans
▶ Pain Treatment, Intracranial Ablative Procedures
▶ Thalamo-Amygdala Interactions and Pain

Linkage Disequilibrium

Definition

Linkage disequilibrium is the condition in which the number of closely linked loci on a chromosome (haplotype frequencies) in a population, deviate from the values they would have if the genes at each locus were combined at random.

▶ NSAIDs, Pharmacogenetics

Lipophilic

Definition

Chemically lipophilic or hydrophobic species are electrically neutral and nonpolar, and thus prefer other neutral and nonpolar solvents or molecular environments such as lipids.

▶ Rest and Movement Pain

Lissauer's Tract

Definition

Lissauer's tract is a pathway formed from the proximal end of small unmyelinated and poorly myelinated fibers in peripheral nerves, which enter at the lateral aspect of the dorsal horn and ascend and descend up to four segments, and terminate in Rexeds laminae I through to VI (principally I, II, and V) of the ipsilateral dorsal horn.

▶ Acute Pain Mechanisms
▶ DREZ Procedures
▶ Somatic Pain

List of Diagnoses and their Definitions

▶ Taxonomy

LLLT

▶ Laser

Load

Definition

The total load imposed on a structure, consisting of the whole of stressors seeking to disrupt the initial integrity of the structure. Load is determined by various factors such as strength, repetitiveness, etc.

▶ Ergonomic Counseling

Load-Bearing Capacity

Definition

The capacity of the structure to resist the destructive, negative impact of loading. Structures with a high load-bearing capacity can resist more load before damage occurs than structures with a low load-bearing capacity.

▶ Ergonomic Counseling

Local Anaesthetics

MARK JOHNSON, NIKOLAI BOGDUK
Musculoskeletal Physician, Hibiscus Coast Highway, Orewa, New Zealand
markjohn@ihug.co.nz, nik.bogduk@newcastle.edu.au

Synonyms

"Local"

Definition

Local anaesthetics are drugs with the unique property of being able to block conduction along peripheral nerves.

Characteristics

Local anaesthetics are perhaps the most powerful and most valuable drug used in Pain Medicine. They are the only ones known to be able to stop pain completely. Their effect, however, is not lasting. They exert only a temporary effect, measured in hours. Their application, therefore, is limited to diagnostic tests.

Chemistry

Local anaesthetics are drugs formed by aromatic and amino residues linked by either an amide or an ester (Fig. 1). The agents most commonly used in Pain Medicine are lignocaine and bupivacaine from amongst the amides, and procaine from the esters. The differences in chemistry underlie the differences in duration of action and metabolism of these drugs.

Mechanisms

Local anaesthetics act on sodium channels in nerve membranes to prevent or impede sodium flux, but their binding and duration of action depends on whether the channels are resting, open, closed, or inactivated (Butterworth and Strichartz 1990; Strichartz 1988). In turn, these states of the channels depend on whether the membrane is being depolarised and the frequency of depolarisation. In nerves that are actively conducting, local anaesthetics have a greater affinity for the channel than they have in resting nerves.

This difference in affinity underlies certain quantitative properties of local anaesthetics that pertain to the interpretation of diagnostic blocks. The duration of action of local anaesthetics has been determined by observation in subjects who were not experiencing ongoing or chronic pain. What was tested was cutaneous anaesthesia in patients undergoing minor operative procedures or during childbirth. Accurate figures are difficult to ascertain because some investigators added adrenaline to the local anaesthetic, whereas others did not. Nevertheless, representative figures for lignocaine would be mean duration of 2–4 h, with a standard deviation of 1–3 h (Moore et al. 1970a; Moore et al. 1970b; Rubin and Lawson 1968; Watt et al. 1968). A duration of up to 7 h is not unusual, and periods longer than 10 h have been reported (Watt

L

Local Anaesthetics, Figure 1 The structural formulae of three common local anaesthetics, illustrating how aromatic and amino residues are linked by either an amide or an ester.

et al. 1968). For bupivacaine, a mean duration of 4–8 h with a standard deviation of 2–3 h would be representative (Moore et al. 1970a; Moore et al. 1970b; Rubin and Lawson 1968; Watt et al. 1968). Periods of anaesthesia up to 12 h are not unusual.

These figures should be understood to apply to individuals about to experience pain. They may not, and do not necessarily, apply to patients with persistent or chronic pain. Indeed, patients with neuropathic pain often exhibit extraordinarily prolonged responses to lignocaine (Arner et al. 1990), probably because the agent is able to bind strongly and persistently to open and changing sodium channels. What the "normal" duration of action of local anaesthetics is in patients with chronic pain has not been determined.

Pharmacology

As local anaesthetics are weak bases, they have an affinity to hydrogen ions, but are subject to dissociation. The affinity and dissociation are described by the Henderson-Hassellbach equation. Different components of that equation govern the various pharmacological properties of local anaesthetics (Fig. 2).

The difference between the ambient pH and the equilibrium constant (Ka) determines the fraction of the local anaesthetic available in the base form. That form is the active form. Being more lipid soluble, it is the base form that penetrates cell membranes to get to the active site. The lipid solubility of the base form determines the potency of the agent. Its protein binding determines its duration of action.

Meanwhile, the acid form of the local anaesthetic is its soluble form. Local anaesthetic agents are prepared and stored in their soluble form. In order to permit storage in the soluble form, local anaesthetic agents are stored at a low pH (e.g. 4.0). For most agents the pKa is about 7.9. In a pH environment of 4.0, the difference between pH and pKa is 4.0–7.9 = –3.9. In which case, the fraction of the agent in the non-soluble form is $10^{-3.9}$, i.e. 1 in 10,000. That means that virtually all of the agent is in the soluble form.

When the agent is injected into tissues of pH 7.4, the difference between pH and pKa is 7.4–7.9 = –0.5. Under those conditions, the fraction of the active, insoluble form is $10^{-0.5}$, i.e. 31% is in the active form.

Metabolism

The amides and esters differ in how they are metabolized. Both are rapidly distributed through the blood stream, and pass to tissues of high vascularity (Fig. 3). The amides are metabolized by the liver, after which they are excreted by the kidneys. The esters are metabolized in the blood by plasma cholinesterase. The products are excreted by the kidneys.

Once absorbed into the bloodstream, all local anaesthetic agents reach the heart and the brain. At these sites they can exert their toxic effects.

Toxicity

At toxic concentrations, local anaesthetics can suppress electrical activity in the heart. In the central nervous system they suppress inhibitory neurons, which results in excitation of disinhibited systems. This is manifest clinically as fitting.

The toxic doses required to produce these effects, however, are considerably higher than the amounts used for most clinical purposes in Pain Medicine. For bupivacaine, the total body dose that is typically toxic is about 150 mg; for lignocaine the dose is 200 mg (Rosenberg et al. 2004).

Applications

In PainMedicine, local anaesthetics are used in three main ways. Most commonly they are used to perform di-

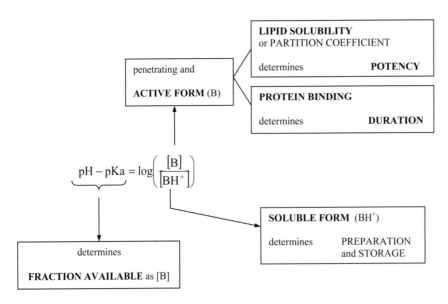

Local Anaesthetics, Figure 2 The relationship between the equilibrium equation of local anaesthetics and their pharmacological properties.

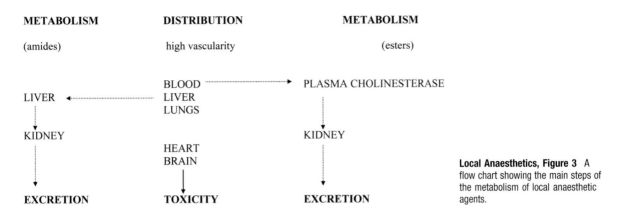

METABOLISM	DISTRIBUTION	METABOLISM
(amides)	high vascularity	(esters)

BLOOD ·······························▶ PLASMA CHOLINESTERASE
LIVER ◀·························· LIVER
LUNGS

KIDNEY   KIDNEY

HEART
BRAIN

EXCRETION   TOXICITY   EXCRETION

Local Anaesthetics, Figure 3 A flow chart showing the main steps of the metabolism of local anaesthetic agents.

agnostic blocks of peripheral nerves or of spinal nerves (See: Peripheral Nerve Blocks). These blocks are used to identify either the source of pain or the nerves that are mediating the pain (Bogduk 2002). Local anaesthetic agents can also be administered intravenously, for the diagnosis or treatment of neuropathic pain or central pain. Occasionally they are administered orally for the treatment of neuropathic pain.

References

1. Arner S, Lindblom U, Meyerson BA et al. (1990) Prolonged Relief of Neuralgia after Regional Anaesthetic Blocks. A Call for Further Experimental and Systematic Clinical Studies. Pain 43:287–297
2. Bogduk N (2002) Diagnostic Nerve Blocks in Chronic Pain. Best Pract Res Clin Anaesthesiol 16:565–578
3. Butterworth JF, Strichartz GR (1990) Molecular Mechanisms of Local Anesthesia: A Review. Anesthesiology 72:711–734
4. Moore DC, Bridenbaugh LD, Bridenbaugh PO et al. (1970a) Bupivacaine for Peripheral Nerve Block: A Comparison with Mepivacaine, Lidocaine, and Tetracaine. Anesthesiology 32:460–463
5. Moore DC, Bridenbaugh LD, Bridenbaugh PO et al. (1970b) Bupivacaine: A Review of 2,077 Cases. JAMA 214:713–718
6. Rosenberg PH, Veering BT, Urmey WF (2004) Maximum Recommended Doses of Local Anesthetics: A Multifactorial Concept. Reg Anesth Pain Med 29:564–575
7. Rubin AP, Lawson DIF (1968) A Controlled Trial of Bupivacaine: A Comparison with Lignocaine. Anaesthesia 23:327–331
8. Strichartz GR (1988) Neural Physiology and Local Anesthetic Action. In: Cousins MJ, Bridenbaugh PO (eds) Neural Blockade in Clinical Anesthesia and Management of Pain, 2nd edn. JB Lippincott, Philadelphia, pp 25–45
9. Watt MJ, Ross DM, Atkinson RS (1968) A Double Blind Trial of Bupivacaine and Lignocaine. Anaesthesia 23:331–337

Local Anesthetic Agents/Drugs

Definition

Local anesthetic agents are drugs that prevent excitable tissues from being excited, and are usually administered in the region of spinal structures or peripheral nerves. These drugs are used to allow procedures to be carried out painlessly, but are also used as an aid to determine

the diagnosis, prognosis or treatment of painful conditions.Local anesthetics are commonly used as part of spinal or epidural anesthesia.

▶ Analgesia During Labor and Delivery
▶ Cancer Pain Management, Anesthesiologic Interventions, Neural Blockade
▶ Local Anaesthetics
▶ Pain Treatment, Spinal Nerve Blocks
▶ Postoperative Pain, Local Anaesthetics

Local Anesthetic Motor Blockade

Definition

Skeletal muscles paralyzed by local anesthetic interruption of nerve impulses to muscle cells.

▶ Postoperative Pain, Acute Pain Team

Local Anesthetics/Antiarrhythmics

Definition

Local anesthetics/antiarrhythmics are sodium-channel modulators that depress the action potential and enhance repolarization of primary afferent neurones.

▶ Drugs Targeting Voltage-Gated Sodium and Calcium Channels

Local-Circuit Cells

Definition

Neurons in the brain are divided into two major groups, projection neurons and interneurons, local neurons, or local-circuit neurons.

▶ Trigeminal Brainstem Nuclear Complex, Anatomy

Local Circuit Interneuron

Definition

Neuron with axonal arborization located in the area occupied by its own dendritic tree.
▶ Spinothalamic Tract Neurons, Morphology

Local Field Potential

Synonyms

LFP

Definition

Synchronized extracellular currents of a few hundred cells generate a LFP that reflects the average input to individual neurons. The LFP can be recorded with a microelectrode with impedance up to 0.5 MΩ. The signal is analyzed for frequencies up to 100 Hz.
▶ Thalamotomy for Human Pain Relief

Local Twitch Response

Synonyms

LTR

Definition

A transient, poorly synchronized, prolonged twitch-like contraction of the group of taut band fibers that is associated with a myofascial trigger point, MTrP. The response is a polysynaptic spinal reflex with its afferent limb commonly arising from mechanical stimulation of sensitized nociceptors in the trigger point, and the efferent limb begins as an activation of alpha motor neurons that supply the involved nerve terminals of taut band fibers in the same or sometimes in functionally related muscles. It can be easily elicited when the needle tip encounters a sensitive locus in the MTrP region during high-pressure stimulation.
▶ Dry Needling
▶ Myofascial Trigger Points

Local-Twitch-Response Locus

▶ Sensitive Locus

Localized Muscle Pain

▶ Myofascial Pain

Locus Coeruleus

Definition

A noradrenergic nucleus that is located in the ponto-mesencephalic junction, and is involved in the regulation of vigilance and descending feedback control of pain. Many neurons in this region contain the neurotransmitter norepinephrine.
▶ Descending Modulation and Persistent Pain
▶ Vagal Input and Descending Modulation

Locus of Control

Definition

Beliefs about whether certain outcomes in life are a result of ones' efforts (internal) or a result of luck, fate, or the actions of others (external).
▶ Psychological Treatment of Headache

Longitudinal Myelotomy

▶ Midline Myelotomy

Longitudinal Study

Synonyms

Cohort study

Definition

A cohort study is an epidemiological method identifying a study population by age, or by using other means or traits of grouping individuals for the purpose of research (Timmreck, 2002).
▶ Pain in the Workplace, Risk factors for Chronicity, Job Demands
▶ Prevalence of Chronic Pain Disorders in Children

Long-Lasting Acute Pain

▶ Postoperative Pain, Acute-Recurrent Pain

Long-Term Depression in the Spinal Cord

▶ Long-Term Potentiation and Long-Term Depression in the Spinal Cord

Long-Term Effects of Pain in Infants

RUTH ECKSTEIN GRUNAU
Centre for Community Child Health Research, Child
and Family Research Institute and the University of
British Columbia, Vancouver, BC, Canada
rgrunau@cw.bc.ca

Synonyms

Infant Pain; long-term effects

Definition

Humans and non-human mammals are born with the
ability to display reflex responses to injury or noxious stimulation. Exposure to pain is generally rare
in the neonatal period. However, with the advent of
neonatal intensive care units (NICU), infants born very
prematurely or with serious medical complications
are exposed to repeated invasive procedures. Survival
of the tiniest infants, who are born at extremely low
gestational age (i.e. ≤ 28 weeks) and are thereby physiologically very immature, has increased significantly
in recent years. Medical intensive care of these infants
involves prolonged exposure to procedures that result in
▶ stress and ▶ pain at a time of very rapid brain development.

Characteristics

Tissue injury induces numerous behavioral, physiological and endocrine changes in neonates, which are consistent with pain responses in older children and adults
under similar circumstances. Long-term functional and
structural changes in ▶ nociception can occur, related to
pain in the neonatal period (Fitzgerald 2005). Moreover,
there is a growing body of evidence suggesting that cumulative neonatal pain and stress may contribute to long-
term alterations of pain systems, and perhaps to multiple
aspects of behavior and development in the most vulnerable infants (Anand 2000; Grunau 2002). A model
for conceptualizing long-term effects of pain in human
neonates has been proposed recently (Grunau 2002).

Neurobiology of Infant Pain

Pain perception is functional by mid-gestation in human
infants (Fitzgerald 2005). Due to advances in knowledge of the developmental neurobiology of pain, it is
now clear that the immature nervous system responds
differently to tissue damage and pain. In experimental
animal studies with rats, pain induced in the neonatal
period (comparable timing in rats to human premature
birth) can induce changes to pain systems, which are
not seen when the pain is applied at later ages. This
"critical window" suggests that the long-term effects of
pain are potentially greatest in premature infants.
In premature human infants and immature rat pups,
reflex responses to touch show greater sensitivity compared to those of older infants and children (Fitzgerald
and Beggs 2001). With repeated stimulation, even at
innocuous levels, the thresholds for touch and pain
responses drop even further, indicating that these immature infants become even more sensitive. It is noteworthy that the phenomenon of sensitization is greatest
at 28–33 weeks postconceptional age and is gone by
42 weeks. Sensory neurons in the spinal cord and brainstem become hyperexcitable following inflammation,
which is referred to as ▶ central sensitization. Activation of these central cells by repetitive pain results in
hypersensitivity to low-level input of non-skin breaking
handling. For example, due to greater tactile (touch)
sensitivity in very immature mammals, frequent pain
alters touch ▶ thresholds so that even non-invasive handling such as diaper changes elicits pain-like responses
in extremely premature infants. In this way, repetitive
pain may lay the groundwork for chronic pain and
discomfort in the NICU.

Neonatal Prolonged Pain and Re-programming of Stress Systems

The process of maintaining physiological stability involves numerous behavioral, autonomic and hormonal
adjustments. The very immature developing organism is
not yet capable of fine-tuning these multiple dimensions
in a balanced fashion; thus premature neonates born
at extremely low gestational age are potentially more
sensitive to external stress than infants born at term (i.e.
≥ 37 weeks). Of all the environmental input, the stress
induced by invasive skin breaking procedures over a
prolonged period is thought to be primary. Cortisol is
the main stress hormone in humans. While infants are
still in the NICU, higher cumulative stress related to
procedural pain since birth is associated with lower
capacity to mount a stress response both behaviorally
and hormonally (Grunau et al. 2005). Of greater concern, however, are findings that basal cortisol is higher
in extremely preterm infants much later in infancy,
at 8 months "corrected age" (CA, age corrected for
prematurity) (Grunau et al. 2004a). Furthermore, in another study also at 8 months, infants born at extremely
low birth weight (ELBW ≤800 g) displayed higher
resting heart rates. Together these findings suggest a
possible long-term "resetting" of basal physiological regulation following prolonged cumulative stress
and pain exposure associated with extreme prematurity.
In experimental animal studies, neonatal stress (e.g.
due to maternal separation) can permanently reprogram
stress responses in the hypothalamic-pituitary-adrenal
(H-P-A) systems. In contrast, in studies of long-term
effects of pain applied in the neonatal period, no changes
were found to H-P-A responses subsequently in adult
rats (Anand et al. 1999; Walker et al. 2003). Walker
et al. showed that in rats, the frequency of maternal
licking and grooming increased in those pups exposed

L

to pain; this maternal care behavior appeared to prevent the reprogramming of the H-P-A axis. There is some evidence that specific mother-infant interaction in humans that may moderate effects of neonatal pain can be identified. However, a great deal remains to be learned.

Animal Studies of Long-Term Effects of Neonatal Pain Exposure

Most of the evidence for long-term effects of neonatal pain on the developing nervous system is from experimental research on rats. Although we cannot extrapolate directly to human infants, these studies are useful because with humans there are multiple factors that cannot be controlled experimentally. Rats are most often studied because the central nervous system of rat pups at birth is very immature, providing an approximation to the central nervous system of a 24 week gestation, extremely premature human infant. Very early exposure to pain in immature organisms has effects that are not observed when pain exposure occurs at later ages. Long-term changes to pain systems have been found using repeated pin pricks or high doses of long-lasting inflammatory agents. However, it is very important to note that with shorter-acting inflammatory agents only short-term reversible changes were found, not long-term changes. Pain induces long-term effects only when applied in the neonatal period, not in more mature animals and the direction (hypersensitivity or reduced sensitivity) and extent of effects varies depending on the type of pain stimulus and whether pain is short lasting or is ongoing (Ren et al. 2004).

Pain and Stress in the NICU Environment

The medical care of "high risk" preterm infants in the NICU involves exposure to frequent invasive procedures. From birth to discharge from the NICU, infants undergo an average of about 50 procedures, which reflects approximately 2–8 procedures per day. However, some of the tiniest, sickest infants can have 200 procedures or more from admission through discharge, the majority of which are heel lances for blood tests. While infants are in the NICU, their tactile and pain responses are altered depending on the context, including their immediate and cumulative pain experience, gestational age at birth and postnatal age. Increased reactivity is typical in infants who are handled immediately before a procedure or who have had more skin breaking procedures the day before, consistent with sensitization. Conversely, however, cumulatively over time, those infants who had more total exposure to prior pain since birth show decreased behavioral and stress hormone reactivity to invasive procedures later while they are still exposed to ongoing stress in the NICU. This is consistent with animal studies of more prolonged pain. Behavioral responses to pain may be dampened over time in both human infants and animal pups that have had more intense early pain exposure.

Pain Responsivity Later in Infancy and Childhood

Preterm Infants

Few studies have directly compared pain reactivity of extremely premature infants with that of healthy infants born full-term. Contrary to expectation, ELBW infants showed little difference in reactivity to pain at 4 months CA compared to full-term infants, except for a subset who had spent the longest time in the NICU. Then surprisingly, pain responses were more divergent in the ELBW children at 8 months corrected age. The pattern was complex, in that the ELBW infants initially showed very brief behavioral hyper-reactivity to a finger lance, followed by significantly faster behavioral and autonomic recovery (see Grunau 2003). Later at 18 months CA, parents rated their ELBW toddler's pain sensitivity to everyday bumps and scrapes significantly lower than parents of heavier preterm and full-term infants (see Grunau 2002). Overall, the findings suggest dampened pain reactivity in the long run for young children born extremely preterm, when they are very young; however, this may predominantly reflect faster recovery.

While somatization (pain of no known cause) was reported to be higher in ELBW children at age 4–5 years, there were no longer any differences at age 9 years (see Grunau 2002), or 17 years (Grunau et al. 2004b). In a study of health status, ELBW teenagers reported more functional limitations, including pain, than full-term teens (Saigal et al. 1996). Furthermore, in late adolescence internalizing behaviors related to anxiety and depression are more prevalent in ELBW than full-term teens. However, there are multiple possible reasons in addition to early pain exposure for such differences. There is wide variation in long-term outcomes of extreme prematurity for children exposed to comparable amounts of pain in the neonatal period.

Full-term Infants

Tissue damage without anesthetic during circumcision in newborn boys can lead to sensitization apparent months later during immunization (Taddio et al. 1997). However, following surgery in toddlers with appropriate pain management, no differences were found in later pain responses (Peters et al. 2003).

Developmental Outcomes in Preterm Infants

Learning, academic and behavior problems are prevalent in children born extremely prematurely, persisting to late adolescence (Grunau et al. 2004b; Hack et al. 2002). For the tiniest, most fragile infants, the period of pain exposure is prolonged, during the last trimester of "fetal" life, which is a time of very rapid and complex brain development. It is known that immature neurons are more sensitive to toxic influences, and brain volumes are smaller in preterm compared to full-term children (Bhutta and Anand 2002). At this time there is no direct evidence for a causal connection between neonatal pain and later developmental and behavioral difficulties in preterm infants. However, there are concerns that chronic neonatal pain may contribute to alterations in the developing brain.

Sex Differences

In animal studies, sex differences in vulnerability to early stress and effects on long-term pain reactivity have been reported. However, sex has rarely been examined in human infant studies of long-term effects of pain, therefore no conclusions can be drawn at this point.

Maternal-Infant Factors

Multiple interacting intrinsic and extrinsic factors potentially ameliorate or exacerbate effects of neonatal experience on developmental trajectories. Later in childhood and as adults, pain perception and / or expression is affected by multiple interacting factors including social modeling, family variables, child temperament, culture and sex. However, this work has been conducted almost entirely on older children born at term.

Maternal verbalizations that promoted coping in full-term human infants at age 6 months, but not general maternal sensitivity, were associated with altered infant behavior during immunization. Moreover, in former extremely preterm infants, child and family factors predicted ▶ somatization at age 4½ years, and positive maternal responsivity was associated with normalized pain response in infancy (see Grunau 2002). Furthermore, in animal studies, it is very important to note that increased maternal behaviors appear to prevent negative effects of early pain on stress hormone response (Walker et al. 2003). Together these studies suggest that in mammals, alterations to pain systems may be modulated, at least to some extent, by ongoing caregiving.

Memory for Pain

There are different types of memory, other than declarative recall for events, which is generally accepted as only accessible after age 2 years. However, conditioned learning begins very early in life, which implies memory at some level. In addition, physiological changes after repeated pain experiences implies "biological memory." Thus, although infants cannot recall early experiance, their central nervous system may retain a type of memory that is manifested later in altered responses to pain in new situations (Taddio et al. 1997; Grunau 2003).

Summary

In human preterm infants, pain reactivity is altered while infants are in the NICU. There is also evidence that reactivity and recovery to pain is different in extremely preterm infants for many months after hospital discharge; however evidence is limited to a small number of studies. In preterm infants, the findings of enhanced pain response in the neonatal period in the presence of ongoing stress and pain but reduced sensitivity in the longer run, are consistent with recent animal studies.

Adaptation of an organism to the environment occurs through multiple processes during the prenatal and neonatal periods, infancy and childhood. The mammalian brain is characterized by its plasticity, namely the ability to adjust to changes in the internal or external environment, which especially applies to the developing nervous system. The extent to which human infants can compensate over time for the adverse early experiences of prolonged pain exposure in the NICU is unknown. The most long-lasting changes may be to generalized stress systems rather than specifically to pain. The extent to which sensitive and responsive parenting may modulate such effects is unknown.

References

1. Anand KJS (2000) Effects of perinatal pain and stress. Progress in Brain Research 122:117–129
2. Anand KJS, Coskun V, Thrivikraman KV et al. (1999) Long-term behavioral effects of repetitive pain in neonatal rat pups. Physiol Behav 66:627–637
3. Bhutta AT, Anand KJS (2002) Vulnerability of the developing brain: Neuronal mechanisms. Clin Perinatol 29:357–372
4. Fitzgerald M (2005) The development of nociceptive circuits. Nature Reviews Neuroscience 6:507–520
5. Grunau RE (2002) Early pain in preterm infants. A model of long-term effects. Clin Perinatol 29:373–394
6. Grunau RE (2003) Self-regulation and behavior in preterm children: effects of early pain. In: McGrath P, Finley GA (eds) Pediatric Pain: Biological and Social Context. IASP Press, Seattle, pp 23–51
7. Grunau RE, Weinberg J, Whitfield MF (2004a) Neonatal procedural pain and preterm infant cortisol response to novelty at 8 months. Pediatrics 114:77–84
8. Grunau RE, Whitfield MF, Fay TB (2004b) Psychosocial and academic characteristics of extremely low birth weight (<800 g) adolescents who are free of major impairment compared with full-term control subjects. Pediatrics 114:725–732
9. Grunau RE, Holsti L, Haley DW et al. (2005) Neonatal procedural pain exposure predicts lower cortisol and behavioral reactivity in preterm infants in the NICU. Pain 113:293–300
10. Hack M, Flannery DJ, Schluchter M et al. (2002) Outcomes in young adulthood for very-low-birth-weight infants. N Engl J Med 346:149–157
11. Peters JW, Koot HM, de Boer JB et al. (2003) Major surgery within the first 3 months of life and subsequent biobehavioral pain responses to immunization at later age: a case comparison study. Pediatrics 111:129–35
12. Ren K, Anseloni V, Zou S-P et al (2004) Characterization of basal and re-inflammation-associated long-term alteration in pain responsivity following short-lasting neonatal local inflammatory insult. Pain 110:588–596
13. Saigal S, Feeny D, Rosenbaum P et al. (1996) Self-perceived health status and health-related quality of life of extremely low-birth-weight infants at adolescence. JAMA 276:453–459
14. Taddio A, Katz J, Ilersich AL et al. (1997) Effect of neonatal circumcision on pain response during subsequent routine vaccination. Lancet 349:599–603
15. Walker CD, Kudreikis K, Sherrard A et al. (2003) Repeated neonatal pain influences maternal behavior, but not stress responsiveness in rat offspring. Dev Brain Res 140:253–261

Long-Term Potentiation

Synonyms

LTP

Definition

This is a long-lasting increase in synaptic efficacy resulting from repetitive activation of the synapse. This process was first described in hippocampus, whereby high-frequency stimulation of afferent pathways leads to a potentiated post-synaptic response that can last for hours to days. It is a form of activity-dependent plasticity. LTP may increase the efficiency of pain transmission for weeks to months or longer.

▶ Alternative Medicine in Neuropathic Pain
▶ Opioids in the Spinal Cord and Central Sensitization
▶ Spinothalamic Tract Neurons, Role of Nitric Oxide

Long-Term Potentiation and Long-Term Depression in the Spinal Cord

JÜRGEN SANDKÜHLER
Department of Neurophysiology, Center for Brain Research, Medical University of Vienna, Vienna, Austria
juergen.sandkuehler@meduniwien.ac.at

Synonyms

Long-Term Potentiation in the Spinal Cord; Long-Term Depression in the Spinal Cord

Definition

Hyperalgesia may result from an acute noxious event such as trauma, inflammation or nerve injury and may persist long after the primary cause for pain has disappeared. Altered processing of sensory information in the central nervous system may contribute to these forms of hyperalgesia. The long-term potentiation of synaptic strength in nociceptive pathways is a cellular model of pain amplification.

Long-term potentiation (LTP) and long-term depression (LTD) of synaptic strength are long-lasting changes in synaptic efficiency irrespective of the type and the location of chemical synapse. Activity dependent forms outlast conditioning pre- and/or post-synaptic stimulation by at least 30 min. Shorter lasting forms of synaptic plasticity are short-term potentiation or depression, post-tetanic potentiation and paired-pulse facilitation or depression. LTP and LTD may be induced and maintained by pre- and/or by post-synaptic mechanisms such as changes in transmitter release or receptor sensitivity or density. LTP and LTD are divided into at least two phases; the early phase up to 6 h is caused solely by posttranslational changes. In contrast, maintenance of the late stage (more than 6 h after conditioning) requires *de novo* protein synthesis. The signal transduction pathways involved depend upon the induction protocol, type of synapse, types of pre- and post-synaptic neurons, direction of synaptic plasticity and developmental stage. While synaptic plasticity cannot be studied by recording action potential firing or polysynaptic or behavioural responses, evaluation of these parameters is indispensable to show that synaptic plasticity is relevant to information processing downstream in the transmission path.

Characteristics

Synaptic Models for Learning and Memory in Pain Pathways

LTP and LTD were first described for synapses in the hippocampus and are now considered the major cellular models for learning and memory. The final proof is, however, still lacking, mainly since the neuronal elements and their activity patterns involved in cognitive or motor learning are largely unknown (Barnes 1995). Fortunately, in the nociceptive system our knowledge is considerably more advanced: The primary afferent nerve fibres as well as their activity patterns that lead to pain are known. Recently, 2nd order neurons in superficial spinal dorsal horn were identified that mediate hyperalgesia and allodynia. In particular, neurons in lamina I that express the NK1 receptor for substance P are essential for full expression of hyperalgesia in various animal model of inflammation and neuropathy (Nichols et al. 1999). These neurons are all nociceptive specific, most project to the parabrachial area and/or periaqueducatal grey and receive input from primary afferent, peptidergic C-fibres.

Conditioning stimulation of primary afferent C-fibres leads to LTP at C-fibre synapses with these lamina I projection neurons, but not other lamina I neurons (Ikeda et al. 2003). Several independent and convergent lines of evidence suggest that synaptic LTP in superficial spinal dorsal horn is a cellular mechanism of afferent induced hyperalgesia (reviewed in (Sandkühler 2000a; Willis 2002; Moore et al. 2000), see also additional original work cited in the text):

a) Protocols that Induce LTP also Cause Hyperalgesia in Animals and Humans

1. Continuous electrical stimulation of C-fibres at low frequencies (1–5 Hz for 2 or 3 min) or high frequency burst-like stimulation (three to five 100 Hz bursts of 1 sec duration) induce LTP in various spinal cord-dorsal root slice preparations under different recording conditions (Ikeda et al. 2000; Ikeda et al. 2003; Randic et al. 1993) and in intact animal models (Liu and Sandkühler 1997) (Fig. 1). LTP at the first nociceptive synapse apparently affects downstream events in nociceptive pathways. Action potential firing in deep dorsal horn, wide dynamic range neurons (Svendsen et al. 1999) and pain rating in human volunteers (Klein et al. 2004) are also potentiated by similar conditioning stimuli (Fig. 1).

2. Natural patterns of afferent barrage during noxious stimuli (subcutaneous injections of capsaicin

or formalin) in intact (i.e. not spinalised) animals also induce LTP in spinal cord and hyperalgesia in behaving animals.

b) Time Courses for LTP and Hyperalgesia are similar

3. LTP and hyperalgesia are induced within minutes after conditioning stimulation, excluding any time consuming processes such as sprouting of nerve fibres. LTP and hyperalgesia may outlast the conditioning stimulation by hours.
4. LTP and hyperalgesia may spontaneously reverse within hours or days or may persist for longer periods depending upon induction protocols and the context of conditioning.

c) Shared Pharmacology and Signal Transduction Pathways for LTP and Hyperalgesia

5. Co-activation of NMDA-, group I mGlu- and NK^{1}-receptors is required.
6. Activation of voltage-gated calcium channels is required.
7. Ca^{2+}-dependent signal transduction pathways are involved.
8. Activation of protein kinase C, calcium-calmodulin-dependent protein kinase II and nitric oxide synthase (in some cases) is necessary.

d) LTP and Hyperalgesia Can Be Prevented by the Same Means

9. Activity in descending inhibitory pathways raises the threshold for induction of both LTP and hyperalgesia.
10. Opioids can pre-empt induction of LTP (Benrath et al. 2004) and hyperalgesia (Katz et al. 2003).

Not all details of signal transduction pathways that have been explored in one model have also been investigated in the other. All presently known cellular key elements are, however, shared by spinal LTP and afferent induced, centrally expressed hyperalgesia. This strongly suggests that LTP at synapses of primary afferent C-fibres is a cellular mechanism of hyperalgesia. However, until now LTP has only been found at synapses of primary afferent C-fibres, but not at synapses of Aβ- or Aδ-fibres. Thus, neither Aδ-fibre mediated hyperalgesia, nor Aβ-fibre induced allodynia can presently be explained by synaptic LTP in superficial spinal dorsal horn.

Synaptic Long-Term Depression in Pain Pathways

Conditioning stimulation of primary afferent Aδ-fibres but not Aβ-fibres at low frequencies (1 Hz for 15 min) induces a homosynaptic LTD at Aδ-fibres synapses *in vitro* (Sandkühler et al. 1997; Chen and Sandkühler 2000; Randic et al. 1993) and a heterosynaptic LTD at synapses of C-fibres in intact animals (Liu et al. 1998).

Similar stimulation parameters lead to long-term depression of primary afferent induced EPSCs in deep dorsal horn neurons (Garraway and Hochman 2001), of the jaw-opening reflex in mice (Ellrich 2004) and of human nociceptive skin senses (Nilsson et al. 2003; Klein et al. 2004). High intensity, low frequency forms of transcutaneous electrical nerve stimulation (TENS) can alleviate clinical pain in some human pain patients. (Electro-) Acupuncture, which leads to the "d Q" sensation, probably also induces a low frequency afferent barrage in Aδ-fibres. When effective, pain relief outlasts the duration of these forms of TENS and acupuncture for hours or days. This is compatible with synaptic LTD in pain pathways if counterirritation is applied closely to the painful area. In contrast, TENS given at high frequencies, but at low (Aβ-fibre) intensity, does not lead to long-lasting analgesia and cannot be explained by synaptic LTD in pain pathways. This low intensity-high frequency form of TENS most probably involves excitation of spinal inhibitory interneurons as described in the "gate-control" theory (reviewed in Sandkühler 2000b). In conclusion convergent evidence suggest that long-term potentiation at or near the first central synapse in pain pathways is relevant to some forms of hyperalgesia (synaptic long-term potentiation) and can also be used therapeutically to treat and perhaps prevent chronic pain states (synaptic long-term depression).

References

1. Barnes CA (1995) Involvement of LTP in memory: are we "searching under the street light"? Neuron 15:751–754
2. Benrath J, Brechtel C, Martin E et al. (2004) Low doses of fentanyl block central sensitization in the rat spinal cord *in vivo*. Anesthesiology 100:1545–1551
3. Chen J, Sandkühler J (2000) Induction of homosynaptic long-term depression at spinal synapses of sensory Aδ-fibers requires activation of metabotropic glutamate receptors. Neuroscience 98:141–148
4. Ellrich J (2004) Electric low-frequency stimulation of the tongue induces long-term depression of the jaw-opening reflex in anesthetized mice. J Neurophysiol 1:1–2
5. Garraway SM, Hochman S (2001) Serotonin increases the incidence of primary afferent-evoked long-term depression in rat deep dorsal horn neurons. J Neurophysiol 85:1864–1872
6. Ikeda H, Asai T, Murase K (2000) Robust changes of afferent-induced excitation in the rat spinal dorsal horn after conditioning high-frequency stimulation. J Neurophysiol 83:2412–2420
7. Ikeda H, Heinke B, Ruscheweyh R et al. (2003) Synaptic plasticity in spinal lamina I projection neurons that mediate hyperalgesia. Science 299:1237–1240
8. Katz J, Cohen L, Schmid R et al. (2003) Postoperative morphine use and hyperalgesia are reduced by preoperative but not intraoperative epidural analgesia: implications for preemptive analgesia and the prevention of central sensitization. Anesthesiology 98:1449–1460
9. Klein T, Magerl W, Hopf HC et al. (2004) Perceptual correlates of nociceptive long-term potentiation and long-term depression in humans. J Neurosci 24:964–971
10. Liu X, Sandkühler J (1997) Characterization of long-term potentiation of C-fiber-evoked potentials in spinal dorsal horn of adult rat: essential role of NK1 and NK2 receptors. J Neurophysiol 78:1973–1982
11. Liu XG, Morton CR, Azkue JJ et al. (1998) Long-term depression of C-fibre-evoked spinal field potentials by stimulation of

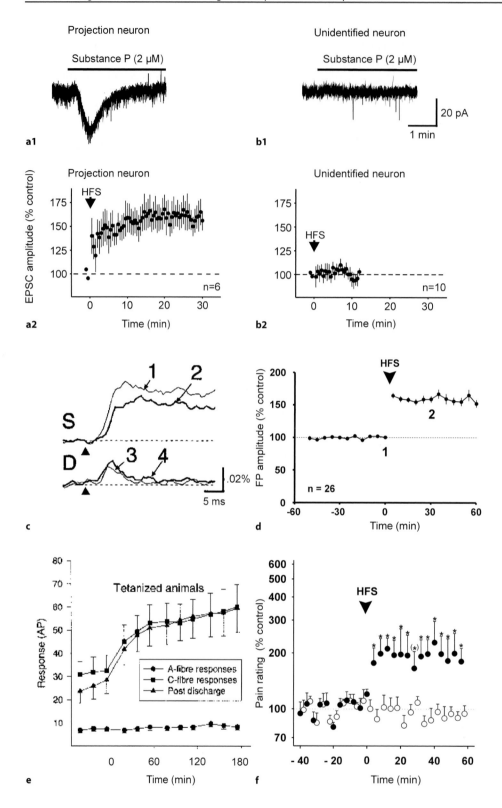

◄ **Long-Term Potentiation and Long-Term Depression in the Spinal Cord, Figure 1,** Long-term potentiation (LTP) of synaptic strength in nociceptive pathways can be demonstrated under a wide range of experimental conditions *in vitro* (a-c) and *in vivo* (d-f) including human subjects (f). (a) In a rat spinal cord-dorsal root slice preparation, conditioning stimulation of dorsal root at C-fibre strength induces LTP at synapses of primary afferent C-fibres with lamina I projection neurons that express NK1 receptors for substance P. A1 illustrates an inward current elicited by bath application of substance P in the presence of tetrodotoxin. A2 shows the mean time course of peaks of monosynaptically, C-fibre-evoked postsynaptic currents before and after conditioning stimulation at time zero. (b) The same conditioning stimulation failed to induce LTP in unidentified neurons of lamina I that did not respond to substance P. Modified from Ikeda et al. 2003. (c) LTP can also be demonstrated by optical recording of C-fibre-evoked responses in superficial spinal dorsal horn in a spinal cord slice preparation. Superimposed time courses of optical responses immediately before (thin lines) and 75 min after (bold lines) high-frequency stimulation at two different locations in the dorsal horn, lamina II "S" and deeper dorsal horn "D". These responses are spatial averages recorded in all pixels present in the area ($\approx$ 60 pixels). Modified from Ikeda et al. 2000. (d) C-fibre-evoked field potentials recorded in superficial spinal dorsal horn of intact, deeply anaesthetized rats are potentiated throughout the recording period of up to 17 h by conditioning high-frequency stimulation of sciatic nerve at C-fibre strength (modified from Benrath et al. 2004). (e) C-fibre but not A-fibre-evoked firing responses of deep dorsal horn neurons and post discharge in spinalised rats are potentiated by a tetanic sciatic nerve stimulation at time zero (mean $\pm$ S.E.M. $n = 8$), modified from Svendsen et al. 1999. (f) Heterotopic effects of conditioning high frequency electrical stimulation of peptidergic cutaneous nerve fibres on pin prick-evoked pain. Conditioning HFS induced a significant enhancement of pin prick-evoked pain adjacent to the conditioning electrode (●) but not adjacent to the control electrode (○). This secondary hyperalgesia occurred after conditioning stimulus intensities of $10\times$ the detection threshold. Mean $\pm$ S.E.M. values across eight subjects are shown. Modified from Klein et al. 2004.

primary afferent A delta-fibres in the adult rat. Eur J Neurosci 10:3069–3075

12. Moore KA, Baba H, Woolf CJ (2000) Synaptic transmission and plasticity in the superficial drosal horn. In: Sandkühler J, Bromm B, Gebhart GF (eds) Nervous system plasticity and chronic pain. Elsevier, Amsterdam, Lausanne, New York, pp 63–81

13. Nichols ML, Allen BJ, Rogers SD et al. (1999) Transmission of chronic nociception by spinal neurons expressing the substance P receptor. Science 286:1558–1561

14. Nilsson HJ, Psouni E, Schouenborg J (2003) Long term depression of human nociceptive skin senses induced by thin fibre stimulation. Eur J Pain 7:225–233

15. Randic M, Jiang MC, Cerne R (1993) Long-term potentiation and long-term depression of primary afferent neurotransmission in the rat spinal cord. J Neurosci 13:5228–5241

16. Sandkühler J (2000a) Learning and memory in pain pathways. Pain 88:113–118

17. Sandkühler J (2000b) Long-lasting analgesia following TENS and acupuncture: Spinal mechanisms beyond gate control. In: Devor M, Rowbotham MC, Wiesenfeld-Hallin Z (eds) Proceedings of the 9th World Congress on Pain, Progress in Pain Research and Management, vol 16. IASP Press, Seattle, pp 359-369

18. Sandkühler J, Chen JG, Cheng G et al. (1997) Low-frequency stimulation of afferent Adelta-fibers induces long-term depression at primary afferent synapses with substantia gelatinosa neurons in the rat. J Neurosci 17:6483–6491

19. Svendsen F, Tjolsen A, Gjerstad J et al. (1999) Long term potentiation of single WDR neurons in spinalized rats. Brain Res 816:487–492

20. Willis WD (2002) Long-term potentiation in spinothalamic neurons. Brain Res Rev 40:202–214

Long-Term Potentiation in the Spinal Cord

▶ Long-Term Potentiation and Long-Term Depression in the Spinal Cord

Loss of Consciousness Associated with Fentanyl

Definition

Loss of consciousness associated with fentanyl occurs at mean serum concentrations of 34 ng/ml.

▶ Postoperative Pain, Fentanyl

Loss of Olfactory Function

Definition

Also called dysosmia; anosmia describes the total loss of the sense of smell, and hyposmia describes a partial loss of olfactory function.

▶ Nociception in Nose and Oral Mucosa

Low Back Pain

Definition

Low back pain affects almost everyone at some point in their lives. It can be acute or chronic in nature and is a primary cause of functional disability in the working population. Multiple causes exist for low back pain including degeneration of the lumbar spine and associated intervertebral discs; intervertebral disc herniation; strain of associated muscles, ligaments, and tendons; and referral from other organs and tissues.

▶ Chronic Low Back Pain, Definitions and Diagnosis
▶ Evoked and Movement-Related Neuropathic Pain
▶ Low Back Pain, Epidemiology
▶ Low Back Pain Patients, Imaging

Low Back Pain, Epidemiology

J. MOCCO, RICARDO J. KOMOTAR, CHRISTOPHER J. WINFREE
Department of Neurological Surgery, Neurological Institute, Columbia University, New York, NY, USA
cjw12@columbia.edu

Synonyms

Pervasiveness of low back pain; Prevalence of low back pain; Incidence of Low Back Pain; Frequency of Low Back Pain; Factors Associated with Low Back Pain

Definition

The word ▸ epidemiology comes from the Greek words epi, "on or upon", demos, "the common people", and logy, "study." Taken from these roots one can extrapolate epidemiology to be the study of that which is upon the people. According to the American College of Epidemiology, epidemiology is "the study of the distribution and determinants of disease risk in human populations." Therefore, the epidemiology of ▸ low back pain is the study of the distribution and determinants of low back pain.

Characteristics

Disability from back pain is more common than any other cause of activity limitation in adults of less than 45 years, and second only to arthritis in people aged 45–65 years (Frank et al. 1996). Additionally, not only is low back pain (LBP) one of the most common causes of missed workdays but it is becoming a bigger problem every year. In fact, over the past 50 years, the number of workdays missed secondary to LBP has increased more than ten-fold (Clinical Standards Advisory Group 1994). A recent review found that 2% of the US work force is compensated for back injuries each year (Andersson 1999). Therefore, efforts to better understand the epidemiology of low back pain are critical.

▸ Prevalence is the number of people in a defined population who have a specific disease or condition at a particular time (Jekel and Katz 1996). Unfortunately, because of the recurrent nature and variable definitions of LBP that are used from study to study, traditional epidemiological concepts are difficult to apply to the experience of low back pain. A recent comprehensive methodological review of the body of literature concerning the prevalence of LBP found that the 1-year prevalence ranged from 3.9–63% with a mean of 32%, and the prevalence at a single point in time ranged from 4.4–33% (Loney and Stratford 1999). If only the highest quality studies were used then the range narrowed to 13.7–28.7% (Loney and Stratford 1999).

▸ Incidence is the occurrence of new cases of disease in a candidate population over a specific time period (Aschengrau 2005). True incidence is essentially impossible to determine for LBP, since onset is often difficult to determine and recurrent episodes confound investigators ability to identify true "new cases." The incidence of LBP has been estimated to vary between 4 and 15% annually in most industrialized countries (Leighton and Reilly 1995; Office of National Statistics 1996).

After attempting to understand the general distribution of LBP, the next step is to better establish the determinants of LBP. Said another way, what factors are associated with the occurrence of LBP? There have been many studies undertaken to attempt to tease out the relevant factors associated with LBP in both patients' workplace and personal environments. Unfortunately, much of this literature is poorly designed and/or contains conflicting results.

Personal risk factors associated with LBP include obesity, smoking, severe scoliosis, and depression (Devereaux 2003a; Devereaux 2003b). An individual's general physical fitness has not been shown to reduce the occurrence of acute LBP, but it has been shown to lower the incidence of chronic LBP and reduce the time needed to recover from episodes of acute LBP (Devereaux 2004). Despite some debate, the greater weight of evidence supports no association between gender and LBP (Devereaux 2004).

In the workplace, a number of characteristics have been identified as risk factors for the occurrence of LBP or a worse disease course. These can be divided into physical and psychosocial characteristics. Accepted physical risk factors include heavy physical labor, long static work postures, and excessive vibration (Devereaux 2003a; Devereaux 2003b). Psychosocial aspects of the workplace that affect LBP were reviewed by Hoogendoorn et al. in a systematic review of the literature, in which there was strong evidence for low workplace social support and low job satisfaction being associated with back pain (Hoogendoorn et al. 2000). In contrast, other commonly held risk factors, such as a high work pace, job autonomy, and long periods of attentiveness, were not strongly associated with LBP, despite some weak supporting literature. Finally, a study by Leino et al. found that monotonous work with few possibilities to learn new skills was associated with LBP in blue-collar workers (Leino and Hanninen 1995).

A final risk factor for LBP recurrence and conversion from acute to chronic status is the presence of litigation and/or workman's compensation claims. Litigation deserves special consideration as multiple studies have been performed in order to elucidate the association between LBP and litigation and/or workman's compensation claims, and the majority of these have found a positive association (Blake and Garrett 1997; Rainville et al. 1997; Valat et al. 1997). These include a well-designed ▸ prospective observational cohort study of 192 individuals, determining that patients with compensation involvement appear to have worse depression and disability before and after rehabilitation interventions (Rainville et al. 1997).

In conclusion, the study of the epidemiology of low back pain has determined that roughly a third of the adult population will suffer low back pain over the course of a year. Many of these individuals will be obese, smoke, suffer from depression, or be employed in careers that expose them to physical labor, long static work postures, excessive vibration, low workplace social support, or low job satisfaction. Of those who suffer low back pain, those with either litigation or workers' compensation involvement are more likely to have a chronic course with worse outcomes and more workdays missed.

References

1. Andersson GB (1999) Epidemiological Features of Chronic Low-Back Pain. Lancet 354:581–585
2. Aschengrau S (2005) Essentials of Epidemiology in Public Health. Jones and Bartlett, Sudbury
3. Blake C, Garrett M (1997) Impact of Litigation on Quality of Life Outcomes in Patients with Chronic Low Back Pain. Ir J Med Sci 166:124–126
4. Clinical Standards Advisory Group (1994) Epidemiology Review: The Epidemiology and Cost of Back Pain. London, UK
5. Devereaux MW (2003a) Approach to Neck and Low Back Disorders. ERW Saunders Manual of Neurologic Practice. Elsevier, Philadelphia, pp 745–751
6. Devereaux MW (2003b) Neck and Low Back Pain. Med Clin North Am 87:643–662
7. Devereaux MW (2004) Low Back Pain. Prim Care 31:33–51
8. Frank K, Brooker et al. (1996) Disability Resulting from Occupational LBP: I: What do we know About Primary Prevention? A Review of the Scientific Evidence on the Prevention before Disability Begins. Spine 21:2908–2917
9. Hoogendoorn WE, Poppel MN van, Bongers PM et al. (2000) Systematic Review of Psychosocial Factors at Work and Private Life as Risk Factors for Back Pain. Spine 25:2114–2125
10. Jekel E, Katz (1996) Epidemiology, Biostatistics, and Preventative Medicine. WB Saunders Co, Toronto, Canada, pp 20–22
11. Leighton DJ, Reilly T (1995) Epidemiological Aspects of Back Pain: The Incidence and Prevalence of Back Pain in Nurses Compared to the General Population. Occup Med 45:263–267
12. Leino PI, Hanninen V (1995) Psychosocial Factors at Work in Relation to Back and Limb Disorders. Scand J Work Environ Health 21:134–142
13. Loney PL, Stratford PW (1999) The Prevalence of Low Back Pain in Adults: A Methodological Review of the Literature. Phys Ther 79:384–396
14. Office of National Statistics (1996) Omnibus Survey. Social Survey Division. Department of Health, London, UK
15. Rainville J, Sobel JB, Hartigan C et al. (1997) The Effect of Compensation Involvement on the Reporting of Pain and Disability by Patients Referred for Rehabilitation of Chronic Low Back Pain. Spine 22:2016–2024
16. Valat J P, Goupille P, Vedere V (1997) Low Back Pain: Risk Factors for Chronicity. Rev Rhum Engl Ed 64:189–194

Low Back Pain Patients, Imaging

PRAMIT PHAL, DANIEL RIRIE, GARY NESBIT
Department of Radiology, Oregon Health and Science University, Portland, OR, USA
nesbitg@ohsu.edu

Synonyms

Lumbar Pain; diagnostic studies

Definition

Diagnostic evaluation of pain localized to the lower back, often associated with radiation in a radicular distribution.

Characteristics

The differential diagnosis for low back pain is broad, including mechanical, compressive, neoplastic, infectious, and referred visceral disease as causes. Only after thorough history and physical examination should one consider the use of imaging studies. For most adult patients under age 50 who do not exhibit signs or symptoms of systemic illness, conservative therapy without imaging is considered appropriate.

The choices available for imaging of back pain are also quite broad and often complimentary. They include: plain radiographs, cross sectional imaging such as computed tomography (CT) (see ▶ Single Photon Emission Computed Tomography) and ▶ magnetic resonance imaging (MRI), myelography, discography, and radionuclide bone scan. The selection of which modality is best suited for a given patient is based on what are the major considerations, such as bone or soft tissue, and what degree of detail is needed.

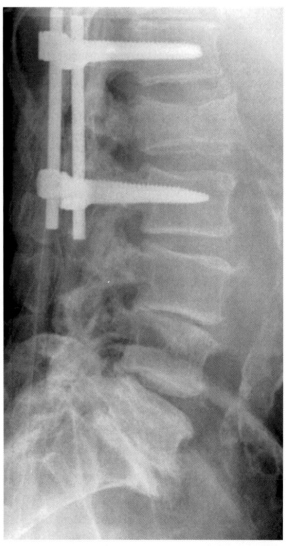

Low Back Pain Patients, Imaging, Figure 1   Lateral radiograph of the lumbar spine demonstrates a burst fracture of L1 with posterior spinal fusion with bilateral paraspinal rods and pedicle screws in T12 and L2. Severe degenerative disc changes are seen in the lower lumbar spine L3 through S1 with loss of disc height, subchondral sclerosis and osteophyte formation.

Plain Films

Plain radiographs are generally the first test performed, perhaps related to their ease of accessibility and low cost. A full lumbar spine series includes an antero-posterior (AP) and lateral projection, along with a spot lateral of the lumbosacral junction and bilateral oblique views. AP and lateral views allow assessment of overall alignment, disc and vertebral body heights and a gross assessment of bony density. Oblique views allow assessment of the pars interarticularis and facet joints, but are often dispensed with due to concerns of excessively irradiating gonadal tissue, particularly in females of reproductive age. If there are concerns of instability or ligamentous injury, lateral views in flexion and extension can be performed.

Plain radiographs have a limited role in the assessment of back pain. As many of the cases of back pain are due to mechanical causes, plain films suffer due to the inability to visualize soft tissue. Hence, disc protusions and nerve root compression cannot be directly visualized. Only the secondary effects of disc degeneration on the adjacent vertebral body, namely subchondral sclerosis and cysts, osteophytosis, disc space narrowing and vacuum phenomenon, are observed. In spinal canal stenosis, only bony narrowing of the spinal canal can be seen. Plain films generally lack sensitivity in diagnosing metastatic disease, as 50% of the bony trabeculae must be destroyed before these lesions are visible (Sartoris et al. 1986).

The current role of plain films in assessment of lower back pain includes that of a screening test in trauma and limited dynamic assessment, by performing flexion and extension views. They are a useful screening test combined with lab tests for symptoms suggesting systemic illness, and can demonstrate specific findings to complement the more sensitive but less specific studies such as MRI and radionuclide bone scan. Plain films have limited usefulness in radiculopathy, only showing bony narrowing of neural exit foramina. They do, however, remain useful in the post-operative patient, particularly in the presence of metallic hardware.

Cross-Sectional Imaging

With the advent of cross-sectional imaging, computed tomography (CT) and magnetic resonance imaging (MRI) have rapidly become mainstays in the imaging of chronic low back pain. CT utilizes x-rays and a series of detectors to measure density in an axial or helical cross-sectional envelope, whereas MRI utilizes magnetic fields and radiowaves to evaluate water concentrations and interactions within tissue. Multiplanar capabilities using either technique provide the ability to interrogate the spine in sagittal, coronal, and even 3-dimensional methods. This, combined with improved contrast resolution over plain radiography, make both techniques superior in evaluating the spinal canal, neural foramina, and paraspinal soft tissues. CT or MRI is usually reserved for those patients

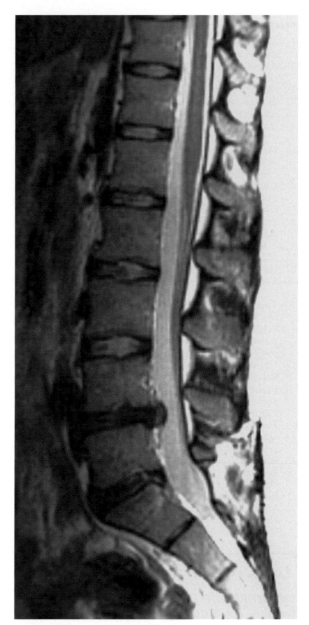

Low Back Pain Patients, Imaging, Figure 2   A sagittal T2 weighted MRI image of the lumbar spine. A bulge of the L4/5 disc encroaches on the central spinal canal. The relative decreased signal in the L4/5 and L5/S1 intervertebral discs is due to decreased water content, a finding of disc degeneration.

with lower back pain who are considering surgery, or in whom neoplastic disease is strongly suspected (Jarvik and Deyo 2002). Additional indications include those with progressive neurologic deficit, suspected cauda equina syndrome, or those who have failed to improve after 6–8 weeks of conservative management (Hicks et al. 2002). The indiscriminate use of MRI and CT may result in unnecessary intervention, which is, in part, due to the extremely high sensitivity of MRI. There is a relatively high prevalence of

L

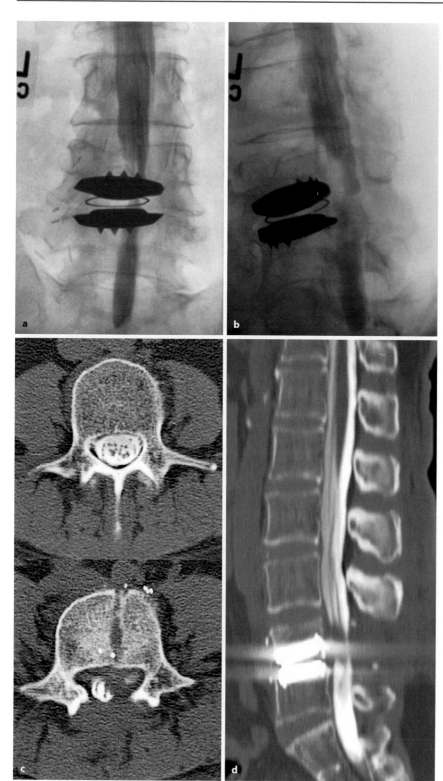

Low Back Pain Patients, Imaging, Figure 3 A frontal (a), and oblique (b) projection of the lumbar spine is shown following the intrathecal injection of contrast for a myelogram. The nerve roots of the cauda equina are well visualized. Surgical changes of posterior laminectomy and intervertebral disc prosthesis at L4-L5 is present. Extrinsic compression of the contrast-filled thecal sac is noted above the L4-L5 disc level. A CT scan of the same patient at L3 (c, upper) shows contrast outlining the normal nerve roots in the canal and L4 (c, lower) there is a midline fracture, bilateral laminectomy and the compression of the thecal sac. A sagittal reconstruction of the CT scan (d) delineates the disc prosthesis, thecal sac and soft-tissue compression of the cauda equina.

disk bulges, protrusions, and facet arthropathy in the asymptomatic population, and the presence of these pathologies in patients with back pain may, in many cases, be coincidental (Gaensler 1999). These findings underscore the need for judicious use of diagnostic imaging when evaluating any patient with low back pain.

Pediatric patients, in contrast, rarely have degenerative disease. These patients usually have more serious underlying disease that should be assessed differently and often involves advanced imaging (Osborne 1994).

Determining whether to use CT or MRI in a given patient is usually by physician preference, however, there are situations when one modality is favored over another. Patients with certain implanted devices or claustrophobia may prohibit the use of MRI, although metallic artifacts from spinal surgical implants are often worse on CT than MRI. CT provides greater bone detail than MRI and is excellent for evaluating neural foraminal and central canal stenosis (Gaensler 1999). The sensitivity and specificity of disk herniation is slightly higher with MRI than CT, but the two modalities are essentially equally effective in evaluating the degree of spinal stenosis (Jarvik and Deyo 2002). MRI has demonstrated superiority in evaluating for neoplasm, with sensitivity and specificity ranging from 0.83–0.93 and 0.9–0.97, respectively (Jarvik and Deyo 2002). Infection is also best evaluated by MRI with sensitivity of 0.96 and specificity of 0.92 (Jarvik and Deyo 2002). In patients who have had prior surgery, MRI is the preferred modality. These patients should always be imaged with gadolinium contrast material to help distinguish scar tissue from recurrent disc herniation (Helms 1999). MRI has also been shown to be particularly useful as a screening tool in evaluating patients with symptomatic discs by identifying tears of the annulus fibrosus with high sensitivity; the relative low specificity, however, cannot replace the need for discography (Yoshida et al. 2002).

Myelography

When intrathecal contrast material is administered for myelography, the contents of the spinal canal and neural foramina are more clearly visualized. When combined with CT, the additional anatomic information can provide a crucial supplement in the evaluation of nerve root impingement in the lateral recess as a cause for radiculopathy, because MRI tends to underestimate the degree of stenosis in this location (Bartynski and Lin 2003). Although myelography is invasive, and its use has decreased with the advent of MRI, it still remains an important technique when other modalities remain equivocal.

Nuclear Medicine

A radionuclide bone scan involves intravenous injection of a radionuclide taken up by bone, most commonly bound to a compound containing phosphate. Imaging is performed with a gamma camera and the use of cross sectional techniques such as SPECT (single photon emission computed tomography) can increase sensitivity and anatomic localization. Early imaging in the blood flow and blood pool phases, detect areas of hyperemia. Delayed images demonstrate bony uptake. This imaging modality is most useful in conditions where there is increased bony turnover: osteoblastic metastases, infection, fractures, in particular in the

diagnosis of stress fractures, and differentiating acute from chronic vertebral body compression fractures (Avrahami et al. 1989). While radionuclide bone scan has excellent sensitivity for detection of these conditions, it suffers from a lack of specificity, and involves exposure to ionizing radiation.

Discography

Discography is a semi-invasive procedure that involves placement of a needle into the central nucleus pulposis of the disc and injection of iodinated contrast material directly into the nucleus.

Information gained from this procedure includes a morphological assessment of the disc. The procedure is most often done under fluoroscopy during which spot images are taken. CT of the lumbar spine is often performed after the procedure, including sagittal and coronal reformatted images. Degenerative change can range from fissures and clefts in the nucleus pulposus, annular tears with contrast extending to the disc periphery and disc rupture with leakage of injected contrast (Anderson 2004; Sachs et al. 1987).

The patient's pain response during the procedure is also assessed. During the procedure the patient is asked to grade the severity pain (usually out of 5) and also the similarity of the pain to their usual symptoms.

Discography is very sensitive for detection of annular tears of the intervertebral disc, a common cause of back pain not confidently detected on MRI. Disparity between MRI and clinical presentation is a major indication for discography. Discography should only be performed on surgical candidates who have failed a period of conservative therapy of around 6 months. Other indications for discography include determining the symptomatic level in multilevel degenerative disease, preoperative planning and evaluation of the postoperative patient.

Due to the semi-invasive nature of the procedure, potential risks of discography include infection, bleeding, neural damage, accentuation of pain and post procedural headache if the dura is traversed. The other main disadvantage of discography is its high false positive rate, which is likely to be around 10% (Saal 2002).

References

1. Anderson MW (2004) Lumbar Discography: An Update. Semin Roentgenol 39:52–67
2. Avrahami E, Tadmor R, Dally O et al. (1989) Early MR Demonstration of Spinal Metastases in Patients with Normal Radiographs and CT and Radionuclide Bone Scans. J Comput Assist Tomogr 13:598–602
3. Bartynski WS, Lin L (2003) Lumbar Root Compression in the Lateral Recess: MR Imaging, Conventional Myelography, and CT Myelography Comparison with Surgical Confirmation. Am J Neuroradiol 24:348–360
4. Gaensler E (1999) Nondegenerative Diseases of the Spine. In: Brant W (ed) Fundamentals of Diagnostic Radiology. Williams and Wilkins, Baltimore, pp 233–280

5. Helms C (1999) Lumbar Spine Disc Disease and Stenosis. In: Brant W (ed) Fundamentals of Diagnostic Radiology. Williams and Wilkins, Baltimore, pp 281–288
6. Hicks GS, Duddleston DN, Russell LD et al. (2002) Low Back Pain. Am J Med Sci 324:207–211
7. Jarvik JG, Deyo RA (2002) Diagnostic Evaluation of Low Back Pain with Emphasis on Imaging. Ann Intern Med 137:586–597
8. Osborne A (1994) Nonneoplastic Disorders of the Spine and Spinal Cord. Neuroradiology. Mosby, St. Louis, pp 820–875
9. Saal JS (2002) General Principles of Diagnostic Testing as Related to Painful Lumbar Spine Disorders: A Critical Appraisal of Current Diagnostic Techniques. Spine 27:2538–2546
10. Sachs BL, Vanharanta H, Spivey MA et al. (1987) Dallas Discogram Description. A New Classification of CT/Discography in Low-Back Disorders. Spine 12:287–294
11. Sartoris DJ, Clopton P, Nemcek A et al. (1986) Vertebral-Body Collapse in Focal and Diffuse Disease: Patterns of Pathologic Processes. Radiology 160:479–483
12. Yoshida H, Fujiwara A, Tamai K et al. (2002) Diagnosis of Symptomatic Disc by Magnetic Resonance Imaging: T2-Weighted and Gadolinium-DTPA-Enhanced T^1-Weighted Magnetic Resonance Imaging. J Spinal Disord Tech 15:193–198

Low First Pass Metabolism

Definition

Oral oxycodone undergoes low first pass metabolism and is among those opioids possessing a short elimination half-life.

▶ Postoperative Pain, Oxycodone

Low Frequency Oscillations

Definition

Oscillatory activity described in the brain when the organism is not attentive or drowsy.

▶ Corticothalamic and Thalamocortical Interactions

Low Intracranial Pressure Headache

▶ Headache Due to Low Cerebrospinal Fluid Pressure

Low Threshold Calcium Spike

Synonyms

LTS

Definition

A membrane depolarization resulting from an inflow of Ca^{++} ions through T-type channels. The LTS occurs when the membrane potential is sufficiently hyperpolarized to cause de-inactivation of the T-channels.

▶ Burst Activity in Thalamus and Pain

Low Threshold Calcium Spike Burst

Synonyms

LTS burst

Definition

Bursting discharges produced by thalamic and reticular cells, when their membranes are hyperpolarized by either disfacilitation or overinhibition. They are due to the deinactivation of calcium T-channels causing the appearance of a large calcium spike, itself inducing a burst of sodium action potentials.

▶ Burst Activity in Thalamus and Pain
▶ Thalamotomy for Human Pain Relief

Low Threshold Neuron

Synonyms

LT neurons

Definition

LT neurons are best activated by innocuous mechanical stimuli.

▶ Functional Changes in Sensory Neurons Following Spinal Cord Injury in Central Pain
▶ Postoperative Pain, COX-2 Inhibitors
▶ Spinothalamic Input, Cells of Origin (Monkey)

Lower Back Pain, Acute

T. SHAH, STEPHAN A. SCHUG
Royal Perth Hospital and University of Western Australia, Crawley, WA, Australia
schug@cyllene.uwa.edu.au

Synonyms

Acute Lumbago; Acute Sciatica; Acute Backache; Bad Back

Definition

Acute lower back pain refers to spinal pain of sudden onset originating from lumbar, sacral or lumbosacral areas. It may also be referred pain from other areas such as the sacro-iliac joints (www.emia.com.au/MedicalProviders/EvidenceBasedMedicine/overview.html). Although often used to mean lower back pain, sciatica specifically refers to pressure on the sciatic nerve causing pain passing down the posterior medial aspect of the leg.

Characteristics

Lower back pain is extremely common, with 60–80 % of adults experiencing it at some time. It is the most common reason cited for absence from work, and its management, therefore, has strong socioeconomic implications. Ninety percent of acute lower back pain, however, will resolve within 6 weeks (www.emia.com.au/MedicalProviders/EvidenceBasedMedicine/overview.html, http://www.acc.co.nz/acc-publications/pdfs/ip/acc1038-col.pdf, http://www.health.gov.au/nhmrc/publications/synopses/cp94syn.htm). The underlying diagnosis is often unknown. There is level I evidence that common findings in patients with lower back pain (e.g. osteoarthritis, spondylosis or spinal canal stenosis) may also be present in asymptomatic patients, and do not necessarily represent the cause of the pain (http://www.health.gov.au/nhmrc/publications/synopses/cp94syn.htm).

Due to its frequent occurrence, it is essential to identify early those rare causes of lower back pain that may have an underlying serious pathology or be non-biomechanical in origin. These should prompt early referral to appropriate treatment that might be urgent. A thorough history and simple examination largely identify these so-called 'red flags'. Red flags include neurological signs and symptoms, a history of significant trauma, weight loss and other signs of systemic illness and severe unrelenting pain, especially in those at risk of pathological fractures. Conditions identified in such cases include cauda equina syndrome, fractures (traumatic or pathological), tumours and infection. In patients with no red flags imaging is largely unnecessary. 'Yellow flags' are also discussed with respect to acute lower back pain. These are behavioural and psychosocial factors that make progression to chronic back pain more likely, and that make rehabilitation from acute back pain difficult, and, or undesirable. Problems such as depression, poor job satisfaction and a belief that physical activity can cause further damage fall under this heading. Early identification and intervention can alter this course and ultimately reduce chronic disability (www.emia.com.au/MedicalProviders/EvidenceBased Medicine/overview.html).

Management of simple mechanical lower back pain has altered significantly in the last few decades. There is now very good evidence that previous recommendations of prolonged bed rest are detrimental, and that staying active and an early return to work are beneficial (www.emia.com.au/MedicalProviders/Evidence BasedMedicine/overview.html, http://www.acc.co.nz/acc-publications/pdfs/ip/acc1038-col.pdf, http://www.health.gov.au/nhmrc/publications/synopses/cp94syn.htm). Manipulative techniques in the first 4–6 weeks have been shown to improve outcome (http://www.acc.co.nz/acc-publications/pdfs/ip/acc1038-col.pdf, Meade et al 1995), as do simple analgesia (e.g. paracetamol) and heat wraps (http://www.health.gov.au/nhmrc/publications/synopses/cp94syn.htm). The evidence for the use of a non steroidal anti-inflammatory drug is conflicting and side effects (in particular gastric mucosal ulceration) are common with long term use (http://www.health.gov.au/nhmrc/publications/synopses/cp94syn.htm). Manipulation under anaesthesia and the use of muscle relaxants (e.g. diazepam) have been shown to be harmful (http://www.acc.co.nz/acc-publications/pdfs/ip/acc1038-col.pdf). Use of oral opioid analgesia may be necessary to relieve pain in acute stages. If used, a short acting regular drug is preferable for as brief a period as possible. The ongoing need for use should prompt a reassessment of the patient (http://www.health.gov.au/nhmrc/publications/synopses/cp94syn.htm).

Patients should have a time frame for their progress and be educated about what to expect. They should be aware that they play an active role in their rehabilitation and should take this on as their responsibility. Those not responding to treatment at 4–12 weeks should be reassessed and considered for specialist referral. They might constitute a group of patients with increased risk of chronification and subsequent complex biopsychosocial consequences.

References

1. Evidence-Based Management of Acute Musculoskeletal Pain-Australian Acute Musculoskeletal Pain Guideline Group. http://www.health.gov.au/nhmrc/publications/synopses/cp94syn.htm
2. Meade TW, Dyer S, Browne W et al. (1995) Randomised Comparison of Chiropractic and Hospital Outpatient Management for Low Back Pain: Results from Extended Follow-Up. BMJ 311:349–351
3. Overview of Clinical Guidelines for the Management of Acute Lower Back Pain. www.emia.com.au/MedicalProviders/EvidenceBasedMedicine/overview.html
4. The New Zealand Acute Lower Back Pain Guide. http://www.acc.co.nz/acc-publications/pdfs/ip/acc1038-col.pdf

Lower Back Pain, Physical Examination

PATRICK B. SENATUS, CHRISTOPHER J. WINFREE
Deptartment of Neurological Surgery, Neurological Institute, Columbia University, New York, NY, USA
cjw12@columbia.edu

Synonyms

Distraction Signs; Inflammatory Syndrome; Lumbago; Lumbosacral; Mechanical Syndrome; Myofascial syndrome; Neural Compressive Syndrome; Neurogenic Claudication; Neuropathic Syndrome; Paravertebral Muscle; Provocative Maneuver; Psychosocioeconomic Syndrome; Radiculopathy; Sacroiliac joint; Schrober's Test; Sciatic Notch; Spondylolisthesis; Straight-Leg-Raising Sign

Definition

Component of the clinical evaluation focusing on the region between L1 above and S1 below and the paravertebral erector spinae muscles laterally (Merskey 1994), relying on inspection palpation, and physical maneuvers to elicit signs and reproduce symptoms in the diagnosis of low back pathology.

Characteristics

Goals

The physical examination of the lower back is an essential part of the evaluation of disorders stemming from this region, particularly lumbago and sciatica. The diagnosis of back pain is complex and must distinguish among disparate entities such as ► myofascial syndrome, in which pain is derived from ligamentous and muscular soft tissue; mechanical syndrome, in which instability and abnormal motion across joints and ligaments causes pain; neural compressive syndrome, in which pain derives from pressure on individual nerve roots or the cauda equina; ► inflammatory syndrome, in which pain is derived from inflammatory diseases such as osteomyelitis, diskitis, or ankylosing spondylitis; osteogenic syndrome, in which pain is derived from bone itself such as with compression fractures and bony metastasis; neuropathic syndrome, in which pain is of neural origin arising from permanent injury to peripheral nerves, nerve roots, or spinal cord; and finally ► psychosocioeconomic syndrome, in which a major contributor to pain is personality dysfunction, depression, or secondary gain. Therefore, when presented with a patient for evaluation the clinician must keep in mind the broad differential diagnosis from which to select the etiology of the patient's ailment (Kirkaldy-Willis 1983).

After a focused detailed history of present illness is obtained, a directed physical examination is undertaken. It should proceed in a fashion as to test, rule out, and distinguish among items on the differential diagnosis. Moreover, it should be used in conjunction with the history to guide and justify further examination including static and dynamic imaging, serological studies, and invasive provocative tests such as discography.

Inspection

The examination begins with a general inspection to determine the patient's overall state of comfort, pain, posture, and gait. The inability to achieve a stable comfortable position while standing or seated may speak to the intensity and nature of the cause of the disease. A persistent flexed posture may be reflective of neural compressive syndrome, as that would tend to alleviate pressure on neural elements that would be exacerbated by hyperextension. Asymmetric gait, or favoring of one extremity, may point to lateralizing ► radiculopathy. Neurogenic claudication, manifesting as bilateral diffuse leg pain on standing or walking, is indicative of spinal stenosis.

From a lateral vantage point, the transition from the thoracic ► kyphotic curve to the lumbar lordotic curve must be assessed. Deviation from the expected degrees of curvature may be indicative of pathology. Loss of lumbar lordosis may be a sign of lumbar spondylopathy as the lumbar spine attempts to straighten itself to minimize neural compression and deleterious force vectors. Exaggerated lumbar lordosis may indicate ► spondylolisthesis. From a posterior vantage point, any lateral or scoliotic curve should be noted. The spinous processes for T1 down should lie along a straight line that should extrapolate through the gluteal cleft. Disparities with respect to shoulder level, the level of the iliac crests, and symmetry of gluteal folds may result from scoliosis or other vertebral abnormalities. Asymmetry of ► paraspinal musculature may indicate spasm or underlying scoliosis.

Tufts of hair, ► melanotic or vitiliginous patches, lipomas, skin dimples, or draining sinuses should raise the suspicion for occult spinal ► dysraphism that may require further investigation.

Inspection under dynamic conditions can yield important diagnostic data. As a patient rotates the shoulder with respect to the hips, bends forward, backward, and laterally, the range of motion, smoothness, symmetry, and changes in the lumbar curvature should be noted. Decreased mobility may point to ankylosing spondylitis, osteoarthritis, or paravertebral muscle spasm as causes of pain.

Schrober's test, in which the change in distance between two points (one 10 cm above S1 and one 5 cm below S1) during maximal forward bending, can be used to quantify restricted mobility. An increased distance of less than 5 cm is abnormal and may point to ankylosing spondylitis (Karnath 2003).

Exacerbation of symptoms on forward bending may point to myofascial syndrome as an etiology. ► Amelioration of symptoms on forward bending and exacerbation on hyperextension suggest spinal stenosis. Asymmetric exacerbation on lateral bending or rotation may point to paracentral or laterally herniated disk.

Palpation

Palpating the lower back in standing, sitting, and prone positions can be informative. Feeling the spines and spinous interspaces can help discern relationships between adjacent vertebrae. Unusual prominence of a spinous process may be a sign of spondylolisthesis or retrolisthesis of one body with respect to the other. Unusual prominence of an interspace may signal disruption or incompetence of posterior spinal elements. If palpation or gentle percussion of the spine causes pain, this raises the specter of fracture, malignancy, diskitis, or osteomyelitis, which may require further work up. Tenderness of the paravertebral muscle, spinous process, intervertebral joint and sacroiliac notch, may be indicative of intervertebral disc herniation.

Provocative Maneuvers

Provocative maneuvers are helpful in determining the etiology of low back pain. The ipsilateral and crossed straight leg raising (iSLR and cSLR) tests should be performed in patients in whom radiculopathy is suspected. With the patient lying supine, a positive iSLR sign is obtained if elevation of the ipsilateral lower extremity to between 30 and 60 degrees reproduces sciatica. With the patient in the same position, a positive cSLR sign is obtained if elevation of the contralateral lower extremity reproduces sciatica in the ipsilateral lower extremity. Ipsilateral SLR sign has high sensitivity but low specificity whereas the crossed SLR has both high sensitivity and specificity. These tests can be performed in the seated position to elicit distraction signs used to rule out overlay.

Psychosocioeconomic Syndrome

As depression, personality dysfunction, somatization, and secondary gain can affect the experience of disease and how it is expressed, the clinician should be cognizant of inconsistencies and non-physiologic findings that suggest supratentorial overlay or psychosocioeconomic syndrome. Overreaction during physical examination, inappropriate tenderness that is too generalized or too superficial, pain on simulated but not actual rotation of the spine or on simulated axial loading, regional impairment of strength or sensation that fails to conform to radicular or dermatomal distributions, and positive distraction signs, such as inconsistent performance during distracting maneuvers, can help the clinician identify psychosocioeconomic syndrome (Waddell et al. 1980).

References

1. Bates B (1995) The Musculoskeletal System. In: Bates B (ed) A Guide to Physical Examination and History Taking, 6th edn. JB Lippincott Company, Philadelphia, pp 477–478
2. Karnath B (2003) Clinical Signs of Low Back Pain. Hospital Physician 39:39–44
3. Kirkaldy-Willis WH (1983) The Pathology and Pathogenesis of Low Back Pain. In Kirkaldy-Willis WH (ed), Managing Low Back Pain. Churchill Livingstone, Philadelphia, pp 23–44
4. Merskey H, Bogduk N (1994) Classification of Chronic Pain: Descriptions of Chronic Pain Syndromes and Definitions of Pain Terms. 2nd edn. IASP Press, Seattle, pp 11–36
5. Sypert G, Arpin-Sypert E (2004) Evaluation and Management of the Failed Back Syndrome. In: Winn HR (ed) Youmans Neurological Surgery, 5th edn. Saunders, Philadelphia, pp 4327–4345
6. Waddell G, McCulloch JA, Kummel E et al. (1980) Nonorganic Physical Signs in Low-Back Pain. Spine 5:117–125

Lower Gastrointestinal Tract Pain Models

▶ Visceral Pain Model, Lower Gastrointestinal Tract Pain

Low-Level Laser Therapy

▶ Laser

Low-Threshold Calcium Channels

▶ Calcium Channels in the Spinal Processing of Nociceptive Input

Low-Threshold VDCCs

▶ Calcium Channels in the Spinal Processing of Nociceptive Input

Low-Voltage Calcium Channels

▶ Calcium Channels in the Spinal Processing of Nociceptive Input

LSN

▶ Lateral Spinal Nucleus

LSP

▶ Laser Silent Period

LT Neurons

▶ Low Threshold Neuron

LTP

▶ Long-Term Potentiation

LTR

▶ Local Twitch Response

LTR Locus

▶ Sensitive Locus

LTS

▸ Low Threshold Calcium Spike

LTS Burst

▸ Low Threshold Calcium Spike Burst

Lumbago

Definition

Pain in the back occasionally radiating into the buttocks.
▸ Chronic Back Pain and Spinal Instability
▸ Lower Back Pain, Physical Examination
▸ Radiculopathies

Lumbar Disc Stimulation

▸ Lumbar Discography

Lumbar Discogram

▸ Lumbar Discography

Lumbar Discography

DAVID DIAMANT
Neurological and Spinal Surgery, Lincoln, NE, USA
ddiamant@neb.rr.com

Synonyms

Lumbar Discogram; provocation discography; provocative discography; Lumbar Disc Stimulation

Definition

Lumbar discography is a diagnostic procedure designed to test if a patient's pain arises from a lumbar intervertebral disc. It involves injecting contrast medium into the disc in an effort to reproduce the patient's pain.

Characteristics

Principles

Since they are innervated, the lumbar intervertebral disc can be a source of low back pain (Bogduk 1983). However, there are no conventional means, such as ▸ musculoskeletal examination or medical imaging, whereby it can be determined if a particular disc is painful or not. For this reason, lumbar discography was adopted and used as the only available means to test if a disc was painful.

The test is analogous to palpation for tenderness, but because lumbar discs are inaccessible to palpation, needles must be used. The needle is used to stress the disc by injecting contrast medium into its nucleus. Contrast medium will outline the internal structure of the disc. This process is described as discography. It verifies that the disc has been correctly injected, but is not the critical component of the test. Critical, is whether or not stressing the disc reproduces the patient's accustomed pain. This phase is called disc stimulation.

Technique

With the patient prone on the x–ray table, and their lumbar area prepped in sterile fashion, a needle is inserted into the target disc via a posterolateral approach through the skin and muscles of the back. Once the needle has been correctly placed (Fig. 1), a pressure transducer is connected to the needle, and contrast dye, mixed with antibiotic, is injected into the nucleus pulposus in a relatively rate controlled fashion (Fig. 2). The flow of contrast medium, the pressure within the disc during injection, and the patient's response to injection are all simultaneously monitored. The nucleus pulposus of a typical lumbar disc may contain between 1.5–2.5 cc of such solution (Aprill 1991). Spread of contrast medium from the nucleus pulposus into the anulus fibrosus may be associated with the onset of pain. It is the pain response, in accordance with a visualized anular spread of dye, which is of critical importance when interpreting the study. When diagnosing the lumbar disc as the pain generator, injection of the disc must provoke reproduction of the patient's typical pattern of pain (concordant pain). Stimulation of an asymptomatic disc will typically not cause such pain, or it will cause pain in an atypical (non-concordant) pattern. Pain patterns may be isolated to the lumbar area, or they may encompass areas that are topographically separated from the site of pathology, such as the buttock and/or lower limb. The manner in which contrast medium spreads within the disc is salient for interpretation of the study. Although visualization of such spread can be attained fluoroscopically, it is best appreciated by computerized tomography (CT) scan. In order to accept a disc as the pain generator, not only must concordant pain have been elicited during disc stimulation, but an internal tear extending at least to the outer one third of the

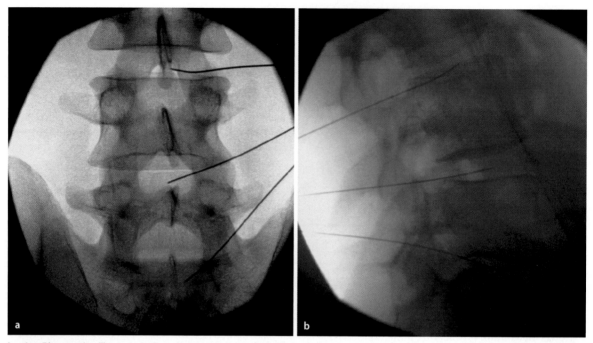

Lumbar Discography, Figure 1 Radiographs of needles placed for L3, L4, and L5 discography. (a) AP view. (b) Lateral view. Reproduced courtesy of the International Spinal Intervention Society (2004).

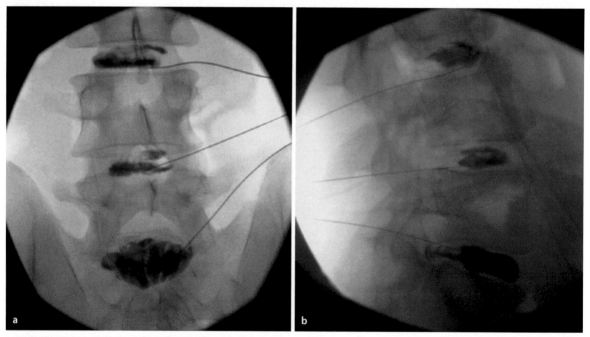

Lumbar Discography, Figure 2 Radiographs of an L3, L4, and L5 discogram, after injection of contrast medium. (a) AP view. (b) Lateral view. Reproduced courtesy of the International Spinal Intervention Society (2004).

posterior or posterolateral disc must be evident on the CT scan. These features correlate significantly with the reproduction of pain (Moneta et al. 1994). Some 70% of fissured discs are painful, and some 70% of painful discs exhibit radial fissures (Vanharanta et al. 1987). If fissures are evident, the diagnosis becomes one of internal disc disruption (Merskey and Bogduk 1994;

Bogduk and McGuirk 2002). However, further data is necessary from this procedure in order to accept a particular disc as a pain generator.

Although reproduction of concordant pain is a necessary step in the diagnosis of discogenic pain, discographic study of an adjacent disc or discs is not ideally associated with concordant pain reproduction. According to the standards of the International Spinal Intervention Society (2004), the diagnosis of lumbar discogenic pain is most robust if stimulation of a single disc reproduces concordant pain, while stimulation of two adjacent discs does not. Furthermore, the intensity of concordant pain must be of moderate or severe magnitude in order to consider that disc a significant pain generator. In diagnosing lumbar discogenic pain, observation of the pressure within the disc, at the development of moderate to severe concordant pain, is of importance. A certain amount of pressure (known as opening pressure) is necessary to induce flow of contrast dye into the nucleus pulposus. Once this is ascertained, then the pressure at which concordant pain is reproduced is determined and recorded. If concordant pain occurs at relatively low pressure, e.g.15 pounds per square inch (psi) or less above the opening pressure, then the response is considered positive. If concordant pain occurs at a pressure of 15–50 psi above opening pressure, then the pain response is indeterminate, possibly being positive. If concordant pain occurs at greater than 50 psi over opening pressure, then such a concordant pain response cannot be considered positive, since there is no way to reliably differentiate whether pain occurred from significant mechanical stimulation, which may cause pain in a normal disc (Carragee et al. 2000), or from pain as a result of internal disc disruption.

Therefore, according to standard (International Spinal Intervention Society 2004), the intervertebral disc is deemed to be the generator of an individual's pain if the following criteria are met:

1. Stimulation of the target disc reproduces the patient's accustomed pain.
2. Stimulation of adjacent discs does not reproduce their pain.
3. Pain is produced at a pressure of injection of not greater than 50 psi, and preferably at a pressure less than 15 psi.
4. The evoked pain has an intensity estimated by the patient as greater than 6, on a 10–point numerical pain rating scale.

Validity

In order for lumbar provocation discography to be valid, it must be demonstrated that the four criteria previously listed are adhered to. If these criteria are satisfied, the diagnosis becomes one of discogenic pain. False-positive results can occur due to technical errors, neurophysiological phenomena and/or psycholological factors. Some investigators have warned that discography can be false-positive, on the grounds that discs can be painful when stimulated in asymptomatic volunteers (Carragee et al. 2000). However, the false-positive rate can be kept to less than 10% if the diagnostic criteria are strictly observed (International Spinal Intervention Society 2004).

Stimulation of the anulus fibrosus, either by injecting into it or by moving the needle within it, can be painful. Accepting a concordant pain response secondary to such an event would be inappropriate in the context of this procedure, as injection must be within the nucleus pulposus while the needle is not otherwise being manipulated. Acceptance of concordant pain that is of mild intensity does not necessarily implicate that disc as one's pain generator, as one of the principal diagnostic tenets for symptomatic internal disc disruption is moderate to severe concordant pain reproduction. Acceptance of concordant pain reproduction at manometric pressures greater than 50 psi above opening pressure would be inappropriate, as high intradiscal pressures have been noted to evoke pain in asymptomatic individuals (Carragee et al. 2000). Acceptance of concordant pain without significant anular disruption would violate the principles of this test, as only the outer one-third of the anulus fibrosus is definitively known to be innervated. Lastly, in those with somatisation disorder, it has been noted that lumbar provocation discography may result in false-positive responses (Carragee et al. 2000).

Applications

The cardinal purpose of provocation discography is to establish if a patient's back pain is due to discogenic pain (internal disc disruption). The diagnostic utility is to provide a diagnosis, and thus help the clinician in planning treatment of such pain. Treatment options include palliative care or surgical management, such as interbody fusion, disc replacement, or ▶ intradiscal electrothermal therapy. It has been shown that provocation discography in the lumbar spine can assist in predicting outcomes of surgical and non-surgical management of symptomatic internal disc disruption (Derby et al. 1999).

References

1. Aprill CN (1991) Diagnostic Disc Injection. In: Frymoyer JW (ed) The Spine: Principle and Practice. Raven Press, New York, pp 45–84
2. Bogduk N (1983) The Innervation of the Lumbar Spine. Spine 8:286–293
3. Bogduk N, McGuirk B (2002) Causes and Sources of Chronic Low Back Pain. In: Bogduk N, McGuirk B (eds) Medical Management of Acute and Chronic Low Back Pain. An Evidence-Based Approach. Elsevier, Amsterdam, pp 113–125
4. Carragee EJ, Truong T, Rossi M, Hagle C (2000) The Rates of False-Positive Lumbar Discography in Select Patients without Low Back Symptoms. Spine 25:1373–1981
5. Derby R, Howard MW, Grant JM, Lettice JJ, Van Peteghem PK, Ryan DP (1999) The Ability of Pressure-Controlled Discography to Predict Surgical and Non-Surgical Outcomes. Spine 24:364–372
6. International Spinal Intervention Society (2004). Lumbar Disc Stimulation. In: Bogduk N (ed) Practice Guidelines for Spinal Diagnostic and Treatment Procedures. International Spinal Intervention Society, San Francisco
7. Merskey H, Bogduk N (eds) (1994) Classification of Chronic Pain. Descriptions of Chronic Pain Syndromes and Definitions of Pain Terms, 2nd edn. IASP Press, Seattle, p 179
8. Moneta GB, Videman T, Kaivanto K, Aprill C, Spivey M, Vanharanta H, Sachs BL, Guyer RD, Hochschuler SH, Raschbaum

RF, Mooney V (1994). Reported Pain during Lumbar Discography as a Function of Anular Ruptures and Disc Degeneration. A Re-Analysis of 833 Discograms. Spine 17:1968–1974

9. Vanharanta H, Sachs BL, Spivey MA, Guyer RD, Hochschuler SH, Rashbaum RF, Johnson RG, Ohnmeiss D, Mooney V (1987) The Relationship of Pain Provocation to Lumbar Disc Deterioration as Seen by CT/Discography. Spine 12:295–298

Lumbar Epidural Steroids

▶ Epidural Steroid Injections

Lumbar Facet Denervation

▶ Lumbar Medial Branch Neurotomy

Lumbar Facet Rhizolysis

▶ Lumbar Medial Branch Neurotomy

Lumbar Lordosis

Definition

The lumbar lordosis is the anterior concavity in the curvature of the lumbar spine as viewed from the side.
▶ Lumbar Traction

Lumbar Medial Branch Blocks

PAUL VERRILLS
Metropolitan Spinal Clinic, Prahran, VIC, Australia
verrills@bigpond.net.au

Definition

Lumbar medial branch blocks are a diagnostic procedure used to determine if a patient's pain arises from a lumbar zygapophysial joint. They involve anaesthetising the nerves that innervate the joint or joints suspected of being the source of pain.

Characteristics

The lumbar zygapophysial joints are a common source of chronic low back pain. In younger aged, injured workers with chronic low back pain the prevalence of lumbar zygapophysial joint pain is about 15% (Schwarzer et al. 1994). In older, non-injured patients, the prevalence may be as high as 40% (Schwarzer et al. 1995). This pain, however, cannot be diagnosed by ▶ medical history, ▶ musculoskeletal examination, or medical imaging. Diagnostic blocks are the only means by which to establish the ▶ diagnosis.

Validity

Although lumbar zygapophysial joint pain can be diagnosed by intra-articular blocks, that type of block has not been validated. Nor have they been shown to have therapeutic utility. In contrast, ▶ lumbar medial branch blocks have been validated.

Of the structures innervated by the medial branches of the lumbar dorsal rami, the zygapophysial joints are the only ones known to be possible sources of chronic pain. There is no evidence to support the competing proposition, that chronic pain can arise from the specific segments of the muscles innervated by individual medial branches (Bogduk et al. 1982).

Lumbar medial branch blocks are target specific, provided that precise target points are accurately accessed with needles introduced under fluoroscopic control (Dreyfuss et al. 1997). That is, structures other than the targeted nerves are not anaesthetised by lumbar medial branch blocks.

In 89% of cases, normal volunteers are protected from experimentally induced lumbar zygapophysial joint pain if the appropriate medial branches are anaesthetised (Kaplan et al. 1998). The 11% false-negative rate may be due local vascular puncture and repositioning of the needle (Kaplan et al. 1998).

Lumbar medial branch blocks are preferable to performing intra-articular injections, as they are easier to perform, safer and more expedient. They are also more easily subjected to pharmacological controls.

Medial branch blocks do have therapeutic utility, for they lead to the target–specific treatment of ▶ radiofrequency neurotomy, which has independently been validated as appropriate treatment for lumbar zygapophysial joint pain.

Control Blocks

Control blocks are essential to minimise false-positive responses. To this end, comparative local anaesthetic blocks are used with a short-acting and a long-acting agent (Barnsley et al. 1993, Lord et al. 1995, International Spine Intervention Society 2004). In clinical practice, these would be lidocaine 2% and bupivacaine 0.5%.

A concordant response would be that the patient reports complete relief of pain for a shorter duration when the short-acting agent is used, and a longer duration of relief when the long-acting agent is used (see ▶ Peripheral Nerve Blocks). These criteria provide for a highly specific diagnosis of zygapophysial joint pain, but may lack sensitivity. Due to the paradoxically prolonged durations of action of lignocaine, some patients with genuine zygapophysial joint pain may be excluded if these criteria are applied.

More generous criteria would require complete relief of pain on each of the two occasions that the nerves are blocked, irrespective of the duration of relief obtained. These criteria will result in a higher sensitivity but a lesser specificity, i.e. more patients will be diagnosed as having zygapophysial joint pain, but this will include false-positive cases. Since the treatment of lumbar zygapophysial joint pain is considered safe and otherwise relatively innocuous, false-positive responses are tolerable. Patients are not put at risk, for lack of a correct diagnosis, but may fail to benefit from the treatment. Although placebo-controlled blocks would secure the most valid results, they require three blocks (Lord et al. 1995, International Spine Intervention Society 2004), and are not readily implemented in conventional practice. Meanwhile, comparative local anaesthetic blocks have been shown to be cost-effective (Bogduk and Holmes 2000).

Patient Selection

Medial branch blocks are not indicated for acute pain. They are appropriate only for patients with persisting low back pain, for whom a diagnosis is required. A fundamental prerequisite is that serious possible causes of back pain, such as infection, tumours, vascular disease and metabolic disease, have been excluded by careful and thorough ► medical history, ► musculoskeletal examination, ► neurological examination, laboratory tests, and medical imaging if necessary. The working diagnosis should be that of lumbar spinal pain of unknown origin.

Contraindications

Absolute contra-indications include bacterial infection, either systemic or localised, in the region that blocks are to be performed, bleeding diatheses or possible pregnancy. Relative contra-indications include allergy to contrast media or local anaesthetics.

Technique

The patient lies prone, and the target points are identified under a C–arm fluoroscope. The target points for the L1 to L4 medial branches are best approached from an oblique view. They lie where the target nerve crosses the junction of the superior articular process and the transverse process, midway between the superior border of the transverse process and the location of the mamillo-accessory notch (Fig. 1).

Correct placement of the needle is confirmed by obtaining a posterior anterior view. A small dose of contrast medium is injected to ensure that there is no venous uptake. Following this, 0.3 ml of local anaesthetic is injected onto the target nerve.

At the L5 level, it is the dorsal ramus proper that is blocked. The target point lies opposite the middle of the base of the superior articular process, and, hence, slightly below the silhouette of the top of the ala of the sacrum. An injection point higher or lower than this has an increased risk of foraminal or epidural spread. (Dreyfuss et al. 1997).

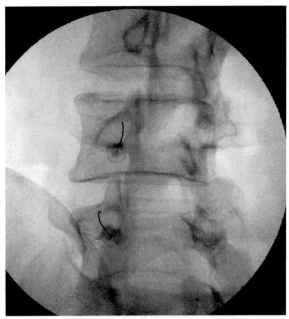

Lumbar Medial Branch Blocks, Figure 1 An oblique view of the lumbar spine, showing needles in correct position on the roots of the L4 and L5 transverse processes, to block the L3 and L4 medial branches. Reproduced, courtesy of the International Spinal Intervention Society (2004).

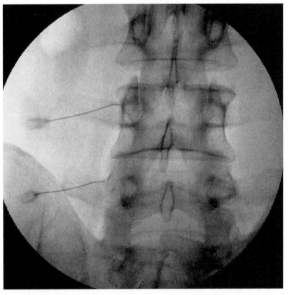

Lumbar Medial Branch Blocks, Figure 2 A postero-anterior view of the lumbar spine, showing needles in correct position on the roots of the L4 and L5 transverse process, to block the L3 and L4 medial branches. Reproduced, courtesy of the International Spinal Intervention Society (2004).

Each zygapophysial joint is innervated from above and below by the medial branch of dorsal rami. Therefore, two nerves need to be blocked for any one joint. For example, an L4 medial branch and L5 dorsal ramus block, anaesthetises the L5/S1 zygapophysial joint; an L3 and L4 medial branch block, anaesthetises the L4/5 zygapophysial joint.

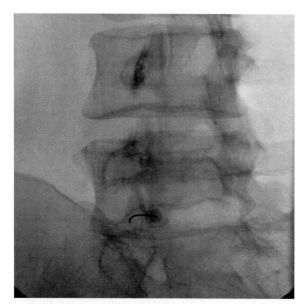

Lumbar Medial Branch Blocks, Figure 3 An oblique view of the lumbar spine, showing a needle in correct position on the ala of the sacrum, to block the L5 dorsal ramus. Reproduced, courtesy of the International Spinal Intervention Society (2004).

Evaluation

The optimal means of reducing error and securing reliable diagnostic information is real time assessment. The response to the diagnostic block is evaluated immediately after the block, and for some time afterwards, at the clinic at which the block was performed, and by an independent observer using validated and objective instruments or tools.

Visual analogue scores are recorded before the block, immediately afterwards, at 30 minutes and then hourly. The patient is instructed to monitor the extent and duration of any relief that ensues. Further, if relief occurs, the patient should carefully attempt movements and activities that are usually restricted by pain, to assess their response during the anaesthetic phase.

If the block is negative, then zygapophysial joint pain can effectively be ruled out at the level tested. It is, therefore, common to perform an initial screening block at the L3, L4 and L5 levels, either unilaterally or bilaterally, depending on clinical pain patterns. If such a screening block is negative, one procedure serves to rule out zygapophysial joint pain at the segmental levels most commonly affected.

If the screening block is positive, then further blocks can be undertaken to identify the particular segment or segments responsible. These blocks can target the L5–S1 joint, in the first instance, and subsequently L4–5, if necessary. If the patient has a concordant response for controlled local anaesthetic medial branch blocks, then the putative diagnosis of zygapophysial joint pain is confirmed and the patient can be considered for

▶ radiofrequency neurotomy treatment (International Spine Intervention Society 2004).

References

1. Barnsley L, Lord S, Bogduk N (1993) Comparative Local Anaesthetic Blocks in the Diagnosis of Cervical Zygapophysial Joints Pain. Pain 55:99–106.
2. Bogduk N, Holmes S (2000) Controlled Zygapophysial Joint Blocks: The Travesty of Cost–Effectiveness. Pain Med 1:25–34
3. Bogduk N, Wilson AS, Tynan W (1982) The Human Lumbar Dorsal Rami. J Anat 134:383–397
4. Dreyfuss P, Schwarzer AC, Lau P, Bogduk N (1997) Specificity of Lumbar Medial Branch and L5 Dorsal Ramus Blocks: A Computed Tomographic Study. Spine 22:895–902
5. International Spine Intervention Society (2004). Lumbar Medial Branch Blocks. In: Bogduk N (ed). Practice Guidelines for Spinal Diagnostic and Treatment Procedures. International Spinal Intervention Society, San Francisco (in press)
6. Kaplan M, Dreyfuss P, Halbrook B, Bogduk N (1998) The Ability of Lumbar Medial Branch Blocks to Anesthetize the Zygapophysial Joint. Spine 23:1847–1852
7. Lord SM, Barnsley L, Bogduk N (1995) The Utility of Comparative Local Anaesthetic Blocks versus Placebo–Controlled Blocks for the Diagnosis of Cervical Zygapophysial Joint Pain. Clin J Pain 11:208–213
8. Schwarzer AC, Aprill CN, Derby R, Fortin J, Kine G, Bogduk N (1994) Clinical Features of Patients with Pain Stemming from the Lumbar Zygapophysial Joints. Is the Lumbar Facet Syndrome a Clinical Entity? Spine 19:1132–1137
9. Schwarzer AC, Wang S, Bogduk N, McNaught PJ, Laurent R (1995) Prevalence and Clinical Features of Lumbar Zygapophysial Joint Pain: A Study in an Australian Population with Chronic Low Back Pain. Ann Rheum Dis 54:100–106

Lumbar Medial Branch Neurotomy

PAUL DREYFUSS
Department of Rehabilitation Medicine, University of Washington, Seattle, WA, USA
pauldspine@aol.com

Synonyms

Lumbar Facet Denervation; Lumbar Facet Rhizolysis; Lumbar Radiofrequency Neurotomy

Definition

Lumbar medial branch neurotomy is a treatment for low back pain stemming from one or more of the zygapophysial joints of the lumbar spine. It involves coagulating the nerves that innervate the painful joint, or joints, with an electrode inserted through the skin. A generator delivers a high-frequency electrical current to the tip of the electrode, which causes the tissues immediately around the tip of the electrode to be heated and, thereby, denatured. Back pain is relieved because nerves incorporated into the heat lesion are made to be unable to conduct nociceptive information from the painful joint or joints (see ▶ Radiofrequency Neurotomy, Electrophysiological Principles).

Characteristics

Indications

Lumbar medial branch neurotomy is not a treatment for any form of back pain. It is explicitly and solely designed to relieve pain from the zygapophysial joints. Therefore, the singular indication for the procedure is complete, or near complete, relief of pain following controlled, ► diagnostic blocks of the nerves innervating the painful joint or joints, i.e. ► lumbar medial branch blocks. These blocks must be controlled, because the false-positive rate of uncontrolled blocks is such that responses to single blocks will be false in up to 60% of patients, and those patients will not benefit from the denervation procedure (Schwarzer et al. 1994a; Bogduk and Holmes 2000).

Setting

The procedure is conducted in a procedure room equipped with a fluoroscope and the necessary apparatus to generate the heat lesion. The procedure is performed under local anesthesia, and no premedication or sedation is required. The patient should be substantially alert in order to report any problems that might occur which threatens their safety. Sedation would be indicated only if the patient is particularly anxious and cannot be relaxed by explanation and assurance; but in that event, the patient must nevertheless always remain conscious.

Typically, the patient will lie face down on a radiolucent table. The physician will cleanse the skin of the back. An x-ray will be taken, using the fluoroscope, in order to identify the target points at which the nerves will be coagulated.

Technique

Exactly what happens in the procedure depends on the type of electrode used. If a blunt electrode is used, the physician will first place a needle onto the target nerve as for a medial branch block. This is used to anaesthetize the nerve and the surrounding tissues, so as to render painless the heating phase of the procedure. That needle is left in place in order to guide the insertion of the electrode. If a hollow electrode is used, this first step can be circumvented, for the electrode can be used to anaesthetize the nerve prior to producing the heat lesion.

In order to maximize the effect on the nerve and to optimize the relief of pain, the electrodes should be inserted so as to lie parallel to the nerve. This requires inserting the electrode upwards and slightly medially through the skin and back muscles, until it reaches the target position. This lies on the root of the superior articular process (Fig. 1). Once the electrode has been correctly placed, the heating current is gradually increased by about 1°C per second. Raising the temperature slowly provides time for both the patient and the physician

to react if any untoward sensations arise. This could occur if the electrode has dislodged, or the target site was not adequately anaesthetized. The physician can respond before any injury occurs to the patient. Once a temperature of 80° – 85°C has been achieved, it is maintained for about 90 seconds to ensure adequate coagulation of the nerve.

Depending on the patient's anatomy, the physician may readjust the electrode to accommodate variations in the possible location of the target nerve, and will produce another lesion in that new location.

The procedure is repeated for all nerves that were anaesthetized, in order to produce relief of pain during the prior conduct of diagnostic lumbar medial branch blocks.

Variants

The optimal technique requires that the electrode be placed parallel to the target nerves (Dreyfuss et al. 2000). Under this condition, a maximal length of the nerve is coagulated, which produces a lasting effect on the pain. Some operators, however, use variants in which the electrode is not placed parallel to the nerve, but at some angle to it. This behavior can be traced to older versions of the procedure (Shealy 1975; Shealy 1976; Ogsbury et al. 1977; Mehta and Sluijter 1979; Sluijter and Mehta 1981; Gallagher et al. 1994), which were used before the nature of radiofrequency lesions was fully appreciated (Bogduk et al. 1987). These techniques are suboptimal, for they can fail to coagulate the target nerve, or coagulate only a small section of it. In which case, the nerve regenerates rapidly and pain recurs.

Efficacy

A controlled trial has shown that the effects of lumbar medial branch neurotomy cannot be attributed to a ► placebo response (van Kleef et al. 1999). When correctly performed, the ► efficacy of lumbar medial branch neurotomy is genuine.

Provided that patients are correctly selected using controlled lumbar medial branch blocks, good outcome can be expected from lumbar medial branch neurotomy. Relief of pain is not permanent. In time, the coagulated nerves regenerate and may again transmit nociceptive information from the painful joint or joints. The time that it takes for this regeneration to occur depends on how accurately and how thoroughly the nerves were coagulated. If suboptimal techniques are used, little of the target nerve may be coagulated, and it recovers rapidly. If a substantial length of nerve is coagulated, relief of pain may last up to and beyond 12 months. Pain may return gradually; it may not return to its former intensity. In some patients the pain never returns.

If the optimal technique is used, 60% of patients can expect at least 80% relief of their pain, and some 80% of patients can expect at least 60% relief of their pain at 12 months after treatment (Dreyfuss et al. 2000).

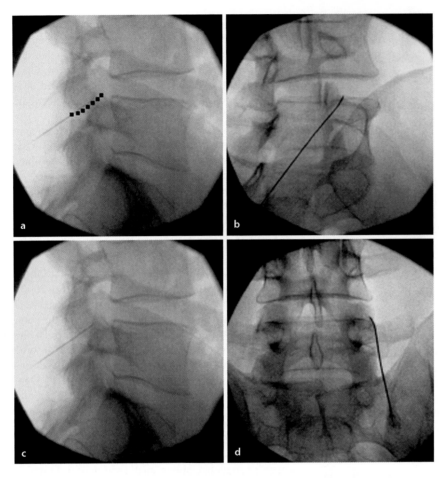

**Lumbar Medial Branch Neurotomy,
Figure 1** Radiographs showing an
electrode in position to coagulate
an L4 medial branch. (a) Lateral
view showing the course of the
nerve depicted by a dotted line. (b)
Oblique view. (c) Lateral view. (d)
Antero-posterior view.

If pain recurs, and becomes sufficiently intense again as
to warrant treatment, lumbar medial branch neurotomy
can be repeated in order to reinstate relief. Patients have
been successfully treated two, three, and more times,
to reinstate and maintain prolonged relief of their pain
(Schofferman, in press).

Complications

Provided that the correct technique is used, no complications are associated with this procedure. Such complications that are known to be associated with lumbar medial
branch neurotomy, incurred in medicolegal proceedings
but not published in the literature, have been due to mis-
placement of the electrode and the use of general anesthesia, which prevented the patient from reporting the
onset of complications.

Whereas it may be believed by some that denervating a
joint will create a neuropathic joint (Charcot's arthropathy), there is no evidence that this occurs, and no grounds
for believing that it would occur. Charcot's arthropathy
occurs in limbs that have been completely denervated,
in which potentially unstable joints are not protected by
muscle activity. In contrast, the zygapophysial joints are
intrinsically stable; they are stabilized further by the intervertebral disc, and most of the muscles that act on the
affected segment remain functional.

Utility

Lumbar medial branch neurotomy is the singular means
by which pain from lumbar zygapophysial joints can
be eliminated. No other forms of treatment have been
shown to be as effective for the treatment of proven lumbar zygapophysial joint pain. Given that the prevalence
of lumbar zygapophysial joint pain is about 15% in
some populations (Schwarzer et al. 1994b), and as high
as 40% in others (Manchikanti et al. 1999; Schwarzer
et al. 1995), this procedure has a possible application
in a substantial proportion of patients with chronic low
back pain.

References

1. Bogduk N, Holmes S (2000) Controlled Zygapophysial Joint
    Blocks: The Travesty of Cost-Effectiveness. Pain Med 1:25–34
2. Bogduk N, Macintosh J, Marsland A (1987) Technical Limita-
    tions to the Efficacy of Radiofrequency Neurotomy for Spinal
    Pain. Neurosurgery 20:529–535.
3. Dreyfuss P, Halbrook B, Pauza K, Joshi A, McLarty J, Bogduk N
    (2000) Efficacy and Validity of Radiofrequency Neurotomy for
    Chronic Lumbar Zygapophysial Joint Pain. Spine 25:1270–1277
4. Gallagher J, Petriccione di Valdo PL, Wedley JR, Hamann W,
    Ryan P, Chikanza I, Kirkham B, Price R, Watson MS, Grahame
    R, Wood S (1994) Radiofrequency Facet Joint Denervation in the
    Treatment of Low Back Pain: A Prospective Controlled Double-
    Blind Study to Assess its Efficacy. The Pain Clinic 7:193–198

5. Manchikanti L, Pampati V, Fellows B, Bakhit CE (1999) Prevalence of Lumbar Facet Joint Pain in Chronic Low Back Pain. Pain Physician 2:59–64.
6. Mehta M, Sluijter ME (1979) The Treatment of Chronic Back Pain. Anaesthesia 34:768–775
7. Ogsbury JS, Simon RH, Lehman RAW (1977) Facet Denervation in the Treatment of Low Back Syndrome. Pain 3:257–263
8. Schofferman J Spine (in press)
9. Schwarzer AC, Aprill CN, Derby R, Fortin J, Kine G, Bogduk N (1994a) The False-Positive Rate of Uncontrolled Diagnostic Blocks of the Lumbar Zygapophysial Joints. Pain 58:195–200
10. Schwarzer AC, Aprill CN, Derby R, Fortin J, Kine G, Bogduk N (1994b) Clinical Features of Patients with Pain Stemming from the Lumbar Zygapophysial Joints. Is the Lumbar Facet Syndrome a Clinical Entity? Spine 19:1132–1137
11. Schwarzer AC, Wang S, Bogduk N, McNaught PJ, Laurent R (1995) Prevalence and Clinical Features of Lumbar Zygapophysial Joint Pain: A Study in an Australian Population with Chronic Low Back Pain. Ann Rheum Dis 54:100–106
12. Shealy CN (1975) Percutaneous Radiofrequency Denervation of Spinal Facets. J Neurosurg 43:448–451
13. Shealy CN (1976) Facet Denervation in the Management of Back Sciatic Pain. Clin Orthop 115:157–164
14. Sluijter M E, Mehta M (1981) Treatment of Chronic Back and Neck Pain by Percutaneous Thermal Lesions. In: Lipton S, Miles J (eds) Persistent Pain. Modern Methods of Treatment, vol 3. Academic Press, London, pp 141–179
15. van Kleef M, Barendse GAM, Kessels A, Voets HM, Weber WEJ, de Lange S (1999) Randomized Trial of Radiofrequency Lumbar Facet Denervation for Chronic Low Back Pain. Spine 24:1937–1942

Lumbar Pain

▶ Low Back Pain Patients, Imaging

Lumbar Plexus

Definition

A network of nerves originating from the spinal nerves of the 2nd through 4th lumbar nerves. This network provides motor and sensory function to a large portion of the proximal leg, such as knee.

▶ Postoperative Pain, Regional Blocks

Lumbar Puncture

Definition

An invasive diagnostic test, in which a needle is inserted into the spinal column at the level between the 3rd and the 5th lumbar vertebra, to examine cerebrospinal fluid, and measure intracranial pressure.

▶ Headache due to Low Cerebrospinal Fluid Pressure

Lumbar Radiofrequency Neurotomy

▶ Lumbar Medial Branch Neurotomy

Lumbar Traction

JUDY CLARKE[1], ANDREA D. FURLAN[1, 2],
MAURITS VAN TULDER[3]
[1]Institute for Work & Health, Toronto, ON, Canada
[2]Institute for Work & Health, University of Toronto, Toronto, ON, Canada
[3]Institute for Research in Extramural Medicine, Free University Amsterdam, Amsterdam, The Netherlands
jclarke@iwh.on.ca, mw.vantulder@vumc.nl

Definition

Traction is one of a wide variety of treatments used for low back pain (LBP). Lumbar traction is applied to stretch the lumbar segment of the spine, generally by putting harnesses around the lower rib cage and around the iliac crest. Traction can be applied through different techniques. The forces can be applied using a motorized pulley (mechanical traction) or by forces exerted by the therapist (manual traction). There are also variations depending on how the forces are applied; the patient may control the forces by grasping pulling bars (auto-traction), traction may be performed with the patient fixed perpendicularly in a deep pool and grasping a bar under the arms (underwater traction) or traction may be given in the bed rest position with forces exerted by a pulley and weights (gravitational traction). Duration and level of force exerted can be varied and force can be applied in a continuous or intermittent mode. Only in mechanical and gravitational traction can the force be standardized.

Characteristics

It has been suggested that the mechanism by which traction works involves spinal elongation, which through decreasing lordosis and increasing intervertebral space, inhibits nociceptive impulses, improves mobility, decreases mechanical stress, reduces muscle spasm or spinal nerve root compression, releases ▶ luxation of a disc or capsule from the ▶ zygo-apophysial joint and releases adhesions around the zygo-apophysial joint and the ▶ annulus fibrosus (van der Heijden et al. 1995). Proponents of traction claim that LBP patients with radiating symptoms are the ones most likely to benefit from traction (Krause et al. 2000). Some also advise lumbar traction for muscle spasm using appropriately applied traction of adequate force (Geiringer et al. 1993). There is discussion about what constitutes adequate technique and forces for lumbar traction. It has been suggested (Beurskens et al. 1995) that forces below 25% of the body weight are ▶ placebo treatment, whereas others (Krause et al. 2000) argue that even low force traction can be expected to produce positive results.

L

Systematic Review of Lumbar Traction as a Treatment for LBP

A ▶ systematic review of ▶ randomized controlled trials (RCTs) involving traction was performed in order to determine whether this modality is effective for LBP with or without radiating symptoms. The review was an update of a previous review (van der Heijden et al. 1995) and was conducted under the framework of the Cochrane Collaboration Back Review Group. Detailed information on the methods of the review and the specific RCTs is available in the Cochrane Library (Clarke et al. 2006). The RCTs that were selected involved adults treated for ▶ non-specific low back pain (acute, sub-acute or chronic), with or without symptoms radiating below the knee (including radicular pain). Trials could involve any type of traction. The primary outcome measures were pain, global well-being, functional status and return to work. Reported side effects were also considered.

The methodological quality of the RCTs was independently assessed by two reviewers, using Cochrane Collaboration guidelines (van Tulder et al. 2003). Because the studies did not provide sufficient data to enable statistical pooling, we performed a qualitative analysis, summarizing the results of the studies in terms of the strength of the scientific evidence. "Strong evidence" indicates consistent findings among multiple high quality RCTs. "Moderate evidence" means consistent findings among multiple low quality RCTs and / or one high quality RCT. "Limited evidence" means only one low quality RCT. "Conflicting evidence" means inconsistent findings among multiple RCTs. "No evidence" means no RCTs. High quality studies were defined as RCTs that fulfilled 5 or more of the 11 ▶ internal validity criteria.

The systematic review included 24 RCTs, 17 of these involved patients with radiating symptoms and in the remaining eight there was a mix of patients with and without such symptoms. Seven studies included solely or primarily patients with chronic LBP (more than 12 weeks); in one study patients were all in the sub-acute range (4–12 weeks); in 12 studies the duration of LBP was a mix of acute, sub-acute and chronic; in five studies duration was not specified. In general, the methodological quality of the RCTs was low. Only five studies were classified as "high quality" studies.

For patients with radiating symptoms, the evidence indicated that continuous or intermittent lumbar traction is not better than placebo, ▶ Sham, no treatment or other treatments (e.g. spinal manipulation, exercise, corset or infra-red lamp). For mixed groups of patients (with and without radiating pain), the conclusions were the same as stated above; however the strength of the evidence was stronger due to more high quality RCTs in this group. In the trials classifying their control groups as "sham traction" the force applied varied from 1.8–9.1 kg or from 10–20% of body weight. No significant differences were demonstrated in any of these trials.

Although it has been argued that some subgroups of patients may benefit from traction, such as patients with acute radicular pain with concomitant neurological deficit (Krause et al. 2000), the preponderance of evidence on the efficacy of traction comes from studies with methodological problems and potential ▶ bias, which do not distinguish between subgroups of patients (for example, with differing pain duration and radicular symptoms).

Conclusion of the Systematic Review

Two recent high-quality studies have strengthened the findings that traction is not indicated in the treatment of LBP. Based on the RCTs currently available in the literature, there is moderate to strong evidence that traction is not an effective treatment for LBP patients, and some suggestion that patients receiving continuous traction are more likely to experience adverse effects, such as increased pain and subsequent surgery.

Regarding side effects, in our systematic review we found one study that mentioned there were no adverse effects, six studies reported some adverse effects (increased pain and more subsequent surgeries) and the remaining studies made no mention of this issue. However, most trials had small sample sizes that were not adequate to evaluate side effects. The few available case reports published in the literature suggest that there is some danger for nerve impingement in heavy traction (i.e. with forces exceeding 50% of body weight). Other potential risks include respiratory constraints due to the traction harness or increased blood pressure during inverted positional traction.

▶ Lumbar Traction

References

1. Beurskens AJHM, van der Heijden GJMG, de Vet HCW et al. (1995) The Efficacy of Traction for Lumbar Back Pain: Design of a Randomized Clinical Trial. J Manipulative Physiol Ther 18:141–147
2. Beurskens AJHM, de Vet HCW, Köke AJA et al. (1997) Efficacy of Traction for Nonspecific Low Back Pain: 12-Week and 6-Month Results of a Randomized Clinical Trial. Spine 22:2756–2762
3. Clarke JA, van Tulder MW, Blomberg SEI et al. (2006) Systematic Cochrane review of traction for low back pain with or without radiating symptoms. Cochrane Collaboration Back Group, Toronto, Ontario (submitted)
4. Geiringer SR, Kincaid CB, Rechtien JR. (1993) Traction, Manipulation, and Massage. In: DeLisa JA (ed) Rehabilitation Medicine: Principles and Practice, 2nd edn. JB Lippincott Company, Philadelphia, pp 440–462
5. Krause M, Refshauge KM, Dessen M et al. (2000) Lumbar spine traction: evaluation of effects and recommended application for treatment. Man Ther 5:72–81
6. van der Heijden GJMG, Beurskens AJHM, Koes BW et al. (1995) The efficacy of traction for back and neck pain: a systematic, blinded review of randomized clinical trial methods. Phys Ther 75:93–104
7. van Tulder M, Furlan A, Bombardier C et al. and the Editorial Board of the Cochrane Collaboration Back Review Group (2003) Updated method guidelines for systematic reviews in the Cochrane Collaboration Back Review Group. Spine 28:1290–1299

Lumbar Transforaminal Injection of Steroids

JAMES M. BOROWCZYK

Department of Orthopaedics and Musculoskeletal Medicine, Christchurch Public Hospital, Christchurch Clinical School of Medicine and Health Sciences, Christchurch, New Zealand
jmbor@clear.net.nz

Synonym

Transforaminal Steroids

Definition

Lumbar transforaminal injection (TFI) of corticosteroids, is a procedure whereby an aliquot of a given corticosteroid preparation is delivered into the immediate vicinity of a lumbar spinal nerve and its respective roots, by way of the corresponding intervertebral foramen. The procedure is designed as a treatment for lumbar radicular pain.

Characteristics

Background

The first description of the 'epidural' injection of corticosteroid was via the transforaminal route (Robecchi and Capra 1952). This became the standard route of administration in the 1950's and 1960's, but was superseded by the caudal and interlaminar routes in the United States and in Britain in the 1960's, and later in Europe and Scandinavia. These latter routes became the standard for common practice.

In the late 1900's, the beginning of a reversion to the transforaminal route was prompted by a number of factors. These include, among others; reviews suggesting that caudal and interlaminar routes were not as effective as had previously been claimed; an increasing use of transforaminal nerve root injection for radicular pain diagnosis; and subsequently, reports of successful outcomes for transforaminal injection in both observational studies, and later in controlled trials (Vad et al. 2002).

Rationale

There is circumstantial evidence that inflammatory processes may play a major role in the production of at least some of the clinical symptoms experienced when a lumbar nerve root is compromised by an intervertebral disc herniation (McCarron et al. 1987; Olmarker et al. 1995; Kang et al. 1995). Corticosteroid delivery to this site of putative inflammation then becomes a logical intervention. This offers a theoretical advantage, in that it targets the site of such inflammation, and may reduce the supposed inflammatory process, presumably through inhibition of phospholipase-A and cellular inflammatory mechanisms (see ▶ Radicular Pain). A competing interpretation is that the steroid preparation may exert a long-lasting local anaesthetic effect (Johansson et al. 1990) on the nerve root, and the dura that surrounds it.

Efficacy

Observational studies have demonstrated statistical benefits from lumbar TFI. With respect to the conservative and non-surgical management of radicular pain, several authors have reported a benefit from transforaminal epidural injection (Weiner and Fraser 1997; Lutz et al. 1998). Prospective, randomised, controlled, double-blinded studies have also suggested a surgery-sparing effect for lumbar TFI, particularly for the corticosteroid component of the injectate (Riew et al. 2000).

Indications

Lumbar TFI is advocated for patients with lumbar radicular pain:

- who require pain relief, and
- who have not responded to other non-surgical (conservative) interventions, or
- for whom other non-surgical interventions are deemed inappropriate, and
- whose pain may have an inflammatory basis

Patient Selection

According to the guidelines set out by the International Spinal Injection Society (2004), selected patients should have symptoms consistent with lumbar or sacral radicular pain that may be amenable to lumbar TFI. Specific signs and symptoms compatible with this include:

- Numbness or paraesthesiae in a dermatomal distribution
- Weakness in a myotomal distribution
- Inhibition of straight-leg raising to 30^0 or less

Additional confirmatory investigations should ideally include:

- Medical imaging demonstrating a cause of the radicular pain consistent with the clinical findings.
- Medical imaging as above that would theoretically be amenable to lumbar TFI.

Imaging findings which do not constitute intervention with LTFI would include:

- Tumour
- Angioma
- Cysts (with the possible exception of zygapophyseal synovial cysts)
- Arachnoiditis

Absolute Contraindications

- The (fully informed) patient is unable or unwilling to consent to the procedure
- The use of contrast media is contra-indicated
- There is evidence of an untreated localized infection in the procedural field

- The patient has a bleeding diathesis
- The patient is unable to co-operate during the procedure
- Adequate imaging of the target is difficult or impossible

Relative Contra-Indications

- Allergy to any of the administrable drugs
- Concurrent use of anticoagulants, or relative anticoagulants
- Anatomical or surgical derangements within the procedural field
- Systemic infection
- Significant co-existing disease
- Immunosuppression
- Pregnancy

Technique

Full details of the technique are provided elsewhere (International Spinal Intervention Society 2004). In essence, the procedure requires placing the injectate as close as possible to the target nerve.

This is first facilitated by visualising the appropriate intervertebral foramen under image intensification. Appropriate adjustments of the imaging apparatus are necessary to maximise the ease of approach to the injection site (International Spinal Intervention Society 2004). The point of needle placement should be in the so-called 'safe triangle' (Bogduk et al. 1995a; Bogduk et al. 1995b) (Fig. 1).

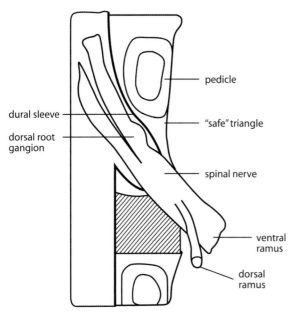

Lumbar Transforaminal Injection of Steroids, Figure 1 A sketch of a lumbar intervertebral foramen, showing the "safe triangle" in relation to the spinal nerve. Reproduced, courtesy of the International Spinal Intervention Society (Riew et al. 2000).

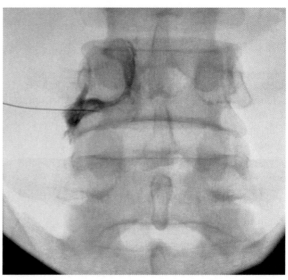

Lumbar Transforaminal Injection of Steroids, Figure 2 An antero-posterior radiograph of the lumbar spine showing a transforaminal injection at L4–5. Contrast medium outlines the course of the L4 spinal nerve and its roots. Reproduced, courtesy of the International Spinal Intervention Society (Riew et al. 2000).

Upon successfully accessing the target point, needle placement is confirmed by visualisation of the needle tip position against the posterior aspect of the vertebral body, in a lateral radiographic view. Proximity to the nerve is then confirmed in the AP projection by the injection of contrast medium so as to obtain a 'radiculogram', and to confirm that there is no intravascular loss of the contrast medium in 'real-time' imaging (Fig. 2). Having satisfied these criteria, the transforaminal corticosteroid injection may be placed.

Complications

Lumbar TFIs are subject to all the possible complications of trans-dermal injection procedures. These include infection, local bleeding, the puncture of adjacent structures, allergy to the various components of the injectate, and adverse vaso-vagal reactions of the injection recipient. With respect to the local anatomy, specific complications include epidural abscess, epidural haematoma, and puncture of the dural sac. Careful and aseptic technique will minimise these risks. Allergic reactions and induced haematomata remain a risk, even with careful patient screening and practised technique. Of the few studies reporting adverse reactions to the procedure, one cited non-positional headache in 4.8% of patients, increased back pain in 4.8%, increased leg pain in 1.6%, and facial flushing (thought to be due to the effect of the corticosteroid component of the injectate) in a further 1.6% (Botwin et al. 2000). Another report cited three patients who suffered paraplegia following the procedure, thought to be due to the inadvertent intravascular injection of colloid corticosteroid into a radicular artery supplying the distal end of the spinal cord (Houten and

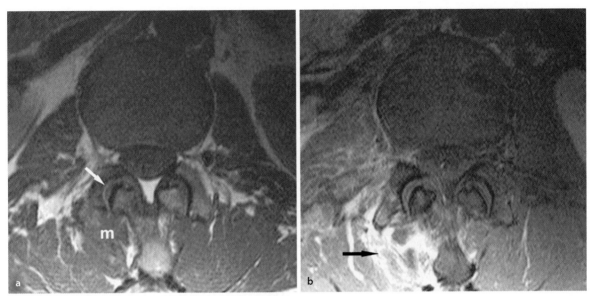

Magnetic Resonance Imaging, Figure 2   Axial MRI scans of a septic arthritis of a right L1-2 zygapophysial joint. (a) The joint on the right exhibits a slightly bright signal in its cavity (arrow) compared with the opposite side. In addition, the architecture of the multifidus (m) is distorted compared with the other side. (b) Administered intravenously, gadolinium enhances the oedema in the multifidus behind the infected joint, rendering it bright white (arrow).

M

reserved for research purposes, but recently, 3 Tesla units have become commercially available. The drive to higher field strength magnets is driven by higher signal to noise ratios and greater speed of imaging. As field strength increases however, safety issues increase. These include not only the need for greater magnetic shielding but also possible adverse biological effects, although to date, there have been no significant reported clinical side-effects. Body heating and possible superficial burns have been reported, but these have been attributed to faulty equipment such as surface coils and unsuspected internal metallic objects, rather than to the magnetic field itself (Shellock 2000).

Applications

Of all medical imaging tests, MRI has the highest sensitivity and highest specificity. It can detect lesions, such as tumours, infections and osteonecrosis, early in their evolution (Figs. 1, 2). Moreover, it allows these lesions to be specifically identified. No other imaging test has these properties. MRI defines soft tissue lesions as clearly as, or better than, ultrasound. For these reasons MRI has assumed a paramount position in imaging for general medical conditions. Its relevance in pain medicine, however, is more limited.

The cardinal application of MRI in pain medicine is as a screening test to detect occult or cryptic lesions that do not manifest distinctive clinical features. Such lesions, however, are unusual and rare. Consequently, when MRI is used as a screening test, the default expectation is that it will not reveal lesions. Under those conditions, MRI is used to clear patients of serious disorders such as tumours, infection or osteonecrosis.

In neurology, headache is a common clinical problem. Some 10–15% of MR studies are undertaken for headache but fewer than 1% of these investigations reveal significant pathology. Apart from tumours and infections, subarachnoid haemorrhage due to a leaking aneurysm in the circle of Willis can be demonstrated by MRI and by MR-angiography. This has the advantage of being non-invasive and avoids the complications of a more invasive procedure such as four-vessel cerebral angiography. MRI can be used to diagnose headaches due to changes in pressure of cerebrospinal fluid (CSF), benign intracranial hypertension, idiopathic low CSF pressure and post-traumatic CSF leakage.

In musculoskeletal medicine, MRI is the best way to detect osteonecrosis (Fig. 3). For this condition, MRI is both sensitive and specific and is able to detect changes earlier than plain radiography or CT or even bone scan. MRI is also able to measure the size of the osteonecrotic bone fragment.

Because of its better resolution of nerves and its ability to provide coronal and sagittal images as well as axial images, MRI is the preferred means of investigating radiculopathy (Fig. 4). The dorsal root ganglion, the spinal nerve roots and nerve-root sleeves can be clearly differentiated from the adjacent dura and the CSF in the spinal canal, making assessment of nerve root compression more reliable than is possible by CT.

Its ability to demonstrate the internal structure of intervertebral disks accords MRI a unique role in the investigation of chronic back pain. Some 30% of patients with low back pain exhibit a high intensity zone in one of their disks (April and Bogduk 1992). This zone is a bright spot located in the posterior anulus fibrosus (Fig. 5). The

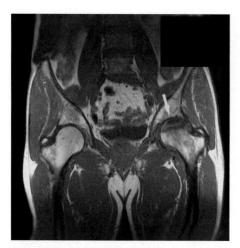

Magnetic Resonance Imaging, Figure 3   A coronal MRI scan of the pelvis and hips, showing avascular necrosis of the head of the left femur. The necrosis appears as a darkened area (arrow).

zone corresponds to a collection of fluid in a circumferential fissure crossing the posterior anulus and correlates strongly with that disk being the source of pain. When present, this sign has positive likelihood ratio of about 6 for incriminating the affected disc as the source of pain (Bogduk and McGuirk 2002).

For other lesions and abnormalities affecting the spine, the utility of MRI is far more questionable. Lesions such as disc bulges, disc herniations and degenerative disc disease occur very commonly in patients with no pain and increasingly with age (Jensen et al. 1994). Consequently, they are not diagnostic signs of back pain.

MR neurography can be used to enhance the appearance of nerves, such as the brachial plexus and lumbar plexus and large peripheral nerves such as the sciatic nerve, radial and ulnar nerves. However, unless there is gross lesion, such as tumour infiltration or neuroma, MR neurography has no proven role in detecting causes of pain arising in nerves.

The ability of MRI to resolve connective tissues makes it the premier means of assessing joints and periarticular structures. In some instances, MRI has an established and valid role. In others, the validity of various MR findings has not been established. In patients with chronic knee pain, MRI can detect meniscal tears, anterior cruciate or posterior cruciate ligament tears and is replacing direct arthroscopy as the preferred, primary diagnostic test. For the assessment of acute knee injury, a short MRI examination following radiography has been shown to save costs and improve quality of life after injury, in terms of time absent from work, additional investigations and time required to recover (Nikken et al. 2003). Although MRI can demonstrate the structure of the shoulder in great detail, tears of the rotator cuff and other lesions occur in totally asymptomatic subjects and increasingly with age. Therefore, demonstrating these lesions by MRI is not diagnostic of the cause of shoul-

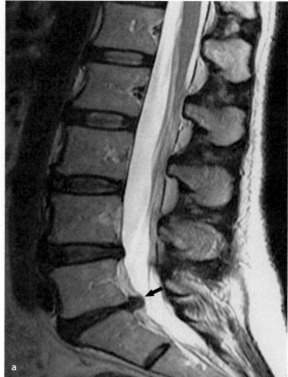

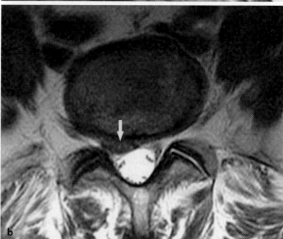

Magnetic Resonance Imaging, Figure 4   MRI scans of a herniation of an L5-S1 intervertebral disc. (a) Sagittal scan. The disc herniation (arrow) protrudes beyond the posterior margin of the L5 vertebral body. (b) Axial scan. The herniation (arrow) protrudes posteriorly to the right, towards the zygapophysial joint.

der pain. Pains in the elbow, wrist, ankle or foot are common problems encountered by sportspeople, either after acute injury or as a result of chronic repeated stress. In such individuals, MRI is being used increasingly to detect bone bruises and chronic enthesopathy or to rule out these conditions so that the athlete may resume activities.

Muscles pain and muscle imaging, however, remain an enigma. Signal changes, due to tissue disruption and

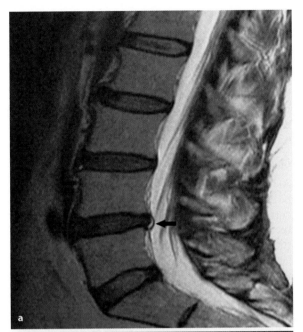

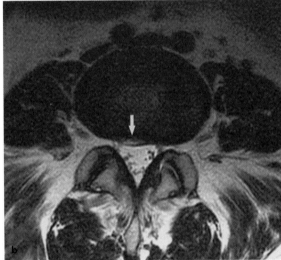

Magnetic Resonance Imaging, Figure 5 MRI scans of a high-intensity zone (HIZ) in an L4-5 intervertebral disc. (a) Sagittal scan. In T2-weighted images, the HIZ appears as a bright signal in the posterior anulus fibrosus (arrow). (b) Axial scan. The HIZ corresponds to a circumferential tear (arrow), which appears as a bright crescentic signal in the posterior anulus.

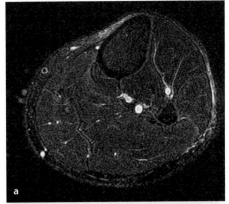

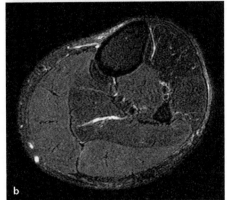

Magnetic Resonance Imaging, Figure 6 Axial MRI scans of the calf showing the effects of strenuous exercise. (a) Before exercise. (b) After exercise. The gastrocnemius muscles exhibit a faint increase in signal intensity, making them appear slightly whiter than the soleus and anterior tibial muscles and whiter than they were before exercise.

oedema, can be seen in patients with muscle strains or tears or with overuse and compartment syndromes (Fig. 6). However, no role for MRI has been established for more common entities such as myofascial pain and fibromyalgia. No features have been identified that allow these conditions to be diagnosed or studied by MRI.

There is work in progress on MR elastography (MRE), which may throw some imaging light on the elastic biomechanical property of muscles in health and disease. MRE is a non-invasive, phase-contrast MRI technique used to spatially map and measure displacement patterns in the muscle fibres in response to an external harmonic shear wave. Amplitude changes are detectable at the level of microns or less.

▶ Amygdala, Pain Processing and Behavior in Animals
▶ fMRI
▶ Headache Due to Arteritis
▶ Motor Cortex (M1)
▶ Secondary Somatosensory Cortex (S2) and Insula, Effect on Pain Related Behavior in Animals and Humans

References

1. April C, Bogduk N (1992) High intensity zone: a diagnostic sign of painful lumbar disc on magnetic resonance imaging. Br J Radiol 65:361–369
2. Bogduk N, McGuirk (2002) Medical Management of Acute and Chronic Low Back Pain. An Evidence Based Approach. Elsevier, Amsterdam, p 136
3. Jensen MC, Brant-Zawadzki MN, Modic MT et al. (1994) Magnetic resonance imaging of the lumbar spine in people without back pain. N Eng J Med 331:69–73
4. Nikken J, Edwin O, Hunink M (2003) A short low-field MRI examination in all patients with recent peripheral joint injury: is it worth the costs? 89th Annual Meeting of the Radiological Society of North America. Chicago, Illinois, November 2003
5. Shellock FG (2000) Radiofrequency energy-induced heating during MR procedures: a review. J Magn Res Imag 12:30–36

Magnetoencephalography

Synonyms

MEG

Definition

Synchronized extracellular currents in a few square centimeters of cortex generate magnetic fields measurable with sensors on the surface of the scalp. The biggest advantage of MEG, as compared with electroencephalography (EEG), is its high spatial resolution due to less of an effect of cerebrospinal fluid, skull and skin, since magnetic fields are not affected by electric current conductivity.

▶ Insular Cortex, Neurophysiology and Functional Imaging of Nociceptive Processing
▶ Magnetoencephalography in Assessment of Pain in Humans
▶ Thalamotomy for Human Pain Relief

Magnetoencephalography in Assessment of Pain in Humans

RYUSUKE KAKIGI, KOJI INUI,
MINORU HOSHIYAMA, SHOKO WATANABE,
DAISUKE NAKA, KENSAKU MIKI,
HIROSHI YAMASAKI, DIEP TUAN TRAN,
YUNHAI QIU, XIAOHONG WANG
Department of Integrative Physiology, National
Institute for Physiological Sciences, Okazaki, Japan
kakigi@nips.ac.jp

Synonyms

Topography; Source Analysis; magnetoencephalogram; Superconducting Quantum Interference Device; Gradiometer; Biomagnetometer; Magnetometer

Definition

Cortical neurons are excited by the signals conducted through thalamo-cortical fibers from the thalamus. After signals are received, electric currents are conducted through apical dendrites of pyramidal cells of the cerebral cortex. The electric currents generate magnetic fields. The electric currents are recorded as electroencephalography (EEG) and magnetic fields are recorded as ▶ magnetoencephalography (MEG). There are two kinds of postsynaptic potentials (PSP), excitatory ones (EPSP) and inhibitory ones (IPSP). EPSP are considered to be the main generators for both EEG and MEG. There are two kinds of cellular currents, intra-cellular and extra-cellular. MEG mainly records intra-cellular currents. EEG records both, but mainly extra-cellular currents.

To record clear MEG, at least 20000 or 30000 neurons must be activated simultaneously, which causes the same directed intra-cellular currents. A summation of the currents of many neurons with the same positive-negative direction can be mimicked as one strong dipole. Since it is easy and simple to imagine it present in the cortex, we hypothesized it by naming the ▶ equivalent current dipole (ECD).

Characteristics

At first, the advantages of MEG compared with EEG will be introduced. When electric currents generated in the cortex are recorded using scalp electrodes, there are effects of cerebrospinal fluid, skull and skin, whose electric conductivities vary markedly. In contrast, since magnetic fields are not affected by current conductivity, the recorded MEG is theoretically unchanged. Therefore, the spatial resolution of MEG is higher than that of EEG. The advantages and disadvantages of MEG compared with positron emission tomography (PET) and functional magnetic resonance imaging (fMRI) are listed below.

Advantages of MEG

1. Completely non-invasive.
2. Measures neuronal activity rather than blood flow changes or metabolic changes.
3. ▶ Temporal resolution is much larger, in the order of ms.
4. Stimulus evoked or event related responses can easily be measured in detail.
5. Frequency response (brain rhythm) analysis can be done, which means physiological changes can be analyzed spatiotemporally.
6. Results in an individual subject can be analyzed in detail, so that averaging results in a number of subjects is not necessary. In other words, one can analyze interindividual differences.

Disadvantages of MEG

1. Spatial resolution is lower than for PET and fMRI, particularly when the ▶ signal-to-noise ratio is low.
2. An inverse problem solution program is necessary. In other words, measuring results are indirectly or artificially induced.
3. The quality of algorithms (solution programs) is not good enough at present when multiple areas are activated simultaneously. Therefore, it is sometimes difficult to use MEG to analyze long-latency components mainly relating to emotional and / or cognitive functions. However, this is an endless game, since users always want new and improved software.
4. It is difficult to detect magnetic fields generated in deep areas. Therefore, the smaller the distance between activated regions and detecting coils the better.

5. It is impossible to record activities generated in white matter and pathways, since EPSPs are not generated there.
6. It is difficult or impossible to record activities in some regions such as the thalamus showing a so-called physiological closed field.
7. Activated location measured by MEG must be overlaid on CT or MRI, but the location can change, though the change must be very small.

Considering the advantages and disadvantages of MEG outlined above, the temporal characteristics of primary components just after the period when signals ascending through ► Aδ fibers and ► C Fiber reach the cortex are the best indication for MEG and later activities relating to cognition are mainly analyzed by PET and fMRI.

Methods

Various methods are used to record pain-related SEP and SEF (see review by Kakigi et al. 2000a,b; 2003a; 2005). The first study was reported by Hari et al. based on dental pulp stimulation (Hari et al. 1983). Then, CO_2 gas was applied to the nasal mucosa, a painful impact stimulation (Arendt-Nielsen et al. 1999), and epidermal electrical stimulation was applied (see review by Kakigi et al. 2000a,b; 2003a; 2005). Each method has its own advantages and disadvantages, but the ideal pain stimulation is pain-specific, controllable, safe and repeatable. At present, there are two main methods for recording pain-related SEP (SEF); (1) SEP (SEF) following high-intensity painful electrical stimulation (see review by Kakigi et al. 2000a,b) and (2) SEP (SEF) following painful CO_2 ► laser beam stimulation (see reviews by Bromm and Lorentz 1998; Kakigi et al. 2000a,b; 2003a; 2005). Since the latter method, which is usually called pain-related SEP (SEF), or laser evoked potential (LEP) or magnetic field (LEF), has several advantages as described below, it is more popular.

1. Other methods causing pain or heat sensation such as needle stimulation of the skin activate not only nociceptive receptors but also mechanoreceptors. Therefore, for example, the SEP waveform recorded following needle stimulation is very similar to that following electrical stimulation. In contrast, since a CO_2 laser beam is light, it does not activate mechanoreceptors of the skin, i.e. it is a purely noxious stimulation.
2. For analyzing temporal information in the order of msec, the time difference (lag) between the stimulus timing and the beginning of the sweep of the computer should be very stable and short, less than 1 ms. Figure 1 shows the procedure using our MEG device. A laser beam is applied to the subject's hand through optical fibers.

One interesting method reported recently is electrical stimulation of a very short needle, whose tip is located

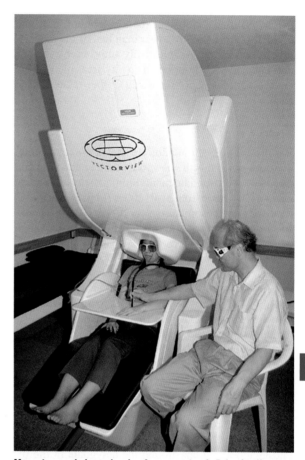

Magnetoencephalography in Assessment of Pain in Humans, Figure 1 The procedure using our MEG device (VectorView 306-channels, Elekta Neuromag Oy, Helsinki). The laser stimulator is set outside the shielded room because of its large magnetic artifacts and the laser beam is applied to the subject's hand through optical fibers. The laser beam can be applied any part of the body except the eyes, so both the experimenter and the subject must wear special glasses or swimming goggles.

in the epidermis where only free nerve endings are present, named ► ES stimulation (Inui et al. 2003a,b). The biggest advantages of this method are: (1) Only Aδ and C fibers are stimulated. (2) When the needle is inserted, subjects feel no uncomfortable painful feeling and show no bleeding. (3) Since a small intensity with a short duration is enough for recording Aδ fiber-related MEG, subjects feel only a tolerable jingling pain. (4) No special device is necessary except for a hand-made short needle, which is easily made.

One of the biggest recent topics in this field is the MEG response to the signals ascending through unmyelinated C fibers (see review by Kakigi et al. 2003a; 2005). Several methods have been reported to selectively stimulate C fibers, but they were difficult to record and the responses obtained were not consistently recorded. Our method was based on that reported by Brussels's group (Bragard et al. 1996). Since the number of polymodal receptors of C fibers relating to second pain is larger than

M

that of Aδ fibers, and since the temperature threshold of the former is slightly lower than that of the latter, C fiber receptors can be selectively activated by using a low-intensity CO_2 laser beam on tiny areas of skin. We made a new device for recording C fiber-related MEG responses.

Results

Results using ES stimulation are shown as a representative case, since it is the newest method in this field and the results were fundamentally similar to those obtained using a CO_2 laser (Inui et al. 2003) (Figs. 2, 3).

First, the primary somatosensory cortex (SI) in the hemisphere contralateral to the stimulation was activated, whose peak latency was approximately 100 ms. It is very small in amplitude and the generator is considered to be area 1 in SI. This long latency is, of course, due to the slow conduction velocity of Aδ fibers (10–20 m / s). Then, ► secondary somatosensory cortex (SII) and insula in the bilateral hemispheres were activated simultaneously as the primary major component, even after stimulation applied to other sites, i.e. bilateral function. Their peak latencies were approximately 150 ms, but ipsilateral responses were significantly longer than contralateral ones, probably through the corpus callosum. SI component in the contralateral hemisphere was also recorded by laser stimulation (Kanda et al. 2000; Ploner et al. 1999). Then, cingulate cortex and mid-temporal regions around the amygdala in the bilateral hemispheres were activated; peak latencies of the first negative and second positive components were approximately 200 and 300 ms, respectively. We believe that MEG is the most appropriate method for a detailed spatio-temporal analysis of these early activities within 300–400 ms after stimulation, which PET and fMRI cannot do.

Factors that Affect the Waveforms of Pain

One frequently sustains an injury while playing sport, but does not notice it until after the game. This clearly indicates that psychological conditions affect pain perception. These interesting findings were also confirmed by MEG (see reviews by Kakigi et al. 2000a,b; 2003b; Kakigi 2005; Kakigi and Watanabe 1996). When subjects paid close attention to a mental activity such as a calculation or memorization (distraction task), MEG responses, particularly the later components generated in limbic systems, were much reduced in amplitude or disappeared and a mental pain rating (► visual analogue scale, VAS) showed a positive correlation with the MEG changes. In contrast, early responses in SI and SII were reduced but still present. Therefore, early components seem important for primary functions such as the localization of stimulus points, but later components are very related to cognitive functions of pain perception. This pattern was more remarkable after C fiber than Aδ stim-

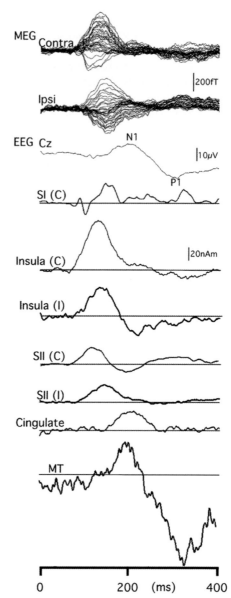

Magnetoencephalography in Assessment of Pain in Humans, Figure 2 MEG waveforms measured using the ES method (intra-epidermal electrical needle stimulation) for primary pain perception in humans by activating Aδ fiber stimulation. C and I: Hemispheres contralateral and ipsilateral to the stimulation, respectively. SI and SII: Primary and secondary somatosensory cortices, respectively. MT Mid-temporal region around amygdala. (Applied from Inui et al. 2003).

ulation. Therefore, second pain may be more related to cognitive functions than the first pain.

During sleep, we usually do not notice pain, unless it is very strong, so what happens in the brain while receiving painful sensations during sleep (see review by Kakigi et al. 2003b)? Most of the MEG responses, particularly later components, were much reduced in amplitude or disappeared. This finding is very similar to the changes in the distraction task, but more remarkable. Interestingly, MEG responses during sleep

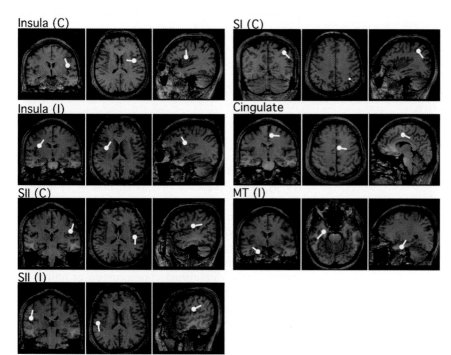

Insula (C)

Insula (I)

SII (C)

SII (I)

SI (C)

Cingulate

MT (I)

Magnetoencephalography in Assessment of Pain in Humans, Figure 3 Activated regions using the ES method (intra-epidermal electrical needle stimulation) for primary pain perception in humans by activating Aδ fiber stimulation. The calculated equivalent current dipole (ECD) of each region was overlaid on the MRI of this subject. See also legend of Fig. 2. (Applied from Inui et al. 2003).

M

to other modalities, such as touch, auditory or visual stimuli were enhanced, probably due to an inhibition of the inhibitory system while awake. Therefore, pain perception seems very different from other kinds of sensations.

MEG and EEG changes and VAS were also significantly reduced in amplitude by other kinds of sensations such as touch, vibration, cooling and movements (see review by Kakigi et al. 2000a; Kakigi et al. 2000b; Kakigi et al. 2003a; Kakigi et al. 2005; Kakigi and Watanabe 1996). The effects of pain relief by tactile stimulation applied to painful areas simultaneously is utilized in transcutaneous electric nerve stimulation (TENS). I think "movement" is most effective for pain relief, since we automatically move painful regions to reduce pain. For example, if we touch a very hot object with our hand, we involuntary shake that hand strongly. We are now trying to clarify the underlying mechanisms by MEG.

Clinical Application

Unfortunately, the clinical application of MEG for pain relief is not very popular at present. Most interesting studies were reported from Germany on MEG responses following tactile stimulation in patients with ► phantom limb pain after amputation (Flor et al. 1995). They confirmed a plasticity of the somatosensory cortex using MEG. These interesting and important issues are described in detail in another chapter.

The following 3 review articles are recommended on the basic physiological and clinical background of pain including MEG (Bromm and Lorentz 1998; Treede et al. 1999, 2000).

References

1. Arendt-Nielsen L, Yamasaki H, Nielsen J et al. (1999) Magnetoencephalographic responses to painful impact stimulation. Brain Res 839:203–208
2. Bragard D, Chen ACN, Plaghki L (1996) Direct isolation of ultra-late (C-fibre) evoked brain potentials by CO_2 laser stimulation of tiny cutaneous surface areas in man. Neurosci Lett 209:81–84
3. Bromm B, Lorentz J (1998) Neurophysiological evaluation of pain. Electroencephalogr Clin Neurophysiol 107:227–253
4. Flor H, Elbert T, Knecht S et al. (1995) Phantom-limb pain as a perceptual correlate of cortical reorganization following arm amputation. Nature 375:482–484
5. Hari R, Kaukoranta E, Reinikainen K et al. (1983) Neuromagnetic localization of cortical activity evoked by painful dental stimulation in man. Neurosci Lett 42:77–82
6. Inui K, Tran TD, Qiu Y et al. (2003a) A comparative magnetoencephalographic study of cortical activations evoked by noxious and innocuous somatosensory stimulations. Neuroscience 120:235–248
7. Inui K, Wang X, Qiu Y et al. (2003b) Pain processing within the primary somatosensory cortex in humans. Eur j Neurosci 18:2858–2866
8. Kakigi R, Watanabe S (1996) Pain relief by various kinds of interference stimulation applied to the peripheral skin in humans: pain-related brain potentials following CO_2 laser stimulation. J Peripher Nerv Syst 1:189–198
9. Kakigi R, Watanabe S, Yamasaki H (2000a) The pain-related somatosensory evoked potentials J Clin Neurophysiol 17:295–308
10. Kakigi R, Hoshiyama M, Shimojo M et al. (2000b) The somatosensory evoked magnetic fields. Prog Neurobiol 61:495–523
11. Kakigi R, Tran TD, Qiu Y et al. (2003a) Cerebral responses following stimulation of unmyelinated C-fibers in humans: Electro- and magneto-encephalographic study. Neurosci Res 45:255–275
12. Kakigi R, Naka D, Okusa T et al. (2003b) Sensory perception during sleep in humans: A magnetoencephalographic study. Sleep Med 4:493–507
13. Kakigi R, Inui K, Tamura V (2005) Electrophysiological studies on human pain perception. Clin Neurophysiol 116:743–763

14. Kanda M, Nagamine T, Ikeda A et al. (2000) Primary somatosensory cortex is actively involved in pain processing in human. Brain Res 853:282–289
15. Ploner M, Schmitz F, Freund HJ et al. (1999) Parallel activation of primary and secondary somatosensory cortices in human pain processing. J Neurophysiol 81:3100–104
16. Treede RD, Kenshalo DR, Gracely RG et al. (1999) The cortical representation of pain. Pain 79:105–111
17. Treede RD, Apkarian AV, Bromm B et al. (2000) Cortical representation of pain: functional characterization of nociceptive areas near the lateral sulcus. Pain 87:113–119

Magnetometer

▶ Magnetoencephalography in Assessment of Pain in Humans

Magnification

Definition

The tendency to exaggerate the threat value associated with a particular symptom, situation or outcome.
▶ Catastrophizing

Magnocellular Neurons

Definition

Magnocellular neurons are neurons with soma of a large size located in the paraventricular and supraoptic hypothalamic nuclei. These neurons synthesize vasopressin and oxytocin and transport them via their axons to the posterior neurohypophysis.
▶ Hypothalamus and Nociceptive Pathways

Maintenance

Definition

A readiness to change stage, in which a person has made a behavior change and has maintained that change for long enough that relapse is unlikely.
▶ Motivational Aspects of Pain
▶ Operant Perspective of Pain

Maitland Mobilisation

▶ Passive Spinal Mobilisation

Major Depressive Disorder

Synonyms

MDD

Definition

Major Depressive Disorder (MDD), as defined by the Diagnostic and Statistical Manual of Mental Disorders 4th ed. (DSM-IV)(American Psychiatric Association, 1994), is the presence of a collection of symptoms that must include depressed mood or loss of interest or pleasure in most activities lasting at least 2 weeks. Additional symptoms include fatigue, feelings of excessive or inappropriate worthlessness or guilt nearly every day, significant weight loss or gain, insomnia or hypersomnia, diminished concentration or ability to make decisions, frequent thoughts of death, suicidal ideation or suicide attempt. In order to meet criteria for MDD, symptoms must cause distress or impairment in functioning.
▶ Depression and Pain

Maladaptive Coping

▶ Catastrophizing

Maladaptive Thoughts

Definition

Cognitions that interfere with successful coping and adaptation to noxious stimuli or aversive events, or contribute to inappropriate behavior.
▶ Multiaxial Assessment of Pain

Malalignment Syndromes

Definition

Malalignment syndromes are abnormal body alignments (for example, an abnormally pronated rear foot) thought to predispose overuse syndromes.
▶ Stretching

Malignant Bone Pain

▶ Adjuvant Analgesics in Management of Cancer-Rated Bone Pain

Malignant Bowel Obstruction

Definition

A mechanical obstruction of the gastrointestinal tract secondary to a malignant tumor that occurs in 5% to 43% of all terminally ill patients. The obstruction may be partial or complete and at one site or multiple sites, however, the small bowel is more commonly involved than the large bowel. It is associated with colorectal, pancreatic, endometrial, gastric, mesothelial, breast, and prostatic cancers, but may develop with any cancer predisposed to metastases to the gastrointestinal tract. Malignant bowel obstruction may occur secondary to extrinsic compression of the bowel lumen, intraluminal occlusion, intramural occlusion, intestinal motility disorders, and miscellaneous causes such as fecal impaction.

▶ Cancer Pain Management, Adjuvant Analgesics in Management of Pain Due To Bowel Obstruction

Malignant Pain

Definition

Pain associated with cancer.
▶ Cancer Pain
▶ Pain Treatment, Implantable Pumps for Drug Delivery

Malingerer

Definition

A malingerer is an individual who consciously and deliberately feigns incapacitation. Malingering is a form of fraud.
▶ Impairment, Pain-Related

Malingering

Definition

A conscious decision to deliberately fake or lie about having pain in order to fool someone.
▶ Credibility, Assessment
▶ Pain in the Workplace, Risk factors for Chronicity, Job Demands

Malingering, Primary and Secondary Gain

David A. Fishbain
University of Miami School of Medicine and The Rosomoff Pain Center at South Shore Hospital, Miami Beach, FL, USA
dfishbain@miami.edu

Synonyms

Sick role; reinforcers

Definitions

Primary gain (Fishbain 1994; Fishbain et al. 1995): A decrease in anxiety (gain) from an unconscious defensive operation, which then causes a physical or conversion symptom, e.g. an arm is voluntarily paralyzed because it was used to hurt somebody, thereby allaying guilt and anxiety.
Secondary gain (Fishbain 1994; Fishbain et al. 1995): The gain achieved from the physical or conversion symptom, which enables the patient to avoid a particularly noxious activity or which enables the patient to get support from the environment (gain) not otherwise forthcoming.
Malingering (Fishbain et al. 1999; Fishbain et al. 2002): It is the intentional production of false or grossly exaggerated physical or psychological symptoms motivated by external incentives (secondary gain), such as avoiding military duty or work or criminal prosecution and obtaining financial compensation or drugs.

Characteristics

Primary and Secondary Gain

Sigmund Freud was the first to define primary and secondary gain and apply these concepts to illness behavior, which was not medically explained. Since then, the concept of secondary gain has infiltrated the nomenclature of every medical specialty, usually being applied in case of medically unexplained symptoms, and/or illness affirming states. The following is a list of previously described secondary gains: gratification of dependency or revengeful strivings; fulfillment of needs for sympathy, concern, solicitousness, or attachment; maintenance of family status, love or domination; desire for financial rewards and to prove entitlement for disability; avoidance of hazardous work conditions; permission to withdraw from an unsatisfactory life or socioemotional role; need for the ▶ sick role; acquisition of drugs; manipulation of spouse; and contraception. It is not clear whether secondary gains are the same as reinforcers. Operationally, some are equivalent; the gain may be the reinforcer. Secondary gains, however, are the more unconscious motivation for the observed behaviors.

▶ Secondary losses has been described as follows: economic; inability to now relate to others through work;

M

loss of family life, social support, and recreational activities; loss of community approval and resultant social stigma of being disabled; guilt over disability; negative sanctions from family and those in the helping roles (e.g. doctors; and loss of a clearly defined role). In general, the secondary losses far outweigh the secondary gains. Yet, patients act in spite of this economy. This problem with the economy of secondary gains and losses is a direct challenge to the integrity of the secondary gain concept and its importance to some of the Illness Affirming States.

Scientifically, there are also major problems with the secondary gain concept. It is poorly defined and rests on psychoanalytic concepts, which are difficult to prove or disprove. Fishbain et al. (1995) recently reviewed the scientific evidence for this concept. They found that results of studies relating to this issue were in conflict, and many had methodological flaws relating to how the presence of secondary gain was established. However, the presence of a secondary gain agenda did change patient behaviors.

The secondary gain concept is also clinically abused. The presence of financial incentives, such as disability payments if associated with treatment failure, results in the accusation of secondary gain, which in turn is utilized as a rationalization for the treatment failure. Clinicians in this paradigm usually focus on the secondary gains and ignore the secondary losses. In addition, clinicians ignore two facts. The alleged presence of a secondary gain does not necessarily mean that the gain has had an etiological or reinforcing effect on the illness, and there is a significant amount of evidence that indicates that physician practices are influenced by secondary gain agendas (Fishbain et al. 1995).

Malingering

Malingering can be divided into the following types (Fishbain et al. 1999): Pure malingering is the feigning of disease or disability when it does not exist. Positive malingering (simulation) is the feigning of symptoms that do not exist. Partial malingering is the conscious exaggeration of symptoms that do exist. False imputation is the ascribing of actual symptoms to a cause consciously recognized to have no relationship to the symptoms. Dissimulation, also a form of malingering, is the concealment or minimization of symptoms for secondary gain reasons. Two other types of malingering may also occur: genuine symptoms formerly present may cease to exist but may be fraudulently alleged to continue, or genuine symptoms may be fraudulently attributed to a cause other than the actual one.

There are no reliability studies on malingering, as these can only be generated if someone admits to being a malingerer. This is rarely the case. As such, three unique approaches for the study of malingering/disease simulation have evolved. In the first approach, a patient suspected of malingering is assigned a task that impacts on this alleged impairment or symptoms. This task is such that the patient is forced to make a choice (e.g. the patient complaining of sensory loss will be asked to close his or her eyes and guess which hand was being touched for a large number of trials). This is called a forced choice technique. In this case the patient has a 50% chance of being correct if he has a sensory impairment. However, hysterical and malingering patients usually will perform at significantly below chance levels, indicating that they may be deliberately providing false answers.

The second approach involves a volunteer group performing a task such as completing a psychological test battery pretending to fake an illness (e.g. fake insanity). The resultant volunteer "faking scores" can be used in two ways. First, the "the faking scores" can be compared with normal scores for differences and for the development of a "faking" profile. Second, the "faking scores" can be compared with authentic patient scores for differences and perhaps for the selection of similar faking profiles.

The third approach involves actual patients. In this case, a patient or groups of patients are asked to complete a task (e.g. a psychological battery) in such a way as to simulate an illness.

These faking patient scores may then be compared with scores from a new group of patients for identification of similar or different profiles. Fishbain et al. (1999) recently reviewed these different approaches in reference to pain. Their findings/conclusions were as follows. Malingering and dissimulation do occur within the chronic pain patient setting. Malingering may be present in 1.25% to 10.4% of chronic pain patients. However, because of poor study quality, these prevalence percentages are not reliable. The study evidence also indicated that facial expression testing, questionnaire, sensory testing, or clinical examination were not reliable ways of identifying malingering. There was no acceptable scientific information on symptom magnification syndrome. Hand-grip testing using the Jamar Dynamometer and other types of isometric strength testing did not reliably discriminate between a submaximal/malingering effort and a maximal/best effort. However, isokinetic strength testing appeared to have potential for discriminating between maximal and submaximal effort, and between best and malingered efforts. Repetitive testing with the coefficient of variation was not a reliable method for discriminating a real/best effort from a malingered effort. It was concluded that as yet there is no reliable method for detecting malingering within chronic pain patients, although isokinetic testing shows promise.

A final issue relating to malingering is that of ► Waddell Signs. These are 8 physical signs frequently found in chronic pain patients. Historically, there has been disagreement on what these signs indicate. However, in a recent evidence-based structured review, Fishbain et al. (2003) concluded the following about Waddell signs:

- They do not discriminate organic from nonorganic problems
- May represent an organic phenomenon
- Are associated with poorer treatment outcome
- Are associated with greater pain levels
- Are not associated with secondary gain; and as a group
- Studies demonstrate methodological problems

In a further evidence-based review, specifically addressing the issue of whether Waddell signs indicate malingering, Fishbain et al. (2004) concluded the following: there is little or no evidence that Waddell signs are associated with malingering.

References

1. Fishbain DA (1994) The Secondary Gain Concept: Definition Problems and Its Abuse in Medical Practice. Am Pain Soc J 3:264–273
2. Fishbain DA, Rosomoff HL, Cutler RB, Rosomoff RS (1995) Secondary Gain Concept: A Review of the Scientific Evidence. Clin J Pain 11:6–21
3. Fishbain DA, Cutler R, Rosomoff HL, Rosomoff RS (1999) Chronic Pain Disability Exaggeration/Malingering and Submaximal Effort Research. Clin J Pain 15:244–274
4. Fishbain DA, Cutler R, Rosomoff HL, Rosomoff RS (2002) Does the Conscious Exaggeration Scale Detect Deception within Patients with Chronic Pain Alleged to have Secondary Gain? Pain Medicine 3:39–46
5. Fishbain DA, Cole B, Cutler RB, Lewis J, Rosomoff HL, Rosomoff RS (2003) A Structured Evidence-Based Review on the Meaning of Nonorganic Physical Signs: Waddell signs. Pain Medicine 4:141–181
6. Fishbain DA, Goldberg M, Rosomoff RS, Rosomoff H (1991) Chronic Pain Patients and the Nonorganic Physical Sign of Non-Dermatomal Sensory Abnormalities (NDSA). Psychosomatics 32:294–303
7. Fishbain DA, Cutler RB, Lewis J, Cole B, Rosomoff RS, Rosomoff HL (2003) Is the Location of Nondermatomal Sensory Abnormalities (NDSAs) Related to Pain Location? Pain Med 4:238–243
8. Fishbain DA, Cutler RB, Lewis J, Cole B, Rosomoff RS, Rosomoff HL (2004) Do Waddell Signs Indicate Malingering? An Evidence-Based Structured Review. Clin J Pain 20:399–408

Malnutrition

► Metabolic and Nutritional Neuropathies

Managed Care

Definition

A board term used to describe various health care payment systems that attempt to contain costs by controlling the type and level of services provided.
► Disability Management in Managed Care System

Management of Postoperative Pain

► Postoperative Pain, Appropriate Management

Mandibular Dysfunction

► Orofacial Pain, Movement Disorders

Manipulation Without Impulse

► Passive Spinal Mobilisation

Manipulation Without Thrust, Oscillatory Mobilisation

► Passive Spinal Mobilisation

Manual or Continuous Traction

► Lumbar Traction

Manual Therapy

Definition

Manipulation of body tissues to restore movement.
► Chronic Pain in Children, Physical Medicine and Rehabilitation

MAO

► Monamine Oxidase Inhibitors

MAPK

► Mitogen-Activated Protein Kinase

Marital Status and Chronicity

► Pain in the Workplace, Risk Factors for Chronicity, Demographics

M

Marstock Method

Definition

The Marstock method is a threshold determination protocol for the thermal senses. This is a reaction time-dependent protocol that was originally developed by Drs. Heinrich Fruhstorfer and W. Schmidt of Marburg, and Dr. Ulf Lindblom of Stockholm, hence the name.

▶ Threshold Determination Protocols

Massage and Pain Relief Prospects

MICHAEAL QUITTAN

Department of Physical Medicine and Rehabilitation, Kaiser-Franz-Joseph Hospital, Vienna, Austria
michael.quittan@wienkav.at

Synonyms

Effleurage; Petrissage; friction; Tapotement; vibration

Definition

The English word 'massage' is derived from the Arabic word "mass'h" which means to press gently. At its most basic, massage is a simple way of easing pain, while at the same time aiding relaxation, promoting a feeling of well being and a sense of receiving good care. Scientifically, massage may be defined as group of systematic and scientific manipulations of body tissues best performed with the hands, for the purpose of affecting the nervous and muscular system and the general circulation.

Although massage techniques may vary considerably between therapists, classical massage consists of a number of basic techniques that have remained essentially unchanged for centuries. Per Henrik Ling is considered the founder of modern massage and subsequently these techniques are referred to as Swedish massage. Five elemental techniques are used in classical massage named effleurage, petrissage, friction, tapotement and vibration. Specific purposes are attributed to each technique.

Effleurage

Effleurage (or stroking) is a deep stroking performed in the direction of venous or lymph flows. It is used to accustom the subject to the following massage procedures.

Petrissage

Petrissage (or kneading) is a deeper technique than effleurage and consists of repeated rolling, grasping and lifting. The technique is directed towards muscles and connective tissue.

Friction

Friction (or rubbing) should be done in a slow elliptical or circular movement with the fingertips or the thenar eminence. It is a deep penetrating technique to relieve trigger points. There may be pain from the application of deep friction massage so this technique is optional. It should not be confused with deep transverse frictions.

Tapotement

Tapotement (or hacking) is a series of blows that may also be described as slapping, tapping, clapping, hacking or cupping, depending on the positioning of the hands.

Vibration

Vibration (or shaking) consists of small tremulous movements with the hands and fingers and in some cases with a electromechanical device. The vibration is performed rhythmically in an attempt to enhance relaxation or stimulation.

Before initiating massage, the patient's individual preferences and responsiveness to touch and massage should be assessed. Cultural and social feelings towards massage should be considered, as well as the patient's ability to communicate concerns or express unwillingness to receive massage therapy. Deep transverse friction massage is a technique popularised by Dr. James Cyriax for pain and inflammation relief in musculoskeletal conditions (Cyriax 1975). It is a technique that attempts to reduce abnormal fibrous adhesions and makes scar tissue more mobile in sub-acute and chronic inflammatory conditions by realigning the normal soft tissue fibres. The technique has been advocated to enhance normal healing conditions by breaking cross bridges and preventing abnormal scarring. Its mechanical action causes hyperaemia, which results in increased blood flow to the area. Beside these classic techniques there are numerous other procedures claiming specific effects. Reflexologists propose that there are reflex points on the feet corresponding to organs and structures of the body and that pain may be reduced by gentle manipulation or pressing certain parts of the foot. Pressure applied to the feet has been shown to result in an anaesthetizing effect on other parts of the body (Ernst and Koeder 1997).

Characteristics

Analgesic Mechanisms

Classical massage is thought to improve physiological and clinical outcomes by offering the symptomatic relief of pain through different mechanisms. Massaging a particular area stimulates large diameter nerve fibres, thus mechanisms described by the gate-control theory. Additionally, a moderate elevation of serum beta-endorphin levels lasting 1 h after cessation of massage has been demonstrated (Goats 1994). Motoneuron activity may be attenuated during application of massage thus beneficially influencing the "pain-spasm-pain" cycle. It is noteworthy that massage both affects the motoneuron pool of the massaged muscles and lasts solely during application of massage (Dishman and Bulbulian 2001). It has recently been shown that intramuscular temperature in superficial layers of the m.vastus laterals is increased after application of massage, mainly due to mechanical manipulation of the skin (Drust et al. 2003). Blood flow is increased, predominantly by dilatation of superficial blood vessels. Vigorous massage techniques enhance these effects by additional histamine release, which may then last as long as 1 h (Goats 1994). Finally, massage promotes physical and mental relaxation contributing to pain relief.

Indications and Outcomes

Despite definitions described above, there have been many variations, with differences in masseur expertise and time of application. This lack of standardisation renders comparison of studies difficult. Nevertheless, massage has been increasingly investigated in the pain management area, for its potential to be a functional, nonpharmacological intervention for reducing chronic pain.

Back Pain

Massage therapy is among the most popular therapeutic strategies used by back pain patients. A survey of an urban rehabilitation medicine outpatient office in New York, addressing the use of alternative therapy and its perceived effectiveness indicated that 29% of the subjects had used one or more alternative medical therapies in the past 12 months and the most common therapy cited was massage (Wainapel et al. 1998). This evidence is confirmed by European data indicating that up to 87% of back pain patients received massage as one form of treatment (Wiesinger et al. 1997).

Until recently, massage was included in RCTs only as a control treatment for various physical treatments. These massage control treatments were poorly described and often involved superficial massage techniques, brief treatment sessions of 10–15 min or few sessions (<5) (for reviews see Ernst 1999; Furlan et al. 2002). Recent published trials therefore address the effectiveness of massage therapy for back pain. Preyde randomly assigned 104 patients with low back pain (lasting 1 week to 8 months) to comprehensive massage therapy including stretching exercises, soft tissue manipulation alone, remedial exercise with posture education and sham laser therapy. Over a 1 month period, all patients received 6 therapies. At 1 month follow-up 63% of subjects in the comprehensive massage therapy group reported no pain as compared with 27% of the soft tissue manipulation group, 14% of the remedial exercise group and 0% of the sham laser therapy group. Clinical significance was evident for the comprehensive massage therapy group and the soft tissue manipulation group on the measure of function (Preyde 2000).

Another RCT compared massage therapy with progressive muscle relaxation (Hernandez-Reif et al. 2001). Twenty-four adults with low back pain of nociceptive origin with a duration of at least 6 months were randomly assigned to a massage therapy or a progressive muscle relaxation group. Sessions were 30 min long twice a week for 5 weeks. By the end of the study, the massage therapy group, as compared to the relaxation group, reported experiencing less pain, depression and anxiety and improved sleep. They also showed improved trunk and pain flexion performance. Furthermore, their serotonin and dopamine levels were higher. The authors conclude that massage therapy is effective in reducing pain, stress hormones and symptoms associated with chronic low back pain. Finally, Cherkin et al. randomly assigned 262 patients with low back pain to receive therapeutic massage compared to acupuncture or self-educational material. After the 10 week treatment period massage was found to be superior both to acupuncture (function) and self education (function and symptoms). At 1 year follow-up massage remained superior to acupuncture regarding function and symptoms (Cherkin et al. 2001).

Cancer-related Pain

At present, evidence exists from multiple time series with or without the intervention that massage is beneficial in pain relief in cancer patients (Pan et al. 2000). In their review, Pan and co-workers identified two studies evaluating massage as single treatment for pain in palliative care patients and 1 study in combination with aromatherapy. In an unblinded randomised controlled trial, 28 patients (mean age 61.5 years) with cancer were assigned to either Swedish massage therapy or a visitor for 10 min. Men experienced immediate pain relief (VAS from 4.2–2.9, P <0.01), but this effect subsided by 1 h after the massage. There was no significant benefit in women (Weinrich and Weinrich 1990). In a case series, 9 male cancer patients (mean age 56.6 years) who received two consecutive 30 min evening massages reported significant reductions in pain as compared to baseline, lasting for 2 days. There was also a reduction in anxiety and enhanced feelings of relaxation (Ferrell-Torry and Glick 1993). In a case series involving 103 patients with cancer, a combination of massage and aromatherapy promoted pain relief in 33% of patients who completed the study (47%) (Wilkinson 1995).

Massage and Critical Care

A recent review identified as many as 19 research articles evaluating the effect of back massage on pain, relaxation and sleep in patients in various forms of critical care settings (Richards et al. 2000). The authors conclude that the most consistent effect of massage is a significantly decreased anxiety or perception of tension. Massage is therefore advocated as an effective treatment for promoting relaxation as indicated by significant changes in the expected direction in one or more physiological indicators. Additionally, massage was found to be effective in reducing pain. Further investigations of the beneficial effects of massage therapy comprise the incidence of chronic tension headache (Quinn et al. 2002) and post exercise muscle pain (Weber et al. 1994).

Contraindications and Safety Considerations

Massage is recognised as a safe therapeutic modality, with little risk or adverse effects. However there are contraindications such as applying massage over an area with acute inflammation, skin infection, non-consolidated fracture, burn, deep vein thrombosis or over sites of active cancer tumour (Vickers and Zollman 1999). Caution should be used in patients with advanced osteoporosis regarding applying only a little pressure on the tissue and the underlying bones.

References

1. Cherkin DC, Eisenberg D, Sherman KJ et al. (2001) Randomized trial comparing traditional Chinese medical acupuncture, therapeutic massage, and self-care education for chronic low back pain. Arch Intern Med 161:1081–1088
2. Cyriax J (1975) Textbook of Orthopaedic Medicine, vol 2, 9th edn. Williams and Wilkins, Baltimore
3. Dishman JD, Bulbulian R (2001) Comparison of effects of spinal manipulation and massage on motoneuron excitability. Electromyogr Clin Neurophysiol 41:97–106
4. Drust B, Atkinson G, Gregson W et al. (2003) The effects of massage on intra muscular temperature in the vastus lateralis in humans. Int J Sports Med 24:395–399
5. Ernst E (1999) Massage therapy for low back pain: a systematic review. J Pain Symptom Manage 17:65–69
6. Ernst E, Koeder K (1997) An overview of reflexology. Eur J Genl Pract 97:52–57
7. Ferrell-Torry AT, Glick OJ (1993) The use of therapeutic massage as a nursing intervention to modify anxiety and the perception of cancer pain. Cancer Nurs 16:93–101
8. Furlan AD, Brosseau L, Imamura M et al. (2002) Massage for low-back pain: a systematic review within the framework of the Cochrane Collaboration Back Review Group. Spine 27:1896–1910
9. Goats, G. C. (1994) Massage-the scientific basis of an ancient art: part 2. Physiological and therapeutic effects. Br J Sports Med 28:153–156
10. Hernandez-Reif M, Field T, Krasnegor J et al. (2001) Lower back pain is reduced and range of motion increased after massage therapy. Int J Neurosci 106:131–145
11. Pan CX, Morrison RS, Ness J et al. (2000) Complementary and alternative medicine in the management of pain, dyspnea, and nausea and vomiting near the end of life. A systematic review. J Pain Symptom Manage 20:374–387
12. Preyde M (2000) Effectiveness of massage therapy for sub-acute low-back pain: a randomized controlled trial. CMAJ 162:1815–1820
13. Quinn C, Chandler C, Moraska A (2002) Massage therapy and frequency of chronic tension headaches. Am J Public Health 92:1657–1661
14. Richards KC, Gibson R, Overton-McCoy AL (2000) Effects of massage in acute and critical care. AACN Clin Issues 11:77–96
15. Vickers A, Zollman C (1999) ABC of complementary medicine. The manipulative therapies: osteopathy and chiropractic. BMJ 319:1176–1179
16. Wainapel SF, Thomas AD, Kahan BS (1998) Use of alternative therapies by rehabilitation outpatients. Arch Phys Med Rehabil 79:1003–1005
17. Weber MD, Servedio FJ, Woodall WR (1994) The effects of three modalities on delayed onset muscle soreness. J.Orthop.Sports Phys Ther 20:236–242
18. Weinrich SP, Weinrich MC (1990) The effect of massage on pain in cancer patients. Appl Nurs Res 3:140–145
19. Wiesinger GF, Quittan M, Ebenbichler G et al. (1997) Benefit and costs of passive modalities in back pain outpatients: A descriptive study. Eur J Phys Med Rehabil 7 / 6:186
20. Wilkinson S (1995) Aromatherapy and massage in palliative care. Int J Palliat Nurs 1:21–30

Massage, Basic Considerations

SUSAN MERCER
School of Biomedical Sciences, University of Queensland, Brisbane, QLD, Australia
susan.mercer@stonebow.otago.ac.nz

Synonyms

Soft tissue manipulation; Classical Massage; Swedish massage; friction massage

Definition

Massage is the application of force, typically by the hands, to the skin, fascia and muscles of the body. Various techniques, e.g. stroking and gliding (effleurage), kneading (petrissage), tapping, clapping, percussion (tapotement), and deep friction that uses different rates and rhythm, direction, pressure and duration of movements are utilized in an effort to enhance circulation and remove waste products from the soft tissues of the body.

Characteristics

Mechanism

Massage therapy is believed to relieve pain by increasing local circulation, stimulating large diameter nerve fibers, stimulating the release of endorphins, decreasing muscle tone, normalizing the general mobility of muscles, tendons, ligaments, and fascia, reducing swelling and relaxing the mind (Ernst 2003; Furlan et al. 2002; Nicholson and Clendaniel 1989).

Applications

Massage is used for its psychological and physiological effects. Slow to evenly applied strokes of light to medium pressure are used in the direction of muscle fibers if general relaxation is desired. To stretch scarring in skin and subcutaneous tissue, moderate to heavy pressure in all directions is applied at a moderate, even rhythm. If the desired effect is to loosen or stretch connective tissue, a slightly less heavy pressure is applied more slowly. However, if adhesions in ligaments, tendons and muscle are to be broken, a heavy pressure perpendicular to the direction of fibers applied at a moderate, even speed is advocated. Here the therapist's fingers and the patient's skin move as one. To reduce swelling moderate to deep pressure is applied slowly and evenly in the direction of venous return. Tapping is used in desensitizing operative sites e.g. following amputation.

Efficacy

Massage is widely used in the general community for the treatment of painful conditions. It can be provided by professional, remedial massage therapists. Physiotherapists and osteopaths may incorporate it into their treatment regimens. Lay persons, such as spouses, may provide it.

Despite the popularity of massage, the literature provides little evidence of efficacy. Reviews have established that massage has little or no effect in relieving pain (Ernst 2004), headaches (Jensen et al. 1990), post exercise muscle pain (Ernst 1998); Weber et al. 1994), or acute, subacute or chronic low back pain (Ernst 1999; Furlan et al. 2002; Godfrey et al. 1984; Hoehler et al. 1981; Preyde 2000).

Side Effects

Incidences of adverse effects are unknown, but are probably low. Reports include fracture of osteoporotic bone, haematoma, peripheral nerve damage, and hearing loss typically associated with the use of too much force (Ernst 2003a; Ernst 2003b).

References

1. Cherkin DC, Eisenberg D, Sherman KJ et al. (2001) Randomized Trial Comparing Traditional Chinese Medical Acupuncture, Therapeutic Massage, and Self-Care Education for Chronic Low Back Pain. Arch Int Med 161:1081–1088
2. Ernst E (1998) Does Post-Exercise Massage Treatment Reduce Delayed Onset Muscle Soreness? A Systematic Review. Br J Sports Med 32:212–214
3. Ernst E (1999) Massage Therapy for Low Back Pain. A Systematic Review. J Pain Symptom Manage 17:65–69
4. Ernst E (2003a) Massage Treatment for Back Pain. Evidence for Symptomatic Relief is Encouraging but not Compelling. BMJ 326:562–563
5. Ernst E (2003b) The Safety of Massage Therapy. Rheumatology 42:DOI:10.1093
6. Ernst E (2004) Manual Therapies for Pain Control: chiropractic and massage. Clin J Pain 20:8–12
7. Furlan AD, Brosseau L, Imamura M et al. (2002) Massage for Low-Back Pain: A Systematic Review within the Framework of the Cochrane Collaboration Back Review group. Spine 27:1896–1910
8. Jensen OK, Nielsen FF, Vosmar L (1990) An Open Study Comparing Manual Therapy with the Use of Cold Packs in the Treatment of Post-Traumatic Headache. Cephalalgia 10:241–250
9. Godfrey CM, Morgan PP, Schatzker J (1984) A Randomized Trial of Manipulation for Low-Back Pain in a Medical Setting. Spine 9:301–304
10. Hsieh CY, Adams AH, Tobis J et al. (2002) Effectiveness of Four Conservative Treatments for Subacute Low Back Pain: A Randomized Clinical Trial. Spine 27:1142–1148
11. Hoehler FK, Tobis JS, Buerger AA (1981) Spinal Manipulation for Low Back Pain. JAMA 245:1835–1838
12. Nicholson GG, Clendaniel RA (1989) Manual Techniques. In: Scully RM, Barnes MR (eds) Physical Therapy. JB Lippincott, Philadelphia
13. Preyde M (2000) Effectiveness of Massage Therapy for Subacute Low-Back Pain: A Randomized Controlled Trial. Can Med Assoc J 162:1815–1820
14. Weber MD, Servedio FJ, Woodall WR (1994) The Effects of Three Modalities on Delayed Muscle Soreness. J Orthop Sports Phys Ther 20:236–242

Masseter Inhibitory Reflex

Definition

Reflex inhibition of the jaw-closing muscles (masseter, temporalis, or pterygoid) that appears as a double phase of electric silence during voluntary contraction, and is elicited by electrical or mechanical stimuli in the intra- or perioral region.

▶ Jaw-Muscle Silent Periods (Exteroceptive Suppression)

Masseter Muscle

Definition

The jaw-closer muscle. This muscle elevates the mandible for mouth closing and during chewing.

▶ Nociceptors in the Orofacial Region (Temporomandibular Joint and Masseter Muscle)

Masseter Silent Periods

▶ Jaw-Muscle Silent Periods (Exteroceptive Suppression)

Mast Cells

Definition

Mast cells are immune competent cells recruited to regions of injury including the skin. They are resident in most tissues and release proinflammatory mediators including NGF when activated.

▶ Nerve Growth Factor, Sensitizing Action on Nociceptors

Mastery Experience

Definition

Experiences that result in the elevation of an individual's assessment of his or her abilities in a specific skill domain.

▶ Psychology of Pain, Self-Efficacy

M

Mastitis

▶ Gynecological Pain, Neural Mechanisms

Matrix Metalloproteinases

Synonyms

MMP

Definition

Matrix Metalloproteinases (MMP) are a zinc- and calcium-dependent family of proteins that are collectively responsible for the degradation of the extracellular matrix tissues. MMP are involved in wound healing, angiogenesis, and tumor cell metastasis. An imbalance between the active enzymes and their natural inhibitors leads to the accelerated destruction of connective tissue, which is associated with the pathology of diseases such as arthritis, cancer, multiple sclerosis and cardiovascular diseases.

▶ Neutrophils in Inflammatory Pain

McGill Pain Questionnaire

RONALD MELZACK , JOEL KATZ
Department of Psychology, McGill University,
Montreal, QC, Canada
rmelzack@ego.psych.mcgill.ca

Synonyms

Subjective pain measurement; Pain evaluation; MPQ; SF-MPQ

Definition

The ▶ McGill Pain Questionnaire (MPQ) consists of 78 words, obtained from pain-patient interviews and the clinical literature, which describe distinctly different aspects of the experience of pain. The words are categorized into three major classes:

1. Words that describe the sensory qualities of the experience in terms of temporal, spatial, pressure, thermal, and other properties
2. Words that describe ▶ affective qualities in terms of tension, fear, and autonomic properties that are part of the pain experience
3. Evaluative words that describe the subjective overall intensity of the total pain experience.

Each class comprises several subclasses, which contain a group of words that are considered by most subjects to be qualitatively similar.

In addition to the list of pain descriptors, the questionnaire contains descriptors of the overall present pain intensity (PPI). The PPI is recorded as a number from 1 to 5, in which each number is associated with the following words: 1, mild; 2, discomforting; 3, distressing; 4, horrible; 5, excruciating. The mean scale values of these words, which were chosen from the evaluative category, are approximately equally far apart, so that they represent equal scale intervals and thereby provide "anchors" for the specification of the overall pain intensity.

Characteristics

The descriptor lists of the MPQ are read by (or to) a patient, with the explicit instruction that he or she choose only those words that describe his or her feelings and sensations currently, or during a specific period (such as "during the past week." Four major indices are obtained:

1. The pain rating index (PRI) based on the rank values of the words. In this scoring system, the word in each subclass implying the least pain is given a value of 1, the next word is given a value of 2, and so on. The rank values of the words chosen by a patient are summed to obtain a score separately for the sensory (subclasses 1–10), affective (subclasses 11–15), evaluative (subclass 16), and miscellaneous (subclasses 17–20) words, in addition to providing a total score (subclasses 1–20)
2. The PRI-corrected scores, using empirically determined scale values to enhance discriminability
3. The number of words chosen (NWC) in the word sets
4. The PPI, the number-descriptor combination chosen as the indicator of the current overall pain intensity.

Since its introduction in 1975, the MPQ has been translated into more than 25 languages. As pain is a private, personal experience, it is impossible for us to know precisely what someone else's pain feels like. However, the MPQ provides us with an insight into the qualities that are experienced. Recent studies indicate that each kind of pain is characterized by a distinctive constellation of words. There is a remarkable consistency in the choice of words used by patients suffering the same or similar pain syndromes, and there is strong evidence that the MPQ is a valid, reliable tool for ▶ pain measurement. The short-form McGill Pain Questionnaire (SF-MPQ) (Fig. 1) was developed for use in research settings when the time to obtain information from patients is limited, and when more information is desired than that provided by intensity measures such as the VAS or PPI. The SF-MPQ consists of 15 representative words from

▶ **McGill Pain Questionnaire, Figure 1,** The short-form McGill Pain Questionnaire. Descriptors 1–11 represent the sensory dimension of pain experience and 12–15 represent the affective dimension. Each descriptor is ranked on an intensity scale of 0 = none, 1 = mild, 2 = moderate, 3 = severe. The Present Pain Intensity (PPI) of the standard long-form McGill Pain Questionnaire and the visual analogue scale are also included to provide overall pain intensity scores.

SHORT-FORM McGILL PAIN QUESTIONNAIRE
RONALD MELZACK

PATIENT'S NAME: _____   **DATE:** _____

	NONE	MILD	MODERATE	SEVERE
THROBBING	0) _____	1) _____	2) _____	3) _____
SHOOTING	0) _____	1) _____	2) _____	3) _____
STABBING	0) _____	1) _____	2) _____	3) _____
SHARP	0) _____	1) _____	2) _____	3) _____
CRAMPING	0) _____	1) _____	2) _____	3) _____
GNAWING	0) _____	1) _____	2) _____	3) _____
HOT-BURNING	0) _____	1) _____	2) _____	3) _____
ACHING	0) _____	1) _____	2) _____	3) _____
HEAVY	0) _____	1) _____	2) _____	3) _____
TENDER	0) _____	1) _____	2) _____	3) _____
SPLITTING	0) _____	1) _____	2) _____	3) _____
TIRING-EXHAUSTING	0) _____	1) _____	2) _____	3) _____
SICKENING	0) _____	1) _____	2) _____	3) _____
FEARFUL	0) _____	1) _____	2) _____	3) _____
PUNISHING-CRUEL	0) _____	1) _____	2) _____	3) _____

M

NO PAIN |_____| WORST POSSIBLE PAIN

P P I

0	**NO PAIN**	_____
1	**MILD**	_____
2	**DISCOMFORTING**	_____
3	**DISTRESSING**	_____
4	**HORRIBLE**	_____
5	**EXCRUCIATING**	_____

© R. Melzack, 1984

the sensory (n = 11) and affective (n = 4) categories of the standard, long-form (LF) MPQ. The PPI and a VAS are included to provide indices of overall pain intensity. The 15 descriptors making up the SF-MPQ were selected based on their frequency of endorsement by patients with a variety of acute, intermittent, and chronic pains. Each descriptor is ranked by the patient on an intensity scale of 0 = none, 1 = mild, 2 = moderate, 3 = severe. The SF-MPQ correlates very highly with the major PRI indices (sensory, affective, and total) of the LF-MPQ, and is sensitive to traditional clinical therapies-analgesic drugs, ▶ epidural blocks, and ▶ transcutaneous electrical nerve stimulation. The SF-MPQ is now available in over 30 languages. A procedural model for testing the factorial validity of the SF-MPQ, which can be applied to translated versions, is provided by Wright et al. (2001).

▶ Amygdala, Pain Processing and Behavior in Animals
▶ fMRI
▶ Headache Due to Arteritis
▶ Motor Cortex (M1)
▶ Secondary Somatosensory Cortex (S2) and Insula, Effect on Pain Related Behavior in Animals and Humans

References

1. Melzack R, Torgerson WS (1971) On the Language of Pain. Anesthesiology 34:50–59
2. Melzack R (1975) The McGill Pain Questionnaire: Major Properties and Scoring Methods. Pain 1:277–299
3. Melzack R (1987) The Short-Form McGill Pain Questionnaire. Pain 30:191–197
4. Melzack R, Katz J (2001) The McGill Pain Questionnaire: Appraisal and Current Status In: Turk DC and Melzack R (eds) Handbook of Pain Assessment, 2nd edn. Guilford Press, New York
5. Wright KD, Asmundson GJ, McCreary DR (2001) Factorial validity of the short-form McGill pain questionnaire (SF-MPQ). Eur J Pain 5:279–284

MCID

▶ Minimal Clinical Important Difference

Mcl–1

Definition

Human myeloid cell differentiation protein, which is involved in programming of differentiation and concomitant maintenance of viability but not of proliferation. Isoform 1 inhibits apoptosis.

▶ NSAIDs and Cancer

MDD

▶ Major Depressive Disorder

MDdc

▶ Densocellular Subnucleus of the Mediodorsal Nucleus

Measuring Tools

▶ Outcome Measures

Mechanical Allodynia

Definition

Mechanical allodynia is the abnormal sensation of pain from usually non-painful mechanical stimulation and is elicited by, for example, lightly touching.

▶ Cancer Pain
▶ GABA Mechanisms and Descending Inhibitory Mechanisms
▶ Neuropathic Pain Model, Chronic Constriction Injury
▶ Neuropathic Pain Model, Partial Sciatic Nerve Ligation Model
▶ Neuropathic Pain Model, Tail Nerve Transection Model
▶ Spinal Cord Injury Pain Model, Contusion Injury Model

Mechanical Allodynia Test

▶ Allodynia Test, Mechanical and Cold Allodynia

Mechanical Effects of Ultrasound

Definition

The mechanical effect on the target tissue results in an increased local metabolism, circulation, extensibility of connective tissue, tissue regeneration and bone growth.

▶ Ultrasound Therapy of Pain from the Musculoskeletal System

Mechanical Hyperalgesia

Definition

An exaggerated response to a painful mechanical stimulus (e.g. a pin-prick producing severe or prolonged pain). A sign that pain pathways are functioning abnormally and may be damaged.

▶ Diabetic Neuropathies
▶ Freezing Model of Cutaneous Hyperalgesia
▶ Restless Legs Syndrome

Mechanical Low Back Pain

▶ Chronic Back Pain and Spinal Instability

Mechanical Nociceptors

▶ Mechanonociceptors

Mechanical Stimuli

Definition

Input produced by physical forces, such as touch, stretch, pressure, and vibration.
▶ Postsynaptic Dorsal Column Projection, Functional Characteristics

Mechanical Syndrome

▶ Lower Back Pain, Physical Examination

Mechanically-Evoked Itch

Definition

Sensation of itch produced by innocuous mechanical stimulation of the skin.
▶ Spinothalamic Tract Neurons, Central Sensitization

Mechanism-Based Approaches to Pain and Nociception

Definition

A therapeutic approach to the treatment of pain and pain syndromes that is based upon treatment of the underlying mechanisms, as opposed to an empirical approach based on symptoms. The prerequisite to this approach is: 1) knowledge of the mechanisms underlying the pain process or disorder in question; and 2) knowledge of the mechanisms of action of the therapeutic intervention proposed.
▶ Quantitative Sensory Testing

Mechanoheat Nociceptor

▶ Nociceptors in the Orofacial Region (Skin/Mucosa)
▶ Polymodal Nociceptors, Heat Transduction

Mechano-Insensitive C-Fibres, Biophysics

CHRISTIAN WEIDNER
Department of Physiology and Experimental Pathophysiology, University Erlangen, Erlangen, Germany
weidner@physiologie1.uni-erlangen.de

Synonyms

Action Potential Conduction of C-Fibres; Post-Excitatory Effects of C-Fibres

Definitions

Biophysical properties of nerve fibres comprise passive properties of the membrane and nerve (resistance, capacitance and derived measures like ▶ time constant) and active properties of membrane channels. For unmyelinated (C-) fibres i.e. nerve fibres with a functionally accessible receptive field *in vivo* and *in vitro*, these properties can only be derived from indirect measures e.g. with the teased fibre technique in animals or ▶ microneurography in humans.

Characteristics

Directly after an action potential, several phases of after-effects can be distinguished (see Fig. 1). An action potential is immediately followed by the absolute refractory period, which is determined by inactivity of most voltage gated Na^+ channels and a repolarising current through open voltage gated K^+ channels.

M

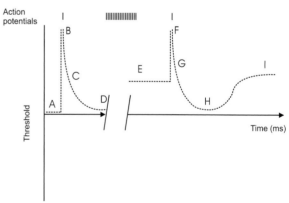

Mechano-Insensitive C-Fibres, Biophysics, Figure 1 Summary of after-effects. Threshold (inversely correlated to conduction velocity) of this exemplified nociceptive nerve fibre starts at an unconditioned level A, increases to an infinite level during the absolute refractory period B followed by a subnormal level during the relative refractory period C. Several seconds after the excitation there is still a remaining subnormality D which cumulates after a series of action potentials to a level E. Starting at level E an action potential of the accommodated nerve fibre again increases threshold during absolute (F) and relative refractory period (G). Thereafter a supernormal period H intermittently renders the nerve more excitable than before the respective action potential (level E) but never more than initially (level A). This relative supernormality is typical for human C-fibres whereas other species can also develop absolute supernormality (exceeding level A). Again a late subnormality I follows this activation.

Thereafter, during the relative refractory period action potentials can be induced at higher than normal stimulus strength and at lower than normal conduction velocity. The refractory periods together last at least 10 ms in all human C-fibre afferents without a difference between receptive classes. In other species they are shorter. After the refractory periods, a supernormal period might briefly turn a nerve fibre hyperexcitable and make action potentials travelling faster than initially. This supernormal period is not constantly observed but varies between species, fibre classes and state of ► accommodation of nerve fibres. While an absolute supernormal period could be observed in different species, in human C-fibres the observed supernormality has always been relative. "Relative" means, that cumulating long-term after-effects must have established an accommodation that slows down all action potentials of the ongoing stimulus train. If a conditioning stimulus is interposed at an inter-stimulus interval adequate to induce supernormality in the conditioned action potential, this supernormality can speed up the conditioned action potential as compared to the conduction velocity it would have had without the conditioning stimulus (relative supernormality). The initial conduction velocity prior to accommodation cannot be exceeded. The supernormal period is directly followed by the subnormal periods. On a cellular basis several subtypes of ► afterhyperpolarisation with different time constants have been suggested as a basis for the late subnormal period. For peripheral nerves, these types are intermingled and a separation using a pharmacological access has not been reported. However, the cumulating long lasting subnormality can most probably be equated with the slow AHP observed in central neurons.

Differences Between Human C-Fibre Classes

Biophysical and receptive properties of human afferent C-fibres are strongly correlated and separate two distinct fibre classes, the mechano-responsive (usually also heat responsive) fibres known as CMH fibres or ► polymodal nociceptors and the mechano-insensitive fibres, with two subclasses, heat responsive (CMi) and heat-insensitive (CMiHi).

Unlike other species, mechano-insensitive fibres of humans do not even respond to the strongest mechanical stimuli but can gain mechanical responsiveness as a result of primary sensitization ("waking up" of a ► Sleeping Nociceptor). Mechano-insensitive fibres have larger ► receptive fields (Schmidt et al. 2002) and higher heat thresholds than CMH fibres (Weidner et al. 1999), sensitise to tonic pressure (Schmelz et al. 1997), respond longer to ► capsaicin injection (Schmelz et al. 2000b) and are responsible for ► neurogenic inflammation (Schmelz et al. 2000a). These properties make mechano-insensitive human afferent C-fibres prominent candidates for an outstanding role in the development of chronic and pathological forms of pain. Besides these receptive differences the two fibre classes also differ with regard to their biophysical properties, in particular to the long-term effects described in the next paragraph.

Long-Term After-Effects

After-effects with time constants in the range of seconds are studied with repetitive pulse protocols. These effects are well known from animal experiments and good evidence is available that the threshold increase and conduction velocity decrease are equivalent measures (Raymond and Lettvin 1978). For experimental ease of assessment, all human studies use conduction velocity decrease as the measure. After the onset of a repetitive stimulation at a certain frequency or the increase to a higher frequency, the conduction latency increases until reaching a plateau. A frequency decrease leads to a velocity increase again. The time constants are in the range of 10–60 s. The amount of activity dependent conduction velocity slowing, but not the time constant clearly separates mechano-insensitive "sleeping" from mechano-responsive afferents (Serra et al. 1999; Weidner et al. 1999). Taking into account the difference in the unconditioned conduction velocities of mechano-insensitive (~0.8 m/s) and mechano-responsive (~1.0 m/s) afferents, the amount of conduction velocity slowing separates the two classes without overlap. A dissociation of these closely linked conductive and receptive properties in patients with pathological pain has been interpreted as "sleeping" nociceptors that "woke up", i.e. have been sensitised in the course of the disease and gained receptive properties like mechano-responsiveness while their conduction velocity slowing remained typical for "sleeping" nociceptors (Orstavik et al. 2003).

Different mechanisms that could influence or account for the accommodation of nerve fibres have been suggested. The Na/K ATPase activity should lead to hyperpolarisation of a nerve fibre and should be activated by Na ions that are brought into the cell by its activity. Hyperpolarisation in turn will slow down action potential propagation by increasing the difference of resting membrane potential and the activation threshold of voltage gated sodium channels. Therefore electrotonic depolarisation of the membrane in front of a fully depolarised (Na channels open) part of the axon will exceed the Na channel threshold over a shorter distance. The effect of ouabain, a blocker of the Na/K pump, on activity dependent threshold increase makes its contribution likely but not necessarily the only factor (Raymond and Lettvin 1978). Changes of K conductance can also modulate the resting membrane potential and have an influence on conduction velocity and activation threshold. An ► apamin insensitive Ca dependant K current is responsible for the slow after-hyperpolarisation (AHP) in central neurons (Wilson and Goldberg 2006). Furthermore the AHP itself can activate the inward rectifying Ih current carried by hyperpolarisation activated cyclic nucleotide gated channels (HCN) that have also been found in peripheral nerves (Takigawa et al. 1998). The Ih current counteracts the AHP and therefore limits the activity dependent conduction velocity slowing. Finally, geometrical reasons could also partly account for the observed differences in accommodation between mechano-responsive and mechano-insensitive C-fibres. The large receptive field of "sleeping" nociceptors is an indication of an extensively branched terminal arborisation with long and thin terminals. In thin fibres with an increased surface to volume quotient (it is indirectly proportional to the radius), all surface bound channels/pumps at a given density (parts per surface-area) will have a higher effect on intracellular concentration (parts per volume).

Short-Term After-Effects

Short-term after-effects with time constants in the range of milliseconds cannot be assessed with the above-mentioned method. The delay between conditioning and conditioned action potential must be in the same range. Therefore, a protocol with a stable ongoing frequency and interposed conditioning action potentials at varying inter-stimulus intervals can be used to assess short term after-effects (Weidner et al. 2000; Weidner et al. 2002; Bostock et al. 2003). Extracellular accumulation of potassium was made responsible for the supernormal period and could explain relative and absolute supernormality. In human C-fibres, however, another mechanism seems to account for the relative supernormality. After an action potential, voltage gated potassium channels repolarise the axon to the resting membrane potential. If accommodation has made the axon hyperpolarised, these potassium channels will only repolarise the fibre to the normal resting membrane potential but not to the hyperpolarised level prior to excitation. After closure of the repolarising potassium channels, the remaining repolarisation back to the accommodated hyperpolarised level is carried out by the "leakage" current, i.e. the current with all gated channels closed. It resembles the time constant to charge or discharge the membrane capacitor. No difference in the supernormal period and the underlying time constant of the axon could be observed for mechano-responsive or mechano-insensitive fibres with the provision that the same amount of accommodation is present. As described above, a higher stimulus frequency is needed for mechano-responsive fibres to yield the same accommodation as mechano-insensitive fibres.

Functional Implications

The most obvious implication of the long-term after-effects is the use dependent desensitisation of nerve fibres. If the threshold to induce an action potential as tested by external electrical stimulation is increased, all receptor potentials will meet the same increased excitation threshold. Paradoxically the maximum frequency that can be reached by a high frequency burst of an accommodated nerve fibre exceeds that in an unused fibre. This is because an unused fibre will only have subnormal after-effects delaying an action potential quickly following another. For an accommodated nerve fibre, the supernormal period can speed up a succeeding action potential. For a train of four action potentials at 50 Hz in the receptive field, this can lead to an "intraburst" frequency of 160 Hz at the knee level. This is an effective contrast enhancement mechanism.

References

1. Bostock H, Campero M, Serra J et al. (2003) Velocity recovery cycles of C fibres innervating human skin. J Physiol (Lond) 553:649–663
2. Orstavik K, Weidner C, Schmidt R et al. (2003) Pathological C-fibres in patients with a chronic painful condition. Brain 126:567–578
3. Raymond SA, Lettvin JY (1978) Aftereffects of activity in peripheral axons as a clue to nervous coding. In: Waxman SG (ed) Physiology and pathobiology of axons. Raven Press, New York, pp 203–225
4. Schmelz M, Schmidt R, Bickel A et al. (1997) Differential sensitivity of mechanosensitive and -insensitive C-fibers in human skin to tonic pressure and capsaicin. Society of Neuroscience Abstract 23:1004
5. Schmelz M, Michael K, Weidner C et al. (2000a) Which nerve fibers mediate the axon reflex flare in human skin? Neuroreport 11:645–648
6. Schmelz M, Schmidt R, Handwerker HO et al. (2000b) Encoding of burning pain from capsaicin-treated human skin in two categories of unmyelinated nerve fibres. Brain 123:560–571
7. Schmidt R, Schmelz M, Weidner C et al. (2002) Innervation territories of mechano-insensitive C nociceptors in human skin. J Neurophysiol 88:1859–1866
8. Serra J, Campero M, Ochoa J et al. (1999) Activity-dependent slowing of conduction differentiates functional subtypes of C fibres innervating human skin. J Physiol (Lond) 515:799–81
9. Takigawa T, Alzheimer C, Quasthoff S et al. (1998) A special blocker reveals the presence and function of the hyperpolarization-activated cation current IH in peripheral mammalian nerve fibres. Neuroscience 82:631–634
10. Weidner C, Schmelz M, Schmidt R et al. (1999) Functional Attributes Discriminating Mechano-Insensitive and Mechano-Responsive C Nociceptors in Human Skin. J Neurosci 19:10184–10190
11. Weidner C, Schmidt R, Schmelz M et al. (2000) Time course of post-excitatory effects separates afferent human C fibre classes. J Physiol (Lond) 527:185–191
12. Weidner C, Schmelz M, Schmidt R et al. (2002) Neural signal processing: the underestimated contribution of peripheral human C-fibers. J Neurosci 22:6704–6712
13. Wilson CJ, Goldberg JA (2006) Origin of the slow afterhyperpolarization and slow rhythmic bursting in striatal cholinergic interneurons. J Neurophysiol 95:196–204

Mechano-Insensitive Nociceptor

▶ Silent Nociceptor

Mechanonociceptors

ELVIRA DE LA PEÑA GARCÍA
Instituto de Neurociencias, Universidad Miguel
Hernández-CSIC, Alicante, Spain
elvirap@umh.es

Synonyms

Mechanical nociceptors; high-threshold mechanoreceptors; C-mechanoreceptor; A Delta(δ)-mechanoreceptor

Definition

Subpopulation of sensory afferents activated only by strong mechanical stimulation, most effectively by sharp objects.

Characteristics

Mechanonociception has been observed in organisms of various evolutionary levels: paramecium, worm, insects and mammals. In mammals, mechano- ▶ nociceptors are peripheral endings of primary sensory neurons that are activated only when harmful mechanical stimuli are applied to their ▶ receptive field, that is located in the skin, superficial mucosa and cornea (Belmonte et al. 1991; Burgess and Perl 1967), in deep tissues, such as joints and muscles (Mense 1977; Schaible and Schmidt 1983) and in the viscera (Cerveró 1994). The force necessary to evoke a nerve impulse discharge in mechanonociceptors is several orders of magnitude higher than the force required for the activation of low-threshold mechanoreceptors, which are the sensory ▶ receptors detecting innocuous mechanical stimuli.

Mechanonociceptor neurons have peripheral axons of variable diameter and degree of ▶ myelination belonging either to the thin myelinated, Aδ (conduction velocity: 2–20 m/s) or to the unmyelinated, C (conduction velocity < 2m/s) fiber type that end as naked nerve endings. Their somas are located in the dorsal root and cephalic sensory ganglia, and are in general of small diameter.

Mechanonociceptors were first described by Burgess and Perl in 1967 in recordings of single ▶ Primary Afferents/Neurons fibres innervating the hind limb of the cat. These authors reported the presence of fibres conducting between 6 and 37 m/s, which were classified as mechanonociceptors because they were activated only by damaging mechanical stimulation of the skin. Burgess and Perl observed that such fibres responded maximally to cutting or pinching the skin with serrated forceps, while noxious heat (50°), noxious cold (20°), acid applied to the receptive fields and ▶ bradykinin injected into skin did not excite this class of sensory afferents. Typically, their receptive fields were 2–5 cm long by 1–2,5 cm wide, and consisted of responsive spots (under 1 mm diameter) separated by unresponsive areas. An example of the ▶ discharge pattern evoked

by noxious mechanical forces in this type of nociceptor is shown in Fig. 1.

The classification of a peripheral sensory afferent as a mechanonociceptor, polymodal nociceptor, cold nociceptors or 'silent' (mechano-insensitive) nociceptor (see nociceptor, categorization), has been established experimentally by applying stimuli of different modality such as mechanical (pressure), thermal (heat or cold), and chemical (acid, inflammatory mediators) stimuli to the receptive field of the fiber. Often, the initial classification of a sensory afferent as nociceptive was defined by its response only to mechanical force of near injurious or injurious intensity. In most cases, strong heating was subsequently used to determine the ▶ polymodality of the nociceptive fiber. Nevertheless, in the skin, C- and A-delta fibres responsive to high intensity mechanical stimuli but also to strong heating, named respectively CMHs, and AMHs, have often been

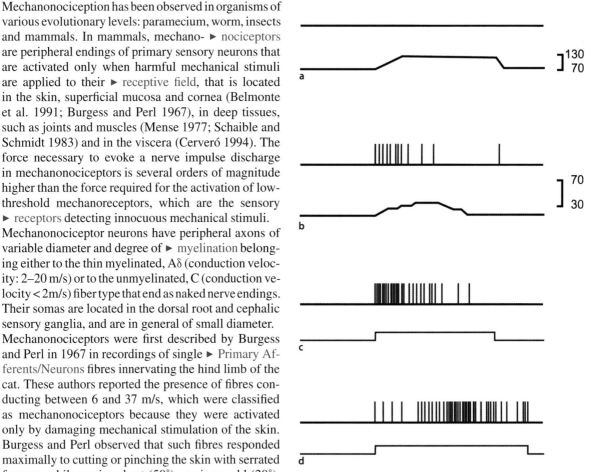

Mechanonociceptors, Figure 1 Responses of a nociceptive fibre to mechanical stimuli. Fibre conduction velocity, 29 m/s. Upper traces in (a), (b), (c) and (d) show the output of a pulse circuit triggered by unitary action potentials. (a) Pressure is used to stimulate the receptive field. (b) Pinching with a needle used as stimuli. (c) Fold of skin in the centre of the receptive field squeezed with serrated forceps used as stimuli. (d) Clip used to pinch the centre of the receptive field used as stimuli. Calibrations on right in g. (Modified from Burgess and Perl 1967).

referred to as mechanonociceptors. This is incorrect, and only those units with high mechanical thresholds, absence of heat response and no initial sensitivity to chemical stimuli (although these have been seldomly tested systematically), can be considered pure mechanical nociceptors, sometimes also called "high threshold mechanoreceptors". The designation as polymodal nociceptor is preferred for CMHs, AMHs and other sensory afferent types that, in addition to their sensitivity to high intensity mechanical forces, also respond to other stimulus modalities (Lynn 1994).

Pure mechanonociceptors have a wide range of sensitivities to mechanical stimuli varying from near noxious to overtly noxious intensities. In this population, A fibres generally respond to equivalent stimuli at higher rates of firing than C fibres (Garell et al. 1996). No background discharges are usually present in mechanonociceptors, which develop partial inactivation after repetitive stimulation of their receptive field. The ▶ adaptation of mechanonociceptors to a sustained stimulus was intermediate, when compared with that of typical phasic or tonic mechanoreceptors (Perl 1967).

With the advent of microneurography in humans (Hallin and Torebjörk 1970), mechanonociceptors have also been identified in the skin of the leg and foot of human subjects (Schmidt et al. 1997). Their receptive fields are not single sensitive spots as classical psychophysical studies had suggested, but cover a relatively large innervation territory.

The cellular and molecular mechanisms by which mechanonociceptors are sensitive only to mechanical stimuli of noxious or near noxious intensity, in contrast with the responsiveness to very light mechanical forces that characterizes low threshold mechanoreceptors, are still unknown.

Mechanotransduction is finally accomplished by opening or closing ▶ ion channels present in the cellular membrane. Many different types of mechanosensitive (MS) channels have been characterized in a wide variety of cell types (García-Añoveros and Corey 1997; Kellenberger and Schild 2002). Also, a variety of extracellular and intracellular proteins have been implicated in the transmission/amplification/modulation of mechanical force to the MS channels present in the cellular

M

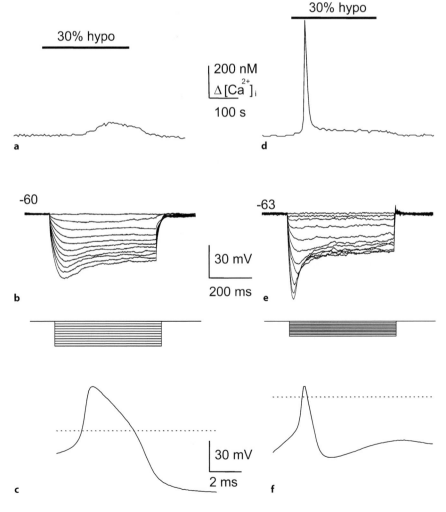

Mechanonociceptors, Figure 2 Electrofisiological properties and $[Ca^{2+}]_i$ responses to hypotonic solution. (a) Time course of the increase in $[Ca^{2+}]$ in response to a 5-min application of a 30% hypotonic solution of a possible mechano nociceptor neuron. (b) Membrane voltage responses of the same neuron to hyperpolarizing current steps of 15 pA. (c) Action potential evoked in the same neuron by depolarizing current pulse at threshold. (d) Time course of the increase in $[Ca^{2+}]$ in response to a 5-min application of a 30% hypotonic solution of a possible mechanosensitive neuron. (e) Membrane voltage responses of the same neuron to hyperpolarizing current steps of 10 pA. (f) Action potential evoked in the same neuron by depolarizing current pulse at threshold. (Modified from Viana et al. 2001)

membrane during the transduction process. CaV3.2, a T-type calcium channel, seems to be required for normal function of D-hair mechanosensory neurons, but it has not yet been directly related with mechanonociception (Dubreuil et al. 2004; Shin et al. 2003). TREK-1, TREK-2 and TRAAK of the 2P domain mechanogated K^+ channels exhibit mechanosensitivity, but there is no experimental proof of their relationship with mechanonociception (Patel et al. 2001). The role played by ASICs, the mammalian homologues of MEC-4 and MEC-10 that mediate mechanotransduction in Caenorhabditis elegans, appears to be minor in mechanical sensibility in mammals (Drew et al 2004). TRPV4, an ▶ osmosensitive channel in mammalian cells, has also been implicated in mechanotransduction (Alessandri-Haber et al. 2003). P2X3 receptors are present in small primary sensory neurons and respond to strong mechanical stimuli when expressed in oocytes of Xenopus. Thus, their implication in the mechanical sensitivity of nociceptor neurons has also been suggested (Cook et al. 1997; Nakamura and Strittmatter 1996).

However, the nature of the MS channels and of the extra- and intracellular matrix proteins involved in the different types of mechanotransduction in mammalian sensory neurons is still unsolved. Whether differences in mechanical threshold between low- and high threshold mechanosensory neurons are due to the expression of different MS channels, to differences in channel density, or to the presence of different associated proteins has been ignored. Cho et al (2002) identified two types of mechanosensitive (MS) channels in isolated membrane patches of cultured neurons of the dorsal root ganglion, with different pressure thresholds as well as distinct biophysical properties, that they named Low-threshold Mechanosensitive (LT-MS) and High-threshold Mechanosensitive channels (HT-MS). The reversal potential of these MS channels was near zero, as occurs with non-selective cationic channels, and they were blocked by the MS channels blocking agent Gd^{3+}. HT-MS channels were present only in small sensory neurons (10–17,5 μm), and were activated only by high pressures and sensitized by PGE2, suggesting their implication in nociceptive transduction.

Neurons with low and high sensitivity to mechanical stimuli appear to have distinct electrophysiological properties. Viana et al. (2001), in cultured trigeminal neurons of the mouse, mechanically stimulated with hypoosmotic solutions, described a small fraction of neurons (12%) that exhibited narrow action potentials and marked time dependent inward rectification, which responded to hypoosmotic solution with fast and prominent elevations of intracellular calcium (Fig. 2), and were classified as low threshold mechanosensitive neurons. In contrast, they identified another group of neurons (19%) showing large and wide action potentials, with an inflexion in the falling phase and no rectification, which

produced smaller and slower elevations of intracellular calcium in response to hypoosmotic stimuli and were classified as mechano nociceptor neurons.

In spite of the progress made in the last years, the molecular and cellular basis of mechanotransduction in mammalian mechano and polymodal nociceptors, and the molecular basis of their differences with low-threshold mechanoreceptors, require further research.

▶ Nociceptors in the Orofacial Region (Skin/Mucosa)
▶ Sensitization of Visceral Nociceptors

References

1. Alessandri-Haber N, Yeh JJ, Boyd AE (2003) Hypotonicity Induces TRPV4-Mediated Nociception in Rat. Neuron 39:497–511
2. Belmonte C, Gallar J, Pozo MA et al. (1991) Excitation by Irritant Chemical Substances of Sensory Afferent Units of the Cat's Cornea. J Physiol 437:709–725
3. Burgess PR, Perl R (1967) Myelinated Afferent Fibres Responding Specifically to Noxious Stimulation of the Skin. J Physiol 190:541–562
4. Cerveró F (1994) Sensory Innervation of the Viscera: Peripheral Basis of Visceral Pain. Physiol Rev 74:95–138
5. Cho H, Shin J, Shin CY et al. (2002) Mechanosensitive Ion Channels in Cultured Sensory Neurons of Neonatal Rats. J Neurosci 22:1238–1247
6. Cook SP, Vulchanova L, Hargreaves KM et al. (1997) Distinct ATP Receptors on Pain-Sensing and Stretch-Sensing Neurons. Nature 387:505–508
7. Dubreuil AS, Boukhaddaoui H, Desmadryl G et al. (2004) Role of T-Type Calcium Current in Identified D-Hair Mechanoreceptor Neurons Studied In Vitro. J Neurosci 24:8480–8484
8. Drew LJ, Rohrer DK, Price MP et al. (2004) Acid-Sensing Ion Channels ASIC2 and ASIC3 Do Not Contribute to Mechanically Activated Currents in Mammalian Sensory Neurones. J Physiol 556:691–710
9. García-Añoveros J, Corey DP (1997) The Molecules of Mechanosensation. Annu Rev Neurosci 20:567–594
10. Garell PC, Mcgillis SL, Greenspan JD (1996) Mechanical Response Properties of Nociceptors Innervating Feline Hairy Skin. J Neurophysiol 75:1177–1189
11. Hallin RG, Torebjork HE (1970) C-Fibre Components in Electrically Evoked Compound Potentials Recorded from Human Median Nerve Fascicles In Situ. A Preliminary Report. Acta Soc Med Ups 75:77–80
12. Kellenberger S, Schild L (2002) Epithelial Sodium Channel/Degenerin Family of Ion Channels: A Variety of Functions for a Shared Structure Physiol Rev 82:735–767
13. Lynn B (1994) The Fibre Composition of Cutaneous Nerves and the Classification and Response Properties of Cutaneous Afferents, with Particular Reference to Nociception. Pain Reviews 1:172–183
14. Mense S (1977) Muscular Nociceptors. J Physiol 73:233–240
15. Nakamura F, Strimatter SM (1996) P2Y1 Purinergic Receptors in Sensory Neurons: Contribution to Touch-Induced Impulse Generation. PNAS 93:10465–10470
16. Patel AJ, Lazdunski M, Honoré E (2001) Lipid and Mechano-Gated 2P Domain K^+ Channels. Curr Op Cell Biol 13:422–427
17. Perl ER (1968) Myelinated Afferent Fibres Innervating the Primate Skin and their Response to Noxious Stimuli. J Physiol 197:593–615
18. Schaible HG, Schmidt RF (1983) Activation of Groups III and IV Sensory Units in Medial Articular Nerve by Local Mechanical Stimulation of Knee Joint. J Neurophysiol 49:35–44
19. Schmidt R, Schmelz M, Ringkamp M et al. (1997) Innervation Territories of Mechanically Activated C Nociceptor Units in Human Skin. J Neurophysiol 78:2641–2648
20. Shin JB, Martinez-Salgado C, Heppenstall PA et al (2003) A T-Type Calcium Channel Required for Normal Function of a Mammalian Mechanoreceptor. Nat Neurosci 6:724–730

6. Fortin JD, Dwyer AP, West S, Pier J (1994) Sacroiliac Joint: Pain Referral Maps upon Applying a New Injection/Arthrography Technique; Part 1: Asymptomatic Volunteers. Spine 19:1475–1482
7. Fukui S, Ohseto K, Shiotani M, Ohno K, Karasawa H, Naganuma Y, Yuda Y (1996) Referred Pain Distribution of the Cervical Zygapophyseal Joints and Cervical Dorsal Rami. Pain 68:79–83
8. Fukui S, Ohseto K, Shiotani M, Ohno K, Karasawa H, Naganuma Y (1997) Distribution of Referred Pain from the Lumbar Zygapophyseal Joints and Dorsal Rami. Clin J Pain 13:303–307
9. Hassett G, Barnsley L (2001) Pain Referral from the Sternoclavicular Joint: A Study in Normal Volunteers. Rheumatology 40:859–862
10. Huskisson EC (1974) Measurement of Pain. Lancet 2:1127–1131
11. Lethem J, Slade PD, Troup JDG, Bentley G (1983) Outline of a Fear Avoidance Model of Exaggerated Pain Perception – I. Behav Res Ther 21:401–408
12. Merskey H, Bogduk N (1994) Classification of Chronic Pain. Descriptions of Chronic Pain Syndromes and Definitions of Pain Terms, 2nd edn. Seattle, IASP Press, pp 3, 11–12
13. Mooney V, Robertson J (1976) The Facet Syndrome. Clin Orthop 115:149–156

Medical Hydrology

▶ Spa Treatment

Medical Misadventures

▶ Postoperative Pain, Adverse Events (Associated with Acute Pain Management)

Medical Mishaps

▶ Postoperative Pain, Adverse Events (Associated with Acute Pain Management)

Medical Outcomes Study 36-Item Short-Form Health Survey (SF-36)

Definition

The Medical Outcomes Study 36-Item Short-Form Health Survey (SF-36) is a 36 item general measure of perceived health status that is usually self-administered.
▶ Pain Inventories

Medical Signs

Definition

Anatomical, physiological, or psychological abnormalities that can be observed, apart from a person's statements (symptoms). Signs must be shown by medically acceptable clinical diagnostic techniques. Psychiatric signs are medically demonstrable phenomena that indicate specific psychological abnormalities, e.g. abnormalities of behavior, mood, thought, memory, orientation, development, or perception. They must also be shown by observable facts that can be medically described and evaluated.
▶ Disability Evaluation in the Social Security Administration

Medically Incongruent Symptoms and Signs

▶ Non-Organic Symptoms and Signs

Medication-Induced Headaches

▶ Headache Attributed to a Substance or its Withdrawal

Mediodorsal Nucleus (MD)

Definition

The main medial nucleus of the thalamus, limited by the intralaminar nuclei.
▶ Spinothalamic Terminations, Core and Matrix
▶ Thalamus, Visceral Representation

Mediolongitudinal Myelotomy

▶ Midline Myelotomy

Meditation

Definition

Meditation is a means of narrowing the focus of one's attention to a simple activity (e.g. awareness of the breath) or word (e.g. a mantra), thereby quieting and calming the mind.
▶ Relaxation in the Treatment of Pain

Medullary Dorsal Horn

Definition

The medullary dorsal horn is a caudal portion of the sub-nucleus caudalis of the spinal trigeminal nucleus, which has laminated cytoarchitecture analogous to the dorsal horn of the spinal cord. The medullary dorsal horn plays a major role in the processing of nociceptive information from the head, face and mouth regions.
► DREZ Procedures
► Trigeminothalamic Tract Projections

Medullary Lateral Reticular Formation

Definition

Lying dorso-medially to the spinal trigeminal nucleus, it contains the interneurons that mediate the long-latency trigeminal reflexes.
► Jaw-Muscle Silent Periods (Exteroceptive Suppression)

MEG

► Magnetoencephalography
► Pain in Humans, EEG Documentation

Meissner Receptor

Definition

Encapsulated cutaneous mechanosensory receptors specialized for the detection of fine touch and pressure. Meissner receptors transmit information about the velocity of the stimulus. They belong to the moderately rapid adapting detectors.
► Perireceptor Elements

Melanotic

Definition

Melanotic refers to a high level of blackish pigmentation that produces a very dark or black color.
► Lower Back Pain, Physical Examination

Melatonin

Definition

Melatonin is a substance secreted by the pineal gland associated with circadian rhythms such as the sleep-wake cycle.
► Hypnic Headache

Membrane Capacitance

Definition

The ability of a cell membrane to store ionic charge.
► Demyelination

Membrane Potential

Definition

The electric potential difference across the membrane of living cells at rest, due to a differential distribution of ions (particularly Na^+, K^+ and Cr) consecutive to the variable permeability of the membrane and the active transport of ions.
► Nociceptor Generator Potential

Membrane Resistance

Definition

A measurement of how easily ions cross the cell membrane.
► Demyelination

Membrane Stabilising Agents

► Postoperative Pain, Membrane Stabilising Agents

Membrane Stabilizers

Definition

Pharmacological agents that reduce the electrical excitability of neurons. Typical membrane stabilizing drugs are local anesthetics and other Na^+ channel blockers.
► Pain Paroxysms
► Tic and Cranial Neuralgias

Membrane-Stabilizing Drugs

▶ Drugs Targeting Voltage-Gated Sodium and Calcium Channels

Memory Decision Theory

Definition

Memory decision theory refers to the application of signal detection theory to judgments concerning whether a descriptor is "old", that is, previously used to describe a symptom, or „new", that is, not previously used.
▶ Statistical Decision Theory Application in Pain Assessment

Meningeal Afferents

▶ Nociceptors in the Orofacial Region (Meningeal/Cerebrovascular)

Meningeal Carcinomatous

Definition

This is wide spread infiltration of the meninges with cancer. Symptoms and signs may reflect involvement of multiple sites in the central nervous system and may include altered mental status, headache and pain. Carcinomatous meningitis occurs in two to three percent of patients with adenocarcinoma of the lung and small cell lung cancer. The median survival of patients with carcinomatous meningitis is two to four months.
▶ Cancer Pain Management, Overall Strategy

Meningeal Layer

Definition

The protective membranes that encase the central nervous system.
▶ Motor Cortex (M1)
▶ Secondary Somatosensory Cortex (S2) and Insula, Effect on Pain Related Behavior in Animals and Humans

Meningeal Nociceptors

▶ Nociceptors in the Orofacial Region (Meningeal/Cerebrovascular)

Meningoencephalitis

Definition

Of the brain stem and cerebellum: neurologic manifestation of Behçet's disease.
▶ Headache Due to Arteritis

Meniscus

Definition

Flattened cartilaginous plate found in certain joints, including the knee. The meniscus serves to maintain the apposition of the opposed surfaces in their various motions, to ease the gliding movement of the joint, and to decrease the effects of pressure and sudden impact on the joint.
▶ Arthritis Model, Osteoarthritis

Mensendieck System

Definition

A pedagogically designed system of functional exercises based on an analysis of human anatomy, physiology, and biomechanics, developed by MD Bess M. Mensendieck, in the early 1900s. The aims are to better the individual's functional capacity in daily life by increasing understanding of anatomically and physiologically correct movements, and improving the ability to interpret body signals.
▶ Body Awareness Therapies

Menstrual Suppression

Definition

The use of hormonal or anti-hormonal medication such as combined hormonal contraception, high dose progestins, androgens or GnRH agonists for prolonged periods of time in order to obviate or minimize menstrual flow and pain.
▶ Dyspareunia and Vaginismus

Mental Disorders, Diagnostics and Statistics

▶ Diagnostic and Statistical Manual of Mental Disorders

Mental Pain

▶ Pain, Psychiatry and Ethics

Menthol

Definition

Menthol is a natural substance (2-isopropyl-5-methyl-cyclohexanol) obtained from plant leaves of the genus *Mentha*, widely used in products such as common cold medications, toothpastes, confectionery and cosmetics. l-menthol evokes a sensation of coolness by stimulation of oral, nasal and skin cold thermoreceptors. Menthol can also act as an irritant involving capsaicin-sensitive pathways. A cold and menthol receptor, named TRPM8, was cloned from peripheral sensory neurons.

▶ Nociceptors, Cold Thermotransduction

Meralgia Paresthetica

Definition

Meralgia Paresthetica is a painful mononeuropathy of the lateral femoral cutaneous nerve due to focal entrapment in the inguinal ligament. It results in pain in the lateral thigh.

▶ Neuralgia, Assessment
▶ Sciatica

Merkel Receptor

Definition

Encapsulated cutaneous mechanosensory receptors specialized for the detection of fine touch and pressure. Merkel receptors transmit information about the intensity of the stimulus. They belong to the slowly adapting detectors.

▶ Perireceptor Elements

Mesencephalic Nucleus

Definition

Mesencephalic nucleus, containing the cell bodies of primary afferents innervating the jaw muscle spindles or periodontal ligaments.

▶ Trigeminal Brainstem Nuclear Complex, Anatomy

Mesencephalic Tractotomy

▶ Pain Treatment, Intracranial Ablative Procedures

Mesencephalon

Definition

The narrow short part of the brain stem above the pons and below the thalamus. An operation to interrupt a pathway at the level of the mesencephalon is called a mesencephalotomy.

▶ Pain Treatment, Intracranial Ablative Procedures

Mesencephalotomy

▶ Pain Treatment, Intracranial Ablative Procedures

Mesmerism

▶ Therapy of Pain, Hypnosis

Meta-Analysis

Definition

Meta-analysis is a statistical technique for combining the findings from independent studies. It is a systematic review that uses quantitative methods to summarize the results. It is most often used to assess the clinical effectiveness of healthcare interventions. Meta-analysis is an effective means of correcting both for bias and lack of power in individual randomized controlled studies. It provides a precise estimate of treatment effect, providing due weight to the size of the studies included. The validity of meta-analysis depends on the quality of the systematic review. A meta-analysis may also allow the investigator to explore whether features associated with studies influence the magnitude of the effects observed, e.g. do studies using skilled therapists obtain better effect than those using relatively unskilled ones?

▶ Operant Treatment of Chronic Pain
▶ Postoperative Pain, Preoperative Education
▶ Psychology of Pain, Efficacy
▶ Transition from Acute to Chronic Pain

Metabolic and Nutritional Neuropathies

ALEX BARLING, JOHN B. WINER
Department of Neurology, Birmingham Muscle and
Nerve Centre, Queen Elizabeth Hospital, Birmingham,
UK
corisanderoad@aol.com, j.b.winer@bham.ac.uk

Synonyms

Vitamin Neuropathy; Beri Beri Disease; Malnutrition;
Alcoholism; Cuban Neuropathy Fabry's Disease; Para-
proteinemic Neuropathies; Nutritional Neuropathies;
Metabolic Neuropathies

Definition

Neuropathy encompasses conditions occurring with
systemic organ failure as well as inherited or acquired
metabolic defects. Nutritional neuropathies are those
related to malnutrition and resulting vitamin deficiency.
Neuropathy related to alcoholism is also discussed in
this section as a toxic metabolic cause that has been
suggested for the axonal injury, it is also frequently
related to malnutrition. Axonal neuropathies usually
result in damage to the nerve cell body and lead to a
dying back of the longest axons.

Characteristics

Alcohol

Alcohol remains the second most common cause of neuropathy after diabetes mellitus and affects a third of alco-
holics (Neundorfer 2001). It is unclear whether alcohol
is toxic itself or simply associated with malnutrition that
results in neuropathy. A recent study by Koike suggested
a direct causal role (Koike 2003).
The neuropathy typically manifests as burning feet
with distal, symmetrical loss of pain sensation and
▶ allodynia in the lower limbs. As the neuropathy progresses distal weakness occurs, initially in the legs and
then the arms. These features can be accompanied by
ataxia from joint position loss or cereballar degeneration, Wernick-Korsakoff encephalopathy and stigmata
of chronic liver disease. Impotence and postural hypotension from autonomic nerve involvement are often
under diagnosed (Monforte 1995).
There are no diagnostic investigations, but the clinical signs in conjunction with a history of alcohol
consumption, typically greater than 3 litres of beer
or 300 ml of spirits per day for three years, are suggestive (Behse 1977). A red cell macrocytosis, elevated
transaminase and gamma glutamyltransferase are also
pointers. Analysis of cerebral spinal fluid should be
normal, although the protein may be minimally elevated. The nerve conduction studies, (NCS), mirror the
clinical findings and show distal, predominantly lower
limb, symmetrically, reduced sensory nerves action

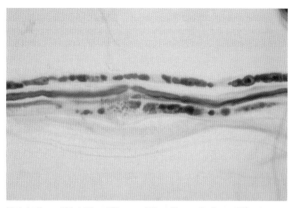

Metabolic and Nutritional Neuropathies, Figure 1 Teased fibre preparation of a peripheral nerve showing axonal degeneration as seen in alcoholic neuropathy.

potentials. Histology demonstrates axonal loss in fibres
of all sizes in the absence of inflammation (Fig. 1).
Treatment of alcoholic neuropathy requires abstinence
and multivitamins including thiamine. Sensory symptoms may initially worsen on treatment.

Nutritional Neuropathies

Nutritional neuropathies occur predominantly in developing countries where crop failure and malnutrition are
common. The last major outbreak was in Cuba in 1992
(Roman 1994). In developed countries nutritional neuropathies are rare but still occur in the context of alcoholism, malignancy, chronic infection and pregnancy.
They are important to recognise, as prompt treatment
can halt the progression and sometimes improve the neuropathy.

Thiamine Deficiency, B_1

Thiamine deficiency causes the syndrome of Beri Beri,
which encompasses peripheral neuropathy (dry Beri
Beri) and congestive cardiac failure (wet Beri Beri).
Initially recognised early in the 19th century, it was associated with a diet of processed rice or during sea voyages.
Thiamine deficiency should be suspected in any mal-
nourished patient. The symptoms and signs are similar to
alcoholic neuropathy with burning ▶ dysaesthesia in the
legs. The condition progresses over weeks and months,
with the sensory symptoms spreading proximally followed by weakness. Less commonly, the cranial nerves
can be affected e.g. laryngeal weakness, facial weakness
and tongue deviation.
Laboratory studies of thiamine levels are unreliable. Numerous studies have looked at pyruvate which accumulates in thiamine deficiency, however the sensitivity is
poor. Assay of erythrocyte transketolase levels, a vitamin B_1 dependant enzyme, is more helpful if measured
prior to any supplementation as it reflects B_1 stores. NCS
are similar to that of alcoholic neuropathy with predominantly distal, symmetrical axonal loss. The pathology
shows distal axonal degeneration.

M

Metabolic and Nutritional Neuropathies, Table 1 Features of Metabolic and Nutritional Neuropathy

Cause	Symptoms	Pain	Examination	Specific Investigations	Pathology
Alcohol	burning feet	+++	distal, symmetrical, loss of pain and hyperasthesia to light touch	raised red cell mean cell volume raised transaminase raised gamma glutamyltransferase	sensory axonal
thiamine deficiency	burning Feet	+++	distal, symmetrical, loss of pain and hyperasthesia to light touch	raised erythrocyte transketolase	axonal
pyridoxine deficiency	Distal numbness and tingling		distal, symmetrical sensory loss		sensory axonal
cobalamine deficiency	Distal tingling and numbness +/- ataxia &weakness		distal loss of vibration followed by joint position sense Absent ankle reflexes	low B_{12}, raised homocysteine and methionine variable increase in haemoglobin &mean cell volume	axonal
vitamin E deficiency	ataxia and weakness		distal areflexia and loss of vibration +/- ataxia	vitamin E level (in presence of normal lipid levels)	axonal
uraemia	Distal paraesthesia	+	distal sensory loss	raised urea	axonal
hepatic dysfunction	variable		variable	deranged liver function tests +/- vitamin E deficiency	demyelinating or axonal
thyroid disease	Distal paraesthesia	++	distal sensory loss	TSH and T4	sensory axonal
Porphyria	Distal paraesthesia &proximal weakness	+	distal paraesthesia &proximal weakness +/- Respiratory muscle weakness	urinary porphobilinogens	axonal
Amyloid	Distal paraesthesia		distal, symmetrical loss of pain and temperature +/- autonomic dysfunction	Congo red staining of nerve biopsy	Axonal
Refsums Disease	Distal paraesthesia	+	distal, symmetrical loss of vibration and proprioception Mild distal weakness	raised plasma phytanic acid and pipecolic acid	demyelinating
Fabrys Disease	burning hands &feet	+++	progressive or episodic sensory loss	α-galactosidase levels in fibroblasts	axonal

The treatment of polyneuropathy is with oral thiamine, 300 g per day. In the presence of heart failure or Wernicke's encephalopathy, thiamine should be administered parenterally (see ► Wernicke-Korsakoff Syndrome). Supplementation with multivitamins is recommended as the neuropathy is often not the result of a single vitamin deficiency state.

Pyridoxine Deficiency, B_6

Pyridoxine deficiency is rare and usually secondary to treatment with isoniazid or hydralazine. These drugs inhibit the phosphorylation of pyridoxine to the active coenzyme pyridoxal phosphate. Distal, symmetrical numbness with tingling is the common presentation. Discontinuing the offending drug usually reverses the symptoms. A daily oral dose of 50–100 mgs of pyridoxime is generally advised. Doses above 180 g per day are toxic to nerves, leading to a pyridoxime induced neuropathy.

Cobalamine Deficiency, B_{12}

The most common cause of B_{12} deficiency is malabsorption secondary to pernicious anaemia. In this condition, antibodies to intrinsic factor prevent absorption of B_{12} specifically. A deficiency state is also well documented in patients post gastrectomy or resection of the terminal ileum. Less frequent causes of deficiency include tropical sprue, severe steatorrhoea, drugs such as colchicine which reduce absorption and rarely a strict vegan diet. Occasionally general anaesthesia with nitrous oxide can precipitate a deficit; this is because nitrous oxide can interfere with the B_{12} dependant conversion of homocysteine to methionine. B_{12} is stored in the liver and many years of deficiency are needed to deplete the stores.

B_{12} deficiency usually begins insidiously and progresses over weeks and months. Practically it is very difficult to separate the symptoms or neuropathy from the myelopathy of sub-acute combined degeneration of the spinal cord as they usually coexist. In the early stages ▶ paraesthesia and numbness are the most common symptoms. Lower limb weakness and ataxia then ensues. Other symptoms include impotence, memory loss and mental slowing.

Examination typically reveals loss of vibration sensation in the early stages followed by loss of joint position sense and then light touch. The ankle reflexes are reduced or absent. The myelopathy leads to pyramidal motor dysfunction, hyperreflexia at the knee and a positive Babinski sign.

Serum B_{12} levels can be measured but the methods of assay varies, and all are prone to inaccuracy, as B_{12} is predominantly protein bound. This means that a normal B_{12} concentration does not exclude a deficiency state. Also, falsely elevated levels are seen in myeloproliferative and hepatic disorders and falsely low levels are seen in pregnancy. B_{12} deficiency is also associated with a macrocytic anaemia. There is debate about whether significant neurological dysfunction from B_{12} deficiency can occur in the presence of a normal haemoglobin level. Significant reduction of the B_{12} concentration will cause an elevation in B_{12} dependant metabolites, homocysteine and methionine. Measuring the levels of these metabolites can be useful in cases of borderline deficiency, to help establish those with neurology resulting from their deficiency. Ninety percent of patients with significant neurological disease have elevated levels (Yuen 2001). NCS show reduced sural nerve action potentials resulting from presumed axonopathy. The pathological studies in this area are limited and inconclusive (Windebank 1993).

Vitamin B_{12} deficiency is treated with intramuscular injections. Partial neurological improvement is usually seen predominantly in the first six months, but recovery can continue for up to a year or more.

Vitamin E Deficiency

Vitamin E is a fat soluble vitamin and absorption is dependent on bile salts and pancreatic esterases in the small bowel. Causes of the deficiency include cystic fibrosis, bile salt deficiency from congenital cholestasis and small bowel resection, a rare inherited defect of chylomicrons and lipoprotein synthesis known as abetalipproteinaemia, and defects in alpha-tocopherol transfer protein genes which are inherited in an autosomal recessive manner.

There are significant reserves of vitamin E in the adipose tissue; this means that deficiency states in adults take many years or decades to become clinically significant. Deficiency of vitamin E leads to spinocerebellar dysfunction with variable peripheral nerve involvement; affected patients usually complain of an unsteady gait and weakness. Examination reveals distal areflexia, prominent loss of vibration and joint position sense with minimal weakness. Other sensory modalities such as light touch are seldom affected. Ataxia can be a feature of both joint position loss and cerebellar involvement. The clinical picture can be confounded by proximal muscle weakness and a positive Babinski sign.

Vitamin E assays are accurate in the presence of normal lipid levels as vitamin E is primarily located in lipoprotein, however, hyperlipidaemic patients with normal vitamin E assays, may still have a deficiency. In general, levels need to be undetectable to be able to attribute neurological disease to vitamin E deficiency. NCS demonstrate a reduction in sensory nerve action potentials with preservation of conduction velocity. Motor nerves are usually unaffected. ▶ Somatosensory evoked potentials and visually evoked potentials (▶ visual evoked potentials) are often delayed due to spinal or central nerve involvement. Electromyography can show mild denervation. CSF examination is normal.

The role of vitamin E as an antioxidant and free radical scavenger are well documented, but the mechanism by which vitamin E deficiency affects the nervous system is not established.

Treatment of vitamin E deficiency involves large doses of oral vitamin E, 1–4 g/day (Sokol 1990). Every case should be carefully monitored and the dose individually tailored. In cases of severe damage to the nervous system, regression is unlikely and treatment would aim to halt the progress of the disease. If conditions such as abetaliproteinaemia are diagnosed early enough, the condition may be prevented by supplementing vitamin E.

Metabolic

Chronic uraemia causes a progressive sensory motor, axonal neuropathy which can be painful (Wolfe 2002). The frequency has decreased over the last ten years due to improved management with dialysis and renal transplant (Said 1987; Lagueny 2002), although the exact mechanism underlying this neuropathy is unknown.

Toxins can effect both the peripheral nerve and liver, but some neuropathies do occur as a consequence of hepatic dysfunction alone: Chronic hepatic failure can lead to an asymptomatic demyelinating neuropathy, and neuropathy is detectable in 93% of patients pre liver transplant (McDougall 2003); An acute demyelinating polyneuropathy similar to Guillian Barre can accompany viral hepatitis. A sensory neuropathy is associated with Primary Biliary Cirrhosis, while childhood cholystatic liver disease can cause a sensory neuropathy secondary to vitamin E deficiency.

A mild chronic sensory motor neuropathy can be seen in both hyperthyroidism and hypothyroidism.

Acute intermittent porphyria can cause an axonal neuropathy which is preceded by the first attack of abdom-

Metabolic and Nutritional Neuropathies, Table 2 Paraproteinemic Neuropathies

Condition	Systemic Symptoms	Neuropathy	Pain	Examination	Specific Investigations	Pathology
MGUS	Nil	Distal numbness, paraesthesia and pain with ataxia. Can resemble chronic inflammatory demyelinating polyneuropathy, CIDP	+++	Predominantly sensory loss Weakness occurs late	IgG or IgM-K paraprotein <3g/dl Bone marrow biopsy < 5% plasma cells	Predominantly demyelinating
Multiple Myeloma	Fatigue, bone pain	Distal weakness and dysaesthesia		Distal, symmetrical, weakness and numbness	IgM or IgG-K paraprotein >3g/dl. Low haemoglobin Raised calcium Renal impairment Skeletal survey	Predominantly axonal
Waldenstrom's macroglobulin-aemia	Fatigue, weight loss, bleeding and hyper-viscosity	Numbness in the feet followed by foot drop	+	Distal, symmetrical paraesthesia and numbness followed by distal weakness initially in the lower limbs	IgM-K paraprotein Full blood count	Demyelinating
Amyloidosis (usually systemic)	Autonomic symptoms, e.g. postural hypotension, diarrhoea and impotence Weight loss cardiac and renal dysfunction can occur	Numb feet initially progressing to lancinating pain and loss of temperature sensation.	+++	Symmetrical, distal, predominantly sensory disturbance.	IgG or IgA- λ paraprotein Biopsy of sural nerve, rectum or bone marrow with congo red staining	Axonal
POEMS Syndrome (osteoscle-rotic myeloma)	Polyneuropathy Organomegaly Endocrinopathy M protein Skin changes +/- plasmacytoma	Progressive distal sensory disturbance and weakness	+/-	Symmetrical, distal, allodynia, numbness, loss of joint position sensation and weakness.	IgG or IgA-λ paraprotein Skeletal survey	Demyelinating
Castleman's Disease	Lymphadenopathy +/- POEMS syndrome	Variable: can resemble motor neurone disease or CIDP	+/-	Variable	IgM or IgG paraprotein Lymph node biopsy looking for angiofollicular hyperplasia	Axonal
Cryoglobulin-aemia	Raynaud's phenomenon Evidence of lymphoproliferative disorders, collagen vascular or chronic inflammatory disease	Pain in the early stages Generalized or multi-focal weakness Paraesthesia can be precipitated by the cold	+++	Symmetric or asymmetric sensorimotor disturbance	IgM or IgG paraprotein, but can be polyclonal Precipitation of cryoglobulins from serum.	Axonal

inal pain. Motor involvement is typically proximal and can affect the respiratory muscles; sensory involvement is mild, distal and symmetrical. The neuropathy can also affect the autonomic system leading to tachycardia, labile blood pressure, urinary retention and diarrhoea. Amyloid neuropathy occurs in twenty percent of patients with light chain disease. This axonal neuropathy is predominantly sensory, distal and symmetrical. Pain and temperature loss occurs initially, but distal weakness can develop in the later stages. Involvement of the autonomic nerves leads to orthostatic hypotension, impotence, bladder dysfunction, hypohydrosis and meiotic pupils. A multifocal neuropathy also oc-

curs and frequently presents as carpal tunnel syndrome.

Refsums disease is an autosomal recessive condition caused by a defect in phytanoyl-CoA-hydroxylase that causes ataxia, retinal damage and deafness. The associated demyelinating neuropathy causes a slow, progressive, distal, symmetrical loss of vibration and proprioception. Weakness also occurs and progresses proximally. Painful paraesthesia can be a feature.

Fabry's disease, caused by α Galactosidase deficiency, is a X linked condition that affects the peripheral nervous system, the central nervous system, the heart and the kidneys. The associated neuropathy is particularly painful. Patients describe burning in the hands and feet which can be episodic or chronic and progressive. Neurophysiology demonstrates an axonal neuropathy which affects the small fibres initially.

Paraproteinemic Neuropathies

Paraproteins are associated with ten percent of peripheral neuropathies, and they can be detected by immunoelectrophoresis or immunofixation of blood or urine. The identified proteins are usually the product of a single clone of plasma cells and are therefore termed monoclonal, M proteins.

Paraproteinaemic neuropathies can precede or be associated with a number of systemic disorders.

Monoclonal gammopathy of undetermined significance, MGUS, is the most common (Kelly 1981). In this condition the paraprotein level is less that 3 g/dl in the serum, the paraprotein usually possesses a kappa light chain component. IgG is the most common paraprotein found in patients with MGUS and no neuropathy, but when MGUS accompanies a neuropathy the IgM isotype is more frequent. MGUS is distinguished from Myeloma by the lower level of paraprotein and the absence of systemic features. The condition typically affects men over the age of fifty and presents with distal numbness and paraesthesia. Fifty percent of patients develop lancinating pains, dysaesthesia or aching discomfort in the limbs; light touch, joint position sense and vibration sensation are also affected (Ropper 1998). In advanced cases distal weakness can occur. Investigations usually reveal a demyelinating but occasional axonal neuropathy. Cerebral spinal fluid protein is typically elevated.

The treatment of MGUS is not established but intravenous immunoglogulin, plasma exchange, steroids and immunosuppresion have all been used with variable success. A number of recent small studies have reported beneficial effects treating MGUS with rituximab, this is a humanized monoclonal antibody directed against CD20 antigens. (Pestronk 2003; Renaud 2003) These studies have not been as promising as originally anticipated, large randomised control trials are awaited to further assess the efficacy of rituximab. In addition to managing the neuropathy, it is important to monitor the paraprotein level in patients with MGUS, as 30% will develop a malignant plasma-cell disorder within 25 years (Veneri 2004). The risk of progression of MGUS to malignancy is, on average, 1.5% per year (Kyle 2003).

Other paraproteinaemic disorders associated with a neuropathy are listed in Table 2. These conditions are important to recognise, as treatment can lead to remission of the condition and improvement in the neuropathy. Therefore, immunoelectrophoresis and immunofixation should be an essential part of the investigations of any unexplained neuropathy.

References

1. Behse F, Buchthal F (1977) Alcoholic Neuropathy: Clinical, Electrophysiological and Biopsy Findings. Ann Neurol 2:95
2. Kelly JJ, Kyle RA, O'Brien PC et al. (1981) Prevalence of Monoclonal Protein in Peripheral Neuropathy. Neurology 31:1480-1483
3. Koike H, Iijima M, Sugiura M et al. (2003) Alcoholic Neuropathy is Clinicopathologically Distinct from Thiamine-Deficiency Neuropathy. Ann Neurol 54:19-29
4. Kyle RA, Therneau TM, Rajkumar SV et al. (2003) Long-Term Follow-up of IgM Monoclonal Gammopathy of Undetermined Significance. Semin Oncology 30:169-171
5. Lagueny A (2000) Metabolic and Nutritional Neuropathies. Rev Prat 50:731-5
6. McDougall AJ, Davies L, McCaughan GW (2003) Autonomic and Peripheral Neuropathy in End Stage Liver Disease and following Liver Transplant. Muscle Nerve 28:595-600
7. Monforte R, Estruch R, Valls-Sole J et al. (1995) Autonomic and Peripheral Neuropathies in Patients with Chronic Alcoholism. Arch Neurol 52:45-51
8. Neundorfer B (2001) Alcohol Polyneuropathy. Fortschr Neurol Psychiatr 69:341-5
9. Pestronk A, Florence J, Miller T et al. (2003) Treatment of IgM Associated Polyneuropathies using Rituximab. J Neurol Neurosurg Psychyatry 74:485-489
10. Renaud S, Gregor M, Fuhr P et al. (2003) Rituximab in the Treatment of Anti-MAG Associated Polyneuropathy. Muscle Nerve 27:611-615
11. Roman GC (1994) An Epidemic in Cuba of Optic Neuropathy, Sensorineural Deafness, Peripheral Sensory Neuropathy and Dorsolateral Myeloneuropathy. J Neurol Sci 127:11-28
12. Ropper AH, Gorson KC (1998) Neuropathies Associated with Paraproteinemia. N Engl J Med 338:1601-1607
13. Said G (1987) Acquired Metabolic Neuropathies (2): Kidney Failure, Hypothyroid and Hypoglycaemia. Rev Neurol 143:785-90
14. Sokol RJ (1990) Vitamin E and Neurologic Deficits. Adv Pediatr 37:119-148
15. Veneri D, Aquel H, Franchini M et al. (2004) Malignant Evolution of Monoclonal Gammopathy of Undetermined Significance: Analysis of 633 Consecutive Cases with Long-Term Follow-Up. Haematologica 89:876-878
16. Windebank A (1993) Polyneuropathy due to Nutritional Deficiency and Alcoholism. In: Peripheral Neuropathy 3rd edn. W B Saunders Company, Philadelphia, pp 1310-1321
17. Wolfe GI, Barohn RJ (2002) Painful Peripheralneuropathy. Curr Treat Options Neurol 4:177-188
18. Yuen T (2001) Nutritional and Alcoholic Neuropathies. In: Peripheral Neuropathy: A Practical Approach to Diagnosis and Management. Lippincott Williams and Walkins, Philadelphia, pp 223-232

M

Metabolic Neuropathies

▶ Metabolic and Nutritional Neuropathies

Metabolism

Definition

The metabolism of a drug describes its biotransformation into other substances due to chemical conversion.

▶ NSAIDs, Pharmacokinetics

Metabotropic Glutamate Receptors

Synonyms

mGlu Receptors; mGluRs

Definition

Family of G-protein-coupled glutamate receptors (mGluRs) that are coupled to intracellular second messenger (G-Protein) systems. There are eight known mGlu receptor subtypes (mGlu1 - mGlu8), and some of these are known to form homo-dimers. The eight receptors can be placed into three groups (Groups I, II, III) on the basis of sequence homology and pharmacology. They trigger long-lasting intracellular processes and mediate slow synaptic components, s. also Glutamate Receptor.

- ▶ Inflammation, Role of Peripheral Glutamate Receptors
- ▶ Metabotropic Glutamate Receptors in the Thalamus
- ▶ Molecular Contributions to the Mechanism of Central Pain
- ▶ Nociceptive Neurotransmission in the Thalamus
- ▶ Nociceptive Processing in the Amygdala, Neurophysiology and Neuropharmacology

Metabotropic Glutamate Receptors in Spinal Nociceptive Processing

VOLKER NEUGEBAUER
Department of Neuroscience & Cell Biology,
University of Texas Medical Branch, Galveston, TX,
USA
voneugeb@utmb.edu

Synonyms

Spinal Cord Nociception, Glutamate Receptor (Metabotropic)

Definition

G-protein-coupled receptors that are activated by glutamate and are linked to a variety of signal transduction pathways to regulate neuronal excitability and synaptic transmission in normal nervous system functions as well as in neurological and psychiatric disorders. They also modulate nociceptive processing at different levels of the pain neuraxis, including the spinal dorsal horn.

Characteristics

Metabotropic glutamate receptors (mGluRs) (see ▶ metabotropic receptor) belong to family 3 of G-protein-coupled receptors, which can trigger long-lasting intracellular processes and "metabolic" changes and mediate synaptic plasticity. They are characterized by a seven transmembrane domain topology and a large N-terminal extracellular domain, which contains important residues for ligand binding and forms two lobes that close like a Venus' flytrap upon ligand binding (Bockaert and Pin 1999). The second intracellular loop determines G-protein specificity and the intracellular C-terminal interacts directly with intracellular proteins such as Homer proteins (Bhave et al. 2003; Bockaert and Pin 1999; De Blasi et al. 2001). Eight mGluR subtypes have been cloned to date and are classified into groups I (mGluRs 1 and 5), II (mGluRs 2 and 3) and III (mGluRs 4, 6, 7 and 8) based on their sequence homology, signal transduction mechanisms and pharmacological profile (De Blasi et al. 2001; Gasparini et al. 2002; Neugebauer 2001; Schoepp et al. 1999; Varney and Gereau 2002) (see Table 1). Several splice variants have been identified which may differ with regard to their pharmacology and G-protein coupling.

Signal Transduction

Group I mGluRs couple through $G_{q/11}$ proteins to the activation of phospholipase C (PLC), resulting in phosphoinositide (PI) hydrolysis, release of calcium from intracellular stores and protein kinase C (PKC) activation (Anwyl 1999; Gasparini et al. 2002; Neugebauer 2001; Schoepp et al. 1999). Tyrosine kinase activation is another signaling pathway of group I mGluRs. The PKC- and tyrosine kinase-dependent pathways are two major signal transduction mechanisms that can activate the mitogen-activated protein kinases (MAPKs) such as the extracellular signal-regulated kinase 1/2 (ERK1/2) (Karim et al. 2001). Group II and group III mGluRs are negatively coupled to adenylyl cyclase (AC) through G_i/G_o proteins, thereby inhibiting cyclic AMP (cAMP) formation and cAMP-dependent protein kinase (PKA) activation (Anwyl 1999; Gasparini et al. 2002; Neugebauer 2001; Schoepp et al. 1999).

Modulation of Voltage- and Ligand-Gated Ion Channels

In general, the predominant effect of group I mGluR activation is enhanced neuronal excitability and synaptic transmission, whereas activation of groups II and III typically produces inhibitory effects. Exceptions exist however, and different subtypes within one group (e.g. mGluR1 and mGluR5) may exert opposing effects. mGluRs can regulate neuronal excitability through direct or indirect effects on a variety of voltage sensitive ion channels, including high voltage-activated Ca^{2+} channels, K^+ channels and nonselective cationic channels (Anwyl 1999; Neugebauer 2001; Schoepp et al. 1999). The modulation of ligand-gated ion channels by mGluRs includes the group I mGluR-mediated enhancement of ionotropic glutamate receptor (see ▶ ionotropic receptor) function, which probably involves receptor phosphorylation (Anwyl 1999; Neugebauer 2001). Group I mGluRs also potentiate the function of the capsaicin/vanilloid receptor (VR1) (Neugebauer 2001). Convincing evidence suggests that mGluRs interact

Metabotropic Glutamate Receptors in Spinal Nociceptive Processing, Table 1 Classification and pharmacology of mGluRs

Group	Group I	Group II	Group III
Subtype	mGluR1, 5	mGluR2, 3	mGluR4, 6, 7, 8
Agonist	S-DHPG (1,5) CHPG (5)	LY354740 LY379268 2R,4R-APDC	LAP4 LSOP
Antagonist	CPCCOEt (1) LY367385 (1) BAY36-7620 (1) MPEP (5) SIB-1757 (5) SIB-1893 (5)	EGLU LY341495	UBP1112 MSOP MAP4
Effector	G_q-protein (G_s-protein) PLC ↑ ERK ↑ (PLD ↑) (AC ↑) tyrosine kinase ↑	$G_{i/o}$-protein AC ↓	$G_{i/o}$-protein AC ↓

with the opioid system and play a role in the development of opioid tolerance and dependence (Fundytus 2001). mGluRs can also modulate the release of transmitters by acting as autoreceptors (glutamate) or heteroreceptors (GABA, substance P, serotonin, dopamine and acetylcholine)(Cartmell and Schoepp 2000).

Pharmacology and Modulation of mGluRs

Several potent and mGluR subgroup/subtype selective compounds have been developed in recent years (see Table 1). Presently available agonists are subgroup-selective; the only subtype-selective agonist is CHPG (for mGluR5). LY367385 is a competitive mGluR1 subtype-selective antagonist. Other subtype-selective group I antagonists that distinguish between mGluR1 (CPCCOEt, BAY36-7620) and mGluR5 (MPEP, SIB-1757, SIB-1893) are ► non-competitive antagonist s or ► inverse agonist s. ► Competitive antagonists that are selective for group II and group III mGluRs are available (Gasparini et al. 2002; Schoepp et al. 1999; Varney and Gereau 2002).

The intracellular C-terminal of group I mGluRs is also the target of interacting proteins, such as the Homer proteins, which can regulate subcellular receptor localization, G-protein coupling and constitutive (basal) activity of mGluR1 and mGluR5 (Gasparini et al. 2002). Receptor phosphorylation is another important mechanism for modulating mGluR function, including PKC-mediated desensitization of group I mGluRs and uncoupling of groups II and III mGluRs from G proteins by PKC and PKA (Karim et al. 2001; Neugebauer 2001; Varney and Gereau 2002).

Spinal Nociception

The important role of group I mGluRs in spinal nociceptive processing, ► central sensitization and spinally mediated pain behavior is now well established. The functions of groups II and III mGluRs are less well known

(Fundytus 2001; Neugebauer 2001; Neugebauer 2002; Varney and Gereau 2002). The current focus of research is on the role of individual mGluR subtypes and signal transduction pathways.

Group I mGluRs

Both mGluR1 and mGluR5 are functionally expressed in the spinal dorsal horn. Anatomical and recent electrophysiological data further suggest that mGluR1 and mGluR5 are localized pre- as well as post-synaptically (Neugebauer 2002; Neugebauer 2001; Park et al. 2004; Varney and Gereau 2002).

Agonists

Activation of spinal group I mGluRs generally produces pro-nociceptive effects in behavioral and electrophysiological assays, although mixed excitatory and inhibitory effects have been reported (Fundytus 2001; Neugebauer 2001; Varney and Gereau 2002). Intrathecal administration of group I agonists such as S-DHPG evokes spontaneous nociceptive behavior, thermal ► hyperalgesia (cold and heat), mechanical hyperalgesia, mechanical ► allodynia and enhanced formalin-induced nociception in the second phase (Fundytus 2001; Neugebauer 2001; Varney and Gereau 2002). These effects are mediated through mGluR1 as well as mGluR5 since they were blocked with antagonists or antibodies for mGluR1 or mGluR5, where tested (Fundytus 2001; Neugebauer 2001; Varney and Gereau 2002).

In electrophysiological studies in anesthetized animals *in vivo,* intraspinally administered group I mGluR agonists, including S-DHPG, had excitatory effects on spinal dorsal horn neurons and increased their responses to ► Innocuous Input/Stimulus and, less consistently, to ► noxious mechanical stimulation of cutaneous or deep tissue (Neugebauer et al. 1999; Neugebauer 2001). In addition, dual excitatory-inhibitory effects of group I

M

mGluR activation have been observed *in vivo* as well as in spinal cord slices *in vitro* (Chen et al. 2000, Gerber et al. 2000; Neugebauer 2001). The facilitatory effects of group I agonists can be blocked with antagonists selective for mGluR1 (CPCCOEt) or mGluR5 (MPEP) whereas the inhibitory effects are mimicked by an mGluR5 agonist (CHPG), suggesting that mGluR1 and mGluR5 are involved in excitation whereas inhibition is mediated through mGluR5 (Neugebauer 2001; Neugebauer 2002; Park et al. 2004).

The functional differences between mGluR1 and mGluR5 may be due to differences in their pre- and postsynaptic distribution, localization on excitatory and inhibitory synapses, regulation of excitatory and inhibitory transmission and different cellular effects, including signal transduction mechanisms and effectors.

Inhibition

The endogenous activation of spinal group I mGluRs, particularly mGluR1, in prolonged nociception and persistent pain states is well documented in behavioral and electrophysiological studies using antagonists, antibodies and antisense oligonucleotides in models of inflammatory (second phase of formalin test; intradermal capsaicin; intraplantar carrageenan; kaolin/carrageenan knee joint arthritis; complete Freund's adjuvant-induced inflammation) and neuropathic pain (Fundytus 2001; Karim et al. 2001; Neugebauer et al. 1999; Neugebauer 2001; Neugebauer 2002; Varney and Gereau 2002; Zhang et al. 2002). The role of group I mGluRs in brief nociception and acute phases of pain remains unclear. Some studies suggested that the block of spinal group I mGluRs reduced noxious heat responses and the first phase of the formalin test whereas several other studies were unable to detect such effects (Fundytus 2001; Neugebauer 2001; Varney and Gereau 2002).

Electrophysiological studies of spinal dorsal horn neurons, including spinothalamic tract cells, in anesthetized animals *in vivo* further emphasize the important role of spinal group I, particularly mGluR1, in nociceptive transmission and pain-related central sensitization in the capsaicin model of central sensitization and mustard oil-induced spinal hyperexcitability and in the kaolin/carrageenan-induced knee joint arthritic pain model (Fundytus 2001; Neugebauer 2001; Neugebauer et al. 1999; Varney and Gereau 2002). The involvement and intrinsic activation of mGluR5 during brief and prolonged nociceptive processing in spinal neurons remains to be investigated.

Groups II and III mGluRs

The roles of group II and group III mGluRs in spinal nociceptive processing are less clear. Both group II mGluR2/3 and group III mGluR4 and 7, but not mGluR6 and 8, are present in the spinal cord. Group III mGluRs

are localized predominantly on presynaptic terminals in the dorsal and ventral horns whereas group II mGluRs have been detected on presynaptic terminals in the superficial dorsal horn as well as on postsynaptic elements in deeper laminae (Neugebauer 2001; Varney and Gereau 2002).

Behavioral studies showed antinociceptive effects of group II or group III mGluR activation (Neugebauer 2002; Neugebauer 2001; Varney and Gereau 2002). Intrathecal administration of a nonselective group II mGluR agonists increased withdrawal thresholds to noxious mechanical cutaneous stimuli in the absence of tissue damage or inflammation, and this effect was blocked by a group II antagonist (EGLU). Intrathecal administration of a group III agonist (LAP4) produced antinociceptive effects both early and late in the second phase of the formalin test. Effects of group II activation are less well documented, but preliminary data suggest that selective group II agonists (LY354740, LY379268) can inhibit nociceptive behavior in the formalin test and carrageenan-induced thermal hyperalgesia.

Electrophysiological studies in anesthetized animals *in vivo* measured inhibitory effects of group II and group III agonists on spinal nociceptive processing (Neugebauer 2001; Varney and Gereau 2002). Activation of spinal group II mGluRs inhibited electrically evoked C-fiber responses of nociceptive dorsal horn neurons in carrageenan-induced hind paw inflammation, whereas mixed effects (inhibition and facilitation) were observed in control rats. Similarly, intraspinal administration of a selective group II agonist (LY379268) inhibited central sensitization of primate spinothalamic tract cells in the capsaicin pain model, but had no effect on normal transmission in non-sensitized neurons (Neugebauer et al. 2000). A group III agonist (LAP4) inhibited the responses of spinothalamic tract cells to brief noxious and innocuous mechanical cutaneous stimuli as well as capsaicin-induced central sensitization (Neugebauer et al. 2000). These data suggest a dramatic change in the functional role of group II, rather than group III, mGluRs in central sensitization associated with prolonged pain.

References

1. Anwyl R (1999) Metabotropic glutamate receptors: electrophysiological properties and role in plasticity. Brain Res Brain Res Rev 29:83–120
2. Bhave G, Nadin BM, Brasier et al. (2003) Membrane topology of a metabotropic glutamate receptor. J Biol Chem 278:30294–30301
3. Bockaert J, Pin JP (1999) Molecular tinkering of G protein-coupled receptors: an evolutionary success. EMBO J 18:1723–1729
4. Cartmell J, Schoepp DD (2000) Regulation of neurotransmitter release by metabotropic glutamate receptors. J Neurochem 75:889–907
5. Chen J, Heinke B, Sandkuhler J (2000) Activation of group I metabotropic glutamate receptors induces long-term depression

at sensory synapses in superficial spinal dorsal horn. Neuropharmacology 39:2231–2243

6. De Blasi A, Conn PJ, Pin, J et al. (2001) Molecular determinants of metabotropic glutamate receptor signaling. Trends Pharmacol Sci 22:114–120

7. Fundytus ME (2001) Glutamate receptors and nociception. Implications for the drug treatment of pain. CNS Drugs 15:29–58

8. Gasparini F, Kuhn R, Pin JP (2002) Allosteric modulators of group I metabotropic glutamate receptors: novel subtype-selective ligands and therapeutic perspectives. Curr Opin Pharmacol 2:43–49

9. Gerber G, Youn DH, Hsu CH et al. (2000) Spinal dorsal horn synaptic plasticity: involvement of group I metabotropic glutamate receptors. Prog Brain Res 129:115–134

10. Karim F, Wang CC, Gereau RW (2001) Metabotropic glutamate receptor subtypes 1 and 5 are activators of extracellular signal-regulated kinase signaling required for inflammatory pain in mice. J Neurosci 21:3771–3779

11. Neugebauer V (2001) Metabotropic glutamate receptors: novel targets for pain relief. Expert Rev Neurotherapeutics 1:207–224

12. Neugebauer V (2002) Metabotropic glutamate receptors - important modulators of nociception and pain behavior. Pain 98:1–8

13. Neugebauer V, Chen PS, Willis WD (1999) Role of metabotropic glutamate receptor subtype mGluR1 in brief nociception and central sensitization of primate STT cells. J Neurophysiol 82:272–282

14. Neugebauer V, Chen P-S, Willis WD (2000) Groups II and III metabotropic glutamate receptors differentially modulate brief and prolonged nociception in primate STT cells. J Neurophysiol 84:2998–3009

15. Park YK, Galik J, Ryu PD et al. (2004) Activation of presynaptic group I metabotropic glutamate receptors enhances glutamate release in the rat spinal cord substantia gelatinosa. Neurosci Lett 361:220–224

16. Schoepp DD, Jane DE, Monn JA (1999) Pharmacological agents acting at subtypes of metabotropic glutamate receptors. Neuropharmacology 38:1431–1476

17. Varney MA, Gereau RW (2002) Metabotropic glutamate receptor involvement in models of acute and persistent pain: prospects for the development of novel analgesics. Current Drug Targets 1:215–225

18. Zhang L, Lu Y, Chen Y et al. (2002) Group I Metabotropic glutamate receptor antagonists block secondary thermal hyperalgesia in rats with knee joint inflammation. J Pharmacol Exp Ther 300:149–156

Metabotropic Glutamate Receptors in the Thalamus

THOMAS E. SALT
Institute of Ophthalmology, University College London, London, UK
t.salt@ucl.ac.uk

Synonyms

Metabotropic glutamate receptor; mGlu receptor; mGluR; G-Protein-coupled glutamate receptor; Thalamus, Metabotropic Glutamate Receptors

Definition

Metabotropic glutamate (mGlu) receptors are ▶ glutamate receptors that are coupled to intracellular second messenger (G-protein) systems.

Characteristics

Eight metabotropic glutamate receptor subtypes (mGlu1–mGlu8) have been characterised to date. They can be placed into three Groups (I, II, III) on the basis of their sequence homology, their pharmacological characteristics and the types of intracellular transduction cascade to which they may couple in *in vitro* expression systems (Conn and Pin 1997). In such expression systems, Group I (mGlu1, mGlu5) receptors typically couple to postsynaptic inositol phosphate metabolism, while Group II (mGlu2, mGlu3) and Group III (mGlu4, mGlu6–8) receptors may couple to an inhibitory cyclic-AMP cascade. All of these receptors can be activated by L-glutamate with a variety of affinities. This amino acid is assumed to be the endogenous ligand, but the receptors may also be activated by other endogenous ligands (e.g. sulphur-containing amino acids such as L-homocysteic acid or dipeptides such as N-acetyl-aspartyl-glutamate or NAAG). A variety of synthetic agonists and antagonists have been developed, some of which show selectivity for mGlu receptor groups or even subtypes (Table 1).

The Group I receptors have been thought to predominantly mediate postsynaptic actions, whereas the Group II receptors and Group III receptors have been found to have presynaptic actions, regulating transmitter release. It is however becoming evident that the situation is more complex than this and that receptors of all three groups can have pre-, post- or extra-synaptic actions (Conn and Pin 1997). The complexity introduced by the variety of glutamate receptor types is compounded by their non-uniform distribution within the brain and within the neuropil, synapses and extra-synaptic areas. Within the thalamus, the distribution of a considerable number of the various mGlu receptors has been described in some detail (Martin et al. 1992; Petralia et al. 1996; Godwin et al. 1996; Liu et al. 1998; Mineff and Valtschanoff 1999; Neto et al. 2000; Tamaru et al. 2001).

Group I Receptors

There is expression of the mRNA for the group I mGlu receptors (mGlu1 and mGlu5) in the thalamus (Martin et al. 1992; Abe et al. 1992), with both mGlu1 and mGlu5 receptor-like immunoreactivities being found on the distal dendrites of ▶ thalamocortical neurons opposed to the corticothalamic axon terminals (Martin et al. 1992; Godwin et al. 1996; Liu et al. 1998) and also on the dendrites of local circuit interneurons pre-synaptic to thalamocortical neurons (Godwin et al. 1996). A particular focus has been the function of mGlu1 receptors, as these have been localised postsynaptically predominantly beneath terminals of cortico-thalamic fibres (Martin et al. 1992; Godwin et al. 1996). Activation of mGlu receptors in thalamic relay neurones causes a slow depolarising response associated with an increase in membrane resis-

Metabotropic Glutamate Receptors in the Thalamus, Table 1   Metabotropic Glutamate Receptor Subtypes

Group		Receptor	Transduction Mechanism	Agonists		Antagonists		
subtype-selective	group-selective		subtype-selective	group-selective				
I		mGlu1	IP3 /Ca^{++} cascade		DHPG	LY367385, CPCOOEt		4CPG
		mGlu5		CHPG		MPEP		
II		mGlu2	Inhibitory cAMP		LY354740, CCG-1,			LY341495
		mGlu3	cascade	NAAG	APDC			
III		mGlu4	Inhibitory cAMP		L-AP4,			MAP4,
		mGlu6	cascade		L-SOP			CPPG
		mGlu7						
		mGlu8		DCPG				

Abbreviations
APDC, 2R,4R-4- aminopyrrolidine-2,4-decarboxylate; CCG-1, (2S,1'S,2'S)-2-(2-carboxycyclopropyl)glycine; CHPG, 2-chloro-5-hydroxyphenylglycine; CP-COOEt, 7-(hydroxyimino)cyclopropa[b]chromen-1a-carboxylate; 4CPG, (S)-4-carboxyphenylglycine; CPPG, *alpha*-cyclopropyl-4-phosphonophenylglycine; DCPG, (S)-3,4-dicarboxyphenylglycine; DHPG, 3,5-dihydroxyphenylglycine; L-AP4, L-2-amino-4-phosphonobutyric acid; L-SOP, L-serine-O-phosphate; LY341495, 2S-2-amino-2 (1S,2S-2-carboxcyclopropyl-$^{1-}$yl)-3-(xanth-9-yl)propanoic acid; LY354740, (+)-2-aminobicyclo [3.1.0]hexane-2,6dicarboxylate; LY367385, (+)-2-methyl-4-carboxyphenylglycine; MAP4, (S)-2-amino-2-methyl-4-phosphonobutanoic acid; MPEP, 2-methyl-6-(phenylethynyl)-pyridine; NAAG, N-Acetyl-aspartyl-glutamate

tance, as seen in many other parts of the brain, probably due a reduction in a potassium conductance. This has been shown to be mediated specifically *via* mGlu1 receptors, which can be synaptically activated by stimulation of cortico-thalamic afferents (Turner and Salt 2000; Hughes et al. 2002). A specific synaptic role for mGlu5 receptors in the thalamus remains to be demonstrated, although these receptors do appear to be activated under physiological conditions (Salt and Binns 2000).

Group II Receptors

High levels of mRNA and protein for Group II receptors have been found in the ► thalamic reticular nucleus (TRN), and much of this may be attributable to mGlu3 receptors, some of which may be localised in glial cells as well as neuronal bodies and dendrites (Petralia et al. 1996; Neto et al. 2000; Tamaru et al. 2001). Intriguingly, it has been shown that activation of these receptors can lead to an inhibition of TRN neurone activity (Cox and Sherman 1999). Ultrastructural information from rodent ventrobasal thalamus (VB) suggests that Group II receptors are localised in glial processes, some of which appear to be surrounding GABAergic terminals (Liu et al. 1998; Mineff and Valtschanoff 1999). More recently mGlu3 receptors have been found to be concentrated on GABAergic axons in VB arising from TRN (Tamaru et al. 2001). Thus Group II receptors may modulate GABAergic transmission within VB, a notion supported by the finding that activation of Group II receptors within VB results in a reduction of TRN-originating inhibition onto relay cells (Turner and Salt 2003).

Group III Receptors

Of the Group III receptors, only mGlu7-like immunoreactivity has been demonstrated in the thalamus (Kinoshita et al. 1998). However, the mRNAs for mGlu4, mGlu7 and mGlu8 receptors are expressed throughout the thalamus-TRN-cortex network (Ohishi et al. 1995; Saugstad et al. 1997; Neto et al. 2000). This suggests that these receptors may be involved in the control of transmission at cortico-thalamic and TRN-thalamic synapses. Consistent with this are electrophysiological data, which suggest that Group III (probably mGlu7) receptors mediate a presynaptic reduction of the corticothalamic excitatory postsynaptic potential (Turner and Salt 1999) and a presynaptic reduction of the TRN-mediated inhibition of VB neurone responses to sensory stimuli *in vivo* and *in vitro* (Turner and Salt 2003).

Functional Considerations

There is little evidence to suggest that mGlu receptors are directly involved in ascending sensory transmission to the thalamic relay nuclei; rather it seems that such fast transmission is mediated *via* ► ionotropic glutamate receptors of the ► NMDA and ► AMPA variety (Salt and Eaton 1996). The characteristics of mGlu receptors are more suited to slow synaptic transmission or modulation (Conn and Pin 1997) and the roles in thalamic function that have been determined fit into this category.

The cortico-thalamic projection has been the subject of many studies. It has been speculated that the influence of the cortical input may operate *via* ► NMDA receptors or mGlu receptors (Sherman and Guillery 2000), largely because transmission *via* these receptor types would allow non-linear amplification of excitatory inputs mediated *via*, for example, ▶ AMPA receptors. This is a particularly attractive hypothesis in the case of mGlu1 receptors, as these are restricted to corticothalamic synapses and because NMDA-receptor mediated responses have been shown to be modulated by activation of Group I (i.e. mGlu1 / mGlu5) receptors in several brain areas. In the VB, activation of mGlu1 receptors potentiates responses mediated *via* either AMPA or NMDA receptors *in vivo* (Salt and Binns 2000). It is probable that this is due to the direct effects of mGlu1 activation on neuronal membrane potential and resistance rather than a specific interaction at the receptor level, or that the potentiation that is seen is a combination of these factors (Salt and Binns 2000). Thus, although the isolated cortico-thalamic synaptic potential which can be attributed to mGlu1 receptors *in vitro* appears to be rather small, it would be able to exert a large influence on ionotropic receptor mediated responses, if the sensory stimulus was appropriate to recruit activity in the cortico-thalamic output. Conditions where this might come into play are, for example, during the processing of nociceptive information in the thalamus (Salt and Binns 2000).

The GABAergic inhibitory output from the TRN onto relay cells is a major contributor to the overall response profile of the relay cells, and thus the control of this inhibition by mGlu receptors is potentially of great functional significance. The location of Group II receptors and the effects of their activation in this circuit suggest they play a pivotal role in these mechanisms. All of these receptors are in locations removed from sites of synaptically released glutamate. Thus this raises the possibility that these receptors are activated by glutamate which spills out of the conventional synaptic area, possibly under conditions of intense synaptic activity. This concept of "synaptic spillover" has been postulated on the basis of *in vitro* experiments from a number of non-thalamic brain areas (Kullmann 2000). This raises the possibility that the Group II (and possibly Group III) receptors may be activated by glutamate via a synaptic spillover mechanism. This glutamate could be released from terminals of sensory or cortical afferents or from astrocytes. This might occur under conditions of intense synaptic activation, perhaps during nociceptive processing or seizure activity. An intriguing further possibility is that mGlu3 receptors could be activated by the endogenous mGlu3 agonist NAAG, which is co-localised with GABA in TRN neurones and within the neuropil within VB (Henderson and Salt 1988). This raises the possibility that NAAG may be released from GABAergic TRN terminals so as to down-regulate GABA release, thus reducing IPSP amplitude. Thus it may be that NAAG has a function as a co-transmitter to regulate GABAergic transmission from TRN to VB, possibly coming into play at higher stimulus frequencies.

References

1. Abe T, Sugihara H, Nawa H et al. (1992) Molecular characterization of a novel metabotropic glutamate receptor mGluR5 coupled to inositol phosphate/Ca^{2+} signal transduction. J Biol Chem 267:13361–13368
2. Conn PJ, Pin JP (1997) Pharmacology and functions of metabotropic glutamate receptors. Annu Rev Pharmacol Toxicol 37:207–237
3. Cox CL, Sherman SM (1999) Glutamate Inhibits Thalamic Reticular Neurons. J Neurosci 19:6694–6699
4. Godwin DW, Van Horn SC, Erisir A et al. (1996) Ultrastructural localization suggests that retinal and cortical inputs access different metabotropic glutamate receptors in the lateral geniculate nucleus. J Neurosci 16:8181–8192
5. Henderson Z and Salt TE (1988) The effects of N-acetyl-aspartylglutamate and distribution of N-acetyl-aspartylglutamate-like immunoreactivity in the rat somatosensory thalamus. Neurosci 25:899–906
6. Hughes SW, Cope DW, Blethyn KL, Crunelli V (2002) Cellular Mechanisms of the Slow (< 1 Hz) Oscillation in Thalamocortical Neurons in Vitro. Neuron 33:947–958
7. Kinoshita A, Shigemoto R, Ohishi H et al. (1998) Immunohistochemical localization of metabotropic glutamate receptors, mGluR7a and mGluR7b, in the central nervous system of the adult rat and mouse: a light and electron microscopic study. J Comp Neurol 393:332–352
8. Kullmann DM (2000) Spillover and Synaptic Cross Talk Mediated by Glutamate and GABA in the Mammalian Brain. Prog Brain Res 125:339–351
9. Liu XB, Munoz A, Jones EG (1998) Changes in subcellular localization of metabotropic glutamate receptor subtypes during postnatal development of mouse thalamus. J Comp Neurol 395:450–465
10. Martin LJ, Blackstone CD, Huganir RL et al. (1992) Cellular localization of a metabotropic glutamate receptor in rat brain. Neuron 9:259–270
11. Mineff E, and Valtschanoff J (1999) Metabotropic Glutamate Receptors 2 and 3 Expressed by Astrocytes in Rat Ventrobasal Thalamus. Neurosci Lett 270:95–98
12. Neto FL, Schadrack J, Berthele A et al. (2000) Differential distribution of metabotropic glutamate receptor subtype mRNAs in the thalamus of the rat. Brain Res 854:93–105
13. Ohishi H, Akazawa C, Shigemoto R et al. (1995) Distributions of the mRNAs for L-2-amino-4-phosphonobutyrate-sensitive metabotropic glutamate receptors, mGluR4 and mGluR7, in the rat brain. J Comp Neurol 360:555–570
14. Petralia RS, Wang YX, Niedzielski AS, Wenthold RJ (1996) The metabotropic glutamate receptors, mGluR2 and mGluR3, show unique postsynaptic, presynaptic and glial localizations. Neurosci 71:949-976
15. Salt TE, Binns KE (2000) Contributions of mGlu1 and mGlu5 receptors to interactions with N-methyl-D-aspartate receptor-mediated responses and nociceptive sensory responses of rat thalamic neurones. Neurosci 100:375–380
16. Salt TE, Eaton SA (1996) Functions of ionotropic and metabotropic glutamate receptors in sensory transmission in the mammalian thalamus. Prog Neurobiol 48:55–72
17. Saugstad JA, Kinzie JM, Shinohara MM et al. (1997) Cloning and Expression of Rat Metabotropic Glutamate Receptor 8 Reveals a Distinct Pharmacological Profile. Mol Pharmacol 51:119–125
18. Sherman SM, Guillery RW (2000) Exploring the Thalamus. Academic Press, New York
19. Tamaru Y, Nomura S, Mizuno N, Shigemoto R (2001) Distribution of Metabotropic Glutamate Receptor mGluR3 in the Mouse CNS: Differential Location Relative to Pre- and Postsynaptic Sites. Neurosci 106:481-503
20. Turner JP, Salt TE (1999) Group III metabotropic glutamate receptors control corticothalamic synaptic transmission in the rat thalamus *in vitro*. J Physiol 519:481–491
21. Turner JP, Salt TE (2000) Synaptic activation of the Group I metabotropic glutamate receptor mGlu1 on the thalamocortical

M

neurones of the rat dorsal lateral geniculate nucleus *in vitro*. Neurosci 100:493–505

22. Turner JP, Salt TE (2003) Group II and III metabotropic glutamate receptors and the control of the TRN input to rat thalamocortical neurones *in vitro*. Neurosci 122:459–469

Metabotropic Receptor

Definition

A Metabotropic Receptor is a G-protein-coupled receptor. The term reflects the fact that transmitter binding results in the production of intracellular metabolites. Metabotropic receptors that couple to G-proteins are a complex of three proteins. Transmitter binding to the receptor results in a conformation change in the receptor, thereby activating the G-protein. One subunit of the G-protein may modulate ion channels, other subunits may increase or decrease the activity of enzymes that produce intracellular messengers that modulate the activity of kinases. Small molecule neurotransmitters such as glutamate, acetylcholine, and serotonin activate metabotropic receptors as well as ionotropic receptors; mammalian peptides generally activate only metabotropic receptors.

▶ Amygdala, Pain Processing and Behavior in Animals
▶ GABA Mechanisms and Descending Inhibitory Mechanisms
▶ Metabotropic Glutamate Receptors in Spinal Nociceptive Processing
▶ Spinothalamic Tract Neurons, Peptidergic Input

Metalloproteases

Definition

Metalloproteases are peptide hydrolases using a metal in the catalytic mechanism, and are implicated in many inflammatory processes.

▶ Vascular Neuropathies

Metastasis

Definition

Metastasis means the spread of cancer cells from the tissue of origin to distant organs. Cancer cells can break out of the primary tumor, penetrate into lymphatic and blood vessels, circulate through the bloodstream, and form a new focus (metastasize) within normal tissues elsewhere in the organism.

▶ NSAIDs and Cancer

Methadone

▶ Postoperative Pain, Methadone

Method of Adjustments

Definition

A psychophysical procedure used in a discrimination (or detection) experiment and in which the subjects adjust the value of the stimulus (e.g. by turning a dial) and sets it to apparent equality with a standard or reference stimulus. Repeated applications of the procedure yields an empirical distribution of stimulus intensities that is used to estimate the just-noticeable-difference (or threshold).

▶ Pain Evaluation, Psychophysical Methods

Method of Constant Stimuli

A psychophysical procedure used in a discrimination (or detection) experiment, which consists of repeatedly presenting the same set of stimuli (between 5 and 9 different intensities each presented a large number of times) in a random order throughout the experiment. The proportion (p) of "yes" responses is recorded and graphed as a psychometric function of stimulus intensity. Critical values (e.g. p=0.5) of the psychometric function are then estimated from the data.

▶ Pain Evaluation, Psychophysical Methods

Method of Limits

Definition

A psychophysical procedure used in a discrimination (or detection) experiment, which consists in varying on each successive trial the intensity of the stimulus, in small ascending or descending steps. At each step the subject reports whether the stimulus appears smaller or larger than the reference stimulus (or is perceived or not). The values of the stimulus at which the subject's response shifts from one category to another is recorded and the threshold is estimated by averaging these values.

▶ Pain Evaluation, Psychophysical Methods

Methotrexate

Definition

Methotrexate is a steroid sparing agent in cranial arteritis.

▶ Headache Due to Arteritis

Methyl-2-(2,6-Xylyloxy)-Ethylamine-Hydrochloride

▶ Postoperative Pain, Mexiletine

Methylprednisolone

Definition
Steroid drug.
▶ Whiplash

Methysergide

Serotonin antagonist.
▶ Migraine, Preventive Therapy

Metopropol

Definition
Beta-blocker.
▶ Migraine, Preventive Therapy

Mexiletine/Mexitil

▶ Postoperative Pain, Mexiletine

mGLu Receptors/mGluRs

▶ Metabotropic Glutamate Receptors
▶ Metabotropic Glutamate Receptors in the Thalamus

MH, HTM, PMN

Definition
Nociceptors are often designated as mechanoheat (MH), high threshold mechanoreceptive (HTM), or polymodal (PM). These designations refer to their capacity to respond to mechanical, thermal or chemical stimuli. The designation HTM implies that the nociceptor responds only to mechanical stimuli. The designation MH, implies that the nociceptor responds to both mechanical and heat stimuli. The designation PMN, implies that the nociceptor responds to mechanical thermal and at least one kind of chemical stimulus (e.g. bradykinin).
▶ Nociceptors in the Orofacial Region (Skin/Mucosa)

Micro-Arousal

Definition
An increase in EEG and heart rate frequency with a possible rise in muscle tone. It should last more than 3 sec. but less than 10 seconds. The subject is unaware of such physiological activity.
▶ Orofacial Pain, Sleep Disturbance

Microdialysis

Definition
Microdialysis is a technique that allows the administration of drugs or sampling of substances in the extracellular fluid by means of a small dialysis fiber of the type used for renal dialysis. The semi-permeable dialysis membrane has pores of a certain size, and molecules smaller than these pores diffuse across the dialysis membrane due to concentration gradients, either into the extracellular space or into the dialysate. The dialysis fluid is continually pumped through the fiber. Microdialysis allows minimal invasive insights into tissue metabolism. Drugs can be dissolved in the dialysate for tissue administration, or samples of the dialysate can be taken for analysis of extracellular fluid concentrations of substances.
▶ Amygdala, Pain Processing and Behavior in Animals
▶ GABA Mechanisms and Descending Inhibitory Mechanisms
▶ Spinal Dorsal Horn Pathways, Dorsal Column (Visceral)
▶ Spinothalamic Tract Neurons, Role of Nitric Oxide
▶ Sympathetically maintained Pain and Inflammation, Human Experimentation

Microglia

Definition
Microglia are considered to be the resident immune cells of the CNS. These cells release classical immune proteins, respond to immunogenic stimuli, and express cell surface receptors characteristic of peripheral phagocytic cells. Blocking microglial activation inhibits the onset of exaggerated pain.
▶ Cord Glial Activation

Microglia Activation

▶ Cord Glial Activation

M

Microinjection

Definition

Microinjection is a common technique in behavioral neuroscience in which micro- or nanoliter amounts of a liquid is directly infused into a specific brain region.

▶ Cingulate Cortex, Nociceptive Processing, Behavioral Studies in Animals

Microiontophoresis

Definition

Microiontophoresis is a technique for releasing active agents near a neuron from which recordings are made. A multibarreled array of micropipettes is generally used. The central barrel records the activity of a neuron, whereas the other barrels are filled with solutions that contain agonist or antagonist drugs or other substances. The dissolved agents are usually charged, and so they can be released from the micropipette by passing a current of the appropriate sign through the micropipette. A current of the opposite sign is generally used to restrain the agent when its release is not desired.

▶ GABA Mechanisms and Descending Inhibitory Mechanisms

Microneurography and Intraneural Microstimulation

Definition

Microneurography is a sophisticated neurophysiological technique for recording electrical activity from an intact peripheral nerve using a sharp tungsten microelectrode inserted into the nerve percutaneously. It allows *in vivo* action potential recording (single or multifiber-recordings) from sympathetic efferent and nociceptive afferent neurons in awake human subjects.

▶ Mechano-Insensitive C-Fibres, Biophysics
▶ Nociceptors, Action Potentials and Post-Firing Excitability Changes
▶ Painless Neuropathies
▶ Polymodal Nociceptors, Heat Transduction
▶ Sympathetically maintained Pain and Inflammation, Human Experimentation

Microneuroma

Definition

A neuroma is the proximal cut end of a peripheral nerve branch or nerve fascicle. Severed axons form swollen terminal endbulbs, and there is usually aborted sprouting. If these regenerative sprouts are not able to elongate they often form a tangled mass at the nerve end. If only a part of the cross-section of the nerve is cut, the cut axons form a neuroma-in-continuity adjacent to their intact neighbors. Transection of small groups of axons scattered throughout a nerve trunk, or of tiny nerve fascicles or tributary yields microneuromas.

▶ Neuroma Pain
▶ Peripheral Neuropathic Pain

Microstimulation

Definition

Low current stimulation (μA) through a small diameter electrode, either intraoperatively or during experiments.

▶ Central Pain, Human Studies of Physiology

Microsurgical DREZotomy

▶ Brachial Plexus Avulsion and Dorsal Root Entry Zone
▶ DREZ Procedures

Microswitch

Definition

A microswitch is a very small switch that acts by the movement of a small lever and is sensitive to minute motions.

▶ Assessment of Pain Behaviors

Microvascular Decompression

Synonyms

MVD

Definition

Neurosurgical procedures to relieve cranial nerve compression by intracranial arteries or veins as described under 'vascular compression syndromes'. The main indication is for pain relief in cranial nerve neuralgias.

▶ Pain Paroxysms
▶ Tic and Cranial Neuralgias
▶ Trigeminal, Glossopharyngeal, and Geniculate Neuralgias

Microwaves

▶ Therapeutic Heat, Microwaves and Cold

Midazolam

Definition

Midazolam is a benzodiazepine drug with an imidazole structure, commonly used as an anxiolytic, amnesic, and sedative/hypnotic. Spinal administration has recently been advocated in the management of complex pain syndromes.

▶ Postoperative Pain, Appropriate Management

Midline Commissural Myelotomy

Definition

Dividing the spinal cord longitudinally in the midline to ablate nerve fibers at the point where they cross the spinal cord.

▶ Cancer Pain Management, Neurosurgical Interventions

Midline Epidural Steroid Injection

▶ Epidural Steroid Injections for Chronic Back Pain

Midline Myelotomy

H. J. W. Nauta
University of Texas Medical Branch, Galveston, TX, USA
hjnauta@utmb.edu

Synonyms

Longitudinal Myelotomy; mediolongitudinal myelotomy; dorsal longitudinal myelotomy. Related terms include commissural myelotomy; Punctate Midline Myelotomy; extralemniscal myelotomy; Bischof Myelotomy; Pourpre Myelotomy; myelotomy

Definition

Midline myelotomy refers to surgical procedures that involve an incision in the dorsal midline of the spinal cord. More recently, the term has come to include derived procedures that continue to include an intervention through the dorsal midline of the spinal cord.

Characteristics

Background

The spinal cord is commonly characterized by both its segmental organization, and the long tracts that link the segments to each other and to the brain. Surgical interventions on the spinal cord similarly can be characterized by their effects on segmental components, long tracts, or both. The distinction is important. If the goal is to interrupt a long ascending tract, then a single lesion should suffice. If the goal is an intervention at the segmental level, then typically several spinal levels must be accessed, and an incision made in the spinal cord over several segments.

Myelotomy – Origin from Procedures Directed at Segmental Structures, not Long Tracts

The original myelotomy procedures were directed at the segments of the spinal cord for treatment of pain or spasticity. The long spinal cord incision distinguished myelotomy from "cordotomy", where a single rostrocaudal level lesion is made, which interrupts longitudinal pathways. The distinction between myelotomy and cordotomy has blurred over time. It is now fairly safe to say that while the anterolateral cordotomy procedure continues to be understood as interrupting ascending tracts related to the conduction of pain, only the Bischof myelotomy (Bischof 1951; Bischof 1967), still occasionally used to treat painful spasticity, continues to be understood as a procedure directed at the segmental level, and therefore requiring a long incision into the spinal cord. The original myelotomy procedures used to treat pain have mutated into much more concise procedures, and are now understood to be effective through their interruption of ascending pain tracts near the midline of the dorsal columns (Nauta et al. 2002). Due to their history, however, these procedures continue to be described as myelotomies, although they no longer require a long incision into the spinal cord.

Impetus to Develop Myelotomy and Original Concepts of Benefit

Anterolateral cordotomy for interruption of the long tract system related to pain has evolved into an elegant fluoroscopic-guided percutaneous procedure at the C1-C2 level, which is effective for all levels below the lesion. The principal disadvantage of the anterolateral cordotomy was the unavoidable concomitant interruption of descending pathways in the anterolateral quadrant related to respiration and bladder control. The potential for the loss of automatic respiration (Ondine's curse) and development of incontinence required special strategies, if bilateral anterolateral cordotomy was contemplated for the all too common bilateral, midline or visceral pain. These problems with bilateral cordotomy led to the proposal in 1926, by the neuropathologist Greenfield, that a longitudinal midline incision of the spinal cord could interrupt the crossing

M

fibers of the spinothalamic pathway bilaterally, near their segmental level of origin and before these fibers assemble into a long ascending tract. The longitudinal midline myelotomy required definition of segmental levels of pain origin, and a large enough exposure to incise the cord deeply over enough levels to bracket the levels of pain origin.

Clinical Observation at Odds with the Original Concept

The long midline myelotomy for pain was first performed by Armour in 1926 (Armour 1927), and while there were several early advocates, the procedure as originally conceived required a big operation which limited its wider acceptance. However, it became clear that the procedure was effective, even when a short myelotomy was performed at a level well above the segmental origin of the treated pain, and that pain relief extended to levels caudal to the zone of decreased pin sensation. Hirshberg et al. (1996) and Hitchcock (1974) originally attempting to treat neck and upper extremity pain, made lesions of only limited rostro-caudal extent near the midline at C1, and observed relief of pain with analgesia extending into the legs. Such observations suggested that the midline myelotomy procedure was interrupting an ascending pain conducting system, perhaps a multisynaptic pathway separate from the spinothalamic tract, as proposed by Hitchcock (Hitchcock 1969; Hitchcock 1974) and others (Davis et al. 1929; Noordenbos 1959). Surprisingly, the midline myelotomy procedure remained effective even if a short midline incision was made above and not deep enough to reach either the commissural fiber systems or the central grey matter (Hirshberg et al. 1996).

Laboratory Evidence of a Dorsal Column Pain Pathway

The literature concerning myelotomy for pain shows an interesting progression, with late recognition that there is a pain pathway ascending near the midline of the dorsal columns (Hirshberg et al. 1996; Nauta et al. 2002). The old concept is that there are two pathways carrying somatic sensation to the brain: the spinothalamic system described as conducting crude or "protopathic" sensations such as pain and temperature, the dorsal column pathway conducting the "epicritic" sensations, such as vibration and proprioception. Recent evidence demonstrates that the dorsal columns do contain a post-synaptic pain pathway (Rustioni et al. 1979; Uddenberg 1968; Willis and Coggeshall 1991), but its role in somatic pain conduction was considered minor. Berkley and Hubscher (1995) gave evidence that neurons in the dorsal column nuclei can respond to innocuous and noxious stimulation of both pelvic viscera and skin. Finally, Al Chaer and others (1996b) demonstrated that the post synaptic dorsal column pain pathway predominated in the conduction of visceral pain. Microdialysis fiber infusion of neurotransmitters or antagonists (morphine or CNQX) into the spinal cord suggested the presence of a synapse in the pathway (Al Chaer et al. 1996a; Al Chaer et al. 1996b). Retrograde tracer studies, depositing a marker in the nucleus gracilis (Christensen et al. 1996), revealed the likely cell bodies of origin of the pathway to reside at the medial base of the dorsal horn just above the central canal, an area known from earlier experiments to receive primary visceral fiber input. Injection of anterograde tracers into the same cell territory (Wang et al. 1999) resulted in fiber labeling ascending near the dorsal column midline, to end in the medial part of the nucleus gracilis. Further studies by this group defined a somatotopic organization within the postsynaptic dorsal column pathway, wherein the fibers originating in the lumbosacral cord ascend near the midline of the dorsal columns, while fibers originating in the thoracic cord terminate in the lateral part of nucleus gracilis and adjacent medial parts of nucleus cuneatus (Wang et al. 1999; Willis et al. 1999).

Subsequent Clinical Observations

Once the basis for the benefit from midline myelotomy was better understood, Nauta et al. (1997, 2000) made very small transverse (rather than sagittal longitudinal) midline incisions in the dorsal columns, well above the segmental level of pain origin, to treat medically intractable pelvic pain. The incisions, later crush, across the midline of the dorsal columns extended only 1mm to either side of the exact midline, and only to a depth of 5 mm. The effective lesion was so small that it was dubbed "punctate myelotomy" since the original lesions were made with what amounted to a puncture across the spinal cord midline with a 16 gauge hypodermic needle. Pain relief from these tiny lesions confirmed that an ascending pathway in the dorsal column was being interrupted. The lesions were effective without reaching the commissures or the central grey, demonstrating that these latter structures were not essential to the benefit. Surprisingly, postoperative neurological examination in these patients by an independent neurologist failed to reveal any new deficit, emphasizing an important distinction between the consequences of small midline lesions of the dorsal columns and tabes dorsalis, in which a pathologic process effects the dorsal root ganglia in a widespread manner and results not only in visible changes in the dorsal columns, but less visible changes in other sensory pathways as well. While Nauta et al. (1997, 2000) treated only pelvic origin visceral pain, more recent reports (Kim and Kwon 2000) suggest that more rostral visceral origin pain related to gastric cancer can also be treated effectively by punctate midline myelotomy at an upper thoracic level. Since it is now understood that the benefit depends on the interruption of an ascending pathway, there are good theoretical reasons to believe that it would be worthwhile to revive the percutaneous procedure described by Hitchcock (1970, 1974) and

Schvarcz (1984), only modified to emphasize the medial dorsal columns rather than the subjacent central grey. Clearly the term "extralemniscal myelotomy" used by Schvarcz (Kanpolat 2002) would no longer apply to such an operation, because the dorsal columns are well known to contribute to signaling within the medial lemniscus.

The Bischof myelotomy and its variants can be used to treat severe, medically intractable, often painful, lower limb spasticity, usually in quadri- or paraplegic or paretic patients (Livshits et al. 2002; Putty and Shapiro 1991). The goal of the procedure is to interrupt the segmental reflex arcs underlying spasticity that pass between the dorsal horn and the motor neurons in the ventral horn. The goal is also to preserve as much residual function as possible and, above all, the anterior horn cells and their continuity with the muscles so that atrophy is minimized, and padding over boney prominences maintained to protect against the development of pressure sores. The latter can be a significant problem following ventral root section or neurectomy. The myelotomy method also offers an advantage over simple dorsal rhizotomy where recurrence of spasticity is more common. Since the availability of intrathecal Baclofen infusion pumps (Penn and Kroin 1987), the procedure is performed less frequently, but still remains a reasonable option for cases where severe problems with the pump are experienced or anticipated.

Since the Bischof myelotomy is directed at the segmental level, there is no alternative to an exposure of the spinal cord by laminectomy (typically, vertebral levels T10-L1) to gain access to those levels determined preoperatively to give rise to the worst spasticity (typically T12-S1). The required spinal cord incision is made in the longitudinal plane, perpendicular to the midsagittal plane. This plane passes through the central canal and dentate ligament of either side, thus filleting the spinal cord into a dorsal and ventral half. The incision along this plane was originally described from the lateral aspect of the cord (Bischof 1951) on either side, and was typically performed with an angled triangular ophthalmology knife inserted just posterior to the dentate ligament and directed towards the central canal. Great care is required to minimize injury to the spinal cord vasculature. Pourpre (Pourpre 1960), who proposed a Myelotomy en croix, in which the cord is entirely bisected into a right and left half. (Bischof 1967), modified his original lateral approach making an upside down "T" incision instead, beginning with a long myelotomy in the midsagittal plane to a depth reaching the center of the cord but sparing the anterior white commissure. An angled triangular ophthalmology knife is then passed laterally along the depth of the midline incision aimed at the pia just above the dentate ligament of either side, thereby separating the dorsal horn from the ventral horn of each side. The lateral limbs of this myelotomy are intended to pass through the grey matter, but not far into

the lateral funiculus containing whatever corticospinal fibers may still be functional.

▶ Postsynaptic Dorsal Column Neurons, Responses to Visceral Input
▶ Spinal Dorsal Horn Pathways, Dorsal Column (Visceral)

References

1. Al Chaer ED, Lawand NB, Westlund KN et al. (1996a) Pelvic Visceral Input into the Nucleus Gracilis is Largely Mediated by the Postsynaptic Dorsal Column Pathway. J Neurophysiol 76:2675–2690
2. Al Chaer ED, Lawand NB, Westlund KN et al. (1996b) Visceral Nociceptive Input into the Ventral Posterolateral Nucleus of the Thalamus: A New Function for the Dorsal Column Pathway. J Neurophysiol 76:2661–2674
3. Armour D (1927) Surgery of the Spinal Cord. Lancet 2:691
4. Berkley KJ, Hubscher CH (1995) Are There Separate Central Nervous System Pathways for Touch and Pain? Nat Med 1:766–773
5. Bischof W (1951) Die Longitudinale Myelotomie. Zentralbl Neurochir 11:79–88
6. Bischof W (1967) Zur Dorsalen Longitudinalen Myelotomie. Zentralbl Neurochir 28:123–126
7. Christensen MD, Willis WD, Westlund KN (1996) Anatomical Evidence for Cells of Origin of a Postsynaptic Dorsal Column Visceral Pathway: Sacral Spinal Cord Cells Innervating the Medial Nucleus Gracilis. Society for Neuroscience Abstract 22:109
8. Davis L, Hart JT, Crain RC (1929) The Pathway for Visceral Afferent Impulses within the Spinal Cord. II. Experimental Dilatation of the Biliary Ducts. Surg Gynecol Obstet 48:647–651
9. Hirshberg RM, Al Chaer ED, Lawand NB et al. (1996) Is There a Pathway in the Posterior Funiculus that Signals Visceral Pain? Pain 67:291–305
10. Hitchcock E (1969) Stereotaxic Spinal Surgery. A Preliminary Report. J Neurosurg 31:386–392
11. Hitchcock E (1970) Stereotactic Cervical Myelotomy. J Neurol Neurosurg Psychiatry 33:224230
12. Hitchcock E (1974) Stereotactic Myelotomy. Proc R Soc Med 67:771–772
13. Kanpolat Y (2002) Percutaneous Stereotactic Pain Procedures: Percutaneous Cordotomy, Extralemniscal Myelotomy, Trigeminal Tractotomy-Nucleotomy. In: Burchiel KJ (ed) Surgical Management of Pain. Thieme, New York, pp 745–762
14. Kim YS, Kwon SJ (2000) High Thoracic Midline Dorsal Column Myelotomy for Severe Visceral Pain due to Advanced Stomach Cancer. Neurosurg 46:85–90
15. Livshits A, Rappaport ZH, Livshits V et al. (2002) Surgical Treatment of Painful Spasticity after Spinal Cord Injury. Spinal Cord 40:161–166
16. Nauta HJ, Hewitt E, Westlund KN et al. (1997) Surgical Interruption of a Midline Dorsal Column Visceral Pain Pathway. Case Report and Review of the Literature. J Neurosurg 86:538–542
17. Nauta HJ, Soukup VM, Fabian RH et al. (2000) Punctate Midline Myelotomy for the Relief of Visceral Cancer Pain. J Neurosurg 92:125–130
18. Nauta HJW, Westlund KN, Willis WD (2002) Midline Myelotomy. In: Burchiel KJ (ed) Surgical Management of Pain. Thieme, New York, pp 714–731
19. Noordenbos W (1959) Pain: Problems Pertaining to the Transmission of Nerve Impulses Which Give Rise to Pain. Elsevier, Amsterdam
20. Penn RD, Kroin JS (1987) Long-Term Intrathecal Baclofen Infusion for Treatment of Spasticity. J Neurosurg 66:181–185
21. Pourpre MH (1960) Traitement Neuro-Chirurgical des Contractures chez les Paraplegiques Posttraumatiques. Neurochirurgie 6:229–236
22. Putty TK, Shapiro SA (1991) Efficacy of Dorsal Longitudinal Myelotomy in Treating Spinal Spasticity: A Review of 20 Cases. J Neurosurg 75:397–401

M

23. Rustioni A, Hayes NL, O'Neill S (1979) Dorsal Column Nuclei and Ascending Spinal Afferents in Macaques. Brain 102:95–125

24. Schvarcz JR (1984) Stereotactic High Cervical Extralemniscal Myelotomy for Pelvic Cancer Pain. Acta Neurochir 33:431–435

25. Uddenberg N (1968) Functional Organization of Long, Second-Order Afferents in the Dorsal Funiculus. Exp Brain Res 4:377–382

26. Wang CC, Willis WD, Westlund KN (1999) Ascending Projections from the Area around the Spinal Cord Central Canal: A Phaseolus Vulgaris Leucoagglutinin Study in Rats. J Comp Neurol 415:341–367

27. Willis WD, Coggeshall RE (1991) Sensory Mechanisms of the Spinal Cord. Plenum Press, New York

28. Willis WD, Al Chaer ED, Quast MJ et al. (1999) A Visceral Pain Pathway in the Dorsal Column of the Spinal Cord. Proc Natl Acad Sci USA 96:7675–7679

Migraine

Definition

Migraine is an common, episodic neurovascular headache disorder characterized by unilateral pulsating moderate to severe headache, typically lasting 4 to 72 hours, of throbbing quality and with associated symptoms of light and sound sensitivity, nausea and vomiting, phono-and/or photophobia. The headache may be preceded by visual disturbances (aura).

► Calcitonin Gene-Related Peptide and Migraine Headaches
► Human Thalamic Response to Experimental Pain (Neuroimaging)
► Migraine, Preventive Therapy
► New Daily Persistent Headache

Migraine Accompagnee

► Clinical Migraine with Aura

Migraine Aphasic

► Clinical Migraine with Aura

Migraine, Childhood Syndromes

ERIC M. PEARLMAN
Pediatric Education, Mercer University School of Medicine, Savannah, GA, USA
pearlmane@aol.com

Synonyms

Childhood Migraine; Pediatric Migraine; Periodic Disorders of Childhood that are Precursors to Migraine; Migraine Variants of Childhood

Definitions

There are many paroxysmal disorders of childhood that have been associated with migraine. The link to migraine is very strong for some of these childhood syndromes, and more tenuous for others. The International Headache Society (The International Classification of Headache Disorders 2004) considers the following to be linked to migraine:

● Abdominal migraine
● Cyclic vomiting syndrome
● Benign paroxysmal vertigo
● Alternating hemiplegia of childhood
● Familial hemiplegic migraine

Benign paroxysmal torticollis is probably associated with migraine, based on genetic links. ► Ophthalmoplegic migraine, originally considered to be linked to migraine, is probably not actually a migraine variant. Other disorders probably represent unusual auras of migraine rather than separate entities. These include acute ► confusional migraine, ► basilar-type migraine and ► Alice in Wonderland syndrome.

Characteristics

Migraine with or without aura may differ slightly between children and adults. The diagnostic criteria proposed by the International Classification of Headache (IHS) Disorders II for children less than 15 years requires headaches of 1 to 48 hours in duration instead of the 4 to 72 hours in individuals greater than 15 years of age. The remainder of the criteria are similar to the adult diagnostic criteria, including at least five attacks with either photophobia and phonophobia, nausea or vomiting and two symptoms out of unilateral pain, throbbing or pulsatile pain, moderate or severe pain intensity or exacerbation by routine activity (Tab. 1).

There are features of headache in children that are not specifically recognized by the IHS classification, but are commonly noted in adolescents and children (Table 2). The quality of the pain may be described as constant or squeezing instead of throbbing. Children also are more likely to report bilateral, bifrontal or a nondescript location rather than unilateral pain. Adults who have migraine with aura have onset and resolution of their aura before the onset of head pain. When aura occurs in children, it may also overlap with the actual headache in onset. Aura should resolve before the headache phase ends. The onset of the head pain may be quite dramatic in children, with maximal pain achieved within 15 minutes. Pain also may resolve fairly quickly, i.e. in 2–4 hours, and may require just a short period of sleep to achieve resolution.

Abdominal Migraine

Abdominal migraine is an idiopathic disorder characterized by discreet episodes of abdominal pain, is poorly localized, is moderate to severe in intensity

Migraine, Childhood Syndromes, Table 1 Classification of adolescent and pediatric migraine with and without aura (The International Classification of Headache Disorders 2004)

Pediatric Migraine without Aura	Pediatric Migraine with Aura
A. At least 5 distinct attacks	E. Fulfills criteria for migraine without aura
B. Headache attack lasting 1–48 hours	F. At least 3 of the following: 1. One or more fully reversible aura symptoms indicating focal cortical and/or brainstem dysfunction
C. Headache has at least 2 of the following: 1. Bilateral location (frontal/temporal) or unilateral location 2. Pulsating quality 3. Moderate to severe intensity 4. Aggravation by routine physical activity	2. At least one aura developing gradually over more than 4 minutes or two or more symptoms occurring in succession 3. No aura lasting more than 60 minutes 4. Headache follows in less than 60 minutes
D. During headache, at least one of the following: 1. Nausea and/or vomiting 2. Photophobia and/or phonophobia	

Migraine, Childhood Syndromes, Table 2 Differentiating features in childhood *vs.* adult migraine

Duration	1 hour to 48 hours	4 hours to 72 hours
Quality	May or not be described as throbbing	Throbbing/pulsatile
Location	Unilateral, bilateral, whole head	Unilateral; bilateral less likely
Aura	May overlap with head pain	Resolves prior to head pain
Resolution	Resolves with rest or brief sleep	Resolves with longer sleep
Associated Features	Nausea/vomiting, photophobia or phonophobia – may be less prominent	Nausea/vomiting, photophobia, phonophobia – necessary for diagnosis

M

and lasts from 1 to 72 hours. These episodes are often associated with anorexia, nausea, vomiting and pallor. Sometimes headache, photophobia and phonophobia accompany migraine episodes. Eight percent of school children between 5–15 years reported recurrent abdominal pain and 4.1% reported episodes that fulfilled the criteria for the diagnosis of abdominal migraine. Abdominal migraine affects both boys and girls equally with a peak age of onset at 10 years. Affected children are otherwise normal between attacks. Often, children undergo extensive gastrointestinal evaluations before the diagnosis of abdominal migraine is considered. Individual attacks will ultimately resolve spontaneously and the syndrome can last from months to years before abating. In these children, there is a strong family history of migraine and individuals who suffer from abdominal migraine are more likely to develop migraine as adults than the general population.

Cyclic Vomiting Syndrome

Cyclic vomiting syndrome consists of stereotypical attacks of intense nausea and vomiting lasting from 1 hour to 5 days. Vomiting can be quite dramatic, occurring at least 4 times in 1 hour. It can lead to significant dehydration and children often require intravenous rehydration. Associated features include lethargy, pallor, headache, photophobia, phonophobia, vertigo, diarrhea, excess salivation and fever. It is equally distributed between males and females and has a mean age of onset of 5.2 years (Li and Balint 2000). The duration of attacks is usually 2–3 years and is associated with significant morbidity. Children with cyclic vomiting syndrome miss on average 20 days of school each year, and more than 50% will require hospitalization for rehydration. Almost half of the children with a diagnosis of cyclical vomiting will go on to develop migraine later in life.

Both cyclic vomiting syndrome and abdominal migraine have a periodicity to attacks, so that many families can predict when the next attack might occur. Attacks can be triggered by many of the same triggers as migraine, for example, infection, certain foods, menstruation, sleep changes, physical exertion and psychological stress.

Benign Paroxysmal Vertigo

Benign paroxysmal vertigo is another paroxysmal disorder linked to migraine. It is characterized by attacks of vertigo, dizziness or unsteadiness lasting minutes to hours. These attacks occur in toddlers or preschoolers and are associated with nystagmus, irritability, pallor, nausea and vomiting. Children will describe an unreal sense of movement. Younger children will often refuse to walk, sit down or cling to a parent until the episode subsides. Attacks are usually brief and do not require any treatment. The key in distinguishing these attacks from seizures or metabolic disturbances is the sparing of consciousness. Attacks often resolve with sleep and can occur in clusters. As with the other paroxysmal disorders, individuals often go on to develop migraine.

Alternating Hemiplegia of Childhood

Alternating hemiplegia of childhood is another rare, perplexing paroxysmal disorder of childhood with a recently identified genetic link to migraine. This syndrome consists of repeated, frequent attacks of hemiparesis, monoparesis or diparesis usually beginning before 18 months of age. Episodes can last from hours to days and may include dystonia or athetosis along with the weakness, which can be on either side of the body or shift from side to side during an attack. There also can be bulbar dysfunction leading to swallowing and respiratory difficulties, which may result in respiratory failure. All these features disappear during sleep. Attacks may increase in frequency, plateau and eventually decrease in frequency, often resolving after 5–7 years. The syndrome may occur in the setting of mild developmental delays and can rarely be associated with developmental regression. The exact etiology is unknown but inborn errors of metabolism, mitochondrial dysfunction and channelopathy have all been suggested. Recently, a genetic link with familial hemiplegic migraine has been identified. In a family with alternating hemiplegia of childhood; affected individuals had a mutation in the ATP1A2 gene, which is an ▶ ATP-dependent Na/K pump (Bassi et al. 2004). Interestingly, mutations in this gene are also associated with familial hemiplegic migraine.

Familial Hemiplegic Migraine

Familial hemiplegic migraine is a rare autosomal dominant disorder characterized by an aura that has more stroke-like qualities than typical aura. The aura consists of motor weakness, usually unilateral, along with other neurological changes. These include positive visual changes (e.g. scintillating lights, colors or lines) or vision loss, sensory changes (e.g. pins and needles sensation or numbness) or speech difficulties. The aura develops gradually, lasts between 5 minutes and 24 hours and may or may not be associated with headache fulfilling the criteria for migraine. Identification of a first or second degree relative with similar attacks completes the diagnostic criteria. While there is no diagnostic testing for familial hemiplegic migraine, specific causative gene mutations have been identified. A missense mutation in ▶ P/Q type calcium channel _gene (CACNA1A) on chromosome 19p13 is responsible for the disorder in about 50% of the families (Kors et al. 2003). Mutations in this gene are also responsible for acetazolamide responsive episodic ataxia and benign paroxysmal torticollis (Ducros et al. 2001). Other families with familial hemiplegic migraine have been identified with mutations in the ATP1A2 gene, which is an ATP-dependent Na/K pump found on chromosome 1q31. This suggests that there may be multiple mechanisms for the neuronal instability that leads to these unusual auras.

Benign Paroxysmal Torticollis

Benign paroxysmal torticollis is an uncommon disorder occurring in infants. This syndrome consists of recurrent attacks of head tilt, truncal ataxia and occasionally vomiting. The attacks last from several hours to days. Attacks may be associated with some irritability but no alteration in consciousness. The differential diagnosis for this condition includes congenital torticollis, disorders of the craniocervical junction, intracranial abnormalities, especially in the posterior fossa and metabolic disorders. A completely normal interictal examination and repeated pattern of attacks is reassuring, but further diagnostic evaluations are certainly appropriate. A strong family history of migraine and tendency to develop migraine later in life suggested a link between benign paroxysmal torticollis and migraine. Recently, a genetic link has been suggested. Giffin and colleagues have found mutations in the CACNA1A gene in 4 cases of benign paroxysmal torticollis. Mutations in this P/Q-type calcium channel gene have been linked to familial hemiplegic migraine, a rare migraine phenotype (Giffin et al. 2002).

References

1. Abu-Arafeh I, Russell G (1995) Prevalence and clinical features of abdominal migraine compared with those of migraine headache. Archives of Disease in Childhood 72:413–417
2. Bassi MT, Bresolin N, Tonelli A et al. (2004) A novel mutation in the ATP1A2 gene causes alternating hemiplegia of childhood. J Med Genet 41:621–628
3. Ducros A, Denier C, Joutel A et al. (2001) The clinical spectrum of familial hemiplegic migraine associated with mutations in a neuronal calcium channel. N Engl J Med 345:17–24
4. Giffin NJ, Benton S, Goadsby PJ (2002) Benign paroxysmal torticollis of infancy: four new cases and linkage to CACNA1A mutation. Dev Med Child Neurol 44:490–493
5. Kors EE, Haan J, Giffen NJ et al. (2003) Expanding the phenotypic spectrum of the CACNA1A gene T666M mutation: a description of 5 families with hemiplegic migraine. Arch Neurol 60:684–688
6. Li BU, Balint JP (2000) Cyclic vomiting syndrome: evolution in our understanding of a brain-gut disorder. Adv Pediatr 47:117–60
7. Ophoff RA, Terwindt GM, Vergouwe MN et al. (1997) Familial hemiplegic migraine: involvement of a calcium neuronal channel. Neurologia 12:31–37
8. Proceedings of the 2nd International Scientific Symposium on Cyclic Vomiting Syndrome (1999) Dig Dis Sci 44:1S–119S
9. The International Classification of Headache Disorders: 2nd edn (2004) Cephalalgia 24:9–160
10. Thomsen L, Eriksen M, Roemer S et al. (2002) A population-based study of familial hemiplegic migraine suggests revised diagnostic criteria. Brain 125:1379–1391

Migraine Epidemiology

RICHARD B. LIPTON[1], MARCELO E. BIGAL[2]
[1]Departments of Neurology, Epidemiology and Population Health, Albert Einstein College of Medicine and Montefiore Headache Unit, Bronx, NY, USA
[2]Department of Neurology, Albert Einstein College of Medicine, The New England Center for Headache,

Stamford, CT, and Montefiore Headache Unit, Bronx, NY, NY, USA
rlipton@aecom.yu.edu

Definition

Migraine is a prevalent under-diagnosed and under-treated medical disorder, associated with a severe impact on the quality of life of the sufferers and their families as well as an enormous economic impact on society. This essay reviews the epidemiology and burden of migraine in population studies. Epidemiological studies often focus on the ► incidence and ► prevalence of disease in defined populations.

Characteristics

The Incidence of Migraine

The incidence of migraine has been investigated in a limited number of studies (Fig. 1). Stewart et al found that in females, the incidence of migraine with aura peaked between ages 12 and 13 (14.1 / 1000 person-years); migraine without aura peaked between ages 14 and 17 (18.9 / 1000 person-years). In males, the incidence of migraine with aura peaked several years earlier, around 5 years of age at 6.6 / 1000 person-years; the peak for migraine without aura was 10 / 1000 person-years between 10 and 11 years. New onset of migraine was uncommon in men in their twenties. This study suggests that migraine begins earlier in males than in females and that migraine with aura begins earlier than migraine without aura (Stewart et al. 1993).

Three other studies assessed the incidence of migraine. A study performed in a random sample of young adults (21–30 years), found that the incidence of migraine was 5.0 per 1,000 person-years in males and 22.0 in females (Breslau et al. 1994), supporting the findings reported above (Stang et al. 1992). A second study using a linked medical records system showed a lower incidence (probably because many people with migraine do not consult doctors or receive a medical diagnosis) (Breslau et al. 1994). In this study, the average annual incidence rate per 1,000 person-years was 3.4 (4.8 in women and 1.9 in men). In women, incidence rates were low at the extremes of age and higher among those aged between 10 and 49 years, with a striking peak at the age of 20 to 29 years. In this study, incidence also peaked later than in other studies, probably because medical diagnosis may occur long after the age of onset. Finally, in the Danish population, the annual incidence of migraine in those aged 25 to 64 years old was 8 / 1,000, being 15 / 1,000 in males and 3 / 1,000 in females (Lyngberg et al. 2003).

The Prevalence of Migraine

The published estimates of migraine prevalence have varied broadly, probably because of differences in the methodology. The studies presented herein primarily used the IHS definition.

Prevalence by Age

Before puberty, as suggested by the incidence data, migraine prevalence is higher in boys than in girls; as adolescence approaches, incidence and prevalence increase more rapidly. As a consequence, at all post-pubertal ages, migraine is more common in girls than in boys. The prevalence increases throughout childhood and early adult life until approximately age 40, after which it declines (Fig. 2) (Scher et al. 1999). Overall, prevalence is highest from 25–55, the peak years of economic productivity. The gap between peak inci-

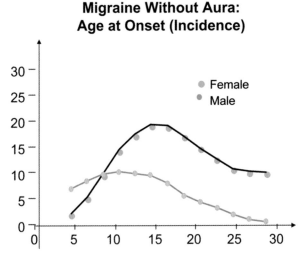

Migraine Epidemiology, Figure 1   Incidence of migraine, by age and sex (from Stewart et al. 1993).

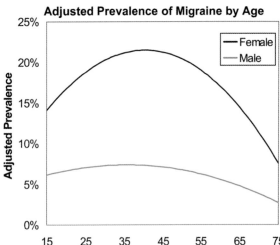

Migraine Epidemiology, Figure 2   Adjusted prevalence of migraine by age from a meta-analysis of studies using IHS criteria. (from Scher et al. 2001).

Migraine Epidemiology, Table 1 Prevalence of headache and migraine by age in selected community and school based-studies

Author(Y) Country	Type of Population	Sample Size	Age Range (Years)	Time Frame	Migraine Definition	Headache Prevalence			Migraine Prevalence		
						Males	Females	Overall	Males	Females	Overall
Ayatollahi (2002) Iran	School teenage girls	1,868	11–18	?	IHS					6.1%	
Al Jumah M (2002) Saudi Arabia	School Children	1,400	6–18	?	IHS				6.4%	7.7%	7.1%
Abu-Arafeh (1994)		1,754	5–15	1 year	IHS[1]						10.6
Bille (1962) Sweden	School Children	8,993	7–15	Lifetime	Vahlquist[1]	58.0	59.3	-	3.3	4.4	-
Linet (1989) USA	Community	10,132	12–29	1 year	2 of NV/U/VA	90	95	-	5.3	14	-
Mortimer (1992) UK	General Practice	1,083	3–11	1 year	IHS[1]	40.6*	36.9*	38.8*	4.1	2.9	3.7
Raielli (1995) Italy	School Children	1,445	11–14	1 year	IHS[1]	19.9	28.0	23.9	2.7	3.3	3.0
Sillanpaa (1976) Finland	School Children	4,825	3 7	? ?	Vahlquist[1]		4.3		3.2	3.2	3.2
Sillanpaa (1983) Finland	School Children	3,784	13	1 year	Vahlquist[1]	79.8	84.2	-	8.1	15.1	-

* age adjusted

N, nausea; U, unilateral; V, vomiting; VA, visual aura

dence in adolescence and peak prevalence in middle life indicates that migraine is a condition of long duration. Despite suggestions to the contrary, the prevalence of migraine is probably not increasing. According to the Centers for Disease Control, self-diagnosed migraine prevalence in the U.S. increased 60%, from 25.8 / 1000 to 41 / 1000 persons, between 1981 and 1989 (MMWR 1991). Because this study relies on self-reported migraine, an increase in diagnosis or disease awareness could be mistaken for an increase in prevalence. Numerous population studies in the U.S. show that prevalence is stable, while consultation and diagnosis have increased (Lipton et al. 2001). It may be that these increases in medical consultation and diagnosis have caused an apparent rather than a real increase in migraine prevalence.

Prevalence in Children and Adolescents

The prevalence of headache in children, as investigated in a number of school and population-based studies shows that by age 3, headache occurs in 3–8% of children. At age 5, 19.5% have headache and by age 7, 37 to 51.5% have headaches. In 7 to 15 year-olds, headache prevalence ranges from 57–82%. The prevalence increases from ages 3–11 in both boys and girls, with higher headache prevalence in 3–5 year old boys than in 3–5 year old girls. Thus, the overall prevalence of headache increases from preschool age children to mid-adolescence, when examined using various cross-sectional studies (Bille 1989).

Recent studies report the prevalence of pediatric migraine in the Asian Middle East. The first one, performed in the southern Iran, evaluated a random sample of 1868 teenaged girls (aged 11 to 18 years). The overall prevalence rate for migraine was 6.1% (95% CI, 5.0 to 7.2). The second study evaluated 1,400 randomly selected Saudi children in grades 1 through 9. Overall, the headache prevalence was 49.8%. The prevalence of migraine was 7.1%. There was a sharp increase in the prevalence rate (from around 2% to around 9%) at aged 10 to 11, in both boys and girls. Age adjusted prevalence for migraine between aged 6 and 15 was 6.2% (for references on the original studies the reader is referred to Bigal et al. 2004).

Another recent study evaluated the evolution of juvenile migraine without aura in adolescents over 5 years. Sixty-four subjects out of 80 previously selected were re-evaluated. Thirty two (50%) had migraine without aura. After 5 years, migraine without aura persisted in 56.2%, converted to migrainous disorder or non-classifiable headache respectively in 9.4% and 3.1% of cases, changed to episodic tension-type headache in 12.5% and remitted in 18.8%.

Prevalence by Gender in Adults

Estimates of migraine prevalence range from 3.3 to 21.9% for women and 0.7% to 16.1% for men. In the United States, the American Migraine Study II found that the prevalence of migraine was about 18% in women and 6% in men (Lipton et al. 2001). Table 1 summarizes several prevalence studies conducted in the last 12 years. The prevalence of migraine in different geographic locations, overall and by gender is presented. The female to male gender ratio is about 3 to 1 in most places where it has been studied.

Prevalence of Migraine by Socioeconomic Status

The relationship between migraine prevalence and socioeconomic status is uncertain. In physician- and clinic-based studies, migraine appears to be associated with high intelligence and social class. In his studies of children, Bille did not find an association between migraine prevalence and intelligence (Bille 1989). Similarly, in adults, epidemiological studies do not support a relationship between occupation and migraine prevalence (Lipton et al. 2001). In both the American Migraine Studies I and II, migraine prevalence was inversely related to household income (i.e. migraine prevalence fell as household income increased) (Lipton et al. 2001). This inverse relationship between migraine and socioeconomic status was confirmed in another U.S. study based on members of a managed care organization and in the National Health Interview Study. In Europe, results are contradictory. While one large study failed to demonstrate an association between migraine and socioeconomic status (Launer et al. 1999), a second recent study in England showed this relationship (Steiner et al. 2003).

The higher prevalence in the lower socioeconomic groups may be a consequence of a circumstance associated with low income and migraine, such as poor diet, poor medical care or stress. It may also reflect social selection, that is migraineurs may have lower incomes because migraine interferes with educational and occupational function, causing a loss of income or the ability to rise from a low-income group. The relationship of migraine and socioeconomic status, especially in children and adolescents, requires further study.

Prevalence of Migraine by Geographical Distribution

Migraine prevalence also varies by race and geography. In the U.S., it is highest in Caucasians, intermediate in African Americans and lowest in Asian Americans (Scher et al. 1999). Similarly, a meta-analysis of prevalence studies suggests that migraine is most common in North and South America, similar in Europe, but lower in Africa and often lowest in studies from Asia (Fig. 3) (Scher et al. 1999). The data suggest that race related differences in genetic risk may contribute.

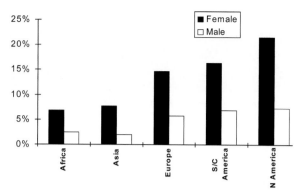

Migraine Epidemiology, Figure 3 Adjusted prevalence of migraine by geographical area and gender in a meta-analysis of studies using IHS criteria (from Scher et al. 2001).

The Burden of Migraine

The Impact of Migraine on the Individual

The burden of migraine is significant both to the individual sufferer and to the society. In the American Migraine Study II, 92% of women and 89% of men with severe migraine had some headache related disability (Lipton et al. 2001). About half were severely disabled or needed bed rest. In addition to the attack related disability, many migraineurs live in fear, knowing that at any time an attack could disrupt their ability to work, care for their families or meet social obligations. Abundant evidence indicates that migraine reduces health related quality of life.

The World Health Organization (WHO) has recently released a report on the burden of diseases (The World Health Report 2001). The WHO report defines the "burden" of a disease to include the economic and emotional difficulties that a family experiences as a result of migraine, as well as the lost opportunities – the adjustments and compromises that prevent other family members from achieving their full potential in work, social relationships and leisure. The global burden of disease (GBD) is an analysis of the onset of disorders and the disability caused by them. Using the GBD methodology, migraine is estimated to account for 2.0% years of life lost due to a disability in women of all ages. In both sexes of all ages, migraine is responsible for 1.4% of total years of life lost due to a disability and ranks within the top 20 most disabled studied disorders (Table 2).

The Impact of Migraine on the Family

The impact of migraine extends to household partners and other family members. In a recent study, one half of the participants believed that, because of their migraine, they were more likely to argue with their partners (50%) and children (52%), while majorities (52–73%) reported other adverse consequences for their relationships with their partner and children and at work. A third (36%) believed they would be better partners but for their headaches. Participating

M

Migraine Epidemiology, Table 2 Gender-Specific Prevalence Estimates of Migraine from 25 Population-Based Studies Using IHS Diagnostic Criteria

Author (Year of Publication)	Country	Source	Method	Sample Size	Time Frame	Age Range	Migraine Prevalence (%)			Comments
							Female	Male	Total	
Abu-Arefeh (1994)	Scotland	School	Clin Interview	1,754	1 Year	5–15	11.5	9.7	10.6	Prevalence is higher in boys prior to age 12 (1.14:1). After age 12, more common in girls (2.0:1).
al Rajeh (1997)	Saudi Arabia	Community	Face to face/ Clin Interview	22,630		All	6.8	3.2	5.0	
Alders (1996)	Malaysia	Community	Face to face	595	1 Year	5+	11.3	6.7	9.0	
Arregui (1991)	Peru	Community	Clin Interview	2,257		All	12.2	4.5	8.4	
Bank et al (2000)	Hungary	Community	Questionnaire	813	1 Year	15–80			9.6	
Barea (1996)	Brazil	School	Clin Interview	538	1 Year	10–18	10.3	9.6	9.9	2-48 hour duration allowed
Breslau (1991)	US	Community	Face to face/ Telephone	1,007	1 Year	21–30	12.9	3.4	9.2	
Cruz (1995)	Ecuador	Community	Clin Interview	2,723	Lifetime	All	7.9	5.6	6.9	Community endemic for cysticercosis
Cull (1992)	UK	Community	Face to face	16,002		16+	11.0	4.3	7.8	Without aura only
Dahlof et al (2003)	Sweden	Community	Telephone interview	1,668	1 Year	18–74	16.7	9.5	13.2	
Deleu et al (2002)	Saudi Arabia	Community	Face to face	1158	1 Year	10+	5.6	4.5		
Göbel (1994)	Germany	Community	Mail SAQ	4,061	Lifetime	18+	15.0	7.0	11.0	
Hagen et al (2000)	Norway	Community	Clin Interview	51,833	1 Year	20+	16.0	8.0	12.0	
Haimanot (1995)[	Ethiopia	Community	Face to face/ Clin Interview	15,000	1 Year	20+	4.2	1.7	3.0	
Henry, P (1992)	France	Community	Face to face	4,204	1 Year	15+	11.9	4.0	8.1	
Henry et al (2002)	France	Community	Face to face	10,585	1 Year	15+	11.2	4.0	7.9	
Jabbar, A (1997)	Saudi Arabia	Community	Face to face	5,891	Lifetime	15+			8.0	
Jaillard (1997)[	Peru	Community	Clin Interview	3,246	1 Year	15+	7.8	2.3	5.3	
Kececi et al (2002)	Turkey	Community	Face to face'	1320	1 Year	All	17.1	7.9		
Lamp et al (2003)	Sweden	Community	Fade to face	997	1 Year	15+	13.8	6.1	10.2	
Lenore et al (1999)	Netherlands	Community	Questionnaire and telephone	6,491	Lifetime 1 Year	18-65	33 25	13.3 7.5		
Lipton et al (2001)	United States	Community	Telephone	29 727	1 Year	12+	18.2	6.5		
Lipton et al (2002)	United States	Community	Telephone	11,863	1 Year	18–65	17.2	6		

Migraine Epidemiology, Table 2 (continued)

Author (Year of Publication)	Country	Source	Method	Sample Size	Time Frame	Age Range	Migraine Prevalence (%)			Comments
							Female	Male	Total	
Merikangas (1993)	Switzerland	Community	Clin Interview	379	1 Year	28–29	32.6	16.1	24.5	Weighted prevalence
Michel (1995)	France	Community	Mail SAQ	9,411	3 Month	18+	18.0	8.0	13.0	
Miranda et al (2003)	Puerto Rico	Community	Telephone	1610	1 Year	All	6	16.7	13.5	
O'Brien (1994)	Canada	Community	Telephone	2,922	1 Year	18+	21.9	7.4	15.2	
Raieli (1994)	Italy	School	Clin Interview	1,445	1 Year	11–14	3.3	2.7	3.0	
Rasmussen (1992)	Denmark	Community	Clin Interview	740	1 Year	25–64	15.0	6.0	10.0	
Russell (1995)	Denmark	Community	Clin Interview	3,471	Lifetime	40	23.7	11.7	17.7	
Sakai (1996)	Japan	Community	Mail SAQ	4,029	1 Year	15+	12.9	3.6	8.4	Female:Male prevalence ratio=3.6. Regional differences
Steiner et al (2003)	England	Community	CATI	4,007	1 Year	18–65	14.3	7.6	18.3	
Stewart (1992)	US	Community	Mail SAQ	20,468	1 Year	12–80	17.6	5.7	12.0	
Stewart (1996)	US	Community	Telephone	12,328	1 Year	18–65	19.0	8.2	14.7	Racial differences
Takeshima et al (2004)	Japan	Community	Questionnaires and telephone	5758	1 year	18+	9.1	2.3	6	Study done in the rural area of western Japan
van Roijen (1995)	Netherlands	Community	Face-to-face	10,480	1−Year	12+	12.0	5.0	9.0	
Wang (1997)	China	Community	Clin Interview	1,533	1 Year	65+	4.7	0.7	3.0	
Wong (1995)	Hong Kong	Community	Telephone	7,356	1 Year	15+	1.5	0.6	1.0	
Zivadinov et al (2001)	Croatia	Community	Telephone and face to face	5173	Lifetime 1 Year	15–65	22.9 18	14.8 12.3	19	

M

partners partly confirmed these findings; 29% felt that arguments were more common because of headaches and 20–60% reported other negative effects on relationships at home. Compared with subjects who did not have migraine, regarding their work performance, a statistically significantly higher proportion of migraine partners were unsatisfied with work demands placed on them, with their level or responsibilities and duties and with their ability to perform (Lipton et al. 2003). Results from this study show that the impact of migraine extends to household partners and other family members (impact beyond the individual).

The Societal Impact of Migraine

Migraine has an enormous impact on society. Studies have evaluated the indirect costs of migraine as well as the direct costs (Lipton et al. 2001). Indirect costs include the aggregate effects of migraine on productivity at work (paid employment), for household work and in other roles. The largest components of indirect costs are the productivity losses caused by absenteeism and reduced productivity while at work. Hu et al estimated that productivity losses due to migraine cost American employers 13 billion dollars per year (Hu et al. 1999). In an UK study, 5.7 working days were lost per year for every working person or student with migraine, although the most disabled 10% accounted for 85% of the total, projecting a lost 25 million days from work or school each year (Steiner et al. 2003).

Migraine's impact on healthcare utilization is marked as well. Studies show that 4% of all visits to physicians' offices are for headache (Bigal et al. 2004). Migraine also

Migraine Epidemiology, Table 3 Global burden of migraine. Leading causes of years of life lost due to a disability according to the global burden of disease initiative (modified from Lipton et al. 2003)

Females All Ages		% Total	Both Sexes All Ages	% Total
1	Unipolar depressive disorders	1	Unipolar depressive disorders	11.9
2	Iron-deficiency anemia	2	Hearing loss, adult onset	4.6
3	Hearing loss, adult onset	3	Iron-deficiency anemia	4.5
4	Osteoarthritis	4	Chronic obstructive pulmonary disease	3.3
5	Chronic obstructive pulmonary disease	5	Alcohol use disorders	3.1
6	Schizophrenia	6	Osteoarthritis	3.0
7	Bipolar affective disorder	7	Schizophrenia	2.8
8	Falls	8	Falls	2.8
9	Alzheimer's and other dementias	9	Bipolar affective disorder	2.5
10	Obstructed labor	10	Asthma	2.1
11	Cataracts	11	Congenital abnormalities	2.1
12	Migraine	12	Perinatal conditions	2.0
13	Congenital abnormalities	13	Alzheimer's and other dementias	2.0
14	Asthma	14	Cataracts	1.9
15	Perinatal conditions	15	Road traffic accidents	1.8
16	Chlamydia	16	Protein-energy malnutrition	1.7
17	Cerebrovascular disease	17	Cerebrovascular disease	1.7
18	Protein-energy malnutrition	18	HIV/AIDS	1.5
19	Abortion	19	Migraine	1.4
20	Panic disorder	20	Diabetes mellitus	1.4

results in major utilization of emergency rooms and urgent care centers (Bigal et al. 2004). Vast amounts of prescription and over the counter medications are taken for headache disorders. OTC sales of pain medication (for all conditions) were estimated to be 3.2 billion dollars in 1999 (U.S.) and headache accounts for about one third of OTC analgesic use (Bigal et al. 2004).

References

1. Bigal ME, Lipton RB, Stewart WF (2004) The epidemiology and impact of migraine. Curr Neurol Neurosci Rep 4:98–104
2. Bille B (1989) Migraine in children: prevalence, clinical features, and a 30-year follow-up. In: Ferrari MD, Lataste X (eds) Migraine and other headaches. Parthenon, New Jersey
3. Breslau N, Davis GC, Schultz LR et al. (1994) Joint 1994 Wolff Award Presentation. Migraine and major depression: a longitudinal study. Headache 34:387–393
4. Hu XH, Markson LE, Lipton RB et al. (1999) Burden of migraine in the United States: disability and economic costs. Arch Intern Med 159: 813–818
5. Launer LJ, Terwindt GM, Ferrari MD (1999) The prevalence and characteristics of migraine in a population-based cohort: the GEM Study. Neurology 53:537–542
6. Lipton RB, Stewart WF, Diamond S et al. (2001) Prevalence and Burden of migraine in the United States: data from the American Migraine Study II. Headache 41:646–657
7. Lipton RB, Bigal ME, Kolodner K et al. (2003) The family impact of migraine: population-based studies in the USA and UK. Cephalalgia 23:429–440
8. Lyngberg A, Jensen R, Rasmussen BK et al. (2003) Incidence of migraine in a Danish population-based follow-up study. (abstract). Cephalalgia 23:596
9. MMWR (1991) Prevalence of chronic migraine headaches – United States, 1980–89. MMWR 40:331–338
10. Ozge A, Bugdayci R, Sasmaz T et al. (2002) The sensitivity and specificity of the case definition criteria in diagnosis of headache: a school-based epidemiological study of 5562 children in Mersin. Cephalalgia 22:791–798
11. Scher AI, Stewart WF, Lipton RB (1999) Migraine and headache: a meta-analytic approach. In: Crombie IK (ed), Epidemiology of Pain. IASP Press, Seattle, Washington, pp 159–170
12. Stang PE, Yanagihara T, Swanson JW et al. (1992) Incidence of migraine headaches: A population-based study in Olmstead County, Minnesota. Neurology 42:1657–1662
13. Stang PE, Sternfeld B, Sidney S (1996). Migraine headache in a pre-paid health plan: ascertainment, demographics, physiological and behavioral factors. Headache 36:69–76
14. Steiner T, Scher A, Stewart W et al. (2003)The prevalence and disability burden of adult migraine in England and their relationships to age, gender and ethnicity. Cephalalgia 23:519–527
15. Stewart WF, Linet MS, Celentano DD et al. (1993) Age and sex-specific incidence rates of migraine with and without visual aura. Am J Epidemiol 34:1111–1120

16. The World Health Report 2001: Mental health, new understanding, new hope. Available at www.who.int/en/

Migraine, Genetics

ANNE DUCROS

Headache Emergency Department and Institut National de la Santé et de la Recherche Médicale (INSERM), Faculté de Médecine Lariboisière, Lariboisière Hospital, Paris, France
anne.ducros@lrb.ap-hop-paris.fr

Synonyms

Inherited Factors Implicated in the Mechanisms of Migraine

Definition

Migraine is a primary headache disorder. It is a complex disease in which environmental factors interact with genetic factors. The major goal of genetic studies is the identification of susceptibility genes that may give clues to the mechanisms underlying migraine, and may help to identify new therapeutic targets.

Characteristics

Migraine is a primary headache disorder responsible for recurrent attacks of disabling pain lasting a few hours to a few days. This condition is characterized by the repetition of such attacks in the absence of any disorder causing secondary headaches. The International Headache Society (IHS) classification distinguishes different varieties of migraine attacks, the most frequent being migraine without aura (MO) and migraine with typical aura (MA). In MO attacks, the headache is the most prominent and disabling symptom. In MA attacks, the headache phase is preceded or accompanied by transient neurological signs including visual, sensory and language troubles. Some patients have only MO, others have only MA, and some have both types of attacks. In addition, hemiplegic migraine is a rare variety of MA characterized by the presence of a motor deficit during the aura, in addition to one or more of the typical aura symptoms. In familial hemiplegic migraine (FHM), the index case has at least one first- or second-degree relative who also has migraine with aura including motor weakness. In sporadic hemiplegic migraine, there is no such familial history. Migraine is a highly frequent condition affecting about 15% of the western population. Familial aggregation has long been known, and was even classically used as a diagnosis criterion. Genetic epidemiological surveys have demonstrated that this familial aggregation was not observed purely by chance, but was due to the existence of genetic factors.

Twin studies have shown that the 'pairwise' concordance rates were significantly higher among monozygous than dizigous twin pairs for MO (Gervil 1999) and for MA (Ulrich 1999), demonstrating the existence of genetic factors in migraine that interact with environmental factors to produce the phenotype. Family studies provided further evidence in favor of the existence of genetic factors in MO and MA, those factors being more important in MA than in MO (Russell and Olesen 1995). In addition, segregation analysis showed that both MO and MA have a non-mendelian polygenic mode of inheritance (Russell 1995). The possible number of genetic susceptibility loci is still unknown. FHM is the only variety of migraine in which a monogenic mendelian mode of inheritance has been clearly established. Two clinical forms of FHM have been described: pure FHM (80% of the families), and FHM with permanent cerebellar symptoms in which some affected subjects have nystagmus and/or ataxia. In addition to usual attacks, patients may have severe attacks with confusion, coma, fever and prolonged hemiplegia. Genetic tools are more powerful to identify the genes responsible for monogenic conditions than genes responsible for polygenic conditions. Thus, the only known migraine genes have been identified in FHM. FHM is genetically heterogeneous, with at least three responsible genes of which two have been identified. The first gene, CACNA1A, located on chromosome 19p13, was identified in 1996 (Ophoff 1996). CACNA1A encodes the pore-forming α1A-subunit of voltage-gated neuronal $Ca_v2.1$ (P/Q type) Ca^{2+} channels. CACNA1A is implicated in about 50% of unselected FHM families and in the vast majority of families with permanent cerebellar symptoms. The second gene, ATP1A2, located on chromosome 1q21-q23, was identified in 2003 (De Fusco 2003). ATP1A2 is implicated in about 20–30% of unselected FHM families, and encodes the catalytic α2-subunit of a transmembrane NA^+/K^+ ATPase. Both known FHM genes encode proteins regulating ion translocation, FHM is thus a channelopathy.

$Ca_v2.1$ channels are found exclusively in neurons including central and peripheral neurons at the neuromuscular junction. They play a major role in neurotransmitter release (mainly glutamate) and in the control of neuronal excitability. CACNA1A is a large gene containing 47 exons. Thus far, a total of 17 CACNA1A mutations have been identified in 41 FHM1 families (33 affected by FHM and cerebellar symptoms and 8 by pure FHM), and in 4 sporadic cases affected by HM and cerebellar symptoms. Five of these mutations are recurrent, i.e. they have been detected in two or more unrelated families. The most frequent mutation T666M has been detected in 19 families and 2 sporadic cases. All mutations are missense mutations, changing only one of the 2550 amino-acids of the predicted protein. They are located in important functional domains of the subunit, near the ionic pore or within the voltage sensor. Mutations causing FHM1 with cerebellar symptoms are distinct from those causing pure FHM1, and all recurrent mutations are causing FHM1 with cerebellar

M

symptoms. Mutations have been detected in sporadic cases, including a de novo mutation, demonstrating that sporadic HM is due to CACNA1A mutations in at least a part of the cases.

Different kinds of CACNA1A mutations have been identified in two other autosomal dominant neurological disorders. Episodic ataxia type 2 is a paroxysmal neurological condition producing recurrent attacks of major cerebellar ataxia, which is due to CACNA1A mutations (Ophoff 1996). Spinocerebellar ataxia type 6 (SCA6) is a progressive cerebellar disease characterized by an adult onset ataxia, which is due to small expansions of the CAG repeat contained within exon 47 of CACNA1A. Electrophysiological studies of CACNA1A mutations causing FHM1 have shown that all mutations analyzed so far modify the density and the gating properties of $Ca_V 2.1$ currents (Pietrobon and Striessnig 2003). Mutated single $Ca_V 2.1$ channels display lower activation thresholds and increased opening probabilities. FHM1 mutations are thus gain-of-function mutations. On the contrary, EA2 mutations have been shown to be loss-of-function mutations, the mutated allele generating no current when expressed in heterologous cells.

Knockout mice that do not have the CACNA1A gene are born with a severe ataxia and die within a few days. Mice carrying different spontaneous mutations within CACNA1A display distinct phenotypes called tottering, leaner, or rocker, characterized by various paroxysmal manifestations (absence epilepsy, motor attacks) always associated with a permanent cerebellar ataxia of variable severity. Leaner mice have lower levels of voltage-dependant glutamate release measurable by cerebral microdialysis. They also have an elevated threshold for initiating cortical spreading depression (CSD) and a slower velocity of CSD propagation. Knockin mice carrying the human pure FHM1 mutation R192Q display multiple gain-of-function phenotypes: increased $Ca_V 2.1$ current density in cerebellar neurons, enhanced neurotransmission at the neuromuscular junction, and, in the intact animal, a reduced threshold and increased velocity of cortical spreading depression (van den Maagdenberg 2004). This mouse is the first animal model for FHM. These various abnormalities strongly suggest that FHM1 mutations in the $Ca_V 2.1$ channel modify the cortical excitability and increase the susceptibility to CSD, which is the mechanism underlying the aura.

ATP1A2 encodes the catalytic α-2subunit of a transmembrane NA^+/K^+ ATPase. This protein hydrolysis ATP to extrude Na^+ ions and pump K^+ ions into the cell. This active pumping maintains the Na^+ transmembrane gradient that is essential for the transport of amino-acids, neurotransmitters (including glutamate) and Ca^{2+}. In neonates, the α-2subunit is mainly expressed in neurons. In adults, it is mainly expressed in astrocytes. ATP1A2 contains 23 exons. So far, 14 mutations have been identified in 14 families and one sporadic case.

These mutations are missense mutations responsible for the substitution of one of the 1020 amino-acids of the protein. Only one mutation (R763H) was found in two unrelated families. In the family with the R689Q mutation, FHM cosegregates with benign familial infantile convulsions. In another family with the T378N mutation, the phenotypic spectrum includes features characteristic of FHM and of alternating hemiplegia. Electrophysiological studies initially suggested that ATP1A2 mutations are loss of function mutations leading to haploinsufficiency. Further studies suggest that the mutations are gain of function mutations leading to an abnormal function of the pump.

FHM is characterized by an important clinical variability. The age of onset, the frequency and duration of attacks, the aura features and the headache characteristics may vary from one patient to another, even among affected members from a given family who are carrying the same mutation in the same gene. This variability suggests complex interactions between the consequences of the FHM causing mutation and environmental factors or modifying genetic factors. However, several studies have shown that the various genotypes play a role in producing this clinical variability. FHM1, due to CACNA1A mutations, is characterized by a higher penetrance of FHM and of permanent cerebellar symptoms, the vast majority of families with permanent cerebellar symptoms being linked to CACNA1A (Ducros 2001). FHM2, due to ATP1A2 mutations, is characterized by a lower penetrance of FHM. Cerebellar symptoms are rarely part of the clinical spectrum of FHM2 (2 families published). In addition, striking correlations between genotype and phenotype have been shown in patients with CACNA1A mutations, including the fact that the most frequent FHM1 causing mutation, T666M, had the highest penetrance of hemiplegic migraine, severe attacks with coma and nystagmus (Ducros 2001). The existence of different CACNA1A mutations partly accounts for the clinical variability.

The implication of CACNA1A in the more frequent varieties of migraine has been analyzed by the mean of linkage and association studies with contradictory results, 3 studies concluding in favor and 5 against. None of the positive studies provided a direct analysis of the CACNA1A gene in order to detect pathogenic mutations. CACNA1A is thus probably not a susceptibility gene for the more common varieties of migraine. Moreover, a subsequent study showed that the 19p13 region does indeed contains a susceptibility locus for MA that is distinct from CACNA1A. The same group showed an association between migraine and five polymorphisms within the insulin receptor (INSR) gene located in 19p13.3/2 (McCarthy 2001). These five polymorphisms had no effect on INSR transcription, translation, and protein expression, and INSR-mediated functions. The nature of the implication of the INSR gene in migraine remains to be understood.

With regards to the FHM2 gene, a linkage analysis conducted in a single family suggested the presence of a possible migraine susceptibility locus in 1q31, distinct from the ATP1A2 locus in 1q21-q23. An ATP1A2 mutation (R548H) was found in a small family in which the two affected subjects had migraine with basilar, non-hemiplegic, aura. This mutation was not found in 100 healthy controls, or in 77 migrainous controls. Actual data do not permit a conclusion regarding the implication of ATP1A2 in MO/MA.

Three linkage analyses, each conducted in a large panel of MA families, have permitted the mapping of three susceptibility loci for MA: the first on 4q24 (in 50 Finnish families) (Wessman 2002), the second on 11q24 (in 43 Canadian families) (Cader 2003), and the last on 15q11-q13 (in 10 Italian families) (Russo 2004). An important linkage analysis in a group of 289 Icelandic patients with MO identified a susceptibility locus on 4q21 (Bjornsson 2003). This genetic interval overlapped the genetic region identified in the Finnish families on 4q24, suggesting an implication of this chromosome 4q region both in MO and MA. Finally, several linkage analyses, each conducted in a single family, suggested the existence of other migraine susceptibility loci on 1q21-q23, 6p12.2-p21.1, 14q21.2-q22.3 and Xq24-q28 (Estevez and Gardner 2004). None of the results have been replicated.

Finally, numerous association studies have been performed in migraine. A wide range of candidate polymorphisms have been tested in migraine. Association studies compare the frequency of alleles of a polymorphic genetic marker between cases and controls. In the absence of methodological shortcomings, a significant difference means that the polymorphism is located within the susceptibility gene or is in linkage disequilibrium with the susceptibility gene. Association studies do not provide any demonstration of the implication of the tested gene, or of an abnormal function of the tested gene in the pathophysiology of the studied disease. Positive associations have been found between migraine and polymorphisms within the dopamine receptor D2 (DRD2) gene, the human serotonin transporter gene, the catechol-o-methyltransferase gene, the endothelin type A gene, the dopamine beta-hydroxylase (DBH) gene, and the 5,10-methylenetetrahydrofolate reductase (MTHFR). These various candidate polymorphisms have been chosen based on the hypothesis that the genes containing them encode proteins that are suspected to be involved in migraine. However, additional studies are needed to determine if the alleles associated with migraine have any biological effect.

References

1. Bjornsson A, Gudmundsson G, Gudfinnsson E et al. (2003) Localization of a Gene for Migraine without Aura to Chromosome 4q21. Am J Hum Genet 73:986–993
2. Cader ZM, Noble-Topham S, Dyment DA et al. (2003) Significant Linkage to Migraine with Aura on Chromosome 11q24. Hum Mol Genet 12:2511–2517
3. De Fusco M, Marconi R, Silvestri L et al. (2003) Haploinsufficiency of ATP1A2 Encoding the Na+/K+ Pump Alpha2 Subunit Associated with Familial Hemiplegic Migraine Type 2. Nat Genet 33:192–196
4. Ducros A, Denier C, Joutel A et al. (2001) The Clinical Spectrum of Familial Hemiplegic Migraine Associated with Mutations in a Neuronal Calcium Channel. N Engl J Med 345:17–24
5. Estevez M, Gardner KL (2004) Update on the Genetics of Migraine. Hum Genet 114:225–235
6. Gervil M, Ulrich V, Kaprio J, Olesen J, Russell MB (1999) The Relative Role of Genetic and Environmental Factors in Migraine without Aura. Neurology 53:995–999
7. Maagdenberg AM van den, Pietrobon D, Pizzorusso T et al. (2004) A Cacna1a Knockin Migraine Mouse Model with Increased Susceptibility to Cortical Spreading Depression. Neuron 41:701–710
8. McCarthy LC, Hosford DA, Riley JH et al. (2001) Single-Nucleotide Polymorphism Alleles in the Insulin Receptor Gene are Associated with Typical Migraine. Genomics 78:135–149
9. Ophoff RA, Terwindt GM, Vergouwe MN et al. (1996) Familial Hemiplegic Migraine and Episodic Ataxia Type-2 are Caused by Mutations in the Ca2+ Channel Gene CACNL1A4. Cell 87:543–552
10. Pietrobon D, Striessnig J (2003) Neurobiology of Migraine. Nat Rev Neurosci 4:386–398
11. Russell MB, Iselius L, Olesen J (1995) Inheritance of Migraine Investigated by Complex Segregation Analysis. Hum Genet 96:726–730
12. Russell MB, Olesen J (1995) Increased Familial Risk and Evidence of Genetic Factor in Migraine. Bmj 311:541–544
13. Russo L, Mariotti P, Sangiorgi E et al. (2004) A New Susceptibility Locus for Migraine with Aura in the 15q11-q13 Genomic Region Containing Three GABA-A Receptor Genes. Am J Hum Genet 76:2
14. Ulrich V, Gervil M, Kyvik KO et al. (1999) Evidence of a Genetic Factor in Migraine with Aura: A Population-Based Danish Twin Study. Ann Neurol 45:242–246
15. Wessman M, Kallela M, Kaunisto MA et al. (2002) A Susceptibility Locus for Migraine with Aura, on Chromosome 4q24. Am J Hum Genet 70:652–662

Migraine Hemiparesthetic

► Clinical Migraine with Aura

Migraine Hemiplegic

► Clinical Migraine with Aura

Migraine Ophthalmic

► Clinical Migraine with Aura

Migraine Optical

► Clinical Migraine with Aura

Migraine, Pathophysiology

PETER J. GOADSBY
Institute of Neurology, The National Hospital for
Neurology and Neurosurgery, London, UK
peterg@ion.ucl.ac.uk

Introduction

An understanding of the pathophysiology of migraine
should be based upon the anatomy and physiology of
the pain producing structures of the cranium integrated
with knowledge of central nervous system modulation
of these pathways. Headache in general, and in particular migraine (Goadsby et al. 2002) and cluster headache
(Goadsby 2002b), is better understood now than has
been the case for the last four millennia (Lance and
Goadsby 2005). This chapter will set out the current
understanding of migraine.

Migraine — Explaining the Clinical Features

Migraine is in essence a familial episodic disorder
whose key marker is headache with certain associated
features (Table 1). It is these features that give clues to
its migraine pathophysiology and will ultimately provide insights leading to new treatments.

The essential elements to be considered are:

- Genetics of migraine;
- Physiological basis for the ▶ aura
- Anatomy of head pain, particularly that of the
  ▶ trigeminovascular system
- Physiology and pharmacology of activation of the
  peripheral branches of ophthalmic branch of the
  trigeminal nerve;
- Physiology and pharmacology of the trigeminal
  nucleus, in particular its caudal most part, the
  ▶ trigeminocervical complex
- ▶ Brainstem and diencephalic modulatory systems
  that influence trigeminal pain transmission and
  other sensory modality processing.

Migraine involves a form of sensory processing disturbance with wide ramifications within the central
nervous system, while pain pathways will be used as an

Migraine, Pathophysiology, Table 1 International Headache Society
defined features of migraine (Headache Classification Committee of The
International Headache Society 2004) Repeated episodic headache (4–
72 h) with the following features:

Any two of	Any one of
unilateral throbbing worsened by movement moderate or severe	nausea / vomiting photophobia and phonophobia

example, it is useful to remember that migraine is not
simply a pain problem.

Genetics of Migraine

One of the most important aspects of the pathophysiology of migraine is the inherited nature of the disorder. It is clear from clinical practice that many patients have first degree relatives who also suffer from
migraine (Lance and Goadsby 2005; Silberstein et al.
2002). Transmission of migraine from parents to children has been reported as early as the seventeenth century (Willis 1682) and numerous published studies
have reported a positive family history (Russell 1997).

Genetic Epidemiology

Studies of twin pairs are the classical method to investigate the relative importance of genetic and environmental factors. A Danish study included 1,013
monozygotic and 1,667 dizygotic twin pairs of the
same gender, obtained from a population based twin
register (Ulrich et al. 1999). The pairwise concordance
rate was significantly higher among monozygotic than
dizygotic twin pairs ($P < 0.05$). Several studies have attempted to analyze the possible mode of inheritance in
migraine families and conflicting results have been obtained (Lalouel and Morton 1981; Mochi et al. 1993;
Russell et al. 1995). Both twin studies and population based epidemiological surveys strongly suggest
that migraine without aura is a multifactorial disorder,
caused by a combination of genetic and environmental
factors.

Familial Hemiplegic Migraine (FHM)

In approximately 50% of the reported families, FHM
has been assigned to chromosome 19p13 (Joutel et al.
1994; Ophoff et al. 1994). Few clinical differences have
been found between chromosome 19 linked and unlinked FHM families. Indeed, the clinical phenotype
does not associate particularly with the known mutations (Ducros et al. 2001). The most striking exception is cerebellar ataxia, which occurs in approximately
50% of the chromosome 19 linked, but in none of the
unlinked families (Haan et al. 1994; Joutel et al. 1993,
1994; Ophoff et al. 1994; Teh et al. 1995). Another less
striking difference includes the fact that patients from
chromosome 19 linked families are more likely to have
attacks that can be triggered by minor head trauma or
are that associated with coma (Terwindt et al. 1996).
The biological basis for the linkage to chromosome 19
is mutations (Ophoff et al. 1996) involving the $Ca_V 2.1$
(P / Q) type ▶ voltage gated calcium channel (Ertel
et al. 2000) *CACNA1A* gene. Now known as FHM-I,
this mutation is responsible for about 50% of identified
families. Mutations in the *ATP1A2* gene (De Fusco et

al. 2003; Marconi et al. 2003) have been identified to be responsible for about 20% of FHM families. Interestingly, the phenotype of some FHM-II families involves epilepsy (Jurkat-Rott et al. 2004; Vanmolkot et al. 2003), while it has also been suggested that alternating hemiplegia of childhood can be due to *ATP1A2* mutations (Swoboda et al. 2004). The latter cases are most unconvincing for migraine.

Taken together, the known mutations suggest that migraine, or at least the neurological manifestations currently called the aura, are caused by a ▶ channelopathy (Goadsby and Ferrari 2001). Linking the channel disturbance for the first time to the aura process has demonstrated that human mutations expressed in a knock-in mouse produce a reduced threshold for ▶ cortical spreading depression (van den Maagdenberg et al. 2004), which has some profound implications for understanding that process (Goadsby 2004).

Migraine Aura

Migraine aura is defined as a focal neurological disturbance manifest as visual, sensory or motor symptoms (Headache Classification Committee of The International Headache Society 2004). It is seen in about 30% of patients (Rasmussen and Olesen 1992) and it is clearly neurally driven (Cutrer et al. 1998; Olesen et al. 1990). The case for the aura being the human equivalent of the cortical spreading depression (CSD) of Leao (1944a, 1944b) has been well made (Lauritzen 1994). In humans, visual aura has been described as affecting the visual field, suggesting the visual cortex and it starts at the centre of the visual field and propagates to the periphery at a speed of 3 mm / min (Lashley 1941). This is very similar to spreading depression described in rabbits (Leao 1944b). Blood flow studies in patients have also shown that a focal hyperemia tends to precede the spreading oligemia (Olesen et al. 1981) and again this is similar to what would be expected with spreading depression. After this passage of oligemia, the cerebrovascular response to hypercapnia in patients is blunted, while autoregulation remains intact (Harer and Kummer 1991; Lauritzen et al. 1983; Sakai and Meyer 1979). Again this pattern is repeated with experimental spreading depression (Kaube and Goadsby 1994; Kaube et al. 1999; Lambert et al. 1999). Human observations have rendered the arguments reasonably sound that human aura has cortical spreading depression as its equivalent in animals (Hadjikhani et al. 2001). An area of controversy surrounds whether aura in fact triggers the rest of the attack and is indeed painful (Moskowitz et al. 2004). Based on the available experimental and clinical data this author is not at all convinced that aura is painful (Goadsby 2001), but this does not diminish its interest, or the importance of understanding it. Indeed therapeutic developments may shed even further light on these relationships.

Tonabersat is a CSD inhibitor that has entered clinical trials in migraine. Tonabersat (SB-220453) inhibits CSD, CSD induced nitric oxide (NO) release and cerebral vasodilation (Read et al. 1999; Smith et al. 2000). Tonabersat does not constrict isolated human blood vessels (MaassenVanDenBrink et al. 2000), but does inhibit trigeminally induced craniovascular effects (Parsons et al. 2001). Remarkably, topiramate, a proven preventive agent in migraine (Brandes et al. 2004; Diener et al. 2004; Silberstein et al. 2004), also inhibits CSD in cat and rat (Akerman and Goadsby 2004). Tonabersat is inactive in the human NO model of migraine (Tvedskov et al. 2004a) as is propranolol (Tvedskov et al. 2004c), although valproate showed some activity in that model (Tvedskov et al. 2004b). Topiramate inhibits trigeminal neurons activated by nociceptive intracranial afferents (Storer and Goadsby 2004), but not by a mechanism local to the trigeminocervical complex (Storer and Goadsby 2005) and thus CSD inhibition may be a model system to contribute to the development of preventive medicines.

Headache Anatomy

The Trigeminal Innervation of Pain-Producing Intracranial Structures

Surrounding the large cerebral vessels, pial vessels, large venous sinuses and dura mater is a plexus of largely unmyelinated fibers that arise from the ophthalmic division of the trigeminal ganglion (Liu-Chen et al. 1984) and in the posterior fossa from the upper cervical dorsal roots (Arbab et al. 1986). Trigeminal fibers innervating cerebral vessels arise from neurons in the trigeminal ganglion that contain substance P and ▶ calcitonin gene related peptide (CGRP) (Uddman et al. 1985), both of which can be released when the trigeminal ganglion is stimulated either in humans or the cat (Goadsby et al. 1988). Stimulation of the cranial vessels, such as the superior sagittal sinus (SSS), is certainly painful in humans (Feindel et al. 1960; Wolff 1948). Human dural nerves that innervate the cranial vessels largely consist of small diameter myelinated and unmyelinated fibers (Penfield and McNaughton 1940) that almost certainly subserve a nociceptive function.

Headache Physiology — Peripheral Connections

Plasma Protein Extravasation

Moskowitz (1990) has provided a series of experiments to suggest that the pain of migraine may be a form of sterile neurogenic inflammation. Although this seems clinically implausible, the model system has been helpful in understanding some aspects of trigeminovascular

M

physiology. Neurogenic plasma extravasation can be seen during electrical stimulation of the trigeminal ganglion in the rat (Markowitz et al. 1987). Plasma extravasation can be blocked by ergot alkaloids, indomethacin, acetylsalicylic acid and the serotonin-5HT$_{1B/1D}$ receptor agonist, sumatriptan (Moskowitz and Cutrer 1993). The pharmacology of abortive anti-migraine drugs has been reviewed in detail (Cutrer et al. 1997). In addition there are structural changes in the dura mater that are observed after trigeminal ganglion stimulation. These include mast cell degranulation and changes in post-capillary venules including platelet aggregation (Dimitriadou et al. 1991, 1992). While it is generally accepted that such changes and particularly the initiation of a sterile inflammatory response would cause pain (Burstein et al. 1998; Strassman et al. 1996), it is not clear whether this is sufficient of itself or requires other stimulators or promoters. Preclinical studies suggest that cortical spreading depression may be a sufficient stimulus to activate trigeminal neurons (Bolay et al. 2002), although this has been a controversial area (Ebersberger et al. 2001; Goadsby 2001; Ingvardsen et al. 1997; Ingvardsen et al. 1998; Moskowitz et al. 1993).

Although plasma extravasation in the retina, which is blocked by sumatriptan can be seen after trigeminal ganglion stimulation in experimental animals, no changes are seen with retinal angiography during acute attacks of migraine or cluster headache (May et al. 1998b). Clearly, blockade of neurogenic plasma protein extravasation is not completely predictive of anti-migraine efficacy in humans, as evidenced by the failure in clinical trials of substance P, neurokinin-1 antagonists (Connor et al. 1998; Diener and The RPR100893 Study Group 2003; Goldstein et al. 1997; Norman et al. 1998), specific PPE blockers, CP122,288 (Roon et al. 1997) and 4991w93 (Earl et al. 1999), an endothelin antagonist (May et al. 1996) and a neurosteroid (Data et al. 1998).

Sensitization and Migraine

While it is highly doubtful that there is a significant sterile inflammatory response in the dura mater during migraine, it is clear that some form of sensitization takes place during migraine, since allodynia is common. About two-thirds of patients complain of pain from non-noxious stimuli, allodynia (Burstein et al. 2000a, b; Selby and Lance 1960). A particularly interesting aspect is the demonstration of allodynia in the upper limbs ipsilateral and contralateral to the pain. This finding is consistent with at least third order neuronal sensitization, such as sensitization of thalamic neurons and firmly places the pathophysiology within the central nervous system. Sensitization in migraine may be peripheral, with local release of inflammatory markers, which would certainly activate trigeminal nociceptors (Strassman et al. 1996). More likely in migraine is a form of central sensitization, which may be classical central sensitization (Burstein et al. 1998) or a form of disinhibitory sensitization with dysfunction of descending modulatory pathways (Knight et al. 2002).

Neuropeptide Studies

Electrical stimulation of the trigeminal ganglion in both humans and the cat leads to increases in extracerebral blood flow and local release of both CGRP and SP (Edvinsson and Goadsby 1998). In the cat, trigeminal ganglion stimulation also increases cerebral blood flow by a pathway traversing the greater superficial petrosal branch of the facial nerve, again releasing a powerful vasodilator peptide, vasoactive intestinal polypeptide (VIP) (May and Goadsby 1999). Interestingly, the VIPergic innervation of the cerebral vessels is predominantly anterior rather than posterior (Matsuyama et al. 1983) and this may contribute to this regions vulnerability to spreading depression, explaining why the aura is so very often seen to commence posteriorly. Stimulation of the more specifically vascular pain producing superior sagittal sinus increases cerebral blood flow and jugular vein CGRP levels. Human evidence that CGRP is elevated in the headache phase of migraine (Gallai et al. 1995; Goadsby et al. 1990), cluster headache (Fanciullacci et al. 1995; Goadsby and Edvinsson 1994) and chronic paroxysmal hemicrania (Goadsby and Edvinsson 1996) supports the view that the trigeminovascular system may be activated in a protective role in these conditions. It is of interest in this regard that compounds which have not shown activity in human migraine, notably the conformationally restricted analogue of sumatriptan, CP122,288 (Knight et al. 1999), and the conformationally restricted analogue of zolmitriptan, 4991w93 (Knight et al. 2001), were both ineffective inhibitors of CGRP release after superior sagittal sinus stimulation in the cat. The recent development of non-peptide, highly specific CGRP antagonists (Doods et al. 2000) and the announcement of proof of concept for a CGRP antagonist in acute migraine (Olesen et al. 2004), firmly establishes this as a novel and important new emerging principle for acute migraine.

Headache Physiology — Central Connections

The Trigeminocervical Complex

Fos immunohistochemistry is a method for looking at activated cells by plotting the expression of Fos protein. After meningeal irritation with blood, Fos expression is noted in the trigeminal nucleus caudalis (Nozaki et al. 1992), while after stimulation of the superior sagittal sinus, Fos-like immunoreactivity is seen in the trigeminal nucleus caudalis and in the dorsal horn at the C$_1$

and C_2 levels in the cat (Kaube et al. 1993c) and monkey (Goadsby and Hoskin 1997; Hoskin et al. 1999). These latter findings are in accord with similar data using 2-deoxyglucose measurements with superior sagittal sinus stimulation (Goadsby and Zagami 1991). Similarly, stimulation of a branch of C_2, the greater occipital nerve, increases metabolic activity in the same regions, i.e. trigeminal nucleus caudalis and $C_{1/2}$ dorsal horn (Goadsby et al. 1997). In experimental animals, one can record directly from trigeminal neurons with both supratentorial trigeminal input and input from the greater occipital nerve, a branch of the C_2 dorsal root (Bartsch and Goadsby 2002). Stimulation of the greater occipital nerve for 5 min results in substantial increases in responses to supratentorial dural stimulation, which can last for over an hour (Bartsch and Goadsby 2002). Conversely, stimulation of the middle meningeal artery dura mater with the C-fiber irritant mustard oil sensitizes responses to occipital muscle stimulation (Bartsch and Goadsby 2003). Taken together these data suggest convergence of cervical and ophthalmic inputs at the level of the second order neuron. Moreover, stimulation of a lateralized structure, the middle meningeal artery, produces Fos expression bilaterally in both cat and monkey brain (Hoskin et al. 1999), a finding that is consistent with the fact that up to one third of patients complain of bilateral pain. This group of neurons from the superficial laminae of trigeminal nucleus caudalis and $C_{1/2}$ dorsal horns should be regarded functionally as the trigeminocervical complex.

These data demonstrate that trigeminovascular nociceptive information comes by way of the most caudal cells. This concept provides an anatomical explanation for the referral of pain to the back of the head in migraine. Moreover, experimental pharmacological evidence suggests that abortive anti-migraine drugs, such as ergots (Hoskin et al. 1996), acetylsalicylic acid (Kaube et al. 1993b), sumatriptan after blood-brain barrier disruption (Kaube et al. 1993a), eletriptan (Goadsby and Hoskin 1999; Lambert et al. 2002), naratriptan (Cumberbatch et al. 1998; Goadsby and Knight 1997), rizatriptan (Cumberbatch et al. 1997) and zolmitriptan (Goadsby and Hoskin 1996) can have actions at these second order neurons that reduce cell activity and suggest a further possible site for therapeutic intervention in migraine. This action can be dissected out to involve each of the 5-HT_{1B}, 5-HT_{1D} and 5-HT_{1F} receptor subtypes (Goadsby and Classey 2003). Interestingly, ▶ triptans also influence the CGRP promoter (Durham et al. 1997) and regulate CGRP secretion from neurons in culture (Durham and Russo 1999). Furthermore, the demonstration that some part of this action is post-synaptic with either 5-HT_{1B} or 5-HT_{1D} receptors located non-presynaptically (Goadsby et al.

2001; Maneesi et al. 2004) offers a prospect of highly anatomically localized treatment options.

Higher Order Processing

Following transmission in the caudal brain stem and high cervical spinal cord information is relayed rostrally.

Thalamus

Processing of vascular nociceptive signals in the thalamus occurs in the ventroposteromedial (VPM) thalamus, medial nucleus of the posterior complex and in the intralaminar thalamus (Zagami and Goadsby 1991). Zagami and Lambert (1991) have shown by application of capsaicin to the superior sagittal sinus that trigeminal projections with a high degree of nociceptive input are processed in neurons particularly in the ventroposteromedial thalamus and in its ventral periphery. These neurons in the VPM can be modulated by activation of $GABA_A$ inhibitory receptors (Shields et al. 2003) and, perhaps of more direct clinical relevance, by propranolol through a β_1-adrenoceptor mechanism (Shields and Goadsby 2005). Remarkably, triptans can also inhibit VPM neurons locally through 5-$HT_{1B/1D}$ mechanisms, as demonstrated by microiontophoretic application (Shields and Goadsby 2004), suggesting a hitherto unconsidered locus of action for triptans in acute migraine. Human imaging studies have confirmed activation of the thalamus contralateral to pain in acute migraine (Afridi et al. 2005a; Bahra et al. 2001), cluster headache (May et al. 1998a) and SUNCT (short-lasting unilateral neuralgiform headache with conjunctival injection and tearing) (May et al. 1999).

Activation of Modulatory Regions

Stimulation of nociceptive afferents by stimulation of the superior sagittal sinus in the cat activates neurons in the ventrolateral periaqueductal grey matter (PAG) (Hoskin et al. 2001). PAG activation in turn feeds back to the trigeminocervical complex with an inhibitory influence (Knight and Goadsby 2001). PAG is clearly included in the area of activation seen in PET studies in migraineurs (Weiller et al. 1995). This typical negative feedback system will be further considered below as a possible mechanism for the symptomatic manifestations of migraine.

Another potential modulatory region activated by stimulation of nociceptive trigeminovascular input is the posterior hypothalamic grey (Benjamin et al. 2004). This area is crucially involved in several primary headaches, notably cluster headache (Goadsby 2002b), short-lasting unilateral neuralgiform headache attacks with conjunctival injection and tearing (SUNCT) (May et al. 1999) and hemicrania continua (Matharu et al. 2004b). Moreover, the clinical features of the premonitory phase (Giffin et al. 2003)

M

and other features of the disorder (Bes et al. 1982; Peroutka 1997) suggest dopamine neuron involvement. Orexinergic neurons in the posterior hypothalamus can be both pro- and anti-nociceptive (Bartsch et al. 2004), offering a further possible region whose dysfunction might involve the perception of head pain.

Central Modulation of Trigeminal Pain

Brain Imaging in Humans

Functional brain imaging with positron emission tomography (PET) in studies during migraine without aura has demonstrated activation of the dorsal midbrain including the periaqueductal grey (PAG) and in the dorsal pons near the locus coeruleus (Weiller et al. 1995). Dorsolateral pontine activation is seen with PET in spontaneous episodic (Afridi et al. 2005a) and chronic migraine (Matharu et al. 2004a) and with nitroglycerin triggered attacks (Afridi et al. 2005b; Bahra et al. 2001). These areas are active immediately after successful treatment of the headache but are not active interictally. The activation corresponds with the brain region that Raskin et al. (1987) initially reported and Veloso confirmed (Veloso et al. 1998) to cause migraine-like headache when stimulated in patients with electrodes implanted for pain control. Similarly, Welch and colleagues (2001) have noted excess iron in the PAG of patients with episodic and chronic migraine and chronic migraine can develop after a bleed into a cavernoma in the region of the PAG (Goadsby 2002a) or with a lesion of the pons (Afridi and Goadsby 2003). What could dysfunction of these brain areas lead to?

Animal Experimental Studies of Sensory Modulation

It has been shown in the experimental animal that stimulation of the nucleus locus coeruleus, the main central noradrenergic nucleus, reduces cerebral blood flow in a frequency dependent manner (Goadsby et al. 1982) through an α_2-adrenoceptor linked mechanism (Goadsby et al. 1985). This reduction is maximal in the occipital cortex (Goadsby and Duckworth 1989). While a 25% overall reduction in cerebral blood flow is seen, extracerebral vasodilatation occurs in parallel (Goadsby et al. 1982). In addition the main serotonin containing nucleus in the brain stem, the midbrain dorsal raphe nucleus can increase cerebral blood flow when activated (Goadsby et al. 1991). Furthermore, stimulation of PAG will inhibit sagittal sinus evoked trigeminal neuronal activity in the cat (Knight and Goadsby 2001), while blockade of P / Q-type voltage-gated Ca^{2+} channels in the PAG facilitates trigemino-vascular nociceptive processing (Knight et al. 2002) with the local GABAergic system in the PAG still intact (Knight et al. 2003).

Electrophysiology of Migraine in Humans

Studies of evoked potentials and event related potentials provide some link between animal studies and human functional imaging (Kaube and Giffin 2002). Authors have shown changes in neurophysiological measures of brain activation but there is much discussion as to how to interpret such changes (Schoenen et al. 2003). Perhaps the most reliable theme is that the migrainous brain does not habituate to signals in a normal way (Afra et al. 2000; Proietti-Cecchini et al. 1997; Schoenen et al. 1995; Wang and Schoenen 1998). Similarly, contingent negative variation (CNV), an event related potential, is abnormal in migraineurs compared to controls (Schoenen and Timsit-Berthier 1993). Changes in CNV predict attacks (Kropp and Gerber 1998) and preventive therapies alter and normalize such changes (Maertens de Noordhout et al.

Migraine, Pathophysiology, Table 2 Neuroanatomical processing of vascular head pain

	Structure	Comments
Target innervation: Cranial vessels Dura mater	Ophthalmic branch of trigeminal nerve	
1st	Trigeminal ganglion	Middle cranial fossa
2nd	Trigeminal nucleus (quintothalamic tract)	Trigeminal n. caudalis and C_1 / C_2 dorsal horns
3rd	Thalamus	Ventrobasal complex Medial n. of posterior group Intralaminar complex
Modulatory	Midbrain Hypothalamus	Periaqueductal grey matter Posterior and lateral nuclei
Final	Cortex	insulae frontal cortex anterior cingulate cortex basal ganglia

1985). Attempts to correlate clinical phenotypes with electrophysiological changes (Gantenbein et al. 2004), may enhance further studies in this area.

What Is Migraine?

Migraine is an inherited, episodic disorder involving sensory sensitivity. Patients complain of pain in the head that is throbbing, but there is no reliable relationship between vessel diameter and the pain (Kruuse et al. 2003; Olesen et al. 1990) or its treatment (Limmroth et al. 1996). They complain of discomfort from normal lights and the unpleasantness of routine sounds. Some mention otherwise pleasant odors are unpleasant. Normal movement of the head causes pain and many mention a sense of unsteadiness as if they have just stepped off a boat, having been nowhere near the water!

The anatomical connections of, for example, the pain pathways are clear, the ophthalmic division of the trigeminal nerve subserves sensation within the cranium and explains why the top of the head is headache and the maxillary division is facial pain. The convergence of cervical and trigeminal afferents explains why neck stiffness or pain is so common in primary headache. The genetics of channelopathies is opening up a plausible way to think about the episodic nature of migraine. However, where is the lesion, what is actually the pathology?

If one considers what patients say, then perhaps they tell us the answer to this question. Migraine aura cannot be the trigger, there is no evidence at all after 4,000 years that it occurs in more than 30% of migraine patients, it can be experienced without pain at all and is seen in the other primary headaches. There is not a photon of extra light that migraine patients receive over others, so for that symptom and phonophobia and osmophobia, the basis of the problem must be abnormal central processing of a normal signal. Perhaps electrophysiological changes in the brain have been mislabeled as hyperexcitability whereas dyshabituation might be a simpler explanation. If migraine was basically an attentional problem with changes in cortical synchronization (Niebur et al. 2002) or hypersynchronization (Angelini et al. 2004), all its manifestations could be accounted for in a single over-arching pathophysiolog-

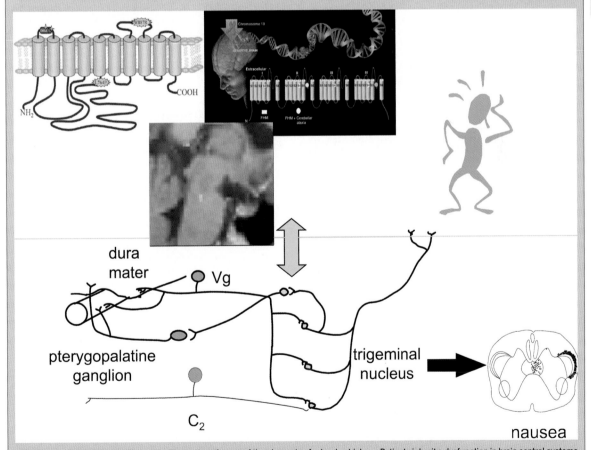

Migraine, Pathophysiology, Figure 1 Illustration of some of the elements of migraine biology. Patients inherit a dysfunction in brain control systems for pain and other afferent stimuli, which can be triggered and are in turn capable of activating the trigeminovascular system as the initiating event in a positive feedback of neurally driven vasodilatation. Pain from cervical inputs that terminate in the trigeminocervical complex accounts for the non-trigeminal distribution of pain in many patients. Migraine has thus a pain system for its expression and brain centers and modulatory systems that define the associated symptoms and periodicity of the clinical syndrome. Brain stem changes after Bahra and colleague (2001).

ical hypothesis of a disturbance of sub-cortical sensory modulation systems (Goadsby 2003). While it seems likely that the trigeminovascular system and its cranial autonomic reflex connections, the trigeminal-autonomic reflex (May and Goadsby 1999) act as a feed-forward system to facilitate the acute attack, the fundamental problem in migraine is in the brain. Unraveling its basis will deliver great benefits to patients and considerable understanding of some very fundamental neurobiological processes.

Acknowledgements

The work of the author has been supported by the Wellcome Trust.

References

1. Afra J, Sandor P, Schoenen J (2000) Habituation of visual and intensity dependence of cortical auditory evoked potentials tend to normalise just before and during migraine attacks. Cephalalgia 20:347
2. Afridi S, Goadsby PJ (2003) New onset migraine with a brainstem cavernous angioma. J Neurol Neurosurg Psychiatry 74:680–682
3. Afridi S, Giffin NJ, Kaube H et al. (2005a) A PET study in spontaneous migraine. Arch Neurol 2005 (in press)
4. Afridi S, Matharu MS, Lee L et al. (2005b) A PET study exploring the laterality of brainstem activation in migraine using glyceryl trinitrate. Brain 128:932–939
5. Akerman S, Goadsby PJ (2004) Topiramate inhibits cortical spreading depression in rat and cat: a possible contribution to its preventive effect in migraine. Cephalalgia 24:783–784
6. Angelini L, Tommaso M de, Guido M et al. (2004) Steady-state visual evoked potentials and phase synchronization in migraine patients. Phys Rev Lett 93:038103-1–038103-4
7. Arbab MA-R, Wiklund L, Svendgaard NA (1986) Origin and distribution of cerebral vascular innervation from superior cervical, trigeminal and spinal ganglia investigated with retrograde and anterograde WGA-HRP tracing in the rat. Neuroscience 19:695–708
8. Bahra A, Matharu MS, Buchel C et al. (2001) Brainstem activation specific to migraine headache. Lancet 357:1016–1017
9. Bartsch T, Goadsby PJ (2002) Stimulation of the greater occipital nerve induces increased central excitability of dural afferent input. Brain 125:1496–1509
10. Bartsch T, Goadsby PJ (2003) Increased responses in trigeminocervical nociceptive neurones to cervical input after stimulation of the dura mater. Brain 126:1801–1813
11. Bartsch T, Levy MJ, Knight YE et al. (2004) Differential modulation of nociceptive dural input to [hypocretin] Orexin A and B receptor activation in the posterior hypothalamic area. Pain 109:367–378
12. Benjamin L, Levy MJ, Lasalandra MP et al. (2004) Hypothalamic activation after stimulation of the superior sagittal sinus in the cat: a Fos study. Neurobiol Dis 16:500–505
13. Bes A, Geraud A, Guell A et al. (1982) Dopaminergic hypersensitivity in migraine: a diagnostic test? La Nouvelle Presse Medicale 11:1475–1478
14. Bolay H, Reuter U, Dunn AK et al. (2002) Intrinsic brain activity triggers trigeminal meningeal afferents in a migraine model. Nat Med 8:136–142
15. Brandes JL, Saper JR, Diamond M et al. (2004) Topiramate for migraine prevention: a randomized controlled trial. JAMA 291:965–973
16. Burstein R, Yamamura H, Malick A et al. (1998) Chemical stimulation of the intracranial dura induces enhanced responses to facial stimulation in brain stem trigeminal neurons. J Neurophysiol 79:964–982
17. Burstein R, Cutrer MF, Yarnitsky D (2000a) The development of cutaneous allodynia during a migraine attack. Brain 123:1703–1709
18. Burstein R, Yarnitsky D, Goor-Aryeh I et al. (2000b) An association between migraine and cutaneous allodynia. Ann Neurol 47:614–624
19. Connor HE, Bertin L, Gillies S et al. (1998) The GR205171 Clinical Study Group. Clinical evaluation of a novel, potent, CNS penetrating NK_1 receptor antagonist in the acute treatment of migraine. Cephalalgia 18:392
20. Cumberbatch MJ, Hill RG, Hargreaves RJ (1997) Rizatriptan has central antinociceptive effects against durally evoked responses. European J Pharmacol 328:37–40
21. Cumberbatch MJ, Hill RG, Hargreaves RJ (1998) Differential effects of the $5HT_{1B/1D}$ receptor agonist naratriptan on trigeminal versus spinal nociceptive responses. Cephalalgia 18:659–664
22. Cutrer FM, Limmroth V, Waeber C et al. (1997) New targets for antimigraine drug development. In: Goadsby PJ, Silberstein SD (eds) Headache. Butterworth-Heinemann, Philadelphia, pp 59–72
23. Cutrer FM, Sorensen AG, Weisskoff RM et al. (1998) Perfusion-weighted imaging defects during spontaneous migrainous aura. Ann Neurol 43:25–31
24. Data J, Britch K, Westergaard N et al. (1998) A double-blind study of ganaxolone in the acute treatment of migraine headaches with or without an aura in premenopausal females. Headache 38:380
25. De Fusco M, Marconi R, Silvestri L et al. (2003) Haploinsufficiency of ATP1A2 encoding the Na^+/K^+ pump α2 subunit associated with familial hemiplegic migraine type 2. Nat Genet 33:192–196
26. Diener HC, Tfelt-Hansen P, Dahlof C et al. (2004) Topiramate in migraine prophylaxis —results from a placebo-controlled trial with propranolol as an active control. J Neurol 251:943–950
27. Diener H-C, The RPR100893 Study Group (2003) RPR100893, a substance-P antagonist, is not effective in the treatment of migraine attacks. Cephalalgia 23:183–185
28. Dimitriadou V, Buzzi MG, Moskowitz MA et al. (1991) Trigeminal sensory fiber stimulation induces morphological changes reflecting secretion in rat dura mater mast cells. Neuroscience 44:97–112
29. Dimitriadou V, Buzzi MG, Theoharides TC et al. (1992) Ultrastructural evidence for neurogenically mediated changes in blood vessels of the rat dura mater and tongue following antidromic trigeminal stimulation. Neuroscience 48:187–203
30. Doods H, Hallermayer G, Wu D et al. (2000) Pharmacological profile of BIBN4096BS, the first selective small molecule CGRP antagonist. Br J Pharmacol 129:420–423
31. Ducros A, Denier C, Joutel A et al. (2001) The clinical spectrum of familial hemiplegic migraine associated with mutations in a neuronal calcium channel. N Engl J Med 345:17–24
32. Durham PL, Russo AF (1999) Regulation of calcitonin gene-related peptide secretion by a serotonergic antimigraine drug. J Neurosci 19:3423–3429
33. Durham PL, Sharma RV, Russo AF (1997) Repression of the calcitonin gene-related peptide promoter by 5-HT1 receptor activation. J Neurosci 17:9545–9553
34. Earl NL, McDonald SA, Lowy MT, 4991W93 Investigator Group (1999) Efficacy and tolerability of the neurogenic inflammation inhibitor, 4991W93, in the acute treatment of migraine. Cephalalgia 19:357
35. Ebersberger A, Schaible H-G, Averbeck B et al. (2001) Is there a correlation between spreading depression, neurogenic inflammation, and nociception that might cause migraine headache? Ann Neurol 41:7–13
36. Edvinsson L, Goadsby PJ (1998) Neuropeptides in headache. Eur J Neurol 5:329–341
37. Ertel EA, Campbell KP, Harpold MM et al. (2000) Nomenclature of voltage-gated calcium channels. Neuron 25:533–535

38. Fanciullacci M, Alessandri M, Figini M et al. (1995) Increase in plasma calcitonin gene-related peptide from extracerebral circulation during nitroglycerin-induced cluster headache attack. Pain 60:119–123

39. Feindel W, Penfield W, McNaughton F (1960) The tentorial nerves and localization of intracranial pain in man. Neurol 10:555–563

40. Gallai V, Sarchielli P, Floridi A et al. (1995) Vasoactive peptides levels in the plasma of young migraine patients with and without aura assessed both interictally and ictally. Cephalalgia 15:384–390

41. Gantenbein A, Goadsby PJ, Kaube H (2004) Introduction of a clinical scoring system for migraine research applied to electrophysiological studies. Cephalalgia 24:1095–1096

42. Giffin NJ, Ruggiero L, Lipton RB et al. (2003) Premonitory symptoms in migraine: an electronic diary study. Neurology 60:935–940

43. Goadsby PJ (2001) Migraine, aura and cortical spreading depression: why are we still talking about it? Ann Neurol 49:4–6

44. Goadsby PJ (2002a) Neurovascular headache and a midbrain vascular malformation—evidence for a role of the brainstem in chronic migraine. Cephalalgia 22:107–111

45. Goadsby PJ (2002b) Pathophysiology of cluster headache: a trigeminal autonomic cephalgia. Lancet Neurol 1:37–43

46. Goadsby PJ (2003) Migraine pathophysiology: the brainstem governs the cortex. Cephalalgia 23:565–566

47. Goadsby PJ (2004) Migraine aura: a knock-in mouse with a knock-out message. Neuron 41:679–680

48. Goadsby PJ, Classey JD (2003) Evidence for 5-HT$_{1B}$, 5-HT$_{1D}$ and 5-HT$_{1F}$ receptor inhibitory effects on trigeminal neurons with craniovascular input. Neuroscience 122:491–498

49. Goadsby PJ, Duckworth JW (1989) Low frequency stimulation of the locus coeruleus reduces regional cerebral blood flow in the spinalized cat. Brain Res 476:71–77

50. Goadsby PJ, Edvinsson L (1994) Human *in vivo* evidence for trigeminovascular activation in cluster headache. Brain 117:427–434

51. Goadsby PJ, Edvinsson L (1996) Neuropeptide changes in a case of chronic paroxysmal hemicrania-evidence for trigemino-parasympathetic activation. Cephalalgia 16:448–450

52. Goadsby PJ, Ferrari MD (2001) Migraine: a multifactorial, episodic neurovascular channelopathy? In: Rose MR, Griggs RC (eds) Channelopathies of the Nervous System. Butterworth Heinemann, Oxford, pp 274–292

53. Goadsby PJ, Hoskin KL (1996) Inhibition of trigeminal neurons by intravenous administration of the serotonin (5HT)$_{1B / D}$ receptor agonist zolmitriptan (311C90): are brain stem sites a therapeutic target in migraine? Pain 67:355–359

54. Goadsby PJ, Hoskin KL (1997) The distribution of trigeminovascular afferents in the nonhuman primate brain *Macaca nemestrina*: a c-fos immunocytochemical study. J Anatomy 190:367–375

55. Goadsby PJ, Hoskin KL (1999) Differential effects of low dose CP122,288 and eletriptan on fos expression due to stimulation of the superior sagittal sinus in cat. Pain 82:15–22

56. Goadsby PJ, Knight YE (1997) Inhibition of trigeminal neurons after intravenous administration of naratriptan through an action at the serotonin (5HT$_{1B / 1D}$) receptors. Br J Pharmacol 122:918–922

57. Goadsby PJ, Zagami AS (1991) Stimulation of the superior sagittal sinus increases metabolic activity and blood flow in certain regions of the brainstem and upper cervical spinal cord of the cat. Brain 114:1001–1011

58. Goadsby PJ, Lambert GA, Lance JW (1982) Differential effects on the internal and external carotid circulation of the monkey evoked by locus coeruleus stimulation. Brain Res 249:247–254

59. Goadsby PJ, Lambert GA, Lance JW (1985) The mechanism of cerebrovascular vasoconstriction in response to locus coeruleus stimulation. Brain Res 326:213–217

60. Goadsby PJ, Edvinsson L, Ekman R (1988) Release of vasoactive peptides in the extracerebral circulation of man and the cat during activation of the trigeminovascular system. Ann Neurol 23:193–196

61. Goadsby PJ, Edvinsson L, Ekman R (1990) Vasoactive peptide release in the extracerebral circulation of humans during migraine headache. Ann Neurol 28:183–187

62. Goadsby PJ, Zagami AS, Lambert GA (1991) Neural processing of craniovascular pain: a synthesis of the central structures involved in migraine. Headache 31:365–371

63. Goadsby PJ, Hoskin KL, Knight YE (1997) Stimulation of the greater occipital nerve increases metabolic activity in the trigeminal nucleus caudalis and cervical dorsal horn of the cat. Pain 73:23–28

64. Goadsby PJ, Akerman S, Storer RJ (2001) Evidence for postjunctional serotonin (5-HT$_1$) receptors in the trigeminocervical complex. Ann Neurol 50:804–807

65. Goadsby PJ, Lipton RB, Ferrari MD (2002) Migraine—current understanding and treatment. N Engl J Med 346:257–270

66. Goldstein DJ, Wang O, Saper JR et al. (1997) Ineffectiveness of neurokinin-1 antagonist in acute migraine: a crossover study. Cephalalgia 17:785–790

67. Haan J, Terwindt GM, Bos PL et al. (1994) Familial hemiplegic migraine in The Netherlands. Clinical Neurol Neurosurgery 96:244–249

68. Hadjikhani N, Sanchez del Rio M, Wu O et al. (2001) Mechanisms of migraine aura revealed by functional MRI in human visual cortex. Proc Natl Acad Sci USA 98:4687–4692

69. Harer C, Kummer R (1991) Cerebrovascular CO_2 reactivity in migraine: assessment by transcranial Doppler ultrasound. J Neurol 238:23–26

70. Headache Classification Committee of The International Headache Society (2004) The International Classification of Headache Disorders, 2nd edn. Cephalalgia 24:1–160

71. Hoskin KL, Kaube H, Goadsby PJ (1996) Central activation of the trigeminovascular pathway in the cat is inhibited by dihydroergotamine. A c-Fos and electrophysiology study. Brain 119:249–256

72. Hoskin KL, Zagami A, Goadsby PJ (1999) Stimulation of the middle meningeal artery leads to Fos expression in the trigeminocervical nucleus: a comparative study of monkey and cat. J Anatomy 194:579–588

73. Hoskin KL, Bulmer DCE, Lasalandra M et al. (2001) Fos expression in the midbrain periaqueductal grey after trigeminovascular stimulation. J Anatomy 197:29–35

74. Ingvardsen BK, Laursen H, Olsen UB et al. (1997) Possible mechanism of c-fos expression in trigeminal nucleus caudalis following spreading depression. Pain 72:407–415

75. Ingvardsen BK, Laursen H, Olsen UB et al. (1998) Comment on Ingvardsen et al. (1997) Pain 72 407–415; Reply to Moskowitz et al. (1998) Pain 76:266–267

76. Joutel A, Bousser MG, Biousse V A et al. (1993) A gene for familial hemiplegic migraine maps to chromosome 19. Nat Genet 5:40–45

77. Joutel A, Ducros A, Vahedi K et al. (1994) Genetic heterogeneity of familial hemiplegic migraine. American J Hum Gen 55:1166–1172

78. Jurkat-Rott K, Freilinger T, Dreier JP et al. (2004) Variability of familial hemiplegic migraine with novel A1A2 Na^+ / K^+-ATPase variants. Neurology 62:1857–1861

79. Kaube H, Giffin NJ (2002) The electrophysiology of migraine. Curr Opin Neurol 15:303–309

80. Kaube H, Goadsby PJ (1994) Anti-migraine compounds fail to modulate the propagation of cortical spreading depression in the cat. Eur Neurol 34:30–35

81. Kaube H, Hoskin KL, Goadsby PJ (1993a) Inhibition by sumatriptan of central trigeminal neurones only after blood-brain barrier disruption. Br J Pharmacol 109:788–792

82. Kaube H, Hoskin KL, Goadsby PJ (1993b) Intravenous acetylsalicylic acid inhibits central trigeminal neurons in the dorsal

M

horn of the upper cervical spinal cord in the cat. Headache 33:541–550

83. Kaube H, Keay KA, Hoskin KL et al. (1993c) Expression of c-*Fos*-like immunoreactivity in the caudal medulla and upper cervical cord following stimulation of the superior sagittal sinus in the cat. Brain Res 629:95–102

84. Kaube H, Knight YE, Storer RJ et al. (1999) Vasodilator agents and supracollicular transection fail to inhibit cortical spreading depression in the cat. Cephalalgia 19:592–597

85. Knight YE, Goadsby PJ (2001) The periaqueductal gray matter modulates trigeminovascular input: a role in migraine? Neuroscience 106:793–800

86. Knight YE, Edvinsson L, Goadsby PJ (1999) Blockade of CGRP release after superior sagittal sinus stimulation in cat: a comparison of avitriptan and CP122,288. Neuropeptides 33:41–46

87. Knight YE, Edvinsson L, Goadsby PJ (2001) 4991W93 inhibits release of calcitonin gene-related peptide in the cat but only at doses with $5HT_{1B/1D}$ receptor agonist activity. Neuropharmacology 40:520–525

88. Knight YE, Bartsch T, Kaube H et al. (2002) P/Q-type calcium channel blockade in the PAG facilitates trigeminal nociception: a functional genetic link for migraine? J Neurosci 22:1–6

89. Knight YE, Bartsch T, Goadsby PJ (2003) Trigeminal antinociception induced by bicuculline in the periaqueductal grey (PAG) is not affected by PAG P/Q-type calcium channel blockade in rat. Neurosci Lett 336:113–116

90. Kropp P, Gerber WD (1998) Prediction of migraine attacks using a slow cortical potential, the contingent negative variation. Neurosci Lett 257:73–76

91. Kruuse C, Thomsen LL, Birk S et al. (2003) Migraine can be induced by sildenafil without changes in middle cerebral artery diameter. Brain 126:241–247

92. Lalouel JM, Morton NE (1981) Complex segregation analysis with pointers. Human Heredity 31:312–321

93. Lambert GA, Michalicek J, Storer RJ et al. (1999) Effect of cortical spreading depression on activity of trigeminovascular sensory neurons. Cephalalgia 19:631–638

94. Lambert GA, Boers PM, Hoskin KL et al. (2002) Suppression by eletriptan of the activation of trigeminovascular sensory neurons by glyceryl trinitrate. Brain Res 953:181–188

95. Lance JW, Goadsby PJ (2005) Mechanism and Management of Headache. Elsevier, New York

96. Lashley KS (1941) Patterns of cerebral integration indicated by the scotomas of migraine. Arch Neurol Psychiatry 46:331–339

97. Lauritzen M (1994) Pathophysiology of the migraine aura. The spreading depression theory. Brain 117:199–210

98. Lauritzen M, Skyhoj-Olsen T, Lassen NA et al. (1983) The changes of regional cerebral blood flow during the course of classical migraine attacks. Ann Neurol 13:633–641

99. Leao AAP (1944a) Pial circulation and spreading activity in the cerebral cortex. J Neurophysiol 7:391–396

100. Leao AAP (1944b) Spreading depression of activity in cerebral cortex. J Neurophysiology 7:359–390

101. Limmroth V, May A, Auerbach P et al. (1996) Changes in cerebral blood flow velocity after treatment with sumatriptan or placebo and implications for the pathophysiology of migraine. J Neurol Sci 138:60–65

102. Liu-Chen L-Y, Gillespie SA, Norregaard TV et al. (1984) Colocalization of retrogradely transported wheat germ agglutinin and the putative neurotransmitter substance P within trigeminal ganglion cells projecting to cat middle cerebral. J Comp Neurol 225:187–192

103. MaassenVanDenBrink A, van den Broek RW, de Vries R et al. (2000) The potential anti-migraine compound SB-220453 does not contract human isolated blood vessels or myocardium; a comparison with sumatriptan. Cephalalgia 20:538–545

104. Maertens de Noordhout A, Timsit-Berthier M, Schoenen J (1985) Contingent negative variation (CNV) in migraineurs

before and during prophylactic treatment with beta-blockers. Cephalalgia 5:34–35

105. Maneesi S, Akerman S, Lasalandra MP et al. (2004) Electron microscopic demonstration of pre- and postsynaptic 5-HT_{1D} and 5-HT_{1F} receptor immunoreactivity (IR) in the rat trigeminocervical complex (TCC) new therapeutic possibilities for the triptans. Cephalalgia 24:148

106. Marconi R, De Fusco M, Aridon P et al. (2003) Familial hemiplegic migraine type 2 is linked to 0.9Mb region on chromosome 1q23. Ann Neurol 53:376–381

107. Markowitz S, Saito K, Moskowitz MA (1987) Neurogenically mediated leakage of plasma proteins occurs from blood vessels in dura mater but not brain. J Neurosci 7:4129–4136

108. Matharu MS, Bartsch T, Ward N et al. (2004a) Central neuromodulation in chronic migraine patients with suboccipital stimulators: a PET study. Brain 127:220–230

109. Matharu MS, Cohen AS, McGonigle DJ et al. (2004b) Posterior hypothalamic and brainstem activation in hemicrania continua. Headache 44:462–463

110. Matsuyama T, Shiosaka S, Matsumoto M et al. (1983) Overall distribution of vasoactive intestinal polypeptide-containing nerves on the wall of the cerebral arteries: an immunohistochemical study using whole-mounts. Neuroscience 10: 89–96

111. May A, Goadsby PJ (1999) The trigeminovascular system in humans: pathophysiological implications for primary headache syndromes of the neural influences on the cerebral circulation. J Cerebral Blood Flow Metabolism 19:115–127

112. May A, Gijsman HJ, Wallnoefer A et al. (1996) Endothelin antagonist bosentan blocks neurogenic inflammation, but is not effective in aborting migraine attacks. Pain 67:375–378

113. May A, Bahra A, Buchel C et al. (1998a) Hypothalamic activation in cluster headache attacks. Lancet 352:275–278

114. May A, Shepheard S, Wessing A et al. (1998b) Retinal plasma extravasation can be evoked by trigeminal stimulation in rat but does not occur during migraine attacks. Brain 121:1231–1237

115. May A, Bahra A, Buchel C et al. (1999) Functional MRI in spontaneous attacks of SUNCT: short-lasting neuralgiform headache with conjunctival injection and tearing. Ann Neurol 46:791–793

116. Mochi M, Sangiorgi S, Cortelli P et al. (1993) Testing models for genetic determination in migraine. Cephalalgia 13:389–394

117. Moskowitz MA (1990) Basic mechanisms in vascular headache. Neurologic Clinics 8:801–815

118. Moskowitz MA, Cutrer FM (1993) Sumatriptan: a receptor-targeted treatment for migraine. Ann Rev Med 44:145–154

119. Moskowitz MA, Nozaki K, Kraig RP (1993) Neocortical spreading depression provokes the expression of C-fos protein-like immunoreactivity within the trigeminal nucleus caudalis via trigeminovascular mechanisms. J Neurosci 13:1167–1177

120. Moskowitz MA, Bolay H, Dalkara T (2004) Deciphering migraine mechanisms: Clues from familial hemiplegic migraine genotypes. Ann Neurol 55:276–280

121. Niebur E, Hsiao SS, Johnson KO (2002) Synchrony: a neural mechanism for attentional selection? Curr Opin Neurobiol 12:190–194

122. Norman B, Panebianco D, Block GA (1998) A placebo-controlled, in-clinic study to explore the preliminary safety and efficacy of intravenous L-758,298 (a prodrug of the NK1 receptor antagonist L-754,030) in the acute treatment of migraine. Cephalalgia 18:407

123. Nozaki K, Boccalini P, Moskowitz MA (1992) Expression of c-fos-like immunoreactivity in brainstem after meningeal irritation by blood in the subarachnoid space. Neuroscience 49:669–680

124. Olesen J, Larsen B, Lauritzen M (1981) Focal hyperemia followed by spreading oligemia and impaired activation of rCBF in classic migraine. Ann Neurol 9:344–352

125. Olesen J, Friberg L, Skyhoj-Olsen T et al. (1990) Timing and topography of cerebral blood flow, aura, and headache during migraine attacks. Ann Neurol 28:791–798

126. Olesen J, Diener H-C, Husstedt I-W et al. (2004) Calcitonin gene-related peptide (CGRP) receptor antagonist BIBN4096BS is effective in the treatment of migraine attacks. N Engl J Med 350:1104–1110

127. Ophoff RA, Eijk Rv, Sandkuijl LA et al. (1994) Genetic heterogeneity of familial hemiplegic migraine. Genomics 22:21–26

128. Ophoff RA, Terwindt GM, Vergouwe MN et al. (1996) Familial hemiplegic migraine and episodic ataxia type-2 are caused by mutations in the Ca^{2+} channel gene CACNL1A4. Cell 87:543–552

129. Parsons AA, Bingham S, Raval P et al. (2001) Tonabersat (SB-220453) a novel benzopyran with anticonvulsant properties attenuates trigeminal nerve-induced neurovascular reflexes. Br J Pharmacol 132:1549–1557

130. Penfield W, McNaughton FL (1940) Dural headache and the innervation of the dura mater. Arch Neurol Psychiatry 44:43–75

131. Peroutka SJ (1997) Dopamine and migraine. Neurol 49:650–656

132. Proietti-Cecchini A, Afra J, Schoenen J (1997) Intensity dependence of the cortical auditory evoked potentials as a surrogate marker of central nervous system serotonin transmission in man: demonstration of a central effect for the 5HT1B / 1D agonist zolmitriptan (311C90, Zomig). Cephalalgia 17:849–854

133. Raskin NH, Hosobuchi Y, Lamb S (1987) Headache may arise from perturbation of brain. Headache 27:416–420

134. Rasmussen BK, Olesen J (1992) Migraine with aura and migraine without aura: an epidemiological study. Cephalalgia 12:221–228

135. Read SJ, Smith MI, Hunter AJ et al. (1999) SB-220453, a potential novel antimigraine compound, inhibits nitric oxide release following induction of cortical spreading depression in the anaesthetized cat. Cephalalgia 20:92–99

136. Roon K, Diener HC, Ellis P et al. (1997) CP-122,288 blocks neurogenic inflammation, but is not effective in aborting migraine attacks: results of two controlled clinical studies. Cephalalgia 17:245

137. Russell MB (1997) Genetic epidemiology of migraine and cluster headache. Cephalalgia 17:683–701

138. Russell MB, Iselius L, Olesen J (1995) Investigation of the inheritance of migraine by complex segregation analysis. Hum Genet 96:726–730

139. Sakai F, Meyer JS (1979) Abnormal cerebrovascular reactivity in patients with migraine and cluster headache. Headache 19:257–266

140. Schoenen J, Timsit-Berthier M (1993) Contingent negative variation: methods and potential interest in headache. Cephalalgia 13:28–32

141. Schoenen J, Wang W, Albert A et al. (1995) Potentiation instead of habituation characterizes visual evoked potentials in migraine patients between attacks. Eur J Neurol 2:115–122

142. Schoenen J, Ambrosini A, Sandor PS et al. (2003) Evoked potentials and transcranial magnetic stimulation in migraine: published data and viewpoint on their pathophysiologic significance. Clin Neurophysiol 114:955–972

143. Selby G, Lance JW (1960) Observations on 500 cases of migraine and allied vascular headache. J Neurol Neurosurg Psychiatry 23:23–32

144. Shields KG, Goadsby PJ (2004) Naratriptan modulates trigeminovascular nociceptive transmission in the ventroposteromedial (VPM) thalamic nucleus of the rat. Cephalalgia 24:1098

145. Shields KG, Goadsby PJ (2005) Propranolol modulates trigeminovascular responses in thalamic ventroposteromedial nucleus: a role in migraine? Brain 128:86–97

146. Shields KG, Kaube H, Goadsby PJ (2003) GABA receptors modulate trigeminovascular nociceptive transmission in the ventroposteromedial (VPM) thalamic nucleus of the rat. Cephalalgia 23:728

147. Silberstein SD, Lipton RB, Goadsby PJ (2002) Headache in Clinical Practice. Martin Dunitz, London

148. Silberstein SD, Neto W, Schmitt J et al. (2004) Topiramate in migraine prevention: results of a large controlled trial. Arch Neurol 61:490–495

149. Smith MI, Read SJ, Chan WN et al. (2000) Repetitive cortical spreading depression in a gyrencephalic feline brain: inhibition by the novel benzoylamino-benzopyran SB-220453. Cephalalgia 20:546–53

150. Storer RJ, Goadsby PJ (2004) Topiramate inhibits trigeminovascular neurons in the cat. Cephalalgia 24:1049–1056

151. Storer RJ, Goadsby PJ (2005) Topiramate has a locus of action outside of the trigeminocervical complex. Neurol (in press)

152. Strassman AM, Raymond SA, Burstein R (1996) Sensitization of meningeal sensory neurons and the origin of headaches. Nature 384:560–563

153. Swoboda KJ, Kanavakis E, Xaidara A et al. (2004) Alternating hemiplegia of childhood or familial hemiplegic migraine? A novel ATP1A2 mutation. Ann Neurol 55:884–887

154. Teh BT, Silburn P, Lindblad K et al. (1995) Familial cerebellar periodic ataxia without myokymia maps to a 19-cM region on 19p13. Am J Hum Genet 56:1443–1449

155. Terwindt GM, Ophoff RA, Haan J et al. (1996) The Dutch Migraine Genetics Research Group. Familial hemiplegic migraine: a clinical comparison of families linked and unlinked to chromosome 19. Cephalalgia 16:153–155

156. Tvedskov JF, Iversen HK, Olesen J (2004a) A double-blind study of SB-220453 (Tonerbasat) in the glyceryltrinitrate (GTN) model of migraine. Cephalalgia 24:875–882

157. Tvedskov JF, Thomsen LL, Iversen HK et al. (2004b) The prophylactic effect of valproate on glyceryltrinitrate induced migraine. Cephalalgia 24:576–585

158. Tvedskov JF, Thomsen LL, Iversen HK et al. (2004c) The effect of propranolol on glyceryltrinitrate-induced headache and arterial response. Cephalalgia 24:1076–1087

159. Uddman R, Edvinsson L, Ekman R et al. (1985) Innervation of the feline cerebral vasculature by nerve fibers containing calcitonin gene-related peptide: trigeminal origin and co-existence with substance P. Neurosci Lett 62:131–136

160. Ulrich V, Gervil M, Kyvik KO et al. (1999) Evidence of a genetic factor in migraine with aura: a population based Danish twin study. Ann Neurol 45:242–246

161. van den Maagdenberg AMJM, Pietrobon D, Pizzorusso T et al. (2004) A Cacna1a knock-in migraine mouse model with increased susceptibility to cortical spreading depression. Neuron 41:701–710

162. Vanmolkot KRJ, Kors EE, Hottenga JJ et al. (2003) Novel mutations in the Na^+,K^+-ATPase pump gene ATP1A2 associated with Familial Hemiplegic Migraine and Benign Familial Infantile Convulsions. Ann Neurol 54:360–366

163. Veloso F, Kumar K, Toth C (1998) Headache secondary to deep brain implantation. Headache 38:507–515

164. Wang W, Schoenen J (1998) Interictal potentiation of passive "oddball" auditory event-related potentials in migraine. Cephalalgia 18:261–265

165. Weiller C, May A, Limmroth V et al. (1995) Brain stem activation in spontaneous human migraine attacks. Nat Med 1:658–660

166. Welch KM, Nagesh V, Aurora S et al. (2001) Periaqueductal grey matter dysfunction in migraine: cause or the burden of illness? Headache 41:629–637

167. Willis T (1682) Opera Omnia. Amstelaedami: Henricum Wetstenium

168. Wolff HG (1948) Headache and Other Head Pain. Oxford University Press, New York

169. Zagami AS, Goadsby PJ (1991) Stimulation of the superior sagittal sinus increases metabolic activity in cat thalamus. In: Rose FC (ed) New Advances in Headache Research: 2. Smith-Gordon, London, pp 169–171

170. Zagami AS, Lambert GA (1991) Craniovascular application of capsaicin activates nociceptive thalamic neurons in the cat. Neurosci Lett 121:187–190

M

Migraine, Preventive Therapy

STEPHEN D. SILBERSTEIN
Jefferson Medical College, Thomas Jefferson
University and Jefferson Headache Center, Thomas
Jefferson University Hospital, Philadelphia, PA, USA
stephen.silberstein@jefferson.edu

Definition

▶ Migraine is a primary episodic headache disorder characterized by various combinations of neurologic, gastrointestinal, and autonomic changes. Diagnosis is based on the headache's characteristics and associated symptoms (Silberstein et al. 2001). The International Headache Society's diagnostic criteria for headache disorders were recently revised, and provide criteria for a total of seven subtypes of migraine (Headache Classification Committee 2004). This review relied on the Technical Reports of the Agency for Healthcare Policy and Research (Goslin et al. 1994; Gray et al. 1999) and the US Headache Consortium Guidelines (Ramadan et al. 1999).

Characteristics

Treatment

Migraine treatment begins with making a diagnosis (Silberstein et al. 2001), explaining it to the patient, and developing a treatment plan that considers coincidental or comorbid conditions. Headache calendars record headache duration, severity, and treatment response. ▶ Comorbidity indicates an association between two disorders that is more than coincidental. Conditions that occur in migraineurs with a higher prevalence than would be expected include stroke, epilepsy, Raynaud's syndrome, and affective disorders, which include depression, mania, anxiety, and panic disorder. Possible associations include essential tremor, mitral valve prolapse, and irritable bowel syndrome (Silberstein 2004). ▶ Pharmacotherapy may be acute (abortive) or preventive (prophylactic), and patients may require both approaches. Acute treatment attempts to reverse or stop the progression of a headache once it has started. It is appropriate for most attacks and should be limited to 2–3 days a week. ▶ Preventive therapy is designed to reduce attack frequency and severity.

Preventive Treatment

Preventive medications reduce attack frequency, duration, or severity (Silberstein and Goadsby 2004; Silberstein et al. 2001). According to the US Headache Consortium Guidelines (Ramadan et al. 1999), indications for preventive treatment include:

- Migraine that significantly interferes with the patient's daily routine despite acute treatment;
- Failure of, contraindication to, or troublesome adverse events (AEs) from acute medications;
- Acute medication overuse;
- Very frequent headaches (>2/week) (risk of medication overuse);
- Patient preference;
- Special circumstances, such as hemiplegic migraine or attacks with a risk of permanent neurologic injury.

Preventive medication groups include beta-adrenergic blockers, ▶ antidepressants, ▶ calcium channel antagonists, ▶ serotonin antagonists, ▶ Anticonvulsant (Agent), and ▶ NSAIDs, Survey (NSAIDs). Choice is based on efficacy, AEs, and coexistent and comorbid conditions (Table 5). The medication is started at a low dose and increased slowly until therapeutic effects develop or the ceiling dose is reached. A full therapeutic trial may take 2–6 months. Acute headache medications should not be overused. If headaches are well controlled, medication can be tapered and discontinued. Dose reduction may provide a better risk-to-benefit ratio. Women of childbearing potential should be on adequate contraception.

Behavioral and psychological interventions used for prevention include ▶ relaxation training, thermal ▶ biofeedback combined with relaxation training, electromyography biofeedback, and cognitive-behavioral therapy (Silberstein 2004). These interventions are effective as monotherapy, but are more effective when used in conjunction with pharmacologic management.

Medication

▶ Beta(β) Blockers ▶ Propranolol, ▶ nadolol, ▶ atenolol, ▶ metropropol, and ▶ timolol are effective preventive drugs (Gray et al. 1999). Their relative efficacy has not been established; choice is based on beta-selectivity, convenience, AEs, and patients' reactions (Silberstein et al. 2001). Beta-blockers can produce behavioral AEs, such as drowsiness, fatigue, lethargy, sleep disorders, nightmares, depression, memory disturbance, and hallucinations; they should be avoided when patients are depressed. Decreased exercise tolerance limits their use by athletes. Less common AEs include impotence, orthostatic hypotension, and bradycardia. Beta-blockers are useful for patients with angina or hypertension. They are relatively contraindicated for patients with congestive heart failure, asthma, Raynaud's disease, and insulin-dependent diabetes.

Antidepressants

▶ Amitriptyline (a tricyclic antidepressant) is the only antidepressant with fairly consistent support for efficacy (Gray et al. 1999). AEs include increased appetite, weight gain, dry mouth, and sedation; cardiac toxicity and orthostatic hypotension occasionally occur (Saper et al. 1994). There has been one positive trial for fluoxetine. Sexual dysfunction is a common AE. Antidepressants are especially useful for patients with comorbid depression and anxiety disorders.

Calcium-Channel Blockers

The Agency for Healthcare Policy and Research analyzed 45 controlled trials (Gray et al. 1999). Flunarizine was effective, nimodipine had mixed results, and nifedipine was difficult to interpret. ▶ Verapamil was more effective than placebo in two of three trials, but both positive trials had high dropout rates, rendering the findings uncertain (Silberstein et al. 2001). Its most common AE is constipation. Flunarizine is the most effective drug of this class, but it is not available everywhere. AEs include Parkinsonism, depression, and weight gain.

Anticonvulsant Medications

Divalproex sodium (500–1000 mg) and sodium valproate are effective, as is the extended release formulation (Gray et al. 1999). The most frequent AEs were nausea (42%), alopecia (31%), tremor (28%), asthenia (25%), dyspepsia (25%), somnolence (25%), and weight gain (19%) (Silberstein and Collins1999). Hepatotoxicity and pancreatitis are the most serious AEs, but irreversible hepatic dysfunction is extremely rare in adults. Baseline liver function studies should be obtained, but follow-up studies are probably not needed in adults on monotherapy. Divalproex carries a high risk of congenital abnormality.
▶ Gabapentin (1800–2400 mg) showed efficacy in a placebo-controlled, double-blind trial only when a modified intent to treat analysis was used. Migraine attack frequency was reduced by 50% in about one-third of patients (Mathew et al. 2001). The most common AEs were dizziness or giddiness and drowsiness.
▶ Topiramate, a D-fructose derivative, has been associated with weight loss, not weight gain. In two large, double-blind, placebo-controlled, multicenter trials, topiramate, both 100 and 200 mg, was effective in reducing migraine attack frequency by 50% in half of the patients (Brandes et al. 2004; Silberstein et al. 2004). Dropouts due to AEs were common in the topiramate groups, but did not affect statistical significance.
Divalproex and topiramate are useful in patients with epilepsy, anxiety disorder, or manic-depressive illness. They can be used in patients with depression, Raynaud's disease, asthma, and diabetes, circumventing the contraindications to beta-blockers.

Serotonin Antagonists

▶ Methysergide is effective (Gray et al. 1999; Silberstein 1998). AEs include transient muscle aching, claudication, abdominal distress, nausea, weight gain, and hallucinations. The major complication is rare (1/2500) retroperitoneal, pulmonary, or endocardial fibrosis (Silberstein 1998). To prevent this, a 4-week medication-free interval is recommended after 6 months of continuous treatment (Silberstein 1998; Silberstein et al. 2001). Pizotifen, a benzocycloheptathiophene derivative, is effective (Ramadan et al. 1999). AEs include drowsiness, increased appetite, and weight gain. It is not available in the US.

Natural Products

Feverfew (*Tanacetum parthenium*) is a medicinal herb whose effectiveness has not been totally established. Riboflavin (400 mg) was effective in one placebo-controlled, double-blind trial, with over half the patients responding. *Petasites hybridus* root (butterbur) is a perennial shrub. A standardized extract (75 mg bid) was effective in a double-blind, placebo-controlled study. The most common AE was belching (Silberstein 2004).

Newer Treatments

Botulinum toxin type A (Botox^R 0, 25, or 75 U) showed promising results in one placebo-controlled, double-blind trial. It was injected into glabellar, frontalis, and temporalis muscles. The 25 U treatment group was significantly better than the placebo group in reducing mean frequency of moderate to severe migraines during days 31–60, incidence of 50% reduction in all migraine at days 61–90, and reduction in all migraine at days 61–90 (Silberstein et al. 2000).

Setting Treatment Priorities (Table 1)

The preventive medications with the best documented efficacy are the beta-blockers, amitriptyline, divalproex, and topiramate. Choice is made based on a drug's proven efficacy, the physician's informed belief about medications not yet evaluated in controlled trials, the drug's AEs, the patient's preferences and headache profile, and the presence or absence of coexisting disorders (Silberstein et al. 2001). Coexistent diseases have important implications for treatment. In some instances, two or more conditions may be treated with a single drug. If individuals have more than one disease, certain categories of treatment may be relatively contraindicated.

Summary

Migraine is an extremely common neurobiologic headache disorder that is due to increased CNS excitability. It ranks among the world's most disabling medical illnesses. Diagnosis is based on the headache's characteristics and associated symptoms. The economic and societal impact of migraine is substantial. It impacts on sufferers' quality of life and impairs work, social activities, and family life. Increased headache frequency is an indication for preventive treatment. Preventive treatment decreases migraine frequency and improves quality of life. More treatments are being developed, which provides hope to the many sufferers who are still uncontrolled.

References

1. Brandes JL, Saper JR, Diamond M et al. (2004) Topiramate for Migraine Prevention: A Randomized Controlled Trial. JAMA 291:965–973

M

Migraine, Preventive Therapy, Table 1 Choices of Preventive Treatment in Migraine: Influence of Comorbid Conditions

Drug	Relative Contraindication	Relative Indication
Beta–blockers	Asthma, depression, CHF, Raynaud's disease, diabetes	HTN, angina
Antiserotonin Pizotifen	Obesity	
Methysergide	Angina, PVD	Orthostatic hypotension
Calcium channel blockers		
Verapamil Flunarizine	Constipation, hypotension Parkinson's	Migraine with aura, HTN, angina, asthma Hypertension, FHM
Antidepressants		
TCAs SSRIs MAOIs	Mania, urinary retention, heart block Mania Unreliable patient	Other pain disorders, depression, anxiety disorders, insomnia Depression, OCD Refractory depression
Anticonvulsants		
Divalproex/Valproate Gabapentin Topiramate	Liver disease, bleeding disorders Liver disease, bleeding disorders kidney stones	Mania, epilepsy, anxiety disorders Mania, epilepsy, anxiety disorders Mania, epilepsy, anxiety disorders
NSAIDs		
Naproxen	Ulcer disease, gastritis	Arthritis, other pain disorders

CHF, Congestive heart failure; OCD, Obsessive compulsive disorder; HTN, Hypertension; PVD, Peripheral vascular disease; MAOIs, Monoamine oxidase inhibitors; SSRI, Serotonin specific reuptake inhibitor; NSAIDs, Nonsteroidal anti-inflammatory drugs; TCA, Tricyclic antidepressants

2. Goslin R, Gray RN, McCrory DC (1999) Behavioral and Physical Treatments for Migraine Headache. Prepared for the Agency for Health Care Policy and Research, Contract No. 290-94-2025. Available from the National Technical Information Service, Accession No. 127946, 1999
3. Gray RN, Goslin RE, McCrory DC (1999) Drug Treatments for the Prevention of Migraine Headache. Prepared for the Agency for Health Care Policy and Research, Contract No. 290-94-2025. Available from the National Technical Information Service, Accession No. 127953, 1999
4. Headache Classification Committee (2004) The International Classification of Headache Disorders, 2nd edn. Cephalalgia 24:1–160
5. Mathew NT, Rapoport A, Saper J et al. (2001) Efficacy of Gabapentin in Migraine Prophylaxis. Headache 41:119–128
6. Ramadan NM, Silberstein SD, Freitag FG (1999) Evidence-Based Guidelines of the Pharmacological Management for Prevention of Migraine for the Primary Care Provider. Neurology
7. Saper JR, Silberstein SD, Lake AE (1994) Double-Blind Trial of Fluoxetine: Chronic Daily Headache and Migraine. Headache 34:497–502
8. Silberstein SD (1998) Methysergide. Cephalalgia 18:421–435
9. Silberstein SD (2004) Migraine. Lancet 363:391
10. Silberstein SD, Collins SD (1999) Safety of Divalproex Sodium in Migraine Prophylaxis: An Open-Label, Long-Term Study (for the Long-Term Safety of Depakote in Headache Prophylaxis Study Group). Headache 39:633–643
11. Silberstein SD, Mathew N, Saper J (2000) Botulinum Toxin Type A as a Migraine Preventive Treatment. Headache 40:445–450
12. Silberstein SD, Saper JR, Freitag F (2001) Migraine: Diagnosis and Treatment. In: Silberstein SD, Lipton RB, Dalessio DJ (eds) Wolff's Headache and Other Head Pain, 7th edn. Oxford University Press, New York, pp 121–237
13. Silberstein SD, Goadsby PJ (2002) Migraine: Preventive Treatment. Cephalalgia 22:491–512
14. Silberstein SD, Neto W, Schmitt J et al. (2004) Topiramate in the Prevention of Migraine Headache: A Randomized, Double-Blind, Placebo-Controlled, Multiple-Dose Study. For the MIGR-001 Study Group. Arch Neurol 61:490–495

Migraine Type Headache

Definition

Manifestation of SLE, Sjögren's syndrome or systemic vasculitides.

► Headache Due to Arteritis

Migraine Variants of Childhood

► Migraine, Childhood Syndromes

Migraine With Aura

► Clinical Migraine with Aura

Migraine With Pleocytosis, Pseudomigraine With Lymphocyctic Pleocytosis

▶ Transient Headache and CSF Lymphocytosis

Migraine Without Aura

ARNAUD FUMAL, JEAN SCHOENEN
Departments of Neurology and Neuroanatomy,
University of Liège, CHR Citadelle, Liege, Belgium
jschoenen@ulg.ac.be

Synonyms

Common Migraine; Clinical Migraine without Aura; Hemicrania Simplex

Definition

Migraine without aura (MO) is a recurrent headache manifesting in attacks lasting between 4 and 72 h. Typical features of this headache are unilateral location, pulsating quality, moderate or severe intensity, aggravation by routine physical activity and association with nausea and / or photophobia and phonophobia (see Diagnostic criteria according to the International Classification of Headache Disorders, 2nd edition or ICHD-II 2004).

Diagnostic Criteria of Migraine without Aura

1. At least 5 attacks fulfilling criteria 2–4
2. Headache attacks lasting 4–72 h (untreated or unsuccessfully treated)
3. At least 2 of the following pain characteristics:

   a) Unilateral location
   b) Pulsating quality
   c) Moderate or severe intensity
   d) Aggravation by or causing avoidance of routine physical activity (e.g. walking or climbing stairs)

4. During headache at least one of the following:

   a) Nausea and / or vomiting
   b) Photophobia and phonophobia

5. Not attributed to another disorder

Characteristics

Epidemiology

The most recent population-based studies in adults, all using the diagnostic criteria of the IHS (International Headache Society), have reached very similar prevalence rates. Several European and American studies have reported somewhat congruent prevalence figures for migraine in adults (Steiner et al. 2003). The overall 1 year period prevalence of migraine with or without aura in adults is about 15% (7.6% among men and 19.1% among women). The overall 1 year prevalence of migraine with aura is about 5.8% (male 2.6%, female 7.7%). Studies in general populations agree that it is most common for migraineurs to have about one attack a month. In clinic samples the frequency is higher, since high frequency may be a compelling reason for referral. A large number of headache sufferers with features of migraine fail to meet criteria for strict migraine but do meet criteria for probable migraine (attacks and / or headache missing one of the features 1–4 needed to fulfill all criteria for migraine without aura, see above). The 1 year prevalence for probable migraine was 14.6% (15.9% in women, 12.6% in men) in a recent study (Patel et al. 2004).

Phenotype

The heterogeneity of the clinical phenotype of migraine is underestimated. Despite a common diagnostic denominator, some clinical features such as type of aura symptoms, pain intensity, presence of prodromes, coexistence of migraine with and without aura or associated symptoms such as vertigo, may characterize subgroups of patients bearing different underlying pathophysiological and genetic mechanisms. Pain intensity can help to distinguish migraine without aura from tension-type headache (TTH); indeed among subjects in the general population classified as TTH sufferers, clinical features suggestive of migraine, i.e. aggravation by routine physical exercise, pulsating quality, anorexia, photophobia, unilateral headache and nausea may occur in non-negligible proportions. Trigger factors are manifold and may vary between patients and during the disease course. The most common ones are stress, the perimenstrual period and alcohol. Overuse of acute anti-migraine drugs, in particular of combination analgesics and ergotamine is another underestimated aggravating factor. There is a complex interrelation between migraine and depression, which are highly comorbid. It is not determined, however, whether the increased prevalence of depression in patients with frequent migraines is primary or secondary. Episodic vertigo without other signs of ▶ basilar migraine might belong to the migraine phenotype.

Genotype

The common migraine phenotypes appear to be complex genetic disorders, where additive genetic effects (susceptibility genes) and environmental factors are interrelated (Stewart et al. 1997). Some studies suggest different liability loci for migraine headache (Estevez et al. 2004). Migraine is characterized by recurrent attacks. Genetic load can be seen as determining on the one hand a critical threshold for migraine attacks. On the other hand, genetic abnormalities may induce incidental subclinical dysfunctions, such as, for instance, a reduced neuromus-

M

cular junction safety factor (Ambrosini et al. 2001) or subtle cerebellar hypermetria (Sandor et al. 2001). Various gene polymorphisms were found to be more prevalent in migraineurs than in controls (Estevez et al. 2004). Their precise role remains to be determined; some of them may not be specific to migraine, but they could increase susceptibility to the disorder and induce endophenotypic vulnerability markers (see below).

Pathophysiology

The present consensus is that both neuronal and vascular components are relevant in migraine and most probably interrelated (Goadsby et al. 2002). The neuronal structures involved are the cerebral cortex, the brainstem (periaqueductal gray matter, aminergic nuclei) and the peripheral as well as the central components of the ► trigeminovascular system. The sequence of activation and the relative roles of these structures are still controversial.

Possible Role of the Brainstem

During attacks of migraine without aura, an area of increased blood flow has been identified contralaterally in the dorso-lateral part of the brainstem in a positron emission tomography (PET) study (Weiller et al. 1995). This led to the hypothesis of a "migraine generator" in the region of the dorsal raphe nucleus, locus coeruleus and periaqueductal gray which would suggest that migraine is a central pain disorder and explain recurrence after acute antimigraine drug treatment. Considering the well-known projections of second order trigeminal nociceptors on the periaqueductal gray and the fact that activations were found in a similar location after other spontaneous and experimental pains, it cannot be excluded that the brain stem activations found in migraineurs reflect secondary modulation of pain.

► Cutaneous allodynia has been described during the attack, ipsilateral and contralateral to the hemicrania as well as in the forearm, indicating central ► sensitization at the level of 2nd and thereafter of 3rd order nociceptors (Burstein et al. 2000). This may justify the clinical rule that early treatment of the attack is more effective (Burstein et al. 2004).

Possible Role of the Cortex

During the headache-free interval, an abnormal functioning of the migrainous brain can be demonstrated by neurophysiological and metabolic studies. Neurophysiological methods show that cortical information processing in migraineurs is characterized by a deficient ► habituation during repetition of the stimulation (see Schoenen et al. 2003 for a review). This has been demonstrated for event-related and visual ► evoked potentials (VEPs). Moreover, intensity dependence of auditory evoked cortical potentials is increased in migraine patients compared to normal controls. The cortical abnormality is likely to be genetically deter-

mined. Although not confirmed in every study, it may represent an endophenotypic vulnerability marker (see above). It could be due to low activity in raphe-cortical serotonergic pathways, which would reduce preactivation levels of sensory cortices, allowing a wider range for suprathreshold cortical activation and thus enhancing intensity dependence and reducing habituation. During the attack, when brain stem activation has been found (see above), electrophysiological methods demonstrate a "normalization" of event-related and evoked potentials.

► Transcranial magnetic stimulation (TMS) studies to assess excitability of motor and visual cortices have yielded conflicting results, but taken together they suggest normal or increased rather than decreased excitation thresholds between attacks (Schoenen et al. 2003). High frequency repetitive TMS (rTMS), which activates the underlying cortex, is able to normalize interictal VEPs in migraineurs, whereas low frequency rTMS, which has an inhibitory effect, induces in healthy volunteers a VEP potentiation similar to the one found in migraine (Bohotin et al. 2002). These rTMS results favor the hypothesis put forward to explain the habituation deficit found interictally in evoked potentials, i.e. that the preactivation level of sensory cortices is reduced in migraineurs.

Metabolic studies using nuclear magnetic resonance spectroscopy (MRS) have shown a low mitochondrial phosphorylation potential (Welch et al. 1989) in brain and muscles of migraineurs. Nevertheless, none of the known mutations of mitochondrial DNA has been found up to now in the common forms of migraine. It has been hypothesized that the conjunction of a decreased mitochondrial energy reserve and a deficit in habituation of cortical information processing, known to protect against over-stimulation and lactate accumulation, might lead to activation of the trigeminovascular system (Schoenen 1994). It is still to be determined whether the mitochondrial abnormality is an independent pathophysiological component or rather a consequence of other functional deficits.

Role of the Trigeminovascular System

The trigeminovascular system is the major pain signaling structure of the visceral organ brain, but there is still no definite proof that an activation of its peripheral components is necessary to produce a migraine attack. Such activation is indeed suggested by the increase of CGRP (► calcitonin gene related peptide) in external jugular vein blood during the attack and by the effectiveness of most acute anti-migraine medications including ► triptans in the experimental neurogenic inflammation model in the rat. It is not known what activates the trigeminovascular nociceptive pathway in migraine. But a link between the migraine aura (probably due to a cortical ► spreading depression) and the headache is suggested by the experimental finding that cortical spreading depression is able to activate trigeminovascular afferents and to evoke a series of cortical, meningeal and brainstem events consistent with the development of headache (Bolay et al. 2002).

Role of Nitric Oxide

Nitric oxide (NO) donors such as glyceryl trinitrate (GTN) are able to induce attacks in patients suffering from migraine with or without aura. The underlying mechanisms are not well established but there is clinical and experimental evidence that NO may favor central sensitization of trigeminal nociceptors.

Treatment of Migraine

Acute Treatment

During the last decade, the advent of highly effective $5\text{-}HT_{1B/1D}$ agonists, the triptans, has been a major breakthrough in the attack treatment. Triptans are able to act as vasoconstrictors *via* vascular $5\text{-}HT_{1B}$ receptors and to inhibit neurotransmitter release at the peripheral as well as at the central terminal of trigeminal nociceptors *via* $5\text{-}HT_{1D/B}$ receptors. The site of action relevant for their efficacy in migraine is still a matter of controversy; possibly their high efficacy rate is due to their capacity to act at all three sites contrary to other anti-migraine drugs. Sumatriptan, the first triptan, was followed by several second-generation triptans (zolmi-, nara-, riza-, ele-, almo-, frova-triptan), which were thought to correct some of the shortcomings of sumatriptan.

A large meta-analysis of a number of randomized controlled trials performed with triptans (Ferrari et al. 2001) confirms that the subcutaneous auto-injectable form of sumatriptan (6 mg) has the best efficacy, whatever outcome measure is considered. Differences between oral triptans do exist for some outcome measures, but in practice each patient has to find the triptan that gives him the best satisfaction.

At present the major reason for not considering triptans as first choice treatments for migraine attacks is their high cost and, in some patients, their cardiovascular side effects. However, stratifying care by prescribing a triptan to the most disabled patients has been proven cost-effective. In severely disabled migraineurs, the efficacy rate of injectable sumatriptan for pain-free at 2 h is twice that of ergot derivatives or NSAIDs taken at high oral doses and of iv acetylsalicylic acid lysinate. The ▶ therapeutic gain tends to be clearly lower for simple analgesics or NSAIDs such as acetaminophen 1000 mg po, effervescent aspirin 1000 mg or ibuprofen 600 mg than for the oral triptans, when severe attacks are considered. Combining analgesics or NSAIDs to an antiemetic and / or to caffeine or administering them as suppositories increases their efficacy. As expected, the triptans have not solved the patients' problems. There

is room for more efficient and safer oral acute migraine treatments, among which CGRP receptor antagonists are at present most promising (Olesen et al. 2004).

Prophylactic Therapy in Migraine

Prophylactic anti-migraine treatment has to be individually tailored to each patient taking into account the migraine subtype, the ensuing disability, the patient's history and demands and the associated disorders. A major drawback of most classical prophylactics (beta-blockers devoid of intrinsic sympathomimetic activity, valproic acid, Ca^{2+} antagonists, antiserotoninergics, tricyclics.), which have all on average a 50% efficacy score, is the occurrence of side effects.

In recent years some new prophylactics with fewer side effects have been studied. High dose magnesium or cyclandelate are well-tolerated, but poorly effective in comparison to the classical prophylactics (Fig. 1). A novel preventive treatment for migraine is high dose (400 mg / d) riboflavin which has an excellent efficacy / side effect ratio and probably acts by improving the mitochondrial phosphorylation potential (see above). Co-enzyme Q10 (100 mg t.i.d.), another actor in the mitochondrial respiratory chain, is also effective in migraine prophylaxis (see Sandor et al. 2005, also for review of therapeutic gain of different drugs used in migraine prophylaxis). Lisinopril (10 mg bid), an inhibitor of angiotensin converting enzyme and, even more so, candesartan (16 mg bid) an angiotensin II inhibitor well known for the treatment of hypertension, were found useful in migraine. Recent preliminary but encouraging results with novel antiepileptic compounds like gabapentin need to be confirmed in large randomized controlled trials, whereas topiramate was found to be effective in several placebo-controlled trials. Non-pharmacological and herbal treatments are increasingly subject to controlled studies and some, like butterbur, are found to be clearly more effective than placebo.

M

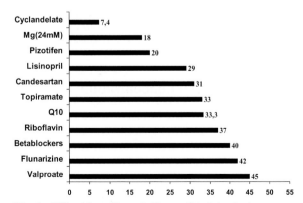

Migraine Without Aura, Figure 1 Therapeutic gain in migraine preventive treatment (% of "responders", with a reduction of minimum 50% of attacks).

References

1. Ambrosini A, Maertens de Noordhout A, Schoenen J (2001) Neuromuscular transmission in migraine: a single fiber EMG study in clinical subgroups. Neurology 56:1038–1043
2. Bohotin V, Fumal A, Vandenheede M et al. (2002) Effects of repetitive transcranial magnetic stimulation on visual evoked potentials in migraine. Brain 125:912–922
3. Bolay H, Reuter U, Dunn AK et al. (2002) Intrinsic brain activity triggers trigeminal meningeal afferents in a migraine model. Nat Med 8:136–142
4. Burstein R, Cutrer MF, Yarnitsky (2000) The development of cutaneous allodynia during a migraine attack clinical evidence for the sequential recruitment of spinal and supraspinal nociceptive neurons in migraine. Brain 123:1703–1709
5. Burstein R, Jakubowski M, Collins B (2004) Defeating migraine pain with triptans: A race against the development of cutaneous allodynia. Ann Neurol 19–26
6. Estevez M, Gardner K (2004) Update on the genetics of migraine. Hum Genet 114:225–235
7. Ferrarri MD, Roon KI, Lipton RB et al. (2001) Oral triptans (serotonin 5-HT(1B / 1D) agonists) in acute migraine treatment: a meta-analysis of 53 trials. Lancet 358:1668–1675
8. Goadsby PJ, Lipton RB, Ferrarri MD (2002) Migraine-current understanding and treatment. N Engl J Med 24:257–270
9. Olesen J, Diener HC, Husstedt IW et al. (2004) BIBN 4096 BS Clinical Proof of Concept Study Group. Calcitonin gene-related peptide receptor antagonist BIBN 4096 BS for the acute treatment of migraine. N Engl J Med 350:1104–1110
10. Patel NV, Bigal ME, Kolodner KB et al. (2004) Prevalence and impact of migraine and probable migraine in a health plan. Neurology 63:1432–1438
11. Sándor PS, Mascia A, Seidel L et al. (2001) Subclinical cerebellar impairment in the common types of migraine: A 3-dimensional analysis of reaching movements. Ann Neurol 49:668–672
12. Sandor PS, Di Clemente L, Coppola G et al. (2005) Effectiveness of Coenzyme Q10 in migraine prophylaxis: A randomized controlled trial. Neurology 64:713–715
13. Schoenen J (1994) Pathogenesis of migraine: the biobehavioural and hypoxia theories reconciled. Acta Neurol Belg 94:79–86
14. Schoenen J, Ambrosini A, Sandor PS et al. (2003) Evoked potentials and transcranial magnetic stimulation in migraine: published data and viewpoint on their pathophysiologic significance. Clin Neurophysiol 114:955–972
15. Steiner TJ, Scher AI, Stewart WF et al. (2003) The prevalence and disability burden of adult migraine in England and their relationships to age, gender and ethnicity. Cephalalgia 23:519–527
16. Stewart WF, Staffa J, Lipton RB et al. (1997) Familial risk of migraine: a population-based study. Ann Neurol 41:166–172
17. The International Classification of Headache Disorders, 2nd edn (ICHD-II) (2004) Cephalalgia 24:1–160
18. Weiller C, May A, Limmroth V et al. (1995) Brain stem activation in spontaneous human migraine attacks. Nat Med 1:658–660
19. Welch KM, Levine SR, D'Andrea G et al. (1989) Preliminary observations on brain energy metabolism in migraine studied by *in vivo* 3^{1-}phosphorus NMR spectroscopy. Neurology 39:538–541

Minimal Alveolar Concentration

Synonyms

MAC

Definition

Alveolar concentration of a volatile anesthetic at 1 atm pressure, which abolishes motor response to a painful surgical stimulus in 50% of patients.

▶ Alpha(α) 2-Adrenergic Agonists in Pain Treatment

Minimal Clinical Important Difference

Synonyms

MCID

Definition

The smallest difference in score in the domain of interest which patients perceive as beneficial.

▶ Oswestry Disability Index

Minimal Sedation

Synonyms

Anxiolysis

Definition

A drug-induced state in which the patient responds normally to verbal commands. Ventilatory and cardiovascular functions are unaffected, although cognitive function and coordination may be impaired.

▶ Pain and Sedation of Children in the Emergency Setting

Minimum Effective Analgesic Serum Concentrations of Fentanyl

Definition

Minimum effective analgesic serum concentrations of fentanyl range from 0.3 – 1.5 ng/ml.

▶ Postoperative Pain, Fentanyl

Minimum Erythema Dose

▶ MED

Minocycline

Definition

Minocycline is used to pharmacologically block microglial activation without directly affecting neurons or astrocytes. As a result, minocycline blocks the production of microglial-derived proinflammatory cytokines. In neuropathic pain, administration of minocycline disrupts exaggerated pain by inhibiting proinflammatory cytokines. Importantly, minocycline has revealed that microglia may be more important in the initiation, rather than the maintenance, of exaggerated pain states.

▶ Cord Glial Activation

ber of familial pain models have been observed in several studies (e.g. Edwards et al. 1985). In children of chronic pain patients, a higher frequency of illness (but not injuries), more days of school absence, more behavioral problems and greater somatic distress have been noted (e.g. Rickard 1988). The specific influence of a parental pain model on the frequency of pain in children has not been addressed systematically. In one study, children of parents with chronic pain indicated a higher frequency of abdominal pain episodes than children of parents without pain (Jamison and Walker 1992). Rather little is known about whether a positive family history of pain determines an individual's response to naturally occurring or injury-related pain. Schrader et al. (1996) questioned a cohort of individuals for the occurrence of neck and other pain 1–3 years after they had experienced a rear-end collision. A positive family history of pain emerged as an important risk factor for the evolution of pain problems subsequent to the injury.

While being consistent with the proposed influence of modeling, mere observation of the co-occurrence of pain problems in families says little about the involved learning processes. From a social learning perspective, one would expect at least some relationship between the model's and the observer's pain behavior, coping behavior and reaction to the pain. Consistent with this assumption, students coming from families with a history of multiple pain problems did not only report more pain sites, but also indicated that their pains interfered more with their daily activities (Lester et al. 1994). Similarly, in a group of mothers with chronic pain, significant correlations were observed between the frequency of pain episodes in the child and the mother's perceived pain intensity, subjective pain-related interference in every-day life and the level of emotional distress (Jamison and Walker 1992). Altogether, these results are well in accordance with previous findings on the impact of parental modeling of illness behavior during childhood on later illness behavior. Growing up with a familial pain model may increase the risk of later experiencing pain problems by learning maladaptive pain and illness behaviors and exacerbating responses to pain. However, the social transmission of specific (maladaptive) pain behaviors, including coping responses, is yet to be clarified. Investigating the role of modeling is complicated by the fact that familial pain models may exert their influence in a sex-dependent manner. Early on, pain models were found to have a greater impact on females than on males (e.g. Edwards et al. 1985). More recently, a higher incidence of familial pain models in a female than a male student population has been noted (Koutantji et al. 1998). Moreover, in females a positive family history of pain was associated with more frequent pain and an enhanced sensitivity to experimental pain stimuli (Fillingim et al. 2000). One explanation has been that females may be more aware of pain in others. Yet, it may also reflect sex-specific

effects of modeling. It is well established that social learning depends on the model's attributes, and the perceived similarity between observer and model. For example, sex-role information is conveyed by observational learning in a sex-selective manner (Bandura 1986). Since more women are affected by chronic pain, girls may be more likely than boys to grow up with a relevant pain model. The possible sex-dependent impact of social learning on pain behavior, and its interaction with sex-related genetically determined differences in pain susceptibility, certainly needs to be further explored.

Experimental Studies

The pioneering experimental work by Kenneth Craig has been most important in accruing empirical support for the hypothesis that social learning can account for individual differences in pain responding (for a review see Craig 1986). Starting in the late 1960s, Craig has conducted a series of experimental studies using variations of the following experimental paradigm. Students were exposed to a series of increasingly painful shocks starting with a noticeable, but not painful stimulus. After each shock, the subject rated pain intensity and then observed a confederate rating the same stimulus as either less (i.e. tolerant model) or more (i.e. intolerant model) painful. This procedure continued for the whole series of shocks. Across studies, subjects exposed to a tolerant model as compared to those exposed to an intolerant model had a higher pain threshold, were less autonomically aroused and indicated less subjective stress. Moreover, ▶ signal detection analyses revealed that subjects showed greater discrimination between painful and non-painful stimuli when they had observed an intolerant model. As Turkat and Guise (1983) noted, the model's behavior served both as an antecedent and a consequence of the subject's pain response in these studies, and therefore may have shaped the subject's response. When this was controlled for, prior exposure to a pain-tolerant or intolerant model again yielded a change of the subjects' ▶ pain tolerance in the expected direction (Turkat and Guise 1983). Recently, first experimental evidence for the influence of maternal modeling on children's pain responses during a ▶ cold pressor test was provided (Goodman and McGrath 2003). Mothers had been instructed to exaggerate their pain display during a cold pressor task, while their children were watching. These children later had a significantly lower ▶ pain threshold as compared to the control children. Minimized maternal pain behavior did not increase the children's pain threshold. Maternal modeling also had no impact on the children's subjective pain intensity ratings during the task.

Overall, experimental studies have consistently demonstrated that modeling can modulate the observer's detection of a stimulus as painful. Whether social learning can also alter the perceived intensity and aversive-

M

ness of a painful stimulus, is less clear. It should be noted that in all experimental studies, the observers could rely either on verbal responses or other overt behavioral responses to infer that the model was detecting pain. Under natural conditions, however, the level of pain experienced by a model is less easily decoded by the observer. Whether vicariously induced emotional arousal in the observer, when observing a person in pain, may shape the intensity and quality of the observer's later pain response, has not been studied systematically. Experimental studies further suggest that individual differences in pain sensitivity may impose constraints on the direction and magnitude of the change of the pain response that can be induced by modeling influences. Moreover, the impact of a tolerant versus an intolerant model may not be symmetrical (e.g. Goodman and McGrath 2003). In one study (Prkachin and Craig 1986), female students were first selected based on whether they had a high or low pain threshold, and were then tested alone or in the presence of another participant with either a high or low pain threshold. Results showed that only women with high pain thresholds lowered their pain threshold when exposed to a low-threshold model. Modeling had no effect on the pain threshold in subjects with a low pain-threshold.

Taken together, there is converging evidence from both correlational and experimental studies that social learning is important in shaping an individual's pain response and pain behavior, even though the exact mechanisms by which this occurs are not fully understood. Data suggest that the effects of social modeling may be modulated by the observer's (and possibly the model's) sex and interindividual differences in pain sensitivity.

▶ Motivational Aspects of Pain
▶ Psychology of Pain and Psychological Treatment

References

1. Bandura A (1986) Social Foundations of Thought and Action: A Social Cognitive Theory. Prentice Hall, Englewood Cliffs, NJ
2. Baranowski T, Nader PR (1985) Family Health Behavior. In: Turk DC, Kerns RD (eds) Health, Illness, and Families: A Life-Span Perspective. Wiley, New York, pp 51–80
3. Craig KD (1986) Social Modeling Influences on Pain. In: Sternbach RA (ed) Chronic Pain: Psychological Factors in Rehabilitation. Williams and Wilkins, Baltimore, pp 73–109
4. Craig KD, Pillai Riddell RR (2003) Social Influences, Culture, and Ethnicity. In: McGrath PJ, Finley GA (eds) Pediatric Pain: Biological and Social Context. IASP Press, Seattle, pp 159–182
5. Edwards PW, Zeichner A, Kuczmierczyk AR et al. (1985) Familial Pain Models: Relationship between Family History of Pain and Current Pain Experience. Pain 21:379–384
6. Fillingim RB, Edwards RR, Powell T (2000) Sex-Dependent Effects of Reported Familial Pain History on Recent Pain Complaints and Experimental Pain Responses. Pain 86:87–94
7. Goodman JE, McGrath PJ (2003) Mothers' Modeling Influences Children's Pain During a Cold Pressor Task. Pain 104:559–565
8. Jamison RN, Walker LS (1992) Illness Behavior in Children of Chronic Pain Patients. Int J Psychiatr Med 22:329–342
9. Koutantji M, Pearce SA, Oakley DA (1998) The Relationship between Gender and Family History of Pain with Current Pain Experience and Awareness of Pain in Others. Pain 77:25–31
10. Lester N, Lefebvre BA, Keefe FJ (1994) Pain in Young Adults: I. Relationship to Gender and Family Pain History. Clin J Pain 10:282–289
11. Prkachin KM, Craig KD (1986) Social Transmission of Natural Variations in Pain Behaviour. Behav Res Ther 24:581–585
12. Rickard K (1988) The Occurrence of Maladaptive Health-Related Behaviors and Teacher-Rated Conduct Problems in Children of Chronic Low Back Pain Patients. J Behav Med 11:107–116
13. Schrader H, Obelieniene D, Bovim G et al. (1996) Natural Evolution of Late Whiplash Syndrome Outside the Medicolegal Context. Lancet 347:1207–1211
14. Turkat ID, Guise BJ (1983) The Effects of Vicarious Experience and Stimulus Intensity on Pain Termination and Work Avoidance. Behav Res Ther 21:241–245
15. Violon A, Giurgea D (1984) Familial Models for Chronic Pain. Pain 18:199–203

Moderate Sedation

Definition

A drug-induced state of depressed consciousness during which the patient responds purposefully to verbal or light tactile stimulation, while maintaining protective airway reflexes and airway patency. Cardiovascular function is usually maintained.

▶ Pain and Sedation of Children in the Emergency Setting

Modifications of Treatment for the Elderly

Definition

The treatment protocol has to take functional, sensory and cognitive restrictions of elderly individuals into account, e.g. by facilitating comprehension and providing more time for a session.

▶ Psychological Treatment of Pain in Older Populations

Modifying Factors

Definition

Pain related factors that may affect the assessment of pain in the newborn include gestational age (number of days since conception), post natal age (number of days of life since birth), behavioral state (sleep/wake state), severity of illness, and gender. Pain expression in infants may also be affected by developmental ability, consolability, chronic pain, environmental stimulation and repeated exposure to pain and stress events, medication, caregiving including direct parent involvement

▶ Pain Assessment in Neonates

Molecular Contributions to the Mechanism of Central Pain

BRYAN C. HAINS

The Center for Neuroscience and Regeneration
Research, Department of Neurology, Yale University
School of Medicine, West Haven, CT, USA
bryan.hains@yale.edu

Synonyms

Central Pain Mechanisms, Molecular Contributions

Definition

Changes in ion channels, neurotransmitters, receptors, signaling pathways and gene expression represent important consequences of disease or ischemic and traumatic injury of the central nervous system that ultimately impact the functional state of neurons at different levels of the neuraxis, leading to the development of central pain.

The molecular organization of the structural and functional components of a neuron endow it with certain electrophysiological properties. After injury to the central nervous system, molecular reconfiguration of ion channels, neurotransmitters and receptors takes place in nociceptive neurons, leading to dysfunctional firing properties and the development and maintenance of central pain syndromes.

Characteristics

The spinal cord dorsal horn contains the primary synapse through which afferent somatosensory information related to touch, pressure, brush, temperature and noxious stimuli is received from the periphery. Dorsal horn sensory neurons receive this information primarily from the skin, perform a degree of processing and transmit signals through distinct tracts within the spinal cord to supraspinal structures where pain is perceived. Within peripheral nerves and spinal cord, pain is thought to exist simply as a signal and is subject to a degree of modulation by circuitry that it passes through.

Experimental spinal cord injury (SCI) induces electrophysiological changes in dorsal horn sensory neurons that contribute to pain-like behaviors in animals (Hains et al. 2003b). These include shifts in proportions of cells responding to evoked noxious stimulation, increases and irregularity in spontaneous ▶ Background Activity / Firing, increased ▶ evoked activity to (formerly) innocuous and noxious stimuli and increases in ▶ afterdischarge activity following stimulation. Since the nature of the applied stimuli does not change, other mechanisms must account for the alterations in stimulus processing that lead to central pain. Central changes in expression of molecules such as ion channels, neurotransmitters and their receptors, contribute to altered sensory processing by changing the electrophysiological excitability and therefore output of sensory neurons. Specific molecular changes shown to contribute to the development of central pain in animal models and specifically to the development of pain following spinal cord injury (SCI) are described below.

Ion Channels

At the most fundamental level, ▶ action potential generation and propagation by sensory neurons relies on multiple isoforms of ▶ voltage gated sodium channels (termed Na_V). The selective expression of ensembles of sodium channels tunes the biophysical properties of each neuron. Within the normal nervous system, properties fundamental to neuronal function such as activation threshold, inactivation and ▶ refractory period, rates of ▶ repriming and the ability to generate and conduct high frequency trains of action potentials all depend on the type(s) of sodium channels expressed within a given neuron (Waxman 2000). Similarly, dysregulation of channel expression can abnormally reconfigure neuronal function in disease states. Ten genes encode molecularly distinct voltage gated sodium channels, at least seven of which are expressed in the rat nervous system. In the adult spinal cord dorsal horn, $Na_V1.1$, $Na_V1.2$ and $Na_V1.6$ are strongly detectable, whereas $Na_V1.3$ expression decreases with development and is down-regulated in adults. In the adult spinal cord, $Na_V1.3$ is expressed at very low levels (Fig. 1a) (Felts et al. 1997). Following SCI, expression of $Na_V1.3$ is up-regulated in the dorsal horn (Fig. 1b) and colocalizes with NK^1-R, a marker of nociceptive neurons. $Na_V1.3$ plays a role in maintaining hyperresponsiveness to peripheral stimulation as well as pain-related behaviors, as evidenced through selective knockdown of $Na_V1.3$ expression via antisense oligodeoxynucleotide administration (Fig. 1c) (Hains et al. 2003a). The $Na_V1.3$ sodium channel produces a rapidly repriming tetrodotoxin sensitive sodium current that permits neuronal firing at higher than normal frequencies (Cummins et al. 2001). Since stimulus intensity is encoded in the dorsal horn by the rate of firing, this change in how neurons process incoming sensory information serves to amplify incoming signals, so that perceived pain thresholds are lowered.

Neurotransmitters and Receptors

Neurotransmitter molecules and their receptors produce signals that cause depolarization of dorsal horn sensory neurons. After SCI, neurotransmitter levels are altered in a way that is facilitative to central pain. ▶ Serotonin (5-HT) is an important molecule that participates in the functional modulation of dorsal horn nociceptive neurons. Released by terminals of fibers descending from cell bodies located within the midline ▶ raphe nuclei of the brain stem, 5-HT can act directly on ion channels or trigger intracellular cascades that cause neuronal depo-

M

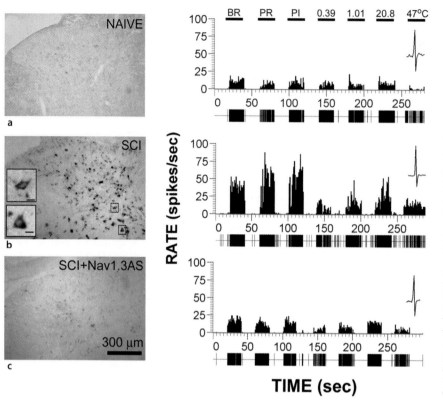

Molecular Contributions to the Mechanism of Central Pain, Figure 1 $Na_V1.3$ mRNA is expressed at low levels in naïve animals, (a) but is upregulated in lumbar dorsal horn neurons after spinal cord injury (SCI). (b) Treatment with antisense oligodeoxynucleotides against $Na_V1.3$ reduces $Na_V1.3$ transcripts after SCI. (c) Corresponding unit recordings show evoked activity to peripheral stimulation (BR = brush, PR = press, PI = pinch, increasing strength von Frey filament stimulation and noxious thermal heating (47° C)), after SCI (b) compared to controls (a). After $Na_V1.3$ antisense delivery, evoked activity of dorsal horn neurons resembles that found in naïve levels (c).

larization and/or regulate intrinsic excitability. SCI results in a loss of the supply of 5-HT within the spinal cord through interruption of descending sources (Hains et al. 2001). After SCI, replacement of interrupted 5-HT reduces abnormal activity of dorsal horn neurons, as well as pain-related behaviors.

Following SCI, 5-HT receptors also undergo changes in expression levels, a change thought to play a role in the development of central pain. The major class of 5-HT receptor found in the dorsal horn is the $5\text{-}HT_1$ family (Zemlan and Schwab 1991). Of this subset of receptors, $5\text{-}HT_{1A}$ represents a high percentage of all high affinity 5-HT binding sites, with highest receptor densities in laminae I and II. $5\text{-}HT_{1A}$ couples an intracellular G-protein cascade and is up-regulated after SCI (Giroux et al. 1999). Also highly represented in the spinal cord, the $5\text{-}HT_3$ receptor, which gates a non-selective monovalent cation channel, has been found in the substantia gelatinosa at all levels of the spinal cord (Hamon et al. 1989). Following SCI, direct activation of both the $5\text{-}HT_{1A}$ and $5\text{-}HT_3$ (Hains et al. 2002) receptors reduces neuronal hyper-responsiveness and/or pain-related behaviors caudal to the injury site. $5\text{-}HT_3$ receptors are thought to be facilitatory to pain after SCI at levels rostral to the injury site (Oatway et al. 2004). The 5-HT transporter protein, which regulates the activity level of 5-HT, undergoes up-regulated expression following SCI (Hains et al. 2001).

Reductions in spinal levels of the inhibitory neurotransmitter gamma-aminobutyric acid (▶ GABA) also support central pain after SCI by decreasing the inhibitory influences within spinal circuitry (Drew et al. 2004). Synthesized locally, GABA is the major inhibitory neurotransmitter and acts *via* ligand gated ion channels ($GABA_A$ receptors) and G-protein coupled ($GABA_B$) receptors. After SCI, reduced GABAergic inhibition results in abnormally exaggerated evoked and spontaneous neuronal firing through the impairment of GABA production or release and/or loss of GABA-releasing cells.

Another mechanism for maintained hyperexcitability of dorsal horn neurons leading to central pain involves changes in the expression of metabotropic glutamate receptors (▶ mGluRs). mGluRs are G-protein coupled receptors that have been subdivided into three groups, based on sequence similarity, pharmacology and intracellular signaling mechanisms. Group I is made up of mGluR1 and 5, Group II is made up of mGluR2 and 3 and Group III is made up of mGluR4, 6, 7, and 8. mGluR1 is found primarily in deeper laminae of the dorsal horn and mGluR5 is found at highest levels in lamina II. mGluR2/3 is also expressed in high levels within lamina II. The differential distribution of mGluRs within laminae associated with sensory processing implicates them in central pain after SCI. In the spinal cord, mGluRs directly modulate neuronal excitability; for example group I mGluRs decrease thresholds of activation, inhibit afterhyperpolarization and induce transient membrane depolarizations. Following SCI, mGluR1 expression increases at the level of injury and mGluR2/3 expression levels are chronically decreased in and around the lesion site. There is also a chronic increase in mGluR1 in all laminae measured and a decrease in mGluR2/3 in laminae IIi, III, IV and V (Mills et al. 2001). SCI produces an increase in mGluR1 expression on spinothalamic tract neurons in both the cervical enlargement and the spinal segment just rostral to the injury site (Mills et al. 2002). Treatment with agonists to group II and III mGluRs affects pain responses following SCI.

Genetic changes that may play a role in pain pathogenesis after SCI have been brought to light by microarray analysis. SCI can lead to altered expression of genes whose transcripts help to determine membrane excitability, including increases in mRNAs for ionotropic glutamate receptors and sodium and calcium channels and decreases in mRNAs for GABA receptors and potassium channels (Nesic et al. 2002).

In summary, molecular events involved in the processing of afferent signals in spinal neurons significantly change following SCI. These changes endow affected neurons with maladaptive functional properties, and provide the substrate to both generate and amplify incorrect signals that ultimately contribute to central pain after SCI. Although the majority of studies related to molecular changes following central injury have focused on changes occurring at the level of the spinal cord (following spinal injury), similar changes are likely to be found at supraspinal levels.

References

1. Cummins TR, Aglieco F, Renganathan M et al. (2001) Nav1.3 sodium channels: rapid repriming and slow closed-state inactivation display quantitative differences after expression in a mammalian cell line and in spinal sensory neurons. J Neurosci 21:5952–5961
2. Drew GM, Siddall PJ, Duggan AW (2004) Mechanical allodynia following contusion injury of the rat spinal cord is associated with loss of GABAergic inhibition in the dorsal horn. Pain 109:379–388
3. Felts PA, Yokoyama S, Dib-Hajj S et al. (1997) Sodium channel alpha-subunit mRNAs I, II, III, NaG, Na6 and hNE (PN1): different expression patterns in developing rat nervous system. Brain Res Mol Brain Res 45:71–82
4. Giroux N, Rossignol S, Reader TA (1999) Autoradiographic study of alpha1- and alpha2-noradrenergic and serotonin1A receptors in the spinal cord of normal and chronically transected cats. J Comp Neurol 406:402–414
5. Hains BC, Fullwood SD, Eaton MJ et al. (2001) Subdural engraftment of serotonergic neurons following spinal hemisection restores spinal serotonin, downregulates serotonin transporter, and increases BDNF tissue content in rat. Brain Res 913:35–46
6. Hains BC, Willis WD, Hulsebosch CE (2002) Serotonin receptors 5-HT1A and 5-HT3 reduce hyperexcitability of dorsal horn neurons after chronic spinal cord hemisection injury in rat. Exp Brain Res 149:174–186
7. Hains BC, Johnson KM, Eaton MJ et al. (2003a) Serotonergic neural precursor cell grafts attenuate bilateral hyperexcitability of dorsal horn neurons after spinal hemisection in rat. Neuroscience 116:1097–1110
8. Hains BC, Klein JP, Saab CY et al. (2003b) Upregulation of sodium channel Nav1.3 and functional involvement in neuronal hyperexcitability associated with central neuropathic pain after spinal cord injury. J Neurosci 23:8881–8892
9. Hamon M, Gallissot MC, Menard F et al. (1989) 5-HT3 receptor binding sites are on capsaicin-sensitive fibres in the rat spinal cord. Eur J Pharmacol 164:315–22
10. Mills CD, Hulsebosch CE (2002) Increased expression of metabotropic glutamate receptor subtype 1 on spinothalamic tract neurons following spinal cord injury in the rat. Neurosci Lett 319:59–62
11. Mills CD, Fullwood SD, Hulsebosch CE (2001) Changes in metabotropic glutamate receptor expression following spinal cord injury. Exp Neurol 70:244–247
12. Nesic O, Svrakic NM, Xu GY et al. (2002) DNA microarray analysis of the contused spinal cord: effect of NMDA receptor inhibition. J Neurosci Res 68:406–423
13. Oatway MA, Chen Y, Weaver LC (2004) The 5-HT3 receptor facilitates at-level mechanical allodynia following spinal cord injury. Pain 110:259–268
14. Waxman SG (2000) The neuron as a dynamic electrogenic machine: modulation of sodium-channel expression as a basis for functional plasticity in neurons. Philos Trans R Soc Lond B Biol Sci 355:199–213
15. Zemlan FP, Schwab EF (1991) Characterization of a novel serotonin receptor subtype (5-HT1S) in rat CNS: interaction with a GTP binding protein. J Neurochem 57:2092–2099

M

Monamine Oxidase Inhibitors

▶ Antidepressant Analgesics in Pain Management

Monoamines

Definition

Classification of neurochemicals based on their chemical structure (usually used to refer to serotonin, norepinephrine and dopamine).

▶ Stimulation-Produced Analgesia

Monocyte/Macrophage

Definition

Monocytes are circulating immune/inflammatory cells that originate in bone marrow and differentiate into macrophages after migrating through blood vessel walls into tissues.

▶ Wallerian Degeneration

Monosynaptic

Definition

Pertaining to a single synapse.

▶ Amygdala, Pain Processing and Behavior in Animals

Mood

Definition

DSM4 APA: Includes mood disorders associated with depression: depressive disorders, bipolar disorders, mood disorders due to a general medical condition and substance-induced mood disorder, as well as anxiety: especially post traumatic stress disorder, acute stress disorder, generalized anxiety disorder, anxiety disorder due to a general medical condition, substance-induced anxiety disorder and anxiety disorder not otherwise specified. Other mood states may include anger, frustration, fear and disappointment.
▶ Pain Assessment in the Elderly

MOP Receptor

Definition

The term μ-opioid (μ from morphine) peptide receptor represents the G-protein coupled receptor that responds selectively to the majority of clinically useful opioid drugs. It is expressed in areas of the nervous system that mediate therapeutic and adverse effects of most opioid drugs. The MOP receptor protein is produced by a single gene. Several mRNA splice variants are known to exist and produce receptor proteins that display different properties when expressed in cells. When activated, the MOP receptor predominantly transduces actions via inhibitory G-proteins. The electrophysiological consequences of MOP receptor activation are usually inhibitory.
▶ Mu(μ)-Opioid Receptor
▶ Opioid Electrophysiology in PAG

MOR–1

Definition

A clone encoding a mu opioid receptor.
▶ Opioid Receptors

Moral Hazard

Definition

When the presence of insurance changes a disability claimant's or health care providers behavior.
▶ Disability Incentives

Morbus Sudeck

▶ Complex Regional Pain Syndromes, General Aspects
▶ Sympathetically Maintained Pain in CRPS I, Human Experimentation

Morning Stiffness

Definition

In arthritis, morning stiffness of joints and muscles may last for several hours.
▶ Muscle Pain in Systemic Inflammation (Polymyalgia Rheumatica, Giant Cell Arteritis, Rheumatoid Arthritis)

Morphine

Definition

Morphine is a strong (potent) naturally-occurring opiate (a phenanterene derivative) produced from extracts of the poppy plant. Morphine undergoes extensive hepatic biotransformation by phase II reactions to Morphine – 3 – glucuronide (70%) and morphine – 6 – glucuronide (5–10%) and the remainder undergoes sulphation.
▶ Forebrain Modulation of the Periaqueductal Gray
▶ Postoperative Pain, Morphine

Morphine and Muscle Pain

▶ Opioids and Muscle Pain

Morphine Sulphate

▶ Postoperative Pain, Morphine

Morphine Tolerance

▶ Glutamate Homeostasis and Opioid Tolerance

Morphology, Intraspinal Organization of Visceral Afferents

YASUO SUGIURA

Nagoya University School of Medicine, Graduate School of Medicine, Department of Functional Anatomy & Neuroscience, Nagoya, Japan

ysugiura@med.nagoya-u.ac.jp

Synonyms

Synaptic Organization of Afferent Fibers from Viscera in the Spinal Cord

Definition

▶ Visceral afferent Aδ- and ▶ C Fiber convey sensory information from the viscera via vagal and spinal nerves. Intraspinal organization of visceral afferents is composed of the large number of sympathetic afferents which mediate pain, and a small number of the vagal afferents. The afferent terminals make synapses with dendrite of the projecting or internuncial neurons or axons of inhibitory neurons in the spinal cord.

Characteristics

Terminal Distribution in the Spinal Cord

Visceral afferent fibers terminate in the superficial (I, II) spinal laminae (see ▶ Spinal cord laminae) and deeper ▶ (IV–V, X) spinal laminae (de Groat et al. 1978). A single visceral afferent C- fiber can project to the dorsal, superficial spinal cord and also in laminae V and X of the contralateral spinal cord (Sugiura et al. 1989). Visceral afferent C-fibers have collateral branches with terminal swellings in the adjacent white mater of ▶ lateral and dorsal funiculi, in addition to terminal branches in the spinal dorsal horn, revealing a distinctly different pattern of termination from somatic afferent C-fiber terminals (Fig. 1). Along the longitudinal axis of the spinal cord, visceral afferent C-fibers terminate with about 20 collateral branches, which are given off at 3–400μm spans in several ▶ spinal segments from rostral and caudal branches. The rostral branch of the C-fiber shown in Figure 2 runs in the surface of the dorsal funiculus, which may project to the dorsal column nucleus (Nucleus gracilis), part of a new tract for visceral pain (Fig. 2) (Al-Chaer et al. 1998). Each collateral branch ramified in a relative narrow sheet consisting of only one or two daughter branches, which did not form a concentrated nest-like termination commonly seen with somatic C-fibers. The collateral branches have 250–300 terminal swellings, forming an array arranged in the orientation of the neuropil of the spinal laminae (Sugiura et al. 1993). The number of terminal swellings is summarized in Table 1. About 5000 to 6000 enlargements (boutons) were identified in visceral afferent C-fibers. Over 60% of visceral terminal swellings are found in the superficial dorsal horn, lamina I and adjacent area, which seems to be the main region of termination. About 10% of terminal swellings are found in deeper dorsal horn (laminae IV and V). A few visceral fiber boutons are in other laminae.

Synaptic Organization

Light microscopic examination gives us some information about the terminal swellings (boutons). The

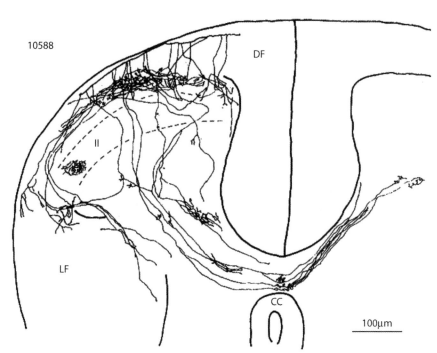

10588

DF

II

LF

CC

100μm

Morphology, Intraspinal Organization of Visceral Afferents, Figure 1 A transverse reconstruction of the central projection of a visceral afferent C-fiber. One of the collaterals could be traced to synaptic enlargements in lamina II. Broken lines indicate borders of Laminae I, II, and III; LF, Lateral funiculus; DF, dorsal funiculus; CC, central canal. (Sugiura et al. 1989)

M

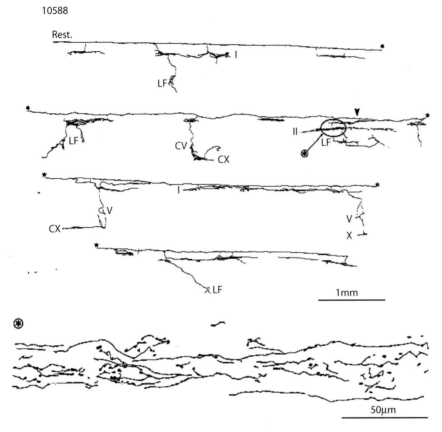

10588

Morphology, Intraspinal Organization of Visceral Afferents, Figure 2 Saggital view of reconstructions of the arborization of visceral afferent C- fibers. On entering the spinal cord (arrow head), the axon bifurcated into rostral and caudal main branches. The main branches ran on the dorsal surface of the dorsal funiculus or in Lissauer's tract, as far rostrally as the 10th thoracic segment (top left) and as far caudally as the 2nd lumbar segment (bottom right). Many collaterals left these parent branches to terminate in laminae I(I) and II(II). Some collaterals also terminated in the lateral funiculus (LF) and the ipsilateral or contralateral laminae V(V, CV) and X(X, CX). The asterisk in a circle (bottom) shows the terminal profiles in lamina II, which is indicated by the circle in the upper view.

Morphology, Intraspinal Organization of Visceral Afferents, Table 1   Number of Terminal Swellings

Case Number	Visceral Fibers*		Somatic Fibers	
	10588	30488	70887	72987
Number of swellings	6099(100)	5370(100)	1482	1450
Number of terminal areas	22	18	1	2
Mean number of areas	277	298	-	725
Dorsal funiculus	359(5.9)	1089(20.3)		
Lamina I	3735(61.2)	2466(45.9)		
Lamina II	240(3.9)	151(2.8)		
Lamina IV and V	391(6.4)	553(10.3)		
Lateral funiculus	276(4.5)	21(0.4)		
Lamina X	171(2.8)	153(2.8)		
Contralateral X	121(2.0)	61(1.1)		
Contralateral VI and V	108(1.8)	142(2.6)		
Total	5401(88.6)	4636(86.3)		

*Number and (percentage).

terminal swellings of visceral afferent C-fibers ranged 1.6 to 1.7μm in diameter and are 4.3 to 5.7μm² in area each, which is smaller than those of somatic afferents. If presented graphically, the distribution of visceral terminal swellings occupy a smaller fraction (one third to one half) of somatic terminal swellings.

In electron microscopy, primary afferent terminals in the spinal cord generally show a central synaptic profile

Morphology, Intraspinal Organization of Visceral Afferents, Table 2 Incidence of Central Terminals of Primary C Afferents

	Fraction	Percentage
Somatic fiber:		
High-threshold mechanoreceptor	24/32	75.0
Polymodal nociceptor	13/16	81.03
Mechanical cold nociceptor	53/63	84.1
Warming receptor	12/38	31.5
Visceral fiber:		
Superficial layer	3/29	10.3
Deeper layer	10/38	26.3

composed of axons and some dendritic spines. In somatic nociceptors, over 75% of terminals show central synaptic profiles, but visceral afferent terminals show a ▶ simple synapse and less than 30% of terminals show central synaptic profiles (Table 2) (reviewed in Sugiura and Tonosaki 1995).

A great number of visceral afferent cell bodies in dorsal root ganglia contain neuropeptides, especially substance P, calcitonin-gene related peptide, somatostatin and vasoactive intestinal peptide, and some are IB–4 positive.

Functional Exploration from Morphological Organization

Visceral afferent C-fibers terminate in spinal lamina I and V, similar to terminals thinly myelinated fibers from somatic nociceptors, which are different from C-fiber terminals of the somatic organ (skin and muscle) (Ling et al. 2003). The laminar arrangement of visceral afferent C-fiber terminals suggests that ▶ somatovisceral convergence on neurons in laminae I and V arise from somatic myelinated and visceral unmyelinated fibers. This system may be committed to referred pain, whereas some somatic unmyelinated afferents may only subserve the transmission of nociceptive information to secondary neurons in the dorsal horn.

Visceral afferent fibers terminate in ▶ single or straight form of terminal branches. Compared with the concentrated focus of somatic terminations, visceral C afferents appear in thin sheets of termination having one or two terminal branches with several enlargements at each terminal focus. These terminal features may reveal the morphological background for the poor localization and possibly vagueness of referred pain (Cervero 1994).

The size of terminal boutons on visceral afferent C fibers is smaller than the boutons found on many kinds of myelinated fiber terminals (Brown et al. 1981) and those of somatic afferent C-fibers (Sugiura et al. 1995). This difference in size may have relevance to the receptor or to the nature of the synaptic transmission in the dorsal horn. The size of terminal swellings of visceral afferent fibers seems to reflect the morphological variety of synaptic ultrastructural profiles (Ribeiro da Silva and Coimbra 1982, Alvarez et al. 1993).

Somatic C-fiber nociceptors make central terminal profiles, which have various shapes according to the adequate noxious stimulus: high threshold nociceptor, cold nociceptor or polymodal nociceptor. These ultrastruc-

M

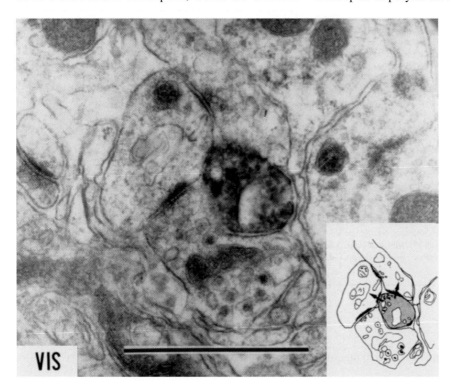

Morphology, Intraspinal Organization of Visceral Afferents, Figure 3 An ultrastructural profile of a visceral afferent C-fiber. A visceral afferent terminal has simple synaptic contacts with post synaptic elements. To easily identify the synaptic relation, a schematic illustration is drawn (right bottom). Bar; 1 μm (modified from Sugiura et al. 1992, Sugiura & Tonosaki 1995).

tural profiles may reveal the possibility of pain modulation at the synaptic site of central terminals (Wall 1989). Contrary to the somatic nociceptors, most visceral afferent C-fiber terminals show simple synaptic profiles. This means that these terminals transmit peripheral inputs to secondary neurons or elements, without modulating the information at the synaptic site. In this interpretation, somatic central terminals may be essential to transmit pain from peripheral somatic tissues to the central nervous system, but visceral pain may be transmitted by other mechanisms or mediated by small numbers of central terminals. If we presume that these central terminals mainly mediate visceral pain, visceral pain would be a ► vague, strange feeling and not definitive for nociception.

References

1. Al-Chaer ED, Feng Y, Willis WD (1998) A Role for the Dorsal Column in Nociceptive Visceral Input into the Thalamus of Primates. J Neurophysiol 70:3143–3150
2. Alvarez FJ, Kavookjian AM, Light AR (1993) Ultrastructural Morphology, Synaptic Relationships, and CGRP Immunoreactivity of Physiologically Identified C-Fiber Terminals in the Monkey Spinal Cord. J Comp Neurol 329:472–490
3. Brown AG (1981) Organization in the Spinal Cord: The Anatomy and Physiology of Identified Neurons. Springer-Verlag, New York, pp 1–138
4. Cervero F (1994) Sensory Innervation of the Viscera: Peripheral Basis of Visceral Pain, Physiol Rev7:495–138
5. de Groat WC, Nadelhaft I, Morgan C, Schauble T (1978) Horseradish Peroxidase Tracing of Visceral Afferent and Primary Afferent Pathways in the Cat's Sacral Spinal Cord using Benzidine Processing. Neurosci Lett 10:103–108
6. Ling L-J, Honda T, Shimada Y, Ozaki N, Shiraishi Y, Sugiura Y (2003) Central Projection of Unmyelinated (C) Primary Afferent Fibers from Gastrocunemus Muscle in the Guinea Pig. J Comp Neurol 461:140–150
7. Ribeiro da Silva A, Coimbra A (1982) Two Types of Synaptic Glomeruki and their Distribution in Laminae I–III of the Rat Spinal Cord. J Comp Neurol 209:176–186
8. Sugiura Y, Terui N, Hosoya Y (1989) Difference in Distribution of Central Terminals between Visceral and Somatic Unmyelinated (C) Primary Afferent Fibers. J Neurophysiol 62:834–840
9. Sugiura Y, Terui N, Hosoya Y, Tonosaki Y, Nishiyama K, Honda T (1993) Quantitative Analysis of Central Terminals Projections of Visceral and Somatic Unmyelinated (C) Primary Afferent Fibers in the Guinea Pig. J Comp Neurol 332:315–325
10. Sugiura Y, Tonosaki Y, Nishiyama K, Honda T, Oda S (1992) Organization of the central projections of unmyelinated primary afferent fibers. In: Inoki R, Shigenaga Y, Tohyama M (eds) Processing and Inhibition of nociceptive information. Excerpta Medica, Amsterdam, pp 9–13
11. Sugiura Y, Tonosaki Y (1995) Spinal Organization of Unmyelinated Visceral Afferent Fibers in Comparison with Somatic Afferent Fibers. In: Gebhalt GF (ed) Visceral pain, Progress in Pain research and Management, vol 5. IASP Press, Seattle, pp 41–59
12. Wall PD (1989) Introduction. In: Wall PD, Merzack R (eds) Text of Pain, 2nd edn. Churchill Livingstone, Edinburgh, pp 1–18

Morris Water Maze

Definition

Morris water maze is a behavioral test used to measure spatial and working memory.

► Cingulate Cortex, Nociceptive Processing, Behavioral Studies in Animals

Morton's Neuroma

Definition

Morton described a painful condition of the fourth toe of the foot, which, over time, has been interpreted as being due to a neuroma of the interdigital nerve to the $3^{rd}/4^{th}$ webspace of the foot. Tradition has called this a neuroma, and the traditional treatment has been to resect this nerve, which creates a true neuroma. Light and electron microscopy has demonstrated that the excised nerve has chronic compression and not neuroma formation. Today, the approach includes a neurolysis, rather than an excision, of this nerve.

► Painful Scars

Motif

Definition

The motif is the region of a protein that is responsible for binding or functional action, which is homologous to other proteins of like function.

► Trafficking and Localization of Ion Channels

Motivation

Definition

Motivation is that which contributes or leads to the initiation, direction, persistence, intensity, or termination of behavior.

► Motivational Aspects of Pain
► Psychology of Pain and Psychological Treatment

Motivational-Affective

Definition

Response to nociceptive stimuli involving the emotional (limbic) and visceral components, including response by homeostatic systems responsible for regulation of blood pressure, respiration rate, and responses involving the hypothalamic-pituitary-adrenal axis.

► Spinomesencephalic Tract
► Spinothalamic Tract Neurons, Descending Control by Brainstem Neurons

Motivational-Affective Aspects/Components of Pain

Definition

The pain experience includes motivational and affective aspects/components, such as negative emotions and arousal.

▶ Parafascicular Nucleus, Pain Modulation
▶ Spinothalamic Input, Cells of Origin (Monkey)
▶ Thalamic Nuclei Involved in Pain, Cat and Rat
▶ Motivational Aspects of Pain

Motivational Aspects of Pain

MARK P. JENSEN
Department of Rehabilitation Medicine, University of Washington, Seattle, WA, USA
mjensen@u.washington.edu

Synonyms

Incentive; drive

Definition

▶ Motivation refers to the initiation, direction, persistence, intensity, and termination of behavior (Landy and Backer 1987). According to most theories of motivation, the primary factors that lead to behavior change can be classified as falling into two categories: (1) the perceived importance of behavior change and (2) the belief that behavior change is possible (i.e. ▶ self-efficacy Bandura 1986).

Characteristics

As the management of chronic pain depends more on what patients do than on what is done to them, patient motivation for pain self-management represents an essential, yet under-studied aspect of clinical care (Jensen et al. 2003). The more that clinicians understand motivation and the factors that contribute to motivation for pain self-management, the better they will be at helping patients learn, practice, and use adaptive pain self-management coping strategies.

Theories of Health Behavior and Health Behavior Change

A number of theories and models have been developed that address the motivational issues that impact on health behavior and health behavior change: the operant model, Cognitive-Behavioral Theory, expectancy-value models, the Transtheoretical Model, and client-centered approaches. The operant learning theory of chronic pain emphasizes the role that environmental ▶ contingencies have on pain behavior (Fordyce 1976). According to this model, patients continue to use maladaptive pain management strategies (such as pain-contingent rest and guarding) because such strategies are followed by reinforcement. Motivation for change therefore results when the contingencies are changed; for example, by encouraging and praising adaptive coping efforts and ignoring maladaptive ones. Cognitive-Behavioral Theory views behavior as a complex interaction of cognitive structures, processes and their consequences. Cognitive-Behavioral Therapy for chronic pain uses various strategies for helping patients change maladaptive cognitions that contribute to both pain and suffering, and also integrates a number of other techniques for modifying, teaching, and encouraging adaptive coping skills (▶ positive reinforcement, ▶ biofeedback, self-control techniques) (Bradley 1996). Expectancy-value models of motivation and health behavior change posit that motivation for behavior and behavior change is determined by patient beliefs (expectancies) and values (incentives) (Bandura 1986; Janz and Becker 1984; Rogers 1983). According to these models, motivation for behavior change increases as people believe that the benefits of change outweigh the costs, and as they increase their beliefs that change is possible. The Transtheoretical Model of behavior change (Prochaska and DiClemente 1984) emphasizes the fact that people vary in their readiness (or motivation) to make change, and classify readiness into five distinct stages: ▶ precontemplation, ▶ contemplation, ▶ preparation, ▶ action, and ▶ maintenance. This model argues that different therapeutic responses may be used to help patients move from one stage of readiness to the next, until the patient is able to maintain the change for good. Although there has been debate concerning whether readiness to change is best thought of as a stage or continuous dimension, few researchers question the importance of the readiness construct, especially when determining the approach best taken with a particular patient (see Jensen et al. 2003). Finally, client-centered approaches to patient motivation, such as Motivational Interviewing and the Patient-Centered Counseling Model, have identified specific therapeutic responses that increase patient motivation for adaptive behavior change, including such responses as developing a collaborative (rather than confrontive) relationship, eliciting and reinforcing patient self-statements consistent with adaptive change, and increasing patient awareness of the risks of maladaptive responses, while at the same time encouraging patient beliefs that adaptive change is possible (Miller and Rollnick 2002; Ockene et al. 1988).

Clinical Implications of the Motivation Models for Enhancing Patient Self-Management

Clinicians may use the motivational models of health behavior change as guides when helping motivate patients with chronic pain make adaptive changes. For example, based on the transtheoretical model, clinicians would

M

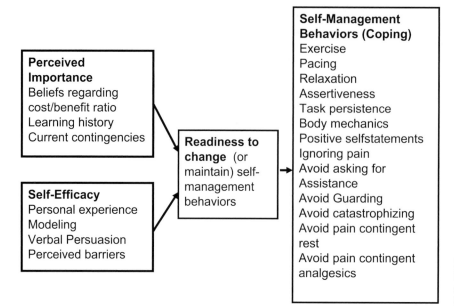

**Motivational Aspects of Pain,
Figure 1** Motivational factors that
contribute to pain self-management
behaviors.

be wise to assess a patient's readiness to participate in whatever specific pain treatment(s) is/are being recommended (e.g. by stating "I think that this intervention is worth trying." and then asking, "What do you think?"). This is particularly important if the treatment involves active patient participation to be effective (such as keeping to a specific medication regimen, relaxation or self-hypnosis training, and active physical or occupational therapy, etc.). If the patient expresses a clear disinterest in the planned treatment approach (i.e. is in the "pre-contemplation stage" concerning this approach), then minimal participation can be expected, leading to few benefits. In this case, specific motivational interventions should be considered to help increase patient readiness to engage in treatment. However, motivational interventions can be useful at all readiness levels, to maximize patient commitment to active participation throughout treatment.

A variety of clinician behaviors and responses will increase patient motivation for engagement in active pain management. Most of these can be classified as interventions that impact either the importance the patient places on participating in treatment, and/or the beliefs that participation is possible (see Fig. 1).

To increase the importance for engaging in regular exercise, for example, clinicians could start with providing patients with information concerning the long-term (negative) effects of inactivity and the benefits of regular exercise. However, information alone is unlikely to produce a change motivation for exercise, or any other adaptive coping behavior, unless patients incorporate this information into their belief system. Merely lecturing patients can, in fact, have a paradoxical effect of pushing patients into the position of defending their current maladaptive (e.g. inactivity, rest) coping responses, caus-

ing them to argue against and therefore resist making adaptive changes (Miller and Rollnick 2002). A more effective strategy is to first provide information, and then encourage the patient to discuss and think through the implications of this information for his or her own pain problem; that is, to elicit from the patient his or her own thoughts concerning the information provided, and especially to pay attention to and reinforce patient statements indicating incorporation of the information. Patients are much more likely to believe what they themselves say than what is told to them (Miller and Rollnick 2002).

The importance that patients place on any particular pain coping response can also be changed by altering the contingencies surrounding that response (Fordyce 1976). Clinicians can, and should, praise and reinforce approximations towards adaptive coping, and seek to ignore coping responses associated with greater dysfunction. Patients' attention on their efforts towards adaptive coping can be emphasized by asking questions about these efforts, and helping the patient come up with solutions to problems associated with the use of new adaptive coping strategies. Such discussion can help focus patients' attention on adaptive coping efforts. Patients, and the people who are close to the patient, can also be taught operant principals, and be encouraged to integrate regular reinforcement for adaptive coping (e.g. exercise contingent rest, praise for regular exercise) (Fordyce 1976).

Self-efficacy for adaptive coping can also be increased in a number of ways. One of these is to simply encourage patients to engage (slowly at first) in new adaptive coping efforts. As the patient sees himself/herself engage in adaptive coping, he/she learns that such coping is possible. Such direct experience is perhaps the most powerful

MPQ

► McGill Pain Questionnaire

MPS

► Myofascial Pain Syndrome

MRI

► Magnetic Resonance Imaging

MRS

Synonyms

Hydrogen Magnetic Resonance Spectroscopy

Definition

1H-MRS (Hydrogen Magnetic Resonance Spectroscopy) is an NMR based technique for assessing function in the brain. MRS takes advantage of the fact that protons (H) possess slightly different resonant properties depending upon the compound. For a given volume of brain (typically > 1 cubic cm), the distribution of these H resonances can be displayed as a spectrum. The area under the peak for each resonance provides a quantitative measure of the relative abundance of that compound.

► Thalamus, Clinical Pain, Human Imaging

MS Contin®

Definition

MS Contin® is a controlled (slow) release tablet formulation of morphine that produces a peak morphine concentration 4-5 hours post dose, and therapeutic concentrations persist for about 12 hours.

► Postoperative Pain, Morphine

MS Contin® Controlled (Slow) Release Morphine Sulphate

► Postoperative Pain, Morphine

MSDs/MSPs

► Disability, Upper Extremity

MTrP

► Myofascial Trigger Point

MTrP Circuit

Definition

An MTrP circuit comprises of the inter-neuronal connections in the spinal cord. The circuit cannot only transfer the nociceptive impulses to the brain, but may also control referred pain patterns via connections to other MTrP circuits. The occurrence of LTRs is also mediated via the MTrP circuit.

► Dry Needling

MTrP Locus

Definition

There are multiple MTrP loci in an MTrP region. An MTrP locus contains two components: the sensitive locus, also known as the local-twitch-response locus (LTR locus), and the active locus, also known as the endplate-noisy locus (EPN locus).

► Dry Needling

Mu(μ)- and Kappa(κ)-Opioids

Definition

Opioids that selectively bind on mu- and kappa- receptors.

► Endogenous Opioid Receptors
► MOP Receptor
► Nitrous Oxide Antinociception and Opioid Receptors
► Psychological Aspects of Pain in Women

Mucosa

Definition

The smooth inner lining of the large intestine that secretes mucus to lubricate the waste materials.

► Animal Models of Inflammatory Bowel Disease

M

Mucosa of Sexual Organs, Nociception

▸ Nociception in Mucosa of Sexual Organs

Mucositis

Definition

Mucous membrane toxicity often occurs shortly after administration of chemotherapy or radiotherapy. Inflammation, ulceration, and infection can then occur on the oral and other mucus membranes.
▸ Cancer Pain Management, Overall Strategy

Mud Therapy

Definition

Mud therapy involves the application of heated mud packs to parts of the body.
▸ Spa Treatment

Multiaxial Assessment of Pain

DENNIS C. TURK
Department of Anesthesiology, University of Washington, Seattle, WA, USA
turkdc@u.washington.edu

Synonyms

Comprehensive Assessment; Multidisciplinary Assessment

Definition

Multiaxial assessment refers to a comprehensive assessment of chronic pain sufferers that addresses biomedical, psychosocial, and behavioral domains, as each of these contribute to the chronic pain and disability (Turk and Rudy 1987).

Characteristics

The ▸ biopsychosocial model of pain proposes that dynamic and reciprocal interactions among biological, psychological, and sociocultural variables shape the pain experience (Turk 1996; Turk et al. 2004). According to this model, the pain experience usually begins when peripheral nociceptive barrage produces physiological changes, although there may be central mechanisms involved in the initiation of pain, and the experience is thoroughly modulated by the unique genetic endowment, learning history, beliefs, affective state, and behavior.

Reports of pain severity and impact will vary depending on a range of contributions, and are not solely the result of physical pathology or perturbations within the nervous system. The biopsychosocial perspective forces an evaluator not only to consider the nature, cause, and characteristics of the noxious stimulation, but the presence of the sensations reflected against a history that preceded symptom onset.

The biopsychosocial model incorporates cognitive-behavioral (CB) concepts (see ▸ Cognitive-Behavioral Perspective) in understanding chronic pain. For example, proponents of this model propose that both the person and the environment reciprocally determine behavior. People not only respond to their environment but elicit environmental responses by their behavior. The person who becomes aware of a physical event and decides the symptom requires attention from a health care provider, initiates a set of circumstances different from the individual with the same symptom who chooses to self-manage symptoms. Another assumption of the CB perspective is that people are active agents and capable of change. The passive role many patients have in traditional physician-patient relationships often reinforces their beliefs that they have minimal ability to impact their own recovery.

To understand and appropriately treat a patient whose primary symptom is pain should begin with a comprehensive history and physical examination. Patients are usually asked to describe the characteristics (for example, stabbing, burning), location, and severity of their pain. Physical examination procedures and sophisticated laboratory and imaging techniques are readily available for use in detecting organic pathology. Physical and laboratory abnormalities, however, correlate poorly with patients' pain reports, and it is often not possible to make any precise pathological diagnosis or even to identify an adequate anatomical origin for the pain. Thus, an adequate pain assessment also requires clinical interviews and utilization of assessment tools to assist in the evaluation of the myriad ▸ Psychosocial Factors and behavioral factors that influence the subjective report.

As there is no pain thermometer that can provide an objective quantification of the amount or severity of pain experienced by a patient, it can only be assessed indirectly based on a patient's overt communication, both verbal and behavioral. However, even a patient's communications make pain assessment difficult, as pain is a complex, subjective phenomenon, comprised of a range of factors, and is uniquely experienced by each individual. Wide variability in pain severity, quality, and impact may be noted in reports of patients attempting to describe what appear to be objectively identical phenomena. Patient's descriptions of pain are also colored by cultural and sociological influences.

A patient's beliefs about the cause of symptoms, their trajectory, and beneficial treatments will have important influences on emotional adjustment and adherence to therapeutic interventions. Clinical attention should focus on the patient's specific thoughts, behaviors, emotions, and physiological responses that precede, accompany, and follow pain episodes or exacerbations, including environmental and temporal conditions, and consequences associated with the patient's responses (cognitive, emotional, and behavioral, including frequency and specificity/generality across situations) in these situations. It is valuable to note any patterns of ▶ maladaptive thoughts, as they may contribute to a sense of hopelessness, dysphoria, and unwillingness to engage in activity. Topics that can be covered in an assessment interview might include: asking what the patient thinks is wrong with him/her, what the patient thinks about the pain (e.g. cause, impact), what worries the patient has (e.g. exacerbation of symptoms, impairment), problems the patient has experienced due to pain (e.g. marital, financial, occupational), how the patient lets others know when pain is present, what effect the patient believes the pain is having on others, in what situations the patient experiences increased pain, what others think about their pain, how others respond to their pain, medications they are taking, strategies they have used to alleviate pain, what treatments they have endured for pain management, and prior and current stressful life events.

Turk and Meichenbaum (1994) have suggested that three central questions should guide assessment of people who report pain: (1) What is the extent of the patient's disease or injury (physical impairment)? (2) What is the magnitude of the illness? That is, to what extent is the patient suffering, disabled, and unable to enjoy usual activities? and (3) Does the individual's behavior seem appropriate to the disease or injury, or is there any evidence of amplification of symptoms for any of a variety of psychological or social reasons or purposes? These three general questions can be conceptualized and address three general domains or axes – biomedical, psychosocial, and behavioral.

A thorough clinical assessment should also involve gathering a detailed history from the patient, including past medical history, drug/alcohol use, history of mental illness, and a list of current medications. It is important for the clinician treating chronic pain patients to understand the use of pain medications, in addition to the side-effects associated with them, so as to avoid misinterpreting symptoms and potential misdiagnosis. Patients may also make use of alcohol and illicit drugs to palliate their symptoms. Patients with histories of substance abuse may be at particular risk of becoming dependent on and abusing pain medications. Reviewing the chart and conducting a detailed history of previous and current prescription and substance use may help ascertain whether this area warrants further inquiry.

In addition to interviews, a number of assessment instruments designed to evaluate patients' attitudes, beliefs, and expectancies about themselves, their symptoms, and the health care system have been developed. Standardized assessment instruments have advantages over semistructured and unstructured interviews. They are easy to administer, can suggest issues to be addressed in more depth during an interview, require less time, and most importantly, they can be submitted to analyses that permit determination of their ▶ reliability and ▶ validity. The poor reliability and questionable validity of physical examination measures has led to the recent development of self-report functional status measures that seek to quantify symptoms, function, and behavior directly, rather than inferring them. Another advantage of self-report instruments is that they enable the assessment of a wide range of behaviors that are relevant to the patient, some of which may be private (sexual relations) or unobservable (thoughts, emotional arousal). Even traditional psychological measures have been used to identify psychosocial characteristics of the pain experience. These measures, however, must be used with caution, as they were usually not developed for or standardized on samples of medical patients. As a result, it is always best to corroborate information gathered from the instruments with other sources, such as interviews with the patient and significant others, and chart review.

In addition to self-report instruments, more valid information may be obtained by asking about current levels of pain or pain over the past week, and by having patients maintain regular ▶ diaries of pain intensity with ratings recorded several times each day for several days or weeks. Through such diaries, patients can also record activities and the amount of time or the number of times they perform specific behaviors such as reclining, sitting, standing, walking, and so forth.

A third use of patient diaries is to record medication use over a specified interval. Diaries not only provide information about the frequency and quantity of medication, but may also permit identification of the antecedent and consequent events of medication use. For example, a patient might note that he took medication after an argument with his wife, and that when she saw him taking the medication she expressed sympathy. Antecedent events might include stress, boredom, or activity. Examination of antecedents is useful in identifying patterns of medication use that may be associated with factors other than pain per se. Similarly, patterns of response to the use of analgesic may be identified. Does the patient receive attention and sympathy whenever he or she is observed by significant others taking medication? That is, do significant others provide positive reinforcement for the taking of analgesic medication, and thereby unwittingly increase medication use?

The multiaxial approach to assessment is designed to assess and integrate physical, psychosocial, and behavior contributors to pain and disability. There are a large number of measures and procedures that can be used to evaluate each axis. The multiaxial approach to assessment

M

does not specify any particular methods for assessment. The evaluator will determine the appropriate methods based on his or her experience with chronic pain sufferers, and specific questions that may be of particular importance for a given patient.

Components of the multiaxial assessment can be summarized as follows:

Biomedical

- Medical History
- Co-morbid medical conditions
- Pain (intensity, quality, duration, location, exacerbating and alleviating factors)
- Physical Examination
- Laboratory Diagnostic Tests
- Imagining Procedures
- Response to previous treatment (both positive and adverse)

Psychosocial

- General history (family composition, education)
- Living status (e.g. married, divorced, romantic relationship)
- Quality of relationships with significant others
- Socioeconomic status
- Work history
- Substance abuse history and current use of drugs and alcohol to control pain as well as recreational.
- Impact of pain on physical, emotional, and social functioning
- Beliefs, attitudes, expectations, and fears about pain, treatment, their plight, and the future
- Prior and current psychiatric status, degree of emotional distress (fear, depression, anger), treatment of patient and family
- Use of stet coping methods (e.g. problem solving, distraction)
- Satisfaction with previous and current treatment(s)

Behavioral

- Use of behavioral methods of coping with pain (e.g. medication, alcohol, exercise, withdrawal)
- Observation of ► pain behaviors (overt communications of pain distress and suffering)
- Response to pain behaviors by significant others
- Physical, social, and recreational activities
- Vocational status
- Adherence to treatment recommendations (e.g. medication, exercise)

References

1. Turk DC, Rudy TE (1987) Toward a Comprehensive Assessment of Chronic Pain Patients. Behav Res Ther 25:237–249
2. Turk DC (1996) Biopsychosocial Perspective on Chronic Pain. In: Gatchel RJ, Turk DC (eds) Psychological Approaches to Chronic Pain Management: Clinical Handbook. Guilford Press, New York, pp 3–33
3. Turk DC, Meichenbaum D (1994) A Cognitive-Behavioural Approach to Pain Management. Wall PD, Melzack R (eds) Textbook of Pain, 2nd edn. Churchill Livingstone, London, pp 1337–1338
4. Turk DC, Monarch ES, Williams AD (2004) Assessment of Chronic Pain Sufferers. In: Hadjistavropoulos T, Craig KD (eds) Pain: Psychological Perspectives. Lawrence Erlbaum, Mahwah NJ, pp 209–243

Multichannel CT

► CT Scanning

Multidimensional

Definition

A pain assessment tool that includes measurement of two or more indicators of newborn pain (behavioral, physiological or biochemical (hormonal). Multidimensional approaches to pain assessment incorporate the use of pain assessment tools that include measurement of two or more indicators of newborn pain, and concurrent consideration of a variety of contextual and modifying factors.

► Pain Assessment in Neonates

Multidimensional Model

► Diathesis-Stress Model of Chronic Pain

Multidimensional Scaling and Cluster Analysis Application for Assessment of Pain

W. Crawford Clark
College of Physicians and Surgeons, Columbia University, New York, NY, USA
clarkcr@pi.cpmc.columbia.edu

Synonyms

Multidimensional scaling; Factor Analysis; Pain Questionnaire; Cluster Analysis; pain; emotion

Definition

Multivariate scaling (MVS), a subset of multivariate statistics, includes a large group of mathematical techniques and data collection procedures. Of particular interest here are multidimensional scaling (MDS), cluster analysis and preference mapping (PREFMAP). These models yield a geometric representation that makes it easier for an investigator to uncover the "hidden structure" of complex data bases. These techniques use similarity judgments or other measures of association to generate proximities among a set of ▶ stimulus objects as input. An object is a thing, or event; a stimulus is the perceived object. Stimulus objects may be words, physical stimuli or concepts. Just as a map yields far more information (distance, direction) than does a list of cities, so MVS procedures yield more information than do scores on rating scales or questionnaires. These procedures yield the ▶ group stimulus space, a configuration of points (stimulus objects) along dimensions in continuous space, or as clusters in discrete space. A ▶ dimension is a characteristic that serves to define a point by its coordinates. Another advantage of these models is that they also quantify individual differences by providing ▶ subject weights in the source or weight space, which quantify the saliency or relative importance that each individual attaches to each cluster or dimension. The subject weight scores can be correlated with other test scores or used to distinguish subpopulations in the sample. Information about individual differences promises to be useful in determining treatment strategies for individual patients. An important aspect of MVS procedures is that the subject is typically asked to make similarity judgments between pairs of a set of stimulus objects. Thus, the MVS procedures are more objective than commonly used procedures that assign scales determined by the investigator, because the participant, not the investigator, determines the dimensions or clusters.

Characteristics

Introduction to Multivariate Scaling

Multidimensional Scaling

Introductions to INDSCAL and other spatial distance models are provided by Carroll and Arabie (1998), Kruskal and Wish (1978), Schiffman (1981), Weinberg and Carroll (1992), and Lattin et al. (2003). Introductions and reviews of applications to pain and emotion are available (Clark 2003).

Of paramount importance to the investigation of sensory pain and emotional suffering is that the stimulus objects may be calibrated physical stimuli (e.g. heat, cold, electrical) or they may be verbal descriptors (e.g. moderate pain, stabbing, anxiety), or both. A variety of data collection procedures and mathematical models are used to obtain and analyze measures of proximity – a number that represents the amount of similarity or difference between a pair of stimulus objects. One of the key ideas in MVS is that these subjective proximity measures, which represent psychological distance, can be used to scale physical distance. MVS models construct a configuration of points as on a map, so that the distances in the group stimulus space systematically model the judged proximities. To obtain direct proximity data, pairs of stimuli are judged with respect to their degrees of similarity or dissimilarity. In general, proximity measures may be obtained from other measures of association such as correlations, joint probabilities, or phi-coefficients. As the number of pairwise comparisons rapidly increases with the number of stimulus objects, less direct procedures, such as pile-sort where the subject partitions the stimulus objects into groups based on similarity, are used.

Interpreting Dimensions

Dimensions are interpreted by examining the stimulus objects at each pole (the remaining central stimulus objects will usually be found at the poles of other dimensions). The stimulus objects at the poles of each dimension should share a common meaning, and the two poles will generally be opposite in nature. The use of PREFMAP in interpreting the meaning of a dimension is described later. Interpretation of the spatial features is somewhat subjective, since, because the sampling distributions are unknown, there are no inferential statistical tests available for determining the number of dimensions. However, Weinberg and Carroll (1992) describe a number of approaches to approximating the true space.

Two-Way, Three-Way and Higher-Way Models

MVS clustering and multidimensional models are classified as two-way, three-way or higher-way (Carroll and Chaturvedi 1995). In these models, the data are organized into a half-matrix, in which rows and columns correspond to stimulus objects and the cells contain some measure of similarity. As two-way models (e.g. KYST) are computed from a single group matrix in which the cells are means averaged over subjects, they yield only the group stimulus space. Three-way, or individual differences scaling, models (e.g. INDSCAL) treat matrices that correspond to individual subjects, or, if desired, to subgroups. Three-way models assume that different individuals perceive stimuli in terms of a common set of dimensions or clusters, but that these features differ in their saliency or importance to different individuals. In addition to the group stimulus space, the three-way models provide a source space that yields individual subject weights on each dimension or cluster. Subject weights measure the importance of each dimension to an individual. They can be used to distinguish among subgroups in the sample population, and may be correlated with psychological and physiological measures. In medicine, where knowledge about the individual patient is essential, the three-way model is essential.

Cluster Analysis

Cluster models represent the structure of a set of stimulus objects as subsets of clusters, where each cluster corresponds to a meaningful group of stimulus objects. Depending upon the model used, the clusters may be non-overlapping or overlapping. Two major types of clus-

M

ter models are the hierarchical and the additive models (Latin et al. 2003).

Relationship between Clustering and Spatial Distance Models

Cluster and MDS (spatial distance) models are similar in many ways: the same pairwise similarity judgment data can be analyzed by either procedure and both are distance models. However, important differences exist. Cluster analysis groups stimulus objects that are most similar, while spatial distance models emphasize ways in which items are different. Cluster analysis is superior to multidimensional scaling when the stimulus objects are discrete and not readily placed on a continuum or when the number of descriptors is large.

Property or Preference Mapping (PREFMAP)

Property or preference mapping (PREFMAP) models (Carroll and Chaturvedi 1995) provide an objective aid to the interpretation of dimensions. Features, that is, the dimensions of the clusters in the group stimulus space, are usually interpreted by inspection. However, if the features are ambiguous, or if specific hypotheses are being tested, it is useful to have additional information that is objectively based on subjects' judgments. The PREFMAP model provides independent information that aids interpretation of the group stimulus.

Relation of MVS to Factor Analysis

Factor analysis, another multivariate procedure, has proven useful for the study of responses to questionnaires by various pain patient populations. However, because the investigator determines the response scales, factor analysis cannot reveal in an unbiased manner the number and types of dimensions that underlie patients' sensory, emotional and other experiences. Schiffman et al. (1981) point out other advantages of the multivariate scaling approach over that of factor analysis. It is easier to interpret the distances between points than angles between vectors, and MVS provides more easily interpretable solutions with fewer and much more homogeneous dimensions.

Pain Studies with MVS Procedures

MVS studies of responses to calibrated sensory stimuli offer a way to discover the dimensions of physical pain and their relationship to pain descriptors. In the first application of INDSCAL to the study of pain, Clark et al. (1986) analyzed judgments made to various intensities of noxious and non-noxious heat stimuli and obtained a two-dimensional solution. In a subsequent study, INDSCAL analysis of pairwise similarity ratings made to electrical stimuli of five intensities (milliwatts) and three frequencies (hertz) yielded a two-dimensional solution with the stimuli ordered with respect to intensity along a Sensory Magnitude dimension and with respect to fre-quency along a Frequency dimension (Janal et al. 1993). The interpretation of the dimensions in the group stimulus space was supported by PREFMAP analysis of subjects' ratings of each of the stimuli with respect to bipolar property scales (e.g. Faint Pain – Severe Pain). As expected, the Pain Magnitude dimension was related to property scales in the Sensory, Emotional and Arousal domains, while the Frequency dimension was identified only with the Fast-Slow property scale.

Studies with Descriptors of Pain and Emotion

The number and composition of the dimensions underlying the sensory, emotional, motivational, and other aspects of pain remain controversial in spite of considerable speculation and some research. These various views concerning the number of dimensions and their composition are based entirely on subjective impressions. Clearly "armchair taxonomy" cannot settle arguments over the number and nature of pain dimensions. Clark et al. (2001) used INDSCAL to study this question. INDSCAL analysis of responses to 16 descriptors of sensations, negative and positive emotions and motivation yielded four dimensions (D) in the group stimulus space. Dimensions are defined by the descriptors at the poles. D-1, Intense to Moderate Experiences, contained two attributes: Strong Pain Sensations (Severe Pain to Slight Sensation) and Strong Emotions (Upsetting to Comforting). D-2, Moderate to Weak Experiences, exhibited two attributes: (i) moderate pain sensations (Faint Pain to No Sensation) and (ii) moderate emotions (Uncomfortable to Comforting). D-3, Motivational State, possessed two attributes: (i) pain (Severe Pain to Faint Pain) and (ii) arousal level (Startling to Indifferent). D-4, Sensory Qualities, exhibited two attributes: (i) pain (Severe Pain to Faint Pain) and (ii) somatosensory qualities (Hammering to Tingling). The interpretation of the dimensions was supported by PREFMAP and by correlations between subject weights and psychological tests. The results clearly demonstrated that pain and other dimensions are not orthogonal to one another, for in each of the four dimensions the sensory pain attribute is inseparable from both the strong and weak emotional attributes, the motivational attribute and the somatosensory qualities attribute. It may be concluded that sensory pain does not exist as an independent dimension separate from other dimensions of pain. The practical implication of this finding is that a score on a unidimensional pain intensity rating scale cannot be a pure measure of the patient's pain experience. That a patient cannot separate these components of pain has been strongly supported by the finding that ratings of pain intense by patients experiencing postoperative pain on a unidimensional numerical pain rating scale are strongly influenced by the patients' emotional state, specifically depression, anxiety, anger and fear (Clark et al. 2002).

Quantifying the Relation between Physical Stimuli and Verbal Descriptors

What is the relationship between sensory experiences induced by physical stimuli and the descriptors of these experiences? In the first study of its kind, we used IND-SCAL to study pairwise similarity responses for a set of stimulus objects containing both electrical stimuli of various intensities, and sensory and emotional descriptors used to describe these sensory experiences (Janal 1995). The subjects made pairwise similarity judgments to all possible pairings of 16 stimulus objects: 8 electro-cutaneous stimuli ranging in intensity from innocuous (3 mW) to noxious (235 mW), and 8 somatosensory and affective descriptors of these sensations which ranged from Slight Sensation, Tingling and Comforting to Severe Pain, Hammering and Upsetting. INDSCAL analysis revealed a 1-dimensional solution with a close relationship between the perceived intensities of the physical stimulus coordinates and the words describing them. While preparing this paper, it occurred to this author that a quantitative relation between the verbal and the physical stimulus weights could be obtained, by plotting the INDSCAL stimulus coordinates of both the verbal and the physical stimulus objects (ordinate) against a scale of intensities in milliwatts (abscissa). A plot of the perceived stimulus coordinates (ordinate) against an objective scale (abscissa) yielded two exponential functions that contain more information than found with magnitude estimation procedures.

Clinical Pain: Identifying Individual Differences in the Saliency of Pain Dimensions

The results of the following study suggest how multidimensional scaling could be used to determine treatment strategies. Clark et al. (1989) used INDSCAL to compare the group stimulus and subject weight spaces of inpatients suffering cancer-related pain with those of healthy volunteers. The question was "Do patients and volunteers differ in whether the emotional or the sensory dimension is more salient?" The participants made pairwise similarity judgments between all possible pairings of a set of nine descriptors of sensory pain, emotional pain and somatosensory qualities. The group stimulus spaces of patients and controls revealed similar 3-dimensional solutions: Sensory Pain Magnitude, Emotional Quality, and Somatosensory Quality. However, the subject weight space, which yields coordinates for each individual on each dimension, demonstrated that the saliency of the various dimensions varied widely among subjects. For some individuals the Pain Magnitude dimension was most important in determining their similarity judgments (high values on the abscissa, low on ordinate); for others the Emotional Quality dimension was most salient, while for yet others the two dimensions were equally important. The coordinates for each subject in the subject weight or source space revealed wide individual differences, but significantly more patients than controls found the Pain Magnitude dimension to be the most salient. The wide individual differences found suggest that the location of a patient in the subject weight space might prove useful in tailoring treatment. For example, a patient who finds the Pain Magnitude dimension to be most salient might profit from a higher analgesic dose, while a patient who weights on the Emotional Quality dimension might experience relief following the addition of a psychoactive medication and, perhaps, a reduction in the analgesic. In brief, the patient's coordinates in the subject weight space can help determine treatment.

Other MDS Applications to Problems of Pain

A number of imaginative applications of various MVS procedures to problems in pain have been pursued: measurement of neural response patterns to noxious stimulation using cluster analysis; pain during activities of daily living; in post-operative myalgia patients by PREFMAP; facial expression of clinical pain and emotion; cross cultural comparison of dental pain and emotional attitudes in Chinese and Western patients and dentists by cluster analysis and cross-cultural comparisons of cancer pain in various European and Asian groups using MDS. Details appear in a review by Clark (2003).

Questionnaire Construction by Cluster Analysis

Another application of MVS is the construction of questionnaires. Clark et al. (1995) used a hierarchical clustering model to analyze pile-sort similarity judgments made by seven experienced pain researchers to 270 descriptors of sensory pain, negative and positive emotions, motivation, illness and health. Analysis by the average-linkage-between-groups clustering model produced a dendrogram with 50 subclusters subsumed within 18 primary clusters. No evidence was found to support the homogeneous status claimed for descriptors in the major Evaluative Class of the MPQ. A large number of the descriptors that were assigned to each of the 22 subgroups of the MPQ were found to be dispersed over a number of different clusters in the dendrogram. In a subsequent study, described by Yang et al. (2000), healthy male and female African-American, Euro-American and Puerto Rican subjects sorted 189 descriptors into similar piles (pile-sort technique), and then sequentially merged their piles on the basis of similarity (merge technique) until only two piles remained. The addition of the merge technique greatly improved the hierarchical structure of the dendrogram. Dendrograms for each of the six groups revealed striking gender and ethnocultural differences in the language of pain. Men and women and ethnocultural groups disagreed on the cluster location, and hence the meaning, of 30 descriptors; 58 other descriptors were found to be very similar (redundant). The remaining 101 descriptors and clusters determined the structure of the Multidimensional Affect and Pain Survey (MAPS). Thus, unlike the MPQ,

M

the MAPS questionnaire is based on the structure of the empirically derived dendrogram that emerged from subjects' views of their sensory-emotional pain spaces.

Validation of MAPS

Factor analysis has demonstrated the validity of MAPS, and hence, the advantage of the cluster analytic approach to test construction (Clark et al. 2003). If MAPS is a valid questionnaire for the quantification of emotion and pain, then factor analysis of cancer patients' ratings should produce factors that correspond uniquely to the clusters and superclusters of the MAPS dendrogram. Almost all of the clusters in the MAPS Somatosensory Pain Supercluster loaded on three sensory-pain related factors. Most of the clusters in the Emotional Pain Supercluster loaded on emotional factors, and the Well-being Supercluster loaded on the good health factor. This correspondence between clusters and factors stands in sharp contrast with factor analytic studies of the MPQ, where subclasses of its sensory, affective and even evaluative classes often load on a single factor. The meanings of such mixed factors are very difficult to interpret. The cause of this factor heterogeneity and the discrepant results obtained by various investigators is probably due to the a priori procedure used by investigators of the MPQ to classify descriptors into its major classes and subclasses.

Conclusions

It is obvious that the MVS models, multidimensional scaling, cluster analysis and PREFMAP, offer original approaches to many theoretical and practical questions in a variety of fields. They identify the underlying structure of the dimensions of the experience and response to pain and emotion, drug induced states, patterns of neural response and facial expressions. These methods can be used to construct new questionnaires and to discover the latent structure of existing questionnaires. In addition, MDS of similarity responses to descriptors and to physical stimuli can be used to quantify the intensity of descriptors at a ratio scale level of measurement. Considering the widespread use of MDS, cluster analysis and PREFMAP in psychology and the social sciences (where it has been used to study visual, auditory and taste perception, language, consumer preferences, kinship patterns, the provenance of ancient pottery, etc.), it is astonishing that these methods have not been applied more extensively to complex medical problems.

Acknowledgements

This essay and much of the research here was supported by the Nathaniel Wharton Fund for Research and Education in Brain, Body and Behavior, NIDR 20248 and NICDR 12725. The author wishes to thank Dr. J.D. Carroll, Board of Governor's Professor, Rutgers University, for his many helpful comments, but the author is responsible for any errors that may remain.

References

1. Carroll JD, Arabie P (1998) Multidimensional Scaling. In: Birnbaum MH (ed) Handbook of Perception and Cognition. Vol 3: Measurements, Judgment and Decision. Academic Press, San Diego, pp 179–250
2. Carroll JD, Chaturvedi A (1995) A General Approach to Clustering and Multidimensional Scaling of Two-Way, Three-Way, or Higher-Way Data. In: Luce RD, D'Zmura M, Hoffman DD (eds) Geometric Representation of Perceptual Phenomena. Erlbaum, Mahwah, pp 295–318
3. Clark WC (2003): Pain, Emotion, and Drug-Induced Subjective States. In: Adelman G, Smith B (eds) Encyclopedia of Neurosciences, 3rd edn. Elsevier, Amsterdam (CD-ROM)
4. Clark WC, Carroll JD, Yang JC et al. (1986): Multidimensional Scaling Reveals Two Dimensions of Thermal Pain. J Exp Psychol (Hum Percept) 12:103–107
5. Clark WC, Ferrer-Brechner T, Janal MN et al. (1989) The Dimensions of Pain: A Multidimensional Scaling Comparison of Cancer Patients and Healthy Volunteers. Pain 37:23–32
6. Clark WC, Janal MN, Hoben EK et al. (2001) How Separate are the Sensory, Emotional, and Motivational Dimensions of Pain? A Multidimensional Scaling Analysis. Somatosens Mot Res 18:31–39
7. Clark WC, Kuhl JP, Keohan ML et al. (2003) Factor Analysis Validates the Cluster Structures of the Dendrogram Underlying the Multidimensional Affect and Pain Survey (MAPS) and Challenges the A Priori Classification of the Descriptors in the McGill Pain Questionnaire (MPQ). Pain 106:357–363
8. Clark WC, Yang JC, Tsui SL et al. (2002) Unidimensional Pain Rating Scales: A Multidimensional Affect and Pain Survey (MAPS) Analysis of What They Really Measure. Pain 98:241–247
9. Janal MN (1995) Concerning the Homology of Painful Experiences and Pain Descriptors: a Multidimensional Scaling Analysis. Pain 64:373–378
10. Janal MN, Clark WC, Carroll JD (1993) Multidimensional Scaling of Painful Electrocutaneous Stimulation: INDSCAL Dimensions, Signal Detection Theory Indices, and the McGill Pain Questionnaire. Somatosens Motor Res 10:31–39
11. Kruskal JB, Wish M (1978) Multidimensional Scaling. Sage, Beverly Hills
12. Lattin JM, Carroll JD, Green PE (2003) Analyzing Multivariate Data. Duxbury Press, Belmont
13. Schiffman SS, Reynolds ML, Young FW (1981) Introduction to Multidimensional Scaling. Academic Press, New York
14. Weinberg SL, Carroll JD (1992) Multidimensional Scaling: An Overview with Applications in Educational Research. Adv Soc Sci Methodology 2:99–135
15. Yang JC, Clark WC, Tsui SL et al. (2000): Preoperative Multidimensional Affect and Pain Survey (MAPS) Scores Predict Post-Colectomy Analgesia Requirement. Clin J Pain 16:314–320

Multidisciplinary

Definition

Medical disciplines working with the same patient.
▶ Physical Medicine and Rehabilitation, Team-Oriented Approach

Multidisciplinary Assessment

▶ Multiaxial Assessment of Pain

Multidisciplinary Pain Centers, Rehabilitation

DENNIS C. TURK
Department of Anesthesiology, University of
Washington, Seattle, WA, USA
turkdc@u.washington.edu

Synonyms

Multidisciplinary pain clinics, Interdisciplinary pain rehabilitation programs, Functional restoration program, Pain clinics

Definition

An organization of health care professionals and basic and applied scientists that includes research, teaching, and patient care related to acute and chronic pain. It includes a wide array of health care professionals including physicians, psychologists, nurses, physical therapists, occupational therapist, and other specialty healthcare providers. Multiple therapeutic modalities are available. These centers provide evaluation and treatment and are usually affiliated with major health science institutions. Multidisciplinary pain clinics are similar to multidisciplinary pain centers (MPC), with the exception being that they do not include basic scientists and may not be involved in conducting research.

Characteristics

Although there is no single format for multidisciplinary pain management or the operations of an MPC, almost every treatment facility of this type has a generic concept and plan.

Concepts of Treatment at Multidisciplinary Pain Clinics

- Reconceptualization of the patient's pain and associated problems from uncontrollable to manageable
- Overt or covert efforts are made to foster optimism and combat demoralization
- Flexibility is the norm with attempts to individualize some aspects of treatment to patient needs and unique physical and psychological characteristics
- Emphasize active patient participation and responsibility
- Provide educational and training in the use of specific skills such as exercise, relaxation, and problem solving
- Encourage patient feelings of success, self-control, and self-efficacy
- Encourages patients to attribute success to their own efforts

These treatment programs also share general features.

General Features of Multidisciplinary Pain Treatment Teams

- Share a common conceptualization of chronic pain patients

- Synthesize the diverse sets of information based on their own evaluations, as well as those of outside consultants, into a differential diagnosis and treatment plan customized to meet the specific need of each patients
- Work together to formulate and implement a comprehensive rehabilitation plan based on available data
- Share a common philosophy of disability management
- Act as a functional unit whose members are willing to learn from each other and modify, when appropriate, their own opinions based on the combined observations and expertise of the entire group

In MPCs, patients are usually treated in groups. Patients work on at least 4 issues simultaneously: physical, pharmacological, psychological, and vocational. Programs usually emphasize helping patients to gain knowledge about pain and how the body functions, physical conditioning, medication management, acquisition of coping and vocational skills. Individual and group counseling address patient's needs. In contrast to traditional Western health care, the emphasis is upon what the patient accomplishes, not on what they say. The providers serve as teachers, coaches, and sources of information and support (Loeser and Turk 2001).

Multidisciplinary pain management requires the collaborative efforts of many healthcare providers, including, but not limited to, physicians, nurses, psychologists, physical therapists, occupational therapists, and vocational counselors. The healthcare providers act as a team, with extensive interaction amongst the team members.

The following list itemizes the goals of multidisciplinary pain management. Every patient will have a different mixture of functional limitations, pain behaviors, affective disturbance, physical disability, and vocational dysfunction. Successful treatment will address each of these general areas.

Goals of Multidisciplinary Pain Management

- Identify and treat unresolved medical issues
- Symptomatic improvement
- Eliminate inappropriate medications, institute desirable medications
- Improve aerobic conditioning, endurance, strength and flexibility (restoration of physical functioning)
- Eliminate excessive guarding behaviors that interfere with normal activities
- Improve coping skills and psychological well-being
- Alleviate depression
- Foster independence
- Assess patient resources and identify vocational and recreational opportunities
- Educate the patient about pain, anatomy, physiology and psychology, discriminating hurt from harm

M

- Educate the patient about prudent health care consumption
- Assist the patient to establish realistic goals and to maintain treatment gains
- Restoration of social and occupational functioning - social reintegration, return to productive employment
- Reduction in use of healthcare system

The original MPCs were inpatient-based. It is now apparent that outpatient programs can be equally successful if they have adequate intensity and duration (for a review see Turk et al. 1993). There are no controlled studies to determine the optimal duration of treatment and hours per day; nor does the literature reveal which aspects of the various components are most important for a treatment program. It is clear, however, that the effects of an MPC are greater than the sum of its parts. Common features of all programs include physical therapy, medication management, education about how the body functions, psychological treatments (e.g. learning coping skills, problem solving, communication skills training), assessment, and therapies aimed at improving function and the likelihood of return to work. Programs usually have a standard daily and weekly format that providers can tailor to individual patient needs. The overall length of a program depends, in part, upon unique patient requirements. Typical programs operate 8 hours per day, 5 days per week and last 3 to 4 weeks, although some programs meet less frequently and are of longer duration.

Roles of the Physician

The physician is responsible for the initial history and physical examination; review of outside records and determination of the need for any further diagnostic tests. Detailed assessment of the patient's medication history is also a key physician contribution. The implementation of medication management, including drug tapering by means of a ▶ pain cocktail technique (described below), is also a physician role. Another important task for the physician is to review with the patient the medical issues and the findings of diagnostic tests and imaging studies. The physician also plays an essential role in the education of the patient, and in legitimating all of the other components of the treatment program.

Roles of the Psychologist

The psychologist typically conducts the initial psychological evaluation, monitors and implements the cognitive and behavioral treatment strategies, teaches the patient coping skills, and educates patients about the relationship between thoughts, feelings, behavior, and physiology. The psychologist usually leads both individual and group educational and counseling sessions for the patients. In addition, the psychologist plays a critical role in helping other members of the treatment team to employ sound behavioral principles in designing patient treatment activities (Turk and Gatchel 2002).

Roles of the Nurse

The nurse is a key part of the treatment program, playing a major role in patient education regarding such topics as medication, diet, sleep hygiene, and sexual activity. Another nursing function is assisting patients in the practice of newly learned skills, assessing medication responses, and acting as the focal point of the communication that keep such a program operational. The roles of nurses vary with their skills and their interaction with other providers. Since the nurses tend to be with the patients throughout their entire treatment course, they play a central role in maintaining continuity during the treatment program.

Roles of Physical and Occupational Therapists

Physical and occupational therapists provide assessment and active physical therapies for patients to improve their strength, endurance and flexibility. They do not provide passive modalities of treatment. They assist the patient in developing proper body mechanics and strategies for coping with the physical demands of a job and everyday life, and function mainly as teachers and coaches.

The occupational therapists review the patient's work history, disabilities, and factors that may play a role in determining who goes back to work and who does not. They help in the establishment of work hardening and training activities. Some programs heavily emphasize ergonomic issues and utilize high technology in physical therapies; however, the need for this type of treatment is unclear.

Role of the Vocational Counselor

The vocational counselor plays a critical role in the treatment of an individual for whom return to work is a treatment goal. Initial assessment occurs as part of the screening process, but in-depth evaluation of interests, education, aptitude, physical capacities, learning capabilities, work experience, transferable skills and vocational goals occurs upon entry into the treatment program. The goals are to identify vocational opportunities and barriers to effective return to work. In addition to occupational counseling, counselors provide job seeking skills training, placement counseling, work hardening, information about educational options and liaison services. Information obtained by the vocational counselor is critical for other team members to establish realistic goals for the patient. In some organizations, rehabilitation nurses provide this service.

Treatment Principles

The goals of multidisciplinary pain management are normally specific, definalble, operationalizable, and realistic in nature (see list 'Goals of Multidisciplinary Pain

Multidisciplinary Pain Centers, Rehabilitation, Table 1 Issues Addressed by Psychologists

Impact of pain on life, significant others	Resourcefulness vs. helplessness
Communication	Problem Solving
Reinforcement and pain behaviors	Relationship between thoughts, feelings, behavior, and physiology
Goal setting, homework, adherence	Coping Skills (relaxation, distraction, positive thoughts)
Self-reinforcement	Fear of activity
Stress and Pain and Homework	Generalization, maintenance, flare-ups,Relapse

Multidisciplinary Pain Centers, Rehabilitation, Table 2 General Educational Topics Covered

Body mechanics, modification of movement patterns	Role of medication
Posture	Sleep hygiene
Energy conservation	Diet
Performance of activities of daily living	Sexuality
Hurt vs. harm	Anatomy &Physiology
Leisure activities	Gate Control Theory
Vocational activities	Home practice
Active vs. passive exercises and modalities	Progressive exercises
Adherence to recommendations	Management of flare-ups

M

Management'). As they have evolved, MPC treatments have become performance based, goal-directed, and outcome driven. Integration of medical evidence related to patientt's pain and physical impairment with information concerning what patients are doing or failing to do because of their pain, how these behaviors influence patientt's physical capacity, how others respond to the patient, the influence of psychosocial factots that contribute directly and indirectly to patientt's physical and emotional status, and the potential for rehabilitation (i.e. disability) are essential. The treatment team must build an alliance with patients to instill a willingness to accept the need for self-management.

Physical therapy employs behavioral medicine principles (Turk et al. 2000) and, as noted, engages few, if any, passive modalities. The emphasis is upon improving strength, endurance and flexibility through the patient's physical activities. The therapists provide instruction, guidance, safety and encouragement. Accomplishments, rather than pain behaviors, receive rewards. Patients maintain graphs of their daily activity and track progress. As patients progress, they enroll in more complex activities that simulate the workplace requirement.

Medications are given on a time contingent basis, so as to uncouple the reinforcement of pain behaviors by medications. In general, patients in an MPC program do not derive adequate pain relief from analgesic medications, and this is why they are usually tapered by means of the pain cocktail technique. This technique is simply a method of converting all opioids to an equivalent dose of methadone, delivered with a masking vehicle. The dose is then tapered over the period of treatment, always with the full knowledge of the patient. Most medications are discontinued; the common exceptions are antidepressants, which often help chronic pain patients. MPCs discourage long-term use of other medications, both because of their potential side effects and because their use undermines the philosophical concept that the patient must learn to control his or her pain, and not depend upon healthcare providers or their prescriptions. Psychological strategies generally target altering behavior rather than changing the patient's personality. Patients learn coping skills because this is frequently a deficiency that has led to the patient's many difficulties (see following list). Couples therapy is sometimes appropriate. Issues that patients bring up receive attention in either the group format or in individual therapy, as needed. As depression is so often a component of the chronic pain problem, it warrants both psychological as well as pharmacological interventions. Psychologists provide relaxation and consolidation sessions that allow the patients to work on newly acquired skills, and explore educational topics and new psychological skills (see Table 1).

Coping Skills Taught

- Relaxation
- Distraction (attention diversion) methods

- Cognitive restructuring – identification and challenging maladaptive thoughts and feelings
- Problem solving
- Anger management
- Desensitization
- Rehearsal and home practice
- Communication skills including assertiveness
- Goal setting
- Pleasant activity planning
- Self-monitoring and Self-reinforcement

An important aspect of MPCs is education. This is an activity that is shared by physicians, psychologists and nurses. Topics cover a wide array of the problems facing those who suffer from chronic pain. Topic selection and content is to some degree a function of the needs of each group of patients, but content always includes a core set of issues (see Table 2).

An important issue is the maintaining of gains that have occurred during the treatment program. Surrounded by a team of supportive healthcare providers and other patients, most patient see some gains by the end of treatment. However, many are unable to maintain their gains when they return to their normal family and occupational activities. Each patient must learn strategies for maintaining his or her gains in a less supportive environment. Most programs have established brief follow-up interactions to try to assist patients to keep up their physical and psychological skills and to prevent relapses.

Outcomes

A substantial body of literature supports the assertion that multidisciplinary pain treatment is effective in reducing pain, the use of opioid medication, the use of health care services; it increases activity, returns people to work, and aids in the closing of disability claims (e.g. Cutler et al. 1994, Guzman et al. 2001). Moreover, treatment at MPCs targets patients with the most recalcitrant problems, yet the benefits appear to exceed those for conventional treatments including surgery and, in contrast to surgery, there are no known iatrogenic complications of treatment at MPCs (Turk 2002). Not only do MPCs appear to be clinically effective, they also appear to be cost-effective, with the potential to provide substantial savings in healthcare and disability payments (Turk 2002).

Conclusions

The team approach to complex chronic pain patients, as found in a multidisciplinary pain treatment facility, has evolved with an underlying set of principles. These include the recognition that Cartesian mind-body dualism is a curse upon effective healthcare. Second, a biopsychosocial model is required to capture all of the relevant factors. Third, the treatment must address the pain itself, and not just be a search for hidden causes and specific remedies for these causes. Fourth, the treatment must address the restoration of well-being and not just aim at the alleviation of symptoms. Finally, the illness is not just chronic pain but is also the failure to work, often ascribed erroneously to the pain instead of the patient or the patient's circumstances.

References

1. Cutler RB, Fishbain DA, Rosomoff HL et al. (1994) Does Nonsurgical Pain Center Treatment of Chronic Pain Return Patients to Work? A Review and Meta-Analysis of the Literature. Spine 19:643–652
2. Guzman J, Esmail R, Karjalinen K et al. (2001) Multidisciplinary Rehabilitation for Chronic Low Back Pain: Systematic Review. BMJ 322:1511–1516
3. Loeser JD, Turk DC (2001) Multidisciplinary Pain Management. In: Loeser JD, Butler SD, Chapman CR, Turk DC (eds) Bonica's Management of Pain, 3rd edn. Lippincott Williams and Wilkins, Philadelphia PA, pp 2069–2079
4. Turk DC (2002) Clinical Effectiveness and Cost Effectiveness of Treatments for Chronic Pain Patients. Clin J Pain 18:355–365
5. Turk DC, Gatchel RJ (2002) Psychological Treatment of Chronic Pain: Clinical Handbook, 2nd edn. Guilford Press, New York
6. Turk DC, Okifuji A, Sherman J (2000) Behavioral Aspects of Low Back Pain. In: Taylor JR, Twomey L (eds) Physical Therapy of the Low Back, 3rd edn. Australia, pp 351–383
7. Turk DC, Rudy T, Sorkin B (1993) Neglected Topics in Chronic Pain Treatment Outcome Studies: Determination of Success. Pain 53:3–16

Multidisciplinary Pain Treatment for the Elderly

Definition

The elderly are underrepresented in multidisciplinary programs, despite the fact that multimodal treatment is a key to successful practice in geriatric medicine.
- ▶ Psychological Treatment of Pain in Older Populations

Multidisciplinary Treatment Program

Definition

Physicians, nurses, physical therapists, and psychologists in one pain-management center. Treatment staff meet weekly to review patient progress in the program, which emphasizes pain reduction and functional outcomes.
- ▶ Complex Chronic Pain in Children, Interdisciplinary Treatment
- ▶ Multimodal Rehabilitation Treatment and Psychiatric Aspects of Multimodal Treatment for Pain
- ▶ Psychological Treatment of Chronic Pain, Prediction of Outcome

Multimodal

Definition

Refers to treatment approaches that use more than one type of therapy (e.g. a combination of drug, psychological and or physical therapies).

▶ Complex Chronic Pain in Children, Interdisciplinary Treatment

Multimodal Analgesia

Synonyms

Balanced analgesia

Definition

Multimodal analgesia (also known as balanced analgesia) occurs from a combination of analgesics (multimodal mixture). The rationale is that each drug exerts its analgesic effect via a different mechanism. Thus, a low-dose combination might offer the best therapeutic effect, while minimizing the risk of the unwanted adverse effects seen with high doses of each of these drugs.

▶ Epidural Infusions in Acute Pain
▶ Multimodal Analgesia in Postoperative Pain
▶ Postoperative Pain, Importance of Mobilisation
▶ Postoperative Pain, Transition from Parenteral to Oral Drugs

Multimodal Analgesia in Postoperative Pain

EDWARD A. SHIPTON
Christchurch School of Medicine and Health Sciences, Department of Anaesthesia, University of Otago, Christchurch, Otago, New Zealand
shiptonea@xtra.co.nz

Synonyms

Balanced analgesia

Definition

▶ Multimodal analgesia is the technique of combining multiple modalities of pain relief to provide more effective analgesia and a lower incidence of adverse effects. Different analgesics act on different receptors, enzymes and ionic channels, creating an additive or synergistic response. There is a concomitant reduction in adverse effects, owing to the lower dose of the individual drugs and differences between drugs in adverse effect profiles (Shang and Gan 2003).

Characteristics

Single analgesics, for example opioids or non-steroidal anti-inflammatory drugs (NSAIDs), are not able to provide effective pain relief without side effects such as nausea, vomiting, sedation, or bleeding (Jin and Chung 2001). The use of multi-drug therapy such as in ▶ neuraxial blocks, is a common and effective example of the multimodal approach, and may help to prevent rapid tolerance to individual medications. Studies of multimodal approaches for postoperative pain control have shown improvements in postoperative pain scores and similar reductions in analgesic requirements (Shang and Gan 2003).

Pharmacological pain relief can be markedly improved by attention to choice of drugs, positive drug interaction, administration route, timing and dosing (Breivik 2002). This may be carried out using the '▶ Acute Pain Service' with anaesthetist-supervised pain nurses.

Commonly, acetaminophen (paracetamol) and NSAIDs are in routine use as components of multimodal analgesia, in combination with opioids or local anaesthetic techniques to modulate this (Power and Barratt 1999). Alpha 2 antagonists (e.g. clonidine) and ▶ N-Methyl-D-Aspartate antagonists (e.g. ketamine to reduce wound secondary mechanical hyperalgesia) can be added either intravenously (in patient controlled analgesia) or epidurally (single shot, constant infusion or by patient controlled epidural analgesia) (Potgatzki et al. 2003). The use of spinal neostigmine and adenosine is currently being investigated (Shipton 1999).

Improved pain control includes the optimal use of acetaminophen (paracetamol) by mouth, rectally or intravenously (as the prodrug proparacetamol). Evidence is now sufficient to recommend that an NSAID be added to acetaminophen for short-term postoperative pain relief, unless there are any known contraindications to NSAIDs (Breivik 2002). These include allergy, gastro-intestinal ulcer disease, potential bleeding problems (due to its irreversible effects on platelet function), renal functional impairment, asthma, hypovolaemia, hyperkalaemia, severe liver disease, circulatory failure, pre-eclampsia or certain drugs (ACE inhibitors, diuretics, beta blockers, cyclosporine, methotrexate) (Breivik 2002).

The new ▶ COX-2 inhibitor ▶ NSAIDs have relative gastric and platelet sparing effects, and can be given orally (e.g. rofecoxib, celecoxib, etoricoxib, valdecoxib) and intravenously (e.g. paracoxib) as a component of multimodal analgesia (Shang and Gan 2003).

Where acetaminophen and NSAIDs result in inadequate pain relief, opioids can be given either orally, rectally, intramuscularly or intravenously (nurse administered or by patient controlled analgesia). Opioid adverse effects such as nausea, vomiting, pruritus and urinary retention are reduced by multimodal analgesia.

M

Local anaesthetic infiltration (in tissue, joints, peritoneal cavity) as part of a multimodal regimen offers a simple, safe and inexpensive alternative to epidural pain control (Schumann et al. 2003). Intra-articularly, local anaesthetics are often combined with opioids (morphine) (Menigaux 2001). Catheters can be used to provide constant infusions of local anaesthetics around peripheral nerves and plexuses (with or without a multimodal mixture).

▶ Regional anaesthesia attenuates the endocrine-metabolic effects (the rise in cortisol, catecholamines, glucagon, hyperglycaemia, insulin resistance and negative nitrogen balance) on stress-induced organ dysfunction, and extends analgesia into the postoperative period (Kehlet and Wilmore 2002). The inhibitory effects on catabolic responses are most pronounced when regional anaesthesia is provided for up to 24–48 hours, preferably as a continuous epidural analgesic technique. After major thoracic or abdominal surgery, patients at risk of postoperative respiratory and cardiac complications are offered optimal analgesia, with thoracic or thoracolumbar epidural infusion of low doses of local anaesthetic (e.g. levobupivacaine, ropivacaine), a lipophilic opioid (e.g. fentanyl, sufentanil) and epinephrine (adrenaline) (Breivik 2002).

Accelerated multimodal postoperative recovery programmes are being developed as a multidisciplinary effort, with the integration of postoperative pain management into a postoperative rehabilitation programme (Kehlet 1999). Multimodal intervention may reduce stress induced organ dysfunction and accompanying morbidity (Kehlet and Wilmore 2002).

An integrated approach to perioperative care (comprising minimally invasive surgical access, optimal pain relief provided by epidural analgesia, early oral nutrition, avoidance of nasogastric tubes, and aggressive active mobilization) decreases time to discharge, readmission rate, and postoperative morbidity with increased patient satisfaction and safety after discharge (Carli et al. 2002). After colonic surgery, as compared to intravenous opioids, epidural analgesia in a multimodal analgesic regimen results in significantly less deterioration in postoperative functional status (lower pain and fatigue scores, earlier mobilization and return of gastro-intestinal function), and health related quality of life at six-week follow-up (Wu and Rajah 2002).

The use of perioperative multimodal techniques may provide long-term benefits to patients.

References

1. Breivik H (2002) Postoperative Pain: Toward Optimal Pharmacological and Epidural Analgesia. In: Giamberardino MA (ed) Pain 2002 – An Updated Review. IASP Press, Seattle, pp 337–349
2. Carli F, Mayo N, Klubien K et al. (2002) Epidural Analgesia Enhances Functional Exercise Capacity and Health-Related Quality of Life after Colonic Surgery: Results of a Randomized Trial. Anesthesiology 97:540–549
3. Jin F, Chung F (2001) Multimodal Analgesia for Postoperative Pain Control. J Clin Anesth 13:524–539
4. Kehlet H (1999) Acute Pain Control and Accelerated Postoperative Surgical Recovery. Surg Clin North Am 79:431–443
5. Kehlet H, Wilmore DW (2002) Multimodal Strategies to Improve Surgical Outcome. Am J Surg 183:630–641
6. Menigaux C, Guignard B, Fletcher D et al. (2001) Intraoperative Small-Dose Ketamine Enhances Analgesia after Knee Arthroscopy. Anesth Analg 93:606–612
7. Pogatzki EM, Niemeier JS, Sorkin LS et al. (2003) Spinal Glutamate Receptor Antagonists Differentiate Primary and Secondary Mechanical Hyperalgesia Caused by Incision. Pain 105:970–1007
8. Power I, Barratt S (1999) Analgesic Agents for the Postoperative Period. Nonopioids. Surg Clin North Am 79:275–295
9. Schumann R, Shikora W, Weis JM et al. (2003) A Comparison of Multimodal Perioperative Analgesia to Epidural Pain Management after Gastric Bypass Surgery. Anesth Analg 96:469–474
10. Shang AB, Gan TJ (2003) Optimising Postoperative Pain Management in the Ambulatory Patient. Drugs 63:855–867
11. Shipton EA (1999) The Future. In: Shipton EA (ed) Pain – Acute and Chronic. Arnold, London, pp 326–365
12. Wu CL, Raja SN (2002) Optimising Postoperative Analgesia. Anesthesiology 97:533–534

Multimodal Analgesics

▶ Drugs with Mixed Action and Combinations, Emphasis on Tramadol

Multimodal Rehabilitation Treatment and Psychiatric Aspects of Multimodal Treatment for Pain

DAVID A. FISHBAIN
Department of Psychiatry and Department of Neurological Surgery and Anesthesiology, University of Miami, School of Medicine and H. Rosomoff Pain Center at South Shore Hospital, Miami, FL, USA
dfishbain@miami.edu

Synonyms

Multidisciplinary treatment; Psychiatric Aspects of Multimodal Treatment for Pain; Multimodal Treatment

Definition

a) Multimodal treatment is defined as applying several treatments simultaneously / concurrently or sequentially (one after another) in order to improve pain and facilitate rehabilitation.
b) Multidisciplinary treatment is defined as treatment involving more than one treatment discipline and as different disciplines usually utilize different treatments, multidisciplinary treatment is by definition multimodal.

Characteristics

Pain Treatment Facilities

Pain treatment facilities developed for a number of reasons. First, people in general put a very high value on living a pain-free life. Second, numerous epidemiological studies determined that a large percentage (2–40%) of the general population suffered from chronic intractable benign pain. And third, the experience of treating continuous severe pain in battle injured World War II soldiers determined that a coordinated team was required to manage the different types of pain (Rosomoff and Steele-Rosomoff 1991).

Multidisciplinary pain clinics or centers evolved from these concepts in the early 1970s. It was observed that a significant percentage of low back pain and neck pain patients did not improve with traditional medical treatment but remained disabled (Rosomoff and Steele-Rosomoff 1991). These patients demonstrated a host of behavioral and psychosocial problems in association with their chronic pain. These problems required the intervention of disciplines besides those of neurosurgery, orthopedic surgery and anesthesiology (Rosomoff and Steele-Rosomoff 1991). In addition, these patients required a concurrent highly integrated multidisciplinary treatment approach that would address all the patient's problems simultaneously, i.e. multimodal treatment (Rosomoff and Steele-Rosomoff 1991).

There were approximately 1500–2000 pain treatment facilities in the US (Rosomoff and Steele-Rosomoff 1991). They differed in their staff composition, size, philosophy and most importantly, treatment approach. Because of this problem, the International Association for the Study of Pain (IASP) developed definitions for four types of pain treatment facilities (see below) (Loeser 1991).

IASP Classification of Pain Facilities (Adapted from Loeser 1991)

Modality-oriented Clinic

- Provides specific type of treatment, e.g. nerve blocks, transcutaneous nerve stimulation, acupuncture, biofeedback.
- May have one or more health care disciplines.
- Does not provide an integrated, comprehensive approach.

Pain Clinic

- Focuses on the diagnosis and management of patients with chronic pain or may specialize in specific diagnoses or pain related to a specific region of the body.
- Does not provide comprehensive assessment or treatment, an institution offering appropriate consultative and therapeutic services would qualify but never an isolated solo practitioner.

Multi-Disciplinary Pain Clinic

- Specializes in the multi-disciplinary diagnosis and management of patients with chronic pain or may specialize in specific diagnoses or pain related to a specific region of the body.
- Staffed by physicians of different specialties and other health care providers.
- Differs from a multi-disciplinary pain center only because it does not include research and teaching.

Multi-Disciplinary Pain Center

- Organization of health care professionals and basic scientists that includes research, teaching and patient care in acute and chronic pain.
- Typically a component of a medical school or a teaching hospital.
- Clinical programs supervised by an appropriately trained and licensed director.
- Staffed by a minimum of physician, psychologist, occupational therapist, physical therapist and registered nurse.
- Services provided integrated and based on interdisciplinary assessment and management.
- Offers both inpatient and outpatient program.

Inspection of the list above indicates that there is a clear distinction between modality-oriented clinics, pain clinics and multidisciplinary facilities. Differences between multidisciplinary pain clinics and multidisciplinary pain centers (MPC) include research and teaching in the MPCs. These definitions also indicate that the MPCs may be more likely to have inpatient and outpatient treatment and to have larger and more diversified multi-disciplinary staffs, including more than one physician specialty. As a consequence, MPCs are likely to offer a wider range of treatments than multidisciplinary pain clinics and thus involve more multimodal treatment. Most of the pain facility treatment outcome studies involve MPCs.

MPC Treatment Outcome Studies

Because MPC developed in the 1970s and because they had to demonstrate treatment efficacy, there are now close to three hundred treatment outcome studies in the literature (Fishbain et al. 1993). As such, this literature has been subjected to a number of meta-analyses (Table 1). It is interesting to note that these meta-analyses (four) were consistent in indicating that MPC treatment or multimodal treatment is effective. This meta-analysis literature has recently been reviewed for meta-analytic procedure quality and found to be of acceptable quality (Fishbain et al. 2000). It is also important to note that this literature now indicates that multidisciplinary (multimodal) treatment is superior to single treatment such as medical therapy or physical therapy (Flor et al. 1992).

Multimodal Rehabilitation Treatment and Psychiatric Aspects of Multimodal Treatment for Pain, Table 1   MPC Chronic Pain Treatment Meta-Analyses

Author / Year	Treatment type and clinical condition	Outcome measure	Author clinical interpretation of meta-analysis data
Malone and Strube (1988)	Pain facility, chronic pain	Activity level. Frequency pain. Index pain. Intensity pain. Medication use. Mood.	Treatment effective, good effect sizes.
Curtis (1992)	Multi-disciplinary pain facility, chronic low-back pain.	Physical fitness. Subjective distress. Daily activity increase. Medication decrease.	Multi-disciplinary treatment programs effective.
Flor et al. (1992)	Multi-disciplinary pain facilities, chronic low-back pain.	Activity level. Pain behavior. Medication use. Return to work.	Multi-disciplinary pain clinics effective at returning chronic back pain patients to work.
Cutler et al. (1994)	Multi-disciplinary pain facility, chronic low-back pain.	Return to work.	Multi-disciplinary pain facilities return chronic low-back pain patients to work.

Which Treatments or Combination Makes MPC Treatment Effective?

For an exhaustive list of treatment by medical specialty available at MPCs, please refer to Fishbain DA et al. (1997). It is to be noted that some of these treatments, e.g. physical therapy, have been studied in a placebo fashion, resulting in a significant number of studies in the literature. There are meta-analysis results available for some of these (Fishbain et al. 2000). Of the non-pharmacological treatments having meta-analyses, physical therapy, cognitive and behavior therapy and educational therapy appear to be effective. Of the psychopharmacological treatments, antidepressants, topical NSAIDs, capsaicin and anticonvulsants are effective (Fishbain et al. 1997; Fishbain et al. 2000).

Yet, in reality MPCs may or may not provide these treatments or may provide a greater range of treatments (Fishbain et al. 1997). Pain facilities generally use multiple treatments simultaneously which are integrated into a treatment package (Fishbain et al. 1997). Thus, it is impossible to say whether the positive MA results for MPCs related to the fact that the specific treatments shown to be effective were provided or that other hitherto untested treatments were utilized. This question awaits further research.

Another issue in relation to which treatments make MPC treatment effective is what outcome variables are examined (Fishbain et al. 1993). As an example, a specific treatment such as capsaicin may decrease pain, but if used alone, it may not be enough to return the patient to work. In other words, for the attainment of some outcome variables, such as return to work, a combination of specific treatments may be required. The evidence indicates that treatments under one category, such as behavior, may have equal efficacy. For example, operant conditioning has been found to be as effective as cognitive-behavior treatment (Turner and

Clancy 1988) and outpatient group cognitive therapy, relaxation training and cognitive therapy have all been demonstrated to be equally efficacious (Turner and Jensen 1993).

In addition, different treatments within one category appear not be additive. When a cognitive component was added to operant pain treatment there was no decrease in patient medical utilization costs or improvement in patient quality of life scores (Goossens et al. 1998). However, treatments from different groups may have an additive effect. The combined package of cognitive-behavioral group pain treatment with physical therapy has been found to be superior to physical therapy alone (Nicholas et al. 1992). This speaks to the apparent advantage of multimodal treatment.

At this time, it is unclear what combination of MPC treatments delivered in a treatment package is effective. It is therefore unclear what combination of treatments is necessary for an effective package. It is also possible that the effectiveness of MPCs rests in their ability to deliver this treatment package and an ability to integrate treatments into a package (Rosomoff and Steele-Rosomoff 1991). This last issue may influence an overall effectiveness that has not been explored in the literature.

Psychiatric Multimodal Treatment within MPCs

Early in the course of development of MPCs it became clear that the vast majority of chronic pain patients suffered from associated psychiatric comorbidity (Fishbain 1999). In addition, it has recently become clear that drugs commonly utilized by psychiatrists, e.g. antidepressants, anticonvulsants, have strong analgesic properties (Fishbain et al. 2000). Finally, it has become recognized that many chronic pain patients have neuropathic pain for which psychopharmacological treatment is becoming increasingly available (Fishbain et al. 2000). This confluence of factors and the fact that psychiatrists by the nature of their specialty have expertise in psychopharmacological treatment and detoxification (Fishbain 2002) has increased the potential impact of this medical specialty on pain treatment outcome.

The list below presents the functions of the psychiatrist within MPCs and the potential treatments that he / she can initiate in a multimodal fashion. With reference to treatments, it is to be noted that these now reflect the major issue of directing psychopharmacological treatment both at pain relief and at the same time psychiatric comorbidity. Thus, the psychiatrist working at an MPC should be very familiar with the literature addressing the psychopharmacological treatment of pain in order to be able to choose an agent for pain, which will also have impact on the psychiatric comorbidity. This concept is very different from 10–15 years ago, when psychiatrists treated psychiatric comorbidity exclusively. In addition, it is to be noted that as there is now a subspecialty psychiatry board in pain management, some psychiatrists are developing expertise in the procedure treatments of chronic pain.

Psychiatric Functions and Multimodal Treatments

Potential Functions

1. Diagnosis of psychiatric comorbidity per DSM-system.
2. Determination presence of psychological difficulties, problems, etc., e.g. suicidal ideation, homicidal ideation, marital / system conflicts, etc.
3. Determination presence of somatic comorbidities, e.g. sleep problems, headaches, dizziness, etc.
4. Develop a psychopharmacological and non-psychopharmacological treatment plan for #1–#3 above.
5. Administer behavioral rating scale testing if necessary.
6. According to the history, physical examination and required laboratory workup determine whether the pain is nociceptive, neuropathic or both.
7. Participate in multidisciplinary case staffing in order to develop a multidisciplinary treatment plan that would encompass the psychiatric treatment plan.
8. Act as consultant to other multidisciplinary staff.
9. Educate members of multidisciplinary staff on psychiatric aspects of chronic pain.
10. Perform clinical research on all aspects of pain.
11. Act as director of the multidisciplinary team.

Multimodal Treatments

1. Psychopharmacological treatment directed at nociceptive pain.
2. Psychopharmacological treatment directed at neuropathic pain.
3. Psychopharmacological treatment directed at psychiatric comorbidity.
4. Detoxify patient if necessary.

5. Provide supportive counseling.
6. Lead behavior rehabilitation groups.
7. Provide program patient education for his / her area of expertise.
8. Participate in the behavior modification (reinforcement) aspects of the multidisciplinary program.
9. If within his / her area of expertise, perform procedures such as trigger point injections, acupuncture, blocks, epidurals, etc.

References

1. Cutler RB, Fishbain DA, Rosomoff HL et al. (1994) Does non-surgical pain center treatment of chronic pain return patients to work? A review and meta-analysis of the literature. Spine 19:643–652
2. Curtis JE (1992) The efficacy of multidisciplinary treatment programs for chronic low back pain: a meta-analysis. Dissertation Abstracts International 53:4948
3. Fishbain DA (1999) Approaches to treatment decisions for psychiatric comorbidity in the management of the chronic pain patient. Med Clin North Am 83:737–759
4. Fishbain DA (2002) Opiate, hynopsedative, alcohol, and nicotine detoxification protocols. In: Tollison CD, Satterthwaite JR, Tollison JW (eds) Practical Pain Management, Lippincott Williams and Wilkins, Philadelphia, pp 314–329
5. Fishbain DA, Rosomoff HL, Goldberg M et al. (1993) The prediction of return to the workplace after multidisciplinary pain center treatment. Clin J Pain 9:3–15
6. Fishbain DA et al. (1997) Pain facilities: a review of their effectiveness and referral selection criteria. Current Review Pain 1:107–115
7. Fishbain D, Cutler RB, Rosomoff HL et al. (2000) What is the quality of the implemented meta-analytic procedures in chronic pain treatment meta-analyses? Clin J Pain 16:73–85
8. Flor H, Fydrich T, Turk DC (1992) Efficacy of multidisciplinary pain treatment centers: a meta-analytic review. Pain 49:221–230
9. Goossens ME, Rutten-Van Molken MP, Kole-Snijders AM et al. (1998) Health economic assessment of behavioural rehabilitation in chronic low back pain: a randomised clinical trial. Health Econ 7:39–51
10. Loeser JD (1991) Desirable characteristics for pain treatment facilities: reports of the IASP taskforce. In: Bond MR, Charlton JE, Woolf CJ (eds) Proceedings of the VI th World congress on Pain. Elsevier, Amsterdam, pp 411–415
11. Malone MD, Strub MJ (1988) Meta-analysis of non-medical treatments for chronic pain. Pain 34:231–244
12. Nicholas MK, Wilson PH, Goyen J (1992) Comparison of cognitive-behavioral group treatment and an alternative nonpsychological treatment for chronic low back pain. Pain 48:339–347
13. Rosomoff HL, Steele-Rosomoff R (1991) Comprehensive multidisciplinary pain center approach to the treatment of low back pain. Neurosurgical Clinics of North America 2:877–890
14. Turner JA, Clancy S (1988) Comparison of operant behavioral and cognitive-behavioral group treatment for chronic low back pain. Clin Psychol 56:261–266
15. Turner JA, Jensen MP (1993) Efficacy of cognitive therapy for chronic low back pain. Pain 52:169–177

Multimodal Treatment

▶ Multimodal Rehabilitation Treatment and Psychiatric Aspects of Multimodal Treatment for Pain

Multiple Sclerosis (MS)

Definition

An idiopathic immune system disease of the central nervous system in which gradual destruction of myelin occurs in patches throughout the brain or spinal cord (or both), interfering with the nerve pathways and causing muscular weakness, loss of coordination and speech and visual disturbances. Sometimes manifests as radiating pain in a similar distribution as the sciatic nerve.
▶ Central Pain, Outcome Measures in Clinical Trials
▶ Sciatica
▶ Trigeminal, Glossopharyngeal, and Geniculate Neuralgias

Multipolar Cells

Definition

Neuron type whose cell body (soma) issues an axon and several primary dendrites forming the dendritic tree.
▶ Trigeminal Brainstem Nuclear Complex, Anatomy

Multiprofessional

Definition

Healthcare professionals working with the same patient
▶ Physical Medicine and Rehabilitation, Team-Oriented Approach

Multireceptive Neuron (MR)

Definition

A neuron that is activated by a variety of innocuous and noxious mechanical and thermal stimuli applied to its receptive field, which is typically widespread and comprises of cutaneous and deep tissue.
▶ Arthritis Model, Kaolin-Carrageenan Induced Arthritis (Knee)
▶ Chronic Pain
▶ Thalamic Bursting Activity
▶ Thalamus, Nociceptive Cells in VPI, Cat and Rat

Multisensory Perceptions

Definition

Perceptions of external objects based on more than one form of sensory input (e.g. sight and smell).
▶ Amygdala, Pain Processing and Behavior in Animals

Munchausen's by Proxy

Definition

A severe type of factitious disorder where the parent consciously causes the child to assume the sick role to satisfy the parent's psychological need.
▶ Somatization and Pain Disorders in Children

Mu(μ)-Opioid Receptor

Synonyms

MOP

Definition

Opioid receptors that preferentially bind endomorphins and morphine-like drugs. It was originally named for the effects of morphine. Also known as OP3 receptors, they are the main sites of action for most opioid drugs. They share the same distribution as kappa receptors with the exception of the hypothalamus. Agonists are associated with analgesia, respiratory depression, euphoria bradycardia, miosis, reduced gut motility and nausea and vomiting.
▶ Opiates During Development
▶ Opioid Receptors
▶ Opioid Rotation in Cancer Pain Management
▶ Postoperative Pain, Appropriate Management
▶ Postoperative Pain, Transition from Parenteral to Oral

Muscle and Joint Pain

▶ Spinal Dorsal Horn Pathways, Muscle and Joint

Muscle Contraction Headache

▶ Headache, Episodic Tension Type

Muscle Cramp

Definition

Involuntary sudden painful muscle contraction. During the cramp, the muscle is visibly and palpably taut and painful, often with abnormal posture of the affected joint, condition which can be relieved by stretching or massage.
▶ Muscular Cramps

Muscle Discrimination

Definition

This refers to a person's ability to accurately sense the current level of tension within the muscles being monitored.

▶ Psychophysiological Assessment of Pain

Muscle Hyperactivity

▶ Orofacial Pain, Movement Disorders

Muscle Nociceptor

Definition

A free nerve ending with high thresholds to mainly mechanical and chemical stimuli (nociceptive); also high-intensity thermal stimuli may excite muscle nociceptors. Their afferents are small-diameter myelinated (Group III) or unmyelinated (Group IV) muscle nerve fibers. Group IV corresponds to cutaneous C-fibers and group III to Aδ-fibers. Conduction velocities for cat muscle afferent fibers are below 2.5 m/s for group IV and 2.5 to 30 m/s for group III fibers.

▶ Exogenous Muscle Pain

Muscle Nociceptors, Neurochemistry

SIEGFRIED MENSE
Institute for Anatomy and Cell Biology III, University Heidelberg, Heidelberg, Germany
mense@urz.uni-heidelberg.de

Definitions

A nociceptor is a receptive ending that specializes in informing the central nervous system (CNS) about the presence of a tissue threatening stimulus. A nociceptor has an elevated stimulation threshold just below the noxious level. (The receptor already has to respond to stimuli below the level that causes tissue damage, because it is supposed to fulfill the function of an alarm system and prevent tissue damage). In addition to an elevated stimulation threshold, a nociceptor has to be able to encode the intensity of a stimulus within the noxious range, i.e. it must not saturate when a stimulus reaches noxious levels.

A receptor molecule is a protein located within the axonal membrane of a receptive ending. It binds sensitizing and stimulating substances in a highly specific manner and is either coupled to an ion channel (which opens after the binding has occurred) or a ▶ G protein, which starts an intracellular cascade of events that – among other effects – leads to the activation of enzymes such as kinases.

Characteristics

Morphology

A nociceptor is an unencapsulated ("free") nerve ending that is connected to the CNS by thin myelinated (group III) or unmyelinated (group IV) nerve fibers. These fibers have a slow conduction velocity, with ▶ group III fibers conducting between 2.5 and approximately 20 m/s and ▶ group IV fibers between 0.5 and 1 m/s. Histologically, the nerve ending is not free in the strict sense but is surrounded by a single layer of ▶ Schwann cells. The Schwann cells leave small patches of the axonal membrane uncovered, the so-called exposed axon areas. These areas are assumed to be the sites of action for the chemical stimuli that are present in a pathologically altered muscle.

Neuropeptide Content

There is no ▶ neuropeptide that can be regarded as specific for sensory fibers from muscle or for muscle nociceptors. Nerve endings in skeletal muscle of the rat have been reported to contain ▶ substance P (SP), calcitonin-gene related peptide (▶ CGRP), ▶ somatostatin (SOM), ▶ vasoactive intestinal polypeptide (VIP) as well as the neurotrophin ▶ nerve growth factor (NGF), and thus presents a neuropeptide pattern similar to that of cutaneous nerves. Of these neuropeptides, SP is of particular interest because, in experiments on fibers from the skin, SP has been shown to be predominantly present in nociceptive fibers (Lawson et al. 1997). The peptides are released during excitation of the ending and influence the chemical milieu of the tissue around the receptor. SP has a strong dilating and permeability increasing action on small blood vessels. By these effects, SP causes an increase in local microcirculation and edema formation at the site of the lesion. In addition to that, SP has a sensitizing action on nociceptors.

Receptor Molecules in the Membrane of a Nociceptive Ending

Data concerning the presence of receptor molecules in muscle nociceptors have not been reported. Based on responsiveness of these endings to intramuscular and intraarterial injections of ▶ Algesic Agent / Algesic Chemical, and existing parallels with cutaneous nociceptors, the following types of receptor molecule are likely to be present (Caterina and David 1999; Mense and Meyer 1985; McCleskey and Gold 1999):

1. Receptors for inflammatory substances. Among these are receptors for ▶ bradykinin (BK; B1 and B2 receptors), 5-hydroxytryptamine (5-HT, ▶ serotonin; e.g. 5-HT3 receptor), and prostaglandins (e.g. PGE2; EP2 receptor). In intact tissue, BK is known to influence the ending via the B2 receptor; in inflamed tissue, the B1 receptor is synthesized in

M

the soma of the nociceptive neuron, transported to the receptive ending and inserted into its membrane. This is an example of a neuroplastic change in the nociceptive ending. In contrast to the 5-HT3 receptor that controls an ion channel, the BKN receptors activate a G protein.

2. Receptors for protons. Besides immunoreactivity (IR) for acid-sensing ion channels (e.g. ASIC1), IR for the transient receptor potential vanilloid receptor (▶ TRPV1) (Caterina and David 1999) is present in somata of the dorsal root ganglion that supply receptive endings in skeletal muscle (U. Hoheisel and S. Mense, unpublished; Fig. 1). The receptor is sensitized by and responds to an increase in H^+-concentration and to heat. The sensitivity of this receptor to protons is important under conditions in which the pH of the tissue is lowered (e.g. exhaustive muscle work, ischemia, inflammation, tonic contraction). A specific stimulant for this receptor molecule is capsaicin, the active ingredient of chili peppers. In inflamed tissue, TRPV1 receptors have been reported to be more frequent than under normal conditions (Carlton and Coggeshall 2001).

3. Purinergic receptors. These receptor molecules bind adenosine triphosphate (ATP) and the products of ATP degradation. The P2X3 receptor (Burnstock 2000; Cook and McCleskey 2002) has been demonstrated to be present in cutaneous nociceptors; it has also been shown to exist in ▶ DRG cells supplying the gastrocnemius-soleus mus-

cle of the rat (U. Hoheisel and S. Mense, unpublished).

4. Receptors for growth factors. In our group, nerve growth factor (NGF; ▶ TrkA receptor) proved to excite muscle nociceptors in concentrations that caused cutaneous pain in humans. ▶ Brain-derived neurotrophic factor (BDNF; TrkB receptor) had no excitatory effect on muscle nociceptors but desensitized the endings to mechanical stimuli (i.e. after i.m. injection of BDNF the response magnitude of the ending to noxious pressure stimuli was reduced).

5. Receptors for excitatory amino acids. Reports in the literature indicate that nociceptors in the deep tissues around the temporomandibular joint are activated by glutamate (Cairns et al. 1998). This means that glutamate receptors must be present in nociceptors of deep somatic tissues.

6. Opioid receptors. These receptors were found on Aδ- and C fibers in cutaneous nerves (Stein et al. 1990). They are upregulated during tissue inflammation.

Other algesic agents may activate muscle nociceptors without binding to specific receptor molecules An example of this are potassium ions which might depolarize and excite nociceptors following muscle trauma if the relatively high intracellular concentration of K^+ is released from muscle cells. High concentrations of Na^+ may likewise have an unspecific mechanism of action. A marked increase in extracellular Na^+ does not occur under (patho)physiologic conditions, but is induced in

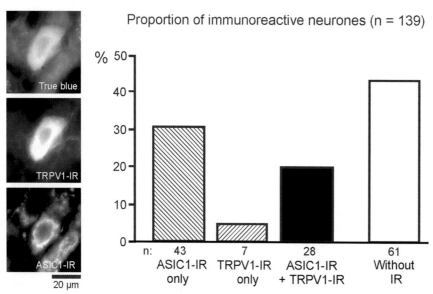

Muscle Nociceptors, Neurochemistry, Figure 1   Neurons in the rat spinal ganglion L5 exhibiting immunoreactivity (IR) for the acid-sensing ion channel 1 (ASIC 1) and the vanilloid receptor 1 (TRPV1), respectively. All evaluated neurons were retrogradely labelled from the gastrocnemius-soleus (GS) muscle with the fluorescent dye True blue. (a) the same neuron labelled with three different stains: Aa, retrograde labelling with True blue from the GS muscle; Ab, fluorescent staining with antibodies to TRPV1; Ac, fluorescent staining with antibodies to ASIC 1. (b) proportion of neurons with IR for ASIC 1 and/or TRPV1. The filled bar shows neurons exhibiting IR for both ASIC 1 and TRPV1 (ASIC 1-IR + TRPV1-IR). Without IR, neurons exhibiting neither ASIC 1-IR nor TRPV1-IR (J. Reinöhl, U. Hoheisel and S. Mense, unpublished).

clinical studies on muscle pain mechanisms when hypertonic saline injections or infusions are injected i.m. (Graven-Nielsen et al. 1997). In these studies, the high Na^+ concentration – and not the hypertonicity of the solution – appears to be the effective stimulus (see essay ▶ muscle pain model, ischemia-induced and hypertonic saline-induced).

Response Properties

Mechanical Stimulation

Upon mechanical stimulation (e.g. by pressure stimuli), a muscle nociceptor has a high stimulation threshold and requires noxious (tissue-threatening, subjectively painful) intensities of stimulation for excitation. In intact muscle, a nociceptor does not respond to everyday stimuli such as physiologic movements or muscle stretch (Mense 1997). Recordings of the activity of single muscle afferent fibers in cats and rats have shown that nociceptors as described in the above definition are present in skeletal muscle (Mense and Meyer 1985). Microneurographic recordings in humans also demonstrated the existence of muscle nociceptors (Marchettini et al. 1996). It is important to note that not all unencapsulated nerve endings in skeletal muscle have nociceptive properties. Many of them can be excited by weak innocuous pressure stimuli and probably mediate subjective pressure sensations.

Chemical Stimulation

BK, 5-HT, and prostaglandin E2 have long been known to excite muscle nociceptors in concentrations that are likely to be present in an inflamed or ischemic muscle (Kumazawa and Mizumura 1977; Mense and Meyer 1985). 5-HT and PGE2 are ubiquitously present in the body and are released under pathologic conditions. BK is cleaved by enzymatic action from kallidin, a plasma protein. Tissue ischemia is a potent stimulus for inducing this cleavage.

In experiments by the author's group, acidic solutions were effective stimulants for muscle receptors with group IV afferent fibers in the rat. Approximately 60% of the tested receptors were excited by intramuscular injections of an acidic phosphate buffer (pH 6; Fig. 2). Such a lowering in pH is known to occur in inflamed or ischemic tissue. The proton-sensitive nociceptors may be of particular importance for the induction of chronic muscle pain. There is evidence indicating that repeated intramuscular administration of acidic solutions results in long-lasting hyperalgesia (Sluka et al. 2001).

In patients, the pain during ▶ bruxism, chronic ▶ dystonia, and some cases of ▶ tension-type headache may be mediated by the TRPV1 receptor or other acid-sensing ion channels, because these conditions are likely to be associated with low tissue pH and ischemia. Due to the ischemia, BK acting on B2 or B1 receptors could also contribute to this pain. In microneurographic recordings from muscle nerves in humans, muscle no-

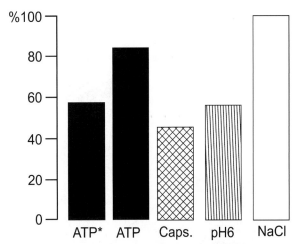

Muscle Nociceptors, Neurochemistry, Figure 2 Proportion of rat muscle nociceptors responding to adenosine triphosphate (ATP), capsaicin (Caps.), acidic phosphate solution (pH 6), and hypertonic saline (NaCl, 5%). The data were obtained in electrophysiological experiments in which the impulses of single group IV afferent fibers from rat muscle were recorded. The stimulating solutions (injection volume 25 μl) were injected intramuscularly into the mechanosensitive receptive field of the ending. ATP*, ATP dissolved in tyrode. The solution had a pH of 5.5. ATP, ATP dissolved in tyrode with the pH adjusted to neutral (7.4). NaCl 5% was the most effective stimulus and activated all of the units tested, the other agents excited at least 40% of the nociceptors (J. Reinöhl, U. Hoheisel and S. Mense, unpublished).

ciceptors with moderate to high mechanical thresholds were found that could be activated by intramuscular injections of capsaicin (Marchettini et al. 1996). The capsaicin injections were associated with strong muscle pain. As capsaicin is assumed to be a specific stimulant for the TRPV1 receptor, these data show that TRPV1 is present in human muscle nociceptors.

Nociceptors of the gastrocnemius muscle in the rat have been shown to respond to ATP in concentrations that are present in muscle cells (Reinöhl et al. 2003). This means that every time a muscle cell is damaged, it releases ATP in amounts that can excite muscle nociceptors. Human muscle nociceptors also appear to be equipped with purinergic receptors, since ATP causes pain when injected i.m (Mörk et al. 2003). In patients, ATP may not only be involved in the pain of muscle trauma, but also in cases of sympathetically maintained pain. The underlying mechanism is that postganglionic sympathetic fibers release ATP as a co-transmitter of norepinephrine.

Among the growth factors studied so far, NGF is of particular interest because data obtained in the author's group indicate that NGF excites nociceptive free nerve endings exclusively, i.e. the low-threshold mechanosensitive (presumably non-nociceptive) endings were not affected. NGF is the only substance known so far that has such an exclusive action on nociceptive free nerve endings. An overview of most of the known receptor molecules in the membrane of a nociceptive ending is given in Fig. 3.

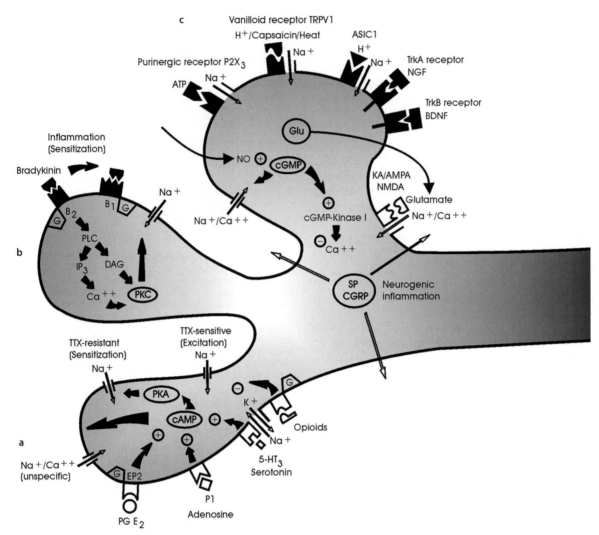

Muscle Nociceptors, Neurochemistry, Figure 3 Receptor molecules in the membrane of a nociceptor. The scheme shows three branches of a free nerve ending. Not all of the receptor molecules included in the figure have been proven to exist in muscle nociceptors, some (e.g. the opioid receptor) are known from studies on nociceptors in the skin. The following processes are of practical importance. Branch (a), sensitization. Sensitization is caused by the binding of sensitizing substances (e.g. prostaglandin E2 (PG E$_2$) or serotonin (5-HT)) to receptor molecules, which induce intracellular cascades of events that~– among other effects – increase the sensitivity of the Na+ channels by phosphorylation (addition of anorganic phosphate to the channel protein) through activated protein kinase A (PKA). Branch (b) , neuroplastic changes of the bradykinin (BKN) receptor. In intact tissue, BKN excites nociceptors by binding to the B2 receptor, in inflamed tissue, it does so by binding to the B1 receptor. Branch (c), other more recently detected receptors. Purinergic receptors (e.g. P2X3) bind adenosine triphosphate (ATP) and its degradation products, and vanilloid receptors (e.g. TRPV1-1) are sensitive to protons (H+), capsaicin, and heat. ASICs are acid-sensing ion channels (e.g ASIC 1) that can be opened by low pH. TrkA is the high-affinity receptor for nerve growth factor (NGF), TrkB for brain derived neurotrophic factor (BDNF). alpha-amino-3-hydroxy-5-methyl-4-isoxazole propionic acid, receptor for glutamate; cAMP, cyclic adenosine monophosphate; cGMP, cyclic guanosin monophosphate; CGRP, calcitonin gene-related peptide; G, Glu, glutamate; G protein; KA, kainic acid; NMDA, N-methyl-D-aspartate, receptor for glutamate; NO, nitric oxide; PKC, protein kinase C; (PLC, IP3, and DAG are steps of the intracellular cascade that leads to the activation of PKC); SP, substance P; TTX, tetrodotoxin.

Interactions between Stimulants at the Receptive Nerve Ending

Interactions between algesic agents have been mainly studied for BK on the one hand, and PGE$_2$ or 5-HT on the other. PGE$_2$ and 5-HT enhance the excitatory action of BK on slowly conducting muscle afferents (Mense 1981). The pain elicited in volunteers by i.m. injection of a combination of BK and 5-HT is likewise stronger than that caused by either stimulant alone (Babenko et al. 1999; Mörk et al. 2003). These interac-

tions are of clinical significance, because the substances are released together in damaged or pathologically altered tissue.

The concentration of PGE$_2$ and 5-HT required for potentiating the action of BK is lower than that for exciting the nociceptors. Therefore, in the course of a tissue inflammation, the receptive endings will first be sensitized and then excited. Clinical observations point in the same direction; in the course of a pathologic alteration, the patient experiences tenderness first (because of nociceptor

Muscle Pain, Fibromyalgia Syndrome (Primary, Secondary),
Table 2 Illnesses Concomitant with Secondary Fibromyalgia Syndrome. With Tests Profile to Characterize the Diagnosis (Russell 1993)*

Illness	Tests
Rheumatic disease	
a. Systemic lupus erythematosus	ANA + ESR or CRP‡
b. Rheumatoid arthritis	RF + ESR or CRP
c. Polymyositis	Creatine phosphokinase
d. Sjögren's syndrome	Labial salivary gland biopsy
Infection/inflammation	
a. Tuberculosis	PPD, ESR, Chest X-ray
b. Chronic syphilis	VDRL, FTA, CSF
c. Subacute bacterial endocarditis	Culture, ESR
d. Lyme disease	Serology
e. Parvovirus	Serology, Change
e. Acquiredimmunodeficiency syndrome	Serology
f. Breast implant	Serology
g. Inflammatory bowel syndromes	Colonoscopy
Endocrine disorders	
a. Hypothyroidism	Thyroxine, TSH
b. Hypopituitary	Prolactin
Obstructive myelopathy	
a. Whiplash C1,2 or subaxial subluxation	CT or MRI of CSpine
b. Chiari malformation	MRI foramen magnum
c. Syringomyelia	MRI of brainstem/Cspine
d. Spinal stenosis	MRI of Cspine

*Adapted with consent
Abbreviations:
ANA=antinuclear antibody; ESR=Westergren erythrocyte sedimentation rate; CRP=C-reactive protein; RF =rheumatoid factor; PPD =purified protein derivative delayed cutaneous test for exposure to tuberculosis bacilli; VDRL =serologic screening test for syphilis; FTA =fluorescent treponemal antibody test for syphilis; CSF =cerebrospinal fluid tests; TSH =thyroid stimulating hormone; C1,2 =cervical spine level 1 and level 2 atlantioaxial; CT =computerized tomography; CSpine =cervical spine; MRI =magnetic resonance tomography

ondary) have elevated spinal fluid (CSF) substance P as an amplifier of afferent pain signals. The distinction seems to be, that only primary FMS patients exhibit elevated concentrations of nerve growth factor as a substance P inducing agent (Giovengo et al. 1999). In secondary FMS, associated with an inflammatory condition, the nerve growth factor levels were found to be normal. The inflammation itself may be responsible for initiating the high CSF substance P levels in those conditions. This concept is important because it provides evidence that there may be a final common pathway (related to the elevated CSF substance P) by which primary FMS and secondary FMS could exhibit the same clinical syndrome (i.e. FMS).

Epidemiology

The FMS exhibits a world-wide distribution. It is viewed as being common, because it affects 2–5 % of the general population. It is female predominant, with 8 of 10 affected individuals being female. It increases in prevalence with age, such that about 10 % of women in the 50–60 years of age decade are affected. About one third of FMS patients are so severely affected by their symptoms that they are unable to maintain their usual occupational activities (Wolfe et al. 1997c). The average annual direct cost of this condition in the United States was estimated to be about $2,250 (Wolfe et al. 1997a). The natural history of FMS is to develop a pattern of severity over a relatively short period of time, and then remain relatively unchanged over a period of many years (Wolfe et al. 1997b). It does not usually become another medical condition like a rheumatic disease.

Comorbidities

In addition to the defining widespread musculoskeletal pain and TePs, people with FMS typically exhibit a constellation of painful symptoms or syndromes that can include insomnia, which occurs in about 70 % (Smythe and Moldofsky 1977), nocturnal myoclonus, cognitive dysfunction, headache, depression in about 40 % (Ahles et al. 1991), anxiety, autonomic neuropathy (Martinez-Lavin 2003), nocturnal bruxism, myofascial pain dysfunction syndrome (the so-called TMJ syndrome), myofascial pain syndrome (particularly involving the piriformis muscles), hypermobility syndrome in about 30 % (Acasuso-Diaz and Collantes-Estevez 1998), biceps tendinitis, pes anserine bursitis, irritable bowel syndrome in about 40 % (Aaron and Buchwald 2001), and irritable bladder syndrome (interstitial cystitis) in about 10 % (Clauw et al. 1997). Despite overlapping features and prevalence, FMS can be distinguished from rheumatic diseases, the complex regional pain syndromes, the chronic fatigue syndrome, and the myofascial pain syndrome affecting a variety of muscles, on the basis of its clinical presentation, its consistent epidemiologic pattern, and its predictable prognosis.

Heterogeneity

How should this heterogeneity of associated manifestations be viewed? Should clinicians caring for FMS patients be lumpers or splitters? It is worthy, in this regard, to consider the established situation with systemic lupus erythematosus (SLE). The ACR supports the concept that 11 diagnostic criteria are important to the clinical diagnosis of SLE, but only four of these criteria are required to diagnose SLE in a given individual (Tan et al. 1982). Lupus subgroups are characterized by their patterns of major organ involvement, critical to the prognosis and management of the disorder (Hughes 1978). For example, in various combinations, about 50 % of SLE patients have renal involvement, 50 % exhibit lung involvement, cardiac involvement is seen in about 40 %, neuropsychiatric manifestations are present in about 60 %, autoimmune hemolysis occurs in about 5 %, and about 30 % have concomitant FMS. The findings from prior psychological studies of FMS, in which two or three distinct clusters (subgroups?) of FMS patients had been identified, were reviewed by Walen and colleagues (Walen et al. 2002). They then conducted extensive evaluations on 600 FMS patients who were members of a health maintenance organization. Cluster analysis on the data from those subjects confirmed the previously described unique clusters of FMS patients that differed from each other with respect to mood disturbance, pain, physical function, and social support. While these subgroup differences were statistically definable, all three subgroups were still much worse than healthy normal controls in the general population.

Electrophysiological assessment methods, such as combinations of quantitative electroencephalography (qEEG) and electromyography (sEMG) have also helped to identify distinct FMS subgroups (Donaldson et al. 2002). Forty patients with FMS, off their usual FMS medications for five half lives, were stratified into three subgroups on the basis of their Symptom Checklist-90-Revised (SCL-90-R) Global Severity Index (GSI) scores (Derogatis 1994). The subgroups were then examined by qEEG activity patterns with the subjects resting, eyes closed. By-subgroup differences in the quantity of the typical qEEG wave forms were found. Across the GSI-defined subgroups, from least to most distressed, alpha brainwave activity (7.5–13 Hertz) progressively decreased, while theta activity (3.5–7.5 Hertz) progressively increased. Beta activity (13 –22 Hertz) was highest in the middle group; while delta activity (0.5–3.5 Hertz) was consistently low across all three subgroups. The addition of sEMG data in this study demonstrated widely dispersed skeletal muscle co-contraction in response to a distant volitional stimulus, but the magnitude of this abnormality did not differ among the three GSI-defined subgroups.

Muscle

The FMS is probably is a central neurological disorder rather than a disorder of skeletal muscle, but there was a time in the history of the disorder when skeletal muscle was the focus of investigation into the pathogenesis of FMS. Indeed, the clinical complaint most consistently reported by FMS patients is deep, aching, body pain. Whether spontaneously, or as learned from their health care providers, FMS patients have tended to interpret these symptoms as muscle pains, muscle fatigue, and muscle stiffness. That may have been what prompted early FMS researchers to seek some specific pathology in affected muscles. Controlled histological examination of FMS muscle tissue sections by light microscopy and electron microscopy have disclosed minor mitochondrial abnormalities, atrophy of type 2 muscle fibers, ragged red fibers, or moth-eaten fibers (Yunus et al. 1989; Lindman et al. 1995), and lower than normal capillary density, but the histological evidence did not support FMS specificity. In addition, lower levels of ATP and phosphoryl creatine were found in the trapezius and the tibialis anterior muscles of FMS patients compared with HNC (Bengtsson et al. 1986). Clearly, skeletal muscle that is at risk could serve as a peripheral pain generator in FMS patients who fail to maintain physical fitness of the very muscle groups needed for usual function, and for critical situations of physiological stress that cause the falling injuries observed to be common among people with FMS.

Biochemistry

Biochemical analysis of fluid samples from patients with FMS has also identified apparent subgroups. For example, 84 % of FMS patients had elevated cerebrospinal fluid levels of substance P (Russell et al. 1994). As noted earlier, patients with "primary" FMS had elevated levels of nerve growth factor not seen in normal controls, or in FMS patients with concomitant rheumatic diseases ("secondary" FMS), or in rheumatic disease patients who do not have FMS (Giovengo et al. 1999). Similarly, blood samples from a subgroup of about 50 % of FMS patients exhibit an antibody to an environmental polymer (Wilson et al. 1999), so the antipolymer antibody assay is being proposed as a way to distinguish these two unique subgroups. A genetic predisposition appears to be a factor in a subgroup of FMS (Iyengar et al. 2003). The current hope is that the findings from objective tests, which are now in active development, can be leveraged to identify pathogenic mechanisms.

Medications

Finally, attempts at diagnostic treatment regimens have disclosed differences in the responses of FMS patients to ketamine, suggesting that the N-methyl-D-aspartic receptor (which ketamine inhibits) in the spinal cord is important to the perceived pain in FMS (Graven-Nielsen et al. 2000). Patient volunteers in one key study (Sorensen et al. 1997) were treated (randomized serial crossover) with brief intravenous infusions of ketamine, morphine sulfate, lidocaine, or saline placebo. Of the 18 FMS patients studied, two patients were placebo responders (responded with improvement to all three agents and the placebo) and three were nonresponders (no improvement with any of the administered agents). The majority (N = 13) responded to one or more of the active medications but not to placebo. Four patients responded to a single drug (morphine-one, ketamine-three), six responded to two drugs (lidocaine and morphine-four, lidocaine and ketamine-two), and three responded to all three active drugs. Since all of the patients were clinically diagnosed as having FMS, this study implies substantial heterogeneity in the response of FMS patients to treatment. It may further help to explain why some patients fail to respond to a clinician's favorite regimen.

From the preceding discussion, it seems likely that the composite of FMS subjects, identified by the 1990 ACR criteria for the classification of FMS (Wolfe et al. 1990), are heterogeneous in several important respects. Walen and colleagues (Walen et al. 2002) concluded their assessment by saying that: "People with FMS may fall into distinct subgroups; . . . (but) the utility of dividing participants into these (sub) groups in planning interventions remains unclear." On the other hand, they also suggest that "the most helpful direction for future research would involve comparing the effects of interventions designed especially for each cluster to a 'nontaylored' intervention." Finally, It always comes back to the hopeful prediction that the better we understand the mechanisms of chronic FMS pain, the more likely we are to find specific and effective therapies.

Pathogenesis

The pathogenesis of FMS is becoming increasingly evident from studies of physiology, pharmacology, neurochemistry, and brain imaging. Available evidence supports the hypothesis that the underlying dysfunction in FMS is within the central nervous system. It is no longer considered to be merely a psychological disorder, a diagnosis to be made by exclusion, or a condition devoid of objective laboratory findings. Patients with FMS exhibit objective abnormalities in ▶ nociception and in neuroendocrine functions, which undoubtedly contribute substantially to their generalized symptoms. Some of the biological participants in this process include: unmyelinated dorsal horn neurons (like A-delta and C-fibers), excitatory amino acids, neuropeptides, zinc, biogenic amines, nitric oxide, wide-dynamic range spinal neurons, the limbic system of the midbrain, and several regions of the cerebral cortex. A lowered pain threshold (ie. allodynia) characterizes the examination findings in FMS. Allodynia can be caused in animal systems by strategic manipulation of nociceptive neurochemicals. Studies of the nociceptive neurochemicals in FMS spinal fluid find them abnormal in concentration and/or correlated with the symptoms. Those observations change the way FMS is viewed, and identify it as a remarkably interesting human syndrome of chronic central neurochemical pain amplification.

Management

Dealing with FMS has been a complicated process for twentieth century medicine, leading to widely conflicting opinions about it. The reasons for the resultant role modeling are buried deep in the fabric of belief system anchoring. Effective contemporary management of FMS requires each of the following (Russell 1996): The unequivocal recognition that pain is always subjective, a willingness to accept FMS as a medical syndrome, the effort to integrate a logical but increasingly complex pathogenesis, and empathetic individualization of increasingly evidence-based therapy. The components of a practical regimen include: accurate diagnosis of the FMS and associated conditions, education about FMS, physical modalities such as exercise, medications for the presenting symptoms, and follow-up assessment to monitor therapeutic progress.

References

1. Aaron LA, Buchwald D (2001) A Review of the Evidence for Overlap among Unexplained Clinical Conditions. Ann Intern Med 134:868–881
2. Acasuso-Diaz M, Collantes-Estevez E (1998) Joint Hypermobility in Patients with Fibromyalgia Syndrome. Arthritis Care Res 11:39–42
3. Ahles TA, Khan SA, Yunus MB et al. (1991) Psychiatric Status of Patients with Primary Fibromyalgia, Patients with Rheumatoid Arthritis, and Subjects without Pain: A Blind Comparison of DSM-III Diagnoses. Am J Psychiat 148:1721–1726
4. Bengtsson A, Henriksson KG, Larsson J (1986) Reduced High Energy Phosphate Levels in the Painful Muscles of Patients with Primary Fibromyalgia. Arthritis Rheum 29:817–821
5. Clauw DJ, Schmidt M, Radulovic D et al. (1997) The Relationship Between Fibromyalgia and Interstitial Cystitis. J Psychiatr Res 31:125–131
6. Derogatis L (1994) SCL-90-R: Administration, Scoring, and Procedures Manual. Clinical Psychometric Research
7. Donaldson M, Donaldson CC, Mueller HH et al. (2002) QEEG Patterns, Psychological Status, and Pain Reports of Fibromyalgia Sufferers. Am J Pain Management (Submitted)
8. Giovengo SL, Russell IJ, Larson AA (1999) Increased Concentrations of Nerve Growth Factor in Cerebrospinal Fluid of Patients with Fibromyalgia. J Rheumatol 26:1564–1569
9. Graven-Nielsen T, Aspregen KS, Henriksson KG et al. (2000) Ketamine Reduces Muscle Pain, Temporal Summation, and Referred Pain in Fibromyalgia Patients. Pain 85:483–491
10. Hughes GRV (1978) Systemic Lupus Erythematosus. In: Scott JT (ed) Copeman's Textbook of the Rheumatic Diseases. T & A Constable Ltd, Edinburgh, pp 901–922
11. Iyengar SK, Arnold LM, Khan MA et al. (2003) Genetic Linkage of Fibromyalgia Syndrome to the Serotonin Receptor 2A Region on Chromosome 13 and the HLA Region on Chromosome 6. In Preparation
12. Lindman R, Hagberg M, Bengtsson A et al. (1995) Capillary Structure and Mitochondrial Volume Density in the Trapezius Muscle of Chronic Trapezius Myalgia, Fibromyalgia and Healthy Subjects. J Musculoske Pain 3:5–22
13. Martinez-Lavin M (2003) Use of the Leeds Assessment of Neuropathic Symptoms and Signs Questionnaire in Patients with Fibromyalgia. Seminars in Arthritis & Rheumatism 32:407–411
14. Russell IJ (1993) A New Journal. J Musculoske Pain 1:1–7
15. Russell IJ (1996) Fibromyalgia Syndrome: Approaches to Management. Bull Rheum Dis 45(3):1–4
16. Russell IJ, Orr MD, Littman B et al. (1994) Elevated Cerebrospinal Levels of Substance P Patients Fibromyalgia Syndrome. Arthritis Rheum 37:1593–1601
17. Smythe HA, Moldofsky H (1977) Two Contributions to Understanding of the "Fibrositis" Syndrome. Bull Rheum Dis 28:928–931
18. Sorensen J, Bengtsson A, Ahlner J et al. (1997) Fibromyalgia – Are there Different Mechanisms in the Processing of Pain?

M

A Double-Blind Crossover Comparison of Analgesic Drugs. J Rheumatol 24:1615–1621

19. Tan EM, Cohen AS, Fries JF et al. (1982) The 1992 Revised Criteria for the Classification of Systemic Lupus Erythematosus. Arthritis Rheum 25:1271–1277

20. Walen HR, Cronan TA, Serber ER et al. (2002) Subgroups of Fibromyalgia Patients: Evidence for Heterogeneity and an Examination of Differential Effects Following a Community-Based Intervention. J Musculoske Pain 10:9–32

21. Wilson RB, Gluck OS, Tesser JR et al. (1999) Antipolymer Antibody Reactivity in a Subset of Patients with Fibromyalgia Correlates with Severity. J Rheumatol 26:402–407

22. Wolfe F, Anderson J, Harkness D et al. (1997a) A Prospective, Longitudinal, Multicenter Study of Service Utilization and Costs in Fibromyalgia. Arthritis Rheum 40:1560–1570

23. Wolfe F, Anderson J, Harkness D et al. (1997b) Health Status and Disease Severity in Fibromyalgia: Results of a Six Center Longitudinal Study. Arthritis Rheum 40:1571–1579

24. Wolfe F, Anderson J, Harkness D et al. (1997c) Work and Disability Status of Persons with Fibromyalgia. J Rheumatol 24:1171–1178

25. Wolfe F, Smythe HA, Yunus MB et al. (1990) The American College of Rheumatology 1990 Criteria for the Classification of Fibromyalgia. Arthritis Rheum 33:160–172

26. Yunus MB, Kalyan-Raman UP, Masi AT et al. (1989) Electron Microscopic Studies of Muscle Biopsy in Primary Fibromyalgia Syndrome: A Controlled and Blinded Study. J Rheumatol 16:97–101

Muscle Pain in Systemic Inflammation (Polymyalgia Rheumatica, Giant Cell Arteritis, Rheumatoid Arthritis)

HENNING BLIDDAL
The Parker Institute, Frederiksberg Hospital, Copenhagen, Denmark
hb@fh.hosp.dk

Synonyms

Arthritogenic Pain; Immuno-Inflammatory Muscle Pain; polymyalgia rheumatica; giant cell arthritis; rheumatoid arthritis

Definition

With the exception of some cases of ► myositis, the inflammatory conditions of joints and muscles have muscle pain as a very prominent symptom. The pain may be caused by changes in the muscles *per se*, including possible referred pain, or be secondary to the inflammatory changes in the joints. Inflammation in both tendon sheaths and tendon insertions may contribute to the condition, which may be quite complex with regard to pain analysis. Due to its frequent involvement, ► giant cell arteritis is often called ► temporal arteritis.

Characteristics

The inflammatory process involves an increased production of ► cytokines e.g. the important pro-inflammatory cytokines TNF-α and Il-1. These cytokines are involved in the pathogenesis of pain (Gotoh et al. 2002) and pain in these conditions is accompanied by tiredness and anemia due to systemic actions of the cytokines as in rheumatoid cachexia (Walsmith and Roubenoff 2002).

In the elderly, it may be very difficult to distinguish between ► rheumatoid arthritis (RA) and ► polymyalgia rheumatica / giant cell arteritis (PMR / GCA) with a possible overlap between the diseases (Lange et al. 2000; Salvarani and Hunder 1999).

PMR / GCA is associated with pain and muscle soreness in the shoulder and head regions. The two diseases have similar symptoms from the muscles but may be distinguished by the finding of vasculitis in a biopsy of the temporal artery in the latter. PMR occurs in the elderly population with an incidence rate of about 0.5 per 10,000 population aged more than 50, while GCA is considerably less frequent, although the incidence may vary over the world.

The muscle pain in PMR / GCA may resemble other conditions in the area and there are no pathognomonic features of the head and ► neck pain with the possible exception of jaw claudication present in about half of the cases (Hall et al. 1983). The diagnosis must be suspected in any person above 50 years of age with unexplained changes in pain patterns in the proximal parts of the upper extremity and to some extent the lower extremity as well. In more than 2 / 3 of the patients, the pain involves the shoulder region as well as headache. The muscles of the shoulder girdle are sore and exhibit exercise intolerance and fatigue. There is often pain at night and decreased range-of-motion of the joints in the affected area. The finding of an elevated erythrocyte sedimentation rate substantiates the diagnosis. The signs of systemic inflammatory action, e.g. light fever, malaise and weight loss may dominate pain as a secondary phenomenon.

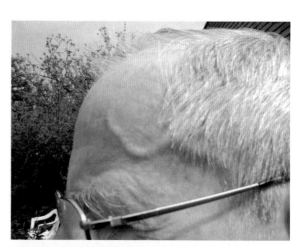

Muscle Pain in Systemic Inflammation (Polymyalgia Rheumatica, Giant Cell Arteritis, Rheumatoid Arthritis), Figure 1 Arteritis temporalis. The artery is abnormally swollen and sore on palpation due to immunoinflammatory changes in the arterial wall. This may eventually lead to obstruction of the lumen and as the process may involve other arteries in the area, including the arteria to the optic nerve, a feared complication is blindness.

Rheumatoid Arthritis (RA)

RA has a prevalence of about 1%, with maximum incidence among the 30–50 year olds and a female / male ratio of 2.5–3. The etiology is unknown, with autoimmune mechanisms involved in the pathogenesis. The disease is most often chronic with fluctuations of disease activity leading to a gradual loss of function. Cardinal symptoms are ▶ morning stiffness of joints, swollen and tender finger joints, symmetrical distribution of arthritis and, depending on severity, joint erosions. The symptoms and signs may differ with the age group. All patients suffer from inflammatory pain in synovial tissues including joints, tendon sheaths and bursae. In the elderly the muscle pain may be very prominent, while all patients have various degrees of muscle fatigue. Some of the medications used for treatment of RA may induce myopathy (Le Quintrec and Le Quintrec 1991). The weakness and the associated activity induced pain in the muscles may not be a primary feature as indicated by the lack of correlation with the muscle strength (Schiottz-Christensen et al. 2001). A specific muscle weakness induced by treatment with ▶ steroids is well described; it is probable, but not fully established, that this may be accompanied by pain (Danneskiold-Samsoe and Grimby 1986). It is possible for patients with RA to train in spite of their joint disease (Bearne et al. 2002; Lyngberg et al. 1994) and exercises to increase muscle strength should be encouraged to maintain general functional abilities.

RA, in 20% of cases, coexists with ▶ Sjögren's syndrome, which, apart from the ▶ sicca-syndrome, is characterized by general muscle pain and fatigue. Myositis may occur in Sjögren's as well and is unrelated to the pain, which is of unknown origin (Lindvall et al. 2002). Finally, RA may – as do other immune-inflammatory diseases - induce a secondary fibromyalgia and the pain quality in the two diseases may be indistinguishable (Burckhardt et al. 1992). In the elderly, an overlap-syndrome exists, with muscle pain in the shoulder region as a common sign between PMR / GCA and RA. In younger women, a similar diagnostic problem arises in the lighter cases of RA, which may resemble fibromyalgia for long periods before a certain diagnosis can be given.

There are aspects of the pain in inflammatory rheumatic diseases, which makes the arthritogenic pain differ from other chronic pain condition.

1. The rheumatic patient is typically well diagnosed with a clear explanation of the pain. Most often the pain correlates with either obvious clinical changes in the joints, e.g. swelling, readily understandable blood tests, e.g. erythrocyte sedimentation rate, ESR or imaging of the inflammatory changes in synovial tissue, e.g. by ultrasound-Doppler or MRI (Terslev et al. 2003). The patients will often have frequent contacts with a specialist, who can reassure them about the nature of the pain. In consequence, unlike other chronic pain conditions, there is less uncertainty associated with the origin or extent of the rheumatic pain.

2. The rheumatic patient has unique possibilities of pain relief by anti-inflammatory agents. The most pronounced effect is the well-documented, almost immediate effect of glucocorticoids in polymyalgia rheumatica (PMR / GCA), which may even be used to substantiate the diagnosis.

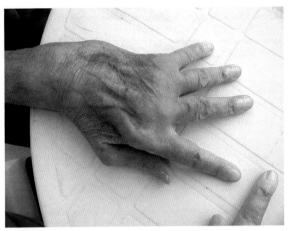

Muscle Pain in Systemic Inflammation (Polymyalgia Rheumatica, Giant Cell Arteritis, Rheumatoid Arthritis), Figure 2 Muscle wasting in rheumatoid arthritis. The inflammation of the joints and the arthritogenic pain affect the whole movement segment with pain-induced muscle wasting. The process is irreversible in cases of joint destruction as in this case where subluxations and ulnar deviation is evident in both wrist joint and fingers.

By such procedures the pain may be explained and even documented to both patients and social contacts, which may save the patients from a deterioration due to an uncertainty of diagnosis, which is otherwise a definite psychological problem in muscle pain of the shoulders (Dyrehag et al. 1998). Nevertheless, the patients with inflammatory diseases may benefit from general therapeutic measures against their pain, including non-medicinal pain management (Evers et al. 2003; Keefe et al. 2001).

Combined muscle and joint pain in a patients involves a number of considerations in internal medicine and in unsettled diagnosis it must be suggested that both clinical examination and blood tests including calcium and thyroid hormones are performed (Table 1).

References

1. Bearne LM, Scott DL, Hurley MV (2002) Exercise can reverse quadriceps sensorimotor dysfunction that is associated with rheumatoid arthritis without exacerbating disease activity. Rheumatology 41:157–166
2. Burckhardt CS, Clark SR, Bennett RM (1992) A comparison of pain perceptions in women with fibromyalgia and rheumatoid arthritis: relationship to depression and pain extent. Arthritis Care Res 5:216–222
3. Danneskiold-Samsoe B, Grimby G (1986) The relationship between the leg muscle strength and physical capacity in patients

M

Muscle Pain in Systemic Inflammation (Polymyalgia Rheumatica, Giant Cell Arteritis, Rheumatoid Arthritis), Table 1   Medical diseases, which may give rise to both joint and muscle pain

Suspected disease	Pain region	Examination
Heart disease	Neck / shoulder / arm	Stethoscopy, EKG
Disease close to diaphragm (e.g. pneumonia, gall-bladder problems)	Neck / shoulder / arm	Stethoscopy, palpation of the abdomen
Thyroid diseases	Diffuse pain in muscles and joints	Palpation of the thyroid –other signs of thyroid disease incl. eye changes
Calcium metabolism	Diffuse pain in muscles and joints	In severe cases, cramps and involuntary muscle contractions

with rheumatoid arthritis, with reference to the influence of corticosteroids. Clin Rheumatol 5:468–474

4. Dyrehag LE, Widerstrom-Noga EG, Carlsson SG et al. (1998) Relations between self-rated musculoskeletal symptoms and signs and psychological distress in chronic neck and shoulder pain. Scand J Rehabil Med 30:235–242
5. Evers AW, Kraaimaat FW, Geenen R et al. (2003) Stress-vulnerability factors as long-term predictors of disease activity in early rheumatoid arthritis. J Psychosom Res 55:293–302
6. Gotoh M, Hamada K, Yamakawa H et al. (2002) Interleukin-[1]-induced glenohumeral synovitis and shoulder pain in rotator cuff diseases. J Orthop Res 20:1365–1371
7. Hall S, Persellin S, Lie JT et al. (1983) The therapeutic impact of temporal artery biopsy. Lancet 2:1217–1220
8. Keefe FJ, Affleck G, Lefebvre J et al. (2001) Living with rheumatoid arthritis: The role of daily spirituality and daily religious and spiritual coping. J Pain 2:101–110
9. Lange U, Piegsa M, Teichmann J et al. (2000) Ultrasonography of the glenohumeral joints –a helpful instrument in differentiation in elderly onset rheumatoid arthritis and polymyalgia rheumatica. Rheumatol Int 19:185–189
10. Le Quintrec JS, Le Quintrec JL (1991) Drug-induced myopathies. Baillieres Clin Rheumatol 5:21–38
11. Lindvall B, Bengtsson A, Ernerudh J et al. (2002) Subclinical myositis is common in primary Sjogren's syndrome and is not related to muscle pain. J Rheumatol 29:717–725
12. Lyngberg KK, Ramsing BU, Nawrocki A et al. (1994) Safe and effective isokinetic knee extension training in rheumatoid arthritis. Arthritis Rheum 37:623–628
13. Salvarani C, Hunder GG (1999) Musculoskeletal manifestations in a population-based cohort of patients with giant cell arteritis. Arthritis Rheum 42:1259–1266
14. Schiottz-Christensen B, Lyngberg K, Keiding N et al. (2001) Use of isokinetic muscle strength as a measure of severity of rheumatoid arthritis: a comparison of this assessment method for RA with other assessment methods for the disease. Clin Rheumatol 20:423–427
15. Terslev L, Torp-Pedersen S, Savnik A et al. (2003) Doppler ultrasound and magnetic resonance imaging of synovial inflammation of the hand in rheumatoid arthritis: a comparative study. Arthritis Rheum 48:2434–2441
16. Walsmith J, Roubenoff R (2002) Cachexia in rheumatoid arthritis. Int J Cardiol 85:89–99

Muscle Pain Model, Inflammatory Agents-Induced

DARRYL T. HAMAMOTO, DONALD A. SIMONE
University of Minnesota, Minneapolis, MN, USA
simon003@umn.edu

Synonyms

Animal Models of Inflammatory Myalgia; Animal Models of Inflammatory Muscle Pain; Nocifensive Behaviors Evoked by Myositis

Definition

Animal models have been recently developed that may allow further elucidation of the underlying mechanisms of pain associated with inflammation of muscle (i.e. ▶ myositis). A better understanding of these mechanisms may lead to the development of novel approaches to treating inflammatory ▶ myalgia (i.e. muscle pain). These animal models also provide methods by which the efficacy and potency of novel pharmacological agents can be examined.

Animal models of inflammatory muscle pain consist of two parts: a method of inducing inflammation in muscle, and a method of evaluating changes in ▶ nocifensive behaviors. Methods of inducing inflammation in muscle include intramuscular injection of substances, such as carrageenan (Kehl et al. 2000), or components of the inflammatory milieu, such as protons (i.e. acidity) (Sluka et al. 2001). Changes in nocifensive behaviors examined by these models are usually described as ▶ hyperalgesia, because they increase the response to stimuli that are normally considered nociceptive. One method of evaluating changes in nocifensive behaviors involves measuring the amount of force that an animal can produce with the inflamed muscle (e.g. ▶ grip force). Another method examines changes in withdrawal responses to controlled mechanical (▶ von Frey monofilaments) stimuli applied to areas of skin, often the hind paw, that are remote from the inflamed muscle.

Characteristics

Protons

Inflammation can result in decreased tissue pH (i.e. acidosis), which activates cutaneous ▶ nociceptors (Steen et al. 1992) and increases withdrawal responses to mechanical stimuli in rats (Hamamoto et al. 2001). In humans, constant infusion of acidic buffer into skin or muscle produces flow-dependent pain that has been shown to correlate with decreased tissue pH, at least

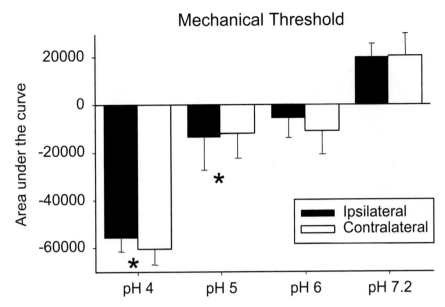

Mechanical Threshold

Muscle Pain Model, Inflammatory Agents-Induced, Figure 1 Decreased mechanical threshold following two injections of acidic saline into the gastrocnemius muscle of one hind limb of a rat. The injections were spaced 2 or 5 days apart. Decrease in the threshold force is expressed as area under the curve for the 6 weeks after the second injection. A significant decrease in mechanical withdrawal threshold occurred bilaterally for rats injected with pH 4 or pH 5 saline, but not for those injected with pH 6 or 7.2. Data are expressed as mean ± SEM, N=8 rats/group, *P < 0.05. Figure modified from Sluka et al. 2001.

in the skin (Steen et al. 1995; Isseberner et al. 1996). Thus, decreased tissue pH may contribute to pain associated with muscle inflammation. Two injections of acidic saline (pH 4.0 – 6.0) administered 2 days apart into the gastrocnemius muscle of one hind limb of a rat, produced cutaneous mechanical hyperalgesia that persisted for up to 4 weeks (Fig. 1) (Sluka et al. 2001). In this model, mechanical hyperalgesia was examined by applying von Frey monofilaments to the plantar surface of the hind paw, a site remote from the site were the acidic saline was injected. The contralateral hind paw also exhibited mechanical hyperalgesia. After mechanical hyperalgesia had developed, neither pharmacological (i.e. intramuscular injection of lidocaine into the site of acidic saline injection) nor physical (i.e. ▶ dorsal rhizotomy) interruption of input from primary afferent innervating the gastrocnemius muscle abolished the contralateral mechanical hyperalgesia. These results suggest that ▶ central sensitization following nociceptive input from muscle may underlie the ▶ secondary hyperalgesia in this model. Interestingly, injection of acidic saline produced histologic evidence of only mild injury and inflammation of the muscle fibers in some rats, which was attributed to the needle penetration and not to the acidic solution. Thus, this model appears to isolate the effects of one component of inflammation, which is tissue acidity. Of interest is the long lasting (i.e. 4 weeks) hyperalgesia produced by two injections of acidic saline. Also, the mechanical hyperalgesia was exhibited in a different tissue (i.e. skin) and at a site remote from the acidified muscle tissue. This pattern of referral from deep structures to remote cutaneous sites has been shown in humans (Marchettini et al. 1990). Thus, this model of acid-induced muscle pain may help to determine the mechanisms by which patients with chronic generalized musculoskeletal pain,

such as fibromyalgia, experience areas of tenderness called tender points (Sluka et al. 2001). This model has subsequently been used to examine the role of excitatory amino acid receptors in the development and maintenance of mechanical hyperalgesia induced by intramuscular injection of acidic saline (Skyba et al. 2002).

Carrageenan

Injection of carrageenan into muscle evokes a localized myositis, as demonstrated by accumulation of leukocytes around the site of injection (Diehl et al. 1988). In electrophysiological studies, injection of carrageenan into muscle sensitizes nociceptors, both increasing their spontaneous activity and lowering their threshold to activation by mechanical stimuli (Berberich et al. 1988; Diehl et al. 1988). Thus, when inflamed muscle is contracted, nociceptors in the muscle would be activated by lower than normal magnitudes of mechanical stimuli. The animal might then react to this nociceptive input by decreasing contraction of the muscle, in order to decrease mechanical activation of muscle nociceptors. This reduction in effort would reduce the force produced by the muscle. Thus, Kehl and colleagues have developed a model of inflammatory muscle pain that involves bilateral injections of carrageenan into the triceps muscles, and examines the grip force produced by the inflamed muscle in rats and mice (Kehl et al. 2000; Wacnik et al. 2003). This appears to be a clinically relevant model, because patients with muscle pain exhibit reduced grip force (Norsdenskiold and Grimby 1993). In this model, grip force is measured using a strain gauge attached to a wire mesh upon which the rodent is allowed to grab with its fore paws (Fig. 2). The rodent is held by the tail and gently pulled until it releases the wire mesh and the maximum force produced by the rodent is

M

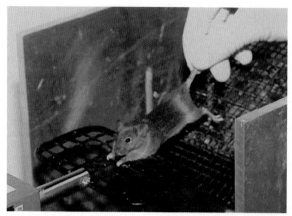

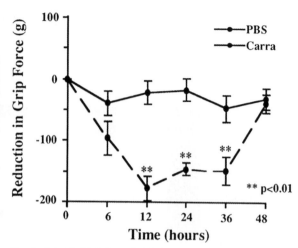

Muscle   Pain   Model,   Inflammatory   Agents-Induced, Figure 2 Measurement of grip force in mice. Mice are positioned and allowed to grasp a wire mesh with their fore paws. Mice are held by the tail and gently moved in a rostral-caudal direction. The wire mesh is attached to a strain gauge and the peak grip force produced by the mouse is determined.

Muscle Pain Model, Inflammatory Agents-Induced, Figure 3 Time-response curve for the reduction in fore limb grip force in rats following injection of carrageenan (4 mg) or an equal volume (75 μl) of PBS into the triceps muscles both fore limbs. Intramuscular carrageenan (Carra) produced a significant treatment- and time-dependent reduction in grip force. Data are expressed as mean ± SEM, N=15 rats/group, **P<0.01. Figure modified from Kehl et al. 2000.

recorded. Grip force is subject to factors, such as hyperalgesia, that influence the behavioral performance of the rodent. Kehl and colleagues have shown that intramuscular injection of carrageenan into the triceps muscle in rodents produces a dose– and time-dependent reduction in grip force (Fig. 3). This reduction in grip force was specific to the inflamed triceps muscles, because the force produced by the hind limbs was not affected. Furthermore, injection of carrageenan into one triceps muscle did not affect the grip force in the contralateral fore limb. Additional support for the clinical relevance of this model of inflammatory muscle pain is the fact that carrageenan-induced reduction in grip force is attenuated by the opioid levorphanol, the nonsteroidal anti-inflammatory drug indomethacin and the steroid dexamethasone. These drugs represent three classes of analgesic agents used clinically to treat muscle pain. Additionally, experimental analgesic agents such as the non-competitive NMDA antagonist MK801 and the cannabinoid agonist WIN 55,212–2 have been shown to have attenuated inflammatory muscle hyperalgesia using this model.

The carrageenan-induced model of muscle pain has several advantages over the model of acidic saline induced hyperalgesia. First, the carrageenan-induced model of muscle pain is a model of pain produced by inflammation in muscle, whereas injection of individual or multiple inflammatory mediators may not be. Second, the carrageenan model is a model of ▶ primary hyperalgesia, because it examines the function of the inflamed muscle. In contrast, models in which the site of hyperalgesia is remote from the site of inflammation or injury are models of secondary hyperalgesia. Third, the grip force assay avoids the potential of misinterpreting drug-induced motor dysfunction or sedation with ▶ antihyperalgesia. Many behavioral assays, such

as paw withdrawal from mechanical or thermal stimuli, are based on the assumption that an animal that withdraws less or withdraws at a higher threshold is exhibiting antihyperalgesia. However, drug-induced motor dysfunction and sedation may produce the same behavioral response. That is, it may take a more intense mechanical or thermal stimulus to elicit a withdrawal response. In contrast, if a drug produces motor dysfunction or sedates an animal then it will produce less grip force, which will not be misinterpreted as antihyperalgesia. Thus, the carrageenan model appears to be useful for further elucidation of the mechanisms associated with inflammatory muscle pain. Furthermore, the grip force assay provides a method by which the analgesic efficacy and potency of novel pharmaceutical agents can be examined in models of inflammatory muscle pain.

References

1. Berberich P, Hoheisel U, Mense S (1988) Effects of a Carrageenan-Induced Myositis on the Discharge Properties of Group III and IV Muscle Receptors in the Cat. J Neurophysiol 59:1395–1409
2. Diehl B, Hoheisel U, Mense S (1988) Histological and Neurophysiological Changes Induced by Carrageenan in Skeletal Muscle of Cat and Rat. Agents Actions 25:210–213
3. Hamamoto DT, Ortiz-Gonzalez XR, Honda JM, Kajander KC (2001) Intraplantar Injection of Hyaluronic Acid at Low pH into the Rat Hindpaw Produces Tissue Acidosis and Enhances Withdrawal Responses to Mechanical Stimuli. Pain 74:225–234
4. Issberner U, Reeh PW, Steen KH (1996) Pain due to Tissue Acidosis: A Mechanism for Inflammatory and Ischemic Myalgia? Neurosci Lett 208:191–194
5. Kehl LJ, Trempe TM, Hargreaves KM (2000) A New Animal Model for Assessing Mechanisms and Management of Muscle Hyperalgesia. Pain 85: 333–343

6. Marchettini P, Cline M, Ochoa J (1990) Innervation Territories for Touch and Pain Afferents of Single Fascicles of the Human Ulnar Nerve. Brain 113:1491–1500
7. Norsdenskiold UM, Grimby, G (1993) Grip Force in Patients with Rheumatoid Arthritis and Fibromyalgia and in Healthy Subjects: A Study with the Grippit Instrument. Scand J Rheumatol 22:14–19
8. Skyba DA, King EW, Sluka KA (2002) Effects of NMDA and Non-NMDA Ionotropic Glutamate Receptor Antagonists on the Development and Maintenance of Hyperalgesia Induced by Repeated Intramuscular Injection of Acidic Saline. Pain 98:69–78
9. Sluka KA, Kalra A, Moore SA (2001) Unilateral Intramuscular Injections of Acidic Saline Produce a Bilateral, Long-Lasting Hyperalgesia. Muscle Nerve 24:37–46
10. Steen KH, Reeh PW, Anton F, Handwerker HO (1992) Protons Selectively Induce Lasting Excitation and Sensitization to Mechanical Stimulation of Nociceptors in Rat Skin, In Vitro. J Neurosci 12:86–95
11. Steen KH, Issberner U, Reeh PW (1995) Pain due to Experimental Acidosis in Human Skin: Evidence for Non-Adapting Nociceptor Excitation. Neurosci Lett 199:29–32
12. Wacnik PW, Kehl LJ, Trempe TM, Ramnaraine ML, Beitz AJ, Wilcox GL (2003) Tumor Implantation in Mouse Humerus Evokes Movement-Related Hyperalgesia Exceeding that Evoked by Intramuscular Carrageenan. Pain 101:175–186

Muscle Pain Model, Ischemia-Induced and Hypertonic Saline-Induced

Siegfried Mense
Institute of Anatomy and Cell Biology III, University Heidelberg, Heidelberg, Germany
mense@urz.uni-heidelberg.de

Synonyms

Ischemia-induced muscle pain: Ischemic muscle pain

Definitions

Ischemia-induced muscle pain: muscle pain during and following muscle exercise under ischemic conditions. In clinical studies, ischemic conditions were induced by occlusion of blood vessels of an entire limb (e.g. by a tourniquet, or by administration of adrenalin to study pain mechanisms in the tooth pulp). In animal experiments, the blood flow was interrupted by occlusion of arteries using a ligature or clamp, by a tourniquet around the tail or by circulatory arrest.

Hypertonic saline-induced pain: muscle pain induced by intramuscular or intraarterial (into the muscle artery) injection of hypertonic saline (NaCl) at a concentration of 5–10% (5.6–11.1 times hypertonic).

Characteristics

Ischemia-Induced Pain

Data from clinical studies and animal experiments indicate that ischemia alone (without muscle contractions) is not an effective stimulus for muscle nociceptors. In clinical studies where a tourniquet was used to induce ischemia in a limb, the pain that occurred after approximately half an hour appeared to be mostly due to the pressure exerted on the nerve by the tourniquet, and not by the ischemia.

Clinical Findings and Results from Studies on Human Subjects

One of the clinically important types of ischemic muscle pain is the pain of ▶ intermittent claudication. It occurs during walking in patients with sclerotic narrowing of the arteries of the lower leg and foot. In earlier clinical studies, a multitude of factors were discussed as being the cause of the pain, e.g. chemical metabolites, accumulation of potassium ions (K^+), and reduced pH due to release of lactic acid. Lactic acid was soon ruled out, because patients with McArdle's disease – who are unable to produce lactic acid due to a gene defect – often present with pain of intermittent claudication or angina pectoris. Another candidate substance was the nonapeptide bradykinin (BKN) that is cleaved by kallikrein – a proteinase – from plasma proteins. The importance of BKN for the pain of intermittent claudication was supported by the finding that administration of a proteinase inhibitor in claudication patients extended the distance the patients were able to walk without pain (Digiesi et al. 1975). Electron microscopic investigations of bioptic material of claudication patients showed that the muscle exhibited signs of inflammation with infiltration by inflammatory cells and muscle fiber necrosis. The latter finding adds adenosine triphosphate (ATP) to the list of candidate substances, because muscle cells contain high concentrations of ATP, which are released into the interstitial space when a muscle fiber is damaged (see below).

Data from Animal Experiments

The results obtained from animal studies indicate that the following agents or factors may be involved in ischemic pain:

1. Potassium ions. The potassium concentration is increased in muscles of experimental animals following contractions with and without occlusion of the blood supply.
2. Proton concentration (pH). The interstitial pH is lowered to approximately 6.5 during prolonged ischemia plus exercise.
3. Kinins such as BKN and kallidin. The kinin-forming activity of muscle tissue is increased after prolonged ischemia.
4. Degeneration and necrosis of muscle fibers. If necrosis is present in a chronically ischemic muscle, the ATP concentrations released from the muscle cells are sufficient to activate muscle nociceptors (Reinöhl et al. 2003).

Electrophysiological recordings from single muscle afferent fibers have shown that in skeletal muscle of cat and rat, receptive endings are present that respond specifically to ischemic contractions, in that they are not excited

M

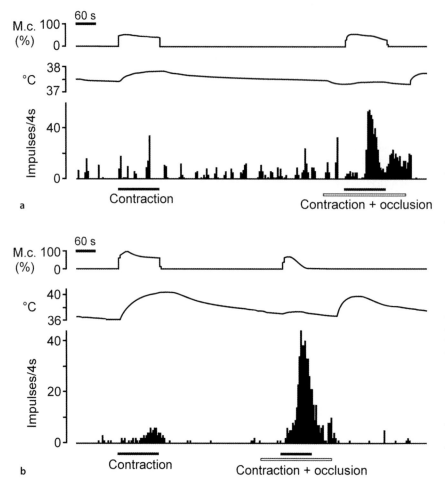

Muscle Pain Model, Ischemia-Induced and Hypertonic Saline-Induced, Figure 1 Impulse activity of single cat muscle receptors with unmyelinated afferent fibers showing exclusive or predominant activation during ischemic contractions. In both panels, the upper trace indicates the force of the contraction of the gastrocnemius-soleus muscle in percent of maximal contraction (M.c.) induced by electrical stimulation of the muscle nerve, the middle trace shows the temperature inside the muscle, and the lower trace is a histogram of the fiber's activity (bin width 4s). Periods of contractions are marked by filled bars underneath the abscissa; occlusion of the muscle artery is marked by open bars. In (a), the force of contraction was adjusted to approximately 50% M.c., and in (b) to 100%. Under the latter condition, the muscle could not maintain the contraction force during occlusion of the muscle artery. Note that in both panels the discharge frequency drops markedly at the end of the contraction period. This indicates that in addition to chemical factors a mechanical component is involved in the activation of the receptors during ischemic contractions. From Mense and Stahnke 1983.

by short-lasting ischemia alone but require ischemia plus contractions for activation (Bessou and Laporte 1958; Mense and Stahnke 1983; Fig 1). This behavior was interpreted as indicating that the units were nociceptors and may mediate the pain of intermittent claudication, but other authors emphasized a possible function in the adjustment of respiration and circulation to the requirements during muscle work (Kaufman et al. 1984).

What Factors Cause the Pain of Intermittent Claudication?

The available data suggest that it is not a single factor that is responsible for ischemic muscle pain but that several stimuli act in combination. Recent findings regarding receptor molecules that are present in the membrane of nociceptors suggest that the following agents could be involved in the induction of ischemic pain:

1. BKN acting on the B2 ▶ bradykinin receptors (unless the nociceptor is sensitized, then BKN stimulates the ending by binding to the B1 receptor).
2. the low pH in an ischemic muscle is likely to sensitize the vanilloid receptor subtype VR 1 (now called ▶ TRPV1), and to activate other acid sensing ion channels (ASICs) (Immke and McCleskey 2003;

for a review on ASICs as channels mediating the pain of angina pectoris, see Sutherland et al. 2000). ▶ Capsaicin is assumed to be a specific ligand for the VR 1 receptor. The fact that intramuscular injection of capsaicin causes strong pain in humans by exciting group IV units (Marchettini et al. 1996) indicates that VR 1 receptors are present in human skeletal muscle.
3. as muscle fibers of claudication patients exhibit necrosis, another likely factor for the activation of muscle nociceptors is ATP, which binds to ▶ purinergic receptors (e.g. the P2X3 receptor) (Burnstock 2000) and activates muscle group IV nociceptors in concentrations that are present in muscle fibers (Reinöhl et al. 2003).

In conclusion, a possible mechanism of activation of muscle nociceptors, in a muscle that contracts under acute ischemic conditions, is that first, BKN or low pH sensitize the ▶ high-threshold mechanosensitive muscle receptors (putative nociceptors) (Mense and Meyer 1985), and subsequently, in the sensitized state, nociceptors are activated by the mechanical force of the contractions. Such a mechanism is suggested by the time

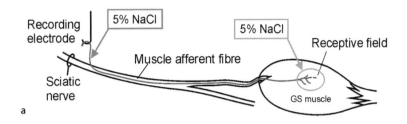

High-threshold
mechanosensitive
group IV unit from
muscle responding to
5% saline

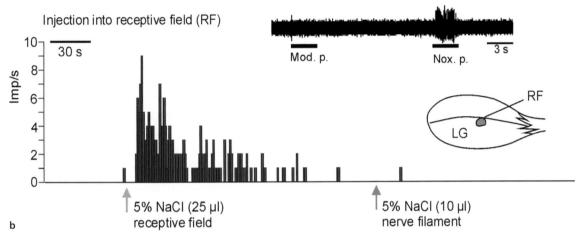

Muscle Pain Model, Ischemia-Induced and Hypertonic Saline-Induced, Figure 2 Effects of hypertonic saline on a single high-threshold mechanosensitive (presumably nociceptive) group IV afferent fiber from rat gastrocnemius-soleus (GS) muscle. (a) Experimental set-up. The impulse activity of a single unmyelinated afferent fiber was recorded from a thin nerve filament dissected from the sciatic nerve. (b) Response of the unit to 5% NaCl injected into that region of the muscle where the receptive ending was located with mechanical stimuli (receptive field, RF). The same NaCl solution that had evoked the strong response when injected i.m. was later put on the nerve filament to show that the axonal membrane was not the site of action of the hypertonic saline. Inset: original recording showing the high mechanical threshold of the receptive ending. Mod.p., moderate, innocuous pressure; Nox.p., noxious, painful pressure.

course of activation of the single group IV unit shown in Figure 1a: the unit was not activated by ischemia or contractions alone, but gave a strong response during ischemic contractions. Moreover, the activity dropped markedly when the contractions were discontinued but the ischemia maintained. The unit in Figure 1b was weakly activated at the end of the contraction period without ischemia (in this case the force of contraction was higher: close to 100% maximal voluntary contraction), but likewise showed a much stronger excitation when the contractions were repeated with the muscle artery occluded.

The release of ATP from damaged muscle fibers appears to occur more under chronic ischemic conditions, but ATP might also be involved in cases of acute ischemic pain, because ATP is a product of any ▶ anaerobic glycolysis (Sutherland et al. 2000).

Hypertonic Saline-Induced Muscle Pain

Studies in human subjects . There are few conditions in which muscle pain is induced by hypertonicity of the tissue in patients. Abscess formation is one of them (Schade 1924), but most cases of myositis

do not exhibit abscesses. In clinical studies, hypertonic saline has been extensively used to induce pain in human subjects. One of the pioneers in this field was Kellgren, who induced pain in muscles and ligaments of volunteers by injecting 0.1 to 0.3 ml of 6% NaCl (Kellgren 1938). Presently, several groups inject or infuse hypertonic NaCl (5–10%) into muscles in healthy subjects and patients to study the mechanisms of muscle pain in humans. With this method, muscle pain of moderate to strong intensity (values around 7 on a VAS with a range from 1 to 10) can be induced. The injected volume is of importance, because the innervation density of muscle with nociceptors is low. Therefore, small injection volumes are likely to yield variable or ill-reproducible pain responses. The results obtained with intramuscular injections of hypertonic saline, suggest that the receptor population mediating ischemia-induced muscle pain is distinct from that mediating hypertonic saline-induced pain (Graven-Nielsen et al. 2003). In human subjects, hypertonic saline appears to excite predominantly group IV muscle afferent units (as opposed to group III units).

Data from animal experiments . Many authors who recorded the activity of single muscle nociceptors used injections of hypertonic saline for receptor activation. Interestingly, 5% NaCl proved to be the only chemical stimulus that excited all of the nociceptors tested, in a recent study (Hoheisel and Mense, unpublished) (Fig. 2) in which the stimulants were injected into the mechanosensitive receptive field of rat group IV receptors. The other agents excited only a fraction of the receptors.

Mechanisms of Nociceptor Activation by Hypertonic Saline

The mechanisms by which muscle nociceptors are excited by hypertonic saline are obscure. Several possibilities exist (for an overview see Kress and Reeh 1996):

1. activation by increased tonicity in the interstitial space. The receptive ending might shrink in the hypertonic environment, and stretch-sensitive Na^+–channels could be opened. However, nothing is known about the water permeability of nociceptive endings, and the high mechanical stimulation threshold of muscle nociceptors speaks against this mechanism.

2. activation by ionic changes. The high Na^+ concentration in the interstitial fluid should have only little influence on the membrane potential of the nociceptive ending, because the Na^+ conductance of an axon is normally low. However, there is evidence indicating that the Na^+ conductance of receptive endings is higher, and therefore the high extracellular Na^+ concentration could cause an effective depolarization with ensuing excitation of the ending. Thus, the high Na^+ concentration could be the decisive factor for hypertonic saline-induced muscle pain. The high Cl^- concentration appears not to be a stimulus, because in peripheral nerve fibers Cl^- channels are rare. An additional unknown factor is that – if shrinking of the ending occurs – the intraaxonal concentrations of all ions increase to an unknown extent.

3. indirect activation of the nociceptor by other algesic agents released from muscle tissue or the nociceptive ending itself. The injection of hypertonic saline has been reported to release glutamate from muscle tissue (Tegeder et al. 2002). Glutamate excites muscle nociceptors and causes muscle pain in humans (Svensson et al. 2003). Hypertonic solutions have also been shown to release substance P from airway sensory cells *in vitro* (Garland et al. 1995).

References

1. Bessou P, Laporte Y (1958) Activation des Fibres Afférentes Amyéliniques d'Origine Musculaire. Compt Rend Soc Biol (Paris) 152:1587–1590
2. Burnstock G (2000) P2X Receptors in Sensory Neurones Br J Anaesth 84:476–488
3. Digiesi V, Bartoli V, Dorigo B (1975) Effect of a Proteinase Inhibitor on Intermittent Claudication or on Pain at Rest in Patients with Peripheral Arterial Disease. Pain 1:385–389
4. Garland A, Jordan JE, Necheles J, Alger LE, Scully MM, Miller RJ, Ray DW, White SR, Solway J (1995) Hypertonicity, but not Hyperthermia, Elicits Substance P Release from Rat C-Fiber Neurons in Primary Culture. J Clin Invest 95:2359–2366
5. Graven-Nielsen T, Jansson Y, Segerdahl M, Kristensen JD, Mense S, Arendt-Nielsen L, Sollevi A (2003) Experimental Pain by Ischaemic Contractions Compared with Pain by Intramuscular Infusions of Adenosine and Hypertonic Saline. Eur J Pain 7:93–102
6. Immke DC, McCleskey EW (2003) Protons Open Acid-Sensing Ion Channels by Catalyzing Relief of $Ca2^+$ Blockade. Neuron 37:75–84
7. Kaufman MP, Rybicki KJ, Waldrop TG, Ordway GA (1984) Effect of Ischemia on Responses of Group III and IV Afferents to Contraction. J Appl Physiol 57:644–650
8. Kellgren JH (1938) Observations on Referred Pain Arising from Muscle. Clin Sci 3:175–190
9. Kress M, Reeh P (1996). Chemical Excitation and Sensitization in Nociceptors. In: Belmonte C, Cervero F (eds) Neurobiology of Nociceptors. Oxford University Press, Oxford, pp 259–297
10. Marchettini P, Simone DA, Caputi G, Ochoa JL (1996) Pain from Excitation of Identified Muscle Nociceptors in Humans. Brain Res 40:109–116
11. Mense S, Stahnke M (1983) Responses in Muscle Afferent Fibres of Slow Conduction Velocity to Contractions and Ischaemia in the Cat. J Physiol 342:383–397
12. Mense S Meyer H (1985) Different Types of Slowly Conducting Afferent Units in Cat Skeletal Muscle and Tendon. J Physiol 363:403–417
13. Reinöhl J, Hoheisel U, Unger T, Mense S (2003) Adenosine Triphosphate as a Stimulant for Nociceptive and Non-Nociceptive Muscle Group IV Receptors in the Rat. Neurosci Lett 338:25–28
14. Schade H (1924) Die Molekularpathologie in ihrem Verhältnis zur Zellularpathologie und zum klinischen Krankheitsbild am Beispiel der Entzündung. Münch Med Woschr 71:1–4
15. Sutherland SP, Cook SP, McCleskey EW (2000) Chemical Mediators of Pain due to Tissue Damage and Ischemia. Prog Brain Res 129:21–38
16. Svensson P, Cairns BE, Wang K, Hu JW, Graven-Nielsen T, Arendt-Nielsen L, Sessle BJ (2003) Glutamate-Evoked Pain and Mechanical Allodynia in the Human Masseter Muscle. Pain 101:221–227
17. Tegeder L, Zimmermann J, Meller ST, Geisslinger G (2002) Release of Algesic Substances in Human Experimental Muscle Pain. Inflamm Res 51:393–402

Muscle Pain, Referred Pain

MARIA ADELE GIAMBERARDINO
Department of Medicine and Science of Aging, G. D'Annunzio University of Chieti, Chieti Scalo, Italy
mag@unich.it

Synonyms

Musculoskeletal Transferred Pain; referred muscle pain

Definition

Pain perceived at muscle level due to a primary algogenic process located at a distance, either in a visceral organ or in a deep somatic structure.

Characteristics

Referred muscle pain can result from an algogenic process in internal organs or in deep somatic structures,

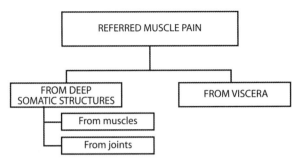

Muscle Pain, Referred Pain, Figure 1 Classification of referred muscle pain.

e.g., another muscle or a joint (referred muscle pain from viscera or from deep somatic structures) (Fig. 1). In both cases, it may or may not be accompanied by secondary hyperalgesia, i.e. increased local sensitivity to pain / decreased pain threshold (referred muscle pain with or without hyperalgesia) (Vecchiet et al. 1999). When present, hyperalgesia is proportional in extent to the degree of activity of the primary algogenic focus and is often accompanied by local trophic changes, i.e. decreased thickness / sectional area of the muscle (Galletti et al. 1990; Giamberardino 2000; Simons and Mense 2003; Vecchiet et al. 1991). Both central (neuronal sensitization) and peripheral (reflex arc activation) mechanisms are likely to be involved in the pathophysiology of referred phenomena at muscle level (Arendt-Nielsen and Svensson 2001; Cervero and Laird 2004; Mense 1994; Procacci et al. 1986).

Referred Muscle Pain from Viscera

Pain referral occurs constantly in visceral nociception (Cervero and Laird 2004). After the transitory phase of "true visceral pain" (midline, vague and poorly defined), the sensation is "transferred" to somatic areas neuromerically connected to the specific viscus (Procacci et al. 1986). Secondary hyperalgesia most often arises at this level, especially if pain episodes are recurrent and / or prolonged; this may involve all three body wall tissues – skin, subcutis and muscle – but is most frequently confined to muscle, often accompanied by sustained contraction (referred muscle pain from viscera without and with hyperalgesia) (Vecchiet et al. 1989). Trophic changes may also occur in the same sites, i.e. increased thickness of subcutis but mostly decreased thickness of muscle (Procacci et al. 1986; Vecchiet et al. 1989). In patients with algogenic conditions from a number of internal organs, muscle hyperalgesia in referred zones has been detected clinically (hypersensitivity to digital compression) and quantified instrumentally (decrease in pain thresholds to different stimuli); in a minor percentage of visceral pain patients, muscle trophic changes have also been measured, using ultrasounds (Giamberardino et al. 1997; Giamberardino et al. 2005; Vecchiet et al. 1989).

Hyperalgesia is accentuated by the repetition of the visceral episodes; although decreasing as they stop, it usually remains significant after cessation of the spontaneous pain and sometimes even after removal of the primary visceral focus. Trophic changes are even more persistent than the hyperalgesia, often remaining unaltered for a long time after extinction of the visceral trigger (Giamberardino et al. 2005).

Clinical Examples

In myocardial infarction, pain is referred to the thoracic region, anteriorly or posteriorly, often extending to the left arm. Hyperalgesia almost always affects the pectoralis major and muscles of the interscapular region and forearm. Trapezius and deltoid muscles are less frequently involved. Dystrophic muscle changes may also occur at the same level. In a low percentage of cases, pain is also referred to the skin, within dermatomes C8-T1 on the ulnar side of the arm and forearm and hyperalgesia is found at the same level (Giamberardino 2000; Procacci et al. 1986). In urinary colics from calculosis, referred pain is perceived in the lumbar region of the affected side, with radiation towards the ipsilateral flank and anteriorly towards the groin. Hyperalgesia and trophic changes characteristically affect muscles of the lumbar and flank area (quadratus lumborum, oblique muscles) (Vecchiet et al. 1989). In biliary calculosis, pain is referred to the upper right quadrant of the abdomen with radiation towards the back. Hyperalgesia and reduced trophism of the rectus abdominis at the cystic point (junction of 10th rib with outer margin of the same muscle) are typical findings (Giamberardino et al. 2005). In dysmenorrhea, pain is referred to the lower abdomen, perineum and sacral region, with radiation towards the groin and upper part of the thighs. Hyperalgesia and trophic changes can be detected in the lowest part of the rectus abdominis and muscles of the pelvic region (Giamberardino et al. 1997).

Referred muscle pain and hyperalgesia are typically enhanced in the case of "viscero-visceral hyperalgesia", when concurrent algogenic conditions affect two viscera which share part of their central sensory projection (Giamberardino 2000). Women suffering from both dysmenorrhea and irritable bowel syndrome (IBS) (common projection for uterus and colon, T10-L1), for instance, frequently report more menstrual pain, intestinal pain and abdominal / pelvic muscle hyperalgesia (in areas of referral from uterus and intestine) than women with dysmenorrhea or IBS only (unpublished observation). Patients with dysmenorrhea / endometriosis plus urinary calculosis (common projection for uterus and upper urinary tract, T10-L1) present with more menstrual pain, urinary colic pain and abdomino-pelvic / lumbar muscle hyperalgesia (in areas of referred pain from uterus and urinary tract) than patients with one condition only (Giamberardino

M

et al. 2001). The phenomenon of "viscero-visceral hyperalgesia" has therapeutic implications. In fact, effective treatment of one condition may significantly improve typical symptoms from the other, e.g. decrease in urinary pain and referred lumbar hyperalgesia after hormonal treatment of dysmenorrhea or decrease in menstrual pain and referred abdomino-pelvic hyperalgesia after urinary stone elimination following lithotripsy (Giamberardino 2000; Giamberardino et al. 2001).

Pathophysiology

"Referred muscle pain from viscera without hyperalgesia" is explained on the basis of the convergence of visceral and somatic afferent fibers upon the same central neurons (convergence-projection theory) (Cervero and Laird 2004; Procacci et al. 1986). Messages from the viscus are "interpreted" by higher brain centers as coming from muscles due to mnemonic traces of previous experiences of somatic pain, more numerous than those of visceral pain in life. "Referred muscle pain from viscera with hyperalgesia" is contributed to by central mechanisms, i.e. a process of sensitization in the central nervous system (CNS), triggered by the massive afferent visceral barrage involving hyperactivity and hyperexcitability of viscero-somatic convergent neurons, as shown by the results of electrophysiological studies on animal models of referred muscle hyperalgesia from viscera (Cervero and Laird 2004; Giamberardino 2000). This process would facilitate the central effect of the normal input coming from the muscle (convergence-facilitation theory). NMDA receptors have been suggested to play an important role in the generation of these central hyperexcitability changes (Cervero and Laird 2004).

In addition to central changes, the afferent visceral barrage probably activates a number of viscero-somatic reflex arcs, whose afferent branch is represented by sensory fibers from the internal organ and whose efferent branch is represented by sympathetic efferences to the skin / subcutis and somatic efferences to the muscle of the referred area (Procacci et al. 1986). Activation of this arc would produce sustained contraction in the skeletal muscle, this, in turn, being responsible for sensitization of nociceptors locally. Studies in a rat model of referred muscle hyperalgesia from artificial ureteric calculosis provide experimental support for this mechanism. Positivity was found for a number of ultrastructural indices of contraction in the hyperalgesic muscle ipsilateral to the affected ureter at lumbar level but not in the contralateral, non-hyperalgesic muscle and the extent of these indices was proportional to the degree of visceral pain behavior and referred hyperalgesia recorded in the animals. In the same model, c-Fos activation was found in the spinal cord not only in sensory neurons but also motoneurons, significantly more on the affected side (refs. in Giamberardino et al. 2005).

Mechanisms underlying enhancement of referred phenomena in "viscero-visceral hyperalgesia" are still hypothetical, but probably involve sensitization of viscero-viscero-somatic convergent neurons. Along with the well-documented viscero-somatic convergence onto the same sensory neurons, extensive viscero-visceral convergence has also been found in the CNS, for instance between the colon / rectum, bladder, vagina and uterine cervix (refs. in Vecchiet et al. 1999). The increased afferent barrage from one visceral organ would thus enhance the afferent signal from the second organ projecting to the same neuron and also from the referred area. This hypothesis needs to be verified in electrophysiological studies on animal models of the condition, such as the model of endometriosis plus ureteral calculosis in the female rat in which an enhancement is observed of both spontaneous pain behavior and referred lumbar muscle hyperalgesia (Giamberardino 2000).

Referred Muscle Pain from Deep Somatic Structures

Clinical Examples

Myofascial pain syndromes (MPSs) are classical examples of "referred muscle pain from muscles". An MPS is characterized by regional muscle pain and dysfunction due to the presence, in muscles or their fascia, of active trigger points (TrPs). A trigger point is a site of tissue hyperirritability included in a taut, palpable band of muscle fibers. When stimulated, it gives rise to pain not only locally, but also at a distance, in an area called "target" because it is often remote from its location (Simons and Mense 2003). The target zone (area of referred pain) is typical and characteristic for each muscle and is the site not only of spontaneous pain, but also of sensory changes. These consist of hyperalgesia, which is a function of the degree of hyperirritability of the trigger point, i.e. the more irritable the TrP, the greater the degree of hyperalgesia in the target and the greater the extension of the tissues involved. Latent trigger points (pre-clinical phase of MPSs) only give rise to muscle hyperalgesia in the target, while active TrPs give rise to hyperalgesia, which extends from the muscle to the overlying subcutaneous / cutaneous tissues also. The dependence of these changes on the presence of the TrPs is testified by their regression after the TrP is extinguished through local infiltration (Vecchiet et al. 1991).

A typical example of "referred muscle pain from joints" is represented by the painful symptomatology in patients with osteoarthritis of the knee (Vecchiet et al. 1999). Pain from this condition is deep, fairly well localized and of varying intensity, sometimes making walking difficult. It spreads upward to the lower part of the thigh and downward as far as the middle of the calf. It begins when walking, increases as walking continues and decreases at rest. The skin appears pale and hypothermic to touch in an area covering the anterior surface of the knee. The underlying subcutis is tender and thickened at pincer palpation; the skeletal muscles connected to the joint are tender and tense. Pain thresholds to electrical stimulation of all three tissues of the parietal wall (but mostly the muscle) in the painful area are decreased (hyperalgesia). The sectional area of periarticular muscles (mostly the vastus medialis), measured *via* ultrasounds, is reduced. The sensory changes in the referred area are reversible when the intraarticular focus is extinguished, testifying their referred nature (Galletti et al. 1990).

Patients with osteoarthritis of the knee have also been shown to present increased pain intensity and larger referred and radiating pain areas after infusion of hypertonic saline into the leg muscles (tibialis anterior) as compared to controls, a finding suggesting the setting up of central sensitization by painful osteoarthritis (Bajaj et al. 2001).

Pathophysiology

As deducible from the two clinical examples provided (MPS and osteoarthritis), referred muscle pain from somatic structures is almost exclusively of the type "referred with hyperalgesia" Similar to what has been described for visceral nociception, referred pain from somatic structures has been attributed mainly to phenomena of central hyperexcitability triggered by the primary algogenic focus (Arendt-Nielsen and Svensson 2001). Animal studies have indeed provided good evidence that dorsal horn neurons become hyperexcitable in response to noxious stimulation of deep tissues (and that NMDA receptors and neurokinin receptors are most probably involved in this mechanism) (Hoheisel et al. 1993; Mense 1994). To account for the phenomenon of referral, however, central hyperexcitability should involve neurons receiving convergent input from the site of injury and the referred zone, whereas it is known that in dorsal horn neurons there is little convergence from deep tissues (Mense 1994). Thus, referred pain from somatic structures is not easily explained by the "convergence-facilitation" theory in its original form. A modified theory has therefore been suggested, especially for referred pain from one muscle to another, based on animal studies. Recordings from dorsal horn neurons reveal that noxious stimuli to a specific receptive field in a muscle generate within minutes new muscle receptive fields at a distance from the original one (Hoheisel et al. 1993). On this basis, the explanation proposed is that convergent connections from deep tissues to dorsal horn neurons are not present from the beginning, but are opened by nociceptive input from skeletal muscle. Referral to myotomes outside the lesion is due to spread of central sensitization to adjacent spinal segments (Mense 1994). Central mechanisms alone, however, are not adequate to account for all referred phenomena, especially the trophic changes. Thus, like the hypothesis for visceral nociception, it has been suggested that the afferent barrage from the deep focus (in muscle or joint) triggers the activation of reflex arcs towards the periphery (area of referral)

via both somatic (towards the muscle) and sympathetic (towards subcutis and skin) efferent fibers, responsible for the local referred changes (Vecchiet et al. 1999).

Diagnosing Referred Muscle Pain

Detection and interpretation of simple referred pain (without hyperalgesia) are relatively easy, as the absence of tenderness at the site of the symptom immediately points out a site of origin of the algogenic impulses at a distance. Correct diagnosis of referred muscle pain with hyperalgesia is, however, much more difficult and represents a major clinical problem, since this form is far more frequent than that of simple referred pain. The problem concerns differentiation from primary muscle pain, i.e. that arising in relation to an algogenic pathology primarily affecting the tissue. Only careful study of the clinical history, accurate physical examination and complete sensory evaluation of the painful areas can help towards diagnostic orientation, an indispensable step in the institution of a therapeutic strategy that is not merely symptomatic (Vecchiet et al. 1999).

References

1. Arendt-Nilesen L, Svensson P (2001) Referred Muscle Pain: Basic and Clinical Findings. Clin J Pain 17:11–19
2. Bajaj P, Bajaj P, Graven-Nielsen T et al. (2001) Osteoarthritis and its association with muscle hyperalgesia: an experimental controlled study. Pain 93:107–114
3. Cervero F, Laird JM (2004) Understanding the signaling and transmission of visceral nociceptive events. J Neurobiol 61:45–54
4. Galletti R, Obletter M, Giamberardino MA et al. (1990) Pain from osteoarthritis of the knee. Adv Pain Res Ther 13:183–191
5. Giamberardino MA (2000) Visceral Hyperalgesia. In: Devor M, Rowbotham MC, Wiesenfeld-Hallin Z (eds) Progress in Pain Research and Management, vol 16. IASP Press, Seattle, pp 523–550
6. Giamberardino MA, Berkley KJ, Iezzi S et al. (1997) Pain threshold variations in somatic wall tissues as a function of menstrual cycle, segmental site and tissue depth in non-dysmenorrheic women, dysmenorrheic women and men. Pain 71:187–197
7. Giamberardino MA, De Laurentis S, Affaitati G et al. (2001) Modulation of pain and hyperalgesia from the urinary tract by algogenic conditions of the reproductive organs in women. Neurosci Lett 304: 61–64
8. Giamberardino MA, Affaitati G, Lerza R et al. (2005) Relationship between pain symptoms and referred sensory and trophic changes in patients with gallbladder pathology. Pain 114:239–249
9. Hoheisel U, Mense S, Simons DG et al. (1993) Appearance of new receptive fields in rat dorsal horn neurons following noxious stimulation of skeletal muscle: a model for referral of muscle pain? Neurosci Lett 153:9–12
10. Mense S (1994) Referral of muscle pain. APS J 3:1–9
11. Procacci P, Zoppi M, Maresca M (1986) Clinical approach to visceral sensation. In: Cervero F, Morrison JFB (eds) Visceral Sensation, Progress in Brain Research. Elsevier, Amsterdam, pp 21–28
12. Simons DG, Mense S (2003) Diagnosis and therapy of myofascial trigger points. Schmerz 17:419–424
13. Vecchiet L, Giamberardino MA, Dragani L et al. (1989) Pain from renal / ureteral calculosis: evaluation of sensory thresholds in the lumbar area. Pain 36:289–295
14. Vecchiet L, Giamberardino MA, Saggini R (1991) Myofascial pain syndromes: clinical and pathophysiological aspects. Clin J Pain 7:16–22

M

15. Vecchiet L, Vecchiet J, Giamberardino MA (1999) Referred Muscle Pain: Clinical and Pathophysiologic Aspects. Curr Rev Pain 3:489–498

Muscle Relaxants

MARK JOHNSON, NIKOLAI BOGDUK
Musculoskeletal Physician, Hibiscus Coast Highway, Orewa, New Zealand
markjohn@ihug.co.nz, nik.bogduk@newcastle.edu.au

Definition

Muscle relaxants are drugs ostensibly designed to relieve pain by reducing painful muscle spasm.

Characteristics

Muscle relaxants have been largely used in the treatment of spinal pain, for it is believed that spasm of the spinal muscles occurs in response to pain, but is itself painful. Most of the literature describes their use for low back pain, but they have also been used and tested for neck pain.

Rationale

The rationale for the use of muscle relaxants is that if they can relieve the spasm, they serve as analgesics by relieving at least part of the pain caused by the muscle spasm. This rationale, however, is not vindicated by the evidence.

There is no evidence that spasm of the back muscles is painful or contributes to the patient's pain. There is no evidence that so-called muscle spasm can be reliably diagnosed. There is no correlation between clinical muscle spasm and any biological parameter such as EMG. Indeed, eminent authorities have decried the wisdom of belief in muscle spasm (Johnson 1989) or lamented its lack of validity (Andersson et al. 1989).

Efficacy

The most recent, systematic review (Van Tulder et al. 2003) concluded that there was strong evidence that muscle relaxants are more effective than placebo for short-term relief of acute low back pain. Inspection of the review revealed that studies included in the tables were not included in the narrative, where the conclusions were drawn. Inspection of the original studies suggests that this conclusion may have been overly generous (Bogduk 2004).

The data are conflicting for orphenadrine (Bogduk 2004). One study found that only nine out of 20 patients treated with orphenadrine had reduced pain at 48 h after treatment, compared to four out of 20 patients treated with placebo. No other, or better, measure of outcome was reported. In contrast, another study found no superiority over placebo.

A low quality study found diazepam to be more effective than placebo at day 5, but a high quality study found it to be no more effective than placebo (Bogduk 2004). Dantrolene was considered more effective than placebo on the grounds that it reduced pain during maximum voluntary movement to a greater extent, but not at other times (Bogduk 2004).

Carisoprodol was considered effective because it reduced pain to a greater extent than placebo at four days (Bogduk 2004). Methocarbamol was as effective as chlormezanone, but chlormezanone was as effective as an NSAID (Bogduk 2004).

Conflicting data concerning tizanidine have been reported by the same investigators in two separate studies. One found no differences in outcome at three and at seven days between patients treated with tizanidine and those treated with placebo (Bogduk 2004). The other study compared tizanidine plus ibuprofen with tizanidine plus placebo (Bogduk 2004). It found no differences in pain scores between the two groups at three days and at seven days. The success attributed to tizanidine was based on a larger proportion of patients having no pain or only mild pain at night, at three days but not at seven days; and a larger proportion of patients having no pain or only mild pain at rest, both at three days and at seven days. The respective proportions in the latter instance were 90% vs. 72% at three days, and 93% vs. 77% at seven days. Two other studies found no differences from placebo (Bogduk 2004).

Baclofen is significantly more effective than placebo in reducing pain, but the magnitude of the difference is about 10% in absolute terms, and 20% in relative terms, but applies only to assessment at ten days after treatment (Bogduk 2004).

Cyclobenzaprine is more effective than placebo in so far as it achieved a reduction in pain, nine days after treatment, of 5.5 points on a 10-point scale, compared with 4 points for placebo (Bogduk 2004). However, cyclobenzaprine is not more effective than NSAIDs (Bogduk 2004). For relieving pain and improving daily activities, it was slightly more effective than placebo at day 7 but not at day 14 (Bogduk 2004). A meta-analysis of studies that compared cyclobenzaprine with placebo (Browning et al. 2003) found that cyclobenzaprine substantially improved local pain and global symptoms when used for four days, but the effect declined considerably after the first week, and was associated with a 25% increase in side-effects such as drowsiness, dry mouth and dizziness compared to placebo. That meta-analysis, however, included studies that were rejected by a systematic review on the grounds that they did not explicitly address low back pain (Van Tulder et al. 2003).

These data indicate that for orphenadrine, diazepam, and tizanidine, the evidence is conflicting as to whether the drugs are more effective than placebo, with the balance favouring no superiority over placebo. Methacarbamol has not been shown to be more effective than placebo. Carisoprodol is more effective than placebo but only at four days. Baclofen and cyclobenzprine are each only slightly more effective than placebo but only for a few days, but not thereafter. Meanwhile, the evidence is strong that muscle relaxants have consistently been associated with a greater incidence of central nervous system side-effects (Van Tulder et al. 2003). This factor, balanced against their limited attributable effect, gives cause to question the propriety of their use for acute low back pain, especially when other interventions are no less effective, or even more effective, with far less risk of troublesome side-effects.

For the treatment of chronic low back pain, the data on muscle relaxants are limited to only a few studies of a few agents. Agents used for acute low back pain have not been studied for chronic low back pain. Those that have been studied, show limited or no superiority of placebo (Bogduk 2004).

Two studies each showed that tetrazepam was significantly more effective than placebo in reducing pain at seven days, but not subsequently (Bogduk 2004). Flupirtin was perceived by physicians as achieving better overall improvement than placebo at seven days, but improvements in pain or muscle spasm were not significantly better (Bogduk 2004). In terms of global impression of efficacy, tolperisone was not significantly better than placebo (Bogduk 2004).

For the treatment of neck pain, diazepam and phenobarbital have been tested, and found to have no greater effect than placebo for the treatment of acute neck pain (Basmajian 1983).

References

1. Andersson G, Bogduk N, Deluca C et al. (1989) Muscle: Clinical Perspectives. In: Frymoyer JW, Gordon SL (eds) New Perspectives On Low Back Pain. American Academy Of Orthopaedic Surgeons, Park Ridge, Illinois, pp 293–334
2. Basmajian JV (1983) Reflex Cervical Muscle Spasm: Treatment by Diazepam, Phenobarbital or Placebo. Arch Phys Med Rehabil 64:121–124
3. Bogduk N (2004) Pharmacological Alternatives for the Alleviation of Back Pain. Expert Opin Phamacother 5:2091–2098
4. Browning R, Jackson JL, O'Malley PG (2001) Cyclobenzaprine and Back Pain: A Meta-Analysis. Arch Int Med 161:1613–1620
5. Johnson EW (1989) The Myth of Skeletal Muscle Spasm (editorial). Am J Phys Med 68:1
6. Van Tulder MW, Touray T, Furlan AD et al. (2003) Muscle Relaxants for Nonspecific Low Back Pain: A Systematic Review within the Framework of the Cochrane Collaboration. Spine 28:1978–1992

Muscle Scanning

Definition

A form of psychophysiological assessment that involves making multiple bilateral recordings of muscle tension levels from varied locations.

▶ Biofeedback in the Treatment of Pain
▶ Psychophysiological Assessment of Pain

Muscle Spasm

▶ Chronic Back Pain and Spinal Instability
▶ Muscle Cramps

Muscle Tension

Definition

Muscle tension refers to the level of tension in a muscle that is usually measured by electromyography and is related to the amount of contraction in muscle fibers.
▶ Muscle Cramps
▶ Respondent Conditioning of Chronic Pain

Muscular Cramps

MARIANO SERRAO
Department of Neurology and Otorinolaringoiatry, University of Rome La Sapienza, Rome, Italy
victor.m@mclink.it

Synonym

Muscle cramps

Definition

▶ Muscle cramps are "spasmodic, painful, involuntary, contractions of the skeletal muscle" (Layzer and Rowland 1971). They represent one of the most common medical complaints. Cramps sometimes occur spontaneously at rest, especially when the muscle is slack (i.e. relaxed and shortened). More often, cramps are triggered by a brief contraction or during exercise of a susceptible muscle (Layzer and Rowland 1971). They can occur in any muscle of the body, though the foot and calf muscles are more frequently involved (Jansen et al. 1991). During the cramp, the muscle is visibly and palpably taut and painful, often with abnormal posture of the affected joint, a condition which can be relieved by stretching or massage (Rowland 1985).

Characteristics

The mechanism of muscle cramps is still speculative, because both their expression and their association with numerous diseases vary. Thus, their pathophysiology awaits clarification. A clear etiological distinction should be made between cramps generically named "▶ contractures", present in metabolic myopathies (e.g. McArdle's disease) and cramps associated with most other pathologies, usually named "▶ ordinary cramps". The former type of cramp is characterized by an absence of activity ("electrical silence") on EMG recordings, suggesting a muscular origin (Layzer 1994); in most cramps, however, the EMG shows brief periodic bursts of high-frequency, high-voltage action potentials (Norris et al. 1957), suggesting a neural origin.

The origin of the pain associated with muscle cramps is not known and there are no consistent studies that have investigated this aspect. The pain present during the muscle cramp seems to be strikingly associated to the muscular contraction, which probably produces a mechanical stimulation of the group III or IV intramuscular fibers (Layzer 1985). Other factors such as an ischemia produced during the muscle contraction, an increase in muscular metabolites or a direct lesion of the muscular fibers have been hypothesized as well.

Muscle cramps have been classified according to their anatomic site of origin, cause or clinical features (Layzer and Rowland 1971; McGee 1990; Rowland 1985). Recently we have proposed a new classification (Parisi et al. 2003) based primarily on their site of pathogenesis and on Layzer's definition of muscle cramp (see below). In accordance with such a definition, the muscle contraction of the cramp must be painful, which therefore excludes involuntary muscle contractions of various origins which are not painful, such as myotonia, stiffness, dystonia and various movement disorders, e.g. myoclonias, chorea, tremors, tics. Furthermore, the muscle contraction must be sudden and sustained for a period of time ranging from a few second to a few minutes. Any pathological conditions such as antalgic contractures, which develop after a muscle injury and last for several days or weeks, should be excluded from this classification because they, unlike cramps, are neither sudden nor transient. In addition, muscular, articular or nervous disorders that induce strong, localized pain but are not associated with a real muscle contraction (e.g. neuralgia, contusion, myalgia) should be distinguished from cramps.

Classification of Muscle Cramps

Paraphysiological Cramps

- Occasional cramps
- Cramps during sporting activity
- Cramps during pregnancy

Idiopathic Cramps

- Familial

  - Autosomal dominant cramping disease
  - Familial nocturnal cramps
  - Continuous muscle fibers activity syndrome

- Sporadic

  - Continuous muscle fiber activity syndrome (Isaac's syndrome, Stiffman syndrome, cramp-

    fasciculation syndrome, myokymia-cramp syndrome)
  - Syndrome of progressive muscle ▶ spasm, alopecia, and diarrhea (Sathoyoshi's syndrome)
  - Idiopathic nocturnal cramps
  - Idiopathic generalized myokymia
  - Myokymia-hyperhidrosis syndrome

- Others (familial insulin resistance with acanthocytosis nigricans and acral hypertrophy, muscle cramps in cancer patients)

Symptomatic Cramps

- Central and Peripheral Nervous System Diseases

  - Motor neuron disease
  - Occupational dystonias
  - Parkinson's disease
  - Tetanus
  - Multiple sclerosis
  - Radiculopathies
  - Plexopathies
  - Peripheral neuropathies (inherited, endocrine-metabolic, infectious, toxic, inflammatory, demyelinating)
  - Others rare (neurolathyrism, familial paroxysmal dystonic choreoathetosis)

- Muscular Diseases

  - Metabolic myopathy (deficiency of myophosphorylase, phosphofructokinase, phosphoglyceromutase, phosphoglycerokinase, lactate dehydrogenase (LDH), adenylate deaminase, G6PDH, phosphorylase b-kinase)
  - Mitochondrial myopathy (carnitine deficiency, CPT1 e 2 deficiency)
  - Endocrine myopathy (Hoffman's syndrome etc)
  - Dystrophinopathies (Duchenne, Becker, others)
  - Myotonia (Thomsen, Becker, rippling syndrome)
  - Inflammatory myopathies (myositis, myopathy with tubular aggregates, rheumatic polymyalgia)
  - Others rare (Lambert-Brody's diseases, Swartz-Jampel syndrome, eosinophilia-myalgia syndrome, type two muscle fiber myopathy)

- Cardiovascular Diseases

  - Venous diseases
  - Arterial diseases
  - Heart diseases
  - Hypertension

- Endocrine-metabolic Disease

  - Hypo-hyperthyroidism

Musculoskeletal Pain

LARS ARENDT-NIELSEN
Laboratory for Experimental Pain Research, Center
for Sensory-Motor Interaction, Aalborg University,
Aalborg, Denmark
lan@hst.aau.dk

The leading causes of disability in people in their working years are musculoskeletal conditions, which are almost exclusively associated with pain. Moreover, the efficacy of treatment of many musculoskeletal pain conditions by currently available pharmacological and non-pharmacological interventions is often less than optimal. Musculoskeletal diseases are one of the most expensive areas for the health system and hence have a substantial socio-economic impact, which leads to suffering for many patients. Musculoskeletal pain is more frequent in the elderly than in the young population with a predominance among females for many of the disorders e.g. joint pain, neck pain, shoulder pain, low back pain, temporomandibular disorders, ▶ fibromyalgia, whiplash and tension type headache. Although musculoskeletal pain is an important factor in many disorders such as injuries, degenerative diseases and cancer, the peripheral and central mechanisms underlying muscle pain are poorly understood. Musculoskeletal disorders can be classified as articular (e.g. ▶ rheumatoid arthritis, osteoarthritis) or non-articular (e.g. low back pain, ▶ myofascial pain syndrome, fibromyalgia) (Mense and Simons 2001).

Basis for Musculoskeletal Pain

In animal studies two major types of Aδ- (type III) and C-fibre (type IV) muscle nociceptors (free nerve endings) have been found, chemo-nociceptors and mechano-nociceptors (Mense 1993). The stimuli for nociceptors are mechanical (e.g. strong pressure, etc.) or chemical (e.g. bradykinin, serotonin, potassium, hypertonic saline and capsaicin) and some of the latter are excited only with particular stimulus configurations like long-lasting contractions during ischaemia. Many of these receptors are notably polymodal, i.e. they respond to stimuli of different modalities (mechanical, thermal, chemical, etc.) or they can be sensitised by one stimulus (e.g. chemical) in order to respond to another stimulus (e.g. mechanical).

Free nerve endings are widely distributed throughout most of the articular structures. The majority remains silent during normal conditions, but become active when the articular tissue is subjected to damaging mechanical deformations and to certain chemical substances. These chemosensitive units are activated by certain ions and inflammatory mediators, such as serotonin, histamine, bradykinin and prostaglandins. Thus they are most probably nociceptors.

Little is known about the peripheral transduction and encoding apparatus for muscle-, ligament-, periosteum- and joint-nociceptive afferents and only very few human microneurographic studies have been published. It seems more difficult to obtain stable recordings from muscle / joint nociceptive afferents than cutaneous nociceptors. The nociceptors can be sensitised by release of neuropeptides from the nerve endings. This may also lead to peripheral sensitisation of the nociceptors and central hyperexcitability of dorsal horn neurones resulting in prolonged neuronal discharges, increased responses to defined noxious stimuli, response to non-noxious stimuli and expansion of the receptive field. A variety of inputs following intense and / or prolonged noxious stimuli and consequent activation of group III and IV fibres increase spinal excitability. Three different pathophysiological processes in the spinal cord can account for the above alterations.

Structural Re-organisation

The synaptic connections between afferent fibres and central (spinal) neurons can be changed structurally and physiologically (or pathophysiologically) in response to a variety of influences (nerve damage, ▶ inflammation, etc.).

Decreased Inhibition

In particular in peripheral neuropathy, the inhibition normally suppressing transmission of nociceptive signals in the spinal cord could be decreased (Woolf and Doubell 1994).

Increased Excitability (Central Sensitisation)

The increased excitability of postsynaptic neurones may in part be due to an increased efficacy of synaptic transmission from afferent nerve fibres onto postsynaptic neurones. Long-term changes in synaptic efficacy can be increases or decreases. Wall and Woolf (1984) showed that muscle nociceptive afferents seem particularly effective at inducing neurofunctional changes in the spinal cord. Peripheral and central muscular related hyperalgesia is assumed to play an important role in musculoskeletal pain disorders.

Manifestations of Musculoskeletal Pain

Musculoskeletal pain is manifested by four main components (1) the effect on the motor system, (2) local and referred pain, (3) increased or decreased muscle sensitivity and (4) somatosensory changes in the referred pain area (Fig. 1).

M

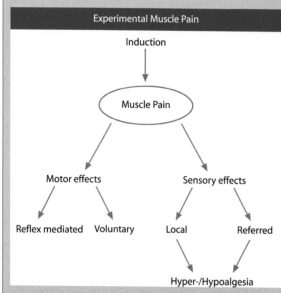

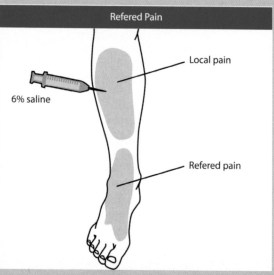

Musculoskeletal Pain, Figure 1 A sketch of how musculoskeletal pain can be manifested. (1) Muscle pain has effects on the motor system. This involves effects on voluntary contractions, endurance and muscle coordination and on reflex mediated pathways (e.g. stretch reflexes, proprioception, and motor unit firing characteristics). (2) Muscle pain may result in local as well as referred pain areas. (3) In the local muscle pain area, the muscle may have changed sensibility (e.g. hypersensitive to pressure). (4) In the referred area, various somatosensory changes can take place.

Musculoskeletal Pain, Figure 3 Examples of local and referred pain patterns in volunteers following intramuscular injections of hypertonic saline (6%, 0.5 ml) into the anterior tibialis muscle. If the area of referred pain is completely blocked by anaesthetic procedures (e.g. a regional block), the referred pain can still be elicited, indicating that referred pain is a central phenomenon. The size of the referred pain area depends on the intensity and duration of the actual muscle stimulus.

In contrast to the localised sharp, burning characteristics of cutaneous pain, muscle pain is described as diffuse aching and cramping. Furthermore, musculoskeletal pain is more complicated to investigate than cutaneous and visceral pain, as muscle pain can consists of both localised pain and referred pain (Fig. 2).

Pain localisation is poor in skeletal muscles and patients may be unable to differentiate it from pain arising from tendons, ligaments and bones as well as from joints and their capsules. The characteristically

referredpain pattern was initially observed by Kellgren (1938), who injected hypertonic saline into many skeletal muscles and ligaments and characterised the referred pain patterns (Fig. 3). Similar characterisation has been performed clinically when activating ▶ trigger points in various muscles (Travell and Simons 1992).

It is obviously important to distinguish the painful tissue, but it may be very difficult, due to poor localisation and ▶ referred pain. Examples can be pain from an arthritic hip, which may refer to the thigh muscles or knee joint, a carpal tunnel syndrome may refer to forearm muscles and cervical spondylosis may refer to

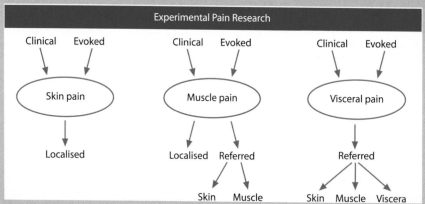

Musculoskeletal Pain, Figure 2 A simple sketch to illustrate the different characteristics and manifestations of cutaneous, muscle and visceral pain. Cutaneous pain is sharp and localised, whereas pain from deep structures is more diffuse. Pain from muscles can be localised to a specific muscle, but can also be referred to another somatic structure. In this referred structure, changes in somatosensibility can occur. Visceral pain is always referred either to somatic structures or via viscero-visceral convergent neurones.

arm muscles. Pain from joints and their capsules tends to be more localised than ▶ myalgia and arthralgia is often worsened by passive joint movements. Capsular pain may be present only in specific joint positions. Bone pain also tends to be poorly localised but, unlike myalgia, usually has a deep, boring quality. Furthermore, bone pain is usually worse at night and tends to be unaffected by either movement or muscle activity (Newham et al. 1994). The manifestations related to musculoskeletal pain can be projected pain, spread of pain and referred pain, somatosensory changes in referred pain areas (Vecchiet et al. 1999) and interaction with the motor system (e.g. muscle coordination and activation, postural stability, movement initiation and reflex pathways). Projected muscle pain is normally used as terminology in relationship to nerve fibre damage (e.g. compression) and felt in the innervation territory / myotome of the damaged nerve.

Spread of muscle pain is not clearly defined, but best described by phenomena related to experimental studies. If the muscle nociceptive afferent is repetitively, electrically stimulated by an intramuscular electrode, the area where the muscle pain is experienced expands or spreads as the stimulation progresses (Laursen et al. 1997). A similar manifestation is seen after repetitive visceral electrical stimulation (Arendt-Nielsen et al. 1997).

Referred muscle pain has been known and described for more than a century and is used extensively as a diagnostic tool. Substantial clinical knowledge exists concerning the patterns of referral from various skeletal muscles and after activation of trigger points (Travell and Simons 1992). The referred pain pattern follows the distribution of sclerotomes (muscle, fascia and bone) more frequently than the classical dermatomes. A clear distinction between spread of pain and referred pain is not possible and these phenomena may also share common pathophysiological mechanisms. Firm neurophysiologically based explanations for referred pain do not exist, but it has been shown that wide dynamic range neurones and nociceptive specific neurones in the spinal cord and in the brain stem of animals receive convergent afferent input from the mucosa, skin, muscles, joints and viscera. This may cause a misinterpretation of the afferent information coming from muscle afferents and reaching high levels in the central nervous system and hence be one reason for the diffuse and referred characteristics.

Referred pain is mainly a central phenomenon as it is possible to induce referred pain to limbs with complete sensory loss due to spinal injury or anaesthetic blockade. The size of the referred area to experimental muscle pain stimulation depends on the intensity and duration of the nociceptive musculoskeletal input and the evoked referred area is significantly enlarged in patients with painful musculoskeletal disorders (fibromyalgia, whiplash, low back pain and osteoarthritis) (Arendt-Nielsen and Svensson 2001; Koelbaek Johansen et al. 1999; Sorensen et al. 1998). Recently it has been emphasised that referred pain and central sensitisation are closely related (Arendt-Nielsen and Graven-Nielsen 2002; Giamberardino 2003).

Somatosensory changes in referred muscle pain areas have been reported – and it seems that the duration and intensity of pain are important for such manifestations. Hypoalgesia as well as hyperalgesia has been reported in referred muscle pain areas. The most consistent finding is muscle hyperalgesia in the referred areas. Referred muscle hyperalgesia can also be a result of visceral pain due to the viscero-somatic convergence. This may occur in e.g. gastrointestinal, gynaecological/urological or in chronic visceral painful conditions without known aetiology (e.g. irritable bowel diseases and endometriosis). It has been shown that the degree of referred muscle hyperalgesia is related to the severity of the visceral pathology and hence the degree of visceral pain. Persistent referred muscle hyperalgesia can be manifested not only by chronic conditions, but also after recurrent painful visceral attacks, such as in dysmenorrheic women where lumbar muscles are hyperalgesic to pressure or after colic attacks following calculosis of the upper urinary tract, where hyperalgesia to pressure is found in muscles in the left lumbar region (Giamberardino 1999).

Exercise-related Painful Musculoskeletal Conditions

Muscle pain in relation to exercise may increase in intensity until the exercise / contractions stop and the blood flow is restored. This is termed ischaemic pain and is the cause of well-known clinical presentations such as intermittent claudication and angina pectoris. Hypoxia was thought to be the cause of ischaemic pain, but it now seems more likely that accumulation of metabolites is responsible, at least in part. Lactic acid was assumed to be the prime algesic substance, but since patients with myophosphorylase deficiency (patients with McArdle's disease do not produce lactic acid) also experience ischaemic muscle pain during ▶ exercise, other substances such as histamine, acetylcholine, serotonin, bradykinin, potassium and adenosine are most likely involved.

Another manifestation of exercise may be ▶ muscle cramps. Muscle cramps are involuntary, painful, sudden contractions of the skeletal muscles and may also appear after overuse of a muscle. Cramps can occur in normal subjects under a variety of conditions (during a strong voluntary contraction, sleep, sports and pregnancy) and in several pathologies such as myopathies, neuropathies, motoneurone diseases, in tetanus, metabolic disorders, hydroelectrolyte imbal-

M

ances or endocrine pathologies (e.g. glycolytic disorders) or as a side effect after certain drugs (salbutamol, phenothiazine, vincristine, lithium, cimetidine and bumetanide). Considerable uncertainty is found in the literature regarding the classification and nomenclature of muscle cramps, both because the term "cramp" is used to indicate a variety of clinical features of muscles leading to its use as an imprecise "umbrella" term that includes stiffness, contractures and local pain and because the spectrum of the diseases in which it appears is wide.

If a muscle is exposed to heavy and unaccustomed and especially eccentric exercise, delayed onset muscle pain may peak 1–2 days later. Delayed onset muscle pain / soreness (post exercise soreness) is associated with tenderness to pressure and pain during movement / contraction. The mechanisms underlying post-exercise muscle pain seem different from those of ischaemic muscle pain, as considerable damage such as structural, biochemical, and radioisotopic changes are found (Friden 1984). Post-exercise pain can be inhibited and treated by NSAIDs suggesting that inflammatory mediators belonging to the arachidonic cycle may be involved in this kind of muscle pain.

Selected Painful Musculoskeletal Disorders

Myofascial pain syndromes are regional muscle pain disorders characterised by localised tenderness and pain and are common causes of persistent regional pain such as back pain, neck pain, shoulder pain, headaches and orofacial pain. The affected muscles often display an increased fatigability, stiffness, subjective weakness, pain in movement and slightly restricted range of motion that is unrelated to joint restrictions. The exact aetiology of myofascial pain syndromes is unclear. The major characteristics of myofascial pain syndromes include tenderness in muscles (trigger points) and local and referred pain. A trigger point is an up to 0.5 cm diameter point of hypersensitivity to pressure in a palpable taut band of skeletal muscle, tendon and ligament. Active trigger points are hypersensitive and display continuous pain in the zone of reference that can be altered with specific palpation. Latent trigger points display only hypersensitivity to pressure with no continuous pain. ▶ Tender points differ from trigger points in the sense that they are tender to pressure, do not cause referred pain by activation and can be identified as one of 18 designated soft tissue body sites.

Widespread pain is defined as pain lasting for longer than 3 months, presenting in both sides of the body, above and below the waist. In addition, axial skeletal pain (cervical spine, anterior chest, thoracic spine or low back pain) must be present. Widespread pain includes classes of syndromes such as fibromyalgia, chronic fatigue syndrome and exposure syndromes (e.g. Gulf War Illnesses). Fibromyalgia is a chronic painful musculoskeletal disorder of unknown aetiology and is defined by chronic widespread pain, involving three or more segments of the body plus the finding of at least 11 out of 18 designated tender points. Physical or emotional trauma, infection or surgery have been reported anecdotally to be precipitating factors in fibromyalgia and it is not uncommon for the patients to report the onset of the syndrome in relation to an accident or an injury. Fibromyalgia and the ▶ whiplash syndrome therefore share some common features.

Studies of the endocrine profile of fibromyalgia patients have indicated elevated activity of corticotropin releasing hormone (CRH) neurones, which could not only explain some symptoms of fibromyalgia, but may also explain alterations observed in the hormonal axes. Hypothalamic CRH neurones may play a role not only in resetting the various endocrine loops, but possibly also nociceptive and psychological mechanisms as well.

The whiplash syndrome is normally associated with car accidents where the car has been hit from the rear or the side and the persistent chronic pain is localised in the neck, shoulder and back. Patients with fibromyalgia and whiplash show accentuated reactions to a variety of stimulus modalities and in general they are hyperalgesic to experimental muscle stimulation (pressure and infusion of algogenic substances). A feature in many of the chronic musculoskeletal disorders is that the referred pain areas to experimentally induced muscle pain are significantly larger than in pain-free volunteers. Both fibromyalgia (Carli et al. 2002) and whiplash (Curatolo et al. 2001) patients show differentiated hyperalgesia to different sensory stimuli indicating that only specific parts of the sensory and nociceptive systems are influenced and that the sensory disturbances are accentuated as the syndrome progresses (Carli et al. 2002). In recent years these generalised chronic musculoskeletal disorders together with work-related muscle-related disorders have become an increasing challenge for the health care system with an increased socio-economic burden on societies.

Myalgia can be related to a variety of medical conditions (see list below) and common terms for the symptom are stiffness, soreness, aching, spasms or cramps. The associated pain is often described as having a dull, aching quality and can be exacerbated by muscle contractions. The manifestation of pain is, however, in some of the myalgias not the most prominent problem, as in ▶ myositis (e.g. ▶ polymyositis and ▶ dermatomyositis) where muscle weakness is often the prominent feature.

Clinical Conditions Associated with Myalgia (Newham et al. 1994)

- Trauma and sports injuries
- Primary infective myositis
- Inflammatory myopathies
  - Polymyositis with and without connective tissue disease
  - Dermatomyositis with and without connective tissue disease
  - Viral myositis
  - Polymyalgia rheumatica
- Myalgia of neurogenic origin
- Muscle cramp
- Impaired muscle energy metabolism
- Drug induced myalgia
- Myalgic encephalomyelitis / chronic fatigue syndrome
- Muscle pain of uncertain cause (repetitive strain injury, fibromyalgia)

Myalgia of neurogenic origin can be difficult to dissociate from other manifestations of neuropathic pain. Examples can be cervical radiculopathy with pain radiating into the myotomal distribution of the roots or nerve compressions (e.g. carpal tunnel syndrome) where the pain radiates into the muscles in the region. Little is known specifically related to muscle sensitisation in relation to neuropathic pain, as normally only the cutaneous manifestations (allodynia, hyperalgesia) are investigated.

Physical Therapies for the Management of Musculoskeletal Pain

A wide range of physical therapies are traditionally used in the repertoire of management regimes offered to patients with chronic musculoskeletal disorders. Such therapies include e.g. ice, heat, massage, acupuncture and ▶ transcutaneous electrical nerve stimulation. The efficacy of these therapies is not known and has rarely been compared in controlled studies. Acupuncture, electro acupuncture and transcutaneous electrical nerve stimulation have been applied in order to inactivate e.g. trigger points, but again the efficacy is not known. The advantage of e.g. transcutaneous nerve stimulation is that the patients feel that they have some control when they can take the device home and switch it on when needed.

A variety of physiotherapeutic management regimes are developed for different musculoskeletal disorders and, for example, the Quebec task force reviewed available literature on the treatment employed by physical therapists in the management of whiplash injuries (Spitzer et al. 1995). Only two of the commonly employed physiotherapy modalities (exercise, mobilisa-

tion) showed an effect. Unfortunately only a few of the physical therapies commonly used in the clinic for the management of musculoskeletal pain are scientifically validated. However, exercise with instruction from physical therapists seems to be the modality most often resulting in good outcome.

Gender Differences in Musculoskeletal Pain

Many musculoskeletal disorders and pains are more prevalent in females than males. Sex (referring to biologically determined aspects of femaleness and maleness) and / or gender (referring to modifiable, socioculturally shaped behaviour and traits such as femininity and masculinity) differences are present, with female predominance in painful musculoskeletal syndromes such as widespread pain, temporomandibular disorders, neck pain, shoulder pain, back pain, joint pain, fibromyalgia, whiplash and headache. Psychological factors operative in chronic painful musculoskeletal disorders cannot be understood within any single frame of reference. It is appropriate to examine emotional, ▶ interpersonal pain behaviour and interpersonal relationships in parallel, not as dichotomous concepts. High rates of comorbidity have been reported between e.g. temporomandibular dysfunctions and other clinical musculoskeletal disorders (e.g. fibromyalgia) and are again more common in women than men.

Fluctuations in hormonal levels have been implicated in symptom severity in women with rheumatoid arthritis, temporomandibular disorders and fibromyalgia. One mechanism by which hormones may affect muscle nociceptors sensitisation could be related to nerve growth factor (NGF) and one of its high-affinity receptors (trkA). The trkA receptor expression is influenced by gonadal hormones (Liuzzi et al. 1999). Injection of NGF into the muscle tissue causes muscle tenderness to pressure which lasts for weeks (Svensson et al. 2003). There has been some speculation that hormone replacement therapy may increase a woman's risk of developing musculoskeletal pain (LeResche et al. 1997). Numerous studies indicate that women have greater sensitivity to experimental muscle pain stimuli than men and the pressure pain threshold is generally lower in females. There are indications in the literature that males and females have different results from some drugs. For musculoskeletal pain, the non-steroidal anti-inflammatory drugs (NSAIDs) are commonly used and some studies have indicated that females experience less pain alleviating effect than males.

Techniques to Assess Sensitivity of Musculoskeletal Structures

Several methods exist to assess the sensitivity of musculoskeletal structures. The methods are based on

M

standardised application or induction of standardised pain to musculoskeletal structures to evaluate how sensitive the structure is to that specific stimulus modality. Such procedures can be applied to healthy volunteers in the laboratory for basic experimental studies or to patients for clinical examinations (Arendt-Nielsen 1997; Arendt-Nielsen et al. 1997). The standardised pain stimulus can be classified as endogenous pain models (the pain arises from muscles without the involvement of external stimuli) or exogenous models (the pain is evoked by external stimuli) (see list below).

Classification of Experimental Stimulus Modalities That Can Be Used to Induce Muscle Pain Experimentally

Endogenous

- Ischaemic
- Exercise-induced

  - Dynamic concentric contraction
  - Isometric contraction
  - Dynamic eccentric contraction

Exogenous

- Electrical
- Mechanical
- Chemical
- Focused ultrasound

Endogenous Models

Ischaemic muscle pain is a classically experimental pain model and has been used as an unspecified pain stimulus. A tourniquet is applied and after a period of voluntary muscle contractions a very unpleasant tonic pain sensation develops. The number of contractions, the level of force and the duration are important determinants for the resulting pain. This is a very efficient model to induce pain in muscles, but skin, periosteum and other tissues will contribute. The model is applicable in experimental studies requiring a general tonic pain stimulus for e.g. PET and fMRI experimental studies. ► Delayed Muscle Soreness is another model used experimentally to investigate endogenous muscle pain and this model is useful for e.g. evaluating drug effect.

Exogenous Models

Intraneural microstimulation of muscle nociceptive afferents can be performed in laboratory studies and can selectively elicit muscle pain accompanied by referred pain, which is dependent on the stimulation time (temporal summation) and the number of stimulated afferents (spatial summation). Repetitive intramuscular electrical stimulation can evoke localised and referred muscle pain. The local and referred pain areas develop during stimulation with the referred area slightly delayed as compared with the local pain area. The ar-

eas are dependent on stimulus intensity and duration (Laursen et al. 1997).

Intramuscular infusion of algogenic substances (e.g. hypertonic saline, capsaicin, bradykinin) causes local and referred pain. In most experimental human studies, manual bolus infusions of hypertonic saline are used, but more advanced models such as standardised infusion of small volumes by computer-controlled infusion pumps have been used. When this advanced model is used, the infusion rate can be controlled by the pain intensity rating feedback so constant pain intensity can be achieved by continuous adjustment of the infusion rate. Muscle pain induced experimentally by intramuscular infusion of algogenic substances causes cutaneous and muscular sensibility changes in referred pain areas. It is not entirely conclusive which somato-sensory changes occur as both hypo- and hyper-aesthesia have been reported. Furthermore, these changes are stimulus modality specific (Graven-Nielsen et al. 1997).

Pressure algometry is the most commonly used technique to induce muscle pain and hence assess tenderness in myofascial tissues and joints such as e.g. tender points, fibromyalgia, work-related myalgia, myofascial pain, strain injuries, myositis, chronic fatigue syndrome, arthritis / orthoses and other muscle / tendon / joint inflammatory conditions (Fischer 1987a; Fischer 1987b). The technique is adequate to quantify and follow the development of given diseases, but has also proven to be instrumental for the documentation of treatment outcome such as local / systemic administration of drugs. Pressure algometry is also suitable for the assessment of joint tenderness.

Assessing Sensory Aspects of Musculoskeletal Pain

Assessing the sensory aspects of musculoskeletal pain involves both evaluation of the muscle pain and of the somatic structures related to the referred pain area (Fig. 1). Clinical and experimentally induced muscle pain intensity and the implications on e.g. physical performance can be assessed quantitatively by various measures (see list below).

Techniques for Assessment of Experimentally Induced Musculoskeletal Pain and for Assessing Clinical Musculoskeletal Pain

Sensory Characterisation

Muscle Sensitivity

- Verbal assessment

  - Visual analogue scales
  - Verbal descriptor scales
  - McGill Pain Questionnaire

- Psychophysical tests

  - Pain thresholds

- Referred pain

  - Distribution of pain
  - Area (size)
  - Somatosensory changes

Motor Effects

- Electromyography

  - Surface electrodes
  - Needle electrodes
  - Indwelling wire electrodes

- Kinetics and kinematics

  - Sirognathograph (jaw movements)
  - Optoelectronic devices

- Force

  - Dynamometers
  - Force platforms
  - Bite force meters

Musculoskeletal pain has implications in many aspects of daily life and questionnaires for assessment of different dimensions have been developed for general and regional (e.g. back pain and neck pain) pain problems (general function score, Roland and Morris disability scale, ▶ Oswestry disability index, West Haven-Yale multidimensional pain inventory, Bournemouth questionnaire, ▶ fear avoidance beliefs, life satisfaction) (Turk and Melzack 1992).

A simple and useful technique is pain drawings where e.g. tender points, trigger points, localised and referred pain areas, hyper- and hypo-algesia are marked. Different colours can eventually be used to characterise different manifestations.

The psychophysical parameters used for the quantification of musculoskeletal pain sensitivity to experimentally applied pressure (pressure algometry) are pain detection, pain tolerance thresholds (Fig. 4) and stimulus-response functions. Stimulus-response functions can provide more information than just a threshold, as sensitisation to low as well as high intensities can be assessed and a shift in parallel of the curve towards the left together with an increased slope as has been found in patients with myofascial pain.

For monitoring purposes quantitative parameters are advantageous as compared with manual palpation. The essence of pressure algometry is that standardised increase in pressure is applied to the part of the body that is being investigated and the outcome is the patient's or volunteer's reaction to the pressure (Fischer 1987a; Fischer 1987b). Pressure rate and pressure area have been shown to be important factors for reliable results. The pressure pain thresholds vary substantially between regions. In some of the commercially available pressure algometers, the pressure application rate can be monitored, which is important for the reliability of the results. For research purposes, advanced computer controlled devices are available where the pressure rate can be pre-defined.

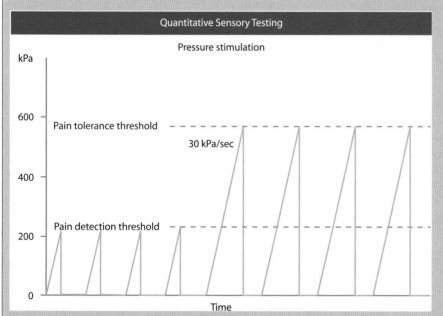

Musculoskeletal Pain, Figure 4 A schematic figure indicating how the psychophysical thresholds related to pressure pain (pressure algometry) are measured. Using a pressure algometer it is possible to control the rate of force increase (e.g. 30 kPa / s to a 1 cm^2 probe) and determine when the volunteer / patient experience the pressure as just painful (pain detection threshold) and when he / she will not tolerate any further increase in stimulus intensity (pain tolerance threshold).

Thresholds from various clinical pressure pain studies are difficult to compare, as different instrumentations have been used with different probe diameters and shapes and different force increase rates. The probe diameter is of utmost importance as there is not necessarily a simple relation between diameter and threshold since spatial summation plays an important role. The shape and contour of the probe are important, as sharp edges may excite more cutaneous receptors due to high shear forces compared with blunt probes.

Verbal assessments of the musculoskeletal pain intensity and other subjective characteristics of the pain are obviously needed in any clinical and experimental muscle pain studies. Visual analogue scales (VAS), verbal descriptor scales (VDS), McGill pain questionnaire (MPQ) and similar scales and questionnaires may be very helpful for the assessment of perceived pain intensity and quality (Turk and Melzack 1992). Musculoskeletal pain is most frequently characterised by descriptors as "drilling" "aching" "boring" and "taut" The intensity of musculoskeletal pain is easily measured using visual analogue scales (VAS). However, this is only a one-dimensional aspect of the experienced pain and additional VAS should be applied to monitor e.g. unpleasantness and soreness. Word descriptors on the VAS are important, as muscle tenderness and muscle pain may not reflect the same mechanisms. In addition to verbal assessments, psychophysical tests are valuable adjuncts for the examination of musculoskeletal pain (Turk and Melzack 1992).

Interaction between Musculoskeletal Pain and Motor Performance

Musculoskeletal pain has implications for motor performance and different electrophysiological and biomechanical methods and disability questionnaires (e.g. Oswestry pain disability index) have been developed to assess this interaction.

After reviewing articles describing motor function in five chronic musculoskeletal pain conditions (temporomandibular disorders, muscle tension headache, fibromyalgia, chronic lower back pain and post-exercise muscle soreness), Lund et al. (1991) concluded that the activity of agonist muscles is often reduced and the activity of the antagonist is slightly increased by musculoskeletal pain. As a consequence of these changes, force production and the range and velocity of movement of the affected body part are often reduced. To explain such changes motor control, Lund et al. (1991) proposed a neurophysiological model based on the phasic modulation of excitatory and inhibitory interneurones supplied by high threshold sensory afferents. They suggested that the "dysfunction", which is characteristic of several types of chronic musculoskeletal pain, is a normal protective

adaptation and is not a cause of pain. This pain adaptation model has also been verified in experimental studies, where motor strategies have been investigated before and after experimentally induced muscle pain. It seems however that the adaptation pattern mainly occurs in relation to gross, high force movements and to a lesser extent for high precision, low force movements. Johansson and Sojka (1991) suggested another pathophysiological model for chronic muscle pain and tension disorders. The model suggests that, under circumstances when chemosensitive group III-IV muscle afferents, joint afferents or certain descending pathways are activated, the activity of both primary and secondary muscle spindle afferents would be increased *via* fusimotor reflexes. This would have several consequences. Initially, an increased activity in γ-motoneurons would reduce the information transmission capacity of muscle spindles. Secondly, an altered activity in the primary muscle spindle afferents would influence proprioception and thereby sensorimotor control at higher levels. This influence could possibly lead to unfavourable work techniques, such as increased co-contractions and insufficient rest periods, which might further increase the interstitial concentration of substances exciting group III–IV afferents. Thirdly, increased levels of these substances might also excite, *via* chemosensitive group III–IV afferents, the sympathetic outflow to skeletal muscles, which may change the balance between sympathetic vasoconstriction and metabolic vasodilation and thus entail a deficiency in oxygen and nutrients with the consequences.

There is so far little clinical evidence to support this model. Experimental human studies have to some degree verified the interaction between γ-motoneuron excitability and the activation of group III–IV nociceptive afferents. Experimentally induced muscle pain causes excitation of the human stretch reflex, which may indicate such facilitatory interaction (Matre et al. 1998). In chronic muscle pain conditions where group III–IV muscle nociceptors are assumed to be active, muscle spindle responses and hence proprioception, should be affected. Indeed, patients suffering from work related myalgia often exhibit reduced proprioception, disturbed motor control and impaired balance.

► Disability, Upper Extremity
► Opioids and Muscle Pain

References

1. Arendt-Nielsen L (1997) Induction and assessment of experimental pain from human skin, muscle and viscera. In: Jensen TS, Turner JA, Wiesenfeld-Hallin Z (eds) Proceedings of the 8th World Congress on Pain. IASP Press, Seattle, pp 393–425
2. Arendt-Nielsen L, Graven-Nielsen T (2002) Deep tissue hyperalgesia. J Musculoskel Pain 10:97–119
3. Arendt-Nielsen L, Svensson P (2001) Referred muscle pain: basic and clinical findings. Clin J Pain 17:11–19

4. Arendt-Nielsen L, Svensson P, Graven-Nielsen T (1997) How to assess muscle pain experimentally and clinically. Eur J Pain 1:64–65

5. Carli G, Suman AL, Biasi G et al. (2002) Reactivity to superficial and deep stimuli in patients with chronic musculoskeletal pain. Pain 100:259–269

6. Curatolo M, Petersen-Felix S, Arendt-Nielsen L et al. (2001) Central hypersensitivity in chronic pain after whiplash injury. Clin J Pain 17:306–315

7. Fischer AA (1987a) Pressure algometry over normal muscles. Standard values, validity and reproducibility of pressure threshold. Pain 30:115–126

8. Fischer AA (1987b) Reliability of the pressure algometer as a measure of myofascial trigger point sensitivity. Pain 28:411–414

9. Friden J (1984) Muscle soreness after exercise: implications of morphological changes. Int J Sport Med 5:57–66

10. Giambierardino MA (1999) Recent and forgotten aspects of visceral pain. Eur J Pain 3:77–92

11. Giambierardino MA (2003) Referred muscle pain / hyperalgesia and central sensitisation. J Rehabil Med 41:85–88

12. Graven-Nielsen T, Arendt-Nielsen L, Svensson P et al. (1997) Stimulus-response functions in areas with experimentally induced referred muscle pain –a psychophysical study. Brain Res 2:121–128

13. Johansson H, Sojka P (1991) Pathophysiological mechanisms involved in genesis and spread of muscular tension in occupational muscle pain and in chronic musculoskeletal pain syndromes: A hypothesis. Medical Hypotheses 35:196–203

14. Kellgren JH (1938) Observations on referred pain arising from muscle. Clin Sci 3:175–190

15. Koelbaek Johansen M, Graven-Nielsen T, Schou Olesen A et al. (1999) Generalised muscular hyperalgesia in chronic whiplash syndrome. Pain 83:229–234

16. Laursen RJ, Graven-Nielsen T, Jensen TS et al. (1997) Quantification of local and referred pain in humans induced by intramuscular electrical stimulation. Eur J Pain 1:105–113

17. LeResche L, Saunders K, Von Korff MR et al. (1997) Use of exogenous hormones and risk of temporomandibular disorder pain. Pain 69:153–160

18. Liuzzi FJ, Scoville SA, Bufton SM (1999) Long term estrogen replacement co-ordinately decreases trkA and beta-PPT mRNA levels in dorsal root ganglion neurons. Exp Neurol 155:260–267

19. Lund JP, Donga R, Widmer CG et al. (1991) The pain-adaptation model: a discussion of the relationship between chronic musculoskeletal pain and motor activity. Can J Physiol Pharmacol 69:683–694

20. Matre D, Sinkjr T, Svensson P et al. (1998) Experimental muscle pain increases the human stretch reflex. Pain 75:331–339

21. Mense S (1993) Nociception from skeletal muscle in relation to clinical muscle pain. Pain 54:241–289

22. Mense S, Simons DG (2001) Muscle pain: Understanding its nature, diagnosis and treatment. Lippincott Williams & Wilkins, Baltimore

23. Newham DJ, Edwards RHT, Mills KR (1994) Skeletal muscle pain. In: Wall PD, Melzack R (eds) Textbook of Pain, 3rd edn. Churchill Livingstone, UK, pp 423–440

24. Sorensen J, Graven-Nielsen T, Henriksson KG et al. (1998) Hyperexcitability in fibromyalgia. J Rheumatol 25:152–1555

25. Spitzer WO, Skovron ML, Salmi LR et al. (1995) Scientific monograph of the Quebec Task Force on Whiplash-Associated Disorders: redefining "whiplash" and its management. Spine 20:1–73

26. Svensson P, Cairns BE, Wang K et al. (2003) Injection of nerve growth factor into human masseter muscle evokes long-lasting mechanical allodynia and hyperalgesia. Pain 104:241–247

27. Travell JG, Simons DG (1992) Myofascial Pain and Dysfunction: The Trigger Point Manual, vol 1, 2. Williams & Wilkins, Baltimore

28. Turk DC, Melzack R (eds) (1992) Handbook of pain assessment. Guilford, New York

29. Vecchiet L, Vecchiet J, Giambierardino MA (1999) Referred Muscle Pain: Clinical and Pathophysiologic Aspects. Curr Rev Pain 3:489–498

30. Wall PD, Woolf CJ (1984) Muscle but not cutaneous C-afferent input produces prolonged increases in the excitability of the flexion reflex in the rat. J Physiol 356:443–458

31. Woolf CJ, Doubell TP (1994) The pathophysiology of chronic pain–increased sensitivity to low threshold A beta-fibre inputs. Curr Opin Neurobiol 4:525–534

M

are required to identify co-morbid conditions or other causes of chronic myalgia.

Associated Symptoms of FMS

FMS is associated with sleep disturbance, fatigue, headache, morning stiffness, irritable bowel syndrome (IBS), interstitial cystitis (IC), dyspareunia and mood disturbance. Some of these symptoms are manifestations of referred muscle pain from ▶ myofascial trigger points (headache, ▶ dyspareunia, morning stiffness) and others, such as IBS and IC are ▶ viscerosomatic pain syndromes (Gerwin) that occur in up to 70% of FMS patients. They are by no means unique to FMS and are usually associated with pelvic floor MPS syndromes. Depression may occur in as many as 30% of FMS patients, but is no more common in FMS than in the general population.

Fibromyalgia: Etiology

Tenderness in FMS is related to central sensitization with amplification of nociception, resulting in a broad array of stimuli perceived as being more painful among FMS patients than they are in control subjects (Russell 2001). Alterations in cardiovascular autonomic nervous system function cause orthostatic hypotension or neurally mediated orthostatic tachypnea (Martinez-Lavin 1997). Neuroendocrine abnormalities in the hypothalamic-pituitary-adrenal system and growth hormone deficiency are hormonal deficiency states that may tie together the symptoms of fatigue, pain and sleep and mood disturbances (Dessein et al. 2000).

Fibromyalgia: Treatment

Treatment of fibromyalgia includes a wide variety of pharmacologic, nutritional, hormonal, behavioral, cognitive, exercise and physical modalities (Goldenberg et al. 2004). The long-term prognosis for FMS is more favorable than initially thought. Symptoms may persist for years, but patients either learn to cope with the chronic pain or the pain does not progress.

Myofascial Pain Syndrome: Characteristics

MPS is a muscular pain syndrome that arises from a primary dysfunction in muscle. It is associated with central sensitization and a segmental spread within the spinal cord to give rise to the phenomenon of referred pain or pain that is felt at a distance (Mense 2001). The clinical picture of MPS is one of musculoskeletal pain, limited mobility, weakness and referred pain (Simons et al. 1999). The trigger point has both a motor abnormality in which an abnormal hardness in muscle (the taut band) is felt on palpation, and a sensory abnormality of exquisite tenderness in the taut band. Identification of the trigger point by physical examination has good interrater reliability (Gerwin et al. 1997). The specifics of a MPS depend on which muscles are involved. For example, TrPs in the muscles of the head, neck and shoulders can cause headache. Local or regional myofascial syndrome can spread through the body and become a widespread myofascial syndrome, but does not become fibromyalgia.

Treatment

Treatment of myofascial pain requires the inactivation of MTrPs by manual trigger point compression or by needling, the restoration of normal muscle length and the elimination or correction of the factors that created or perpetuated the trigger points in the first place. Awareness of ergonomic and postural factors is important in developing a treatment plan. Trigger point needling is done with or with out the injection of local anesthetic (Cummings 2001). Injection of other materials such as steroids or ketorolac is inappropriate. Trigger point inactivation must be accompanied by correction of mechanical or structural stresses and of psychological and medical contributing factors.

Mechanical Causes

Mechanical causes of myalgia include ergonomic, structural and postural pain syndromes.

Hypermobility Syndromes

Hypermobility syndromes produce multiple mechanical stresses. Structural stress occurs as ligamentous laxity results in poor joint stabilization, muscles then being recruited to maintain joint integrity. This can result in a seemingly disproportionate number of hypermobile persons, mostly women, who have focal or generalized myalgia. The affected muscles always have myofascial trigger points. The mechanism of injury appears to be muscular stress or overload that arises from the effort required to maintain joint integrity. The most effective treatment is strengthening.

Forward Head Posture

Forward head posture places stress on the extensor muscles of the neck and shoulder (longissimus cervicis, semispinalis capitis and cervicis, splenius capitis and cervicis, the suboccipital muscles at the base of the skull and the trapezius and levator scapulae muscles). Posterior cervical muscle and shoulder muscle myalgic syndromes are thus frequently associated with head pain and headache.

Pelvic Torsion-related Pain

Pelvic torsion-related pain is associated with pseudo-leg-length-inequality or with trigger point muscular shortening (pseudoscoliosis). It can be caused by, and in turn either cause or aggravate, myalgia in lumbar muscles and in the pelvic floor muscles.

SI joint Dysfunction

Sacroiliac joint dysfunction, or sacro-iliac joint hypomobility can cause pelvic and spine dysfunction that results in painful, widespread axial muscle trigger points. Pain may be felt in the sacroiliac joint region (on either the hypomobile or the normal side), referred to the low back or occur because of the secondary development of paraspinal trigger point up the axial spine to the shoulders and neck.

Static Overload

Static overload occurs when mechanically stressful positions are held for prolonged periods of time, causing fatigue and pain in the persistently activated muscles.

Nerve Root Compression

Nerve root compression can present with acute or chronic myofascial trigger points. Trigger point pain syndromes can develop acutely when there is an acute disc herniation. Muscle pain is in the distribution of the affected nerve root. It can precede any neurological impairment such as weakness, sensory loss, paresthesia or reflex loss.

Delayed Onset Muscle Soreness (DOMS)

Delayed onset muscle soreness (DOMS), as is well known, occurs after eccentric exercise, but has been shown to occur after ischemic exercise as well (Barlas et al. 2000). Exercise under these conditions causes injury to the muscle fiber and consequent pain or soreness.

The second major category is systemic medical illness. The relationship of some of these conditions to myalgia has been difficult to confirm. Yet when such an illness is identified and treated and muscle pain improves or resolves, it is tempting to equate the treatment with a successful outcome. Nonetheless, one must be cautious about assuming a causal relationship. The conditions of interest include autoimmune disorders, infectious diseases, allergies, hormonal and nutritional deficiencies, viscerosomatic pain syndromes and iatrogenic drug induced myalgic pain syndromes.

Autoimmune Disorders

Muscle pain is a common accompanying symptom of many autoimmune disorders, particularly connective tissue diseases like lupus and Sjögren's syndrome.

Polymyalgia rheumatica (PMR) must certainly be considered in any head, neck and shoulder regional muscular pain syndrome in an older (>50 years of age) individual. Chewing-induced pain is an important component of both PMR and MPS, the latter when the temporomandibular joint is involved. Muscle pain may precede other signs of Sjögren's syndrome by several years.

Infectious Diseases

Lyme disease is perhaps the most prevalent of the infectious diseases associated with myalgia and arthralgia. Post-Lyme disease syndrome is characterized by diffuse arthralgia, myalgia, fatigue and subjective cognitive difficulty (Weinstein and Britchkov 2002). Patients diagnosed with this condition do not show evidence of chronic borrelial infection and they do not respond to a 3 month course of antibiotics any better than a control group treated with placebo. Chronic infections that look like Lyme disease and that may co-infect with Lyme disease are babesiosis, ehrlichiosis and *Bartonella*. Other infectious diseases thought to be related to myalgia are *Mycoplasma* pneumonia and *Chlamydia* pneumonia. Interest in these two diseases arises because of a putative association with arthralgia or synovitis and with chronic fatigue. A number of patients with widespread myalgia have parasitic disease, most commonly amebiasis and *Giardia*.

Allergies

Cases of widespread myalgia (myofascial pain syndrome) have been associated with persons who have had untreated allergies. When the myalgic syndrome is limited to the head, neck and shoulders, forward head posture as described above may be related to allergies and obstruction of the nasal passages may play a role.

Viscero-somatic Pain Syndromes

Internal organs are associated with somatic segmental referred pain syndromes. Endometriosis, for example, is associated with abdominal myofascial pain (Jarrell and Robert 2003). Interstitial cystitis and irritable bowel syndrome are associated with chronic pelvic pain syndromes (Hetrick et al. 2003; Weiss 2001). Liver disease can cause local abdominal and referred shoulder myofascial pain syndromes that present as a regional pain syndrome responsive to treatment of the trigger points by needling or by manual therapy.

Brain Tumor and Base of Skull Pain

Posterior fossa mass lesions (primary and metastatic tumors) can present as focal base of skull or upper cervical pain with identifiable myofascial trigger points that transiently respond to trigger point inactivation.

Nutritional Deficiencies

Vitamin D deficiency was found in 89% of the persons in a group with chronic musculoskeletal pain (Plotnikof 2003). This is an astounding figure that indicates that vitamin D deficiency is extremely common among those with myalgia.

Iron Deficiency

This causes a metabolic stress that produces fatigue and muscle pain. Muscle is depleted of iron available for energy-producing enzymatic reactions when serum ferritin levels are 15 ng / ml or less. Treatment with iron supplements in women whose serum ferritin level is 20 ng / ml or less results in less fatigue, less coldness and less muscle pain. Iron insufficiency is also associated with restless leg syndrome (RLS), a cause of sleep disturbance. Sleep deprivation also causes myalgia. Thus, iron deficiency can aggravate muscle pain secondarily by causing RLS.

Drug Induced Myalgia

This is widespread and diffuse, rather than regional. Drug-induced myalgia may or may not be associated with trigger points. Elevation of CK is a marker of muscle tissue breakdown. However, CK is not necessarily elevated when there is drug-induced myalgia. Drugs known to produce myalgia, regardless of whether or not CK is elevated, include propoxyphene and the statin family of cholesterol lowering drugs (Thompson et al. 2003). The risk of acquiring myalgia is increased when a statin drug is taken concomitantly with fibric acid derivatives like gemfibrozil, niacin, cyclosporin, azole B antifungal and macrolide antibiotics, protease inhibitors, nefazodone, verapamil, diltiazem, amiodarone or grapefruit juice (> 1 qt / day).

Conclusion

Muscle pain can be the result of a wide array of clinical conditions. The inflammatory diseases of muscle, such as polymyositis or the inherited myopathies, can also present with pain. Myoadenylate deaminase deficiency is the most common inherited muscle enzyme disorder, but the role that it plays in muscle pain is still no clearer today than it was 10 years ago. In order to treat patients well, the conditions that produce muscle pain must be identified in order to be specifically addressed.

▶ Guillain-Barré Syndrome
▶ Muscle Pain Model, Inflammatory Agents-Induced

References

1. Andreu AL, Hanna MG, Reichman H et al. (1999) Exercise intolerance due to mutations in the cytochrome *b* gene of mitochondrial DNA. N Eng J Med 341:1037–1044
2. Barlas P, Walsh DM, Baxter GD et al. (2000) Delayed onset muscle soreness: effect of a n ischemic block upon mechanical allodynia in humans. Pain 87:221–225
3. Cummings T, White A (2001) Needling therapies in the managementof myofascial trigger point pain: a systematic review. Arch Phys Med Rehabil 82: 986–992
4. Dessein PH, Shipton EA, Joffe BI et al. (2000) Neuroendocrine deficiency-mediated development and persistence of pain in fibromyalgia: a promising paradigm? Pain 86:213–215
5. Gerwin RD (1999) Differential diagnosis of myofascial pain syndrome and fibromyalgia. J Musculoskeletal Pain 7:209–215

M

6. Gerwin RD (2002) Myofascial and visceral pain syndromes: visceral-somatic pain representations. J Musculoskelet Pain 10:165–175
7. Gerwin RD, Shannon S, Hong C-Z et al. (1997) Interrater reliability in myofascial trigger point examination. Pain 69:65–73
8. Goldenberg DL, Burckhardt C, Crofford L (2004) Management of fibromyalgia syndrome. JAMA 292:2388–2395
9. Hetrick DC, Ciol MA, Rothman I et al. (2003) Musculoskeletal dysfunction in men with chronic pelvic pain syndrome type III: a case-control study. J Urology 170:828–831
10. Jarrell J, Robert M (2003) Myofascial dysfunction and pelvic pain. Canadian J CME Feb:107–116
11. Martinez-Lavin MA, Hermosilla AG, Mendoza C (1997) Orthostatic sympathetic derangement in subjects with fibromyalgia. J Rheumatology 24:714–718
12. Mense S, Simons DG (2001) Muscle Pain. Lippincott Williams & Wilkins, Baltimore, pp 205–288
13. Plotnikoff GA, Quigley JM (2003) Prevalence of severe hypovitaminosis D in patients with persistent, nonspecific musculoskeletal pain. Mayo Clin Proc 78:1463–1470
14. Russell IJ (2001) Fibromyalgia Syndrome. In: Mense S, Simons DG (eds) Muscle Pain. Lippincott Williams & Wilkins, Baltimore, pp 289–337
15. Simons DG, Travell JG, Simons LS (1999) Myofascial Pain and Dysfunction: The Trigger Point Manual. Williams and Wilkins, Baltimore
16. Thompson PD, Clarkson P, Karas RH (2003) Statin-associated myopathy. JAMA 289:1681–1690
17. Weinstein A, Britchkov M (2002) Lyme arthritis and post-Lyme disease syndrome. Curr Opin Rheumatol 14:383–387
18. Weiss JM (2001) Pelvic floor myofascial trigger points: manual therapy for interstitial cystitis and the urgency-frequency syndrome. J Urology 166:2226–2231
19. Wolfe F, Smythe H, Yunus MB et al (1990) The American College of Rheumatolgy criteria for the classification of Fibromyalgia. Arthritis Rheum 33:160–172

Mycobacterium Leprae

Definition

Mycobacterium Leprae is the causative agent of Hansen's disease. The bacterium was discovered in 1873 by a Norwegian physician named Gerhard Armauer Hansen.
► Hansen's Disease

Mycobacterium Species

Definition

Mycobacteria are a large genus of class of bacteria that are responsible for a multitude of diseases of many species. The most common mycobacterium used in Freund's complete adjuvant is mycobacterium tuberculosis, the organism responsible for tuberculosis in humans. Mycobacterium butyricum has also been used in FCA.
► Arthritis Model, Adjuvant-induced Arthritis

Myelin

Definition

Myelin is a specialized cell membrane composed of lipids and proteins that ensheathes axons and fosters rapid electrical conduction.
► Demyelination
► Hereditary Neuropathies
► Postsynaptic Dorsal Column Projection, Anatomical Organization
► Spinothalamic Tract Neurons, Morphology
► Toxic Neuropathies

Myelinated

Definition

Medium and large nerve fibers can be wrapped in a variable number of concentric layers of glial membrane that provide for rapid neurotransmission.
► Postsynaptic Dorsal Column Projection, Anatomical Organization

Myelination

Definition

Myelination is a process by which oligodendroglial cells wrap axons with multiple layers of glial cell membrane forming myelin, which electrically insulates the axon increasing axonal conduction velocity.
► Mechanonociceptors

Myelitis

Definition

Myelitis is the inflammation of the spinal cord.
► Viral Neuropathies

Myelopathy

Definition

Myelopathy is the manifestation of systemic vasculitides and the isolated angiitis of the central nervous system.
► Headache Due to Arteritis

Myelotomy

Definition

Myelotomy or midline or commissural myelotomy is useful for the treatment of bilateral pain syndromes caused by cancer and other illnesses. Second order spinalothalamic tract nociceptive track fibers cross the spinal cord, and a myelotomy is intended to cut these fibers as they decussate in the spinal cord.
▶ Cancer Pain Management, Overall Strategy
▶ Midline Myelotomy

Myenteric Plexus

Definition

The myenteric plexus consists of unmyelinated nerve fibers that are spread out in the muscular part of the intestinal wall of the esophagus, stomach, and intestines. The plexus is involved in the regulation of gut motility.
▶ Opioid Therapy in Cancer Pain Management, Route of Administration

Myocardial Ischemia

▶ Visceral Pain Model, Angina Pain

Myoclonus

Definition

Myoclonus refers to Irregular, involuntary contraction of a muscle.
▶ Opioids and Reflexes

Myofascial

Definition

The fascia (the sheath around a muscle).
▶ Lower Back Pain, Physical Examination
▶ Myofascial Pain

Myofascial Manipulation

Definition

Myofascial manipulation is the forceful, passive movement of the musculofascial components through their restrictive direction. Treatment is initiated in the superficial layers and moves into the deeper layers while considering the relationship to the joints involved.
▶ Chronic Pelvic Pain, Physical Therapy Approaches and Myofascial Abnormalities

Myofascial Pain

ROBERT BENNETT
Department of Medicine, Oregon Health and Science University, Portland, OR, USA
bennetrob1@comcast.net

Synonyms

Trigger Point Pain; Soft Tissue Rheumatism; Myotomal Pain; Localized Muscle Pain

Definitions

Myofascial pain: Pain arising from muscles or related fascia.
Active Trigger point: This is a trigger point that results in pain at rest with increased pain on contraction or stretching of the involved muscle.
Latent trigger point: A latent trigger point is a focal area of tenderness and tightness in a muscle that does not result in spontaneous pain. However, a latent trigger point may restrict range of movement and cause weakness of the involved muscle.

Characteristics

Prevalence

Myofascial pain is a universal occurrence commonly developing as a result of muscle injuries, overuse or repetitive strain. In most instances the problem resolves within a few days without any need for medical intervention. When pain persists or worsens, necessitating a medical consultation, it is referred to as a myofascial pain syndrome (Travell and Simons 1983). There have not been any epidemiological studies of myofascial pain problems in the general population. Rather, physicians have reported prevalence figures in specialized situations. For instance, in one internal medicine practice, 30% of patients presenting with pain complaints were diagnosed as having a myofascial pain origin for their symptoms. A report from a clinic specializing in head and neck pain reported a myofascial etiology in 55% of cases. A report from one pain management center attributed a myofascial origin to the symptomatology in 85% of patients. On the other hand, latent trigger points have been found in

M

the shoulder girdle muscles of 54% of female and 45% of male subjects who were completely asymptomatic (Simons 2001).

Diagnosis

The clinical diagnosis of myofascial pain is critically dependent on the physician being aware of this diagnosis as a possible cause for the patient's pain complaint (Travell and Simons 1983). Myofascial pain syndromes may mimic a large number of other disorders, thus there is a necessity to perform a thorough physical examination, with appropriate investigations. Myofascial pain characteristically presents as a dull deep aching sensation, which is aggravated by use of the involved muscles as well as psychological stressors that cause increased muscle tension (Alvarez and Rockwell 2002). The defining clinical characteristic of myofascial pain is the finding of a trigger point. This is a well-defined point of focal tenderness within a muscle. Sometimes firm palpation of this focus elicits pain in a referred distribution that reproduces the patient's symptoms. Importantly, referred pain from a trigger point does not follow a nerve root distribution (i.e. it is not dermatomal). Palpation usually reveals a ropelike induration of the associated muscle fibers, often referred to as the "taut band". Sometimes, snapping this band or needling the trigger point produces a localized twitch response of the involved muscle. This twitch response can only be reproducibly elicited in fairly superficial muscles. Importantly, trigger points produce functional consequences in terms of a restriction of range of movement and weakness (probably a reflex inhibition secondary to pain), which is usually associated with easy fatigability of the involved muscle.

Clinical Syndromes

A myofascial pain syndrome may be due to just one trigger point, but more commonly there are several trigger points responsible for any given regional pain problem. It is not uncommon for the problem to be initiated with a single trigger point, with the subsequent development of satellite trigger points, which evolve over time due to the mechanical imbalance resulting from reduced range of movement and pseudo-weakness. The persistence of a trigger point may lead to neuroplastic changes at the level of the dorsal horn, which results in amplification of the pain sensation (i.e. central sensitization) with a tendency to spread beyond its original boundaries (i.e. expansion of receptive fields) (Graven-Nielsen and Arendt-Nielsen 2002). In some instances segmental central sensitization leads to the phenomena of mirror image pain (i.e. pain on the opposite side of the body in the same segmental distribution), and in other instances a progressive spread of segmental central sensitization gives rise to the widespread pain that characterizes fibromyalgia (Arendt-Nielsen and Graven-Nielsen 2003).

Low Back Pain

Acute low back pain has many causes. Some are potentially serious, such as cancer metastases, osteomyelitis, massive disk herniations (e.g. cauda equina syndrome), vertebral fractures, pancreatic cancer and aortic aneurysms. However, the commonest cause of acute back pain is so-called lumbosacral strain. In 95% of cases this resolves within three months. In those cases that do not resolve, the development of a chronic low back pain syndrome is usually accompanied by the finding of active myofascial trigger points. Simons describes 15 torso and pelvic muscles that may be involved in low back pain (Simons 2001). The most commonly involved muscle group is the quadratus lumborum; pain emanating from trigger points in these muscles is felt in the low back with occasional radiation in a sciatic distribution or into the testicles. Trigger points involving the iliopsoas are also a common cause of chronic low back pain. The typical distribution of iliopsoas pain is a vertical band in the low back region and the upper portion of the anterior thigh. Trigger points at the origin of the gluteus medius from the iliac crest are a common cause for low back pain in the sacral and buttock, with a referral pattern to the outer hip region.

Neck and Shoulder Pain

Latent trigger points are universal findings in many of the muscles of the posterior neck and upper back. Active trigger points commonly involve the upper portion of the trapezius and levator scapula. Upper trapezius trigger points refer pain to the back of the neck and not uncommonly to the angle of jaw. Levator scapula trigger points cause pain at the angle of the neck and shoulder; this pain is often described as lancinating, especially on active use of this muscle. As many of the muscles in this area have an important postural function, they are commonly activated in office workers and developmental problems causing spinal malalignment (e.g. short leg syndrome, hemipelvis and scoliosis). As the upper trapezius and levator scapulae act synergistically with several other muscles in elevation and fixation of the scapula, it is common for a single trigger point in this region to initiate a spread of satellite trigger points through adjacent muscles that are part of the same functional unit.

Hip Pain

Pain arising from disorders of the hip joint is felt in the groin and the lower medial aspect of the anterior thigh. This distribution is uncommon in myofascial pain syndromes except for iliopsoas pain. The great majority of patients complain of hip pain, and in fact localize their pain to the outer aspect of the hip. In some patients this is due to a trochanteric bursitis, but in the majority of cases it is related to myofascial trigger points in the adjacent muscles. By far the commonest trigger points giving rise to outer hip pain are those in the attachments of the gluteus medius and minimus muscles into the greater trochanter.

Pelvic Pain

The pelvic floor musculature is a common sight for myofascial trigger points. There is increasing recognition by gynecologists and urologists that pain syndromes described in terms of prostatitis, coccydnia, vulvodynia and endometriosis are often accompanied by active myofascial trigger points. One of the most commonly involved intrapelvic muscles is the levator ani; its pain distribution is central low buttock.

Headaches

Active myofascial trigger points in the muscles of the shoulder, neck, and face, are a common source of headaches (Borg-Stein 2002). In many instances, the headache has the features of so-called tension headache, but there is increasing acceptance that myofascial trigger points may initiate classical migraine headaches or be part of a mixed tension/migraine headache complex. For instance, sterno-cleido mastoid trigger points refer pain to the anterior face and supraorbital area. Upper trapezius trigger points refer pain to the vertex forehead and temple. Trigger points in the deep cervical muscles of the neck may cause post occipital and retro-orbital pain.

Jaw Pain

There is a complex interrelationship between temporomandibular joint dysfunction and myofascial trigger points (Fricton et al. 1985) Common trigger points involved in jaw pain syndromes are the massetters, pterygoids, upper trapezius and upper sterno-cleido mastoid.

Upper Limb Pain

The muscles attached to the scapula are common sites for trigger points that can cause upper limb pain (Gerwin 1997). These include the subscapularis, infraspinatus, teres major and serratus anterior. It is not uncommon for trigger points in these locations to refer pain to the wrist, hand, and fingers. Extension flexion injuries to the neck often activate a trigger point in the pectoralis minor with a radiating pain, or down the ulnar side of the arm and into the little finger. Myofascial pain syndromes of the upper limbs are often misdiagnosed as frozen shoulder, cervical radiculopathy or thoracic outlet syndrome (Simons 2001).

Lower Limb Pain

Trigger points in the tensor fascia lata and ilio tibial band may be responsible for lateral thigh pain and lateral knee pain, respectively. Anterior knee pain may result from trigger points in various components of the quadriceps musculature. Posterior knee pain can result from trigger points in the hamstring muscles and popliteus. Trigger points in the anterior tibialis and the peroneus longus muscles may cause pain in the anterior leg and lateral ankle, respectively. Myofascial pain syndromes involving these muscles are often associated with ankle injuries or an excessively pronated foot. Sciatica pain may be mimicked by a trigger point in the posterior portion of the gluteus minimus muscle.

Chest and Abdominal Pain

Disorders affecting intrathoracic and intra-abdominal organs are some of the commonest problems encountered in internal medicine. For instance, anterior chest pain is a frequent cause for emergency room admissions, but in the majority of patients a myocardial infarction is not found. In some cases, the chest pain is caused by trigger points in the anterior chest wall muscles (Travell and Simons 1992). Pectoralis major trigger points cause ipsilateral anterior chest pain with radiation down the ulnar side of the arm – thus mimicking cardiac ischemic pain. A trigger point in the sternalis muscle typically causes a deep substernal aching sensation. Trigger points at the upper and lower insertions of the rectus abdominus muscles may mimic the discomfort of gall bladder and bladder infections, respectively. It is important to note that myofascial trigger points may accompany disorders of intrathoracic and intra-abdominal viscera, and thus a diagnosis of an isolated myofascial cause for symptoms should never be made without an appropriate workup.

Pathogenesis

The precise pathophysiological basis for the trigger point phenomena is still not fully understood. There is a general agreement that electromyographic recordings from trigger points show low voltage spontaneous activity resembling endplate spike potentials (Rivner 2001). Simons envisions a myofascial trigger point to be "a cluster of numerous microscopic loci of intense abnormality that are scattered throughout the tender nodule" (Simons 2001). It is thought that these loci result from a focal energy crisis (from injury or repetitive use), which results in contraction of focal sarcomeric units due to calcium release from the sarcoplasmic reticulum. A more detailed coverage of this topic is provided in the essay ▶ myofascial trigger point. Factors commonly cited as predisposing to trigger point formation include deconditioning, poor posture, repetitive mechanical stress, mechanical imbalance (e.g. leg length inequality), joint disorders, non-restorative sleep and vitamin deficiencies.

Prognosis

Uncomplicated myofascial pain syndromes usually resolve with appropriate correction of predisposing factors and myofascial treatment (Alvarez and Rockwell

M

2002). If the symptoms are persistent, due to ineffective management, the development of segmental central sensitization may lead to a stubbornly recalcitrant pain disorder. In some such cases, the spread of central sensitization leads to the widespread pain syndrome of fibromyalgia.

Treatment

For effective management of myofascial pain, syndromes require attention to the following issues (Alvarez and Rockwell 2002; Rudin 2003):

Postural and Ergonomic

The most critical element in the effective management of myofascial pain syndromes is the correction of predisposing factors (see above). These interfere with the ability of the muscle to fully recover and are the commonest reason for treatment failures.

Stretching

The muscles involved in myofascial pain syndromes are shortened due to the aforementioned focal contractions of sarcomeric units. It is thought that these focal contractions result in a prolonged ATP consumption, and that the restoration of a muscle to its full stretch length breaks the link between the energy crisis and contraction of sarcomeric units. Effective stretching is most commonly achieved through the technique of spray and stretch (Rudin 2003). This involves the cutaneous application, along the axis of the muscle, of ethyl chloride spray, while at the same time passively stretching the involved muscle. Other techniques to enhance effective stretching include trigger point to pressure release, post isometric relaxation, reciprocal inhibition and deep stroking massage (Simons 2001).

Strengthening

Muscles harboring trigger points usually become weak due to the inhibitory effects of pain. A program of slowly progressive strengthening is essential to restore full function and minimize the risk of recurrence and perpetuation of satellite trigger points.

Trigger Point Injections

Injection of trigger points is generally considered to be the most effective means of direct inactivation. A peppering technique using a fine needle to inactivate all the foci within a trigger point locus is the critical element of successful trigger point therapy (Hong 1994). Accurate localization of the trigger point is confirmed if a local twitch response is obtained; however, this may not be obvious when needling deeply lying muscles. Successful elimination of the trigger point usually results in a relaxation of the taut band. Although dry needling is effective, the use of a local anesthetic (1% lidocaine or 1% procaine) helps confirm the accuracy of the injection and provides instant gratification for patients (Hong 1994). There is no evidence that the injection of corticosteroids provides any enhanced effect. A beneficial role for botulinum toxin in trigger point injections has not so far been conclusively demonstrated.

Medications

There is currently no evidence that any form of drug treatment of men eighths myofascial trigger points (Rudin 2003). NSAIDs and other analgesics usually provide moderate symptomatic relief. Tricyclic antidepressant drugs, which modulate pain at the central level, are often of benefit, especially in those patients with an associated sleep disturbance. In the author's experience, tizanidine (a muscle relaxant that also ameliorates pain by activating alpha 2 adrenergic receptors) is often a useful adjunct in difficult to treat myofascial pain syndromes.

Psychological Techniques

In severe myofascial pain syndromes that are not responding to treatment, patients often become anxious and depressed. These mood disorders need to be recognized and appropriately treated. Persistent muscle tension exacerbates the pain of myofascial trigger points and can often be effectively managed with EMG biofeedback, cognitive behavioral therapy and hypnotic/meditation relaxation techniques.

References

1. Alvarez DJ, Rockwell PG (2002) Trigger Points: Diagnosis and Management. Am Fam Physician 65:653–660
2. Arendt-Nielsen L, Graven-Nielsen T (2003) Central Sensitization in Fibromyalgia and Other Musculoskeletal Disorders. Curr Pain Headache Rep 7:355–361
3. Borg-Stein J (2002) Cervical Myofascial Pain and Headache: Curr Pain Headache Rep 6:324–330
4. Fricton JR, Kroening R, Haley D et al. (1985) Myofascial Pain Syndrome of the Head and Neck: A Review of Clinical Characteristics of 164 Patients. Oral Surg Oral Med Oral Pathol 60:615–623
5. Graven-Nielsen T, Arendt-Nielsen L (2002) Peripheral and Central Sensitization in Musculoskeletal Pain Disorders: An Experimental Approach. Curr Rheumatol Rep 4: 313–321
6. Gerwin RD (1997) Myofascial Pain Syndromes in the Upper Extremity. J Hand Ther 10:130–136
7. Hong C-Z (1994) Considerations and Recommendations Regarding Myofascial Trigger Point Injection. J Musculoskeletal Pain 2:29–59
8. Hong C-Z (1994) Lidocaine Injection versus Dry Needling to Myofascial Trigger Point. The Importance of the Local Twitch Response. Am J Phys Med Rehabil 73:256–263
9. Rivner, MH (2001) The Neurophysiology of Myofascial Pain Syndrome. Curr Pain Headache Rep 5:432–440
10. Rudin NJ (2003) Evaluation of Treatments for Myofascial Pain Syndrome and Fibromyalgia. Curr Pain Headache Rep 7:433–442
11. Simons DG (2001) Myofascial Pain Caused by Trigger Points In: Mense S, Simons DG, Russel IJ (eds) Muscle Pain: Understanding its Nature, Diagnosis, and Treatment. Lippincott Williams and Wilkins, Philadelphia, pp 205–288
12. Travell JG, Simons DG (1983) Myofascial Pain and Dysfunction: The Trigger Point Manual. Williams and Wilkins, Baltimore
13. Travell J, Simons D (1992) Myofascial Pain and Dysfunction: The Trigger Point Manual, vol 2. Williams and Wilkins, Baltimore

Myofascial Pain Syndrome

Synonyms

MPS

Definition

Myofascial pain syndrome is a muscle disorder characterized by the presence of trigger points (TrPs) within the muscle. There is also pain, muscle spasm, tenderness, stiffness, limited range of motion, weakness and/or autonomic dysfunction. Pressure on the trigger point refers pain to an area distant from the trigger point. However, the trigger point itself could and usually is painful.

► Chronic Back Pain and Spinal Instability
► Chronic Pelvic Pain, Musculoskeletal Syndromes
► Chronic Pelvic Pain, Physical Therapy Approaches and Myofascial Abnormalities
► Muscle Pain, Fibromyalgia Syndrome (Primary, Secondary)
► Myalgia
► Nocifensive Behaviors (Muscle and Joint)
► Opioids and Muscle Pain
► Sacroiliac Joint Pain
► Stretching
► Trigger Point

Myofascial Release

Definition

Myofascial release can be described as a manual soft tissue technique that can be either direct or indirect, and is frequently combined. As a treatment technique, it utilizes the principles of biomechanical loading of soft tissue, and the neural reflex changes by stimulation of mechanoreceptors in the fascia.

► Chronic Pelvic Pain, Physical Therapy Approaches and Myofascial Abnormalities

Myofascial Trigger Points

DAVID G. SIMONS
Department of Rehabilitation Medicine, Emory University, Atlanta, GA, USA
loisanddavesimons@earthlink.net

Synonyms

MTrP

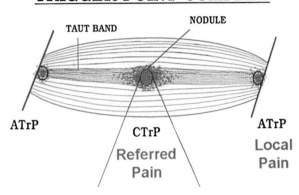

Myofascial Trigger Points, Figure 1 This schematic longitudinal view of muscle illustrates key clinical features of a myofascial trigger point. The central trigger point (CTrP), which is located near the mid-muscle fiber, exhibits outstanding spot tenderness in a palpable taut band and refers pain to a distance. The taut band extends the length of the muscle fibers to its attachments, where the sustained tension of the taut band induces an attachment trigger point (ATrP) enthesopathy (that is sensitive to applied pressure and increased muscle tension). Adapted from Simons et al. (1999).

Definition

Clinically, a central ► myofascial trigger point (MTrP) is characteristically a very tender, circumscribed, nodule-like spot that is located in the mid-portion of a ► taut band of skeletal muscle fibers and can cause referred pain. Application of digital pressure to the spot typically induces referred pain that is characteristic of that muscle, and is familiar to the subject if the MTrP is active. The indurated tender attachments of taut-band muscle fibers are identified as ► attachment trigger points (see Fig. 1).
Etiologically, the central MTrP is associated with ► endplate noise, which originates from a motor endplate that is releasing abnormal amounts of ► acetylcholine. Shortened ► sarcomeres, in the region of endplates, are associated with local release of sensitizing substances (Shah et al. 2005) that cause pain and tenderness.

Characteristics

Myofascial trigger points (MTrPs) are only one part of the complex neuromusculoskeletal pain picture, however, that part is probably as important as the nervous system and is certainly the most neglected and overlooked part. The term myofascial pain is often used with two different meanings. Myofascial pain caused by MTrPs is a specific etiological diagnosis, whereas myofascial pain, used in the general sense of regional pain of unidentified etiology in myofascial structures, is only a symptom, not a diagnosis. Musculoskeletal pain is one of the major causes of common human aches and pains such as low back pain and tension type headache.
In one study, of the 32.5 % of the unselected population who were experiencing chronic pain, 94.5 % identified

it as musculoskeletal (Wolfe et al. 1998). Myofascial trigger points (MTrPs) are often the major cause of the pain, or a major component in association with well-recognized sources of pain. Any of the approximately 500 skeletal muscles can develop MTrPs. For more detailed information on this subject, consult the two latest volumes of The Trigger Point Manual (Simons et al. 1999; Travell and Simons 1992), or the german or spanish editions, and the Muscle Pain book (Mense et al. 2001).

Active MTrPs cause a clinical pain complaint but latent MTrPs do not – an important clinical distinction. One well-designed article (Hsieh et al. 2000) described 520 muscle examinations of muscles commonly causing low back pain (LBP), both in subjects with LBP and in normal pain-free controls. The authors found MTrPs (some active) in 90 % of low back pain subjects' muscles, and found latent MTrPs (not producing a pain complaint) in 70 % of the control subjects' muscles. Latent MTrPs were common in control subjects.

The natural history of MTrPs is unknown; however, a recent study provided a valuable lead. Among 13 healthy, normal, pain-free hospital personnel, only one subject had no latent MTrPs in the eight muscles examined. Two subjects had MTrPs in seven of the eight muscles (see Table 1). Age was not a significant factor. Note subjects 1 and 2. This small sample suggests that most adults have at least some latent MTrPs; a few adults have many and a few have almost none. This needs

verification. If this study is representative, the natural history of MTrPs could be that we are born with the tendency to develop latent MTrPs upon reading adolescence and, during adulthood, life stresses can convert them into active MTrPs. A simple study, by reasonably skilled investigators, could resolve this issue.

The diagnosis of MTrPs can firstly be approached by answering three questions, which require limited manual skill to determine if MTrPs are a viable differential diagnosis. Could MTrPs of muscle be causing the pain? If so, which muscle(s) should be examined? Does an initial screening exam identify active MTrPs? If so, the patient needs further examination and testing by a skilled practitioner who can also treat the MTrPs as listed below. Diagnosis of myofascial trigger points (MTrPs)

- Could MTrPs of muscle be causing the pain?

  - Other possibilities: nerves (radiculopathy), joints (somatic dysfunction), central nervous system (fibromyalgia), viscera (renal calculi), etc.
  - Trigger point pain is initiated by: Sudden, unexpected overload (acute onset from fall or motor vehicle accident)Chronic overload (insidious onset from poor posture, poor ergonomic arrangement, repetitive strain)

- Which muscle(s) should be examined?

  - Which muscles were overloaded (history above)— based on knowledge of muscle functions
  - Distorted posture or movements
  - Pain pattern that fits known patterns of suspected muscle(s).
  - Painful restriction in stretch range of motion of involved muscle(s). Involved muscle shows increased stiffness and tension.

- What is a simple initial muscle examination (differential diagnosis screening)?

  - Localized very tender spot in skeletal muscle+
  - Pressure-evoked referred pain that is characteristic of that muscle= a likely latent myofascial trigger point+
  - Patients' recognition of evoked pain as part or all of the primary pain complaint= a likely active myofascial trigger point

- Confirmatory myofascial trigger point examination (training and skill required)

  - Tender spot feels nodular (if located sufficiently superficial)
  - Tender spot located in a palpable taut band, see Fig. 1
  - Tender attachment TrP (enthesopathy) at attachment of taut band.

Myofascial Trigger Points, Table 1 Distribution of latent myofascial trigger points (MTrPs) in eight muscles of 13 pain-free, healthy normal control subjects. Subjects were numbered to correspond to their relative ages, which ranged between 23 and 59 years. Number 1 was the youngest. Age does not appear to be an important factor among these adults and showed no linear regression.

Subject Number	Number of muscles with MTrPs in each subject
2	7
6	7
10	6
8	5
3	5
12	5
5	4
11	3
13	3
4	2
9	2
7	1
1	0

- Favorable response to specific MTrP treatment
- Occurrence of a local twitch response evoked incidentally by palpation of, or purposely by needle insertion into, the TrP.

The diagnostic process is complicated by the complex neuromusculoskeletal nature of musculoskeletal pain and the lack of a diagnostic gold standard for MTrPs, which are not identifiable by available laboratory or imaging testing. In addition, the appropriate examination depends on the amount and texture of overlying tissue and the skills of the examiner. Different muscles may require quite different examinations.

Initially, the diagnosis depends on medical history, knowledge of MTrP characteristics, and knowledge of muscle anatomy and function. Effective confirmatory examination and treatment depend on clinical skill. A growing body of research studies and clinical experience increasingly substantiates the guidelines presented here.

Could MTrPs of Muscle be Causing the Pain?

Commonly, in patients with chronic myofascial pain, the likely diagnoses, except MTrPs, have already been ruled out, often by numerous expensive tests. Chronic progressive MTrP symptoms are perpetuated by mechanical or systemic factors, which need identification and correction – factors that alone, without the activated MTrPs, often do not cause enough symptoms to demand attention. Without a perpetuating factor, acute onset active MTrPs tend to subside to asymptomatic latent MTrPs with gentle, normal, muscle-stretching daily activities.

Which Muscle(s) Should be Examined?

Patient posture and modified movements is often a key. Special attention should be paid to problems in the feet that commonly reflect dysfunctions, which extend up the body to the head. Active MTrPs of each muscle project a characteristic referred pain pattern that is variable in time and among individuals. Critically important referred pain patterns from active MTrPs throughout the body are described in books (Travell and Simons 1992; Simons et al. 1999; Dejung et al. 2003), also on wall charts and flip charts, and have been updated for masticatory muscles in a journal article (Wright 2000). The pain patterns help greatly to identify the MTrP cause of the pain. The pain that limits stretch is usually located in the involved muscle, rather than in the referred pain zone.

Simple Initial Examination

If palpation with about 3 kilograms of calibrated consistent pressure on a spot of localized tenderness in a suspected muscle elicits referred pain that is familiar to the patient, that spot is likely an active MTrP. MTrPs are then ruled in as a differential diagnosis that requires a confirmatory examination and, if indicated, treatment by a skilled practitioner. Referral may be necessary. Latent MTrPs can cause muscle inhibition, imbalance, and other motor problems.

Confirmatory Myofascial Trigger Point Examination

This examination demands skills that usually require considerable training and clinical practice, and are often critical for effective treatment of MTrPs. Clinically, the taut band is considered by skilled and experienced clinicians to be the most distinctive feature of MTrPs, but was one of the most difficult exams in credible interrater reliability studies because of the skill required (Gerwin et al. 1997; Sciotti et al. 2001). Fortunately, confusingly, similar fascial structures are rarely tender. Taut bands are usually indistinguishable in muscle that lies beneath thick layers of fat, firm subcutaneous tissue and/or overlying muscle tissue. Figure 1 schematically illustrates the relationship between the taut band and its central and attachment ▶ trigger points.

The ▶ local twitch response is a sensory-motor spinal reflex that induces a series of motor unit activations only in taut band fibers. It has high specificity but relatively poor reliability in most hands and can be extremely painful to the patient.

The pathophysiology of MTrPs is not totally unknown, but it is not firmly established and has been controversial. An integrated hypothesis (Simons et al. 1999; Mense et al. 2001; Simons 2004) incorporates the available research studies and explains the clinical features of MTrPs. The hypothesis helps to identify what we do know with confidence and what remains to be clarified. Figure 2 outlines and summarizes the hypothesis.

Clinically, compression (radiculopathy) of the motor nerve can facilitate conversion of latent MTrPs to active ones, which are associated with electromyographic evidence of increased acetylcholine (ACh) release. Excessive spontaneous release can be identified by endplate noise (Simons 2001), which is mistakenly considered a normal finding by many electromyographers – a source of controversy. Endplate noise is significantly associated with MTrPs – a fact not generally recognized by electromyographers – but it is not uniquely diagnostic of MTrPs (Couppe et al. 2001; Simons et al. 2002).

Microscopic changes in muscle fibers in the region of the endplate include localized regions of severe sarcomere shortening (contraction disks and contraction knots), with evidence of increased tension of some fibers. The microscopic picture also suggests the possibility of abnormal calcium permeability of the muscle fiber membrane (sarcolemma). Increased tension of many fibers can account for the taut band. The pathological changes and natural history of MTrPs, suggest the possibility of a genetic aberration of calcium channels of variable penetrance in the sarcolemma, and or neurolemma of the nerve terminal.

M

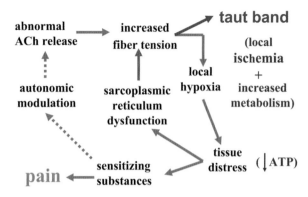

Integrated hypothesis

Myofascial Trigger Points, Figure 2 The integrated hypothesis postulates a positive feedback cycle, which characteristically involves excessive spontaneous release of acetylcholine in a number of motor endplates associated with a myofascial trigger point. Mechanical stress (muscle overload) and increased autonomic activity can cause or increase abnormal spontaneous acetylcholine release. The strong spontaneous local contractile activity increases fiber tension producing the palpable taut band, increased energy demand and local hypoxia. Together, they deplete the supply of adenosine triphosphate (ATP) and produce tissue distress, which releases substances that sensitize nociceptors causing MTrP pain. Shortage of ATP could reduce recovery of calcium into the sarcoplasmic reticulum sustaining contractile activity and increased fiber tension. See text for alternate pathway (broken arrows).

Mechanisms by which the sensitizing substances produce local tenderness and referred pain has been described in detail (Mense et al. 2001) (see Fig. 2). Many substances have been demonstrated histochemically (Shah et al. 2005).

An alternate route to complete the feedback cycle (broken arrows) is presented, because several kinds of studies indicate that increased sympathetic nervous system activity increases the endplate noise (or endplate spikes) of a trigger point. Specific mediators have not been adequately identified for locally modulating autonomic effects, which include release of ACh packets from the nerve terminal. Both routes may occur.

Treatment

Three manual treatments of MTrPs – contract-release, trigger point pressure release, and vapocoolant spray and release – are usually effective (Simons 2002). In addition, injection or dry needling provides another valuable approach (Simons et al. 1999). A quite new and remarkably effective modality that operates on a poorly explored mechanism is frequency specific microcurrent therapy (www.frequentcyspecific.com). This has been demonstrated to be effective for MTrPs (McMakin 2004) and in patients who developed fibromyalgia following a whiplash injury (McMakin 2005) as listed below. The patient benefits when treatment begins with manual therapy rather than dry needling or injection. When patients are shown how to perform the manual therapy on themselves, the experience of immediate

pain relief helps to convince them that muscles are causing the pain, gives them a sense of control, and improves compliance for the important home stretching exercises. When the patient receives only dry needling or injection, treatment becomes the clinician's responsibility, not the patient's. A close physician-therapist relationship permits the physician to concentrate on injections when indicated, while the therapist teaches the patient home stretch exercises specific to the involved muscles. Treatments may cause slight discomfort, but should always be pain-free (not over about 2 or 3 on a 10 point visual analog scale) to avoid plasticity changes in the central nervous system, which enhances and prolongs pain perception.

Treatment of myofascial trigger points (MTrPs)

- Manual techniques

    - Trigger point pressure release—finger pressure applied to the MTrP
    - Contract release—alternate voluntary contraction and passive or active stretching of the muscle with the MTrPs
    - Vapocoolant spray and stretch—application of a stream of vapocoolant, or use of a covered edge of ice, to facilitate release

- Needling techniques (require diagnostic skill)

    - Dry needling (as effective as injection, but leaves more post injection soreness)

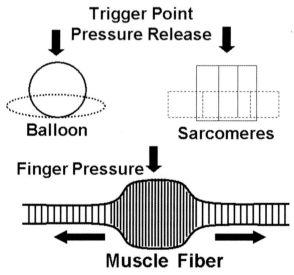

Myofascial Trigger Points, Figure 3 This schematic illustrates the mechanism by which trigger point pressure release can relieve the tension of the taut band by elongating the shortened sarcomeres, which has the effect of localized stretching of the muscle fibers. Like the balloon, a sarcomere has a nearly constant volume, so flattening elongates it. The contracted fibers in the nodular swelling of muscle fibers represent either a contraction knot or contraction disc. The effect of trigger point pressure release is enhanced by including a gentle voluntary contraction of that muscle, while holding it at positions of progressive gentle passive stretch.

- Injection of 1% lidocaine (reduces post-injection soreness)
- Injection of Botulinum toxin (specifically for muscles with spasticity and MTrPs using electromyographic guidance for endplate noise).

- New possibilities
  - Frequency specific microcurrent therapy
  - Shockwave therapy

Figure 3 shows how ▶ trigger point pressure release can be effective. Shortened sarcomeres are a key part of the cause of MTrP symptoms. The constant-volume balloon is analogous to a sarcomere, showing how gentle but firm pressure on contraction knots (or contraction discs) will flatten and lengthen (normalize) the shortened sarcomeres. As their tension releases, digital pressure is increased. This local stretch reduces actin and myosin overlap, which reduces contractile activity, energy consumption, and ischemia – all of which tend to break the TrP feedback cycle.

▶ Contract-release (also post-isometric relaxation) requires only recognition of the painfully restricted stretch range of motion to which this treatment is then applied (see Fig. 4). This can be learned and used by patients. If necessary, additional release can often be obtained with vapocoolant spray and stretch, dry needling, injection of the MTrP with 1% lidocaine (to reduce post-injection soreness) or with reciprocal inhibition. Following treatment, three full cycles of active range of motion help to normalize function of the treated muscle. If relief is still temporary, perpetuating factors must be investigated and resolved.

Effective injection or dry needling require precise location of the MTrP to enter it with the needle. Elicited pain and local twitch responses assure a more effective treatment. Concentration on just injection encourages neglect of home exercises and perpetuating factors, and the patient usually does not understand the cause of the pain as well.

Since Botulinum toxin inactivates ACh release at the motor endplate, it should be a specific therapy for MTrPs and has been effective. However, it is very expensive, lasts about 3 months, can induce an immune reaction, and is unlikely to be more effective than the other techniques described when they are skillfully applied. It is specifically indicated in muscles that are spastic and also have painful MTrPs. Botulinum toxin is most effectively injected under electromyographic guidance.

Application of shockwave technology for the localization and treatment of MTrPs looks promising. (Bauermeister 2005; Müller-Ehrenberg and Licht 2005).

One reason for the neglect of MTrPs as a muscular source of pain is that no medical specialty takes responsibility for research and training in all medical aspects of muscle as an organ. As a result, clinical and basic research on MTrPs is conspicuous for its scarcity, and MTrP training of medical practitioners is rarely adequately covered in schools. It can be very difficult for patients to find practitioners adequately skilled in the diagnosis and treatment of MTrPs.

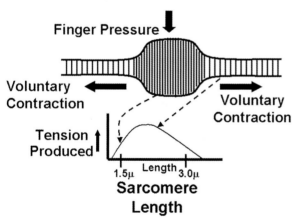

Myofascial Trigger Points, Figure 4 Schematic showing effect of combining trigger point pressure release (Finger Pressure) and contract-release, which takes advantage of the reduction in muscle tightness following a gentle (about 10 % of maximum effort) voluntary contraction. Treatment slowly alternates between gentle voluntary contractions held for several seconds, immediately followed by passive or active stretching of the muscle. This takes up slack that developed following contraction. The contraction-release cycles can be repeated rhythmically, as long as each cycle brings progress. The graph of a characteristic length-tension curve for one sarcomere shows that the strongly shortened sarcomeres produce much less tension than the mid-length sarcomeres throughout the rest of the muscle fiber. The mid-length sarcomeres are both stronger and far outnumber the shortened sarcomeres, so a gentle contraction temporarily increases the length of the shortened sarcomeres. Several cycles of full range of motion help to consolidate treatment gains. The two techniques are combined for increased therapeutic effectiveness.

Myofascial Trigger Points, Table 2 Number of MEDLINE citations (mainstream medical literature) that were indexed in the past 7 years under *low back pain* compared to the number of trigger point citations retrieved by combining *low back pain and trigger points* with a *low back pain and myofascial trigger point* search.

Year of Publication	Low Back Pain Citations	Trigger Point Citations	Percent Trigger Point (%)
1996	552	2	0,4
1997	312	2	0,5
1998	459	2	0,4
1999	561	0	0
2000	527	3	0,6
2001	537	3	0,6
2002	553	5	0,9
1996–2002	3601	17	0,5

Unfortunately, many practitioners were not trained to include MTrPs as a differential diagnosis for musculoskeletal pain. Low back pain (LBP) causes much human suffering and health care costs. However, of the 3,501 LBP citations retrieved from MEDLINE covering the past seven years, less than 1% were also indexed as including MTrPs (see Table 2). Moreover, much LBP is either caused by MTrPs or has a significant MTrP component. A number of papers that do relate MTrPs and LBP describe MTrPs, but do not identify them in the title or abstract. A few articles that identified MTrPs in LBP were published in journals that are not listed by MEDLINE. Most authors writing about LBP do not include MTrPs as part of their routine differential diagnosis.

A recent series of papers by César Fernández of spain and collegues is now appearing in the scientific literature that indicate a strong relationship between MTrPs and several kinds of headache (Fernández et. Al 2005; Fernández et al. 2006).

► Central Trigger Point
► Chronic Pelvic Pain, Physical Therapy Approaches and Myofascial Abnormalities
► Dry Needling
► Myalgia

References

1. Bauermeister W (2005) Diagnose und Therapie des Myofaszialen Triggerpunk Syndroms durch Lokalisierung und Stimulation Sensibilisierter Nozizeptoren mit Focussierten Elektrohydraulischen Stosswellen. MOT 5:65–74
2. Couppé C, Midttun A, Hilden J et al. (2001) Spontaneous Needle Electromyographic Activity in Myofascial Trigger Points in the Infraspinatus Muscle: A Blinded Assessment. J Musculoske Pain 9:7–16
3. Dejung B, Gröbli C, Colla F et al. (2003) Triggerpunkt-Therapie (Trigger Point Therapy). Hans Huber Verlag, Bern
4. Gerwin RD, Shannon S, Hong C-Z et al. (1997) Interrater Reliability in Myofascial Trigger Point Examination.Pain 69: 65–73
5. Hsieh C-Y, Hong C-Z, Adams AH et al. (2000) Interexaminer Reliability of the Palpation of Trigger Points in the Trunk and Lower Limb Muscles. Arch Phys Med Rehabil 81:258–264
6. Mense S, Simons DG, Russell IJ (2001) Muscle Pain: Its Nature, Diagnosis, and Treatment. Lippincott, Williams & Wilkins, Philadelphia
7. Sciotti VM, Mittak VL, DiMarco L et al. (2001) Clinical Precision of Myofascial Trigger Point Location in the Trapezius Muscle. Pain 93:259–266
8. Shah JP, Phillips T, Danoff J et al. (2004) Novel Microanalytical Technique Distinguishes Three Clinically Distinct Groups: 1) Subjects without Pain and without a Myofascial Trigger Point; 2) Subjects without Pain with a Myofascial Trigger Point; 3) Subjects with Pain and a Myofascial Trigger Point. Am J Phys Med Rehabil 83:231
9. Simons DG (2001) Do Endplate Noise and Spikes Arise from Normal Motor Endplates? Am J Phys Med Rehabil 80:134–140
10. Simons DG (2002) Understanding Effective Treatments of Myofascial Trigger Points. J Bodywork and Movement Therapy 6:81–88
11. Simons DG, Hong C-Z, Simons LS (2002) Endplate Potentials are Common to Midfiber Myofascial Trigger Points. Am J Phys Med Rehabil 81:212–222
12. Simons DG, Travell JG, Simons LS (1999) Travell & Simons' Myofascial Pain and Dysfunction: The Trigger Point Manual, vol 1, edn 2. Williams & Wilkins, Baltimore
13. Travell JG, Simons DG (1992) Myofascial Pain and Dysfunction: The Trigger Point Manual, vol 2. The Lower Extremities. Williams & Wilkins, Baltimore
14. Wolfe F, Ross K, Anderson J et al. (1998) The Prevalence and Characteristics of Fibromyalgia in the General Population. Arthritis Rheum 38:19–28
15. Wright EF (2000) Referred Craniofacial Pain Patterns in Patients with Temporomandibular Disorder. JADA 131:1307–1315

Myofibrositis

► Myalgia

Myogelosis

► Myalgia

Myositis

DIETER PONGRATZ
Friedrich Baur Institute, Medical Faculty at the Neurological Clinic and Policlinic, Ludwig Maximilians University, Munich, Germany
dieter.pongratz@fbs.med.uni-muenchen.de

Synonyms

Inflammatory Myopathies

Definition

Inflammatory Myopathies represent a small, but from a therapeutical point of view, important group of acquired muscular disorders. With the exception of infectious causes (viral myositis, bacterial myositis, and parasitic myositis) immunogenic forms have to be considered. There are 4 different forms:

1. Dermatomyostis
2. Overlap Syndromes
3. ► Polymyositis
4. ► Inclusion Body Myositis

Characteristics

The most prominent clinical symptoms of all immunogenic inflammatory myopathies are muscle weakness and muscle atrophy. Muscle pain is common in ► dermatomyositis and overlap syndromes, but is less prominent or even missing in chronic polymyositis and especially inclusion body myositis. From a clinical point of view, there is a predominant involvement of the proximal muscles of the limbs and the arms. Only in inclusion body myositis is the presence of distal muscle weakness, especially of the foot extensors and finger flexors, a diagnostic clue from the beginning.

Negative Reinforcement

Definition

Negative reinforcement is the removal of an aversive stimulus (tangible or non-tangible) following a behavior, with the goal of increasing future incidents of that behavior.
► Impact of Familial Factors on Children's Chronic Pain
► Operant Perspective of Pain

Negative Responding

► Spouse, Role in Chronic Pain

Negative Sensory Phenomenon

Definition

Negative sensory phenomenon is a clinical sign that is interpreted by the patient as less than when compared to normal bodily function and experiences.
► Hypoalgesia, Assessment
► Hypoesthesia, Assessment

Nematode

Definition

Nematode is a roundworm, a non-segmented worm phylum.
► Species Differences in Skin Nociception

Neocortical

Definition

Belonging to the top, approximately 2 mm thick layer of the two hemispheres of the brain.
► Prefrontal Cortex, Effects on Pain-Related Behavior

Neonatal Inflammation

► Visceral Pain Model, Irritable Bowel Syndrome Model

Neonatal Pain

► Visceral Pain Model, Irritable Bowel Syndrome Model

Neonate

► Newborn

Neospinothalamic Tract

Definition

Lateral and phylogenetically younger component of the spinothalamic tract, also known as the lateral spinothalamic tract. It is comprised of the axons nociceptive-specific and wide dynamic range neurons. It projects to the ventral posterolateral nucleus of the thalamus and is responsible for the discriminative aspects of pain (location, intensity, duration).
► Acute Pain Mechanisms
► Parafascicular Nucleus, Pain Modulation
► Somatic Pain

Nerve Blocks by Local Anesthetic Drugs

N

Definition

Nerve blocks by local anesthetic drugs stop nerve impulse conduction in nerve cells, inhibiting pain impulses from reaching the central nervous system (CNS). They will often also make the pain-free body part numb, with weak or paralyzed muscles.
► Cancer Pain Management, Anesthesiologic Interventions
► Epidural Steroid Injections for Chronic Back Pain
► Postoperative Pain, Acute Pain Management, Principles

Nerve Compression

Definition

Nerve compression or nerve entrapment is caused by mechanical obstruction. They usually involve mixed nerves so the symptoms are motor sensory. Compression of pure motor nerves, which carry muscle and joint afferents, may produce deep diffuse discomfort. Pain in the referred territory, numbness, exacerbated by movements are the main symptoms. Nerve compression is more acute than (chronic) nerve entrapment. The treatment of choice is decompression, either pharmacological (dexamethasone) or surgical. Nerve blocks are also useful.
► Cancer Pain

Nerve Conduction

Definition

Nerve conduction is a clinical test of named peripheral nerves, in which all axons are stimulated to threshold, and the responses of the largest cohort of myelinated axons are measured.

▶ Electrodiagnosis and EMG
▶ Hereditary Neuropathies

Nerve Growth Factor

Synonym

NGF

Definition

Nerve growth factor (NGF) belongs to a family of polypeptide growth factors. It consists of alpha, beta and gamma subunits. NGF is a target-derived factor and is essential for survival, differentiation, and maintenance of sympathetic and afferent neurons. In inflamed tissue, NGF biosynthesis is rapidly increased leading to elevated concentrations of NGF in inflamed tissues. It has been shown that NGF is a mediator of inflammatory hyperalgesia and also a modulator of immune cell function. An enhanced retrograde transport of NGF to the DRG leads to an increase in the production of brain-derived neurotrophic factor (BDNF) at the level of gene expression, mainly in trkA-expressing small- and medium-sized neurons. During embryonic and early postnatal stages, sensory neurons are dependent on NGF for survival. Although adult sensory neurons do not depend on NGF for survival, the functional properties of some nociceptive sensory neurons, such as responsiveness to capsaicin or noxious heat, are modulated by NGF. NGF can exert its actions either through the high-affinity trkA receptor or the low-affinity p75 neurotrophin receptor.

▶ Congenital Insensitivity to Pain with Anhidrosis
▶ ERK Regulation in Sensory Neurons during Inflammation
▶ IB4-Positive Neurons, Role in Inflammatory Pain
▶ Immunocytochemistry of Nociceptors
▶ Nerve Growth Factor, Sensitizing Action on Nociceptors
▶ Neutrophils in Inflammatory Pain
▶ Satellite Cells and Inflammatory Pain
▶ Spinal Cord Nociception, Neurotrophins
▶ TRPV1, Regulation by Nerve Growth Factor
▶ TRPV1, Regulation by Protons
▶ Wallerian Degeneration

Nerve Growth Factor Overexpressing Mice as Models of Inflammatory Pain

DEREK C. MOLLIVER, KATHRYN M. ALBERS
Department of Medicine, University of Pittsburgh
School of Medicine, Pittsburgh, PA, USA
kaa2@pitt.edu

Synonyms

Transgenic Mice; NGF-OE mice

Definitions

NGF and Inflammatory Pain

In peripheral tissues, the level of nerve growth factor (NGF) expression is often elevated following inflammation or injury (Heumann et al. 1987; Weskamp and Otten 1987). Studies using rodents have shown that injection of NGF causes behavioral thermal and mechanical ▶ hyperalgesia (Lewin et al. 1993; Lewin et al. 1994). Increased NGF expression is also accompanied by elevation of other inflammatory mediators such as bradykinin, prostaglandins, serotonin, ATP and protons (Bennett 2001). These changes in the periphery are thought to collectively contribute to sensitization of sensory afferents and central pain processing pathways. The link between NGF and inflammatory pain signaling can be examined using a transgenic mouse model (see ▶ Nerve Growth Factor Overexpressing Mice as Models of Inflammatory Pain) in which NGF is overexpressed in the skin, a major target of sensory afferents. In these mice (NGF-OE mice), NGF is overexpressed in basal keratinocytes of stratified, keratinizing tissues such as the skin and oral epithelium, using the human keratin K14 promoter and enhancer region to drive expression of the mouse NGF cDNA (Albers et al. 1994). As described below, the increase in NGF expression causes an increase in the developmental survival of neurons that project to K14-expressing epithelium, altering their physiological properties and the expression of genes related to nociceptive signaling.

Characteristics

Anatomical Characteristics of NGF-OE Transgenic Mice

Mice that overexpress NGF in the skin exhibit hypertrophy of both sensory and sympathetic neurons (Albers et al. 1994; Davis et al. 1994; Davis et al. 1997). NGF–OE mice have an approximate 2-fold increase in the number of trigeminal and dorsal root ganglion (DRG) sensory neurons, and a 2.5-fold increase in the number of sympathetic neurons in the superior cervical ganglia. In addition, preferential increases of unmyelinated and thinly myelinated fibers that project to the skin occur (Davis et al. 1997; Stucky et al. 1999), a finding consistent with the types of axons lost in ▶ ngf -/- mice (Crowley et al.

1994). Immunolabeling of skin and DRG have shown a preferential increase of peptidergic sensory neuron subtypes. For example, the percent of TrkA neurons is doubled, as is the percent of calcitonin gene related peptide-positive neurons (Goodness et al. 1997). The population of sensory neurons that bind the plant lectin IB4 is not increased, consistent with the finding that glial cell line-derived growth factor (GDNF) is a major contributor to the trophic support of these neurons (Molliver et al. 1997).

Electrophysiologic Properties of NGF-OE Cutaneous Afferents

Electrophysiologic properties of cutaneous sensory afferents in the ► saphenous nerve of NGF-OE mice were analyzed using a skin-nerve preparation (Stucky et al. 1999). Large myelinated, low-threshold Aβ fibers showed no change in the proportion of slowly adapting (SA) or rapidly adapting (RA) fibers relative to wildtype animals. In addition, no significant difference in the mechanical stimulus-response properties, or conduction velocity, of SA or RA fibers of NGF-OE mice were found.

In contrast to Aβ fibers, both Aδ and C fiber nociceptors of NGF-OE mice had altered properties. The percent of Aδ mechanosensitive (AM) nociceptors was significantly increased from control values of 65% of all Aδ fibers analyzed to 97% in NGF-OE mice. Individual AM fibers also showed increased mechanical responsiveness, which was particularly evident at suprathreshold stimuli. A 100–300 mN sustained force evoked discharge rates in NGF-OE AM fibers double those of wildtypes. Though mechanically sensitized, AM fibers were unchanged with heat sensitivity. No significant difference was measured in the percent of AM fibers that respond to heat, the threshold for a response, or in the mean spikes per heat stimulus.

C fiber afferents showed a 50% increase in total number in the saphenous nerve of NGF-OE mice (Stucky et al. 1999). Nearly all C fibers (96%) responded to heat and showed a four-fold increase in the number of heat evoked action potentials per C fiber. In addition, C fibers in NGF-OE mice exhibited spontaneous activity that was much higher than C fibers of wildtype mice (60% versus 6.5%, respectively). This increase in sensitivity was not global however, since the response of C fibers to mechanical stimulation was half relative to control fibers. Thus, increased NGF in the skin regulates the receptive properties of cutaneous C and Aδ fibers in differential manners.

Behavioral Phenotype of Naïve NGF-OE Mice

To evaluate the response of NGF-OE mice to inflammatory stimuli, the behavioral response of NGF-OE mice to a focused heat source applied to the foot was measured. Two other types of animals were used for comparison in this analysis: littermate control mice (Blk6/C3H strain) and transgenic mice that overexpress GDNF in the skin (GDNF-OE mice). GDNF-OE mice have an enhancement of GDNF-dependent nociceptor neurons (Zwick et al. 2002). GDNF-dependent neurons are peptide poor neurons, which primarily project to lamina II of the spinal cord (with some overlap in lamina I) and bind the plant lectin IB4 (Vulchanova et al. 2001). During postnatal development, GDNF-dependent neurons switch dependence from NGF to GDNF, and express the

N

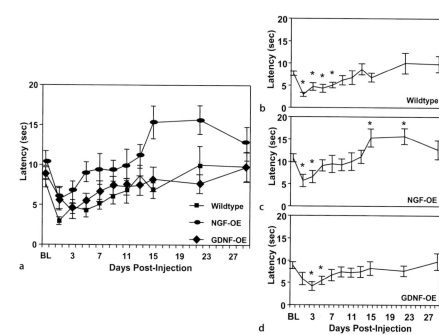

Nerve Growth Factor Overexpressing Mice as Models of Inflammatory Pain, Figure 1 CFA injections did not cause increased hyperalgesia in NGF-OE and GDNF-OE mice. (a) Comparison of all three genotypes. (b) Wildtype, (c) NGF-OE and (d) GDNF-OE mice were injected with CFA and tested for behavioral heat hyperalgesia over a 1 month time period. Each mouse line exhibited significant hyperalgesia within 3 days of being injected. NGF-OE mice recovered first (by day 5), followed by GDNF-OE mice on day 7. Wildtype mice did not fully recover until day 9. NGF-OE mice also exhibited hypoalgesia on days 15 and 22 (relative to their pre-CFA baseline). ν=Wildtype mice; μ=NGF-OE mice; u=GDNF-OE mice; BL=Baseline value.

tyrosine kinase receptor Ret and its coreceptor GFRα1 (Molliver et al. 1997). GDNF dependent neurons have been proposed to primarily modulate responses to ▶ neuropathic pain as opposed to inflammatory pain (Snider and McMahon 1998). To compare NGF and GDNF-dependent nociceptor populations, the behavioral response of NGF-OE, GDNF-OE and wildtype (WT) mice to heat was measured (Fig. 1). This analysis showed NGF-OE mice had slightly longer latencies (they were hypoalgesic) relative to WT and GDNF-OE mice, which had equivalent baselines (Zwick et al. 2003).

Response of NGF-OE and GDNF-OE Mice to Inflammatory Stimuli

The response of NGF-OE, GDNF-OE and WT mice to inflammatory pain was tested by injecting an emulsion of ▶ complete Freund's adjuvant (CFA) subcutaneously into the plantar skin of the hind paw (Zwick et al. 2003). Sets of 10 animals were tested for heat and mechanical hyperalgesia at various timepoints following CFA injection (Fig. 1). WT and NGF-OE mice showed decreased response times 1 day post-injection (Fig. 1b–d). On day 3, all three genotypes displayed hyperalgesic behavior compared to their respective baselines. All groups of animals showed recovery following the 3-day time-point, with WT mice recovering to normal by day 9, GDNF-OE mice recovering by day 7 and NGF-OE mice recovering by day 5. NGF-OE mice not only recovered faster than wildtype and GDNF-OE mice, they became hypoalgesic between days 15 and 22 relative to their starting baseline. Thus, the increased number of nociceptors in NGF-OE and GDNF-OE transgenic mice did not cause a hyperalgesic phenotype in the naïve or inflamed state.

The lack of enhanced behavioral hyperalgesia in NGF-OE and GDNF-OE mice suggested compensatory changes developed in each transgenic mouse line in response to the trophin-induced anatomical and physiological changes. To examine how these analgesic effects could be elicited, mRNA expression for selected genes thought to be involved in nociceptive signaling was analyzed in the L4/L5 dorsal horn and DRG of naïve mice (Tab. 1 and 2) (Zwick et al. 2003). ▶ Real time PCR analysis of reverse transcribed total RNA isolated from the dorsal horn of the spinal cord and lumbar DRG were done. No significant change for any of the genes examined was found in dorsal horn mRNA samples (Tab. 1).

However, in L4/L5 DRG, significant changes were measured for most of the gene products examined (Tab. 2). In NGF-OE DRG, changes were found for the opioid receptors MOR1, DOR1, KOR1 and NR1, NR2B, mGluR1 and the sodium channel Nav1.3. In GDNF-OE DRG, mRNAs encoding DOR1, KOR1 and mGluR1

Nerve Growth Factor Overexpressing Mice as Models of Inflammatory Pain, Table 1 Change in mRNA abundance in mouse dorsal horn

mRNA	WT vs. NGF-OE (fold change)	WT vs. GDNF-OE (fold change)
MOR1	1.0	+1.2
DOR1	1.0	+1.2
KOR1	+1.3	+1.1
NR1	-1.1	1.0
NR2B	+1.3	+1.3
mGluR1	+1.1	+1.1
DREAM	+1.1	+1.1

All values are reported as fold change relative to wildtype (WT) measurements. A value of "1" indicates no change. Negative values indicate a decrease. None of the observed changes were statistically significant

Nerve Growth Factor Overexpressing Mice as Models of Inflammatory Pain, Table 2 Change in mRNA abundance in mouse L4-L5 dorsal root ganglia

mRNA	WT vs. NGF-OE (fold change)	WT vs. GDNF-OE (fold change)
MOR1	+3.2*	-1.1
DOR1	-1.6*	-1.5*
KOR1	+1.5*	+2.1*
NR1	-1.8*	1.0
NR2B	-1.8*	1.0
mGluR1	+3.1*	+3.7*
Nav 1.8	+2.6	+2.1
Nav 1.3	-1.4*	+1.1

All values are reported as fold change relative to wildtype (WT) measurements. Fold change equal to "1" indicates no change. Negative values indicate a decrease. Asterisk indicates $p < 0.05$

were changed. Thus, opioid and glutamate signaling in the primary afferent may contribute to the compensatory changes evoked in transgenic OE animals in the naïve state.

How these selected genes changed on the transcriptional level, following CFA injection into the hind paw, was then examined (Molliver et al. 2005). Genes expressed in lumbar DRG of NGF-OE, GDNF-OE and WT animals were assayed using real time PCR (Fig. 2). Measures were done at 0 (baseline), 1-day, 4-day and 15-day time-points, post CFA treatment. These times coincide with the development, maximal expression and resolution of thermal hyperalgesia, as indicated by the behavioral measures (Fig. 1). This analysis showed that opioid receptor mRNA abundance is changed in DRG following CFA injection (Fig. 2). Following CFA injection in

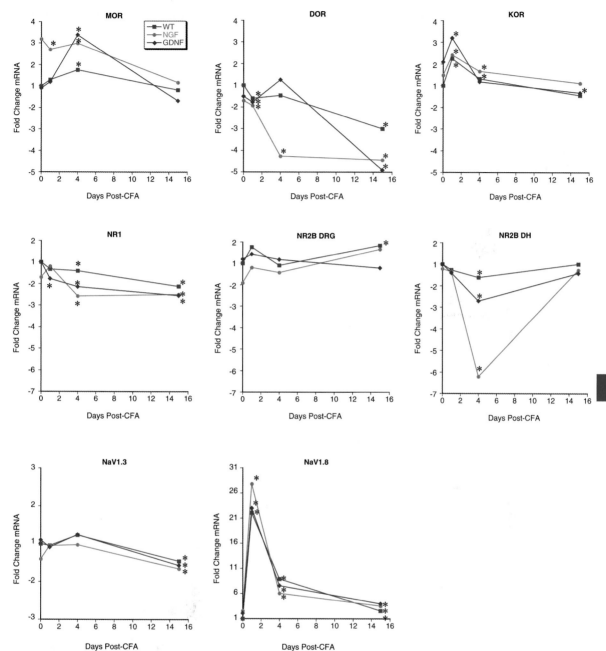

Nerve Growth Factor Overexpressing Mice as Models of Inflammatory Pain, Figure 2 Comparison of the temporal change in mRNA levels of various genes related to nociception in DRG and dorsal horn of wildtype (green line), NGF-OE (red line) and GDNF-OE (blue line) mice following CFA injection in the hind paw. CFA injection was done at day 0 and the relative abundance of mRNAs for each gene determined using real time PCR assays. A significant change from the baseline value determined for each animal type is indicated by an asterisk.

WT mice, MOR mRNA levels were slightly elevated, in contrast to GDNF-OE mice, where a spike at 4 days occurred followed by a decline. Although the abundance of MOR mRNA was increased (3.2 fold) in NGF-OE mice at baseline, a steady decline in MOR levels was also measured in NGF-OE DRG. DOR mRNA was downregulated in WT mice following CFA injection, though an overall greater decline occurred in both OE lines. In all

genotypes, KOR showed a peak rise at 1 day, followed by a decline back to near baseline levels.

For the NMDA receptor subunit NR1, a decrease for all genotypes occurred by the 4-day time-point and continued to the 15-day time-point. The decrease in NR1 in the transgenics is particularly profound, given the increased number of nociceptive neurons in these mice. Notably, both lines of transgenic mice recover from CFA-evoked hyperalgesia early: NGF-OEs by day 5 and GDNF-OEs by day 7 (Fig. 1). The NR2B subunit showed no significant change in NGF-OE or GDNF-OE ganglia, and was only modestly elevated in WT ganglia at the 15-day timepoint. As NR2B may mediate central sensitization, mRNA abundance was assessed in the dorsal horn (DH) of the lumbar spinal cord. In WT mice, NR2B was slightly decreased in the dorsal horn at 4 days, with a return to baseline by 15 days. In the GDNF-OE and NGF-OE samples, this pattern of regulation was exaggerated, particularly for NGF-OE samples, which showed a near 7-fold decrease at 4 days. Similar to WT animals, both transgenic samples had a return to baseline by day 15. This suggests that NGF-OE mice compensate for the increased nociceptor input by downregulation of NR2B, which presumably restricts second messenger potentiation of NMDA currents, and inhibits sensitization of spinal synapses contributing to hyperalgesia.

The regulation of the sodium channel (Nav1.8 and Nav1.3) mRNA level in DRG of NGF-OE and GDNF-OE lines was very similar to the pattern of change in WT mice, i.e., a sharp rise in Nav1.8 is seen at 2 days post CFA, followed by a decline to near normal level by day 4. In contrast to the response in Nav1.8, Nav1.3 mRNA abundance showed a steady decline, which became significantly lower than baseline levels by day 15.

NGF overexpression in skin results in nociceptive primary sensory neurons that are hyperexcitable and present in substantially increased numbers. However, when tested behaviorally, these mice are resistant to inflammatory hyperalgesia and actually become hypoalgesic. Evidence suggests the resistance in each OE line to inflammatory pain is due to compensatory changes in nociceptive signaling, which act to reduce the impact of the increased nociceptive input. Understanding of how these compensatory changes develop and are regulated following injury will provide insight into the role of NGF in inflammatory pain processes. In particular, this model system has allowed identification of genes that are more susceptible to compensatory regulation. For instance, Nav1.8 is essentially the same in all genotypes after CFA, whereas in transgenic mice the opioid receptors and NMDA receptors exhibit striking alteration, relative to WT mice, in their patterns of transcriptional regulation following an inflammatory challenge. This suggests that specific elements in the transcriptional response to injury are particularly amenable to modulation and that their expression may determine the severity of the injury response, whereas other elements show a more fixed transcriptional response to injury. The NGF-OE mice provide a model system in which to examine this hypothesis. In addition, the OE system provides a means in which to determine how different subpopulations of nociceptive neurons respond to inflammatory stimuli. In this manner, a more global visualization of the role of growth factor expression in primary afferent sensitization following injury and their use as therapeutic targets can be constructed.

References

1. Albers KM, Wright DE, Davis BM (1994) Overexpression of Nerve Growth Factor in Epidermis of Transgenic Mice Causes Hypertrophy of the Peripheral Nervous System. J Neurosci 14:1422–1432
2. Bennett DL (2001) Neurotrophic Factors: Important Regulators of Nociceptive Function. Neuroscientist 7:13–17
3. Crowley C, Spencer SD, Nishimura MC, Chen KS, Pitts-Meek S, Armanini MP, Ling LH, MacMahon SB, Shelton DL, Levinson AD et al. (1994) Mice Lacking Nerve Growth Factor Display Perinatal Loss of Sensory and Sympathetic Neurons yet Develop Basal Forebrain Cholinergic Neurons. Cell 76:1001–1011
4. Davis BM, Albers KM, Seroogy KB, Katz DM (1994) Overexpression of Nerve Growth Factor in Transgenic Mice Induces Novel Sympathetic Projections to Primary Sensory Neurons. J Comp Neurol 349:464–474
5. Davis BM, Fundin BT, Albers KM, Goodness TP, Cronk KM, Rice FL (1997) Overexpression of Nerve Growth Factor in Skin Causes Preferential Increases Among Innervation to Specific Sensory Targets. J Comp Neurol 387:489–506
6. Goodness TP, Albers KM, Davis FE, Davis BM (1997) Overexpression of Nerve Growth Factor in Skin Increases Sensory Neuron Size and Modulates Trk Receptor Expression. Eur J Neurosci 9:1574–1585
7. Heumann R, Korsching S, Bandtlow C, Thoenen H (1987) Changes of Nerve Growth Factor Synthesis in Nonneuronal Cells in Response to Sciatic Nerve Transection. J Cell Biol 104:1623–1631
8. Lewin GR, Ritter AM, Mendell LM (1993) Nerve Growth Factor-Induced Hyperalgesia in the Neonatal and Adult Rat. J Neurosci 13:2136–2148
9. Lewin GR, Rueff A, Mendell LM (1994) Peripheral and Central Mechanisms of NGF-Induced Hyperalgesia. Eur J Neurosci 6:1903–1912
10. Molliver DC, Wright DE, Leitner ML, Parsadanian AS, Doster K, Wen D, Yan Q, Snider WD (1997) IB4-Binding DRG Neurons Switch from NGF to GDNF Dependence in Early Postnatal Life. Neuron 19:849–861
11. Molliver DC, Lindsay J, Albers KM and Davis BM (2005) Overexpression of NGF or GDNF alters transcriptional plasticity evoked by inflammation. Pain 113:277–284
12. Snider WD, McMahon SB (1998) Tackling Pain at the Source: New Ideas about Nociceptors. Neuron 20:629–632
13. Stucky CL, Koltzenburg M, Schneider M, Engle MG, Albers KM, Davis BM (1999) Overexpression of Nerve Growth Factor in Skin Selectively Affects the Survival and Functional Properties of Nociceptors. J Neurosci 19:8509–8516
14. Vulchanova L, Olson TH, Stone LS, Riedl MS, Elde R, Honda CN (2001) Cytotoxic Targeting of Isolectin IB4-Binding Sensory Neurons. Neuroscience 108:143–155
15. Weskamp G, Otten U (1987) An Enzyme-Linked Immunoassay for Nerve Growth Factor (NGF): A Tool for Studying Regulatory Mechanisms Involved in NGF Production in Brain and in Peripheral Tissues. J Neurochem 48:1779–1786
16. Zwick M, Davis BM, Woodbury CJ, Burkett JN, Koerber HR, Simpson JF, Albers KM (2002) Glial Cell Line-Derived Neurotrophic Factor is a Survival Factor for Isolectin B4-Positive, but not Vanilloid Receptor [1-]Positive, Neurons in the Mouse. J Neurosci 22:4057–4065
17. Zwick M, Molliver DC, Lindsay J, Fairbanks CA, Sengoku T, Albers KM, Davis BM (2003) Transgenic Mice Possessing Increased Numbers of Nociceptors do not Exhibit Increased Behavioral Sensitivity in Models of Inflammatory and Neuropathic Pain. Pain 106:491–500

Nerve Growth Factor, Sensitizing Action on Nociceptors

LORNE M. MENDELL

Department of Neurobiology and Behavior, State
University of New York at Stony Brook, Stony Brook,
NY, USA
lorne.mendell@sunysb.edu

Definition

The response of the nociceptive system can be sensitized by exposure to a ► neurotrophin molecule called
► nerve growth factor (NGF). This sensitization has 2
components, one peripheral due to an enhanced response
to nociceptive stimuli, and the other central due to increased action of nociceptive impulses in the dorsal horn.

Characteristics

Nerve Growth Factor is a member of a family of
molecules called neurotrophins. Neurotrophins are
best known for their function during development,
specifically in promoting axonal growth and in assuring
cell survival. Cells affected selectively by NGF express
a specific receptor tyrosine kinase called ► trkA to
which NGF binds. Nociceptors express trkA, which
makes them sensitive to NGF during development (reviewed in Lewin and Mendell 1993; Mendell et al.
1999). Recently, however, a postnatal role for NGF has
been established. Administration of NGF to an animal
results in enhanced responsiveness to noxious stimulation (► hyperalgesia), which is partly due to direct
sensitization of nociceptive afferents, i.e. peripheral
sensitization. In addition, exposure of the receptive
field of sensory neurons to NGF and other sensitizing
agents, elicits changes in the cell body in the dorsal
root ganglion that increase the central effect of sensory
impulses, a phenomenon known as central sensitization.
Several findings have established the involvement of endogenous NGF in sensitizing the subsequent response to
nociceptive inputs after injury (reviewed in Lewin and
Mendell 1993; Mendell et al. 1999). First, is the upregulation of NGF in skin and other peripheral tissues after
inflammatory injury. A second is the demonstration that
administration of exogenous NGF can elicit hyperalgesia. The third is the finding that inflammatory pain can
be significantly reduced by interfering with endogenous
NGF action, using either an antibody to NGF or an immunoadhesin (trkA-IgG) which sequesters endogenous
NGF.
The time course of hyperalgesia elicited by systemically
administered NGF ($1\,\mu g/g$) has revealed 2 phases of the
response, an initial thermal component beginning just a
few minutes after NGF administration, and a later one
beginning several hours after NGF administration that
includes mechanical hyperalgesia (Lewin et al. 1994).
The early response can also be elicited by local injec-

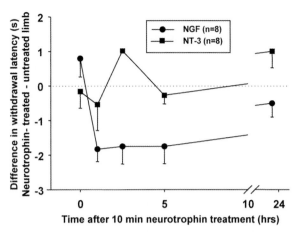

**Nerve Growth Factor, Sensitizing Action on Nociceptors,
Figure 1** Administration of NGF to the foot of the rat makes the
affected paw hyperalgesic to noxious heat as measured by a reduced
latency to withdrawal from a fixed thermal stimulus. The ordinate
represents the mean difference in the latency of response of the affected
limb compared to the contralateral limb (negative value implies that it
took less time for the thermal stimulus to reach noxious threshold on the
treated foot than on the untreated foot). NGF treatment gave a rapid and
consistent thermal hyperalgesia lasting at least 1 day. NT-3 produced no
change in response to noxious heat. (Adapted from Shu et al. 1999).

tions of NGF into the periphery (Fig. 1), suggesting that
exogenous NGF directly sensitizes thermal nociceptive
afferents but not high threshold mechanoreceptors (Shu
et al. 1999). These confirm the results of previous recordings from individual nociceptors using a ► skin-nerve
preparation. In these experiments, it has been found that
the response to noxious heat is sensitized, measured as
a decrease in threshold, whereas there is no systematic
change in the threshold to mechanical stimulation (Rueff
and Mendell 1996). This suggests that mechanical hyperalgesia is of central origin (Lewin et al. 1994; see below) although the possibility of e peripheral contribution
by increased discharge of high threshold mechanoreceptors is not ruled out by currently available data.
NGF has also been shown to operate as a sensitizing
agent in visceral structures such as the bladder or the
gut. As in skin, there is upregulation of NGF message
and protein in painful inflammatory conditions, brought
on by diseases such as interstitial cystitis or in an experimental model of ulcers (e.g. Lamb et al. 2004).
Administration of NGF to the visceral periphery results
in enhanced afferent activity. Experimental models of
arthritis are also characterized by release of NGF into
the synovial fluid, indicating a role in joint hyperalgesia
(Manni et al. 2003).
A difficulty in determining the mechanism of NGF action from these experiments arises from the multiplicity
of cell types in the peripheral target tissues that express
trkA (the high affinity receptor for NGF) or that release
NGF. Many of these cells are non neural, and are believed to interact closely in the inflammatory cascade.
For example, ► mast cells are known to express trkA

N

and to release NGF after injury, and ▶ keratinocytes have been shown to release NGF in response to histamine produced by mast cells (reviewed in Mendell et al. 1999). Degranulation of mast cells can diminish the sensitizing action of exogenous NGF and other inflammatory mediators (Lewin et al. 1994). In order to investigate the effect of NGF directly on nociceptors, small diameter cells acutely dissociated from DRG have been studied in culture. The assumption in carrying out such experiments is that the cell body in culture expresses the same receptors as the peripheral terminals *in situ*. A problem with this approach is that the original target (skin, muscle, viscera) can only be identified if it is prelabeled with a dye transported to the ganglion from the target tissue. However, this still leaves the identity of the receptor type (e.g. for skin: polymodal nociceptor, mechanical nociceptor, D-Hair, etc.) to be determined, since unique molecular identifiers are not yet available at this level of resolution. NGF is now recognized as an inflammatory mediator with a sensitizing action similar to that associated with other inflammatory mediators such as prostaglandin and bradykinin. The sensitizing effect of NGF has been examined most extensively on the response to capsaicin, which is now known to signal via the recently cloned ▶ TRPV1 receptor (also known as VR1). This receptor can also be activated by physiological stimuli, specifically noxious heat and low pH (rev. in Caterina and Julius 2001). Normally, the TRPV[1]-mediated response studied in isolated cells is smaller to the second of 2 capsaicin or noxious heat stimuli (i.e., exhibits tachyphylaxis) that are separated by as much as 10 or 15 min (Galoyan et al. 2003; Shu and Mendell 1999). However, in the presence of NGF (100 ng/ml), tachyphylaxis does not occur in most cells; rather the second response is larger than the first, i.e. it is sensitized (Shu and Mendell 1999) (Fig. 2). These same studies have revealed that the initial response to noxious heat or capsaicin is larger on the average in the presence of NGF than in its absence. Sensitization by NGF is not accompanied by any systematic change in threshold temperature (Galoyan et al. 2003), unlike sensitization measured in the skin-nerve prepara-

tion (Rueff and Mendell 1996). Thus NGF-induced sensitization is not a property of nociceptors alone; other cells in the skin (keratinocytes, mast cells, etc.) are likely to contribute significantly. It is important to note that administration of NGF alone does not elicit any response from the cell; it merely sensitizes the response evoked by noxious heat or capsaicin. Immunohistochemical analysis of these cells reveals that the ability of NGF to sensitize these responses is strongly correlated with expression of trkA (Galoyan et al. 2003), indicating that sensitization to noxious heat by NGF involves an interaction between the ▶ trkA receptor and the TRPV1 receptor. Chuang et al. (2001) have demonstrated that activation of trkA disinhibits TRPV1 via action of phosholipase C (PLC) leading to a reduced level of PIP2 which, at normal levels, maintains a tonic level of inhibition of TRPV1. NGF also sensitizes the response of nociceptors by increasing their membrane gain, as determined by an enhanced action potential firing in response to an imposed current (Zhang et al. 2002). This occurs as a result of augmentation of a TTX-resistant Na^+ current known to be expressed in nociceptors. An additional factor underlying this enhanced response to depolarization is inhibition of a K^+ current. NGF mediates these actions on membrane gain by activating the ▶ p75 receptor, rather than trkA which is responsible for enhancing the inward current through TRPV1. The p75 receptor is coupled to the sphingomyelin signaling pathway, and exposure to ▶ ceramide, an independent intermediate of this signaling pathway, mimics the effect of NGF on membrane gain. Experiments with independent expression of p75 and TRPV1 in heterologous cells suggest that the p75 receptor is unlikely to be crucial for sensitization of the response of TRPV1 to capsaicin (Chuang et al. 2001). However, some modulatory effect of p75 on the response of trkA is not ruled out by these experiments.

Thus, NGF can sensitizes the response of nociceptors to noxious heat both by enhancing the response of the noxious heat sensitive receptor via trkA, and by amplifying the gain of the membrane via the p75 receptor, in effect sensitizing the response of the receptor as well as

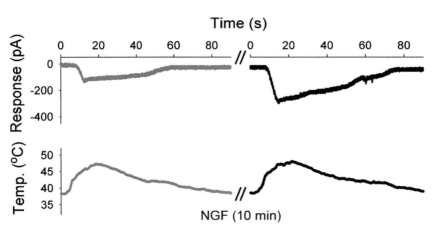

Nerve Growth Factor, Sensitizing Action on Nociceptors,
Figure 2 Response of small diameter DRG cell in acute cell culture to noxious heat stimulation. Note that the response to the second pulse of heat (bottom traces) measured 10 min after the initial response in the continuous presence of NGF (100 ng/ml) during the 10 min interval was a larger inward current (top traces) measured in perforated patch clamp mode. This sensitization is never observed under control conditions. (Adapted from Galoyan et al. 2003).

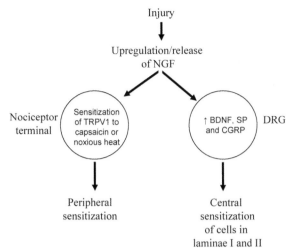

Nerve Growth Factor, Sensitizing Action on Nociceptors, Figure 3 Schematic diagram illustrating some effects of NGF in causing peripheral sensitization by direct action on nociceptive terminals and indirect central sensitization by upregulating peptides such as brain derived neurotrophic factor (BDNF), substance P (SP) and calcitonin gene related peptide (CGRP).

enhancing the gain of the impulse encoder. Longer term exposure to NGF also induces changes in the ▶ P2X3 Receptor composition of sensory neurons. Thus NGF can influence the response of these neurons to ATP which is released by non neural cells after damage or noxious stimuli (Scholz and Woolf 2002).

The central action of nociceptors is also sensitized by inflammatory stimuli including NGF (Scholz and Woolf 2002). NGF has not been shown to have any direct effect on spinal neurons in the superficial dorsal horn that are involved in transmitting nociceptive signals (Kerr et al. 1999). Rather, exposure of the peripheral terminals to NGF results in internalization of the NGF-trkA complex and transport to the cell body, where it stimulates upregulation of several peptides including substance P, CGRP and another neurotrophin, ▶ brain derived neurotrophic factor (BDNF). These peptides are released into the dorsal horn (e.g., Lever et al. 2001) where they can rapidly sensitize the response of dorsal horn neurons in lamina II to subsequent inputs (Garraway et al. 2003). They can also elicit changes in gene expression that are pronociceptive (long term central sensitization, Scholz and Woolf 2002).

Together, these studies indicate that the role of NGF in eliciting sensitization of nociceptors is complex with both direct peripheral and indirect central components (Fig. 3).

References

1. Caterina MJ, Julius D (2001) The Vanilloid Receptor: A Molecular Gateway to the Pain Pathway. Ann Rev Neurosci 24:487–517
2. Chuang HH, Prescott ED, Kong H et al. (2001) Bradykinin and Nerve Growth Factor Release the Capsaicin Receptor from PtdIns(4,5)P2-Mediated Inhibition. Nature 411:957–962
3. Galoyan SM, Petruska J, Mendell LM (2003) Mechanisms of Sensitization of the Response of Single DRG Cells from Adult Rat to Noxious Heat. Eur J Neurosci 18:535–541
4. Garraway SM, Petruska JC, Mendell LM (2003) BDNF Sensitizes the Response of Lamina II Neurons to High Threshold Primary Afferent Inputs. Eur J Neurosci 18:2467–2476
5. Kerr BJ, Bradbury EJ, Bennett DL et al. (1999) Brain-Derived Neurotrophic Factor Modulates Nociceptive Sensory Inputs and NMDA-Evoked Responses in the Rat Spinal Cord. J Neurosci 19:5138–5148
6. Lamb K, Gebhart GF, Bielefeldt K (2004) Increased Nerve Growth Factor Expression Triggers Bladder Overactivity. J Pain 5:150–156
7. Lever IJ, Bradbury EJ, Cunningham JR et al. (2001) Brain-Derived Neurotrophic Factor is released in the Dorsal Horn by Distinctive Patterns of Afferent Fiber Stimulation. J Neurosci 21:4469–4477
8. Lewin GR, Mendell LM (1993) Nerve Growth Factor and Nociception. Trends Neurosci 16:353–359
9. Lewin GR, Rueff A, Mendell LM (1994) Peripheral and Central Mechanisms of NGF-Induced Hyperalgesia. Eur J Neurosci 6:1903–1912
10. Manni L, Lundeberg T, Fiorito S et al. (2003) Nerve Growth Factor Release by Human Synovial Fibroblasts Prior to and Following Exposure to Tumor Necrosis Factor-Alpha, Interleukin–1 Beta and Cholecystokinin–8: The Possible Role of NGF in the Inflammatory Response. Clin Exp Rheumatol 21:617–624
11. Mendell LM, Albers KM, Davis BM (1999) Neurotrophins, Nociceptors and Pain. Microsc Res Tech 45:252–261
12. Rueff A, Mendell LM (1996) Nerve Growth Factor and NT–5 Induce Increased Thermal Sensitivity of Cutaneous Nociceptors *In Vitro*. J Neurophysiol 76:3593–3596
13. Scholz J, Woolf CJ (2002) Can we Conquer Pain? Nat Neurosci 5:1062–1067
14. Shu X, Llinas A, Mendell LM (1999) Effects of trkB and trkC Neurotrophin Receptor Agonists on Thermal Nociception: A Behavioural and Electrophysiological Study. Pain 80:463–470
15. Shu X, Mendell LM (1999) Nerve Growth Factor Acutely Sensitizes the Response of Adult Rat Sensory Neurons to Capsaicin. Neurosci Lett 274:159–62
16. Zhang YH, Vasko MR, Nicol GD (2002) Ceramide, A Putative Second Messenger for Nerve Growth Factor, Modulates the TTX-Resistant Na(+) Current and Delayed Rectifier K(+) Current in Rat Sensory Neurons. J Physiol 544:385–402

Nerve Inflammation

▶ Inflammatory Neuritis

Nerve Injury

▶ Retrograde Cellular Changes after Nerve Injury

Nerve Lesion

Definition

Lesion to/damage of a peripheral nerve.
▶ Causalgia, Assessment

Nerve Ligation

▶ Retrograde Cellular Changes after Nerve Injury

Nerve Pain

▶ Peripheral Neuropathic Pain

Nerve Pain of Joint and Muscle Origin

▶ Neuropathic Pain, Joint and Muscle Origin

Nerve Stump Pain

▶ Neuroma Pain

Nerve Terminals

Definition

These axon endings are found in the dermis around the base of hair follicles and close to the surface of the skin (epidermis) where the hair emerges. These free endings contain specialized receptors that respond to changes in temperature and other events (pH) associated with tissue damage.

▶ Opioid Receptor Localization

Nerve Viral Infection

▶ Viral Neuropathies

Nervus Intermedius, Primary Otalgia

▶ Trigeminal, Glossopharyngeal, and Geniculate Neuralgias

Neural Blockade

▶ Cancer Pain Management, Anesthesiologic Interventions, Neural Blockade

Neural Compressive Syndrome

▶ Lower Back Pain, Physical Examination

Neural Foramen

Definition

Neural foramen is a foramen in the spinal canal which is bounded by the intervertebral disc, the pedicles and facet joints of the vertebrae above and below, and the posterior aspect of the vertebral bodies above and below. The nerve root exits through this foramen and the dorsal root ganglion is situated in the foramen.

▶ Dorsal Root Ganglionectomy and Dorsal Rhizotomy

Neural Plasticity

Definition

The ability of the brain and/or certain parts of the nervous system to change in order to adapt to new conditions such as an injury, and can include changes in synaptic connectivity and strength between cells.

▶ Cytokines, Effects on Nociceptors

Neuralgia

Definition

Neuralgia is pain that occurs along the distribution of a nerve or nerves initiated or caused by a primary lesion or dysfunction in the nervous system. Common usage often implies a paroxysmal quality, but neuralgia should not be reserved for paroxysmal pains.

▶ CRPS, Evidence-Based Treatment
▶ Opioids in Geriatric Application
▶ Orofacial Pain, Taxonomy/Classification

Neuralgia, Assessment

RALF BARON
Klinik für Neurologie, Christian Albrecht University Kiel, Kiel, Germany
r.baron@neurologie.uni-kiel.de

Definition

Neuralgia is defined as a pain in the distribution of a nerve or nerves (IASP Pain Terminology 1994) (Merskey and Bogduk 1994). It is mostly associated with neuropathic pain states that occur after nerve lesion. It is a pure descriptive term that does not imply the etiology of the pain generation, nor the underlying pathophysiological mechanism, nor the characteristic of the pain. According to this definition, neuralgia pain may be located superficially in the skin or also in deep somatic structures, it may be of constant spontaneous type, shooting type or of evoked type ▸ (hyperalgesia, ▸ allodynia).

Note: Common usage, especially in Europe, often implies a paroxysmal quality, but neuralgia should not be reserved for paroxysmal pains.

Although the definition clearly states the fact that the pain of neuralgia occurs within the innervation territories, the symptoms may in individual cases spread to some degree beyond the innervation territories. This is particular true for allodynic pain in for example ▸ postherpetic neuralgia or posttraumatic neuralgia that sometime occurs in formerly unaffected dermatomes or peripheral nerve territories. Thus the symptoms, signs and their distribution can lead to confusion with regard to the diagnosis.

According to the underlying etiology several different terms for neuralgias are commonly used in pain medicine. The following comprises examples of some syndromes without being complete.

Characteristics

Post-traumatic Neuralgia (PTN)

Traumatic mechanical partial injury to a peripheral nerve may lead to PTN. The cardinal symptoms are spontaneous burning pain, shooting pain and hyperalgesia and mechanical and, in some cases severe, cold allodynia. These sensory symptoms are confined to the territory of the affected peripheral nerve, although allodynia may extend beyond the border of nerve territories to a certain degree (Wahren and Torebjörk 1992; Wahren et al. 1991; Wahren et al. 1995).

Special forms of ▸ post-traumatic neuralgias are chronic compression injuries to peripheral nerves, e.g. spermatic neuralgia and ▸ meralgia paresthetica.

Postherpetic Neuralgia (PHN)

PHN is one of the most common types of neuropathic pain. Its etiology is well known; the recrudescence of the varicella zoster virus (VZV) with inflammation and damage to dorsal root ganglion cells. If the pain lasts more than 3–6 months after the acute shingles, the criteria for PHN are fulfilled. It typically occurs in elderly but otherwise healthy individuals with no previous history of chronic pain. The diagnosis is straightforward, based on the history of a dermatomal rash and the dermatomal distribution of the pain. The incidence of PHN in zoster-affected patients of all age groups is about 15%. The pain of PHN appears as the acute viral infection subsides and persists, often indefinitely. The severity is frequently sufficient to completely disrupt the lives of otherwise healthy individuals. Patients with PHN report one or more of the following: a steady, deep aching pain that often has an abnormal quality, a lancinating pain that is brief, intense and often described in terms reminiscent of ▸ trigeminal neuralgia and finally, dynamic mechanical allodynia, which is the induction of a sharp pain by light, moving, cutaneous stimuli. In individual patients, the most unpleasant aspect of their pain may be either a continuous deep aching pain, lancinating pain or allodynia (Dworkin and Portenoy 1994; Fields et al. 1998).

Cranial Nerve Neuralgias (Burchiel 2003; Kapur et al. 2003)

Trigeminal Neuralgia (TN)

Trigeminal neuralgia (tic douloureux) is a disorder of the fifth cranial (trigeminal) nerve that causes episodes of intense, stabbing, electric shock-like pain in the areas of the face where the branches of the nerve are distributed – lips, eyes, nose, scalp, forehead, upper jaw and lower jaw. The disorder is more common in women than in men and rarely affects anyone younger than 50. The attacks of pain, which generally last several seconds and may be repeated one after the other, may be triggered by talking, brushing teeth, touching the face, chewing or swallowing. The attacks may come and go throughout the day and last for days, weeks or months at a time, and then disappear for months or years. Trigeminal neuralgia is not fatal, but it is universally considered to be the most painful affliction known to medical practice (Fields 1996).

Glossopharyngeus Neuralgia (GN)

▸ Glossopharyngeal neuralgia is described as sharp, jabbing, electric or shock-like pain located deep in the throat on one side. It is generally located near the tonsil, although the pain may extend deep into the ear. It is usually triggered by swallowing or chewing.

Facial (Geniculate) Ganglion Neuralgia (FN)

Pain paroxysms are felt in the depth of the ear, lasting for seconds or minutes or intermittently. A trigger zone is present in the posterior wall of the auditory canal. Disorders of lacrimation, salivation and taste sometimes accompany the pain. There is a common association with herpes zoster.

Post-sympathectomy Neuralgia (PSN)

▸ Post-sympathectomy neuralgia is a pain syndrome associated with a lesion at the sympathetic nervous system. 1 to 2 weeks after lumbar or cervicothoracic sympathectomy, up to 35% of the patients develop a deep, boring pain. The pain of PSN characteristically has a proximal location within the innervation territory of the sympathectomized nerves. PNS patients describe a variable degree of deep somatic tenderness in the area of pain, which typically responds to oral cyclooxygenase inhibitors. PSN is often nocturnal and typically remits in a few weeks without specific treatment (Baron et al. 1999).

Meralgia Paresthetica

Meralgia paresthetica, a painful mononeuropathy of the lateral femoral cutaneous nerve, is commonly due to focal entrapment of this nerve as it passes through the in-

N

guinal ligament. It is a purely sensory nerve and has no motor component. Pain associated with paresthesias and numbness in the area of the anterolateral thigh are common symptoms. Rarely, it has other etiologies such as direct trauma, stretch injury or ischemia. It typically occurs in isolation. The clinical history and examination is usually sufficient for making the diagnosis. However, the diagnosis can be confirmed by nerve conduction studies. Treatment is usually supportive.

Differential Diagnoses

Atypical Facial Neuralgia and Post-traumatic Facial Pain

The typical symptom is a continuous, unilateral, deep, aching pain, sometimes with a burning component within the face, most commonly in the area of the second trigeminal branch. More than half the patients with nondescript facial pain report its onset after trauma to the face, often surgical trauma. Orbital enucleations, sinus procedures and complicated dental extractions are the most common procedures that antedate the appearance of pain. Fortunately, for the large majority of the patients, their pain problem is self-limited; within 1–5 years it subsides whether symptomatic treatment is effective or not. The mechanism underlying this disorder presumably involves activation or central pain transmission pathways; how and why this occurs remains to be elucidated (Burchiel 2003; Kapur et al. 2003).

Complex Regional Pain Syndrome type II (CRPS II, Causalgia)

Injury of a peripheral nerve may lead to CRPS II. In contrast to patients with post-traumatic neuralgias, CRPS II patients exhibit a more complex clinical picture. They show marked swelling and a tendency for progressive spread of symptoms in the entire distal extremity. Spontaneous and evoked pains are felt superficially as well as deep inside the extremity and the intensity of both is dependent on the position of the extremity (Baron et al. 2002; Janig and Baron 2003; Wasner et al. 1998).

Assessment of Neuralgia

Since neuralgia is a pure descriptive term defined as a pain that occurs within the innervation territory of a peripheral nerve or a nerve root, there are no objective diagnostic procedures. However, in addition to the pain history and the clinical symptoms clinical signs that are characteristic for neuropathic pain states are also helpful and should be analyzed with quantitative sensory testing to aid the diagnosis of neuropathy (e.g. in postherpetic neuralgia, posttraumatic neuralgia, meralgia paresthetica) (see below) (Baron 2000). However, it should be recognized that in several forms of neuralgia (e.g. idiopathic trigeminal neuralgia) sensory testing does not reveal any abnormalities.

Symptom-based Classification of Neuropathic Pain. I. General Definitions

Negative sensory symptoms

- Loss of sensory quality
- Due to system involved: hypoesthesia, hypoalgesia, thermhypoesthesia, pallhypoesthesia etc...
- Bothering, but not painful

Positive sensory symptoms

- Paresthesias
- Dysesthesias
- Spontaneous pain (burning ongoing pain, shock-like pain)
- Evoked pain (see below)

  - Allodynia: a normally non-painful stimulus evokes pain
  - Hyperalgesia: a painful stimulus evokes pain of higher intensity

Symptom-based Classification of Neuropathic Pain. II. Definition of Different Evoked Pains

- Static mechanical allodynia

  - Gentle static pressure stimuli at the skin evokes pain
  - Present in the area of affected (damaged or sensitized) primary afferent nerve endings (primary zone)

- Punctate mechanical allodynia

  - Normally stinging but not painful stimuli (stiff von Frey hair) evoke pain
  - Present in the primary affected zone and spread beyond into unaffected skin areas (secondary zone)

- Dynamic mechanical allodynia

  - Gentle moving stimuli at the skin (brush) evoke pain
  - Present in the primary affected zone and spread beyond into unaffected skin areas (secondary zone)

- Warm allodynia, heat hyperalgesia

  - Warm or heat stimuli at the skin evoke pain
  - Present in the area of affected (damaged or sensitized) primary afferent nerve endings (primary zone)

- Cold allodynia

  - Cold stimuli at the skin evoke pain
  - Characteristic of post-traumatic neuralgia and some polyneuropathies

- Temporal summation
  - Repetitive application of identical single noxious stimuli (interval <3 s) is perceived as increasing pain sensation

Quantitative Sensory Testing (QST) in Neuralgia

A bedside testing should be part of the physical examination to confirm e.g. loss of afferent function, as well as evoked pain symptoms (e.g. allodynia and hyperalgesia), i.e. dynamic mechanical allodynia (cotton swab). Additionally standardized psychophysical tests (von Frey hairs, thermotest) should be used to detect impairment and changes in warm and cold sensation as well as heat and cold pain thresholds. By these means the function of small myelinated and unmyelinated afferent fibers is assessed.

So far, no characteristic sensoric pattern of patients with neuralgia has been identified. However, the analysis is useful to determine and quantify the individual signs of each patient and to document successful response to treatment.

References

1. Baron R (2000) Peripheral neuropathic pain: from mechanisms to symptoms. Clin J Pain 16:12–20
2. Baron R, Levine JD, Fields HL (1999) Causalgia and reflex sympathetic dystrophy: Does the sympathetic nervous system contribute to the generation of pain? Muscle Nerve 22:678–95
3. Baron R, Fields HL, Janig W et al. (2002) National Institutes of Health Workshop: reflex sympathetic dystrophy / complex regional pain syndromes –state-of-the-science. Anesth Analg 95: 812–816
4. Burchiel KJ (2003) A new classification for facial pain. Neurosurgery 53:1164–1166; discussion 1166–1167
5. Dworkin RH, Portenoy RK (1994) Proposed classification of herpes zoster pain. Lancet 343:1648
6. Fields HL (1996) Treatment of trigeminal neuralgia. N Engl J Med 334:1125–1126
7. Fields HL, Rowbotham M, Baron R (1998) Postherpetic neuralgia: irritable nociceptors and deafferentation. Neurobiol Disease 5:209–227
8. Janig W, Baron R (2003) Complex regional pain syndrome: mystery explained? Lancet Neurol 2:687–697
9. Kapur N, Kamel IR, Herlich A (2003) Oral and craniofacial pain: diagnosis, pathophysiology, and treatment. Int Anesthesiol Clin 2003 41:115–150
10. Merskey H, Bogduk N (1994) Classification of chronic pain: descriptions of chronic pain syndromes and definition of terms, 2nd edn. IASP Press, Seattle
11. Wahren LK, Torebjörk E (1992) Quantitative sensory tests in patients with neuralgia 11 to 25 years after injury. Pain 48:237–44
12. Wahren LK, Torebjörk E, Nystrom B (1991) Quantitative sensory testing before and after regional guanethidine block in patients with neuralgia in the hand. Pain 46:23–30
13. Wahren LK, Gordh T Jr, Torebjork E (1995) Effects of regional intravenous guanethidine in patients with neuralgia in the hand; a follow-up study over a decade. Pain 62:379–385
14. Wasner G, Backonja MM, Baron R (1998) Traumatic Neuralgias: Complex Regional Pain Syndromes (Reflex Sympathetic Dystrophy and Causalgia): Clinical Characteristics, Pathophysiological Mechanisms and Therapy. Neurol Clin 16:851–868

Neuralgia, Diagnosis

JAYANTILAL GOVIND
Department of Anesthesia, Pain Clinic, Liverpool Hospital, University of New South Wales, Sydney, NSW, Australia
jaygovind@bigpond.com

Synonyms

Neurodynia

Definition

Pain in the distribution of a nerve, ostensibly due to an intrinsic disorder of that nerve (Merskey and Bogduk 1994).

Characteristics

The taxonomical distinction between ▶ neuralgia and ▶ neuropathic pain is contentious. The distinction is largely historical, in that the classical neuralgias were named before the entity of neuropathic pain was popularised. Nevertheless, certain semantic, anatomic, and pathologic distinctions apply.

The term – neuralgia – explicitly means pain along a nerve. It neither identifies the aetiology, pathophysiology nor any specific feature e.g. pain quality. Neuropathic pain implies that the affected nerve has a disease, and typically it is associated with features of abnormal nerve function, such as numbness, hyperaesthesia, or allodynia. These latter features are characteristically absent in neuralgias, or are subtle and minor.

Neuralgia should also be distinguished from ▶ radicular pain. Although similar to neuralgia in some respects clinically, radicular pain has certain distinguishing features clinically, and with respect to aetiology and mechanisms (see ▶ radicular pain).

Archetypical Conditions

There are two archetypical conditions that are different from one another in many respects; and each is representative of other, less common conditions. These are: ▶ trigeminal neuralgia, and its relatives glossopharyngeal and vagal neuralgia; ▶ post-herpetic neuralgia, which is probably a unique condition, and which may exemplify other dorsal root ganglionopathies, such as tabes dorsalis, and possibly Guillan-Barre syndrome.

Site of Lesion

In trigeminal neuralgia the lesion is in the sensory root. It is not in the ganglion or in the peripheral nerve.

In post-herpetic neuralgia the lesion is largely in the dorsal root ganglion, but may also extend into the peripheral and central nervous systems.

N

Histopathology

Trigeminal neuralgia is a focal disorder of the cell membrane of the sensory root of the nerve. Focal demyelination is the primary pathology, located between the ganglion and the dorsal root entry zone of the nerve into the brainstem (Kerr 1967). The remainder of the root is normal (Rappaport et al. 1997). In the majority of cases demyelination is due to irritation of the sensory root by an aberrant blood vessel, typically, the superior cerebellar artery (Loeser 2001). Other causes include: aberrant veins, angiomas, and tumours of the posterior cranial fossa. Intrinsic demyelination may occur in patients with multiple sclerosis.

In post-herpetic neuralgia the fundamental pathology is intrinsic inflammation of the affected dorsal root ganglion. In time, inflammation is replaced by axonal degeneration. Demyelination, degeneration, and fibrosis occur in the dorsal root ganglion, associated with atrophy of the dorsal horn and the dorsal root, which may extend distally into the peripheral nerve, with loss of axons and a lymphocytic response (Watson et al. 1991).

Pathophysiology

In trigeminal neuralgia, areas of demyelination act as a site for generation of ectopic impulses ("ectogenesis") and/or abnormal impulse traffic. The ignition hypothesis (Devor et al. 2002) calls for ectopic generation of action potentials. The Calvin model only requires abnormal refractory periods and reflection of normally generated impulses (Calvin et al. 1977). In both models the location of the lesion proximal to the ganglion seems critical. This allows impulses to reflect between the lesion and ganglion, which becomes the basis for the characteristic reverberation of the pain.

In post-herpetic neuralgia, inflammation of the affected nerve may cause pain on the basis of neuritis, but progressive necrosis of peripheral axons and the cell bodies in the dorsal root ganglion may result in deafferentation and disinhibition of dorsal horn neurons. Thereby, post-herpetic neuralgia converts from a peripheral neuropathic pain to a ▶ central pain.

Epidemiology

The incidence of trigeminal neuralgia is estimated to be four per 100,000 persons per year (Katusic et al. 1990). Risk factors include multiple sclerosis and hypertension (Katusic et al. 1990). There is a weak association with multiple sclerosis, but multiple sclerosis could be an incidental finding given that vascular compression of the trigeminal root has been reported in individuals as young as seventeen years (Katusic et al. 1991).

Whilst few children develop post-herpetic neuralgia, the risk of contracting this disorder and the intractability of pain increases with age. This susceptibility is attributed to a selective decline in cellular immunity to varicella virus; and recurrences are strongly related to immuno-suppressive conditions such as HIV and SLE (Head and Campbell 1900).

Clinical Features

Trigeminal neuralgia is characterised by electric shock-like brief stabbing pains, with pain–free intervals between attacks, during which the patient is completely asymptomatic. Onset is usually abrupt. Pain is restricted to the trigeminal nerve distribution, and idiopathic trigeminal neuralgia is not associated with sensory loss. Non-nociceptive triggering of the pain (light touch, hair movement, chewing, speech, wind puffs) is almost ipsilateral to the pain, and usually from the peri-oral region. Intra-oral trigger zones may be accompanied by a decline in general health.

Patients with PHN present with a constellation of painful sensations including burning, dysaesthesia, aching, itching, or severe paroxysmal of stabbing pain. Allodynia or hyperpathia may occur, and the sensitivity to touch is the most distressing feature to patients. These various features are consistent with loss of nerve fibres, of all types, and ultimately with central disinhibition.

Treatment

Although trigeminal neuralgia and post-herpetic neuralgia are both called neuralgias, they differ in pathology and pathophysiology. Consequently, they respond differently to treatment. There is no treatment universally applicable to all neuralgias. To be effective treatment should target the known pathomechanisms.

Since trigeminal neuralgia is a membrane disease, membrane-stabilisers (anti-convulsants) are the treatment of first choice. Classical agents include: phenytoin, clonazepam, and carbamazepine. Of these, only carbamazepine has been vindicated in placebo-controlled trials. Baclofen may be used an adjunct, if required. For resistant cases, gabapentin, and lamotrigine are reputedly effective, as is intravenous lignocaine (Sindrup and Jensen 2002).

When the condition is refractory to pharmaceuticals, various surgical interventions are known to be effective. The choice lies with the preference of the operator. They include ganglionolysis, radiofrequency neurotomy, balloon compression, or injection of glycerine or alcohol; and microvascular decompression (see ▶ Dorsal root ganglionectomy and dorsal rhizotomy).

For post-herpetic neuralgia, amitriptyline is the drug of first choice (Watson and Evans 1985). It is the only agent for which there is consistent and strong evidence of efficacy, from controlled trials. However, only about 60% of patients obtain reasonable benefit. For resistant cases, a large variety of interventions have been recommended, but few with evidence of efficacy (Kingery 1997). Gabapentin and opioids appear to be effective for resistant cases (Watson 2000). In contrast to their efficacy for trigeminal neuralgia, baclofen,

Neuralgia, Diagnosis, Table 1 Similarities and differences between trigeminal neuralgia, post-herpetic neuralgia, and radicular pain

DOMAIN	TRIGEMINAL NEURALGIA	POST-HERPETIC NEURALGIA	RADICULAR PAIN
Anatomical site	sensory root	**dorsal root ganglion**	**dorsal root ganglion**
Key pathology	demyelination	**inflammation**	**inflammation**
Aetiology	**extrinsic**	intrinsic	extrinsic
Mechanism	reverberating impulses	disinhibition	ectopic discharge
Site	pre-central	central	peripheral
Pain	paroxysmal	constant,	intermittent,
		burning	lancinating
Associated	trigger point	allodynia	nil
Neurological	normal	**sensory loss**	**sensory loss**
Treatment	**decompression**		**decompression**
	neuro-ablation		
	anticonvulsants	tricyclics	steroids

Bold text indicates features shared by two of the conditions, otherwise features are unique and distinctive

phenytoin, and carbamazepine are usually not helpful in post-herpetic neuralgia (Kingery 1997).

Topical applications of local anaesthetic or capsaicin can be used to palliate the cutaneous sensory symptoms, but these interventions do not target the fundamental mechanism of post-herpetic neuralgia. Topical capsaicin has been vindicated in a placebo-controlled trial (Watson et al. 1993). In extreme cases, surgical interventions can be undertaken (see ▶ Dorsal root ganglionectomy and dorsal rhizotomy).

Comparison

Whilst the ▶ neuralgias share certain features, they also share some features with radicular pain, but are distinct in others (Table 1). The similarities invite some practitioners to assume that the conditions belong to the same class, and should respond to the same treatments. However, the differences in pathology and mechanisms predicate distinctly different responses to treatment. Appreciating these differences is pivotal to successful management. Treatments that work for one type of neuralgia, will not work for another. Nor do treatments commonly used for neuralgias work for radicular pain.

References

1. Calvin WJ, Loeser JD, Howe JF (1977) A Neurophysiological Theory for the Pain Mechanism of Tic Douloureux. Pain 3:147–154
2. Devor M, Amir R, Rappaport ZH (2002) Pathophysiology of Trigeminal Neuralgia: The Ignition Hypothesis. Clin J Pain 18:4–13
3. Head H, Campbell AW (1900) The Pathology of Herpes Zoster and its Bearing on Sensory Localisation. Brain 23:323–353
4. Katusic S, Beard M, Bergstralh MS, Kurland LT (1990) The Incidence and Clinical Features of Trigeminal Neuralgia. Rochester, Minnesota, 1945-1984. Ann Neurol 27:89–95
5. Katusic S, Williams DB, Beard M, Bergstralh EJ, Kurkland LT (1991) Epidemiology and Clinical Features of Idiopathic Trigeminal Neuralgia and Glossopharyngeal Neuralgia; Similarities and Differences, Rochester, Minnesota, 1945–1984. Neuroepidemiology 10:276–281
6. Kerr SWL (1967) Pathology of Trigeminal Neuralgia: Light and Electron Microscopic Observation. J Neurosurg 26 (suppl 6):151–156
7. Kingery W (1997) A Critical Review of Controlled Trials for Peripheral Neuropathic Pain and Complex Regional Pain Syndromes. Pain 73:123–139
8. Loeser JD (2001) Cranial Neuralgias. In: Loeser JD (ed) Bonica's Management of Pain. Lippincott, Williams & Wilkins, Philadelphia, pp 855–866
9. Merskey H, Bogduk N (1994) Classification of Chronic Pain. Descriptions of Chronic Pain Syndromes and Definitions of Pain Terms. International Association for the Study of Pain. IASP Press, Seattle
10. Rappaport ZH, Govrin-Lippmann R, Devor M (1997) An Electron Microscopic Analysis of Biopsied Samples of the Trigeminal Root taken during Microvascular Decompressive Surgery. Stereotact Funct Neurosurg 68 (1/4 Pt 1):182–186
11. Sindrup SH, Jensen TS (2002) Pharmacotherapy of Trigeminal Neuralgia. Clin J Pain 18:22–27
12. Watson CPN (2000) The Treatment of Neuropathic Pain: Antidepressants and Opioids. Clin J Pain 16:S49–S55
13. Watson CPN, Deck JS, Morshead C, Van der Koog D, Evans RJ (1991) Post-Herpetic Neuralgia: Further Post-Mortem Studies of Cases with and without Pain. Pain 44:105–117
14. Watson CPN, Evans RJ (1985) A Comparative Trial of Amitriptyline and Zimelidine in Post-Herpetic Neuralgia. Pain 25:387–394
15. Watson CPN, Tyler KL, Bicers DR, Millikan LE, Smith S, Coleman E (1993) A Randomized Vehicle-Controlled Trial Capsaicin in the Treatment of Post-herpetic Neuralgia. Clin Ther 15:510–526

Neuralgia of Cranial Nerve V

▶ Tic and Cranial Neuralgias

Neuralgia of Cranial Nerve VII

▶ Tic and Cranial Neuralgias

Neuralgia of Cranial Nerve IX with or without Cranial Nerve X

▶ Tic and Cranial Neuralgias

Neuraxial Blocks

Definition

Neuraxial blocks or central neural blockade comprise of intrathecal (spinal) and epidural (cervical, thoracic, lumbar and caudal) blocks. They are the most widely used regional blocks. The blocks have a well-defined end-point and can be reliably produced with a single injection. Most neuraxial blocks are performed in the lumbar region. The arachnoid membrane is a delicate, non-vascular membrane that is closely attached to the outermost layer, the dura mater. Deep to the arachnoid membrane and between the arachnoid mater and the pia mater lies the intrathecal or subarachnoid space. It contains cerebrospinal fluid, the spinal nerve roots, a trabecular network between the two membranes, blood vessels that supply the spinal cord, and the lateral extensions of the pia mater, the dentate ligaments. The epidural space surrounds the dural mater sac. Anteriorly, it is bound by the posterior longitudinal ligament; posteriorly by the ligamenta flava and the periosteum of the laminae; and laterally by the pedicles and the intervertebral foramina with their neural roots. Cranially, the epidural space is closed at the foramen magnum where the spinal dura attaches with the endosteal dura of the cranium. Caudally, the epidural space ends at the sacral hiatus that is closed by the sacrococcygeal ligament. The epidural space contains loose areolar connective tissue, fat, lymphatics, arteries, a plexus of veins, and the spinal nerve roots as they leave the dural sac and pass through the intervertebral foramina. The epidural space communicates freely with the paravertebral space through the intervertebral foramina.

▶ Multimodal Analgesia in Postoperative Pain

Neuraxial Infusion

Definition

Neuraxial infusion is the delivery of medications via a catheter inserted into the epidural or intrathecal space.

▶ Cancer Pain Management, Anesthesiologic Interventions, Spinal Cord Stimulation, and Neuraxial Infusion

Neuraxial Morphine

Definition

Morphine administered into the cerebrospinal fluid (or epidurally) to reach the spinal cord directly, causing profound analgesia.

▶ Postoperative Pain, Acute Pain Team

Neuraxis

Definition

Neuraxis is the term that refers to the entire nervous system, from receptors in periphery to spinal cord and to the subcortical structures and cortex of the brain.

▶ Hypoalgesia, Assessment
▶ Hypoesthesia, Assessment

Neurectomy

Definition

Neurectomy is the removal of part of a nerve, implying surgery. This usually refers to the distal, or nerve portion farthest from the brain.

▶ Cancer Pain Management, Neurosurgical Interventions
▶ Trigeminal Neuralgia, Diagnosis and Treatment

Neuritis

▶ Inflammatory Neuritis

Neuroablation

Definition

Neuroablation is an irreversible surgical technique that permanently blocks nerve pathways to the brain by destroying nerves and tissues at the source of the pain. This may be caused by various means, such as thermal or chemical, and occur in various places, such as in peripheral nerve or the brain.

▶ Dorsal Root Ganglionectomy and Dorsal Rhizotomy
▶ Trigeminal Neuralgia, Diagnosis and Treatment

Neuroactive Substance

Definition

A substance that can activates cells of the nervous system.
▶ Cytokines, Regulation in Inflammation

Neuroaxial

Definition

The epidural and intrathecal (spinal) spaces. Neuroaxial analgesic/anesthetic techniques involve the administration of agents into these spaces.
▶ Postoperative Pain, Appropriate Management

Neuro-Behçet

Definition

Behçet's disease with neurologic manifestations.
▶ Headache Due to Arteritis

Neurobehavioral Scores

Definition

Neurobehavior testing is a means of assessing neurologic status of the neonate. The United States Food and Drug Administration has mandated the use of a neurobehavior test to assess the neonatal effects of medications on the newborn. The neurologic and adaptive capacity score (NACS) was developed for this purpose and is commonly used in research studies by anesthesiologists.
▶ Analgesia During Labor and Delivery

Neurochemical Markers

▶ Immunocytochemistry of Nociceptors

Neurochemistry

▶ Immunocytochemistry of Nociceptors

Neurodegeneration

Definition

Neurodegeneration is the continuous and progressive dying of neurons.
▶ Viral Neuropathies

Neurodynia

▶ Neuralgia, Diagnosis

Neurofilament Protein NF200

Definition

Neurofilaments are a class of intermediate filaments that are found in neurons. They form the structure of the cytoskeleton and are particularly abundant in axons. DRG neurons express low (68 kD), medium (155 kD) and high (200 kD) molecular weight neurofilament proteins. Large light DRG neurons are rich in expression of neurofilaments, especially the high molecular weight (200 kD) protein, whereas the small dark neurons are poor in expression of neurofilaments. The phosphorylated form, the 200 kD neurofilament, is localized specifically to the large light cell population, and therefore, the presence of immunoreactivity for this protein can be used to distinguish large light cells from small dark cells. Since a low level of non-phosphorylated 200 kD neurofilament is found in small and large neurons, an antibody against the non-phosphorylated form of the 200 kD subunit does not distinguish well between the large light and small dark neurons.
▶ Immunocytochemistry of Nociceptors

Neurogenic Claudication

▶ Lower Back Pain, Physical Examination

Neurogenic Inflammation

Definition

A subset of nociceptive Aδ and C afferents contain pro-inflammatory neuropeptides (mainly "sleeping" nociceptors). If a peptidergic C fiber is activated, it releases neuropeptides from all the nerve terminals, which belong to this C fiber (axonal tree). Since always more than one C fiber will be activated by noxious stimulation, a homogenous area of neurogenic inflammation in the vicinity of the painful stimulus occurs. Release of

N

these neuropeptides upon nociceptive activation causes inflammatory responses consisting of protein ▶ plasma extravasation (edema; mainly induced by substance P and neurokinin A) and vasodilatation (mainly mediated by CGRP). Endothelial activation and secretion, degranulation of perivascular mast cells and the attraction of leucocytes has additionally been observed in some tissues like the dura mater. This reaction was first described as the axon reflex by Thomas Lewis, and underlies the flare and wheal response often seen surrounding local tissue damage.

- ▶ Arthritis Model, Adjuvant-Induced Arthritis
- ▶ Cytokines, Effects on Nociceptors
- ▶ Formalin Test
- ▶ Freezing Model of Cutaneous Hyperalgesia
- ▶ Functional Imaging of Cutaneous Pain
- ▶ Inflammation, Modulation by Peripheral Cannabinoid Receptors
- ▶ Mechano-Insensitive C-Fibres, Biophysics
- ▶ Neurogenic Inflammation and Sympathetic Nervous System
- ▶ Nociceptor, Axonal Branching
- ▶ Nociceptors in the Orofacial Region (Meningeal/Cerebrovascular)
- ▶ Quantitative Thermal Sensory Testing of Inflamed Skin
- ▶ Substance P Regulation in Inflammation
- ▶ Sympathetically Maintained Pain and Inflammation, Human Experimentation

Neurogenic Inflammation and Sympathetic Nervous System

HEINZ-JOACHIM HÄBLER
FH Bonn-Rhein-Sieg, Rheinbach, Germany
heinz-joachim.haebler@fh-bonn-rhein-sieg.de

Synonyms

Neurogenic inflammation, sympathetic nervous system

Definition

There is evidence that ▶ neurogenic inflammation may be influenced by the sympathetic nervous system. This evidence is based on experiments, mainly on animals, in which neurogenic inflammation was elicited by chemical activation of nociceptors, and the extent of either ▶ plasma extravasation (neurogenic edema) or vasodilation (flare) was measured before and after interventions on the sympathetic nervous system. Pharmacological experiments indicate that the interaction between sympathetic neurons and primary afferent neurons, which may be responsible for sympathetic modulation of neurogenic inflammation, can take place proximal and/or distal to the neurovascular junction, i.e. prejunctionally on the nociceptor terminal, and/or

postjunctionally at the level of the blood vessels. Only a prejunctional interaction can specifically modulate ▶ neuropeptide release from small-diameter afferent terminals, whereas at the postjunctional level, the interaction would occur non-specifically and indirectly via changes in blood flow. However, both modes of interaction may be difficult to distinguish in experiments. Here only sympathetic modulation of neurogenic inflammation is considered likely to occur at the prejunctional level.

Characteristics

Capsaicin-Induced Neurogenic Inflammation in Skin

In healthy humans, after topical application of ▶ capsaicin to forearm skin, the area of flare was significantly decreased during whole-body cooling, which enhances sympathetic vasoconstrictor activity to the skin (Baron et al. 1999). However, capsaicin-induced pain and ▶ mechanical hyperalgesia were not changed, indicating an inhibitory effect of sympathetic activity on the signs of neurogenic inflammation, but not on the corresponding pain symptoms.

In contrast, in animal experiments, the flare response after intradermal capsaicin was found to be partially dependent on the sympathetic nervous system. It was reported that capsaicin injected intradermally into the hind paw of rats elicits dorsal root reflexes in peptidergic afferents, which antidromically evoke vasodilation outside the axon reflex area, as far as 20 mm remote from the capsaicin injection site. This part of the flare response was almost abolished by surgical ▶ sympathectomy, unaffected by decentralization of the postganglionic sympathetic neurons supplying the hind paw, and depended on an α_1-adrenoceptor-mediated mechanism (Lin et al. 2003). The sympathetic co-transmitter ▶ neuropeptide Y (NPY) via Y2 receptors also seemed to contribute to the flare (Lin et al. 2004). Vasopressin had no effects on the flare response, ruling out the possibility that sympathetic effects on the flare were indirectly due to the evoked cutaneous vasoconstriction. These findings suggest that sympathetic neurons contribute to neurogenic inflammation, and that the integrity of the sympathetic terminals, but not the ongoing activity of postganglionic neurons, may be the crucial factor. Interestingly, an almost identical sympathetic dependence was reported for mechanical hyperalgesia induced by intradermal capsaicin in the same rat model. Intradermal capsaicin injection led to mechanical hyperalgesia at the injection site (▶ primary hyperalgesia) and in areas remote from the injection site (▶ secondary hyperalgesia). Capsaicin-induced secondary hyperalgesia was blocked by the α_1-adrenoceptor antagonist prazosin but not by the α_2-adrenoceptor antagonist yohimbine. Surgical sympathectomy before capsaicin injection prevented secondary hyperalgesia (Kinnman and Levine 1995), but decentralization of sympathetic postganglionic neurons did not affect mechanical hyperalgesia.

Neurogenic Inflammation of the Rat Knee Joint

Capsaicin injection into the knee joint of rats produces intraarticular plasma extravasation lasting for 30–40 min, which was found to be reduced after chemical or surgical sympathectomy (Coderre et al. 1989). This indicates that small diameter afferent-evoked plasma extravasation in the synovia is in part dependent on the sympathetic nervous system. However, release of norepinephrine from postganglionic sympathetic terminals by joint perfusion with 6-hydroxy-dopamine led to a much larger and prolonged plasma extravasation, which was almost abolished after surgical sympathectomy and after pretreatment with indomethacin, restored in the presence of prostaglandin E_2 but unchanged in rats treated with capsaicin neonatally. Similar results were obtained when bradykinin, instead of 6-hydroxy-dopamine, was injected into the knee joint. Decentralization of postganglionic sympathetic neurons supplying the hind limb left bradykinin-induced plasma extravasation unchanged (Miao et al. 1996). Indirect effects due to changes in blood flow resulting from interventions on the sympathetic nervous system were excluded. These observations led to the concept that neurogenic inflammation in the rat knee joint has two components: a relatively small component depending on primary afferent terminals and in part dependent on sympathetic neurons, and a second larger component depending on the presence of postganglionic sympathetic terminals but not on on-going sympathetic activity nor on capsaicin-sensitive afferents. Inflammatory mediators such as ▶ bradykinin are thought to release prostaglandins, and possibly other mediators from postganglionic terminals, to elicit this so-called sympathetically dependent neurogenic inflammation (Green et al. 1998).

In contrast, knee joint inflammation in rats induced by kaolin and carrageenan was found to depend, in part, on primary afferents, but was unaffected by sympathectomy (Sluka et al. 1994).

Prejunctional Control of Neuropeptide Release from Nociceptive Afferents by Sympathetic Transmitters

It is well established that in the superficial dorsal horn, synaptic release of glutamate from small-diameter afferents is inhibited by α_2-adrenoceptor agonists (e.g. Pan et al. 2002), indicating the presence of presynaptic α_2-adrenoceptors. Presynaptic inhibition of nociceptors via these receptors is thought to be one mechanism by which descending monoaminergic pathways control input from nociceptors at the level of the spinal cord. The evidence that the release of neuropeptides, such as substance P and CGRP, is inhibited in parallel with that of glutamate at spinal synapses is scarce. However, in vitro pharmacological studies on animals indicate

that α_2-adrenoceptors are also present on the peripheral terminals of capsaicin-sensitive afferents (prejunctional receptors), and inhibit stimulation-induced release of neuropeptides.

In the guinea-pig lower airways, capsaicin-sensitive afferents elicit neurogenic inflammation by liberating ▶ substance P, ▶ neurokinin A and ▶ CGRP. Both CGRP release and neurokinin-evoked bronchoconstriction after a low dose of capsaicin or low frequency (1 Hz) antidromic stimulation of the vagus nerve were attenuated by α_2-adrenoceptor agonists (Lou et al. 1992). These inhibitory effects were small when high doses of capsaicin or high frequency (10 Hz) electrical stimulation of afferents were used. Similar experiments provided evidence for the presence of inhibitory prejunctional NPY (Y2) receptors on small-diameter afferents (see Lundberg 1996).The effects of both prejunctional α_2-adrenoceptors and Y2 receptors are likely to be mediated by the opening of large conductance Ca^{++}-activated K^+ channels (Stretton et al. 1992). As these observations were made on vagal rather than spinal afferents, it may be questioned whether these results can be generalized to all peptidergic small-diameter afferents.

However, results obtained in other animal models are similar. In the perfused mesenteric vascular bed of the rat, in vitro perivascular nerve stimulation elicits vasodilation, which depends on CGRP released from capsaicin-sensitive afferents (Kawasaki et al. 1988) that are mainly of spinal origin. Pharmacological experiments in this model indicate that norepinephrine, released from sympathetic postganglionic terminals, can suppress CGRP release from perivascular afferents by activation of prejunctional α_2-adrenoceptors, and that NPY also inhibits CGRP release via prejunctional Y receptors (Kawasaki 2002). Thus, results identical to those obtained in the lower airways of the guinea-pig were found in the rat mesentery, and these were confirmed in a number of in vitro studies on the control of isolated autonomic targets by neuropeptides originating from capsaicin-sensitive afferents.

Taken together, evidence indicates that the release of neuropeptides, which can elicit neurogenic inflammation from the peripheral terminals of capsaicin-sensitive afferents, is inhibited via prejunctional receptors for sympathetic transmitters. However, it remains to be shown that these prejunctional receptors play any functional role in the intact organism under the conditions of physiological or pathophysiological regulation. Rates of on-going activity in sympathetic neurons are normally low, and in particular, the release of NPY from sympathetic terminals requires a high rate of on-going activity that may rarely occur in vivo.

In conclusion, there is evidence that neurogenic inflammation, induced by the liberation of neurokinins and CGRP from peripheral terminals of capsaicin-sensitive afferents, may be influenced by sympathetic

N

postganglionic neurons by a direct action on peripheral afferent terminals. However, the evidence is not yet conclusive. While in some studies capsaicin-induced neurogenic inflammation in the skin and knee joint of the rat was found to depend, in part, on sympathetic neurons, other studies indicate that there are prejunctional α_2-adrenoceptors and NPY receptors on afferent terminals that may inhibit neurogenic inflammation.

References

1. Baron R, Wasner G, Borgstedt R et al. (1999) Effect of Sympathetic Activity on Capsaicin-Evoked Pain, Hyperalgesia, and Vasodilatation. Neurology 52:923–932
2. Coderre TJ, Basbaum AI, Levine JD (1989) Neural Control of Vascular Permeability: Interactions between Primary Afferents, Mast Cells, and Sympathetic Efferents. J Neurophysiol 62:48–58
3. Green PG, Miao FJ, Strausbaugh H et al. (1998) Endocrine and Vagal Controls of Sympathetically Dependent Neurogenic Inflammation. Ann NY Acad Sci 840:282–288
4. Kawasaki H (2002) Regulation of Vascular Function by Perivascular Calcitonin Gene-Related Peptide-Containing Nerves. Jpn J Pharmacol 88:39–43
5. Kawasaki H, Takasaki K, Saito A et al. (1988) Calcitonin Gene-Related Peptide acts as a Novel Vasodilator Transmitter in Mesenteric Resistance Vessels of the Rat. Nature 335:164–167
6. Kinnman E, Levine JD (1995) Involvement of the Sympathetic Postganglionic Neuron in Capsaicin-Induced Secondary Hyperalgesia in the Rat. Neuroscience 65:283–291
7. Lin Q, Zou X, Fang L, Willis WD (2003) Sympathetic Modulation of Acute Cutaneous Flare Induced by Intradermal Injection of Capsaicin in Anesthetized Rats. J Neurophysiol 89:853–861
8. Lin Q, Zou X, Ren Y, Wang J et al. (2004) Involvement of Peripheral Neuropeptide Y Receptors in Sympathetic Modulation of Acute Cutaneous Flare Induced by Intradermal Capsaicin. Neuroscience 123:337–347
9. Lou YP, Franco-Cereceda, Lundberg JM (1992) Variable α_2-Adrenoceptor-Mediated Inhibition of Bronchoconstriction and Peptide Release upon Activation of Pulmonary Afferents. Eur J Pharmacol 210:173–181
10. Lundberg JM (1996) Pharmacology of Cotransmission in the Autonomic Nervous System: Integrative Aspects on Amines, Neuropeptides, Adenosine Triphosphate, Amino Acids and Nitric Oxide. Pharmacol Rev 48:113–178
11. Miao FJ, Jänig W, Levine JD (1996) Role of Sympathetic Postganglionic Neurons in Synovial Plasma Extravasation Induced by Bradykinin. J Neurophysiol 75:715–724
12. Pan YZ, Li DP, Pan HL (2002) Inhibition of Glutamatergic Synaptic Input to Spinal Lamina Lio Neurons by Presynaptic α_2-Adrenergic Receptors. J Neurophysiol 87:1938–1947
13. Sluka KA, Lawand NB, Westlund KN (1994) Joint Inflammation is Reduced by Dorsal Rhizotomy and not by Sympathectomy or Spinal Cord Transection. Ann Rheum Dis 53:309–314
14. Stretton D, Miura M, Belvisi MG et al. (1992) Calcium-Activated Potassium Channels Mediate Prejunctional Inhibition of Peripheral Sensory Nerves. Proc Natl Acad Sci USA 89:1325–1329

Neurogenic Inflammation, Vascular Regulation

HEINZ-JOACHIM HÄBLER
FH Bonn-Rhein-Sieg, Rheinbach, Germany
heinz-joachim.haebler@fh-bonn-rhein-sieg.de

Definition

▶ Neuropeptides, such as ▶ neurokinins (▶ substance P, neurokinin A) and CGRP, are the mediators of ▶ neurogenic inflammation. Their primary targets are blood vessels within the microvasculature where they elicit vasodilation and, by increasing the leakiness of the blood-tissue-barrier, ▶ plasma extravasation. Neurokinin effects may, in part, be mediated indirectly by the activation of mast cells and endothelial cells. At the neurovascular junction, neurokinins and ▶ CGRP interact with sympathetic neurotransmitters, vasoactive hormones and autacoids produced by the endothelium that are involved in the on-going regulation of the vasculature.

Characteristics

Vascular Effects of Neurokinins and CGRP

Both neurokinins and CGRP act primarily on blood vessels, but their efficacy in evoking vasodilation and plasma extravasation is different. The neurokinins substance P and neurokinin A are the main mediators of neurogenic plasma extravasation. They act on neurokinin 1 (NK1) receptors on postcapillary venues, and within seconds lead to the opening of circular gaps of about 1.5 μm diameter between endothelial cells, exposing the basement membrane and permitting the leakage of plasma proteins into the interstitial space (McDonald 1998). In addition, substance P also degranulates mast cells, which enhances plasma extravasation by an indirect mechanism involving histamine. CGRP alone does not elicit plasma extravasation. However, it seems to cooperate with neurokinins, since it potentiates neurokinin-induced plasma extravasation, possibly resulting from its vasodilator action or from its inhibitory effect on substance P degradation (Gamse and Saria 1985, Escott and Brain 1993). Generally, neurogenic edema requires longer-lasting and higher frequency stimulation of small-diameter afferents than vasodilation, probably because neurokinin effects are short-lived and a higher amount of neuropeptides may be necessary.

The main mediator of vasodilation in neurogenic inflammation is CGRP, acting via CGRP 1 receptors. CGRP is one of the most potent vasodilators known, and upon brief stimulation of small-diameter afferents, elicits long-lasting vasodilation by relaxing small arteries, arterioles and precapillary sphincters. Most of the vasodilation, in particular during the later phase, can be blocked by the CGRP 1 receptor antagonist $CGRP_{8-37}$, but part of the vasodilation remains, indicating that CGRP is not the only vasodilator involved. Substance P and neurokinin A applied exogenously also evoke strong but short-lasting vasodilation. Their role in the vasodilation elicited by adequate or electrical stimulation of small-diameter afferents has been disputed, because in animal models NK1 receptor antagonists can block vasodilation evoked by exogenous substance P and neurokinin A, but no clear effects of NK1 receptor antagonists on the vasodilation evoked by stimulation of small-diameter afferents was seen (Rinder and Lundberg 1996; Delay-Goyet et al. 1992). However, in the hairy and hairless skin of the rat, it has been possible to demonstrate that an NK1 receptor antagonist can delay antidromic vasodilation elicited by electrical stimulation of small-diameter afferents by several seconds. Furthermore, the NK1 receptor antagonist potentiated the reduction of the amplitude of antidromic vasodilation by $CGRP_{8-37}$, implying that substance P and/or neurokinin A play a role in the early phase of antidromic vasodilation (Häbler et al. 1999).

Endothelium Dependence of Vascular Neurokinin and CGRP Effects

The effects of substance P and neurokinin A, when applied exogenously, on vasodilation and plasma extravasation, are probably mediated indirectly, at least in part, via NK1 receptors located on vascular endothelium leading to the production of ▶ nitric oxide (NO), because these effects can be reduced by blocking NO synthesis (e.g. Whittle et al. 1989). It is, however, unclear whether the effects of neurokinins released upon adequate or antidromic electrical stimulation of small-diameter afferents are endothelium-dependent and involve NO. As perivascular nerves contact vascular smooth muscle on the adventitial side, it is an open question whether neuropeptides released at the neurovascular junction can penetrate the vascular wall to act on receptors located on the endothelium. Experimental studies addressing this issue are scarce. A study on neurogenic edema elicited by antidromic nerve stimulation in the rat found an involvement of NO in the response, but NO was generated by the neuronal isoform rather than the endothelial isoform of NO synthase (Kajekar et al. 1995). In another study on rats, the NK1 receptor dependent component of antidromic vasodilation was unaffected by blocking NO synthesis (Häbler et al. unpublished).

In contrast to the neurokinins, CGRP, applied exogenously or released from small-diameter afferents, exerts its vascular effects in a manner independent of the endothelium in most vascular beds, including that of the skin. Exceptions are the rat aorta and the gastric microcirculation of the rat, where the vasodilator effects of CGRP are partially inhibited by blocking NO synthesis (Holzer et al. 1995).

Interaction of Sympathetic Efferents and Small-Diameter Afferents in Vascular Regulation

As the vascular bed of most organs, including skin, is regulated under physiological conditions by low-frequency on-going activity in sympathetic vasoconstrictor fibers, the question arises, how this activity interferes with small-diameter afferent-induced vasodi-lation. In human skin, antidromic vasodilation evoked by transcutaneous electrical stimulation was decreased under the conditions of body cooling, which raises sympathetic vasoconstrictor activity to skin. This effect was abolished by an anesthetic block of the proximal nerves supplying the skin territory. Other stimuli that are known to increase sympathetic vasoconstrictor activity to skin, such as deep breaths or emotional stress, also transiently reduced antidromic vasodilation (Hornyak et al. 1990). In rat hairless skin, antidromic vasodilation elicited by brief stimulation of the corresponding dorsal root was able to override the vasoconstriction evoked by electrical stimulation of the sympathetic chain, up to a frequency of 3 Hz. Higher sympathetic frequencies suppressed antidromic vasodilation, but this suppression could be overcome by longer-lasting stimulation of the afferents at high frequency (Häbler et al. 1997). These studies show that the vasodilation elicited by thin afferents is likely to dominate over sympathetic vasoconstriction under almost all conditions of normal regulation, and may be reduced only when sympathetic vasoconstrictor activity is exceptionally high. Pharmacological experiments indicate that the interaction of both neural vasomotor systems occurs mainly at the postjunctional level, but inhibitory prejunctional α_2-adrenoceptors on peripheral terminals of small-diameter afferents may also be involved.

Implication of Neuropeptides Derived from Small-Diameter Afferents in Systemic Vascular Regulation

Neuropeptides are released from small-diameter afferents, not only in the context of noxious stimulation and local neurogenic inflammation, but they also appear in the systemic circulation, where they may be of importance for vascular regulation under physiological and pathophysiological conditions. Without any overt noxious stimulation, CGRP is present in the plasma of humans, and CGRP levels increase during exercise (Lind et al. 1996) and in patients with sepsis (Shimizu et al. 2003) and severe hypertension (Edvinsson et al. 1992). Studies on spontaneously hypertensive rats suggest that CGRP release from perivascular nerves may be impaired, implying a role for peptidergic small-diameter afferents in the long-term control of systemic vascular resistance and blood pressure (Kawasaki 2002).

References

1. Delay-Goyet P, Satoh H, Lundberg JM (1992) Relative Involvement of Substance P and CGRP Mechanisms in Antidromic Vasodilation in the Rat Skin. Acta Physiol Scand 146:537–538
2. Edvinsson L, Erlinge D, Ekman R et al. (1992) Sensory Nerve Terminal Activity in Severe Hypertension as Reflected by Circulating Calcitonin Gene-Related Peptide and Substance P. Blood Pressure 1:223–229
3. Escott KJ, Brain SD (1993) Effect of a Calcitonin Gene-Related Peptide Antagonist (CGRP8-37) on Skin Vasodilatation and Oedema Induced by Stimulation of the Rat Saphenous Nerve. Br J Pharmacol 110:772–776

4. Gamse R, Saria A (1985) Potentiation of Tachykinin-Induced Plasma Protein Extravasation by Calcitonin Gene-Related Peptide. Eur J Pharmacol 114:61–66
5. Häbler HJ, Wasner G, Jänig W (1997) Interaction of Sympathetic Vasoconstriction and Antidromic Vasodilatation in the Control of Skin Blood Flow. Exp Brain Res 113:402–410
6. Häbler HJ, Timmermann L, Stegmann JU et al. (1999) Involvement of Neurokinins in Antidromic Vasodilatation in Hairy and Hairless Skin of the Rat Hindlimb. Neuroscience 89:1259–1268
7. Holzer P, Wachter C, Heinemann A et al. (1995) Sensory Nerves, Nitric Oxide and NANC Vasodilatation. Arch Int Pharmacodyn Ther 329:67–79
8. Hornyak ME, Naver HK, Rydenhag B et al. (1990) Sympathetic Activity Influences the Vascular Axon Reflex. Acta Physiol Scand 139:77–84
9. Kajekar R, Moore PK, Brain SD (1995) Essential Role for Nitric Oxide in Neurogenic Inflammation in Rat Cutaneous Microcirculation. Evidence for an Endothelium-Independent Mechanism. Circ Res 76:441–447
10. Kawasaki (2002) Regulation of Vascular Function by Perivascular Calcitonin Gene-Related Peptide-Containing Nerves. Jpn J Pharmacol 88:39–43
11. Lind H, Brudin L, Lindholm L et al. (1996) Different Levels of Sensory Neuropeptides (Calcitonin Gene-Related Peptide and Substance P) During and After Exercise in Man. Clin Physiol 16:73–82
12. McDonald DM (1998) Endothelial Gaps: Plasma Leakage during Inflammation. News Physiol Sci 13:104–105
13. Rinder J, Lundberg JM (1996) Effects of hCGRP 8-37 and the NK[1]-Receptor Antagonist SR 140.333 on Capsaicin-Evoked Vasodilation in the Pig Nasal Mucosa In Vivo. Acta Physiol Scand 156:115–122
14. Shimizu T, Hanasawa K, Tani T et al. (2003) Changes in Circulating Levels of Calcitonin Gene-Related Peptide and Nitric Oxide Metabolites in Septic Patients during Direct Hemoperfusion with Polymyxin B-Immobilized Fiber. Blood Purif 21:237-243
15. Whittle BJ, Lopez-Belmonte J, Rees DD (1989) Modulation of the Vasodepressor Actions of Acetylcholine, Bradykinin, Substance P and Endothelin in the Rat by a Specific Inhibitor of Nitric Oxide Formation. Br J Pharmacol 98:646–652

Neurogenic Pain

Definition

A pain syndrome arising after damage to the somatosensory pathways, from peripheral nerves and dorsal roots (peripheral neurogenic pain) to the spinal cord, brainstem, thalamus and cortex as well as the fibers inbetween (central neurogenic pain). The denominations deafferentation pain, dysesthetic pain, neuropathic pain (for peripheral type) and central pain are also used. Neurogenic pain is characterized by the following clinical descriptors: 1) pain localization in and around the deafferented body part, 2) pain qualities (pins and needles, electrical discharges, burning, tearing and compressive), and 3) timing of the pain: continuous, intermittent in attacks (lasting a fraction to a few seconds) or in episodes lasting more than a minute. The history and the neurological examination often reveal the evidence and signs of somatosensory damage (hypoesthesia and hypoalgesia). The examination may, however, be normal in some patients if the deficits have been compensated over time. Neurogenic pain responds specifically to antiepileptics and antidepressants, and represents the most frequent indication for pain surgery in the case of chronicity and resistance to non-invasive therapies.

▶ Thalamotomy for Human Pain Relief

Neurogenic Pain of Joint and Muscle Origin

▶ Neuropathic Pain, Joint and Muscle Origin

Neurogenic Pain, Painful Neuropathy

▶ Neuropathic Pain, Diagnosis, Pathology and Management

Neurogenic Vasodilation

▶ Nociceptor, Axonal Branching

Neuroglial Cells

▶ Satellite Cells and Inflammatory Pain

Neuroimaging

Definition

Neuroimaging is the production of images of the brain and/or spinal cord. It can include Computerized Tomography (CT) scanning, Magnetic Resonance Imaging (MRI), Photon Emission Computerized Tomography (SPECT) and Positron Emission Tomography (PET).

▶ Amygdala, Pain Processing and Behavior in Animals

Neuroimmune Activation

Definition

Neuroimmune activation is the adaptive, specific activation of endothelial cells, microglia, and astrocytes leading to the production of cytokines, chemokines, and the expression of surface antigens (Deleo 2001).

▶ Viral Neuropathies

Neuroimmune Interaction

Definition

Interactions between the immune system and the nervous system.
► Cytokines, Regulation in Inflammation

Neuroinflammation

Definition

Following an immune challenge or an injury in the nervous system, immune cells invade from the vascular system. T-lymphocytes enter the central nervous system where the microglia are activated and express major histocompatibility complexes, particularly class II (MHC II). Blood derived macrophages also become activated and encroach the perivascular space. In the dorsal root ganglia and sympathetic ganglia, where the vasculature is leakier and microglia are absent, the inflammatory response involves activation of endogenous macrophages and invasion of hematogenous ones and T-cells. The role of the immune cells is controversial. The macrophages/activated microglia are phagocytic if neuronal death occurs, but T-cells may be neuroprotective.
► Viral Neuropathies

Neurokinin

Definition

The tachykinins are a family of small biologically active peptides whose principle mammalian members are substance P (11 amino acids) and neurokinin (NK) A and B (10 amino acids). These peptides are derived from precursor proteins, the preprotachykinins, which are encoded by two different genes. Three receptors for tachykinins, the so-called neurokinin receptors NK1, NK2, NK3, have been cloned and characterized to have seven transmembrane spanning segments, to be coupled to G proteins and to be linked to the phosphoinosite signaling pathway. Although NK1 receptors are considered to be substance P-preferring, NK2 receptors NKA-preferring, and NK3 receptors NKB-preferring, substance P, NKA and B are full agonists at all three tachykinin receptors.
► Cancer Pain Management, Gastrointestinal Dysfunction as Opioid Side Effects
► Neuropeptide Release in Inflammation
► Neuropeptide Release in the Skin
► Substance P Regulation in Inflammation

Neurological Deficit

Definition

Neurological deficit refers to loss of function related to the nervous system.
► Hypoalgesia, Assessment
► Hypoesthesia, Assessment

Neurolytic Drugs

Definition

Neurolytic drugs (usually 50-96% ethanol or 5-7% phenol) destroy nerve cells and stop pain-impulse transmission for days to months.
► Cancer Pain Management, Anesthesiologic Interventions, Neural Blockade
► Trigeminal Neuralgia, Etiology, Pathogenesis and Management

Neuroma

Definition

When a nerve is cut, the fibers in the nerve distal to the cut die, while the fibers in the nerve that lie closer to the brain survive, and after some time may begin to heal. When both the nerve and its insulation have been cut and the nerve is not fixed, the growing nerve fibers may grow into a ball at the end of the cut, forming a nerve scar or neuroma. A neuroma can be painful and cause an electrical sensation when tapped (Tinel's sign). If the nerve injury was partial such that the insulation was not cut, new fibers may grow down the empty cover of the tissue until reaching a muscle or sensory receptor.
► Ectopia, Spontaneous
► Sympathetically Maintained Pain in CRPS II, Human Experimentation

Neuroma Endbulb

Definition

Severed axons form swollen terminal endbulbs. This usually occurs as a prelude to sprouting, but endbulbs may persist in the absence of sprouting.
► Neuroma Pain

Neuroma Model of Neuropathic Pain

► Anesthesia Dolorosa Model, Autotomy

N

Neuroma Pain

JAMES N. CAMPBELL
Department of Neurosurgery, Johns Hopkins
University School of Medicine, Baltimore, MD, USA
jcampbel@jhmi.edu

Synonyms

Nerve Stump Pain; Pain Associated with Traumatic Nerve Injury; Traumatic Nerve Endbulb Pain

Definition

The peripheral nerve consists of nerve fibers, supporting ▶ Schwann cells and associated elements such as blood vessels, extracellular matrix molecules and the nerve sheaths. The cell body of motor fibers (somatic and sympathetic) is in the anterior or intermedio-lateral part of the gray matter of the spinal cord, whereas the cell body of sensory fibers is contained in the paraspinal, dorsal root ganglion. When the peripheral nerve is cut, the injured fibers form terminal endbulbs and outgrowing sprouts (Fawcett and Keynes 1990; Fried et al. 1991). The nerve fibers distal to the cut are not supported by the cell body and as a result they undergo (Wallerian) degeneration. The Schwann cells survive and begin to divide, a process apparently triggered by denervation. When the denervated Schwann cells are encountered by the sprouting fibers, after nerve repair for example, regeneration proceeds in an orderly fashion. When Schwann cells guides cannot be accessed by the outgrowing sprouts, as for example happens in the event of amputation or if there is a large gap between the two ends of the severed nerve, the fibers entangle into an often bulbous mass at the proximal cut end of the nerve. This nerve end structure is known as a neuroma (Fawcett and Keynes 1990; Sunderland 1978).

Characteristics

Neuromas go through a life-cycle as the nerve fibers continue to grow out into the adjoining tissue. The ultimate appearance of the neuroma depends on milieu, how the nerve was injured and the amount of time that has passed (Campbell 2001). When a nerve is caught by a suture, as may happen inadvertently in surgery, a swollen bulb tends to form at the site, as the outgrowing sprouts are contained by the epineurium and scar tissue. When the nerve is cut and otherwise left alone in a healthy bed of tissue, the neuroma tends to be less discrete, as the outgrowing nerve fibers may advance and spread widely through the host tissue. Variations between full regeneration and a swollen ▶ neuroma endbulb abound, however. These variations may reflect the age of the patient, the nature and point of injury, the nature of the surrounding tissue, vascularization and genetic factors. All of these parameters can affect the fraction of severed nerve fibers that emit sprouts, the number that regenerate successfully, the number that fan out in local tissues at the nerve end and the number that become trapped within the swollen endbulb (Sunderland 1978). They *may* also affect whether the neuroma will be a source of pain. It is likely that most neuromas are not a source of pain.

Most neuromas, painful and non-painful, are due to nerve trauma caused by penetrating injuries, amputations, burns, bone fractures and surgery. Tumors and vascular insufficiency are also common causes. The location of some nerves, and perhaps their intrinsic biological properties, make them particularly prone to generating a (painful) neuroma. Entrapment may cause a neuroma if severe enough to actually sever axons. In these cases, the clinician observes a significant swelling of the nerve just proximal to the entrapment. After the entrapment is relieved the nerve fibers may regenerate. Morton's "neuroma" actually in most cases represents an entrapment neuropathy and may or may involve neuroma formation. Pain is associated with neuromas of cutaneous nerves and of nerves that serve muscles. It is uncertain how frequently pain originating in other deep tissues and viscera is related to neuroma formation.

Causes of Neuroma Pain

Surgeons in the past have followed the logic:

- Nerve injuries lead to neuromas.
- Nerve injuries are painful.
- *Ergo*, neuromas cause pain.

The exploration of this hypothesis has led to a richly complicated understanding of the basis of neuropathic pain. In short what we can say as of now is that yes, the neuroma is an important element in the genesis and perpetuation of pain, but that the biology of this pain goes well beyond the neuroma. A considerable amount of information has been obtained from observations on humans and on animal models, but these studies still leave unanswered questions. Most informative are electrophysiological recordings from injured nerves, from which we can say the following:

- Ectopic impulse activity in C-fibers, presumably nociceptive afferents, arises from the neuroma. Neuroma A-fibers also become abnormally active (Devor 2005).
- Abnormal spontaneous activity also arises in the dorsal root ganglion, though the prevailing data indicate that this activity is primarily in large cells that presumably give rise to A-beta (non-nociceptive) fibers (Devor 2005).
- The nociceptors that share the innervation territory of the injured nerve also become spontaneously active (Ali et al. 1999; Wu et al. 2001).

- Central abnormalities develop (e.g. in the dorsal horn) following nerve injury. It remains unclear to what extent discharges in nociceptive transmission pathways in the spinal cord and brain are dependent on peripheral inputs (Ji et al. 2003).

These considerations leave open the question of how important the neuroma itself is in generating pain. A very simple human experiment can go a long way towards resolving this issue. One may merely anesthetize the nerve injury site and determine whether the pain goes away for the duration of the block. If the pain goes away, then the neuroma generated the relevant neural signals that led to pain. If the pain does not go away, then the pain generator is elsewhere. Amazingly, there remains no comprehensive study of this question. For sure, there are cases where simply anesthetizing the neuroma gives rise to partial if not complete relief of pain. In other cases, however, pain persists (Campbell 2001).

In the instance where the neuroma does indeed directly play a role in generating pain, we still have a question of major clinical significance to consider. The neuroma may induce pain simply by virtue of (Burchiel et al. 1993) inherent spontaneous activity that arises in the nociceptors and/or it may induce pain when activated by virtue of its location. Neuromas have *mechanosensitivity* (Devor 2005; Koschorke et al. 1991; Koschorke et al. 1994). This means that mechanical stimuli applied to the neuroma produce neural activity and pain (the ▶ Tinel sign). Mechanical stimuli can arise in different ways. For example, the neuroma at the end of a stump of an amputated limb may be stimulated by the prosthesis. The neuroma infiltrating muscles or tendons in the hand or adhered to these by scar tissue may be stimulated every time the patient opens and closes his/her hand.

Treatment Approaches

In the clinical situation, where applying a temporary local anesthetic to the neuroma convincingly removes pain, what should be done? One possibility is to simply remove the neuroma. However, neuroma resection is a misguided surgical mission. As long as the sensory nerve fibers in the proximal nerve end are connected to the dorsal root ganglion, the neuroma reforms. Thus, neuroma resection is in fact *neuroma relocation* to the position of the new nerve cut. Will neuroma relocation work? This depends. If the dominant mechanism of pain production from the neuroma is inherent spontaneous activity, relocating the neuroma would not be expected to be effective. If however, the dominant mechanism is ▶ ectopic mechanosensitivity, then neuroma relocation does indeed make sense, if it is moved to a new location less prone to mechanical stimulation. There are numerous results in the literature about neuroma relocation surgery. Reports of efficacy range from 30 to 100% (Burchiel et al. 1993; Dellon et al. 1995).

If a nerve is only partially severed, intact conducting nerve fibers and severed neuroma sprouts may intermingle forming what may be termed a "▶ neuroma-in-continuity". Resection in this case may relieve the neuroma pain, but at the cost of residual nerve function. Nerve grafting may be feasible.

Part of the variability of neuroma pain may be due to unexpected peculiarities of the anatomy associated with the nerve's attempts to regenerate. For example, neuromas may form on the wrong (distal) side of an injured nerve (Belzberg and Campbell 1998). Nerves routinely have nerve branches going back and forth to one another. For example, in the forearm the superficial radial nerve has nerve branches to the lateral antebrachial cutaneous nerve. A nerve branch that makes its way to the distal end of another nerve that has been severed upstream encounters denervated Schwann cells. These denervated Schwann cells appear to attract outgrowing sprouts from the intact nerve. Over time the growing fibers could make their way back upstream along the distal portion of the severed nerve to reach the distal end of the cut nerve. The surgeon would do well to consider the possibility of such scenarios in planning neuroma relocation surgery.

Neuromas may be surgically treated in other ways as well. When a major nerve is involved, the primary approach is to repair the nerve. Clinical experience and some data from experimental animals (Lancelotta et al. 2003) suggest that pain is less when the nerve successfully regenerates. This raises an interesting clinical issue. In the instance where motor recovery is not feasible, for example in the event of proximal lesions involving the lower brachial plexus or sciatic nerve, should nerve repair be considered as a means to relieve pain? The answer is a qualified yes: "qualified" because little data are available to answer this question; "yes" because the rationale is compelling and the other options are less attractive. Painful cutaneous neuromas should be treated with proximal resection (*neuroma relocation surgery*), particularly when diagnostic block indicates that the origin of pain is in the neuroma. This is because the morbidity of the surgical procedure is low, regardless of the fact that efficacy may be as low as 30% (Burchiel et al. 1993; Sunderland 1978).

Other surgical options exist. Surgical sympathectomy may be considered in cases of sympathetically maintained pain. In the case of spinal nerve injury, it might make sense to consider dorsal root rhizotomy or dorsal root ganglionectomy, though these options are notorious for late recurrence of pain. Spinal cord or direct nerve stimulation may have striking palliative benefits. Pain might subside with time. Finally standard pharmacological approaches to neuropathic pain may be useful.

References

1. Ali Z, Ringkamp M, Hartke TV et al. (1999) Uninjured cutaneous C-fiber nociceptors develop spontaneous activity and alpha

N

adrenergic sensitivity following L6 spinal nerve ligation in the monkey. J Neurophysiology 81:455–466

2. Belzberg AJ, Campbell JN (1998) Evidence for end-to-side sensory nerve regeneration in a human. Case report. J Neurosurg 89:1055–7

3. Burchiel KJ, Johans TJ, Ochoa J (1993) The surgical treatment of painful traumatic neuromas. J Neurosurg 78:714–9

4. Campbell JN (2001) Nerve lesions and the generation of pain. Muscle Nerve 24:1261–73

5. Devor M (2005) Response of nerves to injury in relation to neuropathic pain. In: McMahon SL, Koltzenburg M (eds) Wall and Melzack's Textbook of Pain, 5th edn. Churchill Livingstone, London (in press)

6. Dellon AL, Mont MA, Krackow KA et al. (1995) Partial denervation for persistent neuroma pain after total knee arthroplasty. Clin Orthop Relat Res 316:145–50

7. Fawcett Y, Keynes R (1990) Peripheral nerve regeneration. Ann Rev Neurosci 13:43–60

8. Fried K, Govrin-Lippmann R, Rosenthal F et al. (1991) Ultrastructure of afferent axon endings in a neuroma, J Neurocytology 20:682–701

9. Ji RR, Kohno T, Moore KA et al. (2003) Central sensitization and LTP: do pain and memory share similar mechanisms? Trends Neurosci 26:696–705

10. Koschorke G, Meyer R, Tillman D et al. (1991) Ectopic excitability of injured nerves in monkey: entrained responses to vibratory stimuli. J Neurophysiol 65:693–701

11. Koschorke GM, Meyer RA, Campbell JN (1994) Cellular components necessary for mechanoelectrical transduction are conveyed to primary afferent terminals by fast axonal transport. Brain Res 641:99–104

12. Lancelotta MP, Sheth RN, Meyer RA et al. (2003) Severity and duration of hyperalgesia in rat varies with type of nerve lesion. Neurosurg 53:1200–1209

13. Sunderland S (1978) Nerves and Nerve Injuries, 2nd edn. Churchill Livingstone, London

14. Wu G, Ringkamp M, Hartke TV et al. (2001) Early onset of spontaneous activity in uninjured C-fiber nociceptors after injury to neighboring nerve fibers. J Neurosci 21:RC140

Neuroma-in-Continuity

Definition

A bulbous swelling in the nerve formed by sprouting axons that are intermixed with nerve fibers that are in continuity. The nerve appears intact to gross inspection but is swollen at the point of pathology.

▶ Neuroma Pain
▶ Neuropathic Pain Model, Chronic Constriction Injury

Neuromatrix

Definition

Neuromatrix is the term used by Ronald Melzack to describe a proposed cortical/subcortical network of interconnections, including the limbic system, responsible for pain. See Ronald Melzack, "Gate Control Theory: On the Evolution of Pain Concepts," Pain Forum 5 (1996): 128-38.

▶ Ethics of Pain, Culture and Ethnicity

Neuromodulation

Definition

The delivery of an electric current (neurostimulation) or drugs (intrathecal drug delivery systems) directly to targeted nerve fibers to treat pain.

▶ Cancer Pain Management, Anesthesiologic Interventions, Spinal Cord Stimulation, and Neuraxial Infusion
▶ Dorsal Root Ganglionectomy and Dorsal Rhizotomy
▶ Stimulation Treatments of Central Pain

Neuromodulator(s)

Definition

Neuromodulators are signaling molecules that play a role in the alteration of baseline neural activity. These neural effector molecules can increase or decrease baseline membrane activation. Examples are substance P, dynorphin, enkephalin, galanin, cholecystokinin, and bombesin.

▶ Nociceptive Neurotransmission in the Thalamus
▶ Placebo Analgesia and Descending Opioid Modulation
▶ Spinothalamic Tract Neurons, Peptidergic Input
▶ Thalamic Neurotransmitters and Neuromodulators

Neuron

Definition

Peripheral nociceptive neurons are afferent nerve fibers (i.e. A-delta - and C fibers) that transfer nociceptive impulses from the periphery to the dorsal horn. In the central nervous system, nociceptive neurons only respond to stimuli that are noxious or painful.

▶ Allodynia (Clinical, Experimental)
▶ Drugs Targeting Voltage-Gated Sodium and Calcium Channels
▶ Hypoalgesia, Assessment
▶ Lateral Thalamic Pain-Related Cells in Humans
▶ Postherpetic Neuralgia, Pharmacological and Non-Pharmacological Treatment Options

Neuron Restrictive Silencer Factor

Synonyms

NRSF

Definition

Is a repressor that is predominantly expressed in non-neuronal cells. NRSF silences neuronal genes in non-neuronal cells by binding to the NRSE (neuron restrictive silencer element) motif.

▶ Substance P Regulation in Inflammation

Neuronal Architecture

▶ Spinothalamic Tract Neurons, Morphology

Neuronal Dysfunction

Definition

Neuronal dysfunction is a state in which neurons display abnormal properties compared to those observed in normal development. For example, neuronal injuries or various neurodegenerative diseases can change normal neuronal conduction velocity or activation threshold by altering receptor distribution and properties, protein synthesis, activation of secondary messengers, etc.

▶ Dietary Variables in Neuropathic Pain

Neuronal Hyperexcitability

Definition

Increased responsiveness of central neurons; may include increased activity in response to stimulation, reduced threshold, increased afterdischarge, and expansion of receptive field size.

▶ Central Pain, Pharmacological Treatments
▶ Post-Seizure Headache

Neuronal Release

▶ Opioid-Induced Release of CCK

Neuronal Structure

▶ Spinothalamic Tract Neurons, Morphology

Neuronavigation

Definition

A stereotaxic system used for locating internal structures in 3D space without the need for fixing the patient in a stereotaxic frame.

▶ Motor Cortex (M1)
▶ Secondary Somatosensory Cortex (S2) and Insula, Effect on Pain Related Behavior in Animals and Humans

Neuropathic Pain

Definition

Neuropathic pain is pain initiated or caused by a primary lesion or dysfunction in the nervous system. Although neuropathic pain includes a number of different conditions some characteristics are shared: pain is often described as stabbing or burning, sensory abnormalities are common and treatment is difficult. Neuropathic (neurogenic pain) has been described in about 1% of the population. It is caused by functional abnormalities or structural lesions in the peripheral or central nervous system and occurs without peripheral nociceptor stimulation. It is caused by heterogeneous conditions unexplained by a single etiology or anatomic lesion. There are many different causes of neuropathic pain. Neuropathic pain may arise from infection/inflammation (postherpetic neuralgia, HIV-associated neuralgia, postpoliomyelitis, leprosy, interstitial cystitis, spinal arachnoiditis, acute inflammatory polyradiculopathy); non-infectious illness (multiple sclerosis, diabetic neuropathy, thalamic pain syndrome, essential vulvodynia) and pain associated with pressure/entrapment (neoplasia, trigeminal and glossopharyngeal neuralgia, carpal tunnel) and injury/trauma (surgery, complex regional pain syndrome, spinal cord injury). The etiology may be classified as localized (ischemic neuropathy, Complex Regional Pain Syndrome, phantom limb) or diffuse (toxins, AIDS, alcohol). Damage can affect the peripheral nerves, the cranial nerves, the posterior nerve roots, the spinal cord and certain regions within the brain. A variety of pain-related phenomena (mechanisms) may be operative in an individual patient necessitating mechanistic-based treatment. Patients with chronic NP are over-represented amongst those who are refractory to classic analgesic including opioid therapy. Although NP is not always opioid insensitive, the treatment of choice are tricyclic antidepressants (e.g. amitriptyline) and antiepileptic drugs (e.g. gabapentin).

▶ Allodynia (Clinical, Experimental)
▶ Alpha(α) 2-Adrenergic Agonists in Pain Treatment
▶ Amygdala, Pain Processing and Behavior in Animals
▶ Cancer Pain
▶ Cancer Pain Management, Overall Strategy

N

Neuropathic Pain, Diagnosis, Pathology and Management

ROBERT GASSIN

Musculoskeletal Medicine Clinic, Frankston, VIC, Australia

rgassin@pen.hotkey.net.au

Synonyms

Neurogenic Pain, Painful Neuropathy

Definition

▶ Neuropathic pain is pain initiated or caused by a primary lesion or dysfunction in the nervous system (Merskey and Bogduk 1994).

This definition allows neuropathic pain to encompass disorders of either the peripheral nervous system or the central nervous system. In the present context, neuropathic pain refers to pain associated with diseases or injuries of peripheral nerves. Pain associated with disorders of the central nervous system is more specifically referred to as ▶ central pain, and covered separately (see ▶ central pain).

Characteristics

Peripheral neuropathic pain occurs in a variety of diseases of peripheral nerves. These include: painful peripheral neuropathies, such as diabetic neuropathy, alcoholic neuropathy, and postherpetic neuralgia. It can also occur after injuries to peripheral nerves, such as avulsions, stretching or crush injury, or nerve transection.

Diagnosis

The diagnosis of neuropathic pain is suggested by the presence of certain features revealed by the ▶ medical history and neurological examination (see ▶ Diagnosis of Pain, Neurological Examination). The history reveals certain features about the nature of the pain, and may provide a cause. The examination reveals features of loss of neurological function or exaggerated neurological function.

Neuropathic pain is commonly worse at night. It is often described as shooting, stabbing, lancinating, burning, or searing. It can be continuous, but often presents as paroxysms of pain in the absence of any identifiable stimulus. In some conditions, such as nerve entrapment syndromes, the pain follows a nerve distribution, whereas in others such as neuropathies and poststroke pain, the distribution is more diffuse and may affect more than one body region. Pain experienced in a numb or insensate site (anaesthesia dolorosa) is highly suggestive of the diagnosis.

Cardinal to the diagnosis are features of disturbed neurological function. These may be in the form of loss of function, such as numbness, which indicates nerve damage directly; or they may be in the form of exaggerated function, which suggest loss of inhibition, and imply nerve damage. The latter features include: hyperalgesia (increased sensitivity to noxious stimuli), hyperpathia (increase response to minimal noxious stimulation), hyperaesthesia (increased sensitivity to touch), and allodynia (touch or brush is perceived as painful). Sometimes, neuropathic pain can be accompanied by the features of ▶ complex regional pain syndrome, such as temperature changes in the skin, swelling, skin colour changes, and increased or decreased sweating. Patients suffering neuropathic pain commonly suffer insomnia,

splayed laterally to the left and right of the surgeon. The fur is shaved from the left leg and lower back.

Step 3: The exposed skin is cleaned with 70% alcohol-soaked gauze. A small amount of concentrated Exidine-2 surgical scrub solution applied to fresh gauze is then used to further clean the surgical area.

Step 4: A midline incision at the lower back area is then made with either a #10 or #11 surgical scalpel blade and the skin around the cut is separated from its underlying loose connective tissue using blunt dissection scissors. This is done to provide space for subcutaneous implantation of the cc-sleeve (described below).

Step 5: A second incision is made along the lateral aspect of the left thigh and separation of the skin from underlying connective tissue extends beyond the incision site to the midline incision (in Step 4), where the exterior portion of the catheter will be encased by the cc-sleeve.

Step 6: The shaved and cleaned skin surrounding the wound is lightly retracted using small-toothed towel clips and then draped with sterile gauze.

Step 7: Exposure of the sciatic nerve is achieved by blunt dissection, and connective tissue is gently teased apart using glass Pasteur pipette hooks, sterilized in the glass-bead mini-sterilizer before each use.

Step 8: At approximately mid-thigh level, a portion of the sciatic nerve is slightly lifted using a sterile glass Pasteur pipette hook, followed by adding a couple of drops of sterile isotonic, endotoxin-free saline to keep the nerve moist.

Step 9: The gelfoam of the silastic+PE-50+gelfoam assembly is then gently threaded around the sciatic nerve starting from the quadriceps side to maintain a clear view of the implant site (Fig. 2a). The surrounding muscle walls are maneuvered to support the silastic+PE-50+gelfoam assembly upright.

Step 10: The 4-0 silk-suture that is part of the silastic+PE-50+gelfoam assembly (as previously described Chronic Peri-Sciatic Catheter Construction) is used to tie together the proximal and distal ends of the gelfoam once it forms a U-shape around the sciatic nerve. Precise control is best when using 2 pairs of micro-forceps. The surrounding muscle walls are then closed around the gelfoam-enwrapped sciatic nerve, leaving the silastic+PE-50 portion exteriorized (Fig. 2b).

Step 11: The silastic tube is anchored to the muscle by threading a sterile 4-0 silk suture with attached suture needle through the muscle at the most proximal portion of the dissection site, followed by threading the suture through the silastic tube, avoiding the internal PE-50 place-holder tube, and then through the opposing mus-

cle. The remaining overlying muscle is closed with one or two more sutures through the muscle.

Step 12: The exposed portion of the silastic catheter is tunneled subcutaneously to exit through the lower back incision (Fig. 2c).

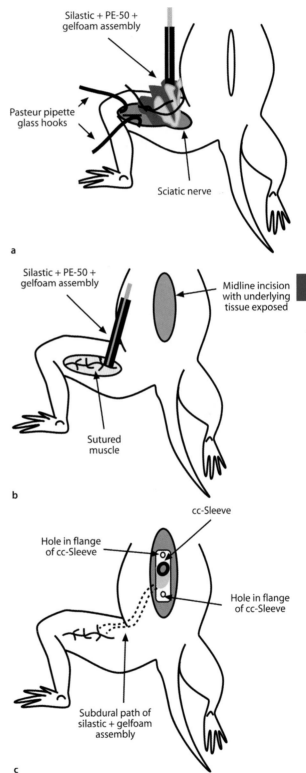

► **Neuropathic Pain Model, Neuritis/Inflammatory Neuropathy, Figure 2,** (a) The process of enwrapping the gelfoam portion of silastic+PE-50+gelfoam assembly around the sciatic nerve. (b) Illustrating the exteriorized portion of the silastic+PE-50 catheter after the gelfoam has been implanted and muscle walls sutured closed. (c) cc-Sleeve attachment to the lower back area after the silastic+PE-50+ gelfoam assembly has been implanted. Reprinted with permission (Milligan et al. in press).

Step 13: The skin overlaying the sutured muscle is closed with wound clips.

Step 14: The PE-50 dummy catheter is carefully removed while holding the silastic catheter in place, to ensure that the gelfoam does not become torn or displaced.

Step 15: The exposed portion of the silastic catheter is threaded through the cc-sleeve. The reader is referred to the methods paper that describes in detail the construction and use of this cc-sleeve (Milligan et al. 1999). The cc-sleeve is then anchored to the muscle overlaying the lumbosacral area, by threading one or two 3-0 silk sutures with attached suture needle through each flange on the cc-sleeve. The overlying skin is then sutured closed with 3-0 silk.

Step 16: The remaining exteriorized portion of the silastic tube is folded into the cc-sleeve and an air-dried concave plug (part of the cc-sleeve) (Milligan et al. 1999) is inserted inside the tip of the sleeve. A small amount of silastic silicon sealant is coated over the end of the plug and cc-sleeve with a moistened Q-tip.

Step 17: The wound area around the hind leg and lower back are lightly cleaned with 0.9% saline. Total surgical time is typically 15–20 minutes.

Step 18: Beginning 4–5 days following surgery, when catheters are used to induce chronic allodynia for extended periods of time, (the wound areas of the hind leg and lower back are cleaned with 0.9% saline every 2 days for as long as 2 weeks). This decreases the amount of inflammation, such as redness, slight bleeding and scabbing of the skin around the surgical sites. The cc-sleeve and the indwelling peri-sciatic silastic catheter are also cleaned with separate single-use peri-sciatic catheter cleaners.

Peri-Sciatic Catheter Injectors

Peri-Sciatic Catheter Injectors are made using the following steps:

Step 1: The beveled end of a sterile 23-gauge, 1-inch hypodermic needle is inserted into one end of a 30 cm PE-50 tube.

Step 2: A mark is made 7.3 cm from the opposite end, using a black permanent fine-tip marker. The mark must line up with the exterior end of the peri-sciatic silastic catheter upon PE-50 tubing insertion. This alignment assures that the interior end of the PE-50 tubing is 3 mm beyond the indwelling silastic catheter within the gelfoam.

Step 3: Prepared peri-sciatic catheter injectors are stored in a sterile, dry place (typically, an autoclavable box) until the time of injections.

Peri-Sciatic Catheter Injection Procedures

Peri-sciatic catheter injections are conducted using the following steps:

Step 1: The 23-gauge needle is attached to a sterile Hamilton 100l micro-syringe.

Step 2: The sterile glass Hamilton micro-syringe and the peri-sciatic catheter injector are flushed with sterile, endotoxin-free water and tightly connected, making the syringe and injector airtight.

Step 3: An air bubble is then created in the 30 cm PE-50 tubing of the peri-sciatic catheter injector by drawing up 1 of air followed by the drug. The length of the injection catheter will vary depending on the volume of drug injection. A 1.0 um volume occupies approximately 0.41 cm of PE-50 tubing.

Step 4: Animals are gently placed in crumpled soft cotton towels and allowed to move freely underneath the towels.

Step 5: The cc-sleeve area is exposed, the indwelling concave rubber plug is removed with a dental probe, and the folded portion of the silastic catheter is exteriorized. The reader is referred to the methods paper that describes in detail the construction and use of this cc-sleeve (Milligan et al. 1999).

Step 6: Fluid that had accumulated in the indwelling silastic catheter is suctioned off with the peri-sciatic catheter cleaner (described below) and discarded.

Step 7: Drug injection is completed using the prepared PE-50 injectors (described above). The PE-50 tubing from the peri-sciatic catheter injector is inserted into the silastic catheter until the 7.3 cm mark on the PE-50 tubing of the peri-sciatic catheter injector is flush with the edge of the silastic catheter. Chronic allodynia is maintained for over 2 weeks by repeated injections every 2 days, which are conducted in steps identical to that described immediately above (steps 1–7).

Peri-Sciatic Catheter Cleaning Procedures

In chronic allodynia, an additional step of cleaning the inside of the cc-sleeve with a separate peri-sciatic catheter cleaner is done, to decrease local inflammation/infection around this foreign body. Peri-sciatic catheter and cc-sleeve cleaning followed by drug injections are done every two days to maintain chronic allodynia. Using this paradigm, unilateral and bilateral allodynia remain stable during the entire testing period, in terms of both pattern (i.e., unilateral does not change to bilateral nor the reverse) and magnitude. Peri-sciatic Catheter Cleaners are used to suction out fluid accumulation within the indwelling silastic catheter starting 4–5 days after surgery and prior to drug injections.

Step 1: The catheter cleaners are made from the same supplies as the injectors, except the Hamilton 100μl micro-syringe is replaced with a sterile 3-cc syringe.

Step 2: The cleaners are constructed in the same way as the injectors (described above) except that the 3-cc syringe is attached to the 23-gauge needle. Prepared peri-sciatic catheter cleaners are stored in a sterile, dry place (typically, an autoclavable box) until the time of injections.

References

1. Bennett GJ, Xie YK (1988) A Peripheral Mononeuropathy in Rat that Produces Disorders of Pain Sensation like those Seen in Man. Pain 33:87–107
2. Bourque CN, Anderson BA, Martin del Campo C, Sima AA (1985) Sensorimotor Perineuritis - An Autoimmune Disease? Can J Neurol Sci 12:129–133
3. Chacur M, Milligan ED, Gazda LS, Armstrong CA, Wang H, Tracey KJ, Maier SF, Watkins LR (2001) A New Model of Sciatic Inflammatory Neuritis (SIN): Induction of Unilateral and Bilateral Mechanical Allodynia Following Acute Unilateral Peri-Sciatic Immune Activation in Rats. Pain 94:231–244
4. DeLeo JA, Coombs DW, Willenbring S, Colburn RW, Fromm C, Wagner R, Twitchell BB (1994) Characterization of a Neuropathic Pain Model: Sciatic Cryoneurolysis in the Rat. Pain 56:9–16
5. Eliav E, Benoliel R, Tal M (2001) Inflammation with no Axonal Damage of the Rat Saphenous Nerve Trunk Induces Ectopic Discharge and Mechanosensitivity in Myelinated Axons. Neurosci Lett 311:49–52
6. Eliav E, Herzberg U, Ruda MA, Bennett G (1999) Neuropathic Pain from an Experimental Neuritis of the Rat Sciatic Nerve. Pain 83:169–182
7. Gazda LS, Milligan ED, Hansen MK, Twining CM, Poulos NM, Chacur M, O'Connor KA, Armstrong CA, Maier SF, Watkins LR, Myers RR (2001) Sciatic Inflammatory Neuritis (SIN): Behavioral Allodynia is Paralleled by Peri-Sciatic Proinflammatory Cytokine and Superoxide Production. J Peripher Nerv Syst 6:111–129
8. Kim SH, Chung JM (1992) An Experimental Model for Peripheral Neuropathy Produced by Segmental Spinal Nerve Ligation in the Rat. Pain 50:355–363
9. Lockwood LL, Silbert LH, Laudenslager ML, Watkins LR, Maier SF (1993) Anesthesia-Induced Modulation of In Vivo Antibody Levels. Anesth Analg 77:769–775
10. Milligan ED, Hinde JL, Mehmert KK, Maier SF, Watkins LR (1999) A Method for Increasing the Viability of the External Portion of Lumbar Catheters Placed in the Spinal Subarachnoid Space of Rats. J Neurosci Methods 90:81–86
11. Milligan ED, Maier SF, Watkins LR (in press) Sciatic Inflammatory Neuropathy in the Rat. In: Luo D (ed) Pain Research: Methods and Protocols. Humana Press, Totowa, NJ
12. Milligan EM, Twining CM, Chacur M, Biedenkap J, O'Connor KA, Poole S, Tracey KJ, Martin D, Maier SF, Watkins LR (2003) Spinal Glia and Proinflammatory Cytokines Mediate Mirror-Iimage Neuropathic Pain. J Neurosci 23:1026–1040
13. Said G, Hontebeyrie-Joskowicsz M (1992) Nerve Lesions Induced by Macrophage Activation. Res Immunol 143:589–599
14. Sato W, Enzan K, Masaki Y, Kayaba M, Suzuki M (1995) The Effect of Isoflurane on the Secreation of TNF-Alpha and IL-1 Beta from LPS-Stimulated Human Peripheral Blood Monocytes. Masui 44:971–975
15. Seltzer Z, Dubner G, Shir Y (1990) A Novel Behavioral Model of Neuropathic Pain Disorders Produced in Rats by Partial Sciatic Nerve Injury. Pain 43:205–218
16. Spataro L, Sloane EM, Milligan ED, Maier SF, Watkins LR (2003) Gap Junctions Mediate Neuropathic Pain Produced by Sciatic Inflammatory Neuropathy (SIN) and Chronic Constriction Injury. In: Journal of Pain, vol 4 (suppl 1). Churchill Livingstone, Philadelphia, p 52

Neuropathic Pain Model, Partial Sciatic Nerve Ligation Model

JIN MO CHUNG

Department of Neuroscience and Cell Biology, University of Texas Medical Branch, Galveston, TX, USA

jmchung@utmb.edu

Synonyms

PSL model; Seltzer Model

Definition

The ▶ partial sciatic nerve ligation (PSL) model of neuropathic pain refers to a rodent ▶ neuropathic pain model that is produced by tightly ligating the dorsal third to half of the common sciatic nerve at the upper-thigh level (Seltzer et al. 1990).

Characteristics

Methods for Producing the PSL Model

Animals

Young adult male rats of various strains are commonly used. Like most other behavioral tests, it is helpful for rats to be acclimated for about a week in the laboratory holding facility with free access to food and water before performing any experiments. It is also convenient to keep rats in a room with a reversed light-dark cycle, allowing behavioral tests to be conducted during their active period.

Surgical Operation

Rats are deeply anesthetized with general anesthetics and placed in the prone position. Under a dissection microscope, the dorsum of the sciatic nerve is freed from surrounding connective tissues at a proximal site just distal to the point where the posterior biceps semitendinosus nerve branches off. An 8-0 silk suture is inserted into the nerve with a 3/8 curved needle, trapping the dorsal third or half of the nerve. The trapped portion of the nerve dorsal to the suture is tightly ligated. The wound is sutured closed. The original developers of the model (Seltzer et al. 1990) emphasized the importance of the site of ligation, which needs to be proximal enough so that the sciatic nerve is not yet fasciculated into individual nerves. Therefore, sciatic injury is made at a site between the branch point of the posterior biceps semitendinosus and a little fat pad (which is located just distally) since the sciatic nerve becomes fasciculated into branches just distal to the fat pad (Schmalbruch 1986; Seltzer et al. 1990).

Extent of Injury and Behavioral Outcome

The number of fibers injured by this procedure varies between animals (Seltzer et al. 1990). It is possible that some fibers in the unligated portion of the nerve may undergo degeneration due to secondary events such as: 1) disruption of the perineurium, 2) interference of local blood flow, 3) focal edema and 4) reaction to the ligature, etc. Therefore, variability in the number of injured fibers after partial sciatic nerve ligation comes from the fact that a variable number of fibers are being ligated and

N

that presumably variable numbers of unligated fibers are being injured by the above secondary causes.

Operated animals normally do not show severe motor deficits, except for the two lateral toes, which are flexed (Seltzer et al. 1990). At rest, the operated rats guard their operated limb somewhat when placing the limb on the floor; yet they show excessive abnormal grooming behaviors on the operated limb, such as repeated licking of the paw. However, none of operated rats show self-mutilating behavior due to the partially deafferented hind paw. During walking, they do not show obvious limping or any other severe locomotive abnormalities. Practically all operated rats show various behavioral signs of neuropathic pain such as ► ongoing pain, ► heat hyperalgesia, and mechanical as well as ► cold allodynia (Seltzer et al. 1990; Kim et al. 1997). Behaviors believed to represent ► mechanical allodynia can be quantified either by measuring foot withdrawal frequency to mechanical stimuli applied to the paw with von Frey filaments (Kim et al. 1997) or by determining the mechanical threshold (Seltzer et al. 1990). Heat hyperalgesia can also be measured by determining the heat threshold of the paw for foot withdrawals or duration of responses to suprathreshold heat stimuli (Seltzer et al. 1990). In addition, behaviors reflecting spontaneous pain have been shown by measuring the duration of foot withdrawals (guarding behaviors) in the absence of any obvious stimuli. Behavior thought to represent cold allodynia was assessed by measuring frequency of foot withdrawals to cold stimuli (e.g. acetone droplet application) applied to the paw (Kim et al. 1997).

Kim et al. (1997) made a comparison between the chronic constriction injury (CCI), spinal nerve ligation (SNL), and PSL models. When magnitudes of behaviors were compared with the CCI and SNL models, the PSL model fell in between the two for mechanical allodynia and spontaneous pain, but the magnitude of cold allodynic behavior was similar in all three models. Behaviors in PSL are partially reversed by sympathectomy (Shir and Seltzer 1991; Seltzer and Shir 1991) suggesting that sympathetic abnormality is involved in producing pain behaviors.

Factors Influencing Variability

Many factors influence neuropathic pain behavior in the PSL model as in other models. As shown in the SNL model (Mogil et al. 1999a; Mogil et al. 1999b; Yoon et al. 1999), genetic factors influence pain behaviors in the PSL model (Shir et al. 2001). Another important factor is diet. The effect of diet on neuropathic pain behavior has been studied in detail using the PSL model (Shir et al. 1998; Shir et al. 2002). Although the mechanisms are not clear, a diet with high soybean content reduces the expression of neuropathic pain behaviors. Finding such factors is important not only in terms of future studies on underlying mechanisms but also for potential therapeutic implications.

Advantages and Disadvantages of the PSL Model Compared to Others

The PSL model has several advantages over other neuropathic pain models. Tight ligation models such as the PSL provide information about the timing of injury better than loose ligation models. The most attractive feature of the PSL model is that it most closely resembles the original description of causalgia patients with injuries produced by high velocity missile impact (Mitchell 1872).

Acknowledgments

This work was supported by NIH Grants NS 31860 and NS 11255.

References

1. Kim KJ, Yoon YW, Chung JM (1997) Comparison of three rodent neuropathic pain models. Exp Brain Res 113:200–206
2. Mitchell SW (1872) Injuries of nerves and their consequences. JB Lippincott, Philadelphia
3. Mogil JS, Wilson SG, Bon K et al. (1999a) Heritability of nociception I: Responses of 11 inbred mouse strains on 12 measures of nociception. Pain 80:67–82
4. Mogil JS, Wilson SG, Bon K et al. (1999b) Heritability of nociception II. "Types" of nociception revealed by genetic correlation analysis. Pain 80:83–93
5. Schmalbruch H (1986) Fiber composition of the rat sciatic nerve. Anat Rec 215:71–81
6. Seltzer Z, Dubner R, Shir Y (1990) A novel behavioral model of neuropathic pain disorders produced in rats by partial sciatic nerve injury. Pain 43:205–218
7. Seltzer Z, Shir Y (1991) Sympathetically-maintained causalgiform disorders in a model for neuropathic pain: a review. J Basic Clin Physiol Pharmacol 2:17–61
8. Shir Y, Seltzer Z (1991) Effects of sympathectomy in a model of causalgiform pain produced by partial sciatic nerve injury in rats. Pain 45:309–320
9. Shir Y, Ratner A, Raja SN et al. (1998) Neuropathic pain following partial nerve injury in rats is suppressed by dietary soy. Neurosci Lett 240:73–76
10. Shir Y, Zeltser R, Vatine JJ et al. (2001) Correlation of intact sensibility and neuropathic pain-related behaviors in eight inbred and outbred rat strains and selection lines. Pain 90:75–82
11. Shir Y, Campbell JN, Raja SN et al. (2002) The correlation between dietary soy phytoestrogens and neuropathic pain behavior in rats after partial denervation. Anesth Analg 94:421–426
12. Yoon YW, Lee DH, Lee BH et al. (1999) Different strains and substrains of rats show different levels of neuropathic pain behaviors. Exp Brain Res 129:167–171

Neuropathic Pain Model, Spared Nerve Injury

ISABELLE DECOSTERD
Anesthesiology Pain Research Group, Department of Anesthesiology, University Hospital (CHUV) and Department of Cell Biology and Morphology, Lausanne University, Lausanne, Switzerland
isabelle.decosterd@chuv.ch

Synonyms

Spared Nerve Injury Model; SNI Model; Sural Spared Nerve Injury Model; sSNI Model

Definition

The rodent spared nerve injury model (SNI) consists of the selective injury of two of the three terminal branches of the sciatic nerve (the tibial and common peroneal nerve), leaving the third branch, the sural nerve, intact (Decosterd and Woolf 2000). Rapid and robust pain hypersensitivity to mechanical and thermal external stimuli is produced in the sural nerve skin territory, similar to stimulus-evoked pain observed in clinical ▶ neuropathic pain syndromes.

Characteristics

Description of the Model

Since the original description of ▶ anesthesia dolorosa by Wall (Wall et al. 1979), several models of transection/ligation-related injury to peripheral nerves have been described, allowing evaluation of the response to an applied external innocuous or nociceptive stimulus (stimulus-evoked pain) (Mosconi and Kruger 1996; Seltzer et al. 1990; Kim and Chung 1992; Bennett and Xie 1988; Vos et al. 1994). Unlike complete denervation of the paw after a sciatic nerve transection, these models enable assessment of pain sensitivity of the spared intact nerve fibers.

However, in the partial sciatic nerve injury (Seltzer et al. 1990) and the chronic constriction injury (Bennett and Xie 1988), the degree of nerve damage is difficult to reproduce, leading to variability within and between laboratories. Developed by Kim and Chung, the tight ligature of L5 and L6 spinal nerves ostensibly leaves all L4 afferents intact, but the surgery itself may damage or produce an inflammatory reaction to the intact L4 spinal nerve. The SNI model has the advantage of a simple surgical procedure and a high degree of reproducibility (Decosterd and Woolf 2000).

Two of the three terminal branches of the sciatic nerve are completely transected, i.e. the tibial and common peroneal nerves, and the sural nerve remains intact. If the surgical procedure is well executed, variability depends only on anatomical variation. Pain hypersensitivity is recorded in the skin territory of the spared sural nerve, preferentially on the plantar surface of the paw. Withdrawal threshold modifications are also present in the dorsal hairy sural nerve skin territory, and to a less extent in the saphenous nerve skin territory. The onset of allodynia- and hyperalgesia-like behavior is rapid (within 3 days post injury), and sensitivity changes last for months (up to 6 months). No change in the contralateral paw is observable when compared to same age sham-injured animal recordings. A crush injury to the tibial and common peroneal nerves induces pain hypersensitivity, but within nine weeks withdrawal thresholds return to baseline value. The original model was described in rats.

Despite technical advantages or disadvantages of each model, a distinct pattern should be distinguished in order to better understand specific mechanisms and possible differences between models. The emerging concept that non-injured fibers may participate in the generation and maintenance of neuropathic pain symptoms, as well as chemical cross talk and non-neuronal cell signaling, makes it important to distinguish models in relation to the co-mingling of injured primary sensory neurons/afferent fibers and uninjured neurons/fibers (see Table 1).

Surgery

Under general anesthesia, the sciatic nerve portion at thigh level is exposed using a longitudinal section through the biceps femoris muscle. The three terminal branches are easily located. Common peroneal and tibial nerves are delicately dissected in order to separate them from the surrounding tissue. The tip of a fine curved forceps is placed under the common peroneal nerve, avoiding any lift up. Five centimeters of 5.0 silk

Neuropathic Pain Model, Spared Nerve Injury, Table 1 Anatomically-related specific patterns of intermingling of primary sensory neuron cell bodies and axons distal to the peripheral nerve injury in animal models of neuropathic pain

Animal model	Sensory ganglia	Peripheral axons distal to injury
Complete sciatic nerve transection (associated or not with femoral nerve transection)[1]	Co-mingling of injured &non-injured neurons in L4 and L5 DRGs	*Injured axons only*
Chronic constrictive injury of the sciatic nerve or the infra-orbital nerve [2]	Co-mingling of injured &non-injured neurons in L4, L5 DRGs or in trigeminal ganglion	Intermingling of injured A-fiber and intact C-fiber axons
Partial sciatic nerve ligation (PSN) [3]	Co-mingling of injured &non-injured neurons in L4, L5 DRGs	Intermingling of injured and intact nerve fibers
Spinal nerve ligation (SNL) [4]	Non-injured neurons in L4 DRG &injured neurons only in L5 and L6 DRGs, no co-mingling	Intermingling of injured and intact axons
Spared nerve injury (SNI) [5]	Co-mingling of injured &non-injured neurons in L4 and L5 DRG	No intermingling of injured and intact axons

[1] Wall et al. 1979. [2] Bennett and Xie 1988; Vos et al. 1994, Mosconi and Kruger 1996. [3] Kim and Chung 1992. [4] Wall et al. 1979. [5] Decosterd and Woolf 2000.

suture is placed into the forceps' tip and slipped under the nerve. Two tight knots are made and the nerve is distally transected, including the removal of a portion of 2–4 mm. The same procedure is repeated for the tibial nerve. Crush injury is performed as above, except that injured nerves are only crushed for 30 seconds by a pair of small arterial clamps (with smooth protective pads). Special care needs to be taken to prevent any lesion to the spared nerve, and especially to avoid lifting up, touching or stretching the spared sural nerve during the surgical procedure.

Experimental Conditions

Genetic and environmental factors influence the course of pain behavioral studies (Chesler et al. 2002), and efforts are needed to standardize study conditions when using the SNI model. We try in our laboratory as much as possible to minimize the major variables:

- The investigator: the same investigator conduct a specific study, and he or she must be blind to the treatment/genotype applied
- Young adult male Sprague-Dawley rats (weighting initially 180–200 g, Charles River Inc) are very docile and all animals develop the neuropathy-related behavior. The same vendor and vendor's strain is recommended for each study
- Behavioral assessment of treated and control animals is performed during the same testing session in order to maintain the same experimental environment in both groups
- The behavioral testing is always performed at the same time of the day, the same order of testing is respected in between testing sessions
- The animals are housed and tested in a room of constant temperature and light cycle, and they have free access to food (same diet) and water. Animal transportation is avoided immediately before the testing session. Recordings are performed in a room devoted only to behavioral testing

Behavioral Assessment

The animals are daily habituated to the environment, testing material and investigator for at least two weeks before the first recordings. Behavioral assessment is performed as described originally (Decosterd and Woolf 2000) before and after SNI surgery. For plantar application, rats are enclosed in a home made transparent Plexiglas observation chamber (22 x 13 x 13 cm) atop a wire mesh floor (mesh of 0.25 cm^2). For dorsal application, rats are placed on a plane neutral floor. The investigator gently holds the animal and has direct access to the dorsal side of the hind paw.

During a study, mechanical and cold sensitivities were tested consecutively, with a 30 minute time interval between modalities tested. Heat assay are performed the next day and the animals are placed in the same obser-

vation chambers, but onto a transparent glass floor (Ugo Basile, Comerio, Italy).

▶ Mechanical allodynia-like behavior: the threshold is determined at the lowest force that evokes a brisk withdrawal response to one of five stimuli. Von Frey monofilaments are applied perpendicularly to the skin, in ascending force order, in the lateral area of the hind paw. Five stimuli cover the area, and contact with footpad or hairs are carefully avoided. The paw withdrawal threshold is recorded, and decreases significantly after surgery in both hairy and glabrous skin territory of the sural nerve (Fig. 1a and Decosterd and Woolf 2000). There is no contralateral effect of SNI.

▶ Cold allodynia-like behavior: a drop of acetone solution (99.6 %) is delicately placed under the plantar lateral side of the paw using a blunt needle. Acetone evaporates and produces a cold sensation. In the affected side, acetone induces long-lasting paw withdrawal as well as paw shaking and licking (Fig. 1b and Decosterd and Woolf 2000). The total duration of paw withdrawal is recorded, with a minimal time at 0.5 s for brief response and a cut-off at 60 s.

▶ Mechanical hyperalgesia-like behavior: a pinprick test is performed in the same skin area, using a safety pin. A single prick was given at a force such that the skin dimpled but was not penetrated. The duration of paw withdrawal was recorded, with a minimal time at 0.5 s for brief response and a maximal cut-off at 60 s. Response duration is increased for the injured paw, but to a lesser extent than after acetone stimulation (Fig. 1b and Decosterd and Woolf 2000).

▶ Heat hyperalgesia-like behavior: a movable radiant infrared heat source enables stimulation of the lateral part of the hind paw (Hargreaves et al. 1988)). Withdrawal reflex latency and duration due to heat stimulation are recorded with a 0.5 s minimal and a 60 s cut-off. Latency of stimulation is not modified by SNI, but the duration of the abnormal response is significantly increased (Fig. 1c and Decosterd and Woolf 2000). Although possible, plantar heat stimulation through transparent plane hard floor is difficult for the SNI lesioned paw. The animals refrained from weight bearing on the affected paw, and the foot is everted due to both pain hypersensitivity and neuro-muscular defects. This may lead to loose contact between the floor surface and the paw, altering the transmission of the thermal stimulus.

In summary, the spared sural nerve SNI model is an easily reproducible model of neuropathic pain. Mechanical and cold pain-hypersensitivity are assessable behaviorally, and, therefore, may provide functional information on mechanisms responsible for stimulus-evoked pain in neuropathic pain conditions.

References

1. Bennett GJ, Xie YK (1988) A Peripheral Mononeuropathy in Rat that Produces Disorders of Pain Sensation Like Those Seen in Man. Pain 33:87–107

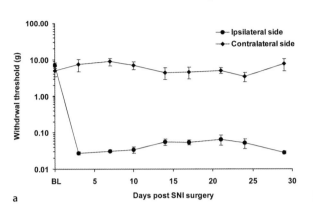

Mechanical allodynia

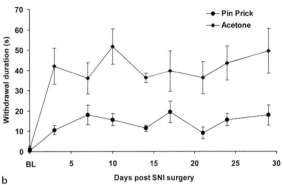

Cold allodynia and Mechanical hyperalgesia

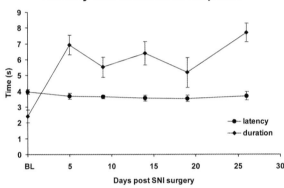

Heat hyperalgesia
Latency and duration of response

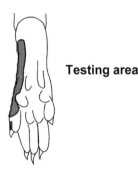

Testing area

N

Neuropathic Pain Model, Spared Nerve Injury, Figure 1   Mechanical and thermal hypersensitivity recorded in the spared sural nerve territory after SNI. (a) Withdrawal threshold in g determined after application of ascending series of von Frey monofilaments. (b) Withdrawal duration in s after application of acetone or pin prick stimulation. (c) Heat sensitivity (withdrawal latency and duration in s). BL, baseline. Representative series of 12 animals tested before (BL) and after SNI surgery. Results are displayed as the mean value ∓SEM.]

2. Chesler EJ, Wilson SG, Lariviere WR et al. (2002) Influences of Laboratory Environment on Behavior. Nat Neurosci 5:1101–1102
3. Decosterd I, Woolf CJ (2000) Spared Nerve Injury: An Animal Model of Persistent Peripheral Neuropathic Pain. Pain 87:149–158
4. Hargreaves K, Dubner R, Brown F et al. (1988) A New and Sensitive Method for Measuring Thermal Nociception in Cutaneous Hyperalgesia. Pain 32:77–88
5. Kim SH, Chung JM (1992) An Experimental Model for Peripheral Neuropathy Produced by Segmental Spinal Nerve Ligation in the Rat. Pain 50:355–363
6. Mosconi T, Kruger L (1996) Fixed-Diameter Polyethylene Cuffs Applied to the Rat Sciatic Nerve Induce a Painful Neuropathy - Ultrastructural Morphometric Analysis Of Axonal Alterations. Pain 64:37–57
7. Seltzer Z, Dubner R, Shir Y (1990) A Novel Behavioral Model of Neuropathic Pain Disorders Produced in Rats by Partial Sciatic Nerve Injury. Pain 43:205–218
8. Vos BP, Strassman AM, Maciewicz RJ (1994) Behavioral Evidence of Trigeminal Neuropathic Pain Following Chronic Constriction Injury to the Rat's Infraorbital Nerve. J Neurosci 14:2708–2723
9. Wall PD, Devor M, Inbal R et al. (1979) Autotomy Following Peripheral Nerve Lesions: Experimental Anaesthesia Dolorosa. Pain 7:103–111

Neuropathic Pain Model, Spinal Nerve Ligation Model

JIN MO CHUNG, KYUNGSOON CHUNG
Department of Neuroscience and Cell Biology,
University of Texas Medical Branch, Galveston, TX,
USA
jmchung@utmb.edu, kchung@utmb.edu

Synonyms

Spinal Nerve Ligation Model; SNL Model; Chung model

Definition

The spinal nerve ligation (SNL) model of ► neuropathic pain, refers to a rodent neuropathic pain model that is produced by tightly ligating the lumbar segmental spinal nerve (L5 alone or both L5 and L6) (Kim and Chung 1992). The lumbar segmental spinal nerve refers to a short length of the peripheral nerve distal to the dorsal root ganglion before it joins with other segmental nerves to form the lumbar plexsus. The lumbar segmental spinal nerve divides into a small dorsal ramus and a large ventral ramus, and the SNL model usually ligates the ventral ramus only since the dorsal ramus is denervated during the surgery.

Characteristics

Methods to Produce the SNL Model

Animals: Most commonly, young adult male rats of various strains are used (see Factors influencing variability). After purchase, rats are normally acclimated for about a week in the Institutional Animal Care Center, with free access to food and water in a room with a reversed light-dark cycle (dark: 8 A.M.-8 P.M.; light: 8 P.M.-8 A.M.) before experimental manipulation.

Surgical Operation: Figure 1 shows the anatomy of the lumbosacral paraspinal region. Rats are anesthetized with either inhalation gas or intraperitoneal injection of sodium pentobarbital and placed in the prone position. Under sterile conditions, a longitudinal incision is made at the lower lumbar/upper sacral level, exposing the paraspinal muscles on the left. Using a pair of small scissors with blunt tips, the paraspinal muscles are isolated and removed from the level of the L5 spinous process to the S1. This opens up the space ventrolateral to the articular processes, dorsal to the L6 transverse process, and medial to the ileum. Connective tissues and remaining muscles are removed with a small scraper. Under a dissecting microscope, the L6 transverse process, which covers the ventral rami of the L4 and L5 spinal nerves, is removed using a small rongeur. Access to the L5 spinal nerve is easier when the transverse process is removed very close to the body of the vertebrae. One can normally visualize the ventral rami of the L4 and L5 spinal

nerves (a thin sheet of connective tissue may cover them in some animals) once the L6 transverse process is carefully removed. The L4 spinal nerve usually runs more laterally (or ventrally in some animals) than the L5, and these two nerves join distally in a common epineurial sheet, however, there is a great deal of individual variability where these two nerves join. Thus, the L4 and L5 spinal nerves need to be separated in some animals to make the L5 spinal nerve accessible for ligation. It is very important not to damage the L4 nerve during this process, because we find that even slight damage to the L4 spinal nerve invariably results in a greatly reduced mechanical sensitivity of the foot. Damage to the L4 spinal nerve can occur with a seemingly mild mechanical trauma (excessive touch, gentle stretch, or slight entrapment within the epineurial sheet). Once enough length of the L5 spinal nerve is freed from the adjacent structure, a piece of 6-0 silk thread is placed around the L5 spinal nerve and the nerve is tightly ligated to interrupt all axons in the nerve. Another option would be to cut the spinal nerve just distal to the ligation to make sure all fibers are interrupted.

The L6 spinal nerve can also be ligated if so desired. The L6 spinal nerve runs underneath the sacrum and is not visible without chipping away a part of the sacrum. Since the sacrum bleeds a lot when chipped, it would be better to approach the L6 spinal nerve blindly without chipping the sacrum. After carefully removing the fascia joining the sacrum to the ileum, one can place a small glass hook underneath the sacrum and gently pull the L6 spinal nerve out into the paravertebral space and ligate it tightly with 6-0 silk thread.

Upon completion of the operation, which normally takes about 10–15 minutes (after some practice), hemostasis is confirmed and the muscles are sutured in layers using silk thread and the skin is closed with metal clips, anesthesia is then discontinued. Animals are then kept in a cage with warm bedding until they completely recover from anesthesia.

Behavioral Outcome of Surgery: Successfully operated animals normally do not show any motor deficits beyond a mild inversion of the foot with slightly ventroflexed toes. The most common and obvious motor deficit of unsuccessfully operated animals is dragging the hind limb of the operated side, a sign of paralyzed proximal muscles. This invariably indicates damage to the L4 spinal nerve, since this nerve innervates many proximal muscles of the hind limb.

A successfully operated rat shows various behavioral signs of neuropathic pain such as ongoing pain, heat ► hyperalgesia, and mechanical as well as cold ► allodynia. Since the SNL model shows a particularly robust sign of mechanical allodynia, one can use the degree of hypersensitivity to gauge the success of the operation. Mechanical sensitivity is quantified either by measuring response frequency to mechanical

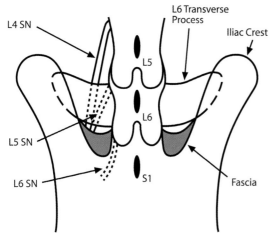

Neuropathic Pain Model, Spinal Nerve Ligation Model, Figure 1 Schematic diagram showing the dorsal view of the bony structures and spinal nerves at the lumbosacral level after removal of paraspinal muscles.

stimuli applied with ▶ von Frey filaments (Kim and Chung 1991; Kim and Chung 1992) or by determining the mechanical threshold (Chaplan et al. 1994). A successful surgical operation will result in a clear sign of mechanical allodynia demonstrated by either: 1) lowering the foot withdrawal threshold below the normal nociceptor activation threshold [below 1.4 g (Leem et al. 1993)], 2) frequent foot withdrawals to mechanical stimulation at a strength below the normal nociceptor activation threshold, or 3) frequent foot withdrawals to obviously innocuous stimulations. On the other hand, sham-operation should not produce any significant changes in mechanical sensitivity, except a mild transient effect lasting one or two days. A significant and long lasting hyperalgesia following sham-operation invariably indicates that the surgery induced damage and/or inflammation to the nerve and is thus an unsuccessful operation.

Factors Influencing Variability

Multiple factors seem to influence the behavioral outcome after SNL and hence contribute to variability of data. The strain of rats is an important variable. Not only do different strains of rats show different levels of neuropathic pain behaviors, but also different levels of pain behaviors can also be seen in different substrains of Sprague-Dawley rats obtained from different suppliers (Yoon et al. 1999). Another important factor that influences the sign of mechanical allodynia is the exact testing spot on the paw where the mechanical stimulation is applied. To represent the most intensely painful area of a human patient, one must measure the threshold at the most sensitive area of the rat. The most sensitive area of the paw after ligation of the L5 or both the L5 and L6 spinal nerves is the base of the 3rd or 4th toe (Xie et al. 1995). The most sensitive spot of the paw after spinal nerve ligation is confined to a small area and does not vary much between rats, presumably due to stereotyped denervation of the foot by the surgical procedure. When measuring in the most sensitive area, the threshold is usually well below the 1 g range, whereas the threshold ranges from 2 to 3 g if one measures it by stimulating the mid-plantar area (Chung et al. 2004).

Advantages and Disadvantages of the SNL Model Compared to Others

The SNL model has several advantages over other models. These include that: 1) the injury is stereotyped, 2) it has successfully adapted to multiple species of animals, and 3) the injured and uninjured afferents are segregated to different spinal segments. Tight ligation is advantageous over loose ligation in terms of knowing the timing of injury, as well as the population of fibers being injured. In addition, a tight ligation of a specific set of nerves in every animal will reduce the variability among animals. Many neuropathic pain models, including the SNL model, which was originally developed using the rat, are now successfully adapted to the mouse (Mogil et al. 1999). The SNL model has also been successfully applied to the monkey (Carlton et al. 1994). The uniqueness of the SNL model, however, is that spinal inputs of injured and uninjured afferents are segregated at separate spinal segments. This feature allows the investigation of the contribution of injured and uninjured afferent fibers to neuropathic pain.

There are also some disadvantages to the SNL model. These include that: 1) the surgical procedure is invasive, and 2) the model is highly artificial. Because the spinal nerves are located deep, the surgery to expose them requires some level of skill and, hence, may be a source of variability. A particularly technically difficult aspect is to preserve the L4 spinal nerve completely undamaged while ligating the L5 spinal nerve since they are located in close proximity. Since it is rare to find a patient with discrete spinal nerve injury, this model is highly artificial.

Different models tend to produce different behavioral outcomes. A previous study compared the behaviors of 3 different models [SNL, chronic constriction injury (CCI), and partial sciatic nerve ligation (PSL) models] (Kim et al. 1997). The CCI model produced the most robust ongoing pain behaviors, whereas mechanical allodynic behaviors were most prominent in the SNL model.

N

References

1. Carlton SM, Lekan HA, Kim SH, Chung JM (1994) Behavioral Manifestations of an Experimental Model for Peripheral Neuropathy Produced by Spinal Nerve Ligation in the Primate. Pain 56:155–166
2. Chaplan SR, Bach FW, Pogrel JW, Chung JM, Yaksh TL (1994) Quantitative Assessment of Tactile Allodynia in the Rat Paw. J Neurosci Methods 53:55–63
3. Chung JM, Kim HK, Chung K (2004) Segmental Spinal Nerve Ligation Model of Neuropathic Pain in Pain Research: Methods and Protocols. In: ZD Luo (ed) Methods in Molecular Medicine series (Serial ed. John M. Walker). The Humana Press Inc, Totowa, NJ (in press)
4. Kim KJ, Yoon YW, Chung JM (1997) Comparison of Three Rodent Neuropathic Pain Models. Exp Brain Res 113:200–206
5. Kim SH, Chung JM (1991) Sympathectomy Alleviates Mechanical Allodynia in an Experimental Animal Model for Neuropathy in the Rat. Neurosci Lett 134:131–134
6. Kim SH, Chung JM (1992) An Experimental Model for Peripheral Neuropathy Produced by Segmental Spinal Nerve Ligation in the Rat. Pain 50:355–363
7. Leem JW, Willis WD,Chung JM (1993) Cutaneous Sensory Receptors in the Rat Foot. J Neurophysiol 69:1684–1699
8. Mogil JS, Wilson SG, Bon K, Lee SE, Chung K, Raber P, Pieper JO, Hain HS, Belknap JK, Hubert L, Elmer GI, Chung JM, Devor M (1999) Heritability of Nociception I: Responses of 11 Inbred Mouse Strains on 12 Measures of Nociception. Pain 80:67–82
9. Xie J, Yoon YW, Yom SS, Chung JM (1995) Norepinephrine Rekindles Mechanical Allodynia in Sympathectomized Neuropathic Rat. Analgesia 1:107–113
10. Yoon YW, Lee DH, Lee BH, Chung K, Chung JM (1999) Different Strains and Substrains of Rats Show Different Levels of Neuropathic Pain Behaviors. Exp Brain Res 129:167–171

Neuropathic Pain Model, Tail Nerve Transection Model

H. S. NA[1], H. J. KIM[2], S. K. BACK[1], B. SUNG[1], Y. I. KIM[1], Y. W. YOON[1], H. C. HAN[1], S. K. HONG[1]
[1]Medical Science Research Center and Department of Physiology, Korea University College of Medicine, Seoul, Korea
[2]Department of Life Science, Yonsei University Wonju Campus, Wonju, Korea
hsna@korea.ac.kr

Definition

The tail nerve transection model is produced by the incomplete injury of the nerves (i.e. the inferior and/or superior caudal trunks) innervating the tail. The model displays chronic neuropathic signs like ▶ mechanical allodynia, ▶ cold allodynia and ▶ warm allodynia in the tail skin.

Characteristics

The tail nerve transection model is one of the ▶ peripheral neuropathic pain animal models. Peripheral nerve injury sometimes results in neuropathic pain. This type of pain is characterized by spontaneous burning pain accompanied by ▶ hyperalgesia and ▶ allodynia lasting variable times. Several experimental animal models for neuropathic pain, produced by a partial injury of the nerves supplying the rat hind paw, were developed by Bennett & Xie (1988), Seltzer et al. (1990) and Kim & Chung (1992), respectively. Although these models display clear signs of neuropathic pain, there are some inherent problems in performing behavioral tests due to foot deformity. To avoid these problems, the tail nerve transection model, produced by transection of interior caudal trunk at the level between the S3 and S4 spinal nerve, was developed (Na et al. 1994; Kim et al. 1995). This model shows neuropathic signs without tail deformity. In addition, modified methods, such as the transection of superior caudal trunk (Back et al. 2002) or both trunks (Kim et al. 2001) also showed similar neuropathic changes.

The tail skin is innervated by the inferior and superior caudal trunks, which are located in the ventral and dorsal parts of the pelvic bone, respectively. The two trunks are composed of the dorsal and ventral divisions, respectively, of the four sacral and the first two caudal spinal nerves. To induce neuropathic pain in the tail skin, the inferior and/or superior caudal trunk(s) is (are) exposed carefully from the surrounding tissues and transected at the level between the S3 and S4 spinal nerves. This surgery eliminates the S^1-S3 spinal nerve innervation of the tail *via* the trunk(s). Figure 1 illustrates schematically how these trunks are composed and the level of the transection of the inferior caudal trunk.

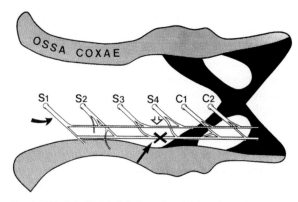

Neuropathic Pain Model, Tail Nerve Transection Model, Figure 1 A schematic diagram (dorsal view) illustrating how the inferior (black arrow) and superior (open arrow) caudal trunks are composed and the level of transection ($\times$) of the inferior caudal trunk. The curved arrow indicates the S1 spinal nerve.

The signs indicative of mechanical allodynia can be sought by applying normally innocuous mechanical stimuli to the tail using ▶ von Frey hairs. For convenient application of the stimuli, the animal is restrained in a transparent plastic tube and the tail is laid on a plate. The most mechanically sensitive spot of the tail is first determined by rubbing various areas of the tail with the shank of the von Frey hair, and then, this area is poked systematically with the von Frey hair to locate the most sensitive spot. An abrupt tail movement of about 0.5–20 cm in response to the von Frey hair stimulation is considered to be an abnormal response, indicative of mechanical allodynia. During repeated trials, the test stimuli are delivered to the same spot without difficulty, since the tail is usually stationary.

Figure 2a and 2b show the data obtained with the von Frey hairs (4.9 mN and 19.6 mN). Prior to the neuropathic surgery, the frequency of the abnormal tail response to von Frey hair stimulation is near 0 percent. However, after the neuropathic surgery, the frequency increases dramatically from 1 day PO (postoperatively) and lasts for at least 4 months, unlike the frequency in sham-operated animals. These results suggest that the partial injury of the nerves innervating the tail leads to mechanical allodynia in the tail.

The signs indicative of cold and warm allodynia can be sought by immersing the tail in 4°C and 40°C water, respectively. The rat is restrained in a plastic tube, and the tail is drooped for convenient application of the thermal stimuli. Following the tail immersion, the investigator measures the latency of the tail withdrawal response with a cut-off time of 15 s. A tail withdrawal response with a latency shorter than the cut-off time is considered to be an abnormal tail response indicative of thermal allodynia. The tail immersion test is repeated 5 times at 5 min intervals to obtain the average tail response latency.

Figure 2c and 2d show the data obtained with the cold (4°C) and warm (40°C) water, respectively. Prior to the

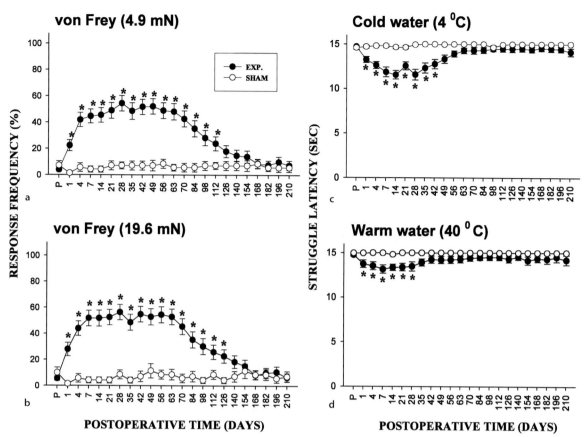

Neuropathic Pain Model, Tail Nerve Transection Model, Figure 2 Tail responses to mechanical (a, b), cold (c) and warm (d) stimuli. The mean (± SEM) response frequency in the case of mechanical stimulation with von Frey hairs (4.9 mN, 19.6 mN) and the mean (± SEM) response latency in the case of cold (4°C) and warm (40°C) stimulation of experimental (Exp, n=44) and sham (n=14) groups are plotted against the experimental days (P: 1 day before nerve injury). Asterisks indicate the scores significantly different from the preoperative value (P<0.05 by the Friedman test followed by a pairwise post-hoc test).

neuropathic surgery, most rats did not show abnormal tail responses to the cold or warm water stimuli. However, after the neuropathic surgery the tail response latency significantly decreased from 1 day PO and lasted for 5–7 weeks. These results suggest that the partial injury of the nerves innervating the tail leads to cold and warm allodynia in the tail. The possibility that the abnormal tail responses to the 4°C or 40°C water immersion are due to the mechanical contact of the tail with the water instead of thermal stimulation is essentially ruled out, since 1) in a vast majority of the cases, 30°C water does not induce any abnormal tail responses and 2) the 4°C or 40°C water-induced responses have latencies greater than at least a few seconds, unlike the von Frey hair-evoked responses which had virtually no latencies. The tail nerve transection model, like the previously developed ones, shows chronic neuropathic signs like mechanical and thermal (cold and warm) allodynia. Furthermore, the model offers several advantages in surgical approach and performing the behavioral tests. First, surgical procedures for the model are so simple that even neonatal rats or mice can be used (Back et al.

2002). In fact, although rat models for neuropathic pain have been applied to the mouse (Malmberg and Basbaum 1998; Mansikka et al. 2000; Mogil et al. 1999), there are some problems from the invasiveness of these approaches. Second, since the inferior and superior caudal trunks are composed of the four sacral and the two caudal spinal nerves, the number of injured fibers or the spinal level of injury can be changed according to the transection site. This advantage was helpful to elucidate of the fact that the extent of ▶ sympathetic fiber sprouting in the ▶ dorsal root ganglion (DRG) was related to the number of injured nerve fibers (Kim et al. 2001) and the distance between the DRG and injury site (Kim et al. 1996). Third, application of both mechanical and thermal stimuli to the partially denervated area (i.e. the tail) is straightforward. For example, tail immersions into cold or warm water make all thermal receptors in the tail receive the same thermal stimulation simultaneously. In addition, since there is no deformity in the tail after the nerve injury, the mechanically sensitive spot is easily located and blind behavioral tests are available.

References

1. Back SK, Sung B, Hong SK et al. (2002) A mouse model for peripheral neuropathy produced by a partial injury of the nerve supplying the tail. Neurosci Lett 322:153–156
2. Bennett GJ, Xie Y-K (1988) A peripheral mononeuropathy in rat that produces disorders of pain sensation like those seen in man. Pain 33:87–107
3. Kim SH, Chung JM (1992) An experimental model for peripheral neuropathy produced by segmental spinal nerve ligation in the rat. Pain 50:355–363
4. Kim YI, Na HS, Han JS et al. (1995) Critical role of the capsaicin-sensitive nerve fibers in the development of the causalgic symptoms produced by transecting some but not all of the nerves innervating the rat tail. J Neurosci 15:4133–4139
5. Kim HJ, Na HS, Nam HJ et al. (1996) Sprouting of sympathetic nerve fibers into the dorsal root ganglion following peripheral nerve injury depends on the injury site. Neurosci Lett 212:191–194
6. Kim HJ, Na HS, Back SK et al. (2001) Sympathetic sprouting in sensory ganglia depends on the number of injured neurons. NeuroReport 12(16):3529–3532
7. Malmberg AB, Basbaum AI (1998) Partial sciatic nerve injury in the mouse as a model of neuropathic pain: behavioral and neuroanatomical correlates. Pain 76:215–222
8. Mansikka H, Sheth RN, DeVries C et al. (2000) Nerve injury-induced mechanical but not thermal hyperalgesia is attenuated in neurokinin-1 receptor knockout mice. Exp Neurol 162:343–349
9. Mogil JW, Wilson SG, Bon K et al. (1999) Heritability of nociception I: Responses of 11 inbred mouse strains on 12 measures of nociception. Pain 80:67–82
10. Na HS, Han JS, Ko KH et al. (1994) A behavioral peripheral neuropathy produced in rat's tail by inferior caudal trunk injury. Neurosci Lett 177:50–52
11. Seltzer Z, Dubner R, Shir Y (1990) A novel behavioral model of neuropathic pain disorders produced in rats by partial sciatic nerve injury. Pain 43:205–218

Neuropathic Pain Models, CRPS-I Neuropathy Model

JEAN-JACQUES VATINE[1], JEANNA TSENTER[2], ZE'EV SELTZER[3]

[1]Outpatient and Research Division, Reuth Medical Center, Tel Aviv, Israel
[2]Department of Physical Medicine and Rehabilitation, Hadassah University Hospital, Jerusalem, Israel
[3]University of Toronto Centre for the Study of Pain, Faculty of Dentistry, Toronto, ON, Canada
vatinejj@reuth.org.il

Synonyms

Reflex Sympathetic Dystrophy; Algodystrohy; Sudeck's Atrophy; CRPS-I neuropathy model

Definition

Complex regional pain syndrome (CRPS) is a neuropathic pain disorder that usually develops after a noxious event. Pain is frequently described as burning and continuous and exacerbated by movement, continuous stimulation or stress. The syndrome includes spontaneous pain and/or stimulus evoked pain (► allodynia and ► hyperalgesia), exceeding in both magnitude and duration the clinical course expected to follow the inciting event. Regardless of the site of injury, the symptoms begin and remain most intense in the distal extremity and are not limited to the distribution of a single peripheral nerve. At some point in time, pain may be associated with edema, changes in skin blood flow and abnormal sudomotor activity in the same area, often resulting in significant impairment of motor function and showing variable progression over time. Two forms of CRPS have been identified. CRPS-I usually develops following trauma with only minor nerve damage or without any demonstrable nerve lesion whereas CRPS-II is associated with a clear nerve injury that can be characterized by abnormal clinical and/or electrodiagnostic findings (Stanton-Hicks et al. 1995). The tetanized sciatic neuropathy (TSN) model is a preparation in rodents that results in allodynia, hyperalgesia and vasomotor disturbances that mimic CRPS-I. This model is produced by activating unmyelinated afferents (C-fibers) at '► wind up' (Mendell 1966) parameters, using a 10 min electrical stimulation (i.e. tetanization) of an intact sciatic nerve.

Characteristics

Harden und Bruehl (2005) recently proposed the following diagnostic algorithm to diagnose CRPS-I in humans. This algorithm is based on presentation of at least one sign in two out of the following four categories: (a) sensory abnormalities; allodynia and/or hyperalgesia, (b) vasomotor abnormalities; temperature asymmetry and/or skin color changes and/or asymmetry, (c) sudomotor abnormalities or edema; swelling and/or altered sweating and/or sweating asymmetry, (d) motor abnormalities or dystrophy; decreased range of motion and/or motor dysfunction (weakness and/or tremor and/or dystonia) and/or trophic changes in hair and/or skin and/or nails. Edema and autonomic dysregulation are usually seen in the early stage of the disease, while movement disorders and trophic changes are more apparent in the later stage. For many decades, sympathetic blockade was the method of choice for the diagnosis and treatment of CRPS-I. Pain relief in response to this procedure has been used as a criterion for diagnosis, hence the term reflex sympathetic dystrophy (RSD). However, it now appears that not all patients may have sympathetically maintained pain in CRPS (Stanton-Hicks et al. 1995). Several animal models have been developed to study the mechanisms underlying neuropathic pain mimicking CRPS-II, including the chronic constriction injury (CCI), partial sciatic ligation (PSL) and spinal nerve ligation (SNL) models. Some of these are described elsewhere in this section. The common denominator of these models is that abnormal sensory responses to stimuli and spontaneous behavior, indicative of neuropathic pain, are produced by partial denervation of a paw, tail or the face. The typical spontaneous pain behaviors include guarding behavior, repeated flicking of the partially denervated paw, excessive licking and holding the paw in the mouth, claw pulling, elevated paw position and antalgic gait, as well as vocalization, reduced appetite, weight loss and self-mutilation (autotomy). The abnormal sensory responses to stimuli include a reduced withdrawal threshold to a stimulus that is normally non-noxious (allodynia), and exaggerated responses to a stimulus that is normally noxious (hyperalgesia). The latter is manifested as increased duration and robustness of nocifensive responses. A wealth of data on the mechanisms that trigger and underlie the pain in CRPS-II has been gathered from these animal models, since they are all produced by some type of nerve injury that partially denervates a limb. However, since in CRPS-I there is no evidence for such a nerve injury, these models may not be relevant to the study of its mechanisms (Jänig and Baron 2001).

The signals that trigger CRPS-I as well as the mechanisms maintaining the abnormalities that characterize this syndrome are still enigmatic. Since the clinical signs of CRPS-I and CRPS–II are similar, they may be produced by the same triggering input. When sensory fibers are injured, 25–33% of transected axons emit a barrage of impulses termed ▶ injury discharge (ID). This is the first neural message to notify the CNS that an injury has occurred (Wall et al. 1974). This message comprises a burst of high frequency discharge in A-fibers and of low frequency firing in C-fibers. This burst decays in most A- and C-fibers within minutes after the injury. However, about 10% of injured fibers continue to fire for many hours and may not stop for days (Baik-Han et al. 1990; Blenk et al. 1996; Sackstein et al. 1996). Muscular afferents emit a clearly more robust ID than cutaneous afferents. ID is a distinct signal in the 'alphabet' of these fibers, unlike their normal response to natural stimuli, since the peak discharge of ID is 2–6-fold higher than the response to maximal normal stimulation (Sackstein et al. 1996). ID is an important signal in triggering neuropathic pain disorders in some animal models and possibly in humans as well (reviewed by Kissin, 2000).

The TSN model has been developed on the basis of the working hypothesis that CRPS I may be caused by a bodily injury that does not result in frank nerve injury but produces a massive nociceptive input that is similar to ID. The following description provides methodological details of the TSN model.

Animals

The original model was developed in the rat but it can easily be adapted to the mouse.

Preparation of the TSN Model

Surgery

Under inhalation anesthesia and aseptic conditions, the sciatic nerve on both sides is exposed at midthigh level and the surgical field is kept widely open with separators, taking care not to pull the posterior biceps semitendi-

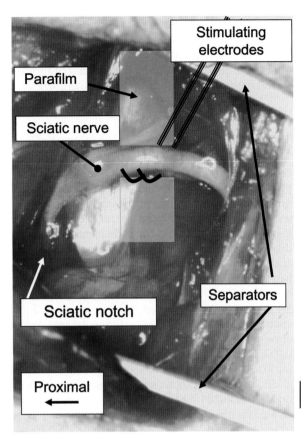

Neuropathic Pain Models, CRPS-I Neuropathy Model, Figure 1 The sciatic nerve is exposed at midthigh level and the surgical field is kept widely open with separators. A sheet of parafilm separates the nerve from neighboring tissues. A pair of stainless steel stimulating electrode hooks is inserted under the nerve.

nosus nerve or other thigh nerves. The sciatic nerve is then carefully separated from neighboring tissues (Fig. 1) and a sheet of parafilm is placed under the nerve. A pair of stainless steel stimulating electrode hooks is inserted under the nerve on both sides. The exposed nerves are covered with mineral oil (37°C) to prevent damage by drying. The side that receives the tetanic stimulation should alternate between individual animals, to minimize the bias of the experimenter when testing.

Tetanization

Electrical stimulation of intact nerves activates leg jerking that may pull the nerves by the hook electrodes. To prevent the injury, both hind paws, the pelvis and the tail are taped to the surgical board. The tetanization includes a train supramaximally activating C-fibers at a wind-up frequency, in addition to A-fibers (shock duration = 0.5 msec, frequency = 0.5 Hz, intensity = 5 mA, train duration = 10 min, n = 300 shocks). It is noteworthy that no sensory disorders were detected when activating A-fibers only (Vatine et al. 1998). Directly observing the surgical field with a dissecting microscope during the tetanization, the experimenter should verify that the nerves are not pulled by the electrodes. The contralateral sciatic nerve receives a sham stimulation at the same time as the ipsilateral nerve is tetanized. A separate control group of bilaterally sham-tetanized animals should optimally be included in every experiment.

Determination of Sensory Disorders

Tactile Allodynia

The animal is placed on top of a metal mesh floor, and covered with an opaque plastic cage. This enables the experimenter to introduce the filaments from underneath, preventing the animal from observing the stimulus approaching. Allodynia is assessed with a set of von Frey hairs. These hairs are nylon monofilaments of different diameters that exert defined levels of force when pressed against the plantar skin with sufficient force to cause the hair to bend. Each hair is indented 5 times at a frequency of about 2 Hz. The testing process begins by using the lowest hair in the set, ascending in the series until the animal responds at threshold by lifting the paw, withdrawing from the filament. The set typically ranges from 0.05 to 25 g and needs to be calibrated weekly using a top load balance. Other methods can be used (Bennett et al. 2002). Figure 2a shows that the average group withdrawal threshold (in g) of TSN rats is significantly decreased for a period of about 40 days, compared to sham tetanized rats.

Heat Hyperalgesia

Several methods can be used, including the Hargreaves instruments or a laser. For the latter method, a painful pulse of infrared energy is beamed from a CO_2 laser (120 msec, 5 W, 150 mCal and 1.5 mm in diameter) to the midplantar area of the hind paw from underneath, targeted by the visual aid of a He/Ne laser beam. This intensity causes sharp stinging pain to humans. Sham tetanized rats respond by a momentary paw flick or paw lift lasting less than a second. When stimulated at the TSN side, rats typically respond by immediate withdrawal followed by prolonged licking, paw lifting and claw pulling lasting on average up to 10 sec, depending on the post tetanization day and genetic and environmental variables. Figure 2b shows that the average group response duration (in sec) to stimulation on the TSN side significantly increased for a period of about 40 days, compared to the sham tetanized side.

Cold Hyperalgesia

A drop of acetone from a syringe is smeared on the plantar surface of the paw through the mesh floor of the testing chamber. As a control stimulus, a drop of tap water at room temperature is likewise applied, alternating between the acetone and water. The response time to each stimulus is recorded, subtracting the water from the acetone and the net result averaged for the group for each stimulated side. Increased response duration indicates cold hyperalgesia.

Mechanical Hyperalgesia

An increased response duration to pinprick applied from underneath to the midplantar area of the hind paw reflects hyperalgesia.

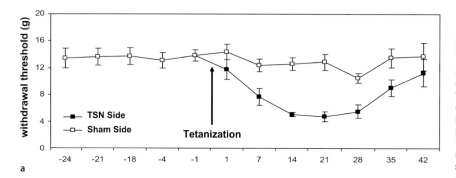

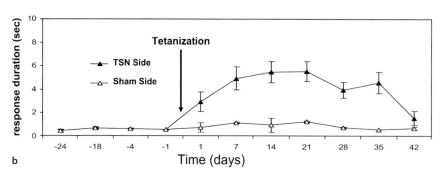

Neuropathic Pain Models, CRPS-I Neuropathy Model, Figure 2 (a) *Tactile allodynia.* Baseline tactile sensitivity was tested with a set of von Frey hairs. The withdrawal thresholds (g) to repetitive touch on the plantar side of both hind paws were tested on 5 sessions prior to nerve stimulation (days -24, -21, -18, -4 and -1). On day 0 the rats underwent unilateral tetanic stimulation of the sciatic nerve for 10 min. Tactile allodynia developed ipsilaterally, but not on the sham side. (b) *Heat hyperalgesia.* Baseline sensitivity to a noxious heat pulse from a CO_2 laser was tested on days -24, -18, -4 and -1 prior to nerve tetanization in intact rats. On day 0, the rats underwent unilateral tetanic stimulation of the sciatic nerve for 10 min. The significantly increased response duration (in sec) to the noxious stimulus, denotes heat hyperalgesia developed ipsilaterally on the tetanized sciatic side but not on the sham side.

Determination of Vasomotor Disorders

Since the temperature of the plantar skin area of conscious animals fluctuates, the paw temperature is measured 2 min after the rat is lightly anesthetized with an inhalation gas and 30 sec after the temperature stabilizes. Plantar hind paw temperature is recorded bilaterally using a remote infrared sensing thermometer, while the rat is lying on its ventral side in a room with an ambient temperature maintained at 21.0±0.5°C. Unilateral tetanic stimulation of the sciatic nerve causes a relative cooling of the tetanized hind paw.

Variables Potentially Affecting the TSN Model

Genetic Considerations

Work done in other animal models of chronic pain showed that the choice of animals might have a critical effect on the outcome, since genetic variation plays an important role. Some lines may develop robust neuropathic pain, while others may develop very weak, short lasting or even undetectable abnormalities. The original experiments on the TSN model were carried out on male Wistar rats (Vatine et al. 1998) and HA and LA rats (Vatine et al. 2001). The latter lines were selected from a stock of out bred rats (Sabra strain) based on contrasting levels of autotomy behavior following hind paw denervation by sciatic and saphenous transection (Devor and Raber 1990). Strain/line-specific differences in levels of allodynia, hyperalgesia and paw temperature abnormalities were noted. Previous reports showed differences in pain levels using the same model on animals from different vendors but also within vendors over time.

Environmental Considerations

The following environmental variables may dramatically affect the levels of neuropathic pain in animal models, including the TSN model. These include organismic variables like age, sex, hormonal status, prior experience with pain or drugs and seizures and variables relating to husbandry, like litter size and sex ratio, age at weaning, caging system, housing density, relation of cage mates, male-male fighting, handling frequency, bedding material, colony health status, prenatal (maternal) stress, maternal deprivation, ambient noise, ambient temperature and illumination. Also important are the circadian phase, circannual phase, meteorological factors, temperature, humidity, barometric pressure, experimenter, testing apparatus, restraint and drug injection method. Variables related to the stimulus can be no less important, including type of noxious stimulus, intensity, location, testing apparatus particularities, dependent measure, repeated testing, data transformation and experimenter proneness to bias. Investigators should exercise extreme care to control these as much as possible.

The TSN model shows similar types and durations of sensory disorders to those produced by intended nerve injury as in the CCI, PSL, SNL and PNI models. But lack of an overt nerve injury in the TSN model, combined with the appearance of mechanical allodynia, mechanical and thermal hyperalgesia and some vasomotor disturbances resembles the abnormalities of CRPS-I in humans (Stanton-Hicks et al. 1995; Baron et al. 1996), support the suggestion that this preparation can be used to study the mechanisms underlying CRPS-I.

References

1. Baik-Han EJ, Kim KJ Chung JM (1990) Prolonged ongoing discharges in sensory nerves as recorded in isolated nerve in the rat. J Neurosci Res 27:219–227
2. Baron R, Blumberg H, Jänig W (1996) Clinical characteristics of patients with complex regional pain syndrome in Germany with special emphasis on vasomotor function. In: Jänig W, Stanton-Hicks M (eds) Reflex Sympathetic Dystrophy: A Reappraisal. Progress in Pain Research and Management, vol 6. IASP Press, Seattle, pp 25–48
3. Bennett GJ, Chung JM, Seltzer Z (2002) Animal models for painful neuropathies. In: Crawley JN, Gerfen C, McKay R et al. (eds) Current Protocols in Neuroscience, Unit 9.14. Wiley Interscience, NY, pp 426–442
4. Blenk KH, Vogel C, Michaelis M et al. (1996). Prolonged injury discharge in unmyelinated nerve fibres following transection of the sural nerve in rats. Neurosci Lett 215:185–188
5. Devor M, Raber P (1990) Heritability of symptoms in an experimental model of neuropathic pain. Pain 42:51–68
6. Harden R, Bruehl S (2005) Diagnostic criteria: The statistical derivation of the four criterion factors. In: Wilson PR, Stanton-Hicks M, Harden RN (eds) CRPS: Current Diagnosis and Therapy. Seattle, IASP Press, pp 45-58
7. Jänig W, Baron R (2001) The value of animal models in research on CRPS. In: Harden RN, Baron R, Jänig W (eds) Complex Regional Pain Syndrome. Progress in Pain research and Management. IASP Press, Seattle, p75–85
8. Kissin I (2000) Preemptive analgesia: how can we make it work? In: Devor M, Rowbotham MC, Wiesenfeld-Hallin Z (eds) Proceedings of 9th World Congress of Pain. Progress in Pain research and Management. IASP Press, Seattle, p 973–985
9. Mendell LM (1996) Physiological properties of unmyelinated fiber projection to the spinal cord. Exp Neurol 16:316–332
10. Sackstein MJ, Ratner A, Seltzer Z (1996) Specific patterns of injury discharge are associated with receptor types in freshly injured sensory myelinated (A-) and unmyelinated (C-) fibers in rat. Abstracts of the 8th World Congress of the International Association for the Study of Pain. IASP Press, Vancouver, Seattle, p 11
11. Stanton-Hicks M, Janig W, Hassenbusch S et al. (1995) Reflex sympathetic dystrophy: changing concepts and taxonomy. Pain 63:127–133
12. Vatine JJ, Argov R, Seltzer Z (1998) Short electrical stimulation of c-fibers in rats produces thermal hyperalgesia lasting weeks. Neurosci Lett 246:125–8
13. Vatine JJ, Tsenter J, Raber P et al. (2001) A model of CRPS I produced by tetanic electrical stimulation of an intact sciatic nerve in the rat: Genetic and Dietary effects. In: Harden RN, Baron R, Jänig W (eds) Complex Regional Pain Syndrome. Progress in Pain research and Management, vol 22. IASP Press, Seattle, pp 53–74
14. Wall PD, Waxman S, Basbaum AI (1974) Ongoing activity in peripheral nerve: Injury discharge. Exp Neurol 45:576–589

Neuropathic Syndrome

▶ Lower Back Pain, Physical Examination

N

Neuropathic Pain of Central Origin

ROBERT P. YEZIERSKI
Department of Orthodontics, Comprehensive
Center for Pain Research and The McKnight Brain
Institute, University of Florida, Gainesville, FL,
USA
ryezierski@dental.ufl.edu

The recognition that disease or injury to the central nervous system (CNS) leads to conditions of chronic pain can be traced back to the 1800s. One of the first descriptions of symptoms, including pain, of a condition later to be called Wallenberg's syndrome was reported by Marchet (1811). A number of later reports further documented severe spontaneous pain associated with vascular lesions of the brainstem and ▶ thalamus. Shortly after the turn of the century Dejerine and colleagues presented their classic papers defining the term thalamic syndrome, which included disturbances of superficial and deep sensibility combined with severe, persistent, paroxysmal, often intolerable pain (Dejerine and Egger 1903; Dejerine and Roussy 1906).

Throughout the early 1900s, reports continued to document the condition of pain following injury or disease in the CNS. Head and Holmes (1911) described spontaneous pain associated with lesions of the spinal cord and brainstem. Several years later the term ▶ central pain was used by Holmes (1919). Although the terms "pain of central origin" and "pain due to lesions of the ▶ central nervous system" were used by a number of authors, it wasn't until 1938 that the definition of central pain was firmly established (Riddoch et al. 1938). By the late 1940s, the concept of central pain was firmly entrenched in the medical literature and was characterized by the presence of ▶ spontaneous pain, ▶ hyperpathia, ▶ hyperalgesia and exaggerated motor and autonomic reactions. Interestingly, many of these symptoms are commonly associated with pain following injury to peripheral nerves. Although comparisons have been made, there are sufficient differences pertaining to incidence, prevalence, time of onset and response to therapy to easily justify separate categories for pain with peripheral-central mechanisms (▶ neuropathic pain) *versus* pain associated solely with disease or injury in the CNS (central pain) (Bonica 1999).

Definition

The term central pain was initially considered synonymous with thalamic pain and for this reason most descriptions have placed both in the same category. Although thalamic lesions are considered to be one of the most common causes of central pain, it is also recognized that central pain can result from lesions anywhere along the neuraxis from the spinal cord to the cerebral cortex (Boivie 1989; Cassinari and Pagni 1969; White and Sweet 1969). In 1994 the International Association for the Study of Pain defined central pain as pain initiated or caused by a primary lesion or dysfunction within the CNS.

Epidemiology

Post-Stroke Pain

The incidence of central poststroke pain (CPSP) was estimated in 1991 to be approximately 750,000–1,000,000 patients worldwide (Bonica 1991). This calculation was based on a figure for poststroke pain of 1–2% as described by Bowsher (1993). Recent reports however, describe this condition as more frequent than previously thought. Andersen et al. (1995) reported that central pain affected 8% of 207 central post-stroke patients with 5% having moderate to severe pain. Kumral et al. (1995) described 9% of patients with thalamic hemorrhage experiencing central pain and CPSP was found in 25% of patients following brainstem infarcts with 49% having somatosensory deficits (MacGowan et al. 1997).

Spinal Cord Injury Pain

The prevalence of pain following ▶ spinal cord injury ranged from 34–94% (mean 69%) in ten studies published between 1947 and 1988 (Bonica 1991) and 36–96% (mean 66%) in studies from 1975–1991 (Yezierski 1996). In recent years the use of more comprehensive pain assessment strategies has raised the overall prevalence of SCI pain to 70–80% (Rintala al. 1998; Widerstrm-Noga et al. 1999). In a recent study Siddall and colleagues (1999) reported 91% of subjects with pain of any type 2 weeks after injury. The percentage decreased to 64% 6 months after injury.

Surgical Lesions

Surgical lesions involving spinal or supraspinal levels of the neuraxis intended to relieve pain can result in the onset of pain. Although Cassinari and Pagni (1969) reported that the incidence of ▶ dysesthesia and central pain following functional neurosurgery was 10–60%, more conservative numbers have been reported following cordotomy (3–5%) (Lipton 1989; White and Sweet 1969). The incidence of pain after medullary tractotomies was described by Bonica (1991) as 30%, with 70–100% of patients experiencing pain after open mesencephalic tractotomy and 5–10% after stereotaxic mesencephalic tractotomy (Bonica 1991).

Other Neurological Disorders

Other central neurological conditions are known to be associated with chronic pain. For example, multiple sclerosis (see ▶ Central Pain in Multiple Sclerosis) causes central pain in 29–75% of patients (Bonica 1991). Although systematic epidemiological studies for pain associated with other types of neurological disorders have not been carried out, other conditions associated with central pain include ▶ epilepsy (Young and Blume 1983), ▶ Parkinson's disease (Koller 1984) and Huntington's disease (Albin and Young 1988).

Clinical Characteristics of Central Pain

Spontaneous, persistent (usually burning), diffuse and / or intermittent, shooting, ice-like, aching, lancinating (with or without evoked elements) sensations, i.e. ▶ hyperesthesia, hyperalgesia, ▶ allodynia and hyperpathia, are characteristics commonly associated with central pain. Dysesthesias, hypersensitivity to somatic stimuli, enhancement of pain by emotion, radiation of sensation, summation of repeated stimuli and prolonged aftersensations have also been described as components of central pain (Pagni 1998).

Central pain can develop explosively and usually continues long after stimulation. Pain intensity can vary during the day, often due to external (e.g. touch, vibration, cold) and frequently emotional factors. Spontaneous pain occurs in a large number of cases, varying from uncomfortable ▶ paresthesias to aching, shooting, burning pain of great intensity. As a rule, spontaneous pains frequently vary in position and may change in character and are aggravated by somatic or visceral stimulation as well as by stress and emotion, especially anxiety. Auditory, visual, olfactory and visceral stimuli can provoke or exacerbate spontaneous pain.

▶ Quantitative sensory testing in a region where pain is localized generally shows a paradoxical lowering of sensitivity to painful stimuli, i.e. ▶ hypoalgesia. Within this hypoesthetic zone, a painful region is most closely correlated with a zone of decreased sensitivity to thermal stimuli (especially cold) with the intensity of pain being proportional to the loss of thermal sensibility. Studies indicate that there may be two recognizable subclasses of central pain, one signaled by loss of cold, warmth and sharpness sensibilities in which burning pain is experienced and one in which the ongoing pain is described as pricking, shooting and aching where tactile allodynia may predominate.

Temporal Profile

Central pain can start at any time after insult, although it usually begins within the first 3 months. The time of onset does not appear to depend on the location of the lesion and there are no definite correlations between the time of onset and associated pathology. In general, central pain following stroke develops gradually as sensory impairment and weakness improve. In cases involving ▶ ischemia or hematomyelia, pain has been reported to appear suddenly after insult. Shieff and Nashold (1987) described patients with pain from the time of initial insult as well as intervals varying up to 2 years. Andersen et al. (1995) described cases with pain 1 month after stroke, at 1–6 months and more than 6 months. In Tasker's series of patients (1991) central pain of brain origin was found to have a delayed onset in two-thirds of the cases, being less than 1 year in 50% of patients. Leijon described patients where pain began within 1 day after stroke, during the first month, after 3–12 months, or after 2–3 years (Leijon et al. 1989). Following spinal injury Siddall and colleagues (1999) reported ▶ at-level neuropathic pain 2 weeks after injury for 53% of subjects and reported ▶ below-level neuropathic pain for 41% of subjects within this same time period. Twenty-four percent of subjects reported neuropathic below level pain 3 months after injury while 18% reported this type of pain 6 months after injury.

Location of Pain

The distribution of central pain is nearly always related to the somatotopic organization of the brain structure damaged by trauma, disease or vascular insult. Because of this, it is possible to identify the location of the lesion in cases of dorsal horn and bulbar lesions, whereas it is difficult to distinguish between cortical, subcortical and thalamic lesions. In the majority of cases, central pain coincides with all or part of the territory in which sensory loss is clinically observed or revealed by quantitative sensory testing. Central pain is generally described as having a diffuse distribution; however, it can involve only one extremity or a portion of an extremity, e.g. hand or side of the face, and is therefore more accurately described as extensive rather than diffuse (Boivie 1994).

Bilateral girdle pain is found in cases of intramedullary tumors or ▶ syringomyelia. Spinal injury to the anterolateral quadrant is often referred to the opposite side of the body below the lesion. Dysesthesias from injury to the posterior column or dorsal column nuclei are typically located on the same side, below the lesion and may be unilateral or bilateral. Pain and dysesthesia due to vascular pontomedullary lesions usually have an alternating distribution, face on the lesion side and limbs and trunk contralateral to the lesion. This distribution is largely due to the fact that bulbar pain syndromes commonly result from the involvement of the posterior inferior communicating artery. Bulbar lesions can give rise to bilateral facial pain when the lesion impinges on the descending root of the trigeminal nerve on one side and on the crossed trigeminothalamic fibers coming from the other side. With pontine lesions, pain in the face is most often on the side opposite the lesion as is pain experienced in the limbs and trunk. Follow-

N

ing mesencephalopontine lesions, pain occurs on the side of the body contralateral to the lesion, typically with a hemiplegic distribution. Pain and dysesthesia due to thalamic lesions also have a hemiplegic distribution and affect the side of the body contralateral to the injured thalamus. Finally, cortical or subcortical lesions result in pain referred to the contralateral distal parts of the body (regions with the most extensive cortical representation).

Central Pain Syndromes

Thalamic Syndrome

The major features of thalamic lesions include severe, often intolerable, persistent or paroxysmal pain on the side opposite the lesion (Dejerine and Roussy 1906). This syndrome is characterized by slight hemiparesis, persistent superficial ► hemianesthesia, mild hemiataxia and astereognosis. While spontaneous pain may be absent in thalamic syndrome, excessive reaction to stimulation of affected body parts is consistent. Pain or discomfort can be evoked by almost any stimulus capable of arousing a sensation and is commonly characterized as intensely disagreeable and unbearable. Aside from spontaneous variations in pain intensity, fluctuations in pain are often exacerbated by environmental changes (especially cold), emotional stress (sudden fear, joy), strong taste or smell, loud noises, bright lights, movements, light touch, smoking and intellectual concentration. Pain is typically prolonged after stimulation and stimuli that normally have no obvious affective qualities may elicit a reaction in patients with thalamic syndrome. Patients with thalamic pain often have signs of autonomic impairment, e.g. vasoconstriction, abnormal sweating, edema (Bowsher et al. 1989).

Post-Stroke Pain

The most common cause of central pain is vascular abnormalities, e.g. ischemic lesions, with an etiology usually including supratentorial thrombotic stroke. Infarcts are not the only vascular disorders causing pain however, as subarachnoid hemorrhage is also associated with the onset of chronic pain (Bowsher et al. 1989; Tasker et al. 1991). The condition associated with thalamic lesions resulting from stroke was redefined by Leijon et al. (1989) as central poststroke pain (CPSP) and pain originating from extrathalamic lesions was referred to as pseudothalamic pain (Boivie 1994). CPSP is characterized by sensory deficits involving cold and warm stimuli, pinprick and to a lesser extent vibration, touch and 2-point discrimination (Verstergaard et al. 1995). There may be spontaneous or evoked sensory disturbances such as paresthesia, dysesthesias, hyperpathia and allodynia to cold.

The majority of patients with post-stroke pain also have more than one kind of pain which can be described as aching, pricking, shooting, stabbing, throbbing, squeezing, stinging, lancinating or lacerating. The pain may be superficial or deep and is typically constant, although it is not uncommon for patients to have intermittent pain and / or pain-free periods lasting a few hours. While there is evidence that a spinothalamic deficit is a necessary condition for post-stroke pain (Andersen et al. 1995; Dejerine and Roussy 1906), it is not a sufficient condition, since spinothalamic deficits are seen in more that 50% of stroke patients who show no signs of pain. However, there is evidence that the development of sensory loss and hyperalgesia in a body part deafferented by stroke is a necessary and sufficient condition for the development of central pain.

Pain Following Spinal Lesions

Painful sensations are a frequent and troublesome sequela of paraplegia and quadriplegia following partial or complete lesions of the spinal cord. Perhaps the most comprehensive classification of spinal injury pain was proposed by Donovon and colleagues who described five pain syndromes based not only on damage to the cord, but also secondary pathological changes, e.g. spinal nerve damage, overuse of muscles and compromised visceral function, that contribute to the onset of various post-injury pain syndromes (Donovon et al. 1982). This list was amended by Davidoff and Roth (1991) with the addition of lesional pain, reflex sympathetic dystrophy and limb pain secondary to compressive mononeuropathies. Recognizing the need for a simpler classification of different SCI pain syndromes Siddall et al. (2002) proposed a taxonomy consisting of two broad categories (a) nociceptive and (b) neuropathic; with subcategories of (1) musculoskeletal and (2) visceral in the nociceptive category and (1) above-level (2) at-level and (3) below-level in the neuropathic category.

Although there is no question concerning the diversity of different pain states associated with spinal injury, of greater importance is the practical impact of SCI pain on a patient's quality of life. Widerstrm-Noga et al. (1999) described 37% of patients rating SCI pain as very hard to deal with (rating of 7–10 on a scale of 0–10). In this study, a cluster analysis of different consequences of injury showed a strong interrelationship among ratings for pain, spasticity, abnormal sensations and sadness further supporting the negative impact of pain on quality of life following injury.

Imaging Central Pain

Central pain patients can be studied with neurometabolic techniques such as ► single photon emission computed tomography (SPECT), ► positron emission tomography (PET), ► functional magnetic resonance imaging (fMRI) and magnetic resonance spectroscopy (MRS), which together with pharmacologic dissection can be helpful in classifying patients according to the pathophysiological mechanism(s) responsible for producing central pain. Unfortunately, there are only a few neurometabolic studies demonstrating the involvement of thalamic and / or cortical hyperactivity associated with central pain (Cesaro et al. 1991; Pagni and Canavero 1995). In PET studies patients with chronic pain show a decrease in thalamic activity (Di Piero et al. 1994). These findings may be compatible with a decrease in thalamic neuronal activity between bursts observed in patients with central pain secondary to spinal injury. Cesaro et al. (1991) in a SPECT study using an amphetamine tracer found hyperactivity in the thalamus contralateral to the pain. In another SPECT study, Canavero et al. (1995) observed hypoactivity in the parietal cortex of a patient with central pain, suggesting that under normal conditions the cortex exerts an inhibitory control over thalamic structures. Consistent with this, four patients with central poststroke pain, two with hyperpathia, showed hyperactivity in the thalamus contralateral to the hyperpathic side. Defining the potential neural and biochemical changes associated with central pain is important in determining the mechanism underlying the onset and maintenance of injury induced pain. Pattany and colleagues (2002) used proton magnetic spectroscopy to study alterations in metabolites resulting from injury induced functional changes in thalamic nuclei following SCI. In patients with pain the concentrations of N-acetyl- and myo-inositol were different compared to those without pain, suggesting anatomical and functional changes in the region of thalamus.

Lesions Causing Central Pain

Central pain can be caused by any lesion of the nervous system that affects either completely, incompletely or subclinically the spinothalamocortical pathway. Based on an extensive review it was concluded that central pain can be due to lesions localized anywhere along this afferent sensory projection system, irrespective of whether cells or fibers are destroyed (Cassinari and Pagni 1969). Lesions leading to central pain are generally slow developing and the highest prevalence of central pain is reported in cases of lesions in the spinal cord, lower brainstem and ventroposterior part of the thalamus (Boivie 1992; Bonica 1991; Tasker 1991). The most severe injury to the spinal cord is a complete spinal transection following which patients can experience phantom limbs and complain of uncomfortable sensations such as tightness or pain. Severe pain may follow hemisection, but remote pains are rare, usually transient, lasting only a few days and are generally referred to the paralyzed, non-analgesic side of the body, but may be bilateral. Holmes attributed the spontaneous pain in these patients to local irritative effects of the lesion. Other lesions of the spinal cord causing central pain include (a) ▶ anterolateral cordotomy (b) dorsal root entry zone coagulation (see also ▶ Junctional DREZ Coagulation) and (c) cordectomy (Pagni 1998). Spinal contusion (see also ▶ Spinal Cord Injury Pain Model, Contusion Injury Model) is the most common cause of spinal injury pain. Spinal tumors can also lead to local pain in the case of extramedullary neoplasms. Local segmental pain with intramedullary tumors is infrequent, but does occur in some cases especially when the tumor arises in the posterior gray matter. One of the most pathologically destructive conditions giving rise to central pain is syringomyelia (Madsen et al. 1994). More than half of patients with delayed onset of central pain following SCI have syringomyelia and it appears that the syrinx rather than the original injury is responsible for the pain (Tasker et al. 1991).

The most common brainstem site for the development of central pain is the medulla. Central pain follows thrombosis of the posterior inferior cerebellar artery (PICA), described as Wallenberg's syndrome and includes analgesia in the trigeminal area on the side of the lesion, which results from damage to the descending nucleus of the fifth nerve and the crossed ascending fibers in the anterolateral system. Garcin (1968) described 56 cases of pain of bulbar origin *versus* 28 of pontine origin. In this analysis the order of frequency of different bulbar lesions included (a) vascular, especially thrombosis of PICA (b) syringobulbia (c) disseminated sclerosis and (d) pontobulbar tumors.

Bulbar spinothalamic tractotomy and bulbar trigeminal tractotomy (Sjoqvist's operation) are also associated with central pain. In general, pain from pontobulbar lesions whether spontaneous or evoked has the same general characteristics as pain of thalamic origin. Pontobulbar pain is aggravated by emotional disturbances and whether facial or remote is often chronic and resistant to ▶ pharmacotherapy. The striking fact that central pain of mesencephalic origin is uncommon may well be due to the absence of sensory nuclei in this region. Except for cases of pontomesencephalic tumors, central pain associated with pure midbrain lesions has not been reported, although surgical lesions following spinothalamic tractotomy at mesencephalic levels have been associated with central pain (Pagni 1998).

Within the thalamus three regions have been implicated in the onset of central pain (a) the ventroposterior part including the posterior and interior nuclei bordering this region (b) the medial-intralaminar region and (c) the reticular nucleus. Damage to the reticular nucleus is thought to release the medial and intralaminar nuclei from their normal control, thereby leading to pain and hypersensitivity (Mauguiere and Desmedt 1988).

N

Leijon et al. (1989) described nine patients with lesions in the ventroposterior thalamus that were associated with central pain. These reports are consistent with the contention that the posterior inferior part of the ventroposterior region is a critical location for lesions causing central pain. Thalamic pain is usually caused by ischemic and hemorrhagic vascular lesions, less frequently by tumors (Tovi et al. 1961), trauma (Riddoch 1938) or A-V malformations (Waltz and Ehni 1966). Lesions restricted to motor thalamus, medial thalamus and pulvinar do not appear to cause the onset of central pain.

Cortical lesions causing central pain are located primarily in the parietal cortex and perhaps the second sensory cortex where the ▶ spinothalamocortical projections are known to terminate. In general pain is rare after cerebral trauma (Marshall 1951), brain tumors, craniotomies or thalamotomies for movement disorders. Whether cortical lesions alone can cause central pain remains controversial, as in most reported cases there is damage to subcortical white matter (Breuer et al. 1981; Sandyk 1985). As a rule pain and hyperpathia occur when both sensory cortex and subcortical white matter are damaged, possibly due to the destruction of inhibitory corticothalamic fibers. Several reports have described patients with combined subcortical and cortical lesions leading to central pain, particularly with lesions in the insular region (Schmahmann and Leifer 1992). These lesions include those caused by infarcts, hematomas, meningiomas and trauma.

Pathophysiology of Central Pain

A number of theories have been proposed to explain central pain (a) irritation of spinothalamic and lemniscal pathways (Dejerine and Roussy 1906) (b) loss of inhibitory mechanisms controlling pain pathways (Head and Holmes 1911; Jeanmonod et al. 1994) (c) switching of importance from primary to secondary pain pathways (Cassinari and Pagni 1969; Tasker et al. 1980) (d) the emergence of abnormal spontaneous and hyperexcitable cells (secondary to ▶ deafferentation) at spinal and/or supraspinal levels of the neuraxis (Pagni 1989) and (e) irritation of the ▶ sympathetic nervous system. Since most central pain patients have abnormal temperature and pain sensibility, but near normal thresholds to touch, vibration and joint movement (Boivie et al. 1989), it was concluded that central pain occurs only after lesions of projections to the ventroposterior thalamic region (Pagni 1998). The fact that thalamic involvement is believed to be at the center of the mechanism responsible for the emergence of pain is underscored by the fact that anatomical and functional abnormalities are found at the termination site of pathways in this region of the brain. For this reason, central pain

is thought to result primarily from surgical or spontaneous lesions that invariably affect afferent sensory pathways. Therefore, it seems reasonable to conclude that lesions sparing fibers and cells of the spinothalamic and dorsal column system are unlikely to give rise to central pain. Cassinari and Pagni (1969) concluded that lesions of the spinothalamic system may give rise to dysesthesias, pain and hyperpathia, while lesions of the dorsal column system give rise to dysesthesias only and not pain. A critical question regarding the mechanism of central pain concerns the location of neurons responsible for this condition. Neurons within the ventroposterior nuclei have been shown to have increased spontaneous activity characterized by bursts of action potentials in the region of the nucleus representing the painful area of the body (Lenz et al. 1989). Bursting is believed to be a fundamental characteristic of central pain and is found in both lateral and medial thalamus. Whether this abnormal burst activity is due to loss of excitatory afferent drive on postsynaptic receptors or increased activity at ▶ NMDA receptors is not known. In patients with thalamic pain, spontaneous neuronal hyperactivity is also found in the mediodorsal, central lateral, central median and parafascicular nuclei (Rinaldi et al. 1991). In patients with central pain secondary to spinal transection, cells without receptive fields due to loss of sensory input show increased bursting, but decreased firing rates between bursts. These findings support the hypothesis that loss of STT input leads to hyperpolarization of these cells with resulting increased burst firing. Since some of these cells are involved in pain signaling pathways, this bursting activity may signal the sensation of pain. Although the hypothesis that abnormal neuronal activity in the ventroposterior thalamic region is important for the onset of central pain, one must reconcile the fact that in some patients this region is completely silent due to existing pathology. In fact some authors contend that this region is precisely where a thalamic lesion must be located in order to precipitate central pain (Leijon et al. 1989). Some thalamic lesions are thought to remove the inhibitory influence exerted by the reticular thalamic nucleus on medial and intralaminar nuclei, thereby releasing abnormal activity leading to pain and hypersensitivity (Cesaro et al. 1991).

The pathophysiology of central pain states may also involve the irritation of cells and fibers of sensory pathways and nuclei that develops at the lesion site. The resulting disruption of normal function is thought to lead to the development of an irritant focus (Dejerine and Roussy 1906; Livingston 1943). This hypothesis however, does not explain pain onset following complete destruction of sensory pathways and nuclei or pain due to section of fiber tracts. One explanation for the sudden disappearance of central pain after focal strokes in the subparietal white matter suggests that central pain is generated by a disturbance in the normal oscillatory mechanisms between cortex and thalamus (Canavero 1994).

Another proposed mechanism of central pain is based on the ▶ disinhibition hypothesis of Head and Holmes (Craig 2002). This thermosensory disinhibition theory proposes that central pain results from the disinhibition of pain resulting from imbalanced sensory integration caused by the loss of temperature sensation. This theory suggests that central pain is a thermoregulatory disorder that produces a thermal distress signal that is modulated by homoeostatic processing. At the heart of this proposal is the fact that loss of input from the lateral spinothalamic tract unmasks a homeostatic spinobulbothalamic pathway to the medial thalamus that is responsible for the development of central pain. This theory proposes that loss of activity in the thermosensory cortex in the dorsolateral mid / posterior insula disinhibits polymodal activation of the medial dorsal nucleus and anterior cingulate cortex, which produces burning pain.

Sympathetic Mechanisms

Sympathetic dysfunction is thought to play a role in central pain because signs of abnormal sympathetic activity, e.g. edema, decreased sweating, lowered skin temperature, changes in skin color and trophic skin changes have been described in many patients (Riddoch 1938). Unfortunately sympathetic blockade, which if effective would support a role of sympathetic mechanisms has shown contradictory results with only a small proportion of patients showing pain relief (Loh et al. 1981).

Spinal Injury: A Model of Central Pain

A major problem with the study of the pathophysiology and central mechanisms of central pain has been the lack of appropriate experimental models. In recent years this has been addressed with regard to the study of central pain following spinal injury with the development of models with pathological and behavioral characteristics consistent with the clinical profile of SCI (Christensen et al. 1996; Siddall et al. 1995; Vierck and Light 1999; Xu et al. 1992; Yezierski et al. 1998). One of the similarities between spinal cord injury and peripheral nerve and / or tissue damage is that both result in an increase in spinal levels of ▶ excitatory amino acids (EAAs). With this in mind, it is easy to envision a scenario whereby the physiological changes associated with SCI are linked to the same central injury cascade initiated by peripheral injury (Yezierski 1996). For example, the hypersensitivity of dorsal horn ▶ wide dynamic range neurons (WDR) described after ischemic and excitotoxic injury of the spinal cord reflects changes similar to those described following peripheral injury. The fact that these effects are blocked by the non-competitive NMDA receptor antagonist MK-801 implicates glutamate in these changes in functional properties. The abnormal bursting patterns and evoked responses of thalamic neurons in patients with SCI supports the hypothesis that the functional changes after spinal injury are not limited to the spinal cord, but as with peripheral injury can also be found at supraspinal sites.

An important factor contributing to changes in functional state of sensory neurons following SCI is believed to be the loss of spinal inhibitory mechanisms (Wiesenfeld-Hallin et al. 1994). Consistent with this is the reversal of the hypersensitivity of WDR neurons after transient spinal cord ischemia with the $GABA_b$ agonist baclofen (Hao et al. 1992). Spinal cord injury may therefore have multiple factors contributing to increased neuronal excitability (a) loss of inhibitory tone due to the loss of inhibitory interneurons and (b) changes in membrane properties due to prolonged periods of depolarization (central sensitization). Not to be ignored in this discussion are the physiological effects of deafferentation, which provide yet another factor capable of influencing the functional state of spinal and especially supraspinal neurons following SCI. Attempts to develop models of experimental thalamic pain have included placing electrolytic lesions in different thalamic nuclei (LaBuda et al. 2000; Saade et al. 1999) or excitotoxic lesions in the lateral thalamus (LaBuda et al. 2000) or giving cortical injections of picrotoxin (Oliveras and Montagne-Clavel 1996). All of these models produce heightened responses to peripheral stimuli, thereby providing support for their use in the study of central pain states.

Treatment of Central Pain

At present a long-term effective treatment for central pain is not available and for this reason the strategy for treatment is to try all available treatment modalities in order to systematically determine the best approach for an individual patient. The realistic goal of central pain treatment is to reduce the intensity of pain intensity to a tolerable level. With this in mind, it is commonly believed that opiate narcotics are totally ineffective in the treatment of central pain, although more systematic studies are needed. Central pain also responds poorly to most conventional analgesics, better to antidepressants, temporarily to sodium thiopental and propofol and may respond to i.v. pentothal. Agents that enhance norepinephrine and dopamine neurotransmission and anticonvulsants have some therapeutic efficacy. A review of controlled studies related to the efficacy of pharmacological treat-

N

ments of neuropathic pain is recommended for additional reading (Sindrup and Jensen 1999). In addition to pharmacotherapy a number of other strategies to treat central pain have been used. These include (1) ▶ peripheral nerve blocks (2) peripheral neurectomy and ▶ rhizotomy (3) ▶ sympathectomy and sympathetic blocks (4) ▶ spinal block and (5) stimulation and ablative procedures.

Conclusion

Chronic pain associated with injury or disease of the central nervous system represents a long-standing enigma that presents a significant challenge to the scientific and health care communities. As a condition that seems to depend on damage to the very substrate required for pain perception, it is one that has defied effective therapeutic intervention and continues to baffle those searching for an underlying mechanism. In spite of efforts to understand the pathophysiology and underlying etiology, there remain many unanswered questions. Parallels between chronic pain states resulting from injury or disease of peripheral and central substrates offers hope for the future. The fact that there are spontaneous and evoked components of central pain suggests multiple mechanisms underlying these and other divergent clinical findings as well as the varied temporal profile and location of pain in patients with different central lesions. The role of disinhibition, sensitization, denervation and other plastic changes in central sensory pathways remain to be addressed. Continued efforts to develop experimental models and strategies to study the human condition will hopefully lead to new insights into the progression of anatomical, chemical and functional changes from the site of injury to higher levels of the neuraxis along with the development of novel treatments.

References

1. Albin RL, Young AB (1988) Somatosensory phenomena in Huntington's disease. Mov Disord 3:343–346
2. Andersen G, Vestergaard K, Ingeman-Nielsen et al. (1995) Incidence of central post-stroke pain. Pain 61:187–193
3. Boivie J (1989) On central pain and central pain mechanisms. Pain 38:121–122
4. Boivie J (1992) Hyperalgesia and allodynia in patients with CNS lesions. In: Willis WD (ed) Hyperalgesia and Allodynia. Raven Press, New York, pp 363–373
5. Boivie J, Central Pain (1994) In: Wall PD, Melzack R (eds) Textbook of Pain. Churchill Livingston, New York, pp 871–902
6. Bonica JJ (1991) Semantic, epidemiologic and educational issues of central pain, In: Casey K (ed) Pain and Central Nervous System Disease: The Central Pain Syndromes. Raven Press, New York, pp 13–29
7. Bowsher D, Foy PM, Shaw MDM (1989) Central pain following subarachnoid hemorrhage. Br J Neurosurg 3:435–442
8. Breuer A, Cuervo H, Selkoe DJ (1981) Hyperpathia and sensory level due to parietal lobe arteriovenous malformation. Arch Neurol 38:722–724
9. Canavero S, Pagni CA, Castellano G et al. (1993) The role of cortex in central pain syndromes preliminary results of a long-term technetium-99 bexamethylpropyleneamineoxime single photon emission computed tomography study. Neurosurgery 32:185–191
10. Cassinari V, Pagni CA (1969) Central Pain. Harvard University Press, Cambridge
11. Cesaro P, Mann MW, Moretti JL et al. (1991) Central pain and thalamic hyperactivity. a single photon emission computerized tomographic study. Pain 47:329–336
12. Christensen MD, Everhart AW, Pickeman J et al. (1996) Mechanical and thermal allodynia in chronic central pain following spinal cord injury. Pain 68:97–107
13. Craig AD (2002) New and old thoughts on the mechanisms of spinal cord injury pain. In: Yezierski RP, Burchiel KJ (eds) Spinal Cord Injury Pain: Assessment, Mechanisms, Management, Progress in Pain Research and Management, vol 23. IASP Press, Seattle, pp 237–261
14. Davidoff G, Roth EJ (1991) Clinical characteristics of central (dysesthetic) pain in spinal cord injury patients. In: Casey KL (ed) Pain and Central Nervous System Disease: The Central Pain Syndromes. Raven Press, New York, pp 77–83
15. Dejerine J, Egger M (1903) Contribution a l'etude de la physiologie pathologique de l'incoordination motrice. Rev Neurol 11:397
16. Dejerine J, Roussy G (1906) Le syndrome thalamique. Rev Neurol (Paris) 14:521–532
17. Di Piero V, Ferracuti S, Sabatini U et al. (1994) A cerebral blood flow study on tonic pain activation in man. Pain 56:167–173
18. Donovan WH, Dimitrijevic MR, Dahm L et al. (1982) Neurophysiological approaches to chronic pain following spinal cord injury. Paraplegia 20:135–146
19. Garcin R (1968) Thalamic syndrome and pain of central origin. In: Soulairac A, Cahn J, Charpentier J (eds) Pain, London, Academic Press, pp 321–541
20. Hao JX, Xu XJ, Yu YX et al. (1992) Baclofen reverses the hypersensitivity of dorsal horn wide dynamic range neurons to mechanical stimulation after transient spinal cord ischemia: implications for a tonic GABAergic inhibitory control of myelinated fiber input. J Neurophysiol 68:392–396
21. Head H, Holmes G (1911) Sensory disturbances from cerebral lesions. Brain 34:102–254
22. Holmes G (1919) Pain of central origin. In: Osler W (ed) Contributions to medical and biological research. Paul B. Hoeber, New York, pp 235–246
23. Jeanmonod D, Magnin M, Morel A (1994) A thalamic concept of neurogenic pain. In: Gebhart GF, Hammond DL, Jensen TS (eds) Proceedings 7th World Congress of Pain, vol 2. IASP Press, Seattle, pp 767–787
24. Koller WC (1984) Sensory symptoms in Parkinson's disease. Neurology 34:957–959
25. Kumral E, Kocaer T, Ertübey NÖ et al. (1995) Thalamic hemorrhage. A prospective study of 100 patients. Stroke 26:964–970
26. LaBuda CJ, Cutler TD, Dougherty PM et al. (2000) Mechanical and thermal hypersensitivity develops following kainite lesion of the ventral posterior lateral thalamus in rats. Neurosci Lett 290:79–81
27. Leijon G, Boivie J, Johansson L (1989) Central post-stroke pain: neurological symptoms and pain characteristics. Pain 36:13–25
28. Lenz FA, Kwan HC, Dostrovsky JO et al. (1989) Characteristics of the bursting pattern of action potential that occurs in the thalamus of patients with central pain. Brain Res 496:357–360
29. Lenz FA, Seike M, Richardson RT et al. (1993) Thermal and pain sensations evoked by microstimulation in the area of human ventrocaudal nucleus. J Neurophysiol 70:200–212
30. Lipton S (1989) Percutaneous cordotomy. In: Wall PD, Melzack R (eds) Textbook of Pain, 2nd edn. Churchill Livingstone, Edinburgh, pp 832–839

pumps. Some of these procedures are characterized by the use of clinical or pharmacologic criteria to identify patients who are candidates for these surgeries. For example, successful pain relief by ► motor cortex stimulation may be predicted if patients have significant pain relief in response to infusions of intravenous thiamylal (Yamamoto et al. 1997). Additionally an intact motor system, but not an intact somatosensory system is required.

The most commonly used stimulation modality is ► spinal cord stimulation (SCS), which is indicated only when pharmacological or surgical treatment options for chronic pain have been exhausted. In general, good results, defined as >50% reduction in chronic pain are reported by 60–70% of the patients (Meyerson and Linderoth 2000; Simpson 1994). Large numbers of retrospective analyses have demonstrated reduction in chronic pain as demonstrated by reduction in analgesic medication and by patient satisfaction.

The most common indication is ► lumbo-sacral rhizopathy, a diagnosis that often represents a mix of nociceptive, neuropathic and inflammatory pain located in the lumbar region. This "low back pain" is less likely to respond to SCS than is the "radiating leg pain" that is amenable to SCS (North et al. 1993). The second common indication is pain following peripheral nerve injury or disease. Of the many forms of neuropathy due to metabolic disease, ► diabetic polyneuropathy is the most common and it is likely to respond to SCS. Pain due to peripheral nerve injury, which sometimes presents as ► complex regional pain syndrome (CPRS) is also considered to be a good indication (Kumar et al. 1997). A recent trend is the treatment of the pain of ► peripheral vascular disease or ► angina pectoris by SCS; this is performed at a small number of centers, mostly in Europe.

Stimulation of the thalamus or midbrain for treatment of chronic pain has a 50-year history. Patient selection for placement of DBS is an important part of current treatment using this modality (Hosobuchi 1986; Levy et al. 1987; Young and Rinaldi 1997). In many published studies, patients have been assessed by intravenous morphine infusion tests, based on the hypothesis that nociceptive but not neuropathic pain responds to opioids. Then ► nociceptive pain is treated by ► periaqueductal gray (PAG) stimulation and ► neuropathic pain is treated with thalamic stimulation.

There are a number of large studies demonstrating that DBS can be effective for both neuropathic and nociceptive pain (Hosobuchi 1986; Levy et al. 1987; Young and Rinaldi 1997). A meta-analysis of 13 studies (1114 patients) evaluating DBS for the treatment of chronic pain reported that 50% of all patients experienced long-term pain relief. Patients with nociceptive pain experienced a 60% long-term relief from pain with PAG stimulation, while those with neuropathic pain experienced a 56% long-term success rate with Vc stimulation.

Stimulation of motor cortex for relief of neuropathic pain of the head, neck or upper extremity has recently emerged as an option for patients with chronic pain. The first series, based on studies in animals was carried out by Tsubokawa who reviewed a series of 11 patients with central pain after putaminal or thalamic hemorrhage treated with ► motor cortex stimulation for 2 years with significant (> 80%) pain relief, sustained in 45% of patients (Tsubokawa et al. 1993). As in the stimulation modalities described above, there are well-described protocols for selection of patients to be treated by motor cortical stimulation. For example, Yamamoto and coworkers (Yamamoto et al. 1997) noted that successful pain relief by motor cortex stimulation could be predicted if patients responded by at least 40% pain relief to incremental infusions of intravenous thiamylal to a maximum dose of 250 mg, but not to morphine in doses of up to 18 gm given over 5 hours (Yamamoto et al. 1997). Additionally, motor cortex stimulation requires an intact motor system to be effective, but not an intact somatosensory system. Thus current stimulation procedures are based upon improved indications and demonstrated efficacy, as in the case of current ablative procedures.

It seems likely that the future will reflect the fact that the conditions we are now treating surgically are all ultimately dependent upon the chemical mechanisms. Surgical treatment of these conditions will be elaborations of the currently available drug pump technology. These therapies will involve selective intrathecal administration to of a drug or drugs (Rainov et al. 2001) specific to the condition being treated (Penn 2003; Weiss et al. 2003). Examples of such tailored drug administration are found in the case of patients with pain due to spasticity (Middleton et al. 1996) or with pain following spinal cord injury or of patients in opiate withdrawal (Lorenz et al. 2002). The possibility of anatomic as well as chemical approaches to surgical targets within the forebrain will shortly be a possibility. Intra-axial administration is becoming practical for delivery of drugs to anatomically or physiologically defined structures. The feasibility of this approach for selectively lesioning neurons but not axons by convection delivery through an intracerebral catheter has been demonstrated in primate models of Parkinson's disease (Lieberman et al. 1999). The intracerebral delivery of neurotransmitters or proteins, such as growth factors or neurotransmitters, into defined structures can also be accomplished by stereotactically placed catheters or by implantation of other novel drug delivery systems (Gouhier et al. 2002; Pappas et al. 1997).

N

These technologies promise to revolutionize the neurosurgical treatment of pain in the future.

Acknowledgement

Supported by grants to FAL from the NIH: NS39498 and NS40059.

References

1. Arner S (1991) Intravenous phentolamine test: diagnostic and prognostic use in reflex sympathetic dystrophy. Pain 46:17–22
2. Boivie J (1999) Central pain. In: Wall PD, Melzack R (eds) Textbook of pain. Churchill Livingstone, Edinburgh, pp 879–914
3. Chabal C, Jacobson L, Russell LC et al. (1992) Pain response to perineuromal injection of normal saline, epinephrine, and lidocaine in humans. Pain 49:9–12
4. Choi B, Rowbotham MC (1997) Effect of adrenergic receptor activation on post-herpetic neuralgia pain and sensory disturbances. Pain 69:55–63
5. Davis KD, Treede RD, Raja SN et al. (1991) Topical application of clonidine relieves hyperalgesia in patients with sympathetically maintained pain. Pain 47:309–317
6. Dreval ON (1993) Ultrasonic DREZ-operations for treatment of pain due to brachial plexus avulsion. Acta Neurochir 122:76–81
7. Drummond PD, Skipworth S, Finch PM (1996) alpha 1-adrenoceptors in normal and hyperalgesic human skin. Clin Sci 91:73–77
8. Friedman AH, Nashold BS Jr, Bronec PR (1988) Dorsal root entry zone lesions for the treatment of brachial plexus avulsion injuries: a follow-up study. Neurosurg 22:369–373
9. Galer BS, Rowbotham MC, Von Miller K et al. (1992) Treatment of inflammatory, neuropathic and sympathetically maintained pain in a patient with Sjögren's syndrome. Pain 50:205–208
10. Gildenberg PL (1973) General and psychological assessment of the pain patient. In: Tindall GT, Cooper PR, Barrow DL (eds) The practice of neurosurgery. Williams and Wilkins, Baltimore, pp 2987–2996
11. Gildenberg PL (1974) Percutaneous cervical cordotomy. Clin Neurosurg 21:246–256
12. Gildenberg PL, DeVaul RA (1985) The chronic pain patient. Evaluation and management. Karger, Basel
13. Gouhier C, Chalon S, Aubert-Pouessel A et al. (2002) Protection of dopaminergic nigrostriatal afferents by GDNF delivered by microspheres in a rodent model of Parkinson's disease. Synapse 44:124–131
14. Gybels JM, Sweet WH (1989) Neurosurgical treatment of persistent pain. Physiological and pathological mechanisms of human pain. Karger, Basel
15. Hassenbusch SJ (1998) Cingulotomy for cancer pain. In: Gildenberg PL, Tasker RR (eds) Stereotactic and functional neurosurgery. McGraw-Hill, New York, pp 1447–1451
16. Hosobuchi Y (1986) Subcortical electrical stimulation for control of intractable pain in humans. Report of 122 cases (1970–1984). J Neurosurg 64:543–553
17. Iskandar BJ, Nashold BS (1998) Spinal and trigeminal DREZ lesions. In: Gildenberg PL, Tasker RR (eds) Textbook of stereotactic and functional neurosurgery. McGraw-Hill, Health professional division, New York, pp 1573–1583
18. Jeanmonod D, Magnin M, Morel A (1993) Thalamus and neurogenic pain: physiological, anatomical and clinical data. Neurorep 4:475–478
19. Kumar K, Nath RK, Toth C (1997) Spinal cord stimulation is effective in the management of reflex sympathetic dystrophy. Neurosurg 40:503–508
20. Levy RM, Lamb S, Adams JE (1987) Treatment of Chronic Pain by Deep Brain Stimulation:Long Term Follow-up and Review of the Literature. Neurosurg 21:885–893
21. Lieberman DM, Corthesy ME, Cummins A et al. (1999) Reversal of experimental parkinsonism by using selective chemical ablation of the medial globus pallidus. J Neurosurg 90:928–934
22. Lorenz M, Hussein S, Verner L (2002) Continuous intraventricular clonidine infusion in controlled morphine withdrawal –case report. Pain 98:335–338
23. McLaughlin MR, Jannetta PJ, Clyde BL et al. (1999) Microvascular decompression of cranial nerves: lessons learned after 4400 operations. J Neurosurg 90:1–8
24. Meyerson BA, Linderoth B (2000) Spinal cord stimulation. In: Loeser JD (ed) Bonica's Management of Pain. Lippincott Williams & Wilkins, Philadelphia, pp 1857–1987
25. Middleton JW, Siddall PJ, Walker S et al. (1996) Intrathecal clonidine and baclofen in the management of spasticity and neuropathic pain following spinal cord injury: a case study. Arch Phys Med Rehabil 77:824–826
26. Nashold BS, El-Naggar AO (1992) Dorsal root entry zone (DREZ) lesioning. In: Rengachary SS, Wilkins RH (eds) Neurosurgical operative atlas. Williams & Wilkins, Baltimore, pp 9–24
27. Nashold BS, Jr., Wilson WP. Slaughter DG (1969) Stereotaxic midbrain lesions for central dysesthesia and phantom pain. Preliminary report. J Neurosurg 30:116–126
28. North RB, Kidd DH, Zahurak M et al. (1993) Spinal cord stimulation for chronic intractable pain: experience over two decades. J Neurosurg 32:384–395
29. Pappas GD, Lazorthes Y, Bes JC et al. (1997) Relief of intractable cancer pain by human chromaffin cell transplants: experience at two medical centers. Neurol Res 19:71–77
30. Patel A, Kassam A, Horowitz M et al. (2002) Microvascular decompression in the management of glossopharyngeal neuralgia: analysis of 217 cases. Neurosurg 50:705–710
31. Penn RD (2003) Intrathecal medication delivery. Neurosurg Clin N Am 14:381–387
32. Peters G, Nurmikko TJ (2002) Peripheral and gasserian ganglion-level procedures for the treatment of trigeminal neuralgia. Clin J Pain 18:28–34
33. Pollock BE, Phuong LK, Gorman DA et al. (2002) Stereotactic radiosurgery for idiopathic trigeminal neuralgia. J Neurosurg 97:347–353
34. Rainov NG, Heidecke V, Burkert W (2001) Long-term intrathecal infusion of drug combinations for chronic back and leg pain. J Pain Symptom Manage 22:862–871
35. Raja SN, Abatzis V, Frank S (1998) Role of α-adrenoceptors in neuroma pain in amputees. Amer Soc Anesthesiologists, Abstracts
36. Raja SN, Treede RD, Davis KD et al. (1991) Systemic alpha-adrenergic blockade with phentolamine: a diagnostic test for sympathetically maintained pain. Anesthesiology 74:691–698
37. Rath SA, Seitz K, Soliman N et al. (1997) DREZ coagulations for deafferentation pain related to spinal and peripheral nerve lesions: indication and results of 79 consecutive procedures. Stereotact Funct Neurosurg 68:161–167
38. Sampson JH, Cashman RE, Nashold BS Jr et al. (1995) Dorsal root entry zone lesions for intractable pain after trauma to the conus medullaris and cauda equina. J.Neurosurg. 82:28–34
39. Simpson BA (1994) Spinal cord stimulation. Pain Rev 1:199–230
40. Sindou M, Mertens P, Wael M (2001) Microsurgical DREZotomy for pain due to spinal cord and / or cauda equina injuries: long-term results in a series of 44 patients. Pain 92:159–171
41. Sindou MP (2002) Dorsal root entry zone lesions. In: Burchiel KJ (ed) Surgical management of pain. Thieme Medical Publishers, New York, pp 701–713
42. Singh B, Moodley J, Shaik AS et al. (2003) Sympathectomy for complex regional pain syndrome. J Vasc Surg 37:508–511
43. Spaic M, Markovic N, Tadic R (2002) Microsurgical DREZotomy for pain of spinal cord and Cauda equina injury origin: clinical characteristics of pain and implications for surgery in a series of 26 patients. Acta Neurochir 144:453–462

44. Tasker RR (1984) Deafferentation. In: Wall PD, Melzack R (eds) Textbook of pain. Churchill Livingstone, Edinburgh, London, Melbourne and New York, pp 119–132
45. Tasker RR (1988) Percutaneous Cordotomy: The Lateral High Cervical Technique. In: Schmidek HH, Sweet WH (eds) Operative Neurosurgical Techniques Indications, Methods, and Results. Saunders WB, Philadelphia, pp 1191–1205
46. Tasker RR, Dostrovsky JO (1989) Deafferentation and Central Pain. In: Wall PD, Melzack R (eds) Textbook of Pain. Churchill Livingstone, Edinburgh London Melbourne and New York, pp 154–180
47. Tasker RR, DeCarvalho GT, Dolan EJ (1992) Intractable pain of spinal cord origin: clinical features and implications for surgery. J Neurosurg 77:373–378
48. Thomas DG, Kitchen ND (1994) Long-term follow up of dorsal root entry zone lesions in brachial plexus avulsion. J Neurol Neurosurg Psychiatry 57:737–738
49. Tsubokawa T, Katayama Y, Yamamoto T et al. (1993) Chronic motor cortex stimulation in patients with thalamic pain. J Neurosurg 78:393–401
50. Weiss N, North RB, Ohara S et al. (2003) Attenuation of cerebellar tremor with implantation of an intrathecal baclofen pump: the role of gamma-aminobutyric acidergic pathways. Case report. J Neurosurg 99:768–771
51. White JC, Sweet WH (1969) Pain and the neurosurgeon: a forty year experience. Charles C Thomas, Springfield
52. Yamamoto T, Katayama Y, Hirayama T et al. (1997) Pharmacological classification of central post-stroke pain: comparison with the results of chronic motor cortex stimulation therapy. Pain 72:5–12
53. Young RF, Rinaldi PC (1997) Brain stimulation. In: North RB, Levy RM (eds) Neurosurgical management of pain. Springer-Verlag, New York, Berlin, Heidelberg, pp 283–301

Neurotransmitter

Definition

A neurotransmitter is a chemical released from a neuron into the synaptic cleft, which can trigger a response in the adjacent neuron on the opposite side of the cleft. Neurotransmitters may excite, inhibit, or otherwise influence the activity of cells.

▶ Cell Therapy in the Treatment of Central Pain
▶ Pain Treatment, Implantable Pumps for Drug Delivery
▶ Somatic Pain

Neurotransmitter Receptors

Definition

Neurotransmitter receptors are membrane proteins to which synaptic transmitters bind, leading to a physiological response in the postsynaptic cell. Neurotransmitter receptors can be ionotropic and cause a change in membrane conductance by an action on membrane channels or they can be metabotropic, causing activation of intracellular second messenger systems. Metabotropic receptors are often coupled to metabolic pathways through G proteins.

▶ Spinothalamic Tract Neurons, Role of Nitric Oxide

Neurotrophic Factors

Definition

Molecules by which tissues or cells affect nerve cell survival and/or phenotype.

▶ Wallerian Degeneration

Neurotrophic Support

Definition

Both developing and mature neurons require the ongoing delivery of a range of factors such as cytokines and neurotrophic factors to facilitate survival and maintain the phenotype of the neuron. This neurotrophic support may be supplied directly by cells of the target organ for the neuron, other cells adjacent to the axon or cell body or via the blood supply. Changes in neurotrophic support can induce changes in phenotype such as altered patterns of neurotransmitter synthesis or potential death of the neuron. Loss of neurotrophic support has been implicated in the etiology of diabetic neuropathy.

▶ Neuropathic Pain Model, Diabetic Neuropathy Model

Neurotrophin

Definition

Neurotrophins are dimeric growth factors that regulate development and maintenance of central and peripheral nervous systems. Members of this protein family include nerve growth factor (NGF), neurotrophin-3 (NT-3), brain-derived neurotrophic factor (BDNF), and neurotrophin-4/5 (NT-4/5). They regulate growth, survival, differentiation of neurons, and many other neuroectoderm tissues. All bind with low affinity to the p75 receptor and with high affinity to three structurally related receptor tyrosine kinases, named Trk receptors. NGF specifically activates TrkA, whereas BDNF and NT-4/5 specifically activate TrkB. NT-3 primarily activates TrkC, but recognizes both TrkA and TrkB to a lesser extent. Trk receptors consist of an extracellular ligand-binding domain, a single transmembrane region and an intracellular tyrosine kinase (TK) domain. Ligand binding to Trk receptors results in dimerization of

N

receptor molecules followed by autophosphorylation of their cytoplasmic tyrosine residues.

► Cell Therapy in the Treatment of Central Pain
► Congenital Insensitivity to Pain with Anhidrosis
► Nerve Growth Factor, Sensitizing Action on Nociceptors
► NGF, Regulation during Inflammation
► Spinal Cord Nociception, Neurotrophins
► Trigeminal Brainstem Nuclear Complex, Immunohistochemistry and Neurochemistry

Neurotrophin Receptors

Definition

Two types of neurotrophin receptors are involved in retrograde neurotrophin signaling, the low affinity p75 (NTR) receptor, also referred to as Nerve Growth Factor Receptor (NGFR), which binds with all the above neurotrophins, and the high affinity tyrosine kinase (Trk) receptors. The tropomyosin receptor kinase TrkA (NTRK1) is the signaling receptor for NGF, TrkB (NTRK2) is the signaling receptor for BDNF and NT-4/-5, TrkC (NTRK3) is the primary receptor for NT-3, although NT-3 also binds to TrkA and TrkB, yet with lower affinity.

► Congenital Insensitivity to Pain with Anhidrosis

References

1. Patapoutian A, Reichardt LF (2001) Trk receptors: mediators of neurotrophin action. Curr Opin Neurobiol 11:272–280
2. Bibel M, Barde YA (2000) Neurotrophins: key regulators of cell fate and cell shape in the vertebrate nervous system. Genes Dev 14:2919-2937
3. Indo Y (2002) Genetics of congenital insensitivity to pain with anhidrosis (CIPA) or hereditary sensory and autonomic neuropathy type IV. Clinical, biological and molecular aspects of mutations in TRKA (NTRK1) gene encoding the receptor tyrosine kinase for nerve growth factor. Clin Auton Res 12 Suppl 1:I20-I32

Neurotrophins in Spinal Cord Nociception

► Spinal Cord Nociception, Neurotrophins

Neutral Cell (RVM)

Definition

Third class of RVM neurons, defined by the lack of reflex-related activity. Neutral cells do not respond to mu-opioid agonists. RVM serotonergic neurons behave as neutral cells, although some authors prefer to consider serotonergic cells as a fourth class of RVM neurons, distinct from neutral cells. Neutral cells as

defined *in vivo* are likely be a subset of primary cells defined *in vitro*.

► Opiates, Rostral Ventromedial Medulla and Descending Control

Neutral Medical Examination

► Independent Medical Examinations

Neutrophils in Inflammatory Pain

RAINER AMANN
Medical University Graz, Graz, Austria
rainer.amann@meduni-graz.at

Definition

The initial stages of the inflammatory response are characterized by the vascular reaction and the local biosynthesis of mediators that sensitize primary afferent neurons. Thereafter, immune cells are attracted to the site of injury, initiating processes that lead to either tissue repair or destruction. Immigration of polymorphonuclear neutrophil granulocytes (PMN), already in the early cellular phase of inflammation, serves to destroy infectious agents and/or cellular debris. In addition, PMNs are sources of various mediators that can affect, directly or indirectly, the sensitivity of primary afferent neurons.

Characteristics

Tissue injury triggers the release of a large number of mediators from neuronal and non-neuronal resident cells, resulting in microvascular changes and increased afferent neuronal sensitivity, effects that provide the basis of key symptoms of inflammation, redness, edema, and pain. Arachidonic acid metabolites are central in this initial response. Conversion of arachidonic acid through the cyclooxygenase pathway leads to enhanced biosynthesis of ► prostanoids, which increase tissue perfusion and sensitize primary afferent neurons. Pharmacological inhibition of cyclooxygenase activity by ► NSAIDs, Survey (NSAIDs) is, therefore, effectively used to alleviate inflammatory pain and edema.

In addition to mediators that serve the initial vascular and neuronal defense reaction, compounds with chemotactic activity are produced by injured tissue. This leads to immigration of PMN to the site of injury, a process that involves a cascade of events, primarily consisting of leukocyte rolling along the endothelial layer, adherence to, and transmigration through the endothelium and vascular wall. This process is under control of various

▶ cytokines, ▶ chemoattractants, and ▶ chemokines (Wagner and Roth 2000).

PMNs can produce a wide range of mediators (e.g. arachidonic acid metabolites, various cytokines, proteases, reactive oxygen intermediaries, and nitric oxide) (Sampson 2000) that serve to initiate the immune response and destroy infectious agents and/or cellular debris. It is evident that, in chronic inflammatory disease, the severity of the cellular inflammatory response and accompanying tissue destruction correlates with inflammatory pain. This provides a rationale for the use of ▶ disease modifying anti-rheumatic drugs (DMARDs), which primarily target immune cell function, in diseases such as rheumatoid arthritis. However, there are reasons to assume that PMNs are involved in the development of inflammatory pain at earlier stages of inflammation, a concept that is primarily based on a number of studies by Levine and associates (Levine et al. 1984; Levine et al. 1986).

With regard to the role of PMN in inflammatory pain, one chemoattractant is of particular interest, ▶ leukotriene (LT) B_4, which has been shown to be present in inflammatory exudates in human inflammatory diseases such as ▶ rheumatoid arthritis (Davidson et al. 1983). LTB_4 is a product of the 5-lipoxygenase pathway of arachidonic acid metabolism; it is a potent chemoattractant for neutrophils, which, in turn, are also major sources of LTB_4. In experimental inflammation, it has been shown that LTB_4 produces ▶ hyperalgesia, which is not prevented by ▶ Cyclooxygenases inhibitors (Levine et al. 1984). In the presence of LTB_4, PMNs release a 15-lipoxygenase product of arachidonic acid, (8R, 15S)-Dihydroxyeicosa-(5E-9,11,13Z)-tetraenoic acid [8R,15S)-diHETE], which directly sensitizes ▶ primary afferent neurons (Levine et al. 1986). Since it has been shown that the hyperalgesic activity of exogenous LTB_4 is dependent on the presence of PMN (Levine et al. 1984), it seems likely that the final mediator of LTB_4-induced hyperalgesia is a product of PMN 15-lipoxygenase. According to this concept, PMNs would promote inflammatory hyperalgesia in a dual fashion, as sources and as targets of LTB_4.

In view of these experimental data, inhibition of LTB_4 biosynthesis would be expected to show analgesic effects. In fact, there are studies showing analgesic effects of 5-lipoxygenase inhibition in some models of experimental inflammation. Thus, it has been shown in rodents, that ▶ nerve growth factor (NGF) elicits ▶ thermal hyperalgesia, which is dependent on PMNs and is blocked by inhibition of the 5-lipoxygenase (Amann et al. 1996, Bennett et al. 1998, Schuligoi 1988). The demonstration of PMN-dependent hyperalgesia induced by NGF may be important, because NGF has been shown to contribute to inflammatory hyperalgesia and bronchial hyperreflexia (Renz 2001). However, the studies mentioned above were conducted using exogenous NGF, and, therefore, did not provide

direct evidence for the presence of a PMN-dependent, 5-lipoxygenase mediated mechanism in inflammatory pain.

In a more recent study, Cunha et al. (2003) have shown that mechanical hypersensitivity, induced by antigen challenge in rats immunized with ovalbumin, is suppressed by inhibition of 5-lipoxygenase and a LTB_4 receptor antagonist. Although in this study the participation of PMNs as sources of LTB_4 was not addressed, the observation that, at later stages of the inflammatory response, LTB_4 was the principal mediator of hyperalgesia points to the involvement of PMNs.

In contrast to these experimental studies in rodents, which are suggestive of involvement of PMN 5-lipoxygenase in inflammatory hyperalgesia, there is no firm evidence that 5-lipoxygenase inhibition can attenuate inflammatory pain in patients, although selective inhibitors of 5-lipoxygenase have been available for a number of years. Therefore, the pathophysiological relevance of PMN lipoxygenases as sources of hyperalgesia-inducing factors in inflammatory pain remains doubtful.

In recent years a novel concept has emerged, suggesting that PMNs play an important role in the generation of lipoxins, lipid mediators that promote the resolution of the inflammatory process (Levy et al. 2001). According to this concept, 15-lipoxygenase products of arachidonic acid [15S-hydroxyperoxyeicosatetraenoic acid (15S-H(p)ETE), or the reduced alcohol form 15S-hydroxyeicosatetraenoic acid (15S-HETE)], derived from epithelial cells, eosinophils or monocytes serve as substrates for PMN 5-lipoxygenase, which results in the generation of lipoxin $(LX)A_4$ and LXB_4. During the synthesis of lipoxins, leukotriene synthesis is blocked at the 5-lipoxygenase level in PMN, resulting in an inverse relationship of lipoxin and LT biosynthesis. An alternative pathway involves an interaction between PMN and platelets, which convert PMN 5-lipoxygenase-derived LTA_2 via 12-lipoxygenase to LXA_4 and LXB_4 (Serhan 1997).

Lipoxins contribute to the resolution of inflammation by inhibiting neutrophil chemotaxis, and transmigration (Takano et al. 1997), stimulation of macrophage clearance of apoptotic PMN from an inflammatory focus (Godson et al. 2000), inhibition of cell proliferation, and modulation of metalloproteinase activity (Sodin-Semrl et al. 2000). Although there are no studies on the possible effects of lipoxins on the nociceptive threshold of primary afferent neurons, it can be expected that, by attenuating the inflammatory response, they can indirectly reduce inflammatory pain.

Since PMN 5-lipoxygenase is a key enzyme in the biosynthesis of lipoxins, pharmacological inhibition of 5-lipoxygenase in PMNs may in fact counteract processes that are involved in the resolution of inflammation. Theoretically, this may also be one possible explanation for the absence of obvious analgesic ef-

N

fects of 5-lipoxygenase inhibition in most types of inflammation.

References

1. Amann R, Schuligoi R, Lanz I, Peskar BA (1996) Effect of a 5-Lipoxygenase Inhibitor on Nerve Growth Factor-Induced Thermal Hyperalgesia in the Rat. Eur J Pharmacol 306:89–91
2. Bennett G, al-Rashed S, Hoult JR, Brain SD (1998) Nerve Growth Factor Induced Hyperalgesia in the Rat Hind Paw is Dependent on Circulating Neutrophils. Pain 77:315–322
3. Cunha JM, Sachs D, Canetti CA, Poole S, Ferreira SH, Cunha FQ (2003) The Critical Role of Leukotriene B4 in Antigen-Induced Mechanical Hyperalgesia in Immunised Rats. Br J Pharmacol 139:1135–1145
4. Davidson EM, Rae SA, Smith MJ (1983) Leukotriene B4, A Mediator of Inflammation Present in Synovial Fluid in Rheumatoid Arthritis. Ann Rheum Dis 42:677–679
5. Godson C, Mitchell S, Harvey K, Petasis NA, Hogg N, Brady HR (2000) Cutting Edge: Lipoxins Rapidly Stimulate Nonphlogistic Phagocytosis of Apoptotic Neutrophils by Monocyte-Derived Macrophages. J Immunol 164:1663–1667
6. Levine JD, Lam D, Taiwo YO, Donatoni P, Goetzl EJ (1986) Hyperalgesic Properties of 15-Lipoxygenase Products of Arachidonic Acid. Proc Natl Acad Sci USA 83:5331–5334
7. Levine JD, Lau W, Kwiat G, Goetzl EJ (1984) Leukotriene B4 Produces Hyperalgesia that is Dependent on Polymorphonuclear Leukocytes. Science 225:743–745
8. Levy BD, Clish CB, Schmidt B, Gronert K, Serhan CN. (2001) Lipid Mediator Class Switching During Acute Inflammation: Signals in Resolution. Nat Immunol 2 612–619
9. Renz H (2001) The Role of Neurotrophins in Bronchial Asthma. Eur. J. Pharmacol.429:231–237
10. Sampson AP (2000) The Role of Eosinophils and Neutrophils in Inflammation Clin Exp Allergy 30 Suppl 1:22–27
11. Schuligoi R (1998) Effect of Colchicine on Nerve Growth Factor-Induced Leukocyte Accumulation and Thermal Hyperalgesia in the Rat. Naunyn Schmiedebergs Arch Pharmacol 358:264–269
12. Serhan CN (1997) Lipoxins and Novel Aspirin-Triggered 15-Epi-Lipoxins (ATL): A Jungle of Cell-Cell Interactions or a Therapeutic Opportunity? Prostaglandins 53:107–37
13. Sodin-Semrl S, Taddeo B, Tseng D, Varga J, Fiore S (2000) Lipoxin A4 Inhibits IL-1 Beta-Induced IL-6, IL-8, and Matrix Metalloproteinase-3 Production in Human Synovial Fibroblasts and Enhances Synthesis of Tissue Inhibitors of Metalloproteinases. J Immunol 164:2660–2666
14. Takano T, Fiore S, Maddox JF, Brady HR, Petasis NA, Serhan CN (1997) Aspirin-Triggered 15-Epi-Lipoxin A4 (LXA4) and LXA4 Stable Analogues are Potent Inhibitors of Acute Inflammation: Evidence for Anti-Inflammatory Receptors. J Exp Med 185:1693–1704
15. Wagner JG, Roth RA (2000) Neutrophil Migration Mechanisms, with an Emphasis on the Pulmonary Vasculature. Pharmacol Rev 52:349–374

New Daily Persistent Headache

TODD D. ROZEN
Michigan Head-Pain and Neurological Institute, Ann Arbor, MI, USA
tdrozmigraine@yahoo.com

Synonyms

Chronic Daily Headache; Daily Persistent Headache

Definition

New daily persistent headache (NDPH) is a form of chronic daily headache along with ▶ chronic migraine, ▶ chronic tension-type headache and ▶ hemicrania continua. The defining symptom of NDPH is a daily headache from onset, typically in an individual with minimal or no prior headache history. The headache will start one day and in most instances continue as daily unremitting pain.

Characteristics

New daily persistent headache (NDPH) was first described by Vanast in 1986 as a benign form of chronic daily headache that improved without therapy. Very little is known about this syndrome and only recently has it been recognized as a distinct entity by headache specialists. It is unique in that the headache begins daily from onset, typically in a patient with no prior headache history and can continue for years, without any sign of alleviation despite aggressive treatment. Proposed diagnostic criteria for NDPH are listed below. It appears that there maybe two subtypes of NDPH, a self-limited form, which typically goes away within several months without any therapy and never presents to a physician's office and a refractory form, which is basically resistant to aggressive outpatient and inpatient treatment schemes.

Proposed Criteria for New Daily Persistent Headache (Rozen)

A Daily head pain for >2 months

B Average headache duration of >4 h per day (if untreated). Frequently constant pain without medication

C No history of migraine or TTH that is increasing in frequency in association with a new daily persistent headache

D Prior history of any headache disorder is uncommon

1. Acute onset of constant unremitting headache (daily from onset)
2. At least 2 of the following pain characteristics
3. Pulsating or pressing/tightening quality
4. Moderate or severe pain intensity
5. Bilateral pain location
6. Aggravation by walking upstairs or similar routine physical activity

E At least one of the following

1. Nausea and / or vomiting
2. Photophobia or phonophobia

F Does not fit the criteria for hemicrania continua

There are only two case series in the literature dedicated to describing the clinical characteristics of NDPH, the largest completed by Li and Rozen in 2002. A retrospective chart review was carried out using a computerized database of patients from the Jefferson Headache Center (a large university based headache specialty unit). All patients who were seen at Jefferson between August 1997 and May 2000 and who met the criteria for NDPH were included. Unique to NDPH is that most patients are able to pinpoint the exact date when their headache started. Headache onset occurs in relation to an infection or flu-like illness in 30%, extracranial surgery (e.g. hysterectomy) in 12% and a stressful life event in 12%. Over one-third of patients cannot identify any precipitating event. NDPH had a female predominance (female to male ratio: 2.5:1). The peak age of onset of NDPH in women is in the second and third decades of life, while the largest incidence of NDPH in men comes in the third to fifth decade. A prior headache history is found in about 40% of patients, with episodic ► migraine being the most common type. In the majority of patients, the pain of NDPH is continuous throughout the day with no pain-free time noted. Baseline average pain intensity is moderate in most, while some patients experience severe pain all of the time. Headache location is typically bilateral and pain can occur anywhere on the head. Headache quality is usually throbbing or pressure-like. With regard to associated symptoms, nausea, photophobia, phonophobia or lightheadedness occur in more than 50% of patients. ► Aura-type symptoms can also occur but are uncommon. A family history of headache is documented in 30% of patients. In almost all instances, general and neurological examinations are normal. Neuroimaging and lumbar puncture are almost always negative studies.

Epidemiology

Even though NDPH has probably been around for centuries, it has only recently been diagnosed as an entity separate from chronic tension-type headache, hemicrania continua and chronic migraine. The prevalence of CDH from population-based studies in the United States, Asia and Europe is about 4% (Silberstein et al. 2001). In those epidemiologic investigations, primary CDH types are sometimes not mentioned in the analysis and NDPH is rarely stratified out from the data. Several studies have documented the prevalence of NDPH; Castillo et al. (1999) looked at the prevalence of CDH in 2,252 subjects in Spain and found that 4.7% of the population has CDH, of which 0.1% had NDPH. Bigal et al. (2002) noted that 10.8% of 638 patients with CDH in a headache specialty clinic had NDPH, while Koenig et al. (2002) found that 13% of a pediatric CDH population, surveyed from selected pediatric headache specialty clinics, had NDPH.

Etiology of NDPH

As at least a third of NDPH patients have a cold or flu-like illness when their headaches begin, an infectious etiology for NDPH has been hypothesized. Some

authors have linked Epstein-Barr virus (EBV) infection with NDPH. Diaz-Mitoma et al. (1987) identified oropharyngeal secretions of EBV in 20 of 32 patients with NDPH compared with 4 of 32 age-and gender-matched controls. A history of mononucleosis was identified in 12 of the patients with NDPH. Almost 85% of the NDPH patients were found to have an active EBV infection as opposed to 8 in the control group. The authors hypothesized that activation of a latent EBV infection may have been the trigger for the development of a chronic daily headache from onset. Santoni and Santoni-Williams (1993) demonstrated evidence of systemic infection in 108 patients with NDPH including *Salmonella*, adenovirus, toxoplasmosis, herpes zoster, EBV and *E.coli* urinary tract infections. How an infection can induce NDPH is unknown. One may hypothesize an activated immune response to a new or reactivated viral or bacterial infection leading to an autoimmune-triggered headache, possibly by setting up a state of continuous neurogenic inflammation. The virus itself could in some way activate and damage the trigeminal system leading to daily pain.

Differential Diagnosis of NDPH

A diagnosis of primary NDPH is made only after secondary causes have been ruled out. Two disorders in particular can mimic the presentation of NDPH, ► spontaneous cerebrospinal fluid leak (CSF) and cerebral venous sinus thrombosis. Spontaneous CSF leaks typically present as a daily headache with a positional component (headache improved in a supine position, worsens in a sitting or standing position). However, the longer a patient suffers with a CSF leak-induced headache the less pronounced the positional component becomes. Thus if a patient is seen in a physician's office months to years after onset of a CSF leak, that patient may not even divulge a history of positional headaches, as that trigger may not have been evident to the patient for a very long time. In this setting, the CSF leak headache may mimic a primary NDPH picture.

In the patient who presents with new daily headache and is subsequently found to have cerebral venous thrombosis, in many instances none of the typical features recognized for cerebral venous thrombosis are present, including no history of new onset seizures, focal neurological deficits, change of consciousness, cranial nerve palsies or bilateral cortical signs and no evidence of papilledema on fundoscopic examination. The patient will just have a new headache that is daily from onset.

The evaluation of an NDPH patient should include neuroimaging, specifically brain MRI without and with gadolinium and MR venography (MRV). Gadolinium must be given to look for the ► pachymeningeal enhancement associated with spontaneous CSF leaks while MRV will help make the diagnosis of cerebral venous thrombosis. If a new daily headache begins after the age of 50 years, then giant cell arteritis must

N

be ruled-out. Headache is the most common reported symptom of the disorder occurring in up to 90% of individuals.

Treatment

NDPH can continue for years to decades after onset and be extremely disabling to the patient. Even with aggressive treatment many NDPH patients do not improve. In many circles, primary NDPH is felt to be the most treatment refractory of all headache disorders. Many patients with NDPH will fail every possible class of abortive and preventive medications without any sign of pain relief. Recently Rozen (2002) presented five patient cases in which successful treatment of NDPH was obtained with gabapentin or topiramate. This was the first ever published study recognizing a positive treatment response for the refractory form of NDPH (the self-limited form will alleviate without any therapy).

▶ Chronic Daily Headache in Children

References

1. Bigal ME, Sheftell FD, Rapoport AM et al. (2002) Chronic daily headache in a tertiary care population: correlation between the international headache society diagnostic criteria and proposed revisions of criteria for chronic daily headache. Cephalalgia 22:432–438
2. Castillo J, Munoz P, Guitera V et al. (1999) Epidemiology of chronic daily headache in the general population. Headache 38:497–506
3. Diaz-Mitoma F, Vanast WJ, Tyrell DL (1987) Increased frequency of Epstein-Barr virus excretion in patients with new daily persistent headaches. Lancet 1:411–415
4. Koenig MA, Gladstein J, McCarter RJ et al. and the pediatric committee of the American Headache Society (2002) Chronic daily headache in children and adolescents presenting to tertiary headache clinics. Headache 42:491–500
5. Li D, Rozen TD (2002) The Clinical Characteristics of New Daily Persistent Headache. Cephalalgia 22:66–69
6. Rozen TD (2002) Successful Treatment of New Daily Persistent Headache with Gabapentin and Topiramate. Headache 42:433
7. Santoni JR, Santoni-Williams CJ (1993) Headache and painful lymphadenopathy in extracranial or systemic infection: etiology of new daily persistent headaches. Intern Med 32:530–533
8. Silberstein SD, Lipton RB (2001) Chronic daily headache, including transformed migraine, chronic tension-type headache and medication overuse. In: Silberstein SD, Lipton RB, Dalessio DJ (eds) Wolff's Headache and other head pain. Oxford University Press, Oxford, pp 247–282
9. Vanast WJ (1986) New daily persistent headaches: Definition of a benign syndrome. Headache 26:317

Newborn

Synonym

Neonate

Definition

Newborn infant who is less than 1 month postnatal age.
▶ Pain Assessment in Neonates

NGF

▶ Nerve Growth Factor

NGF -/- Mice

Definition

Mice that lack a functional gene encoding nerve growth factor, i.e. NGF knockout mice.
▶ Nerve Growth Factor Overexpressing Mice as Models of Inflammatory Pain

NGF-OE mice

▶ Nerve Growth Factor Overexpressing Mice as Models of Inflammatory Pain

NGF, Regulation during Inflammation

RAINER AMANN
Medical University Graz, Graz, Austria
rainer.amann@meduni-graz.at

Definition

In inflamed tissue, there is increased expression of ▶ nerve growth factor (NGF), which affects afferent neuron function, and contributes to the development and resolution of the inflammatory process. Pharmacological tools that can modify inflammation-induced NGF biosynthesis are, therefore, of potential therapeutic value.

Characteristics

Nerve growth factor (NGF) belongs to a family of structurally related ▶ neurotrophins. During inflammation, there is a rapid increase in local NGF biosynthesis. The local increase in NGF in inflamed tissues leads to changes in the phenotype of a subset of ▶ primary afferent neurons, with consequences for the transmission of noxious afferent input (Mendell et al. 1999).

In addition to its neurotrophic properties, NGF has been shown to affect immune cell function (Aloe et al. 1999). Direct neuronal effects (Mendell et al. 1999), as well as effects on immune cells (Bennett et al. 1998; Schuligoi 1998), seem to contribute to NGF-induced sensitization of primary afferent neurons, which manifests itself as inflammatory ▶ hyperalgesia in the skin or bronchial hyperreactivity in the respiratory system (Renz 2001). Furthermore, it has been suggested that, by promoting keratinocyte proliferation and vascular neoangiogenesis, NGF contributes to cutaneous morphogenesis,

14. Quock RM, Mueller JL, Vaughn LK (1993) Strain-dependent differences in responsiveness of mice to nitrous oxide antinociception. Brain Res 614:52–56
15. Quock RM, Vaughn LK (1995) Nitrous oxide: Mechanism of its antinociceptive action. Analgesia 1:151–159
16. Zuniga JR, Joseph SA, Knigge KM (1987) The effects of nitrous oxide on the secretory activity of pro-opiomelanocortin peptides from basal hypothalamic cells attached to cytodex beads in a superfusion *in vitro* system. Brain Res 420:66–72

NK–1 Blockers

Definition

Neurokinin–1 (NK–1) receptor inhibitors lessen emesis after cisplatin, ipecac, copper sulfate, apomorphine, and radiation therapy; e.g. aprepitant.
▶ Cancer Pain Management, Chemotherapy

NK-1 Receptor

Definition

One of the three types of G-protein coupled receptors where tachykinins act. Substance P is the preferred ligand, although neurokinin A (NKA) can also activate the NK1 receptor.
▶ Wind-Up of Spinal Cord Neurons

NMDA

Definition

N-methyl-D-aspartate (NMDA), a chemical analogue of glutamate that gives its name to the receptor. This receptor is formed of at least 4 subtypes, one of which is the NR2B.
▶ GABA and Glycine in Spinal Nociceptive Processing
▶ N-methyl-D-aspartate
▶ Opioids in the Spinal Cord and Central Sensitization

NMDA Glutamate Receptor(s)

Synonyms

N-methyl-D-aspartate receptor; NMDA Receptor

Definition

One of 4 general classes of glutamate receptors. Activated by N-methyl-D-aspartate with high affinity. It is involved in inducing long-term changes in the function of the neurons due to an influx of Ca^{++} through it. This receptor requires a release of glutamate (ligand-gated) and a change in the membrane voltage (voltage-gated) concomitantly to be activated. The NMDA receptor is found in high concentrations in the anterior horn of the spinal cord, where it is associated with the process of central sensitization, one of the precursors of neuropathic pain. Agonists include glutamate and aspartate, and antagonists include ketamine and dextromethorphan, and to a much lesser extent methadone. The receptors may be the site of action of dissociative anesthetics such as ketamine. The NMDA ion channel has a relatively high Ca^{2+} permeability, and this may be important in the initiation of plastic changes necessary for several types of learning and memory.
▶ Acute Pain Mechanisms
▶ Amygdala, Pain Processing and Behavior in Animals
▶ Descending Modulation and Persistent Pain
▶ GABA and Glycine in Spinal Nociceptive Processing
▶ Metabotropic Glutamate Receptors in the Thalamus
▶ Nociceptive Neurotransmission in the Thalamus
▶ NSAIDs, Adverse Effects
▶ Opiates During Development
▶ Opioids in the Spinal Cord and Central Sensitization
▶ Pain Control in Children with Burns
▶ Pain Modulatory Systems, History of Discovery
▶ Postoperative Pain, Transition from Parenteral to Oral
▶ Somatic Pain
▶ Wind-Up of Spinal Cord Neurons

NMDA Receptors in Spinal Nociceptive Processing

HORACIO VANEGAS[1], HANS-GEORG SCHAIBLE[2]
[1]Instituto Venezolano de Investigaciones Cientificas (IVIC), Caracas, Venezuela
[2]Department of Physiology, Friedrich Schiller University, Jena, Germany
hvanegas@ivic.ve,
hans-georg.schaible@mti.uni-jena.de

Synonyms

Glutamate receptors; spinal dorsal horn; calcium channel; ionotropic receptor

Definition

The NMDA receptor is a tetrameric molecule provided with a channel that upon glutamate binding allows the outflow of potassium ions as well as the inflow of sodium and, characteristically, calcium ions across the neuronal membrane. The NMDA receptor is responsible for excitatory synaptic transmission in nociceptive pathways and circuits.

Characteristics

Glutamate is the main excitatory transmitter in the central nervous system. When released by presynaptic terminals, glutamate reaches the postsynaptic membrane, where various types of receptor molecules may be found. Glutamate receptor molecules can be divided in two broad types, the ionotropic type, which possesses an ion channel that opens upon glutamate binding, and the metabotropic type, which has no channel but is coupled to G-proteins that transduce glutamate binding into modifications of intracellular messengers and enzymes.

Molecular Biology and Biophysics of NMDA Receptors

The ionotropic glutamate receptors (Kandel and Siegelbaum 2000) are named after their main pharmacological ligands, that is AMPA (α-amino-3-hydroxy-5-methylisoxazole-4-propionic acid), kainate and NMDA (*N*-methyl-D-aspartate). In all three types, the ion channel permits the flow of sodium and potassium ions. Although a minority of AMPA receptors also permit the flow of calcium ions, a large calcium inflow is characteristic of all NMDA receptors and constitutes the key to their physiological role. NMDA receptors are also characterized by the fact that, at resting membrane potential (*ca.* -65 mV), the entrance to the ion channel is blocked by a magnesium ion. At resting membrane potential, glutamate binding does not lead to any ion current through the NMDA receptor; first the magnesium ion must be dislodged from this channel. The ionotropic glutamate receptors then function in the following manner.

The glutamate released from presynaptic terminals first activates AMPA and kainate receptors (usually called non-NMDA receptors), which leads to a fast flow of sodium and potassium ions and thus to depolarization of the postsynaptic neuron. If (and only if) this depolarization is large enough, the magnesium ion will no longer be attracted into the NMDA channel entrance and the channel will finally become free for sodium and potassium to flow through; this causes a prolonged depolarization. Most importantly, the unblocked NMDA channel now lets large amounts of calcium ions flow into the neuron.

Ionotropic glutamate receptor molecules are made of two pairs of subunits, each subunit in turn with four intramembranous segments. Subunits in NMDA receptors are called NR1, NR2 and NR3. The predominant NR2 subunit is the NR2B. These subunits can be sensitized through phosphorylation by protein kinases (see below). NR1 binds glycine and NR2 binds glutamate (Furukawa et al. 2005). Glycine is essential for the NMDA receptor to function. Normally there is enough glycine in the extracellular fluid and the function of the NMDA receptor then depends only on the glutamate released presynaptically and on the membrane potential of the postsynaptic neuron (Kandel and Siegelbaum 2000).

Involvement of NMDA Receptors in Normal Nociception

Some authors have found that NMDA receptor antagonists, whether given systemically or intrathecally onto the spinal cord, do not modify behavioral baseline responses to acutely painful stimuli (Yaksh 1999). Also, conditional deletion of the NR1 subunit in the spinal cord had no influence upon behavioral responses to tactile stimulation or to acute, high intensity non-damaging thermal stimuli applied to the skin (South et al. 2003). However, recordings from spinal cord nociceptive neurons have shown (Dougherty et al. 1992; Neugebauer et al. 1993a; Neugebauer et al. 1993b) that NMDA receptors participate in responses to various types of cutaneous and deep somatic noxious stimuli. It therefore seems that NMDA receptors will contribute to normal nociception whenever the postsynaptic neurons become sufficiently depolarized for the magnesium ion to be dislodged from the receptor. This will of course be more intense in cases of persistent nociception.

Involvement of NMDA Receptors in Persistent Nociception

In cases of persistent damage to a peripheral tissue, such as during inflammation, trauma or nerve lesions, the continuous and often large barrage of action potentials coming into the spinal cord causes a considerable release of glutamate and this in turn, *via* non-NMDA receptors, causes a sufficiently large neuronal depolarization for the magnesium ion to be evicted from the NMDA channel. Calcium then flows into the postsynaptic neurons and a whole series of events is triggered, which results in a considerable and long lasting increase in spinal neuronal excitability (central sensitization). The hyperalgesia (increased pain upon noxious stimulation) and allodynia (pain elicited by normally non-painful stimuli) of chronic pain conditions are thus thought to arise not only from an increased nociceptive input into the spinal cord, but also from an increased synaptic relay of nociceptive messages towards supraspinal structures.

It must be made clear that activation of NMDA receptors is not the only mechanism whereby central sensitization comes about. Concomitant mechanisms are, for example: (1) activation of receptors for pronociceptive neuropeptides such as ► substance P (NK1), neurokinin A (NK2), ► calcitonin gene related peptide (CGRP receptor), cholecystokinin (mainly CCK$_B$) and vasoactive intestinal peptide (VIP receptor); and (2) induction of cyclooxygenase-2 (Vanegas and Schaible 2001), with the resulting enhancement of the pronociceptive effects of prostaglandins and thromboxanes (► Prostaglandins, Spinal Effects). It must also be made clear that, in addition to the NMDA receptor, there are voltage activated calcium channels (Vanegas and Schaible 2000) through which considerable amounts of calcium can flow into the depolarized neuron (▶ Calcium Channels in the Spinal Processing of Nociceptive Input). Compounds that antagonize NMDA receptors or the other mechanisms just mentioned have been shown to attenuate pain messages and are, of course, potential analgesic agents.

Electrically Induced Spinal Neuronal Hyperexcitability

Two types of electrophysiological manipulation have shown that the NMDA receptor plays a key role in spinal neuronal hyperexcitability. Both of these involve stimulating the primary afferents with electrical pulses whose intensities are generally large enough to fire all fiber types, from Aβ to C. Each stimulus pulse elicits in spinal cord neurons a depolarizing synaptic potential that lasts up to 20 s and is due to the activation of non-NMDA, NMDA and substance P receptors (Woolf 1996). If the pulse is applied about once per second, these potentials summate one on top of the other, thus giving rise to increasingly larger neuronal discharges. This is known as windup and shows that the excitability of neurons may increase as result of previous activity (thus a form of "learning"), that this involves NMDA receptors and that low frequency but persistent discharges in pain afferent fibers may cause increasing pain. Windup is not a product of neuronal plasticity; it happens by virtue of mechanisms that are normally present in the spinal cord. The enhanced excitability quickly returns to baseline if the electrical stimulation is terminated.

On the other hand, an increase in synaptic strength that may last for hours can be obtained if the stimulus pulse is applied about 100 times per second during a few seconds. This is known as long-term potentiation (LTP), and is the most widely and deeply studied form of activity dependent synaptic enhancement (the basis of learning) (Sandkühler 2000). The presence of LTP is shown after the inducing pulse train by applying a single test pulse to the presynaptic axons every few minutes - each test pulse elicits an enhanced excitatory postsynaptic response in the recorded neuron. Antagonists to NMDA, NK1 or glutamate metabotropic receptors prevent induction of LTP.

Induction of Hyperexcitability by Persistent Tissue Damage

In the spinal cord, LTP of responses to electrical pulses can be elicited by strong "natural" noxious stimuli (burning or crushing of paws, crushing of nerves) in anesthetized rats (Sandkühler 2000), provided that the nociceptive inhibition that normally descends from the brain stem is blocked (▶ Long-Term Potentiation and Long-Term Depression in the Spinal Cord). Another way of investigating the role of NMDA receptors in central sensitization and hyperalgesia is to use natural noxious stimuli instead of electrical pulses to test the responses of dor-

sal horn nociceptive neurons in anesthetized animals or the behavioral nociceptive responses in conscious animals. As mentioned above, inflammation or trauma of peripheral tissues or lesions to peripheral nerves induce an enhancement of spinal nociceptive responses in animals that is akin to the hyperalgesia and allodynia of clinical chronic pain conditions.

Plasticity of the NMDA Receptor

During persistent damage or LTP, the key to an increase in neuronal excitability is an increase in intracellular calcium concentration. This is brought about not only by the inflow of calcium through the NMDA receptor channel, but also by inflow through voltage dependent calcium channels or calcium permeable AMPA receptors and by activation of G-protein coupled receptors (to glutamate, prostaglandins, substance P), which results in calcium inflow and/or release from intracellular stores towards the cytosol (Ikeda et al. 2003; Woolf and Salter 2000). The paramount role of NMDA receptor activation, however, has been demonstrated in numerous studies where application of pharmacological antagonists or deletion of the NR1 subunit of the NMDA receptor in the spinal cord completely prevent induction of LTP or central sensitization (Sandkühler 2000; South et al. 2003; Woolf and Salter 2000). Nevertheless, blockade of other receptors, like the NK1 receptor, may also prevent LTP (Ikeda et al. 2003; Woolf 1996).

The increased intracellular calcium leads to activation of calcium-calmodulin dependent protein kinase II (CaMKII), protein kinase A (PKA) and protein kinase C (PKC), as well as nitric oxide synthase and the cyclooxygenases (Sandkühler 2000; Woolf 1996; Woolf and Salter 2000). This in turn leads to several events, including sensitization of both NMDA and non-NMDA receptors.

In spinal cord neurons, one important point of convergence for various intracellular pathways is PKC. CaMKII, another serine/threonine kinase that plays a key role in hippocampal and neocortical plasticity is less important in the spinal dorsal horn (Woolf and Salter 2000). Protein kinases phosphorylate the NMDA receptor and thereby sensitize it and partially dislodge the magnesium ion from the channel (Woolf 1996); as a result, binding of glutamate to the NMDA receptor will more easily cause calcium inflow. Tyrosine kinases such as Src also potentiate NMDA currents (Woolf and Salter 2000). Indeed, Src and PKC are involved in phosphorylation of the NR2B subunit induced by brain derived neurotrophic factor (BDNF) (Guo et al. 2004a), which binds to the tyrosine kinase B (trkB) receptor. Since peripheral inflammation induces expression of BDNF in primary afferents, this would contribute to central sensitization. It must be noted that increases in intracellular calcium as well as other forms of protein kinase activation do not necessarily result from an activation of the NMDA receptor and yet they feed back

N

and sensitize it. Indeed, activation of NK1, glutamate metabotropic and tyrosine kinase receptors may lead to nociceptive neuronal sensitization (Ikeda et al. 2003) and this has been shown to be associated with phosphorylation of the NMDA receptor (Guo et al. 2004a; Guo et al. 2004b).

Activation of spinal neuronal NMDA, glutamate metabotropic, NK1 and trkB receptors as a result of peripheral noxious stimulation and inflammation eventually leads to activation of ERK (extracellular signal regulated protein kinase, a mitogen activated protein or MAP kinase). ERK activation, by way of the cAMP responsive element binding (CREB) protein in the cell nucleus, results in gene expression mediated by the cAMP responsive element (CRE). This may in turn lead to medium- and long-term persistence of central sensitization to painful stimulation (Kawasaki et al. 2004) and to transition to chronicity in clinical pain.

References

1. Dougherty PM, Palecek J, Sorkin LS et al. (1992) The role of NMDA and no-NMDA excitatory amino acid receptors in the excitation of primate spinothalamic tract neurons by mechanical, chemical, thermal, and electrical stimuli. J Neurosci 12:3025-3041
2. Furukawa H, Singh SK, Mancusso R et al. (2005) Subunit arrangement and function in NMDA receptors. Nature 438:185-192
3. Guo W, Wei F, Zou S-P et al. (2004a) Effect of brain-derived neurotrophic factor on N-methyl-D-aspartate receptor subunit NR2B tyrosine phosphorylation in the rat spinal dorsal horn. Abstr View/Itin Plann, Society of Neuroscience, Progr No 864.811
4. Guo W, Wei F, Zou S-P et al. (2004b) Group I metabotropic glutamate receptor NMDA receptor coupling and signaling cascade mediate spinal dorsal horn NMDA receptor 2B tyrosine phosphorylation associated with inflammatory hyperalgesia. J Neurosci 24:9161–9173
5. Ikeda H, Heinke B, Ruscheweyh R et al. (2003) Synaptic plasticity in spinal lamina I projection neurons that mediate hyperalgesia. Science 299:1237-1240
6. Kandel ER, Siegelbaum SA (2000) Synaptic integration. In: Kandel ER, Schwartz JH, Jessell TM (eds) Principles of Neural Science. McGraw-Hill, New York, pp 207-228
7. Kawasaki Y, Kohno T, Zhuang Z-Y et al. (2004) Ionotropic and metabotropic receptors, protein kinase A, protein kinase C, and Src contribute to C-fiber-induced ERK activation and cAMP response element-binding protein phosphorylation in dorsal horn neurons, leading to central sensitization. J Neurosci 24:8310-8321
8. Neugebauer V, Lücke T, Schaible H-G (1993a) Differential effects of N-methyl-D-aspartate (NMDA) and non-NMDA receptor antagonists on the responses of rat spinal neurons with joint input. Neurosci Lett 155:29-32
9. Neugebauer V, Lücke T, Schaible H-G (1993b) N-methyl-D-aspartate (NMDA) and non-NMDA receptor antagonists block the hyperexcitability of dorsal horn neurons during development of acute arthritis in rat's knee joint. J Neurophysiol 70:1365-1377
10. Sandkühler J (2000) Learning and memory in pain pathways. Pain 88:113-118
11. South SM, Kohno T, Kaspar BK et al. (2003) A conditional deletion of the NR1 subunit of the NMDA receptor in adult spinal cord dorsal horn reduces NMDA currents and injury-induced pain. J Neurosci 23:5040-5031
12. Vanegas H, Schaible H-G (2000) Effects of antagonists to high-threshold calcium channels upon spinal mechanisms of pain, hyperalgesia and allodynia. Pain 85:9-18
13. Vanegas H, Schaible H-G (2001) Prostaglandins and cyclooxygenases in the spinal cord. Prog Neurobiol 64:327-363
14. Woolf CJ (1996) Windup and central sensitization are not equivalent. Pain 66:105-108
15. Woolf CJ, Salter MW (2000) Neuronal plasticity: increasing the gain in pain. Science 288:1765-1768
16. Yaksh TL (1999) Spinal systems and pain processing: development of novel analgesic drugs with mechanistically defined models. Trends Neurosci 20:329-337

N-methyl-D-aspartate

Synonym

NMDA

Definition

N-methyl-D-aspartate (NMDA), a chemical analogue of glutamate that gives its name to the receptor. Agonist for the NMDA receptor for glutamate, which is the major excitatory neurotransmitter in the CNS.

▶ GABA and Glycine in Spinal Nociceptive Processing
▶ Opioids in the Spinal Cord and Central Sensitization
▶ Spinal Cord Nociception, Neurotrophins

N-methyl-D-aspartate (NMDA) Antagonist

Definition

There is accumulating evidence to implicate the importance of N-methyl-D-aspartate (NMDA) receptors to the induction and maintenance of central sensitization during pain states. However, NMDA receptors may also mediate peripheral sensitization and visceral pain. NMDA receptors are composed of NR1, NR2 (A, B, C, and D), and NR3 (A and B) subunits, which determine the functional properties of native NMDA receptors. Antagonists acting at the N-methyl-D-aspartate (NMDA) receptor can block the development of tolerance to the analgesic effects of [mu] opioid receptor (MOR) ligands, such as morphine, and can also enhance the analgesic efficacy of opioids. The last decade has seen significant progress in our understanding of the NMDA receptor complex and the site(s) of action of various uncompetitive antagonists. This has led to the development of a family of low-affinity, uncompetitive, cation channel antagonists that seem to offer many of the benefits of the older channel blockers but with a more acceptable adverse effect profile. Drugs such as memantine have shown beneficial effects in clinical trials for Alzheimer's disease and ischemia, with few adverse effects. Likewise, the NMDA receptor NR2B subunit antagonists derived from drugs such as ifenprodil, have proven beneficial in the treatment of neuropathic pain, and are also associated with few adverse effects.

▶ Multimodal Analgesia in Postoperative Pain

N-methyl-D-aspartate (NMDA) Receptor

Definition

Activation of the NMDA receptor sets in motion a series of events that increase the responsiveness of the nociceptive system (central sensitization). NMDA receptors are composed of NR1, NR2 (A, B, C, and D), and NR3 (A and B) subunits, which determine the functional properties of native NMDA receptors. Central sensitization lowers the activation thresholds of spinal neurones and is characterized by wind-up, whereby repeated C-fiber volleys result in a progressive increase in discharge of secondary dorsal horn nociceptive neurones. This contributes to the hyperalgesia. The N-methyl-D–aspartate (NMDA) receptor, at physiological Mg^{++} levels is initially unresponsive to glutamate, but following depolarization at the amino methyl propionic acid (AMPA) receptor by glutamate or the Neurokinin–1 receptor by Substance P, and the trkB receptor by brain-derived neurotropic factor (BDNF), it becomes responsive to glutamate, allowing Ca^{++} influx. The action of glutamate on the metabotropic receptor (modulated by glycine) stimulates G-protein-mediated activation of phospholipase C (PLC), which catalyses the hydrolysis of phophatidylinositol 4,5-biphosphonate (PIP2) to produce inositol triphosphate (IP3) and diacylglycerol (DAG). DAG stimulates production of protein kinase C (PKC), which is activated in the presence of high levels of intracellular Ca^{++}. IP3 stimulates the release of Ca^{++} from intracellular stores within the endoplasmic reticulum. Increased PKC induces a sustained increase in membrane permeability, with Ca^{++} leading to the expression of proto-oncogenes (c-fos, c-jun). The proteins produced encode a number of peptides (enkephalins, dynorphins, tachykinins). Increased intracellular Ca^{++} leads to the activation of calcium/calmodulin-dependent protein kinase (which briefly increases membrane permeability), to the activation of phospholipase A–2 (PLA–2), as well as to the activation of nitric oxide synthetase (NOS) (via a calcium/calmodulin mechanism). The conversion of phosphatidyl choline to prostaglandins and thromboxane is catalyzed by PLA2. The lipooxygenase pathway also produces leukotrienes. NOS catalyses the production of nitric oxide (NO) and L-citrulline from L-arginine. NO activates soluble guanalyte cyclase, increasing the intracellular content of cyclic GMP, leading to the production of protein kinases and alterations in gene expression. NO diffuses out of the cell to the primary afferent terminal, where, via a guanalyte cyclase/cyclic-GMP mechanism, it increases glutamate release. NO is responsible for the cell death demonstrated after prolonged activation of nociceptor afferents. Among NMDA receptor subtypes, the NR2B subunit-containing receptors appear particularly important for nociception, leading to the possibility that NR2B-selective antagonists may be useful in the treatment of chronic pain.

▶ Opioid Responsiveness in Cancer Pain Management
▶ Postoperative Pain, Persistent Acute Pain
▶ Postoperative Pain, Postamputation Pain, Treatment and Prevention
▶ Spinothalamic Tract Neurons, Glutamatergic Input

NMR

▶ Magnetic Resonance Imaging

NNT

Definition

The NNT of oxycodone 15 mg is 2.3.
▶ Number Needed to Treat
▶ Postoperative Pain, Oxycodone

Nocebo

N

Definition

Nocebo (from the Latin: "I shall harm") can be thought of as an agent or intervention that results in harm, either in the form of adverse outcomes or adverse side-effects. A nocebo effect is the effect that such an agent or intervention ostensibly exerts.

The term – nocebo effect, is most commonly used to describe side-effects that occur in response to interventions for which there is no physiological mechanism, such as a placebo. These side-effects are the same as, and may be more prevalent, than those encountered with the active medication. Interestingly, the side-effect profile of placebos mimic the active drug that it is being compared with and also appear to be disease-specific (e.g. dizziness in psychiatric disorders, headache in angina, gastro-intestinal disturbance in peptic disease (Barsky et al. 2002). This is thought to be due to patients being informed, and therefore cued, to expect potential adverse effects of the medication that they might be taking in the research project. Suggestion, expectation and conditioning are the likely reasons. It is commonly seen in clinical practice when some patients assiduously study their consumer product information in their medicine packets, and read about all the possible side-effects of the medicine they have been prescribed. Upon taking the medication, they believe that they experience the expected side-effect.

The nocebo effect can be reduced by some simple steps (Weihrauch and Gauler 1999). Firstly, if patients with negative expectations can be identified, especially in conditions such as anxiety, depression and somatisation, it is worthwhile attempting to shift their cognition to more positive expectations. For example, with serotonin uptake inhibitors, telling patients that the nausea they are likely to experience is a good sign (since it shows serotonin is increasing and, therefore, the drug is working) makes it more likely they will continue taking the medication. Secondly, commencing with low doses and increasing them slowly reduces the risk of side-effects. Thirdly, using other health-care professionals who will reinforce the messages given to the patient lessens the risk of nocebo.

The term – nocebo response, is used in another fashion, to describe the response of patients who know that they have been given or allocated to an inferior treatment. Under those conditions, they report failure to improve in order to indicate indirectly their disaffection with the way that they have been treated.

References

1. Weihrauch T, Gauler T (1999) Placebo – Efficacy and Adverse Effects in Controlled Clinical Trials. Arzneimittelforschung 49:385-393
2. Barsky AJ, Saintfort R, Rogers MP, Borus JF (2002) Nonspecific Medication Side-Effects and the Nocebo Phenomenon. JAMA 287:622-627

Nocebo Effect

Definition

Harmful effects occurring from placebos.
▶ Placebo

Nociceptin

▶ Orphanin FQ

Nociception

Definition

Nociception (from the Latin word *nocere*, to injure) is the transduction, encoding, and transmission of neural information about tissue damage, or impending tissue damage, which would occur if a stimulus was maintained over time. Cognitive central processing identifies the location of the stimulus, its general character, and the severity of the associated tissue injury. Some of the biological participants in this process include: unmyelinated dorsal horn neurons [like A-delta and C-fibers], excitatory amino acids, neuropeptides, zinc, biogenic amines, nitric oxide, wide-dynamic range spinal neurons, the limbic system of the brain, and several regions of the cerebral neocortex cortex. Normal nociception depends on a delicate balance between pronociceptive and antinociceptive forces. Chronic noxious stimulation causes ▶ central sensitization in which there is an increase in sensitivity of nociceptive neurons function nociceptively [recruitment] and new, semi-permanent neural connections develop [neuroplasticity].

▶ Allodynia and Alloknesis
▶ Amygdala, Pain Processing and Behavior in Animals
▶ Consciousness and Pain
▶ Ethics of Pain, Culture and Ethnicity
▶ Forebrain Modulation of the Periaqueductal Gray
▶ Muscle Pain, Fibromyalgia Syndrome (Primary, Secondary)
▶ Nociceptive Withdrawal Reflex
▶ Pain in Humans, Psychophysical Law
▶ Psychological Aspects of Pain in Women
▶ Secondary Somatosensory Cortex (S2) and Insula, Effect on Pain Related Behavior in Animals and Humans
▶ Spinothalamic Tract Neurons, in Deep Dorsal Horn
▶ Spinothalamocortical Projections from SM
▶ Transition from Acute to Chronic Pain

Nociception in Genital Mucosa

▶ Nociception in Mucosa of Sexual Organs

Nociception in Mucosa of Sexual Organs

MARITA HILLIGES
Halmstad University, Halmstad, Sweden
marita.hilliges@set.hh.se

Synonyms

Nociception in Genital Mucosa; Genital Mucosa, Nociception; Mucosa of Sexual Organs, Nociception

Definition

Pain perception and nociceptors in mucosal lining, including epithelium and underlying connective tissue, of human external genital organs. The external genital organs covered by mucosa comprise vulvar vestibule, clitoris and glans penis. The vagina belongs to the internal female genital organs but is included since it has partly somatic innervation.

Characteristics

Pain Perception in Sexual Mucosa

The vestibule is by origin visceral tissue but is considered to have a somatic innervation (Cervero 1994). Sensations for touch, temperature and pain are therefore similar to sensations evoked in skin. Heat pain threshold is approximately 43° C, which is slightly below heat pain thresholds in skin (45–46°C). There are

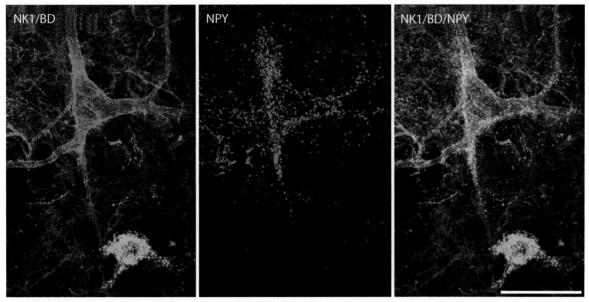

Nociceptive Circuitry in the Spinal Cord, Figure 2   This figure shows selective innervation of one of two different types of projection neuron in lamina III of the dorsal horn by axons belonging to a population of inhibitory interneurons. Two cells can be seen in the left image: the large cell in the upper part of the field is stained with an antibody against the NK1 receptor (green). All cells of this type are projection neurons. The lower cell was retrogradely labelled with biotin dextran (BD; blue) injected into the gracile nucleus and therefore belongs to the post-synaptic dorsal column (PSDC) pathway. The middle image shows the same field scanned to reveal axons that contain neuropeptide Y (NPY), and the image on the right is a merge of the three colours. NPY-containing axons in the dorsal horn are derived from a population of GABAergic interneurons in laminae I and II, and these axons can be seen to form numerous contacts with the NK1 receptor-immunoreactive cell, but not with the PSDC neuron. Scale bar = 50 μm. (Modified from Polgár et al. 1999, J Neurosci 19:2637-2646. Copyright 1999 by the Society for Neuroscience).

N

afferents respond to noxious stimulation (Lawson et al. 1997), this provides a direct route through which nociceptors can activate brain regions involved in pain mechanisms. The nociceptive afferents release both glutamate and substance P and these act through different mechanisms. Glutamate will be released across the synaptic cleft and act on receptors in the postsynaptic membrane, whereas substance P will diffuse to nearby NK1 receptors (▶ volume transmission). Nociceptive primary afferents presumably also form synapses with both excitatory and inhibitory interneurons, although much less is known about these connections.

There is some evidence to indicate that different populations of inhibitory interneurons have specific postsynaptic targets. One group of inhibitory cells in laminae I and II is characterised by the presence of GABA and neuropeptide Y. Axons of these cells form numerous synapses with projection neurons in laminae III and IV that express the NK1 receptor, but not with another population of projection cells that occupy the same laminae, those belonging to the ▶ post-synaptic dorsal column pathway (Polgár et al. 1999) (Fig. 2). As mentioned above, axoaxonic synapses are responsible for presynaptic inhibition of primary afferent terminals. Different classes of primary afferent appear to receive axoaxonic synapses from axons belonging to different types of inhibitory interneuron (Todd and Koerber 2004).

Much less is known about the synaptic connections between different types of interneuron, or between excitatory interneurons and projection neurons. It is likely that these are fairly specific (at least in some cases) and also very complex. Clearly, a great deal of research will be needed to unravel the details of nociceptive circuits in the spinal cord.

▶ Nociceptive Processing in the Spinal Cord

References

1. Grudt TJ, Perl ER (2002) Correlations between neuronal morphology and electrophysiological features in the rodent superficial dorsal horn. J Physiol 540:189–207
2. Lawson SN, Crepps BA, Perl ER (1997) Relationship of substance P to afferent characteristics of dorsal root ganglion neurones in guinea-pig. J Physiol 505:177–191
3. Light AR, Perl ER (1979) Spinal termination of functionally identified primary afferent neurons with slowly conducting myelinated fibers. J Comp Neurol 186:133–150
4. Mantyh PW, Rogers SD, Honore P et al. (1997) Ablation of lamina I spinal neurons expressing the substance P receptor profoundly inhibits hyperalgesia. Science 278:275–279
5. Polgár E, Shehab SAS, Watt C et al. (1999) GABAergic neurons that contain neuropeptide Y selectively target cells with the neurokinin 1 receptor in laminae III and IV of the rat spinal cord. J Neurosci 19:2637–2646
6. Rexed B (1952) The cytoarchitectonic organization of the spinal cord in the cat. J Comp Neurol 96:415–495
7. Spike RC, Puskár Z, Andrew D et al. (2003) A quantitative and morphological study of projection neurons in lamina I of the rat lumbar spinal cord. Eur J Neurosci 18:2433–2448
8. Todd AJ, Puskár Z, Spike RC et al. (2002) Projection neurons in lamina I of rat spinal cord with the neurokinin 1 receptor are

selectively innervated by substance P-containing afferents and respond to noxious stimulation. J Neurosci 22:4103–4113

9. Todd AJ, Koerber R (2004) Neuroanatomical substrates of spinal nociception. In: McMahon S, Koltzenburg M (eds) Melzack and Wall's textbook of pain, 5th edn, Churchill Livingstone, Edinburgh, UK, pp 73–90
10. Villanueva L, Bernard J-F (1999) The multiplicity of ascending pain pathways. In: Lydic R, Baghdoyan HA (eds) Handbook of behavioral state control: cellular and molecular mechanisms. pp 569–585 CRC Press LLC, Boca Raton, FL
11. Willis WD, Coggeshall RE (2004) Sensory mechanisms of the spinal cord, 3th edn. Kluwes Academic Plenum Publishers, New York
12. Yaksh TL (1989) Behavioral and autonomic correlates of the tactile evoked allodynia produced by spinal glycine inhibition: effects of modulatory receptor systems and excitatory amino acid antagonists. Pain 37:111–123

Nociceptive Coding in Lateral Thalamus

▶ Thalamic Nuclei Involved in Pain, Human and Monkey

Nociceptive Masseter Muscle Afferents

▶ Nociceptors in the Orofacial Region (Temporomandibular Joint and Masseter Muscle)

Nociceptive Nerve Endings

Definition

The terminal branches of the peripheral axon of nociceptive neurons located in sensory ganglia.
▶ Nociceptor Generator Potential

Nociceptive Neuroplasticity

Definition

At its most general level, nociceptive neuroplasticity denotes the changes in nervous system processing resulting from nociceptive inputs. Used in this way, the term includes both functional and structural, reversible and irreversible changes. Other groups would use this term in a narrower sense, and only include alterations in nervous system function that are due to structural change.
▶ Central Sensitisation
▶ Quantitative Sensory Testing

Nociceptive Neurotransmission in the Thalamus

THOMAS E. SALT
Institute of Ophthalmology, University College London, London, UK
t.salt@ucl.ac.uk

Synonyms

Chemical Transmitter; neuromodulator; Thalamus, Nociceptive Neurotransmission

Definition

Neurotransmitters are chemical messengers that are released from one neural element (e.g. a nerve terminal) to then act upon a receptor located on or in another neural element (e.g. a dendrite). This transfer of information is neurotransmission, and this contribution describes neurotransmitter mechanisms which mediate the transmission and integration of nociceptive information in the thalamus.

Characteristics

The integrative role of the thalamus in the processing of nociceptive information is complex and diverse. A variety of different neurotransmitters and an array of receptors take part in this process, and it has become clear that the nature of these processes is pivotal to the function of the thalamo-cortico-thalamic circuitry (McCormick 1992; Broman 1994; Salt and Eaton 1996; Millan 1999). The majority of work carried out in the field of thalamic neurotransmitters has been in the so-called relay nuclei, of which the ventrobasal complex (ventroposterolateral and ventroposteromedial nuclei) is the somatosensory representative. Some of this function pertains to nociception, but it is important to remember that the ventrobasal complex (VB) has an important role in the processing of non-nociceptive somatosensory information and that many other thalamic nuclei (whose detailed transmitter functions are much less well studied) also participate in nociceptive functions.

Ascending Sensory Input

There is overwhelming neuroanatomical evidence, at both the light-microscopical and ultrastructural levels, to favour a neurotransmitter role for glutamate in the ascending afferent fibres in several mammalian species including rodents and primates (Broman 1994). These fibres impinge upon ionotropic ▶ glutamate receptors of the ▶ NMDA and ▶ AMPA varieties located upon proximal dendrites of VB thalamic relay neurones (Broman 1994; Liu 1997). Ascending afferents to other thalamic nuclei that may be important in nociception are probably also glutamatergic (Broman 1994). Electrophysiological studies confirm a functional role for these receptor types in somatosensory transmission to the VB in rodents and primates (Salt and Eaton 1991; Dougherty et al. 1996) and it appears probable that, as in many other central synapses, the initial synaptic response is mediated *via* ► AMPA receptors with a following longer duration NMDA receptor mediated component which may become more prominent upon repetitive stimulation (Salt and Eaton 1991).

Cortico-Thalamic Input

The cortical inputs to thalamic relay neurones have been a focus of much study and speculation over many years (Sherman and Guillery 2000). Electrophysiological studies of these pathways have focussed on the role of NMDA receptors and, latterly, ► metabotropic glutamate (mGlu) receptors (Salt 2002). A particular focus has been the function of mGlu1 receptors, as these have been localised postsynaptically beneath terminals of cortico-thalamic fibres (Martin et al. 1992). However, it is also evident that there is a contribution from AMPA receptors to cortico-thalamic transmission (Golshani et al. 2001), a finding supported by ultrastructural evidence which indicates that there are AMPA receptor subunits that are predominantly GluR2/3 and GluR4 located postsynaptically at cortico-thalamic synapses in VB (Golshani et al. 2001). More recently a low level of ► kainate receptor subunits (GluR5/6/7) has been found postsynaptically beneath corticothalamic synapses in VB, although a synaptic role for these receptors has not been detected at this location.

Inhibitory Interneurones

► GABAergic inhibitory interneurones are a prominent feature of thalamic relay nuclei, and it is well known that ► GABAA and ► GABAB receptors play a prominent part in synaptic processing at both the pre- and post-synaptic level (Crunelli and Leresche 1991). There are two major groups of GABAergic neurones in the thalamic relay nuclei: the intrinsic Golgi II type interneurones, and the neurones of the ► thalamic reticular nucleus (TRN) which exert their influence *via* their projection into the relay nuclei (Ralston 1983). In rodents, only the latter population appears to be present (Ralston 1983) and performs a profound gating function upon thalamic transmission (Sherman and Guillery 2000). These GABAergic mechanisms may play an important part in the processing of sensory information in both acute and chronic nociception (Roberts et al. 1992). Intriguingly the GABAergic output from TRN is itself modulated by metabotropic ► glutamate receptors (Salt 2002) and ► kainate receptors (Binns et al. 2003). Such mechanisms indicate that sensory transmission through VB is not only dependent upon excitatory transmission, but that reduction of inhibitory transmission (i.e. functional disinhibition) could also have a significant potentiating influence on transmission.

Glia

The concept that glial cells or astrocytes may be active participants in brain function is supported by several findings, including that astrocytes possess ion channels and neurotransmitter receptors for a variety of neurotransmitters, and that astrocytes contain and can release excitatory amino acids such as glutamate and homocysteate (Haydon 2001). It is known that, in the ventrobasal thalamus, activity in astrocytes can evoke NMDA-receptor mediated responses in thalamic relay neurones *in vitro* (Parri et al. 2001), and that homocysteate can be released from thalamus *in vivo* and activate NMDA receptors (Do et al. 2004). This raises the possibility that astrocytes play a key role in the responses of thalamic neurones to sensory stimuli.

Neurotransmitters and Thalamic Integrative Function in Nociception

A role for NMDA receptors in the signalling of acute thermal and mechanical nociceptive responses in the VB thalamus at the single-neurone and behavioural level is now well established (Salt and Eaton 1996; Millan 1990). However, it is important to note that transmission of non-nociceptive sensory information to the thalamus can also show substantial NMDA receptor involvement (Salt and Eaton 1996). In addition, *both* Group I mGlu (mGlu1 and mGlu5) receptors also participate in the signalling of acute nociceptive information but not in the signalling of non-nociceptive mechanoreceptor input to the VB thalamus (Salt and Binns 2000). This functional distinction is intriguing, as there appears to be remarkable anatomical and neurochemical similarity between lemniscal (which carries non-nociceptive information) and spinothalamic (which carries nociceptive and convergent multimodal somatosensory information) inputs to the ventrobasal thalamus (Ralston 1983; Ma et al. 1987; Liu 1997). In view of this, it is conceivable that the recruitment of additional neural circuitry during noxious stimuli underlies the Group I mGlu receptor involvement in nociceptive responses. A possible source of this additional input could be the dense cortico-thalamic projection (Eaton and Salt 1995), which is known to be glutamatergic and which impinges upon mGlu receptors, particularly mGlu1 (see above). This is a particularly attractive hypothesis in the case of mGlu1 receptors, as these are restricted to corticothalamic synapses and because NMDA-receptor mediated responses have been shown to be modulated by activation of Group I (i.e. mGlu1 / mGlu5) receptors in several brain areas, as has modulation of AMPA-receptor mediated responses. In the VB, activation of mGlu1 receptors potentiates responses mediated *via* either AMPA or NMDA receptors *in vivo* (Salt and Binns 2000). It is probable that this is due to the direct effects of mGlu1 activation on neuronal membrane potential and resistance rather than a specific interaction at the receptor level, or that the potentiation that is seen is a combination of these factors (Salt and Binns 2000). Thus the cortico-thalamic input would be able to exert a profound influence on ionotropic receptor mediated responses, if the sensory stimulus was appropriate to recruit activity in the cortico-thalamic output. This may well be the case for nociceptive stimuli (Eaton and Salt 1995; Millan 1999). A further enabling factor could be the removal of the inhibitory influence arising from the TRN (see above) (Roberts et al. 1992), and in this respect it is interesting to note that TRN neurones are inhibited by noxious peripheral stimulation (Peschanski et al. 1980).

Modulatory Systems

Transmission through the thalamic relay nuclei, including those serving somatosensation and nociception, can be modulated by amine neurotransmitters such as serotonin, noradrenaline or acetylcholine (McCormick 1992). These systems appear to be associated with activating systems that govern states of wakefulness and arousal, and it is unclear to what extent these specifically affect nociceptive processing at the thalamic level. In addition, the nitric oxide (NO) system is associated with some of these activating systems (Vincent 2000), and it has been shown that NO can modulate somatosensory transmission through the thalamus (Shaw and Salt 1997). Similarly, a number of ▶ neuropeptides have been located in thalamic nuclei and afferents, but their function remains unclear (Sherman and Guillery 2000). Of particular interest to nociceptive processing is the finding that ▶ cannabinoid receptors modulate acute nociceptive responses of VB neurones in the rat (Martin et al. 1996). However the precise mechanisms of this action remain to be elucidated.

Thalamic Transmitter Mechanisms and Adaptive Changes

It is known that thalamic neurones change their response and firing characteristics in conditions of chronic pain or chronic pain models, and a role for mGlu receptors and NMDA receptors in models of synaptic plasticity has been known for some time. Thus it is conceivable that changes in thalamic neurone responses may be due to changes in glutamate receptor function and may even be a consequence of activation of these receptors as has been suggested for the spinal cord (Willis 2002). Indeed there is already evidence to suggest that NMDA receptors in the thalamus are involved in inflammation-produced hyperalgesia in the rat. In arthritic rats, decreases in thalamic expression (including VB) of mRNA for mGlu1, mGlu4 and mGlu7 receptors have been observed (Neto et al. 2000). Interestingly, in these same animals, mGlu3 mRNA expression is elevated in the TRN and this expression appears to be both in presumed GABAergic neurones and in glial cells (Neto et al. 2000). Furthermore, injection into TRN of an antagonist for this receptor was found to be anti-hyperalgesic in such rats (Neto and Castro-Lopes 2000). Thus it may be that

thalamic mGlu receptor mechanisms are important in both the induction of hyperalgesia and in the expression of hyperalgesic behaviours. It is noteworthy, however, that changes in other thalamic transmitter systems may also occur in chronic pain conditions, for example in the serotonergic system (Goettl et al. 2002). It is therefore important to note that transmitter systems should not be regarded in isolation.

Conclusions

It is evident that glutamate receptors are of fundamental importance in the transmission of nociceptive and other sensory information through the thalamus. Activation of NMDA receptors and certain mGlu receptors may be particularly important in the signalling and processing of nociceptive information, as well as in the induction of longer-term plastic changes in response to chronic noxious stimulation or injury. Molecular intervention at some of these sites may have considerable therapeutic potential.

References

1. Binns KE, Turner JP, Salt TE (2003) Kainate receptor (GluR5)-mediated disinhibition of responses in rat ventrobasal thalamus allows a novel sensory processing mechanism. J Physiol (Lond) 551:525–537
2. Broman J (1994) Neurotransmitters in subcortical somatosensory pathways. Anat Embryol 189:181–214
3. Crunelli V, Leresche N (1991) A role for GABAB receptors in excitation and inhibition of thalamocortical cells. Trends Neurosci 14:16–21
4. Do KQ., Benz B, Binns KE, Eaton SA, Salt TE (2004) Release of homocysteic acid from rat thalamus following stimulation of somatosensory afferents in vivo: feasability and possible glial participation in synaptic transmission. Neurosci 124:387–93
5. Dougherty PM, Li YJ, Lenz FA, Rowland L, Mittman S (1996) Evidence That Excitatory Amino Acids Mediate Afferent Input to the Primate Somatosensory Thalamus. Brain Res 728:267–273
6. Eaton SA, Salt TE (1995). The role of excitatory amino acid receptors in thalamic nociception. In: Besson JM, Guilbaud G, Ollat H (eds) Forebrain areas involved in pain processing. John Libbey Eurotext, Paris, pp 131–141
7. Goettl VM, Huang Y, Hackshaw KV et al. (2002) Reduced basal release of serotonin from the ventrobasal thalamus of the rat in a model of neuropathic pain. Pain 99:359–366
8. Golshani P, Liu XB, Jones EG (2001) Differences in Quantal Amplitude Reflect GluR4-Subunit Number at Corticothalamic Synapses on Two Populations of Thalamic Neurons. Proceedings of the National Academy of Sciences of the United States of America 98:4172–4177
9. Haydon PG (2001) Glia: listening and talking to the synapse. Nat Rev Neurosci 2:185–193
10. Liu XB (1997) Subcellular distribution of AMPA and NMDA receptor subunit immunoreactivity in ventral posterior and reticular nuclei of rat and cat thalamus. J Comp Neurol 388:587–602
11. Ma W, Peschanski M, Ralston III HJ (1987) The differential synaptic organization of the spinal and lemniscal projections to the ventrobasal complex of the rat thalamus. Evidence for convergence of the two systems upon single thalamic neurons. Neurosci 22:925–934
12. Martin, LJ, Blackstone CD, Huganir RL et al. (1992) Cellular localization of a metabotropic glutamate receptor in rat brain. Neuron 9:259–270
13. Martin WJ, Hohmann AG, Walker JM (1996) Suppression of noxious stimulus-evoked activity in the ventral posterolateral nucleus of the thalamus by a cannabinoid agonist: Correlation be-

tween electrophysiological and antinociceptive effects. J Neurosci 16:6601–6611

14. McCormick DA (1992) Neurotransmitter actions in the thalamus and cerebral cortex and their role in neuromodulation of thalamocortical activity. Prog Neurobiol 39:337–388
15. Millan MJ (1999) The induction of Pain: an integrative review. Progress in Neurobiology 57:1–164
16. Neto FL, Castro-Lopes JM (2000) Antinociceptive effect of a group II metabotropic glutamate receptor antagonist in the thalamus of monoarthritic rats. Neurosci Lett 296:25–28
17. Neto FL, Schadrack J, Platzer S et al. (2000) Expression of metabotropic glutamate receptors mRNA in the thalamus and brainstem of monoarthritic rats. Mol Brain Res 81:140–154
18. Parri HR, Gould TM, Crunelli V (2001) Spontaneous Astrocytic Ca^{2+} Oscillations in Situ Drive NMDA- Mediated Neuronal Excitation. Nature Neuroscience 4:803–812
19. Peschanski M, Guilbaud G, Gautron M (1980) Neuronal responses to cutaneous electrical and noxious mechanical stimuli in the nucleus reticularis thalami of the rat. Neurosci Lett 20:165–170
20. Ralston III HJ (1983). The synaptic organization of the ventrobasal thalamus in the rat, cat and monkey. In: Macchi G, Rustioni A, Spreafico R (eds) Somatosensory Integration in the Thalamus. Elsevier Science Publishers, Amsterdam, pp 241–250
21. Roberts WA, Eaton SA, Salt TE (1992) Widely distributed GABA-mediated afferent inhibition processes within the ventrobasal thalamus of rat and their possible relevance to pathological pain states and somatotopic plasticity. Experimental Brain Research 89:363–372
22. Salt TE (2002) Glutamate Receptor Functions in Sensory Relay in the Thalamus. Philosophical Transactions of the Royal Society of London Series B-Biological Sciences 357, 1759–1766
23. Salt TE, Binns KE (2000) Contributions of mGlu1 and mGlu5 receptors to interactions with N-methyl-D-aspartate receptor-mediated responses and nociceptive sensory responses of rat thalamic neurones. Neuroscience 100:375–380
24. Salt TE, Eaton SA (1996) Functions of ionotropic and metabotropic glutamate receptors in sensory transmission in the mammalian thalamus. Progress in Neurobiology 48:55–72
25. Salt TE, Eaton SA (1991) Sensory excitatory postsynaptic potentials mediated by NMDA and non-NMDA receptors in the thalamus *in vivo*. Eur J Neurosci 3:296–300
26. Shaw PJ, Salt TE (1997) Modulation of Sensory and Excitatory Amino Acid Responses by Nitric Oxide Donors and Glutathione in the Ventrobasal Thalamus of the Rat. Eur J Neurosci 9:1507–1513
27. Sherman SM, Guillary RW (2000) Exploring the Thalamus. Academic Press, New York
28. Vincent SR (2000) The ascending reticular activating system – from aminergic neurons to nitric oxide. J Chem Neuroanat 18:23–30
29. Willis WD (2002) Long-term potentiation in spinothalamic neurons. Brain Res Rev 40:202–214

Nociceptive Pain

Definition

Pain caused by ongoing activation of Aδ and C nociceptors in response to a noxious stimulus of somatic or visceral structures such as inflammation, trauma, or disease.
- ▶ Analgesic Guidelines for Infants and Children
- ▶ Cancer Pain, Goals of a Comprehensive Assessment
- ▶ Cancer Pain Management, Treatment of Neuropathic Components

- ▶ Complex Chronic Pain in Children, Interdisciplinary Treatment
- ▶ Guillain-Barré Syndrome
- ▶ Opioids in Geriatric Application
- ▶ Opioid Responsiveness in Cancer Pain Management

Nociceptive Pathways

Definition

Neural circuits, including long sensory tracts, which convey information related to noxious stimuli are called nociceptive pathways. The consequences of nociceptive processing can include pain sensation, motivational-affective responses, reflex behavior, endocrine changes, and learning and memory of painful events.
- ▶ Nociceptive Circuitry in the Spinal Cord
- ▶ Spinothalamic Tract Neurons, Descending Control by Brainstem Neurons

Nociceptive Primary Afferents

N

Definition

Primary afferent neurons that respond to tissue damaging stimuli.
- ▶ Nociceptive Afferents
- ▶ Opioid receptors at postsynaptic sites

Nociceptive Processing in the Amygdala, Neurophysiology and Neuropharmacology

VOLKER NEUGEBAUER
Department of Neuroscience and Cell Biology, University of Texas Medical Branch, Galveston, TX, USA
voneugeb@utmb.edu

Synonyms

Amygdala, Nociceptive Processing

Definition

The amygdala is an almond-shaped structure in the medial temporal lobe and consists of several functionally and pharmacologically distinct nuclei. The central nucleus of the amygdala (CeA), which has been designated as the "▶ nociceptive amygdala", plays an important role in pain processing and pain modulation.

Characteristics

As part of the limbic system the amygdala plays a key role in attaching emotional significance to sensory stimuli, emotional learning and memory and affective states and disorders. The amygdala receives information from all sensory modalities; it also processes nociceptive information and projects to pain modulatory systems through forebrain and brainstem connections. Accumulating evidence suggests that the amygdala integrates nociceptive information with affective content, contributes to the emotional response to pain and serves as a neuronal interface for the reciprocal relationship between pain and affective states and disorders.

Anatomy and Circuitry

The amygdala includes at least 12 different nuclei. The lateral, basolateral, basomedial and central nuclei of the amygdala (LA, BLA, BMA and CeA, respectively) are of particular importance for the processing and evaluation of sensory information (Fig. 1). The LA is an in-

put region; receiving sensory information from the thalamus; particularly the posterior areas and cortex, including insular cortex and association cortical areas (LeDoux 2000; Neugebauer et al. 2004; Pare et al. 2004; Price 2003). The LA represents the initial site of sensory convergence, processing and associative learning and plasticity in the amygdala (LeDoux 2000; Pare et al. 2004; Shi and Davis 1999). This highly processed information, which is a key element of the fear- and anxiety-related circuitry, is then transmitted to other amygdaloid nuclei, including the CeA (LeDoux 2000; Neugebauer et al. 2004; Pare et al. 2004).

The CeA serves as the output nucleus of major amygdala functions. The CeA integrates inputs from other amygdala nuclei without forming reciprocal intra-amygdaloid connections. Sensory information reaches the CeA from the LA, either directly or indirectly, as well as from the brainstem (parabrachial area, PB) and spinal cord (Bernard et al. 1996; Burstein and Potrebic 1993; Gauriau and Bernard 2002; Neugebauer et al. 2004). Contextual representations are transmitted from the hippocampus to the CeA through the BLA and BMA (LeDoux 2000).

The CeA forms widespread connections with various forebrain and brainstem areas that are involved in emotional behavior and emotional experience and regulate autonomic and somatomotor functions. Targets of CeA projections include the cholinergic basal forebrain nuclei and the ► bed nucleus of the stria terminalis, midline and mediodorsal thalamic nuclei and paraventricular hypothalamus *via* the ► stria terminalis and lateral hypothalamus and brainstem areas such as periaqueductal gray (PAG) and parabrachial area (PB) *via* the ► ventral amygdaloid pathway (LeDoux 2000; Neugebauer et al. 2004; Price 2003).

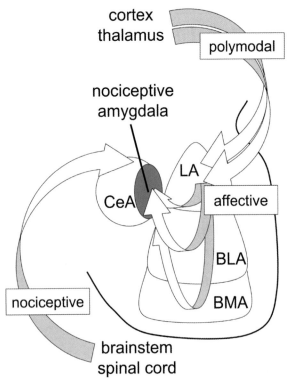

Nociceptive Processing in the Amygdala, Neurophysiology and Neuropharmacology, Figure 1 Circuitry of information processing in the principal sensory nuclei of the amygdala. The lateral nucleus of the amygdala (LA) receives and integrates polymodal information from thalamic and cortical areas. This highly processed information with affective content is then distributed to other amygdaloid nuclei, including the central nucleus (CeA), either directly or through the basolateral (BLA) and basomedial (BMA) nuclei. The CeA is the major output nucleus of the amygdala and forms widespread connections with forebrain and brainstem areas. The latero-capsular division of the CeA represents the "nociceptive amygdala".

Nociception and Nociceptive Plasticity

Within the CeA, the laterocapsular division is defined as the "nociceptive amygdala" because of the high content of neurons that respond exclusively or predominantly to ► noxious stimuli (Bernard et al. 1996; Neugebauer et al. 2004). The latero-capsular CeA receives nociceptive-specific information from the spinal cord and brainstem through the spino-parabrachio-amygdaloid pain pathway (Bernard et al. 1996; Gauriau and Bernard 2002) as well as through direct projections from the spinal cord (Burstein and Potrebic 1993).

Electrophysiological single-unit analysis in anesthetized rats has shown several characteristics of neurons in the nociceptive amygdala (Bernard et al. 1996; Gauriau and Bernard 2002; Neugebauer et al. 2004; Neugebauer and Li 2002). The majority of these neurons (80%) respond either exclusively ("nociceptive-specific" [NS] neurons) or predominantly ("multireceptive" [MR] neurons) to noxious stimuli. More neurons are excited than inhibited by noxious stimuli. A significant number of "non-responsive" (NR) neurons (up to 20%) also exist in the latero-capsular CeA; they do not respond to somatic stimuli. NS and MR CeA neurons have large, mostly symmetrical bilateral receptive fields in the superficial and deep tissue; they respond to mechanical and thermal stimuli. Their stimulus-response functions are not monotonically increasing linearly but sigmoidaly. These properties argue against a sensory-discriminative function of CeA neurons. Among neurons with predominantly cutaneous input, there appear to be more NS than MR neurons whereas a larger percentage of MR neurons can be found among neurons with receptive fields mainly in the deep tissue. It is believed that NS neurons receive input from the spino-parabrachio-amygdaloid pathway whereas MR neurons integrate nociceptive information with affective content from the polymodal LA-BLA circuitry (Fig. 1).

Accumulating evidence now suggests that neurons in the nociceptive amygdala develop plasticity in models of persistent inflammatory pain such as arthritis and colitis (Bird et al. 2005; Han and Neugebauer 2004; Han et al. 2005; Neugebauer and Li 2003; Neugebauer et al. 2003). Extracellular single-unit recordings in anesthetized rats showed that MR neurons and NR neurons, but not NS neurons, become sensitized to afferent inputs in a model of arthritis pain induced in one knee joint by the intraarticular injection of kaolin and carrageenan. Characteristics of the pain-related sensitization of MR neurons are as follows: the processing of mechanical, but not thermal, pain-related information is increased (upward shift of the stimulus-response functions); responses to stimulation of the arthritic knee as well as of non-injured tissue in other parts of the body are enhanced; the total size of the receptive field expands; a constant input evoked by orthodromic electrical stimulation in the PB produces greater activation; background activity is increased. Unlike changes in the peripheral nervous system and spinal cord in this arthritis model, changes in MR amygdala neurons develop with a biphasic time course; the first phase (1–3 h) reflects changes at the spinal cord and brainstem levels whereas the persistent plateau phase (>5 h) involves intra-amygdala plasticity. MR neurons serve to integrate and evaluate sensory-affective information in the context of pain. NS neurons would continue to distinguish between noxious and ▶ Innocuous Input/Stimulus at the stage of plasticity.

Evidence that the sensitization of amygdala neurons involves plastic changes within the amygdala comes from electrophysiological studies in brain slices *in vitro*. Coronal slices containing the amygdala were obtained from normal rats, from rats with a ▶ Kaolin-Carrageenan Induced Arthritis and from rats with a zymosan-induced colitis (Han and Neugebauer 2004; Han et al. 2004; Neugebauer et al. 2003). Whole-cell patch-clamp recordings in slices from rats with arthritis or colitis (6 h post induction) showed enhanced synap-

tic transmission and increased neuronal excitability of CeA neurons with input from the PB and from the BLA (resembling the MR neurons *in vivo*). Synaptic plasticity in the reduced preparation is thus maintained at least in part independently of continuous input from the site of the somatic or visceral inflammation.

Pharmacology of Nociception and Plasticity

The roles of ionotropic and metabotropic glutamate receptors in brief nociceptive processing and persistent pain have been studied in CeA neurons.

Ionotropic Glutamate Receptors (Bird et al. 2005; Li and Neugebauer 2004b)

Extracellular single-unit recordings of CeA neurons in anesthetized animals showed that non-NMDA receptors are involved in the responses to innocuous and brief (15 s) noxious stimuli whereas NMDA receptors contribute only to the processing of nociceptive information. In the kaolin / carrageenan arthritis pain model (6 h post induction), activation of NMDA and non-NMDA receptors is required for the pain-related sensitization of CeA neurons. In these studies, antagonists at NMDA receptors (AP5) and non-NMDA (NBQX) receptors were administered into the CeA by microdialysis.

Pain-related synaptic plasticity recorded (patch-clamp) in the CeA in brain slices from arthritic rats involves enhanced function of postsynaptic NMDA receptors through PKA-dependent phosphorylation of the NR1 subunit.

Metabotropic Glutamate Receptors (Li and Neugebauer 2004a; Neugebauer et al. 2003)

Electrophysiological studies of amygdala neurons *in vivo* and *in vitro* have shown an important role of group I metabotropic glutamate receptors (mGluRs), which include the mGluR1 and mGluR5 subtypes and couple to G-proteins to activate phospholipase C, PKC and MAP kinases such as ERK. Extracellular single-unit recordings of CeA neurons in anesthetized rats suggest a change of mGluR1 function in the amygdala in pain-related sensitization, whereas mGluR5 is involved in brief as well as prolonged nociception. Activation of group I mGluR1 and mGluR5 by the agonist DHPG enhances the responses of CeA neurons to brief (15 s) innocuous and noxious stimuli under normal conditions. This effect can be mimicked by an mGluR5 agonist (CHPG). In the kaolin / carrageenan arthritis pain model (6 h post induction), the facilitatory effects of DHPG, but not CHPG, increased. Block of mGluR1 by CPCCOEt inhibits the responses of sensitized CeA neurons in the arthritis pain state but has no effect under normal conditions before arthritis. An mGluR5 antagonist (MPEP) inhibits both brief nociceptive responses under normal conditions and prolonged nociception in the arthritis pain model. Agonists and antagonists were administered into the CeA by microdialysis. The roles of group II and III mGluRs in nociception and plasticity in the amygdala are not yet clear.

The contribution of group I mGluRs to normal synaptic transmission and pain-related synaptic plasticity in the amygdala was analyzed in brain slices *in vitro* using whole-cell voltage-clamp recordings of neurons in the nociceptive amygdala (Neugebauer et al. 2003). Synaptic transmission was studied at the nociceptive PB-CeA synapse and the polymodal-affective BLA-CeA synapse (Fig. 1). A group I mGluR1 and mGluR5 agonist (DHPG) and a mGluR5 agonist (CHPG) potentiate normal synaptic transmission similarly in CeA neurons in slices from normal rats. In slices from arthritic rats (6 h post induction), the effects of DHPG, but not CHPG, are increased, suggesting an enhanced function of mGluR1 rather than mGluR5. Block of mGluR1 with an antagonist (CPCCOEt) has no effect on synaptic transmission in CeA neurons in slices from normal rats but inhibits synaptic plasticity in slices from arthritic rats. An mGluR5 antagonist (MPEP) inhibits basal synaptic transmission in CeA neurons in slices from normal rats and synaptic plasticity in slices from arthritic rats. Thus, enhanced receptor activation of mGluR1 appears to be a key mechanism of pain-related synaptic plasticity in the CeA. Importantly, these agents had no effect on membrane properties and neuronal excitability but affected paired-pulse facilitation, suggesting a pre- rather than post-synaptic site of action. These data suggest that pain-related plastic changes in the amygdala involve a critical switch of presynaptic mGluR1 function.

Pain Modulation by the Amygdala

As part of the pain system and a key player in affective states and disorders, the amygdala contributes to the emotional response to pain and its modulation by affective state (Fig. 2). The CeA, including the latero-capsular division, forms direct and indirect connections with descending pain-modulating systems in the brainstem (Neugebauer et al. 2004). Descending pain control can be facilitatory (pro-nociceptive) and inhibitory (anti-nociceptive) (Gebhart 2004; Heinricher and McGaraughty 1999). Recent behavioral studies suggest that the consequence of pain-related plasticity in the CeA is increased pain. Pharmacologic inactivation of the CeA with mGluR1, mGluR5 or CGRP1 receptor antagonists inhibited pain behavior of arthritic rats (Han and Neugebauer 2005; Han et al. 2005).

Activity in the amygdala can be modified by negative and positive emotions, which in turn are known to reduce (stress, fear; music) or enhance (anxiety) pain (Fig. 2). The dependence of amygdala activity on affective state and the dual coupling of the amygdala to inhibitory and facilitatory pain control may explain some of the differential effects of amygdala stimulation and / or activation on pain behavior.

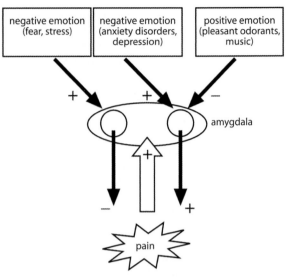

Nociceptive Processing in the Amygdala, Neurophysiology and Neuropharmacology, Figure 2 Pain, emotions, and the amygdala: a hypothetical model. Pain produces plastic changes in the amygdala. Affective states also modify activity in the amygdala; negative emotions generally increase amygdala activity, whereas positive emotions have been shown to deactivate the amygdala. The amygdala is linked to facilitatory and inhibitory pathways to modulate pain. Negative emotions associated with pain reduction (fear and stress) would activate amygdala-linked inhibitory control systems, whereas negative affective states that correlate with increased pain (depression and anxiety disorders) would activate pain-facilitating pathways. Positive emotions inhibit amygdala coupling to pain facilitation. Reprinted with permission of Sage Publications, Inc., from Neugebauer et al. (2004) The amygdala and persistent pain. Neuroscientist 10, p 232.

References

1. Bernard J-F, Bester H, Besson JM (1996) Involvement of the spino-parabrachio -amygdaloid and -hypothalamic pathways in the autonomic and affective emotional aspects of pain. Prog Brain Res 107:243–255
2. Bird GC, Lash LL, Han JS, Zou X, Willis WD, Neugebauer (2005) PKA-dependent enhanced NMDA receptor function in pain-related synaptic plasticity in amygdala neurons. J Physiol 564.3:907–921
3. Burstein R, Potrebic S (1993) Retrograde labeling of neurons in the spinal cord that project directly to the amygdala or the orbital cortex in the rat. J Comp Neurol 335:469–485
4. Gauriau C, Bernard J-F (2002) Pain pathways and parabrachial circuits in the rat. Exp Physiol 87:251–258
5. Gebhart GF (2004) Descending modulation of pain. Neurosci Biobehav Rev 27:729–737
6. Han JS, Neugebauer V (2004) Synaptic plasticity in the amygdala in a visceral pain model in rats. Neurosci Lett 361:254–257
7. Han JS, Neugebauer V (2005) mGluR1 and mGluR5 antagonists in the amygdala inhibit different components of audible and ultrasonic vocalizations in a model of arthritic pain. Pain. 113:211–222
8. Han JS, Bird GC, Neugebauer V (2004) Enhanced group III mGluR-mediated inhibition of pain-related synaptic plasticity in the amygdala. Neuropharmacology 46:918–926
9. Han JS, Li W, Neugebauer V (2005) Critical role of calcitonin gene-related peptide 1 receptors in the amygdala in synaptic plasticity and pain behavior. J Neurosci 25:10717–28
10. Heinricher MM, McGaraughty S (1999) Pain-modulating neurons and behavioral state. In: Lydic R, Baghdoyan HA (eds) Handbook of Behavioral State Control. CRC Press, New York, pp 487–503

11. LeDoux JE (2000) Emotion circuits in the brain. Annu Rev Neurosci 23:155–184
12. Li W, Neugebauer V (2004a) Differential roles of mGluR1 and mGluR5 in brief and prolonged nociceptive processing in central amygdala neurons. J Neurophysiol 91:13–24
13. Li W, Neugebauer V (2004b) Block of NMDA and non-NMDA receptor activation results in reduced background and evoked activity of central amygdala neurons in a model of arthritic pain. Pain 110:112–122
14. Neugebauer V, Li W (2002) Processing of nociceptive mechanical and thermal information in central amygdala neurons with knee-joint input. J Neurophysiol 87:103–112
15. Neugebauer V, Li W (2003) Differential sensitization of amygdala neurons to afferent inputs in a model of arthritic pain. J Neurophysiol 89:716–727
16. Neugebauer V, Li W, Bird GC et al. (2003) Synaptic plasticity in the amygdala in a model of arthritic pain: differential roles of metabotropic glutamate receptors 1 and 5. J Neurosci 23:52–63
17. Neugebauer V, Li W, Bird GC et al. (2004) The amygdala and persistent pain. Neuroscientist 10:221–234
18. Pare D, Quirk GJ, Ledoux JE (2004) New vistas on amygdala networks in conditioned fear. J Neurophysiol 92:1–9
19. Price JL (2003) Comparative aspects of amygdala connectivity. In: Shinnick-Gallagher P, Pitkanen A, Shekhar A et al (eds) The amygdala in brain function. Basic and clinical approaches, vol 985. The New York Academy of Sciences, New York, pp 50–58
20. Shi C, Davis M (1999) Pain pathways involved in fear conditioning measured with fear-potentiated startle: lesion studies. J Neurosci 19:420–430

Nociceptive Processing in the Cingulate Cortex, Behavioral Studies in Animals

▶ Cingulate Cortex, Nociceptive Processing, Behavioral Studies in Animals

Nociceptive Processing in the Cingulate Cortex, Behavioral Studies in Human

▶ Pain Processing in the Cingulate Cortex, Behavioral Studies in Humans

Nociceptive Processing in the Hippocampus and Entorhinal Cortex, Neurophysiology and Pharmacology

SANJAY KHANNA
Department of Physiology, National University of Singapore, Singapore
phsks@nus.edu.sg

Definition

The hippocampus is the simplest part of the cortex, the ▶ allocortex, which, in humans, is arched around the mesencephalon, while in rodents it arches over the thalamus (Amaral and Witter 1995). The various fields of the hippocampus and its layers are illustrated in Figure 1. The principal neurons in the hippocampus are

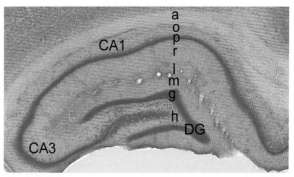

Nociceptive Processing in the Hippocampus and Entorhinal Cortex, Neurophysiology and Pharmacology, Figure 1 Digitized image of Nissl stained transverse section taken through dorsal hippocampus and dentate gyrus (DG) of rat. The hippocampus is sub-divided into various fields, of which the prominent ones are CA1 and CA3. In a dorsal to ventral order in the transverse section, the layers of the hippocampus and DG are: a, alveus (which is as a fiber bundle marking the outer boundary of the hippocampus); o, stratum oriens; p, stratum pyramidale; r, stratum radiatum; l, stratum lacunosum-moleculare; m, stratum moleculare; g, stratum granulosum; h, hilus.

the ▶ pyramidal cells that are localized in the stratum pyramidale (Fig. 1).

Both anatomical and physiological studies suggest that the entorhinal cortex is a major source of afferent input to the hippocampus, either directly or indirectly via the dentate gyrus (Amaral and Witter 1995). Indeed, stimulation of perforant path fibers from the entorhinal cortex evokes both short- and long-latency excitatory responses in CA1, which are suggested to involve direct entorhinal to CA1 projection, and a ▶ sequential relay from the entorhinal cortex to CA1 via the dentate gyrus and CA3, respectively.

Characteristics

Melzack and Casey (1968) proposed that the limbic forebrain structures, including the hippocampus, are involved in 'aversive drive and affect that comprise the motivational dimension of pain'. Indeed, lesions of the hippocampus-dentate gyrus region reduce aversive foot shock-induced ▶ conditioned place avoidance (Selden et al. 1991), while intra-hippocampal administration of a NMDA receptor antagonist attenuated nociceptive behaviors to hind paw injection of the algogen formalin (▶ formalin test), a model of persistent clinical inflammatory pain (McKenna and Melzack 2001). Consistent with a role in affect-motivation, a functional magnetic resonance imaging study reported that the anxiety-induced hyperalgesia in man was associated with bilateral activation in the entorhinal area, which correlated with activity in anterior cingulate cortex and insular cortex (Ploghaus et al. 2001). Furthermore, the hippocampus was also activated on peripheral application of high intensity noxious heat stimulation, relative to similar application of the stimulus at a lower intensity (Ploghaus et al. 2001). Indeed, and consistent with a role as a central intensity monitor, electrophys-

N

Nociceptive Processing in the Brainstem

JONATHAN O. DOSTROVSKY[1],
BARRY J. SESSLE[1, 2]
[1]Department of Physiology, Faculty of Medicine,
University of Toronto, Toronto, ON, Canada
[2]Faculty of Dentistry, University of Toronto,
Toronto, ON, Canada
j.dostrovsky@utoronto.ca,
barry.sessle@utoronto.ca

Introduction

The craniofacial region is principally innervated by the trigeminal (V) nerve, which terminates in the trigeminal brainstem nuclear complex (TBNC). The caudal portion of the TBNC is largely homologous to the spinal cord dorsal horn in terms of anatomy, neurochemistry and physiology and is termed the subnucleus caudalis (Vc) or medullary dorsal horn. It is the major region involved in the processing of pain and temperature sensations from the head. However, the more rostrally located subnuclei interpolaris (Vi) and oralis (Vo) also receive some nociceptive afferents and contain neurons responding to noxious stimuli. There is evidence that these subnuclei contribute to the perception of pain and especially pain of intraoral origin. There is no obvious homologous region in the spinal cord.

The craniofacial region contains several unique structures which include the tooth pulp and the cornea, as well as several other deep and intraoral tissues such as the temporomandibular joint (TMJ), the intracranial meninges and vessels and the intraoral mucosa. Pathological changes in these structures or their central representations can result in several pain conditions unique to the trigeminal region and these are described in the field ► orofacial pain. There is mounting evidence for sex differences in pain and analgesia, e.g. temporomandibular disorders (TMD) and migraine headaches are much more prevalent in females. Experimental studies in both animals and humans are revealing clear sex differences in peripheral and central neural processes underlying craniofacial nociception (e.g. Cairns et al. 2003; Okamoto et al. 2003). For further details see ► trigeminal brainstem nuclear complex, anatomy ► trigeminal brainstem nuclear complex, physiology ► trigeminal brainstem nuclear complex ► immunohistochemistry and neurochemistry ► nociceptors in the dental pulp ► ocular nociceptors ► nociceptors in the orofacial region (temporomandibular joint and masseter muscle) ► nociceptors in the orofacial region (meningeal/cerebrovascular) ► nociceptors in the orofacial Region (skin/mucosa).

Role of the Vc in Orofacial Nociceptive Processing

Several of the essays point out that most of the small diameter trigeminal (V) primary afferents terminate in the Vc, which is a laminated structure with many morphological and functional similarities with the spinal dorsal horn (although see below). There are 7 lines of evidence that the Vc is critical in V brainstem nociceptive processing. These include a direct projection to higher brain centers involved in pain perception and other aspects of pain behavior. In addition, by virtue of these ascending projections, the Vc has recently been documented to be essential for the expression of central sensitization in rostral elements of the V brainstem complex and ventrobasal thalamus (e.g. the Vo) (Chiang et al. 2002; Chiang et al. 2003). The extensive range of convergent afferent inputs to the Vc contributes to the development of the central sensitization that can be induced by inflammation or injury of peripheral tissues or nerves. Moreover, most Vc nociceptive neurons have in addition to a cutaneous receptive field (RF) also a deep RF (e.g. in the TMJ, muscle, tooth pulp, dura). The particular efficacy of deep nociceptive afferent inputs in inducing central sensitization, including an expansion of both their cutaneous and deep RFs, represent neuronal properties that may explain the poor localization of deep pain, as well as contribute to the spread and referral of pains that are typical of deep pain conditions such as TMD, toothaches and headaches (see ► orofacial pain).

The neurons in the Trigeminal Complex (TBNC) and particularly those in the Vc are subject to modulatory influences originating locally within the Vc or in more rostral parts of the complex as well as descending modulatory influences from brainstem, in particular the rostral ventromedial medulla (RVM) (Dubner and Ren 2004). These descending influences are very similar to those directed at the spinal dorsal horn and are described in ► descending modulation of nociceptive processing.

As mentioned above, a unique feature of the V system is the processing of nociceptive inputs from afferents supplying structures not found elsewhere in the body; these include the tooth pulp, periodontal tissues, cornea and nasal mucosa. Another unique feature is the dual organization of the Vc in the representation of some orofacial tissues. Some noxious stimuli (e.g. to cornea or TMJ) evoke a bimodal distribution of c-fos labeled neurons in the Vc that includes c-fos expression in the rostral Vc / caudal Vi transitional zone as well as in the transitional region between the caudal part of the Vc and the upper cervical spinal cord (see Bereiter et al. 2000; Dubner and Ren 2004). These findings are consistent with electrophysiological evidence of neurons responsive to corneal or TMJ inputs in one or both of these regions. The caudal Vc merges without clear boundaries with the cervical dorsal horn, while the rostral Vc forms a distinctive transition region with the Vi. This transition region has a ventral Vi / Vc transition area, which is especially clear in rodents, and a dorsomedial transition area. It is becoming apparent that these 2 areas of the rostral Vc and the caudal Vc each have their own unique morphological and functional features that may be differentially involved in contributing to perceptual, autonomic, endocrine and muscle reflex responses to noxious stimulation of different orofacial tissues, in particular involving ophthalmic structures (Bereiter et al. 2000; Dubner and Ren 2004).

Further investigation of these different areas within the Vc, as well as caudal to the Vc, is needed to determine their specific functional roles in orofacial pain processes. It has been over 50 years since the trigeminal spinal nucleus was divided into Vo, Vi and Vc subdivisions and over 25 years since the structural homologies between the Vc and the spinal dorsal horn were emphasized. These studies have shaped discussions of the special relationship between the Vc and craniofacial pain (see Sessle 2000; Sessle 2005), although this useful homology may need some revision as recent evidence cited above indicates that select portions of the Vc are organized differently from the spinal system. The region ventral to the Vc, which is part of the medullary reticular formation and is outside the main projection area of trigeminal primary afferents, also contains neurons that respond to noxious facial stimulation. Their receptive fields are usually larger than those in Vc, often bilateral and sometimes include the entire body (e.g. see Fujino et al. 1996; Nord and Kyler 1968; Yokota et al. 1991). In the rat, a population of neurons with large nociceptive receptive fields including the face is located in the subnucleus reticularis dorsalis. It has been suggested that this region is involved in circuits mediating ► diffuse noxious inhibitory controls (Villanueva et al. 1996).

Role of Rostral Components of V Brainstem Complex

Morphological, physiological, neurochemical and behavioral evidence support the involvement of more rostral components of the TBNC in orofacial nociceptive processing, especially in the case of the Vo. For example, lesions of rostral components may disrupt some pain behaviors and substantial numbers of NS and WDR neurons exist in the rostral components. These neurons have cutaneous RFs that are usually localized to intraoral or perioral areas and many can be activated by tooth pulp stimulation. These findings have raised the possibility that the rostral nociceptive neurons, particularly those in the Vo, are principally involved in intraoral and perioral nociceptive processing. Moreover, it is probable that their nociceptive afferent inputs are predominantly relayed through more caudal regions, such as the Vc, which exerts a considerable modulatory influence over Vo nociceptive processes. Although some rostral neurons may directly receive primary afferent inputs from the tooth pulp, it is not clear that these inputs are nociceptive. How then can nociceptive phenomena occur in the rostral components when, especially in the case of the Vo, they lack an anatomical and in many instances a neurochemical substrate generally considered necessary for nociceptive processing? One possible explanation is that these substrates, although typical of the Vc and the spinal dorsal horn, are not essential for all types of nociceptive phenomena. In support of this possibility are the observations that nociceptive neurons contributing to nociceptive behavior occur in some spinal cord and brainstem areas devoid of some of these substrates (e.g. lateral cervical nucleus, reticular formation) (Dubner and Bennett 1983).

Another explanation lies in the anatomical and neurochemical framework for nociceptive processing that typifies the Vc and in its ascending projections to the rostral components of the TBNC. Parada et al. (1997) have argued that the cutaneous C fiber related nociceptive responses of Vo cutaneous nociceptive neurons that can be blocked by systemic administration of the NMDA antagonist MK-801 may depend on the well-documented ascending projection from the Vc that exerts a net facilitatory modulatory influence on Vo neurons (for review see Sessle 2000), since the Vc does have the features (NMDA receptors, C-fiber afferent terminals, substantia gelatinosa) considered necessary for these nociceptive phenomena. Furthermore, local application of MK-801 or morphine to the Vc can block the C-fiber related activity of some Vo nociceptive neurons. An analogous argument has also been used as an explanation for the neuroplastic changes that have been documented in the Vo and in the main sensory nucleus subsequent to C-fiber depletion induced by the neonatal application of capsaicin. Nonetheless, MK-801 applied directly to the Vo itself can antagonize Vo nociceptive neuronal changes induced by afferent inputs evoked from the tooth pulp (Park et al. 2001), which suggests that NMDA receptor mechanisms do operate within the Vo (see Sessle 2000 for references and further details).

Collectively, these various findings raise the possibility that, on the one hand, the cutaneous RF and response properties of rostral nociceptive neurons, particularly in the Vo, may be dependent on caudal regions such as the Vc for the relay of nociceptive signals from primary afferents supplying superficial craniofacial tissues. On the other hand, some of the extensive pulp afferent inputs to and effects upon neurons in the rostral TBNC may be dependent on relays in both rostral and caudal components. Such a view, nonetheless, is still largely speculative and the relative roles of the rostral and caudal TBNC components, not only in cutaneous nociceptive mechanisms but also in nociceptive responses to noxious stimulation of deep craniofacial tissues and tooth pulp, represent an important issue requiring further research.

Ascending Projections and Higher Level Processing of Trigeminal Nociceptive Inputs

The nociceptive signals from the TBNC are relayed on to higher levels and in particular to the thalamus and from there to cerebral cortex. The thalamus receives direct contralateral input from each of the TBNC subnuclei (Kemplay and Webster 1989; Mantle-St John and Tracey 1987). The majority of the TBNC neurons projecting to the contralateral thalamus are found in the trigeminal principal nucleus, terminate in the ventroposterior medial nucleus (VPM) and are primarily involved in tactile sensation. The remaining neurons are located in the Vi, the Vo and the Vc. However, the major thalamic projection related to pain and temperature perception arises from neurons in the contralateral Vc and is equivalent to the spinothalamic tract (for references see Discussion in Craig 2004).

The trigeminothalamic neurons in the Vc are located primarily in laminae I and V. Those in lamina V have a major projection to the VPM (or its borders in the cat), but those in lamina I terminate in several other regions, which are species dependent. For example, in the monkey, lamina I neurons project primarily to the posterior ventromedial nucleus (VMpo) as well as to the ventrocaudal medialis dorsalis (MDvc), but have only a sparse projection to the VPM (Craig 2004). In the cat, the main projections of lamina I neurons are to the ventral border of the VPM and adjacent nuclei, the dorsomedial VPM and the nucleus submedius (Craig 2003). In the rat, lamina I neurons project largely to the VPM, the nucleus submedius, the posterior nucleus and the posterior triangular nucleus (Iwata et al. 1992; Jasmin et al. 2004; Yoshida et al. 1991).

The main cortical targets of thalamic nuclei receiving nociceptive inputs are the insula, the primary and secondary somatosensory cortices and the cingulate. There are extensive connections between cortex and thalamus, which play an important although poorly understood role in processing nociceptive inputs. Most of the electrophysiological studies on responses of thalamic and cortical neurons to noxious stimuli have focused on inputs from the limbs and have revealed neurons with both NS and WDR type responses. These responses are generally similar to those of neurons in the spinal dorsal horn and the trigeminal Vc, but tend to have increased and fluctuating spontaneous activity (see reviews by Kenshalo and Willis 1991; Willis

1997). Sections ► Nociceptive Processing in the Thalamus and ► Cortical and Limbic Mechanisms Mediating Pain and Pain-Related Behavior provide further details of the roles of thalamus and cortex in pain.

In addition to the thalamus, TBNC neurons also project to several diencephalic and brain stem areas that are involved in regulation of autonomic, endocrine, affective and motor functions. In the rat, all TBNC subnuclei contain neurons that project directly to the hypothalamus (Malick and Burstein 1998). Most of these hypothalamic tract neurons in the Vc and C1-2 respond preferentially or exclusively to noxious mechanical and thermal stimulation to the facial skin and to electrical, mechanical and chemical stimulation of the dura mater (Burstein et al. 1998). There also are projections from the TBNC to the parabrachial and Kölliker-Fuse nuclei (Bernard et al. 1989; Feil and Herbert 1995; Hayashi and Tabata 1990). In particular, neurons in the Vc, including those in the superficial laminae, project to the external portion of the lateral parabrachial area, where many respond exclusively to noxious stimuli (Hayashi and Tabata 1990). It has been proposed that this projection is part of a trigeminopontoamygdaloid pathway involved in the affective, behavioral and autonomic reactions to noxious stimuli (Bernard et al. 1989). Anatomical studies also have shown that there are projections from the TBNC to the adjacent reticular formation, the RVM, the periaqueductal gray, various brain stem autonomic nuclei, the superior colliculus, the ipsilateral cerebellum, the contralateral inferior olive and the nucleus of the solitary tract (Bruce et al. 1987; Craig 1995; Jacquin et al. 1989; Mantle-St John and Tracey 1987; Marfurt and Rajchert 1991; Keay and Bandler 1998; Renehan et al. 1986). Several of these projections are likely to be important in mediating nonperceptual (e.g. autonomic) effects elicited by nociceptive stimuli.

In summary, a great deal of information regarding the representation and processing of craniofacial nociceptive inputs in the TBNC and higher levels has been gained in recent years. Although there are many similarities between the spinal and trigeminal systems, there are also some important differences and some of these relate to unique structures and likely contribute to these pain conditions that are unique to this region. Nevertheless, there are still important gaps in our knowledge and further experimental studies are necessary to fully understand the mechanisms underlying the normal and pathological processing in the TBNC of nociceptive inputs from the craniofacial region.

References

1. Bereiter DA, Hirata H, Hu JW (2000) Trigeminal subnucleus caudalis: beyond homologies with the spinal dorsal horn. Pain 88:221–224

2. Bernard JF, Peschanski M, Besson JM (1989) A possible spino (trigemino)-ponto-amygdaloid pathway for pain. Neurosci Lett 100:83–88
3. Bruce LL, McHaffie JG, Stein BE (1987) The organization of trigeminotectal and trigeminothalamic neurons in rodents: a double-labeling study with fluorescent dyes. J Comp Neurol 262:315–330
4. Burstein R, Yamamura H, Malick A et al. (1998) Chemical stimulation of the intracranial dura induces enhanced responses to facial stimulation in brain stem trigeminal neurons. J Neurophysiol 79:964–982
5. Cairns BE, Wang K, Hu JW et al. (2003) The effect of glutamate-evoked masseter muscle pain on the human jaw-stretch reflex differs in men and women. J Orofac Pain 17:317–325
6. Chiang CY, Hu B, Hu JW et al. (2002) Central sensitization of nociceptive neurons in trigeminal subnucleus oralis depends on integrity of subnucleus caudalis. J Neurophysiol 88:256–264
7. Chiang CY, Hu B, Park SJ et al. (2003) Purinergic and NMDA-receptor mechanisms underlying tooth pulp stimulation-induced central sensitization in trigeminal nociceptive neurons. Proceedings of the 10th World Congress on Pain. IASP Press, Seattle, pp 345–354
8. Craig AD (1995) Distribution of brainstem projections from spinal lamina I neurons in the cat and the monkey. J Comp Neurol 361:225–248
9. Craig AD (2003) Distribution of trigeminothalamic and spinothalamic lamina I terminations in the cat. Somatosens Mot Res 20:209–222
10. Craig AD (2004) Distribution of trigeminothalamic and spinothalamic lamina I terminations in the macaque monkey. J Comp Neurol 477:119–148
11. Dubner R, Bennett GJ (1983) Spinal and trigeminal mechanisms of nociception. Annu Rev Neurosci 6:381–418
12. Dubner R, Ren K (2004) Brainstem mechanisms of persistent pain following injury. J Orofacial Pain 18:299–305
13. Feil K, Herbert H (1995) Topographic organization of spinal and trigeminal somatosensory pathways to the rat parabrachial and Kolliker-Fuse nuclei. J Comp Neurol 353:506–528
14. Fujino Y, Koyama N, Yokota T (1996) Differential distribution of three types of nociceptive neurons within the caudal bulbar reticular formation in the cat. Brain Res 715:225–229
15. Hayashi H, Tabata T (1990) Pulpal and cutaneous inputs to somatosensory neurons in the parabrachial area of the cat. Brain Res 511:177–179
16. Iwata K, Kenshalo DR Jr, Dubner R et al. (1992) Diencephalic projections from the superficial and deep laminae of the medullary dorsal horn in the rat. J Comp Neurol 321:404–420
17. Jacquin MF, Barcia M, Rhoades RW (1989) Structure-function relationships in rat brainstem subnucleus interpolaris: IV. Projection neurons. J Comp Neurol 282:45–62
18. Jasmin L, Granato A, Ohara PT (2004) Rostral agranular insular cortex and pain areas of the central nervous system: a tract-tracing study in the rat. J Comp Neurol 468:425–440

19. Keay KA, Bandler R (1998) Vascular head pain selectively activates ventrolateral periaqueductal gray in the cat. Neurosci Lett 245:58–60
20. Kemplay S, Webster KE (1989) A quantitative study of the projections of the gracile, cuneate and trigeminal nuclei and of the medullary reticular formation to the thalamus in the rat. Neuroscience 32:153–167
21. Kenshalo DR Jr, Willis WD Jr (1991) The role of the cerebral cortex in pain sensation. In: Jones EG, Peters A (eds) Cerebral Cortex. Plenum, New York, pp 151–212
22. Malick A, Burstein R (1998) Cells of origin of the trigemino-nohypothalamic tract in the rat. J Comp Neurol 400:125–144
23. Mantle-St John LA, Tracey DJ (1987) Somatosensory nuclei in the brainstem of the rat: independent projections to the thalamus and cerebellum. J Comp Neurol 255:259–271
24. Marfurt CF, Rajchert DM (1991) Trigeminal primary afferent projections to "non-trigeminal" areas of the rat central nervous system. J Comp Neurol 303:489–511
25. Nord SG, Kyler HJ (1968) A single unit analysis of trigeminal projections to bulbar reticular nuclei of the rat. J Comp Neurol 134:485–494
26. Okamoto K, Hirata H, Takeshita S et al. (2003) Response properties of TMJ units in superficial laminae at the spinomedullary junction of female rats vary over the estrous cycle. J Neurophysiol 89:1467–1477
27. Parada CA, Luccarini P, Woda A (1997) Effect of an NMDA receptor antagonist on the wind-up of neurons in the trigeminal oralis subnucleus. Brain Res 761:313–320
28. Park SJ, Chiang CY, Hu JW et al. (2001) Neuroplasticity induced by tooth pulp stimulation in trigeminal subnucleus oralis involves NMDA receptor mechanisms. J Neurophysiol 85:1836–1846
29. Sessle BJ (2005) Orofacial pain. In: Merskey H (ed) Pathways of Pain. IASP Press, Seattle
30. Sessle BJ (2000) Acute and chronic craniofacial pain: brainstem mechanisms of nociceptive transmission and neuroplasticity, and their clinical correlates. Crit Rev Oral Biol Med 11:57–91
31. Villanueva L, Bouhassira D, Le BD (1996) The medullary subnucleus reticularis dorsalis (SRD) as a key link in both the transmission and modulation of pain signals. Pain 67:231–240
32. Willis WD Jr (1997) Nociceptive functions of thalamic neurons. In: Steriade M, Jones EG, McCormick DA (eds) Thalamus, Volume II Experimental and Clinical Aspects. Elsevier Science Ltd, Oxford, pp 373–424
33. Yokota T, Koyama N, Nishikawa Y et al. (1991) Trigeminal nociceptive neurons in the subnucleus reticularis ventralis. I. Response properties and afferent connections. Neurosci Res 11:117
34. Yoshida A, Dostrovsky JO, Sessle BJ et al. (1991) Trigeminal projections to the nucleus submedius of the thalamus in the rat. J Comp Neurol 307:609–625

N

iological studies conducted in anaesthetized rat provided evidence that noxious stimulus evoked intensity-dependent changes in ▶ excitability of CA1 pyramidal cells (Khanna and Sinclair 1989, Wei et al. 2000) that were ▶ non-topographic (Khanna and Sinclair 1992). Interestingly, Khanna (1997) reported that following hind paw injection of formalin, a population of dorsal CA1 putative pyramidal cells was selectively excited against the background of widespread pyramidal cell suppression, reflecting 'signal-to-noise' processing by the hippocampal network that enhanced the 'signal' to noxious stimulus relative to 'background' noise. Such processing was observed in correlation with ▶ theta ▶ rhythm (Khanna 1997), which is sinusoidal rhythmic extracellular oscillations that reflect rhythmic oscillations of CA1 neurons in processing of information. Hippocampal theta activation has been linked to ▶ sensorimotor integration and animal motivated behavior (Bland and Oddie 2001). In addition, CA1 'signal-to-noise' processing, in parallel with theta activation, has been linked to ▶ mnemonic function of the hippocampus (Buzsaki 1989). In this context, a noxious stimuli-induced increase in levels of the transcription protein Egr1 has been observed in the hippocampus, especially in field CA1 (Wei et al. 2000). The enhanced level of Egr1 in CA1 was linked to facilitation of ▶ long-term potentiation (LTP) of excitatory synaptic transmission in the region (Wei et al. 2000), LTP being a cellular model of learning and memory.

Consistent with findings from electrophysiological studies, ▶ c-Fos mapping techniques in anaesthetized and behaving rats also indicated that neural changes in hippocampus, especially field CA1 and medial entorhinal cortex, are noxious intensity-dependent (Funahashi et al. 1999, Khanna et al. 2004). The changes in CA1 were bilateral and were observed along the length of the region. However, the noxious stimuli-induced effect in entorhinal cortex was significant only ipsilateral to the stimuli, though a trend was also observed in the contralateral entorhinal cortex (Funahashi et al. 1999).

A role for acetylcholine in hippocampal nociceptive processing has been proposed. In this context, acetylcholine is released in the hippocampus in the formalin test (Ceccareli et al. 1999), and intra-hippocampal administration of the muscarinic antagonist, atropine, attenuates peripheral noxious heat-induced suppression of CA1 pyramidal cell synaptic excitability (Zheng and Khanna 2001). Furthermore, destruction of ▶ cholinergic input to the hippocampus attenuated the pyramidal cell suppression, without an apparent effect on cell excitation to hind paw injection of formalin (Zheng and Khanna 2001). This points to the possibility that the hippocampal cholinergic input influences the background 'noise' of 'signal-to-noise' processing to formalin.

The evidence, that intra-hippocampal administration of NMDA antagonist attenuated animal behavior in the formalin test (McKenna and Melzack 2001), favors a role for glutamate in nociceptive processing in the hippocampus-dentate gyrus. Further, the noxious stimuli-induced increase in Egr1 in hippocampus was blocked by systemic administration of an NMDA receptor antagonist (Wei et al. 2000). Another molecule that has drawn some attention and may be in a position to influence hippocampal processing of noxious information is the cytokine, ▶ tumor necrosis factor-alpha (TNFα). The levels of this molecule are elevated in the hippocampus-dentate gyrus region after the development of thermal ▶ hyperalgesia in the rat chronic constriction nerve injury animal model of neuropathic pain (see ▶ Neuropathic Pain Model, Chronic Constriction Injury) (Ignatowski et al. 1999). Interestingly, TNFα induces thermal hyperalgesia when administered intracerebroventricularly in otherwise normal animals. In summary, the evidence so far suggests that nociceptive processing in hippocampus and the entorhinal cortex is,

at least in part, distributed, non-topographic, and noxious stimulus intensity-dependent, which is in line with the postulated role of these regions in affect-motivation to pain. The processing of noxious information in these regions is likely to be influenced by multiple transmitters/modulators.

References

1. Amaral DG, Witter MP (1995) Hippocampal Formation. In: Paxinos G (ed) The Rat Nervous System. Academic Press, San Diego, pp 443–493
2. Bland BH, Oddie SD (2001) Theta Band Oscillation and Synchrony in the Hippocampal Formation and Associated Structures: The Case for its Role in Sensorimotor Integration. Behav Brain Res 127:119–136
3. Buzsaki G (1989) Two-Stage Model of Memory Trace Formation: A Role for 'Noisy' Brain States. Neurosci 31:551–570
4. Ceccareli I, Casamenti F, Massafra C et al. (1999) Effects of Novelty and Pain on Behavior and Hippocampal Extracellular Ach Levels in Male and Female Rats. Brain Res 815:169–176
5. Funahashi M, He Y-F, Sugimoto T et al. (1999) Noxious Tooth Pulp Stimulation Suppresses C-Fos Expression in the Rat Hippocampal Formation. Brain Res 827:215–220
6. Ignatowski TA, Covey WC, Knight PR et al. (1999) Brain-Derived TNFα Mediates Neuropathic Pain. Brain Res 841:70–77
7. Khanna S (1997) Dorsal Hippocampus Field CA1 Pyramidal Cell Responses to a Persistent versus an Acute Nociceptive Stimulus and their Septal Modulation. Neurosci 77:713–721
8. Khanna S, Chang S, Jiang F et al. (2004) Nociception-Driven Decreased Induction of Fos Protein in Ventral Hippocampus Field CA1 of the Rat. Brain Res 1004:167–176
9. Khanna S, Sinclair JG (1992) Responses in the CA1 region of the rat hippocampus to a noxious stimulus. Exp Neurol 117:28-35
10. Khanna S, Sinclair JG (1989) Noxious Stimuli Produce Prolonged Changes in the CA1 Region of the Rat Hippocampus. Pain 39:337–343
11. McKenna JE, Melzack R (2001) Blocking NMDA Receptors in the Hippocampal Dentate Gyrus with AP5 Produces Analgesia in the Formalin Pain Test. Expl Neurol 172:92–99
12. Melzack R, Casey KL (1968) Sensory, Motivational and Central Control Determinants of Pain. In: Kenshalo DR (ed) The Skin Senses. Thomas, Springfield, IL, pp 423–443
13. Ploghaus A, Narain C, Beckmann CF et al. (2001) Exacerbation of Pain by Anxiety is Associated with Activity in a Hippocampal Network. J Neurosci 21:9896–9903
14. Selden NRW, Everitt BJ, Jarrard LE et al. (1991) Complementary Roles for the Amygdala and Hippocampus in Aversive Conditioning to Explicit and Contextual Cues. Neurosci 42:335–350
15. Wei F, Xu ZC, Qu Z et al. (2000) Role of EGR1 in Hippocampal Synaptic Enhancement Induced by Tetanic Stimulation and Amputation. J Cell Biol 149:1325–1333
16. Zheng F, Khanna S (2001) Selective Destruction of Medial Septal Cholinergic Neurons Attenuates Pyramidal Cell Suppression, but not Excitation in Dorsal Hippocampus Field CA1 Induced by Subcutaneous Injection of Formalin. Neurosci 103:985–998

Nociceptive Processing in the Nucleus Accumbens, Neurophysiology and Behavioral Studies

LINO BECERRA, MARNIE SHAW, DAVID BORSOOK
Brain Imaging Center, McLean Hospital-Harvard Medical School, Belmont, MA, USA
lbecerra@mclean.harvard.edu

in lamina IV and lamina V have long spiny dendrites that pass dorsally, laterally and ventrally. The dorsal dendrites penetrate the substantia gelatinosa to be contacted by axons from interneurons and from fine primary afferents. In addition they receive inputs from terminal ramifications of large myelinated primary afferent fibres that make synaptic contacts to lamina IV cells. There is not much fine primary afferent input directly into lamina IV. Neurons in lamina VI often send dendrites across the width of the dorsal horn but the dendrites do not penetrate laminae I and II. The primary afferent input is from collaterals from primary afferent axons destined to reach ventral horn cells (for references see Willis and Coggeshall 2004).

Output of Neurons in Laminae I–VI

Most neurons are interneurons with axons ending in the same or adjacent laminae. For example, some of the laminae III–V cells are antenna-type neurons that send dendrites to lamina II and are thus output neurons from lamina II. However, lamina I, includes the dendrites to lamina III–VI neurons that form long axons projecting to supraspinal sites (Willis and Coggeshall 2004). Lamina I neurons project to various sites in the brain stem. Within laminae III to VI are spinocervical tract neurons and ▶ postsynaptic dorsal column cells. Neurons in laminae IV to VI send their axons into the lateral white column or across the midline, presumably to the opposite ▶ spinothalamic tract through the anterior white commissure. They may bifurcate before they go to the white matter and collaterals of these axons ramify in laminae III–V and deeper laminae, including the contralateral side and lamina X.

Response Properties
of Nociceptive Spinal Cord Neurons

Recordings have shown responses of spinal cord neurons to electrical stimulation of nerve fibres and to natural innocuous and noxious stimulation (for references see Willis and Coggeshall 2004). Upon electrical nerve stimulation lamina I neurons were excited by cutaneous Aδ fibres and sometimes by volleys in C fibres, in line with the morphological studies. However, some neurons were excited (polysynaptically?) by Aβ fibre stimulation. Neurons in the substantia gelatinosa were activated primarily by C fibres; however, Aβ and Aδ fibre stimulation also activated some of them. Neurons in laminae III to VI respond either to A and C fibre or only to A fibre stimulation. Many neurons show convergence of Aβ, Aδ and C fibre inputs.

It is noteworthy that neurons in laminae I and V in the thoracic and sacral spinal cord also show responses to stimulation of visceral nerves and neurons in the superficial and deep lumbosacral enlargement are activated by cutaneous fibres, muscular group III fibres and joint afferents.

Neuronal responses were also recorded during natural stimulation (for references see Willis and Coggeshall 2004). It appeared that neurons in the different laminae are heterogeneous in their response properties. This is not surprising on the one hand, because each of the Aβ, Aδ and C fibre classes has different modalities (mechanoreception, nociception, thermoreception). On the other hand, the response properties do not seem simply to reflect the input into the laminae. This has to be expected because only about 50% of the synapses are from primary afferent fibres. Lamina I contains neurons that are only activated by intense mechanical stimulation of the skin, neurons that are activated by intense mechanical stimulation of skin and noxious heat applied to the skin and non-nociceptive thermoreceptive neurons that respond to innocuous warming or cooling. Other neurons are wide dynamic range neurons responding weakly to innocuous and strongly to noxious stimulation. Furthermore, neurons in lamina I show convergent inputs from cutaneous and deep tissue or convergence from cutaneous and visceral inputs.

Information on identified lamina II neurons is sparse. Cells were excited by innocuous or noxious mechanical stimuli. However, several authors reported that spontaneously active neurons in this lamina were inhibited by natural stimulation or they were inhibited and then excited by weak mechanical stimuli. Furthermore, neurons showed phenomena such habituation, long afterdischarges following brief stimuli and variable receptive fields.

Neurons in laminae III–VI are of different types. Concerning thresholds and encoding ranges some neurons are low threshold, responding only to innocuous stimulation. Many of these neurons are located in laminae III and IV. Most neurons are wide dynamic range, responding weakly to innocuous stimuli and strongly to noxious stimuli and a further group of neurons are high threshold responding only to noxious intensities. Thus, at least the wide dynamic range neurons seem to receive inputs from non-nociceptive as well as from nociceptive afferents, in line with morphological studies showing projection of non-nociceptive afferents into deep laminae, extension of dendrites of deep cells up to the superficial laminae and interneurons transmitting information from superficial into deeper laminae. Many neurons in laminae III–VI receive inputs from deep tissue. These cells are solely excited by deep tissue stimulation or show convergent inputs from deep tissue and skin, or they are excited from skin and viscera. All neurons with visceral input seem to receive input from the skin as well. Lamina X neurons are also either low threshold, wide dynamic range or high threshold. Many of these neurons respond to visceral stimulation such as colorectal distension, in addition to cutaneous stimuli. Some cells in lamina X have bilateral receptive fields.

Encoding of Noxious Stimuli in the Spinal Cord

The understanding of the encoding of nociceptive information in the spinal cord is not very advanced. On the basis of single neuron recordings both ► wide dynamic range neurons and ► nociceptive specific neurons seem to be suitable to encode the intensity of a noxious stimulus to a specific site. However, wide dynamic range neurons in particular often have large receptive fields and a stimulus of a defined intensity may elicit differently strong responses when applied to different sites in the receptive field. It is questionable whether the activity of a single neuron reflects more the magnitude of a stimulus or the site in the receptive area where a stimulus of a defined intensity is applied. Furthermore, the situation becomes more complicated when inputs from different tissues to a neuron are studied. It seems impossible that e.g. a single wide dynamic range neuron with convergent cutaneous and visceral inputs can unequivocally signal that the skin or a visceral organ has been challenged with a noxious stimulus. This uncertainty in the message of a neuron could in fact be the reason why pain in viscera and to some extent in the deep tissue is often referred to a cutaneous area, namely into a so-called Heat zone. However, it is quite clear that the precise location of a noxious stimulus, its intensity and character cannot be encoded by a single nociceptive neuron. It is assumed therefore, that encoding of a noxious stimulus is only achieved by a population of nociceptive neurons (for further discussion see Price et al. 2003). This topic is addressed in detail in ► encoding of noxious information in the spinal cord. Samples of neurons were studied by the recording of field potentials in the dorsal horn, but these data have not contributed to the understanding of encoding. Furthermore, changes in metabolic activity and the expression of immediate early genes such as ► C-Fos have been used to map regions in the spinal cord that are activated by a noxious stimulus. The expression of FOS protein (► c-fos) has been used extensively because individual neurons can be visualised. The expression of C-FOS in a neuron is thought to show its activation (Willis and Coggeshall 2004). For example, noxious heat stimulation evokes expression of C-FOS in the superficial dorsal horn within a few minutes and staining shifts to deeper laminae of the dorsal horn thereafter (Menetréy et al. 1989; Williams et al. 1990). Noxious visceral stimulation evokes C-FOS expression in laminae I, V and X, thus resembling the projection area of visceral afferent fibres and injection of mustard oil into muscle elicits C-FOS expression in laminae I and IV to VI (Hunt et al. 1987; Menetréy et al. 1989). These data show therefore, in which spinal laminae and segments neurons were activated by noxious stimulation. It should be noted however, that excitatory as well as inhibitory neurons may express C-FOS.

Plasticity in the Nociceptive Processing in the Spinal Cord

Importantly, spinal cord neurons show changes in their response properties, including the size of their receptive fields, when the peripheral tissue is sufficiently activated by noxious stimuli or when thin fibres in a nerve are electrically stimulated. In general, it is thought that plasticity in the spinal cord contributes significantly to clinically relevant pain states.

Wind-up

► Wind-up is the increase in the response of a spinal cord neuron when electrical stimulation of C-fibres is repeated at intervals of about 1 s (Mendell 1966; Mendell and Wall 1965). The basis of wind-up is a prolonged EPSP that builds up as a result of a repetitive C-fibre volley and thus it rests on temporal summation of synaptic potentials within the cord (Sivilotti et al. 1993). Other neurons show wind-down (Alarcon and Cervero 1990; Fitzgerald and Wall 1980; Woolf and King 1987). Wind-up disappears quickly when repetitive stimulation is stopped. Wind-up is likely to contribute to short lasting increases in response to painful stimulation (see ► wind-up of spinal cord neurons).

Long-term Potentiation (LTP) and Long-term Depression (LTD)

These are long lasting changes in synaptic activity after peripheral nerve stimulation (Randic et al. 1993; Rygh et al. 1999; Sandkühler and Liu 1998; Svendsen et al. 1997). They can be observed as increases in field potentials in the superficial dorsal horn. The most pronounced ► LTP with a short latency can be elicited after application of a high frequency train of electrical stimuli that are suprathreshold for C-fibres when the spinal cord has been transected in order to interrupt descending inhibitory influences from the brain stem. However, LTP can also be elicited with natural noxious stimulation, although the time course is much slower (Rygh et al. 1999). By contrast, LTD in the superficial dorsal horn is elicited by electrical stimulation of Aδ fibres. This latter form of plasticity may be a basis of inhibitory mechanisms that counteract responses to noxious stimulation (Sandkühler et al. 1997). LTP and LTD will be addressed in detail in the essay ► long-term potentiation and long-term depression in the spinal cord.

Central Sensitization in the Course of Inflammation and Nerve Damage

Changes in responses of spinal cord neurons have been studied in models of inflammation and neuropathy. Pronounced changes in response properties of neurons in the superficial dorsal horn, the deep dorsal horn and the ventral cord have been described. ▶ Central sensitization, originally described by Woolf (1983), has been observed in neurons with cutaneous input during cutaneous inflammation and other forms of cutaneous irritation such as capsaicin application. Pronounced central sensitisation of spinal cord neurons with deep input has been shown during inflammation in joints, muscle and viscera. Typical changes in responses of individual neurons are (a) increased responses to noxious stimulation of inflamed tissue, (b) lowering of the threshold of spinal cord neurons with an initially high threshold (initially nociceptive spinal neurons will change into wide dynamic range neurons), (c) increased responses to stimuli applied to non-inflamed tissue surrounding the inflamed site and (d) expansion of the receptive field. In particular the enhanced responses to stimuli applied to non-inflamed tissue in the vicinity of the inflamed zone indicate that the sensitivity of the spinal cord neurons is enhanced, so that previously subthreshold input is sufficient to activate the neuron under inflammatory conditions. The sensitisation of individual spinal cord neurons will lead to an increased percentage of neurons in a segment that respond to stimulation of an inflamed tissue. Thus the population of responsive neurons increases. Central sensitisation can persist for weeks judging from the recording of neurons at different stages of acute and chronic inflammation (for review see Coderre et al. 1993; Dubner and Ruda 1992; Mense 1993; Schaible and Grubb 1993).

In ▶ neuropathic pain states, findings in the spinal cord are dependent on the neuropathic model used. Evidence for central sensitisation has been observed in neuropathic pain states in which conduction in the nerve remains present and thus a receptive field of neurons can be identified. In these models, more neurons show ongoing discharges and on average higher responses can be elicited by innocuous stimulation of receptive fields (Laird and Bennett 1993; Palacek 1992 a, b). In some models of neuropathy, neurons with abnormal discharge properties can be observed. For more information see chapters on neuropathic pain.

During inflammation and neuropathy, more neurons that express C-FOS are observed in the spinal cord, supporting the finding that a large number of neurons are activated. At least at some time points, enhanced ▶ metabolism can be seen in the spinal cord during inflammation and neuropathy. Both of these findings underscore the plasticity that occurs in the spinal cord under these conditions (Price et al. 1991; Schadrack et al. 1999).

Transmitters and Receptors Involved in the Spinal Nociceptive Processing

Numerous transmitters and receptors are involved in spinal nociceptive processing. They mediate processing of noxious information arising from noxious stimulation of normal tissue and they are involved in plastic changes in spinal cord neuronal responses when the peripheral tissue is inflamed or when a nerve is damaged in a neuropathic fashion. Other transmitters are inhibitory and control spinal processing. In general, transmitter actions have either fast kinetics (action of glutamate on ionotropic AMPA and kainate receptors, action of ATP at ionotropic purinergic receptors, action of GABA at ionotropic GABA receptors) or slower kinetics (in particular neuropeptides that act through G-protein coupled metabotropic receptors). Actions with fast kinetics evoke immediate and short-term effects on neurons, thus encoding the input to the neuron, whereas actions with slow kinetics rather modulate synaptic processing (Millan 1999; Willis and Coggeshall 2004). The following paragraphs summarize the main findings on synaptic transmission of nociceptive information (for references see Willis and Coggeshall 2004).

Glutamate

This excitatory amino acid is a principal transmitter in the spinal cord that produces fast synaptic transmission. ▶ Glutamate is a transmitter of primary afferent neurons and of dorsal horn interneurons. Many spinal cord interneurons are excited by glutamate and by agonists at glutamate receptors. Glutamate activates ionotropic AMPA / kainate (non-NMDA) and ▶ NMDA receptors as well as ▶ metabotropic glutamate receptors. They are expressed all over the spinal cord grey matter, although differences in regional densities are found. Glutamate receptors are found in both excitatory and inhibitory interneurons.

Glutamate receptors are involved in the excitation of substantia gelatinosa neurons by Aδ and C fibres in slice preparations. Usually these actions are mainly blocked by CNQX, an antagonist at non-NMDA receptors, whereas ▶ NMDA receptor antagonists usually cause a small reduction in EPSPs and reduce later components of the EPSP. *In vivo* recordings showed that both non-NMDA and NMDA receptors are involved in the synaptic activation of neurons by noxious stimuli. In addition, both of these receptors are involved in forms of functional plasticity. For example, both wind-up and central sensitisation by inflammation are blocked by spinal application of NMDA antagonists (and non-NMDA antagonists). Metabotropic glutamate receptors can potentiate the action of ionotropic glutamate receptors (for review see Fundytus 2001; Millan 1999; Willis and Coggeshall 2004). A detailed discussion of glutamate receptors is provided by the essays ► NMDA receptors in spinal nociceptive processing and ► metabotropic glutamate receptors in spinal nociceptive processing.

Adenosine Triphosphate

► ATP depolarises some dorsal horn neurons in the superficial dorsal horn. ATP has been implicated in the fast synaptic transmission of innocuous mechanoreceptive input but evidence has also been provided for an involvement in nociceptive synaptic transmission. Some spinal cord neurons seem to express purinergic receptors for actions of ATP, but other reports rather described presynaptic actions of ATP that caused an enhanced release of glutamate. The latter finding is consistent with the localisation of purinergic receptors in dorsal root ganglion cells. ► P2X3 Receptor immunoreactivity in the inner part of lamina II is reduced following dorsal rhizotomy (for review see Willis and Coggeshall 2004).

GABA and Glycine

► GABA is probably the most important fast inhibitory transmitter in the spinal cord. Application of GABA to neurons causes IPSPs and inhibition of the activity of spinal cord neurons. GABA occurs in inhibitory interneurons throughout the spinal cord. ► GABAergic inhibitory interneurons can be synaptically activated by primary afferent fibres and this explains why strong nociceptive inputs can induce, in addition to excitation, inhibition of neurons (usually following initial excitation) that are under the control of these inhibitory interneurons. Noxious stimuli can cause FOS expression in GABAergic interneurons. Some of the GABAergic interneurons also contain other mediators such as glycine, acetylcholine, enkephalin, galanin, neuropeptide Y or nitric oxide synthase (NOS).

Both the ionotropic ► GABAA receptor and the metabotropic ► GABAB receptor are located presynaptically on primary afferent neurons or postsynaptically on dorsal horn neurons. Responses to both innocuous mechanical and noxious stimuli can be reduced by GABA receptor agonists (for review see Willis and Coggeshall 2004). It is under discussion whether reduced inhibition may be a mechanism of neuropathic pain (Polgár et al. 2004).

Some of the inhibitory effects are due to glycine and indeed, the ventral and the dorsal horn contain numerous glycinergic neurons. Glycine may be colocalized with GABA in synaptic terminals. The roles of GABA and glycine are addressed in more detail in ► GABA and glycine in spinal nociceptive processing.

Acetylcholine

Many small DRG neurons, some large DRG ones and some neurons in the dorsal horn are cholinergic. *Vice versa*, many DRG neurons and neurons in the dorsal horn express nicotinergic and muscarinergic receptors. Application of ► acetylcholine to the skin is pronociceptive (*via* nicotinic and muscarinergic receptors) whereas spinal acetylcholine produces pro- or anti-nociception (for review see Willis and Coggeshall 2004).

Excitatory Neuropeptides

A number of peptides are colocalised with excitatory transmitters, in particular with glutamate. Excitatory neuropeptides evoke EPSPs, but these differ from EPSPs evoked by glutamate in several respects. Usually they occur after a latency of seconds, but they last longer. They may not be sufficient to evoke action potential generation. Because glutamate and excitatory peptides are coreleased from synaptic endings, they are thought to act in a synergistic way (Urban et al. 1994).

Substance P

This excitatory peptide is colocalized with glutamate in a proportion of thin diameter primary afferents and in a proportion of spinal cord interneurons. SP-containing endings are concentrated in laminae I and II and in lamina X. They terminate on cell bodies and dendrites of dorsal horn neurons. SP is released mainly in the superficial dorsal horn following electrical stimulation of unmyelinated fibres and during noxious mechanical, thermal or chemical stimulation of the skin and deep tissues such as the joints. In part, release of SP is dependent on NMDA receptors on primary afferent endings (for review see Willis and Coggeshall 2004).

SP acts on ► neurokinin-1 (NK-1) receptors that are located on dendrites and cell bodies of dorsal horn neurons in laminae I, IV–VI and X. Fewer neurons in laminae II and III have NK-1 receptors. The vast majority of neurons with NK-1 receptors are excitatory, while a few contain GABA and glycine and are thus inhibitory. Some of the neurons with NK-1 receptors are projection neurons including spinothalamic, spinoreticular and spinobrachial neurons. Upon strong activation by SP, NK-1 receptors can be internalized. Such an internalization is blocked by NK-1 receptor antagonists and by NMDA receptor antagonists.

NK-1 receptors are G-protein coupled receptors, i.e. the action of SP on ion channels is indirect. Application of SP evokes a prolonged excitation of nociceptive dorsal horn neurons. These depolarizations are presumably caused by Ca^{2+} inward currents and inhibition of K^+ currents and possibly by other currents. Several second messengers such as PKA and PKC are involved.

There is general agreement that SP and NK-1 receptors are involved in the plasticity of nociceptive processing, whereas the involvement of this system in normal nociception is controversial. Responses of dorsal horn neurons to C-fibre volleys and to noxious stimulation of skin and deep tissue are enhanced by SP and receptive fields can show an expansion. Antagonists at NK-1 receptors reduce responses to C-fibre volleys and to noxious stimulation of skin and deep tissue and they attenuate central sensitisation. Mice with a deletion of preprotachykinin A have intact responses to mildly noxious stimuli but reduced responses to moderate and intensely noxious stimuli. Mice with a deletion of the gene responsible for the production of NK-1 receptors respond to acutely painful stimuli, but lack intensity coding for pain and wind-up (for review see Willis and Coggeshall 2004).

Neurokinin A

In addition to substance P, neurokinin A (NKA) is found in small DRG cells and in the spinal dorsal horn. NKA is released in the spinal cord upon noxious stimulation. Due to its resistance to enzymatic degradation, NKA spreads throughout the grey matter. Interestingly, it has not so far been possible to identify NK-2 receptors immunohistochemically in the dorsal horn, leading to the unresolved question as to where NKA acts. It was proposed that NKA activates NK-1 receptors, because these are internalized after application of both SP and NKA. However, specific NK-2 receptor antagonists suggest that specific binding sites for NKA should be present.

The literature on NKA effects is controversial, because some authors found an involvement of NKA in nociceptive processing whereas others did not. Intrathecal application of NKA produces nocifensive behaviour and iontophoretic application of NKA activates nociceptive and non-nociceptive dorsal horn neurons. NKA facilitates behavioural nociceptive responses to heat stimulation, which are blocked by NK-2 receptor antagonists. While some authors could not antagonize responses of dorsal horn neurons to noxious mechanical stimulation, others were able to show such an effect. Antagonists at NK-2 receptors were able to attenuate central sensitisation during knee inflammation and colon inflammation (for review see Willis and Coggeshall 2004).

Neurokinin B

This peptide is found in synaptic terminals and dendrites in laminae I–III, independently of SP-containing elements and is not contained in dorsal root ganglion cells. NK-3 receptors are found in the most superficial part of the dorsal horn. Their function is unclear.

Calcitonin Gene-Related Peptide (CGRP)

This peptide is found in many small DRG neurons and is often colocalized with substance P. Probably the primary afferent neurons are the only source of CGRP in the dorsal horn. CGRP-containing afferents project mainly to laminae I, II and V. However, CGRP is also contained in motoneurons. CGRP is released in the spinal cord by electrical stimulation of thin fibres and by noxious mechanical and thermal stimulation. During joint inflammation, the pattern of CGRP release changes in that innocuous stimuli to the joint are sufficient to elicit CGRP release.

CGRP binding sites are concentrated in lamina I and in the deep dorsal horn. CGRP enhances actions of substance P. It inhibits enzymatic degradation of SP and it seems to potentiate release of SP. Enhanced Ca^{2+} influx may be important in this respect. CGRP activates nociceptive dorsal horn neurons with a slow time course. Blockade of CGRP effects reduces nociceptive responses and attenuates inflammation evoked central sensitisation. The effects of CGRP are discussed in more detail in the essay ▶ CGRP and spinal cord nociception.

Vasoactive Intestinal Polypeptide (VIP)

▶ Vasoactive intestinal polypeptide is found in small diameter afferent fibres especially in the sacral spinal cord. Terminals with VIP are concentrated in laminae I, II, V, VII and X. In addition, neurons with VIP are located in laminae II–IV and X. VIP bindings sites are concentrated in laminae I and II. VIP excites nociceptive dorsal horn neurons.

Neurotensin

Neurotensin is located in interneurons in lamina I and the substantia gelatinosa and neurotensin binding sites are present in the dorsal horn. The peptide excites neurons in the superficial dorsal horn.

Cholecystokinin (CCK)

▶ Cholecystokinin (CCK) is located in DRG neurons and in neurons in several laminae of the dorsal horn. Binding sites reach their highest concentration in laminae I and II. CCK can excite neurons in laminae I–VII and an antagonist at CCK-B receptors is antinociceptive. Antinociceptive effects of CCK have also been described.

Thyrotropin Releasing Hormone (TRH)

Thyrotropin releasing hormone (TRH) is located in the ventral and dorsal horn. Many TRH-containing neurons also contain GABA. TRH facilitates responses of nociceptive neurons to glutamate at NMDA receptors, wind-up and responses to noxious stimuli.

N

Corticotropin-releasing hormone (CRH)

(CRH)-immunoreactive fibres are present in the sacral spinal cord (laminae I, V–VII, X, intermediolateral column) and CRH immunostaining is abolished after dorsal rhizotomy. CRH binding sites are found in the superficial dorsal horn.

Pituitary Adenylate Cyclase Activating Polypeptide (PACAP)

▶ Pituitary adenylate cyclase activating polypeptide (PACAP) is localized in small DRG cells and many axons in the superficial dorsal horn. PACAP is released after intrathecal capsaicin, and intrathecal PACAP causes nocifensive behaviour. Nociceptive dorsal horn neurons are excited by PACAP (for review see Willis and Coggeshall 2004).

Inhibitory Neuropeptides

Numerous neuropeptides are inhibitory. They may reduce release of transmitters by presynaptic actions or inhibit postsynaptic neurons.

Opioid Peptides

The dorsal horn contains leuenkephalin and metenkephalin, ▶ dynorphin and ▶ endomorphins 1 and 2. Enkephalin containing neurons are particularly located in laminae I and II and dynorphin containing neurons in laminae I, II and V. Endomorphin II has been visualised in terminals of primary afferent neurons in the superficial dorsal horn and in dorsal root ganglia but also in postsynaptic neurons.
▶ Opiate Receptors μ, δ, κ) are concentrated in the superficial dorsal horn and in particular μ and δ receptors are not only located in interneurons but also on primary afferent fibres. The activation of these opiate receptors reduces release of mediators from primary afferents (presynaptic effect). This effect is mediated by inhibition of Ca^{2+} channels. Other opiate receptors are located on intrinsic spinal cord neurons and mediate postsynaptic effects. The activation of a K^+ conductance could be the relevant mechanism. In general, enkephalins are ligands at δ-receptors, endomorphins are ligands at μ-receptors and dynorphin is a ligand at κ-receptors. However, dynorphin may also activate NMDA receptors. Actions of all opiates are antagonized by naloxone. Specific antagonists at different receptors are available (Waldhoer et al. 2004).
Application of opioids into the dorsal horn reduces responses to (innocuous) and noxious stimulation and responses of neurons to iontophoretic application of excitatory amino acids, showing postsynaptic effects of opioids. Depending on the site of application (superficial or deep laminae), μ-, κ- or δ-receptor ligands are more or less effective in producing neuronal effects. In addition many dorsal horn neurons are hyperpolarised by opiates. While agonists at μ- and δ-receptors usually evoke inhibitory effects, dynorphin may produce either inhibitory or excitatory effects.

In addition to these "classical" opiate receptors, nociceptin / orphanin FQ receptors (see ▶ Orphanin FQ) have recently been discovered. These proteins share greater than 90% sequence identity and about 60% homology with the classical opiate receptors (Waldhoer et al. 2004). An endogenous ligand at these receptors is ▶ Nociceptin. This peptide has similar cellular actions to classical opioid peptides. It causes presynaptic inhibition of glutamate release in the spinal cord and reduces FOS expression in the superficial dorsal horn. However, pronociceptive effects have also been described. A related peptide is nocistatin. At present it is unknown at which receptor nocistatin acts (for review see Willis and Coggeshall 2004).

Somatostatin

This peptide is expressed in primary afferent neurons, in dorsal horn interneurons and in axons that descend from the medulla. ▶ Somatostatin is released mainly in the substantia gelatinosa, by heat stimulation. Actions of somatostatin on nociceptive neurons in the dorsal horn are inhibitory. It is an intriguing question as to whether inhibitory somatostatin is released in the spinal cord from primary afferent fibres or from interneurons.

Galanin

This peptide is expressed in a subpopulation of small DRG neurons and galanin binding sites are also expressed on DRG neurons. Both facilitatory and inhibitory effects of galanin have been described in inflammatory and neuropathic pain states.

Neuropeptide Y

This is normally only expressed at very low levels in DRG neurons, but DRG neurons express Y1 and Y2 receptors. It was proposed that Y1 and Y2 receptors contribute to presynaptic inhibition.

Other Mediators

A number of other mediators influence synaptic transmission in the spinal dorsal horn. Most attention has given to ▶ NO, ▶ prostaglandins and ▶ neurotrophins. These mediators have actions in non-neuronal tissues as well as in neuronal tissues in the peripheral and central nervous systems including the spinal cord. They play significant roles in pathophysiological pain states. The role of prostaglandins is addressed in another section, and a recent review (Vanegas and Schaible 2001) provides a comprehensive summary. The role of neurotrophins is addressed in the essay ▶ spinal cord nociception, neurotrophins.

Involvement of Calcium Channels in Release of Transmitter and Postsynaptic Excitability

The release of transmitters is dependent on the influx of Ca^{2+} into the presynaptic ending through ▶ Voltage-Dependent Calcium Channels. In addition Ca^{2+} also regulates excitability of postsynaptic neurons. High voltage activated N-type channels, which are mainly located presynaptically but also on the postsynaptic side and P / Q-type channels that are located on the presynaptic side are important for nociceptive processing. In particular, blockers of N-type channels reduce responses of spinal cord neurons and behavioural responses to noxious stimulation of normal and inflamed tissue and blockade of N-type channels can also reduce neuropathic pain. There is some evidence that P / Q-type channels are mainly involved in the generation of pathophysiological pain states. A role for high voltage activated L-type channels and low voltage activated T-type channels has also been discussed. The role of calcium channels is addressed in detail in the essay ▶ calcium channels in the spinal processing of nociceptive input.

Final conclusions

This review concentrated on spinal cord neurons that are excited by noxious stimuli applied to the peripheral tissue. The significance of particular types of neurons in the transmission of sensory information to supraspinal sites through ascending tracts will be addressed in another section. The modulation of responses of spinal cord cells by descending inhibition and facilitation is described in another section. In addition, the particular aspects concerning deep somatic and visceral pain are also covered elsewhere. As briefly outlined here, the spinal cord is subject to considerable changes during pathophysiological pain states. These changes will also be addressed in other sections. Moreover, the spinal cord is the major site at which antinociceptive compounds work. Again this will be addressed in other sections.

References

1. Alarcon G, Cervero F (1990) The effects of electrical stimulation of A and C visceral afferent fibres on the excitability of viscerosomatic neurones in the thoracic spinal cord of the cat. Brain Res 509:24–30
2. Chung K, McNeill DL, Hulsebosch CR et al. (1989) Changes in dorsal horn synaptic disc numbers following unilateral dorsal rhizotomy. J Comp Neurol 283:568–577
3. Coderre TJ, Katz J, Vaccarino AL et al. (1993) Contribution of central neuroplasticity to pathological pain:review of clinical and experimental evidence. Pain 52:259–285
4. Dubner R, Ruda MA (1992) Activity-dependent neuronal plasticity following tissue injury and inflammation. Trends Neurosci 15:96–103
5. Fitzgerald M, Wall PD (1980) The laminar organization of dorsal horn cells responding to peripheral C fibre stimulation. Exp Brain Res 41:36–44
6. Fundytus ME (2001) Glutamate receptors and nociception. CNS Drugs 15:29–58
7. Laird JMA, Bennett GJ (1993) An electrophysiological study of dorsal horn neurons in the spinal cord of rats with an experimental peripheral neuropathy. J Neurophysiol 69:2072–2085
8. McMahon SB, Wall PD (1983) A system of rat spinal cord lamina I cells projecting through the contralateral dorsolateral funiculus. J Comp Neurol 214:217–223
9. Mendell LM (1966) Physiologial properties of unmyelinated fiber projection to the spinal cord. Exp Neurol 16:316–332
10. Mendell LM, Wall PD (1965) Responses of single dorsal cord cells to peripheral cutaneous unmyelinated fibers. Nature 206:97–99
11. Menetréy D, Gannon JD, Levine JD et al. (1989) Expression of c-fos protein in interneurons and projection neurons of the rat spinal cord in response to noxious somatic, articular, and visceral stimulation. J Comp Neurol 285:177–195
12. Mense S (1993) Nociception from skeletal muscle in relation to clinical muscle pain. Pain 54:241–289
13. Millan MJ (1999) The induction of pain: an integrative review. Progr Neurobiol 57:1–164
14. Palacek J, Dougherty PM, Kim SH et al. (1992b) Responses of spinothalamic tract neurons to mechanical and thermal stimuli in an experimental model of peripheral neuropathy in primates. J Neurophysiol 68:1951–1966
15. Palacek J, Paleckova V, Dougherty PM et al. (1992a) Responses of spinothalamic tract cells to mechanical and thermal stimulation of skin in rats with experimental peripheral neuropathy. J Neurophysiol 67:1562–1573
16. Polgár E, Gray S, Riddell JS et al. (2004) Lack of evidence for significant neuronal loss in laminae I–III of the spinal dorsal horn of the rat in the chronic constriction injury model. Pain 111:144–150
17. Price DD, Mao J, Coghill RC et al. (1991) Regional changes in spinal cord glucose metabolism in a rat model of painful neuropathy. Brain Res 564:314–318
18. Price DD, Greenspan JD, Dubner R (2003) Neurons involved in the exteroceptive function of pain. Pain 106:215–219
19. Randic M, Jiang MC, Cerne R (1993) Long-term potentiation and long-term depression of
20. primary afferent neurotransmission in the rat spinal cord. J Neurosci 13:5228–5241
21. Rexed B (1952) The cytoarchitectonic organization of the spinal cord in the rat. J Comp Neurol 96:415–466
22. Rexed B (1954) A cytoarchitectonic atlas of the spinal cord in the cat. J Comp Neurol 100:297–380
23. Rygh LJ, Svendson F, Hole K et al. (1999) Natural noxious stimulation can induce long-term increase of spinal nociceptive responses. Pain 82:305–310
24. Sandkühler J, Liu X (1998) Induction of long-term potentiation at spinal synapses by noxious stimulation or nerve injury. Eur J Neurosci 10:2476–2480
25. Sandkühler J, Chen JG, Cheng G et al. (1997) Low-frequency stimulation of afferent Aδ-fibers induces long-term depression at primary afferent synapses with substantia gelatinosa neurons in the rat. J Neurosci 17:6483–6491
26. Schadrack J, Neto FL, Ableitner A et al. (1999) Metabolic activity changes in the rat spinal cord during adjuvant monoarthritis. Neuroscience 94:595–605
27. Schaible H-G, Grubb BD (1993) Afferent and spinal mechanisms of joint pain. Pain 55:5–54
28. Scheibel ME, Scheibel AB (1968) Terminal axon patterns in cat spinal cord: II. The dorsal horn. Brain Res 9:32–58
29. Sivilotti LG, Thompson SWN, Woolf CJ (1993) The rate of rise of the cumulative depolarization evoked by repetitive stimulation of small-calibre afferents is a predictor of action po-

tential windup in rat spinal neurons *in vitro*. J Neurophysiol 69:1621–1631

30. Sugiura Y, Lee CL, Perl ER (1986) Central projections of identified, unmyelinated (C) afferent fibres innervating mammalian skin. Science 234:358–361

31. Sugiura Y, Terui N, Hosoya Y (1989) Difference in the distribution of central terminals between visceral and somatic unmyelinated (C) primary afferent fibres. J Neurophysiol 62:834–840

32. Svendsen F, Tjolsen A, Hole K (1997) LTP of spinal Aβ and C-fibre evoked responses after electrical sciatic nerve stimulation. Neuroreport 8:3427–2430

33. Urban L, Thompson SWN, Dray A (1994) Modulation of spinal excitability: cooperation between neurokinin and excitatory amino acid transmitters. Trends Neurosci 17:432–438

34. Vanegas H, Schaible H-G (2001) Prostaglandins and cyclooxygenases in the spinal cord. Progr Neurobiol 64:327–363

35. Waldhoer M, Bartlett SE, Whistler JL (2004) Opioid receptors. Annu Rev Biochem 73:953–990

36. Williams S, Ean GL, Hunt SP (1990) Changing pattern of c-fos induction following thermal cutaneous stimulation in the rat. Neuroscience 36:73–81

37. Willis WD, Cggeshall RE (2004) Sensory Mechanisms of the Spinal Cord 3rd edn. Volume 1, Kluwer Academic / Plenum Publishers. New York

38. Woolf CJ (1983) Evidence for a central component of post-injury pain hypersensitivity. Nature 306:686–688

39. Woolf CJ, King AE (1987) Physiology and morphology of multireceptive neurons with C-afferent inputs in the deep dorsal horn of the rat lumbar spinal cord. J Neurophysiol 58:460–479

Nociceptive System

Definition

Peripheral, spinal and cerebral structures involved in the processing of noxious stimuli. Sensory-discriminative aspect of pain: Perceptual component of pain perception including the perception of location, quality, intensity and duration of the painful stimulus.

► Noxious Stimulus
► Primary Somatosensory Cortex (S1), Effect on Pain-Related Behavior in Humans

Nociceptive Temporomandibular Joint Afferents

► Nociceptors in the Orofacial Region (Temporomandibular Joint and Masseter Muscle)

Nociceptive Threshold

Definition

Nociceptive thresholds in experimental animals are usually defined as the threshold (temperature, mechanical force) at which a withdrawal response is evoked, measured either by active withdrawal of a limb or the tail, for example, or measurement of the electrical activity of a muscle in an anaesthetized animal.

► Arthritis Model, Adjuvant-Induced Arthritis

Nociceptive Transduction

Definition

Generation of the nociceptive information in nociceptors in response to noxious stimuli by generation of depolarizing currents.

► Nociceptor Generator Pontential
► NSAIDs, Mode of Action

Nociceptive Withdrawal Reflex

Definition

Nociceptive withdrawal reflexes denote an integrated reflex to avoid potential tissue injury. The reflex response is dependent on stimulus site, stimulus intensity, and functional context. During standardized experimental conditions, the reflex is correlated to the pain intensity.

► Pain in Humans, Electrical Stimulation (Skin, Muscle and Viscera)

Nociceptor Accommodation

► Nociceptor, Adaptation

Nociceptor Desensitization

Definition

Decreased sensitivity to noxious stimuli elicited by application of capsaicin. Short-term desensitization is due to the inactivation of TRPV1, preventing the generation of action potentials. On the other hand, long-term desensitization evoked by large doses of capsaicin onto polymodal nociceptor endings, is due to the destruction of a subset of small diameter primary afferent fibers and their cell bodies.

► Polymodal Nociceptors, Heat Transduction
► TRPV1 Receptor

Nociceptive Processing in the Thalamus

A. VANIA APKARIAN
Department of Physiology, Northwestern University
Feinberg School of Medicine, Chicago, IL, USA
a-apkarian@northwestern.edu

The thalamus (Jones 1985) is the primary gateway for nociceptive information transmission to the cortex, similarly to most other sensory systems other than olfaction. However, in contrast to other sensory systems, nociceptive information is also transmitted to the cortex through pathways outside of the ► spinothalamic-thalamocortical projections. Recent new advances have pointed to nociceptive inputs to the brainstem, which in turn project to the thalamus and then to the cortex in a very different pattern from that of the spinothalamic inputs. Nociceptive information transmission to the cortex through thalamocortical projections remains the most thoroughly examined, even though substantial gaps remain in current understanding of this system. The thalamus is the only CNS structure that contains ► mast cells. Their exact role remains unclear but they exist in thalamic nuclei with cortical projections and seem to increase or decrease in number under different conditions. They may be involved in regulating the ► blood-brain barrier. They are probably important in neural-endocrine interactions. (see ► spinothalamic projections in rat). The state of current knowledge regarding the properties of nociceptive processing in the thalamus is outlined here, emphasizing the best-established facts, gaps in current knowledge and points of contention.

Cells of Origin and Tracts

► Spinothalamic and ► trigeminothalamic pathways are the main direct source of nociceptive information input to the thalamus. Multi-synaptic projections through the ► brainstem provide additional nociceptive inputs to the thalamus. Specific subpopulations of spinal cord cells within laminae I, V–VI and VII–VIII project contralaterally through the spinothalamic pathway and transmit mainly nociceptive inputs to medial and lateral thalamic nuclei. The axons of the spinothalamic tract show a topographic organization and a dorsoventral segregation, with axons of superficial lamina spinothalamic cells being located more dorsally than axons of deeper lamina spinothalamic cells. The vast majority of spinothalamic cells respond to nociceptive stimuli. These responses may be uniquely nociceptive and thus called nociceptive specific or convergently responding to both noxious and innocuous stimuli, called ► wide dynamic range type. The responses may be to heat, cold or tactile stimuli specifically or convergently. There is little evidence as to the

spinothalamic cell responses to chemical irritants (see ► spinothalamic input, cells of origin (monkey)).

Spinothalamic Targets

The differential projections for innocuous and nociceptive inputs to the thalamus were first noted when the functional distinctions between the dorsal columns and the anterolateral tract were observed in humans following cordotomies, over a 100 years ago. The terminations of the spinothalamic pathway still remain controversial. There is disagreement as to the terminations of the pathway in the lateral and medial thalamus. In 1980s, the ► nucleus submedius (SM) in the medial thalamus was claimed to be the nociceptive specific nucleus of the thalamus (Craig and Burton 1981), since it was thought to receive inputs only from spinal cord lamina I nociceptive neurons. This idea has been mostly discounted, at least in the rat and monkey. However, the primary medial thalamic termination site, which has traditionally been reported to be in ► MD has been put into doubt in recent reports as well; instead it is claimed that the main spinothalamic input is to ► CL. Lateral thalamic terminations have classically been reported to target ► VP, VPI and ► PO and there is ample evidence for this idea. However, this was recently challenged by the claimed existence of another nociception, thermoception and itch specific nucleus ► VMpo within the lateral thalamus, which seems to receive spinal cord and trigeminal lamina I inputs somatotopically and is most evident in the monkey and man (Craig et al. 1994). This notion has recently been questioned as well, by demonstrating that VMpo may simply be part of the periphery of ► VPM. At one level, these disputes seem simply a consequence of disagreements over how one delineates various borders of thalamic nuclei, which are invariably ambiguous and poorly defined, especially the transition zones between nuclei. On the other hand, they reflect philosophical differences as to the rules of the organization of the central nervous system regarding pain perception. The claim of the existence of nociceptive specific nuclei in the thalamus has the consequence of implying that these regions together with their inputs and output targets constitute the pain specific network of the brain. This claim in turn denies the contribution of other thalamic nuclei and their inputs and outputs to pain perception (see ► Spinothalamocortical Projections from SM).

Periphery of VP, Rod and Matrix of VP and VMpo

Staining thalamic tissue for ► cytochrome oxidase (CO) showed that lateral thalamic somatosensory regions, VP and its surrounding nuclei, can be subdivided into two compartments, a region densely la-

N

beled with CO and a surrounding periphery (VPp) labeled weakly with CO. This observation was first made in Kniffki's lab for the cat thalamus, in the late 1980s. Independently, E.G. Jones noted the same CO staining based distinction in the monkey lateral thalamus and extended the parcellation by combining CO staining with two calcium binding proteins (▶ calbindin and ▶ parvalbumin), which preferentially label the CO dense and CO sparse domains of ▶ VP and its periphery. Jones advanced the hypothesis that the CO dense region, dubbed the rod region, was involved in sensory information transmission to the cortex by terminating in layer IV, while the CO weakly labeled region, dubbed the matrix region, projected mainly to layer I of the cortex and was involved in modulating cortical responses. A subsequent study did not substantiate this idea (Shi et al. 1993). Kniffki and colleagues hypothesized, mainly by relating terminations of the spinothalamic tract to the CO sparse region of the cat VP, that neurons in the VP periphery (VPp) are mainly nociceptive, while the CO dense region receives inputs from the medial lemniscus and signals innocuous somatosensory information to the cortex. A series of studies indicated that the cat VP does not have nociceptive cells. However, the opposite claim has been harder to prove since the number of nociceptive cells characterized in the VPp of the cat has remained small (Horn et al. 1999; Martin et al. 1990). To further explore the segregation of VP and its periphery in the monkey, electrophysiological studies contrasted nociceptive neurons in the squirrel monkey VP and VPI (equivalent to VPp in the cat) and observed that most VP nociceptive cells were WDR type while VPI nociceptive cells were both NS and WDR types. Given the distinct white matter localization of spinal cord lamina I vs. deeper spinothalamic cells and the evidence that most NS type cells in the spinal cord are localized to lamina I, it was proposed that the monkey periphery of VP preferentially or exclusively receives inputs from spinal cord lamina I cells, while the VP proper receives inputs from deeper laminae spinothalamic cells. This claim remains unproven and does not match with earlier reports (in the macaque) that VP nociceptive cells are of both NS and WDR types; it also does not match with the prevalences of NS and WDR type spinothalamic cells in the monkey, which do not seem to differ between spinal cord laminae. Craig and colleagues extended these ideas to the extreme and proposed the existence of VMpo, a unique lateral thalamic nucleus that provides pain specific inputs to the insular cortex. The corollary to this idea is that nociceptive inputs to VP proper are modulatory in nature and do not signal nociceptive sensory information. This idea has been criticized by various groups and remains controversial. Human imaging shows robust activation of SII and posterior insula and more variable responses in SI for experimental pain in healthy humans. A recent meta-analysis, however, indicates no significant difference in activation incidence between these structures (Apkarian et al. 2005). Even if one assumes that posterior insular activity is due to inputs from VMpo, nociceptive inputs to SI and SII are undoubtedly from VP and VPI and hence nociceptive inputs to the latter nuclei participate in the cortical activity associated with pain perception (see essays ▶ corticothalamic and thalamocortical interactions; ▶ spinothalamic terminations, core and matrix; ▶ thalamic nuclei involved in pain, human and monkey; ▶ spinothalamic projections in rat; ▶ spinothalamic input, cells of origin (monkey); ▶ thalamic nuclei involved in pain, cat and rat; ▶ spinothalamocortical projections to ventromedial and parafascicular nuclei; ▶ thalamus, nociceptive cells in VPI, cat and rat).

Generally, this debate is the most modern version of specificity vs. pattern theories of coding for pain in the nervous system, a debate that goes back to Helmholz, Von Frey and Goldsheider, who were battling pain representation models based on the discovery of punctate receptive fields on the human skin. In the 1960s, the debate moved from psychophysics to the properties of spinal cord neurons and the contribution of nociceptive specific vs. wide dynamic range type cells to pain perception. One group of scientists staked the claim that the wide dynamic range neurons were necessary and sufficient for pain perception, while another group claimed that nociceptive specific cells were all that was needed for pain perception. There was probably always a silent majority of scientists who simply accepted that both types of neurons are involved in pain perception and that these cell types complement each other in the range of stimuli that could evoke pain perception. Thus, VMpo and its connectivity represent the latest effort in pinpointing a specific group of cells from the skin to the cortex that uniquely signal pain from neurons that are specifically involved in coding noxious, thermal and itch stimuli. The opponents of this idea question whether VMpo exists as a unique thalamic nucleus and argue that there is ample evidence that other spinal cord neurons, thalamic nuclei and cortical regions have repeatedly been demonstrated to have all the necessary characteristics to encode nociceptive information.

Brainstem Inputs

Spinoreticulothalamic projections, which are pathways conveying spinal cord inputs to different brainstem targets and then in turn projecting to the thalamus have been studied best in the rat. Some of these pathways seem specifically involved in conveying whole body nociceptive information to the thalamus. In the medullary brainstem, the subnucleus reticularis dorsalis (SRD) seems to be one of the main nociceptive relays to the thalamus. Neurons from the SRD project to VMl and ► PF in the ► medial thalamus and neurons in VMl in turn project to the layer I of the ventrolateral cortex, while projections from PF project to the ► basal ganglia, the subthalamic nucleus and parts of the motor and parietal cortex (see ► brainstem subnucleus reticularis dorsalis neuron).

Another brainstem-thalamic projection, described in the rat, is through the internal lateral parabrachial nucleus, which receives nociceptive inputs from deep laminae of the spinal cord and projects to medial thalamic nuclei PC, CM and PF. Traditionally, CM and PF have been grouped together and implicated in affective modulation of pain. A large proportion of PF cells respond to nociceptive stimuli and stimulation in the region evokes pain-like reports in humans and pain-like behavior in animals. In humans, medial thalamic stimulation or lesioning has been used for pain relief and has targeted the CM-PF region. Such procedures report a fair incidence of success. PF and amygdala receive serotonergic inputs from ventral PAG and the three structures seem to interact in modulating the affective component of pain. Suppression of rats' affective reaction to noxious stimuli by injection of morphine into the ventral PAG is reversed by serotonin antagonists applied either to PF or amygdala (see ► parafascicular nucleus, pain modulation ► thalamus, nociceptive inputs in the rat (spinal) ► thalamo-amygdala interactions and pain).

Spinothalamo-Cortical Connectivity

Although the suggested role of the nucleus submedius (SM) in nociception has diminished over the years, its projection targets show that SM neurons (in the rat) terminate in the ventrolateral orbital cortex (VLO), a region where nociceptive neurons have been described in the rat. The VLO nucleus also receives inputs from the ventral ► periaqueductal gray (PAG) and dorsal raphe. A similar but smaller brainstem projection seems to exist for the SM as well. The rat SM does not receive spinal cord lamina I inputs as originally claimed; instead its inputs are from deeper laminae. Although a nucleus equivalent to SM was originally described in the monkey, this claim has been repeatedly refuted (see ► thalamus, nociceptive inputs in the rat (spinal); ► spino-thalamocortical projections from SM).

Potential connectivity between thalamocortical projecting neurons and spinothalamic terminations has been studied probabilistically at the light microscopy level (Gingold et al. 1991). Hand primary somatosensory cortex projecting cells are labeled retrogradely with a given marker and spinothalamic terminations from the upper cervical enlargement labeled antero-

gradely with a different marker. Given the known dendritic branching pattern of thalamocortical cells, one can then calculate how many of these cells can potentially receive spinothalamic inputs on their dendritic perimeter. Although such an analysis cannot establish the presence or absence of synapses, it provides quantitative bounds as to the influence of nociceptive inputs through the spinothalamic projections to the cortical target. The analysis shows that 87% of cervical enlargement spinothalamic terminations are localized to VPL, VPI and CL and 24% of the hand region of the primary somatosensory cortex is putatively contacted by these spinothalamic terminations. A more recent study examined connectivity between thalamic cells and spinothalamic afferents by intracellularly labeling individual thalamic neurons and examining the proximity of the labeled dendrites to spinothalamic terminals (Shi and Apkarian 1995). A similar study has also been done electrophysiologically and indicates that the probability of encountering spinothalamic terminations in the vicinity of nociceptive cells in VP is 33% while in VPI it is 73% (Apkarian and Shi 1994).

Synaptic Connectivity

Synaptic morphology, using electron microscopy, has been studied for spinothalamic inputs and contrasted to dorsal column inputs in VP (Ralston 2003). The study examined synapses for spinothalamic projections onto VP proper cells and contrasted them to medial lemniscal synapses. Spinothalamic synapses were found to be mainly on dendrites of projecting cells, in contrast to medial lemniscal synapses that formed triads between terminals and projecting and local GABAergic cells. This distinction between afferent input types and synapses is congruent with physiological connectivity differences observed for VP cell groups with and without nociceptive inputs (see ► thalamus, dynamics of nociception). More recently, similar electron microscopic studies were also done for spinal cord lamina I inputs to VMpo (Beggs et al. 2003). The synaptic profiles in VMpo were almost always triadic. Thus, the lamina I spinothalamic inputs to VMpo are different from spinothalamic inputs to VP. The difference is partly attributed to the targets and partly to inputs. Most likely most of the inputs examined in VP reflected terminations from deeper laminae than lamina I. These differences are consistent with the light microscopic observation regarding proximity of spinothalamic terminations to nociceptive cells in VP *vs.* VPI.

Species Differences

There are important species differences regarding the spinothalamic pathway, its terminations in the thalamus and response properties of thalamic nociceptive cells. The rat spinothalamic tract (see ▶ Spinothalamic Projections in Rat) is composed of a third fewer cells than that of the monkey. Rat lateral thalamic nuclei are devoid of local interneurons. Thus, one can assert that terminations in these nuclei are synapses on cortex projecting cells. Also, the rat VP was not traditionally subdivided into a core and a periphery; as a result there is no doubt that some spinothalamic terminals are on VP cells that project to the primary or secondary somatosensory cortex. Rat spinothalamic terminations in the medial thalamus generally target the same nuclei as in the cat or monkey, perhaps with the exception of SM, which does not seem to receive spinal cord lamina I inputs. In the spinal cord, the lateral cervical nucleus (LCN) seems more prominent in the rat and these cells do project to the thalamus, although their functional role has remained unclear.

More recent studies have unraveled differences in terminations of superficial laminar spinal cord cells and deeper ones as to their targets in the rat thalamus. Lamina I inputs seem to be limited to lateral thalamic targets, where the region is subdivided into VP, VPpc, Po and PoT, where VPpc and PoT probably correspond to different portions of VP periphery. Direct deeper laminae projections in the rat seem to be limited to PoT and CL. (see ▶ thalamus, nociceptive inputs in the rat (spinal) ▶ spinothalamic projections in rat).

Neurotransmitters and Neuromodulators

Like other sensory inputs to the thalamus, ▶ glutamatergic neurotransmission is assumed to transmit nociceptive information. Although such transmission has been demonstrated for other sensory modalities, as in somatosensory transmission, it is not proven in the case of nociception. The thalamocortical efferent pathway is made of neurons that are glutamatergic. Cortical inputs to the thalamus seem to be mediated through ▶ AMPA and ▶ mGLU receptors. ▶ GABAergic inhibitory interneurons and GABAergic thalamic reticular nucleus innervation provide inhibition on projecting neurons through ▶ GABA$_A$ and ▶ GABA$_A$ receptors. Most current knowledge regarding nociceptive neurotransmission is based on studies of VB neuronal properties and indicates that ▶ NMDA receptors signal acute thermal and mechanical responses. There is also evidence that thalamic mGLU receptor mechanisms are important in inflammation-induced hyperalgesia and in the expression of such behavior (see ▶ metabotropic glutamate receptors in the thalamus).

Eight metabotropic glutamate receptor subtypes (mGLU1–mGLU8) have been characterized, are divided into three groups (I, II, III) and are all found in the thalamus. Group I receptors mediate mainly postsynaptic actions, while Groups II and III regulate presynaptic transmitter release. Different subtypes are important in either cortico-thalamic inputs or thalamic reticular neuronal modulating of GABAergic transmission. Thus, mGLU receptors have a minimal role in ascending sensory transmission but are more important in modulating this transmission (see ▶ nociceptive neurotransmission in the thalamus).

Spinothalamic neurons contain glutamate and various ▶ neuropeptides. Of the large list of neuropeptides seen in spinothalamic cells, ▶ substance P (SP) is found abundantly in the medial thalamus, some of which may be due to spinothalamic inputs. Cholinergic, ▶ serotonergic and ▶ noradrenergic inputs from the brainstem are also found in the thalamus, all of which are probably part of the arousal modulatory system. Intrinsic SP neurons are described in thalamic regions receiving spinothalamic inputs. ▶ CGRP neurons are found in the periphery of VP and described as projecting to the amygdala or insula (see ▶ thalamus, visceral representation ▶ parafascicular nucleus, pain modulation ▶ thalamic neurotransmitters and neurochemical effector molecules).

Somatic Representation

Nociceptive representation in the thalamus has been described in multiple species, primarily in rat, cat and monkey and mainly in anesthetized preparations. The overall number of nociceptive cells described remains relatively small and the properties of cells located in medial in contrast to lateral thalamic nuclei seem distinct. Nociceptive cells found in the medial thalamic nuclei tend to have more nociceptive specific responses, with response patterns that are modulated with the sleep-wakefulness cycle, level of anesthesia and attentional manipulations. In contrast, nociceptive cells in the lateral thalamus have more divergent inputs, they can be nociceptive specific or wide dynamic range types, with response properties that seem more reproducible and less dependent on attentional manipulations. The receptive field size, location and properties seem labile in medial thalamic cells, while in lateral thalamic cells they seem more constant and correspond to the properties of similar cells described in the spinal cord or trigeminal nuclei. These response differences are generally consistent with the notion that medial thalamic nociceptive information may be providing cortical signals regarding the affective properties of pain and also providing a more general modulatory signal that may be important in biasing the cortex and in modulating the attentional circuitry of the cortex. In contrast, lateral thalamic nociceptive signals are consistent with the general idea that these are the ▶ sensory-discriminative information being transmitted to cortical regions specifically involved in pain perception. Even though both notions may generally be

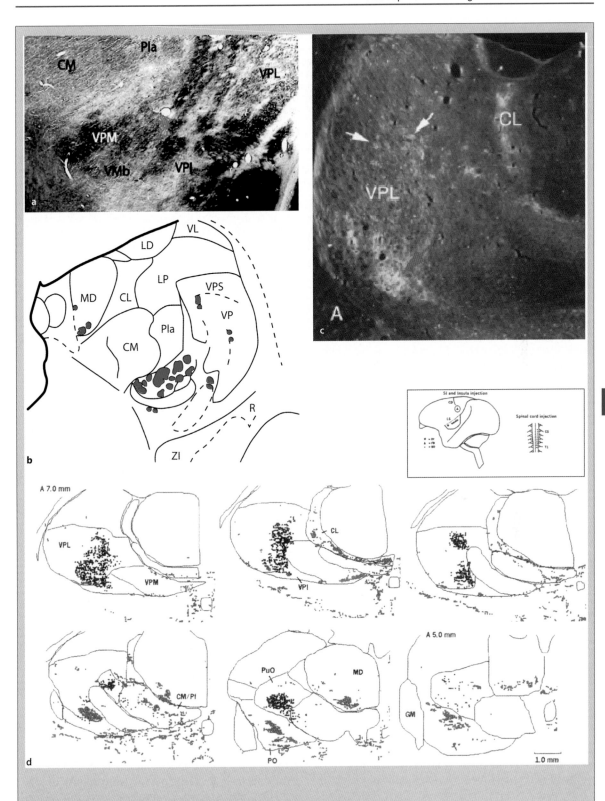

true, there are important deviations regarding input-output properties and response properties of nociceptive cells in specific thalamic nuclei, implying that the medial *vs.* lateral thalamic functional differentiation is most probably too simplistic (see ▶ parafascicular nucleus, pain modulation ▶ thalamus, nociceptive inputs in the rat (spinal) ▶ spinothalamic input, cells of origin (monkey)).

◄ **Nociceptive Processing in the Thalamus, Figure 1,** Spinothalamic inputs to the lateral thalamus. Data are presented from four different labs. (a) A recent study (Graziano and Jones 2004) shows that trigeminothalamic projections in the monkey terminate in the periphery of VP, asserts that these terminations in turn project to primary and secondary somatosensory cortex and thus questions whether VMpo is a unique thalamic nucleus (from Graziano and Jones 2004). (b) An extensive study of spinal and trigeminal lamina I projections to the thalamus shows the location of VMpo and the somatotopic terminations within it (Craig 2004). Terminations from the cervical enlargement are in red, while those from trigeminal nucleus caudalis are in blue (from Craig 2004). (c) Site of dense terminations from cervical enlargement in monkey (Ralston 2003). The spinal cord injection does not distinguish between laminae. The author illustrates that the dense terminations in this case are more lateral and anterior than VMpo (from Ralston 2003). (d) Terminations from cervical enlargement in the monkey, in relation to neurons projecting to the hand region of the primary somatosensory cortex and in relation to neurons projecting to the insula (Apkarian and Shi 1998). Spinothalamic terminations are in red, cells projecting to hand primary somatosensory cortex in blue, cells projecting to insula green. Spinothalamic terminations in slice 4 from the most anterior section show a dense terminal patch at the border of VPL and VPI, closely corresponding to the labeling illustrated in (c). On the other hand, spinothalamic terminals in slice 6 are very similar to the labeling shown in (b), thus matching the VMpo label. At least at this slice location and from the specific insular injection, there is no overlap between these terminations and insular projecting cells. More anteriorly, there is some overlap between spinothalamic terminations and insula projecting cells. However, the overlap between primary somatosensory cortex projecting cells and spinothalamic terminations is more extensive. Comparing the four panels it should be evident that spinothalamic terminations in the lateral thalamus extend from VP proper to VPI and other VP periphery regions and most posteriorly are located at the interface between VP and PO, a region that has been called VMpo. At least in (d) this labeling seems continuous antero-posteriorly, casting doubt on the notion that the VMpo region is a unique nucleus with distinct projections to the insula. Figure from Apkarian and Shi, 1998.

Visceral Representation

Visceral stimulation induced thalamic activity is demonstrated in the thalamus in humans with brain imaging studies and in animals using electrophysiology. Visceral responsive cells are found in and around VP with no evidence for viscerotopy, although visceral topography for baro- and chemo-receptors has been suggested. Visceral responsive cells are also reported in the medial thalamus. However, thalamic regions with inputs from SRD seem to lack visceral inputs (see ► thalamus, visceral representation ► thalamus and visceral pain processing (human imaging) ► thalamus, clinical visceral pain, human imaging ► thalamus, nociceptive cells in VPI, cat and rat ► spinothalamocortical projections to ventromedial and parafascicular nuclei).

Thalamic Lesions in Animals

Thalamic lesions (thalamotomy) are used to relieve chronic pain in humans. On the other hand, stimulation within the human thalamus gives rise to pain sensations. Recent animal studies examined the behavioral effects of thalamic lesions, targeting either the lateral thalamus or both the lateral and medial thalamus. Generally, it seems, at least in the rat, that lesions involving any part of the thalamus give rise to increased sensitivity to mechanical and thermal noxious stimuli, reminiscent of 'thalamic syndrome' outcomes in humans. Moreover, when thalamic lesions are performed in animals with neuropathic pain-like behavior (partial peripheral nerve injury), this behavior is diminished only transiently and when the neuropathic injury is performed after a thalamic lesion, no significant change in neuropathic behavior is observed. These results challenge the idea that the thalamus is the main sensory transmission pathway for nociception, at least in the rat (see ► lateral thalamic lesions, pain behavior in animals ► thalamotomy, pain behavior in animals).

Thalamic Plasticity

Plasticity of thalamic representation of innocuous and noxious inputs has been demonstrated following a variety of deafferentation procedures. The main effect is an expansion of intact adjacently represented regions into the areas of deafferentation. Spinothalamic tract lesions seem to increase spontaneous firing rates and increase sensitivity and bursting of thalamic cells with innocuous inputs. Similar observations have been made in humans with chronic pain (see ► thalamic plasticity and chronic pain).

Dynamics of Thalamic Coding for Nociception

A major function of the thalamus is state dependent modulation of incoming sensory information. Changes in intrinsic response properties of thalamic cells with the sleep and wake cycle have been documented extensively in many regions of the thalamus (Steriade et al. 1990). However, there is minimal such information regarding nociceptive inputs, the difficulty being that most thalamic nociceptive neurons are studied under anesthesia.

Thalamic neurons fire in two distinct modes, tonic and bursting. The bursting mode is due to a T-type calcium channel and such bursting activity is seen in conscious chronic pain patients. During sleep, thalamic neurons are mostly in burst mode and shift to tonic mode with wakefulness. Bursting activity in the conscious state is termed ► thalamocortical dysrhythmia and suggested to be a basis for pain and other neurological disorders (see ► burst activity in thalamus and pain).

A very early report documented that most nociceptive neurons in the thalamus switch response modes with the sleep cycle. Of 8 neurons that were characterized at different states of wakefulness, 5 began to respond to innocuous stimuli as well when the animal was more awake and 3 responded more specifically to noxious stimuli with increased wakefulness (Casey 1966).

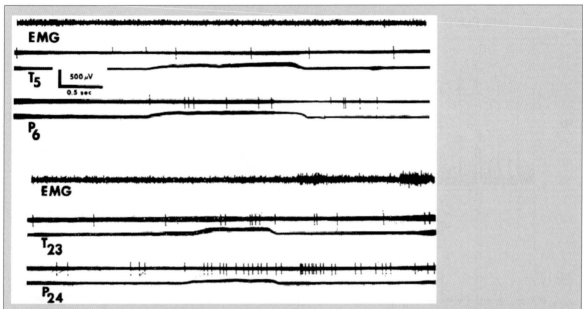

Nociceptive Processing in the Thalamus, Figure 2 Response properties of a neuron recorded in MD, in a conscious monkey (Casey 1966). Responses to innocuous and noxious stimuli are modulated with the wakefulness of the animal. In the top panel the animal is drowsy or lightly asleep, as a result the painful stimulus (delivered to the arm) does not evoke an EMG response. Tactile stimulation (T5) does not activate the neuron, but a painful stimulus does (P6). When the animal becomes more awake, the neuron responds at a higher frequency to both tactile (T23) and painful (P24) stimuli. Figure from Casey 1966.

Moreover, the author noticed and described changes in firing patterns for these nociceptive cells before and after the animal was given either an auditory or visual stimulus, which also changed the responses of the nociceptive cells to the noxious or innocuous somatic stimuli. Casey presented these results as evidence for refuting the notion of specificity of pain processing in the CNS. It is noteworthy that most neurons that changed responses with the state of wakefulness were located in the medial thalamus. Unfortunately, there are no new systematic studies on the topic. The effects of anesthesia on transmission of somatosensory inputs have recently been examined in VP, mainly for somatic innocuous inputs (Vahle-Hinz and Detsch 2002). Simultaneous recordings from groups of neighboring neurons in and around the VP in the anesthetized monkey indicate that the firing patterns of such cells change dynamically with every stimulus (see ▶ thalamus, dynamics of nociception).

Bushnell and colleagues (Bushnell et al. 1993) performed electrophysiological recordings in conscious monkeys trained in a thermal discrimination task on the lip. The recordings were mostly from the medial border region of VPM (which proponents of VMpo now claim was mislabeled and that in fact these were recordings from VMpo). They found 22 cells responding to heat, the majority of which also responded to noxious heat; some responded to mechanical stimuli and / or cooling. Thus, neurons in this region had both NS-type responses and WDR-type responses. The group average of some of the nociceptive responsive cells showed

a well-definedthreshold and a linear increase in firing rate above threshold. Importantly, cells in this region were tested for modulation by attentional shifts and, in contrast to the observations by Casey (Casey 1966), these VPM cells were not affected by attention towards or away from the stimulus.

The most comprehensive physiological study of nociceptive thalamic neurons was done in anesthetized monkeys, where 73 nociceptive cells were characterized in 26 animals (Kenshalo et al. 1980). The study explored neurons in VPL and showed that nociceptive cells' receptive field properties generally matched the somatotopic organization of this nucleus, with nociceptive cells in medial VPL having somatic fields localized to the forelimbs, while nociceptive cells in lateral VPL usually had receptive fields limited to the lower body. They also showed that repeated thermal stimulation of these cells increased their responses, implying that such neurons may participate in perceptions associated with thermal sensitization. Moreover, the authors showed that only spinal cord lesions that severed the ventrolateral white matter ipsilateral to the recording in the thalamus and contralateral to the location of the receptive field on the skin would abolish the responses of these cells to noxious stimuli applied within the receptive field.

The stimulus-response curves for noxious thermal stimuli from Kenshalo et al. (Kenshalo et al. 1980) and from Bushnell et al. (1993) are presented together to emphasize the similarity of the results obtained in anesthetized and conscious monkeys and to show the sim-

N

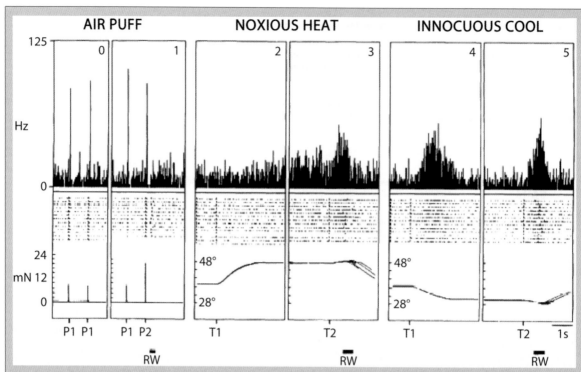

Nociceptive Processing in the Thalamus, Figure 3 Response properties of a neuron recorded from VPM in conscious monkey (Bushnell et al. 1993). The neuron responds to air puffs (a), to noxious heat (b) and to innocuous cooling (c) of the skin on the maxilla. The initial heat response at 4°C is small but increases with continued heating. The second heat change (T2 of 0.4, 0.8 or 1.0°C) results in a robust response. From Fig. 2 of Bushnell et al. 1993.

ilarity of responses for nociceptive cells in VPL and VPM thalamic nuclei. Both group-averaged curves increased positively for stimuli above 47°C at approximately the same rate, although in the conscious preparation, threshold to painful thermal stimulus-responses seemed closer to 47°C than in the anesthetized monkey, where the threshold was around 43–45°C. Thus, in the lateral thalamus, nociceptive cells respond to thermal stimuli within a range that generally corresponds to human psychophysical studies for heat pain perception and at least the threshold of these neurons also corresponds to the heat response thresholds for peripheral nociceptive afferents.

Thalamic physiology, especially for nociception, has traditionally emphasized the response properties of individual neurons. Establishing such properties provides the basis for the kinds of information that different neurons in different parts of the thalamus have access to, but it by no means demonstrates the dynamic properties of such neurons when neurons are considered as part of a population and where interactions between members and modulatory influences from remote sites would change stimulus-response properties in time and space within and across neuronal assemblies. Populational recording studies show that even the notion of a receptive field is a function of the group of neurons and the time point at which the group interactions are considered and neighboring groups of

VP cells with and without nociceptive inputs have distinct spatio-temporal response properties. Such populational coding properties must also be modulated with intrinsic thalamic conditions (burst or tonic mode), as well as modulatory functions of cortical and brainstem inputs (see ▶ thalamus, dynamics of nociception).

At a higher level of integration, one needs to consider the mode of interaction between cortical areas, especially given that a diverse set of cortical regions have been shown to participate in pain perception. The cortico-cortical interactions are usually assumed to be direct. Recent models, however, propose that all such interactions may be mediated through thalamocortical – corticothalamic chained loops. Such models have been advanced mainly for the visual thalamus and cortex and remain to be tested for pain (see ▶ thalamocortical loops and information processing).

Human Imaging Studies — Visceral

The participation of the human thalamus in various innocuous and noxious visceral sensations has now been demonstrated in human brain imaging studies. Thalamic activity in humans has now been observed in angina, silent ischemia and syndrome X, as well as in noxious esophageal stimulation, gastric distension and noxious gastrointestinal distension in healthy

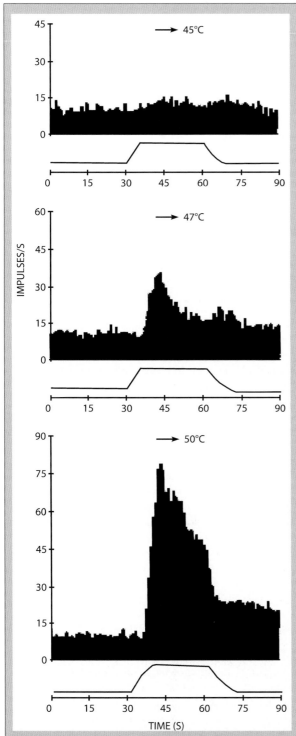

Nociceptive Processing in the Thalamus, Figure 4 Average responses of 10 neurons in anesthetized monkey (Kenshalo et al. 1980). Recordings are from VPL. Responses to 45, 47 and 50°C thermal stimuli are shown. The stimulus time course is shown below each response. Figure from Fig. 5 of Kenshalo et al. 1980.

subjects and in irritable bowel syndrome patients (see ► thalamus and visceral pain processing (human imag-

ing) ► thalamus, clinical visceral pain, human imaging).

Human Imaging Studies — Acute Pain and Clinical Conditions

Thalamic activity has been observed in some of the earliest brain imaging studies of pain (Jones al. 1991). There is now ample evidence that thalamic activity can be reproducibly observed in human studies of acute or experimental conditions. More recent studies have attempted to parcel this activity into lateral and medial activations. Spatial resolution of this technology limits our ability to state the specific thalamic nuclei activated in the human brain (see ► human thalamic response to experimental pain (neuroimaging)).

Inflammatory pain conditions *vs.* neuropathic pain conditions in animals show distinct reorganization of the peripheral and spinal cord circuitry. This has been only minimally studied in the thalamus (Vos et al. 2000) and the results indicate increased rates and more nociceptive responses for VP cells in neuropathic rats. Human brain imaging studies generally show a decreased baseline activity, noxious stimulus evoked activity and atrophy in chronic clinical pain states, but there is no evidence as to whether this pattern is generally applicable for inflammatory pain conditions as well (see ► thalamus, clinical pain, human imaging).

Human Thalamus: Recording, Stimulation and Lesion

Neurosurgical attempts to control chronic pain and tremor by thalamic lesions or stimulation, such as ► thalamotomy, ► deep brain stimulation, ► gamma knife procedures or stereotactic surgeries targeting the thalamus provide the opportunity to study thalamic neuronal properties in conscious humans or to examine the effects of localized electrical stimulation evoked perceptions. In the lateral thalamic ► Vc region, the human equivalent of VP, WDR and NS type nociceptive cells are described. A few nociceptive cells are also found in human medial thalamus. Unfortunately, the human studies cannot pinpoint the exact location of such neurons. In subjects with a history of existing painful conditions, there is now good evidence that incidence of stimulation-evoked pain is enhanced in Vc and this increase may be more prominent in the periphery of Vc (posterior-inferior area) (see ► lateral thalamic pain-related cells in humans; ► human thalamic nociceptive neurons)

Based on different traditions and theoretical ideas, different neurosurgeons have had their preferred targets for thalamic stimulation or lesion for pain relief. Jeanmonod and colleagues have targeted the CL region and within that region especially neurons that exhibit low threshold calcium spike bursts since they believe that

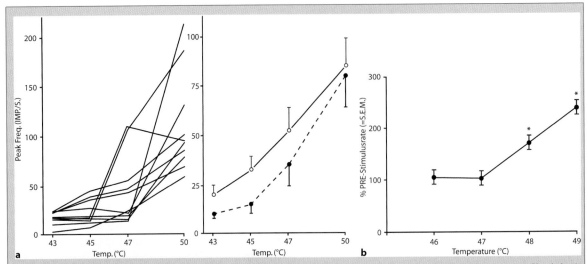

Nociceptive Processing in the Thalamus, Figure 5 (a) Stimulus-response for 10 neurons found in VPL in the anesthetized monkey (Kenshalo et al. 1980). The peak impulses / second are plotted for each corresponding temperature. Left panel are individual neurons, right panel is group average (from Fig. 4 of Kenshalo et al. 1980). (b) Average stimulus-response curve of 6 heat activated and heat / cold activated neurons to temperatures of 46–49°C, as compared to baseline activity (Bushnell et al. 1993). The neurons were characterized in the conscious monkey VPM. Stimulus-responses increase only for 48 and 49°C. Figure from Fig. 6 of Bushnell et al. 1993.

neurogenic pain of central or peripheral origin can be adequately controlled by silencing these neurons with a central lateral thalamotomy (CLT). Other neurosurgeons have targeted the CM-PF region. Lenz and colleagues, on the other hand, have targeted the Vc region and its periphery, based on observing increased bursting activity in the region in chronic pain conditions in humans and in monkey studies. Increased bursting activity seems most prominent in patients with spinal transection or thalamic cells that do not have receptive fields and that are located in the representation of the anesthetic part of the body. Given the location of these bursting cells, their specific role in pain perception remains to be established (see ▶ thalamotomy for human pain relief; ▶ thalamic bursting activity, chronic pain). Electrophysiological mapping of the thalamus during neurosurgical procedures provides the opportunity to characterize the neurons' receptive fields (RF) and compare them to the perceived location and quality of sensations evoked by stimulating these neurons (projected field or PF maps). This method can reveal plasticity of thalamic organization in humans with chronic pain. Such studies have been done mainly for Vc and its periphery. In chronic pain patients, in and around Vc, there is often a mismatch between RF and PF especially at the zone between the anesthetic site, the site of sensory loss and the transition to sites with normal sensations. Moreover, electrical stimulation in and around Vc has a higher probability of evoking pain in patients with chronic pain. These plastic changes probably contribute to the chronic pain condition (see ▶ thalamus, receptive fields, projected fields, human).

Nociceptive responsive cells have been described in and around Vc in humans. Most nociceptive cells in this region are characterized as WDR-type. Some respond to mechanical and heat stimuli, others to mechanical and cold. Microstimulation in the same region of the human thalamus results in sensations of pain and / or heat. Nociceptive neurons in the human CM-PF have also been described, most responding to noxious pinprick but not innocuous touch (see ▶ parafascicular nucleus, pain modulation ▶ human thalamic nociceptive neurons ▶ Lateral thalamic pain-related cells in humans). In a subject suffering from angina, thalamic micro-stimulation evoked a pain 'almost identical' to her angina, which started and ended in exact relationship to the electrical stimulation. The stimulation site was in the periphery of Vc. Thus, this region and its cortical connectivity can access the memory of angina pain (see ▶ angina pectoris, neurophysiology and psychophysics).

Overview

It should be clear from this overview that there remain large gaps in our knowledge regarding the role of the thalamus in nociception. Unfortunately, animal studies of the thalamic physiology of pain have dramatically decreased in the last few years. Perhaps this is due to the success of human brain imaging studies that provide us with information regarding thalamus and cortex in conscious human pain perception. There is no doubt that human brain imaging is providing exciting new insights into the role of the CNS in pain. On the other hand, the spatial and temporal resolution of these techniques severely limit the detailed information on neuronal and glial processes that remain to be uncovered

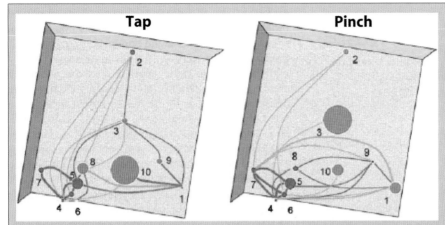

Nociceptive Processing in the Thalamus, Figure 6 Dynamics of nociceptive responses in a group of neurons in the lateral thalamus in the monkey (Apkarian et al. 2000). Responses of 10 neurons studied simultaneously in a 100 micron^3 space are shown. The relative locations are shown by the circles, the size and color indicate stimulus responses (red increased activity, blue decreased activity). Connections between cells indicate strength of correlations (orange positive, green negative). The figure illustrates that response magnitude and connectivity change dynamically with different types of stimuli for a cluster of cells that are involved in coding nociceptive inputs (from Apkarian et al. 2000).

in order to properly understand the functional roles of various thalamic structures and their interconnections with the cortex in pain perception.

References

1. Apkarian AV, Shi T (1994) Squirrel monkey lateral thalamus. I. Somatic nociresponsive neurons and their relation to spinothalamic terminals. J Neurosci 14:6779–6795
2. Apkarian AV, Shi T (1998) Thalamocortical connections of the cingulate and insula in relation to nociceptive inputs to the cortex. In: Ayrapetyan SN, Apkarian AV (eds) Pain mechanisms and management. IOS Press, Amsterdam, pp 212–221
3. Apkarian AV, Shi T, Bruggemann J et al. (2000) Segregation of nociceptive and non-nociceptive networks in the squirrel monkey somatosensory thalamus. J Neurophysiol 84:484–494
4. Apkarian AV, Bushnell MC, Treede RD et al. (2005) Human brain mechanisms of pain perception and regulation in health and disease. Eur J Pain 9:463–484
5. Beggs J, Jordan S, Ericson AC et al. (2003) Synaptology of trigemino- and spinothalamic lamina I terminations in the posterior ventral medial nucleus of the macaque. J Comp Neurol 459:334–354
6. Bushnell MC, Duncan GH, Tremblay N (1993) Thalamic VPM nucleus in the behaving monkey. I. Multimodal and discriminative properties of thermosensitive neurons. J Neurophysiol 69:739–752
7. Casey KL (1966) Unit analysis of nociceptive mechanisms in the thalamus of the awake squirrel monkey. J Neurophysiol 29:727–750
8. Craig AD (2004) Distribution of trigeminothalamic and spinothalamic lamina I terminations in the macaque monkey. J Comp Neurol 477:119–148
9. Craig AD Jr, Burton H (1981) Spinal and medullary lamina I projection to nucleus submedius in medial thalamus: a possible pain center. J Neurophysiol 45:443–466
10. Craig AD, Bushnell MC, Zhang ET et al. (1994) A thalamic nucleus specific for pain and temperature sensation. Nature 372:770–773
11. Gingold SI, Greenspan JD, Apkarian AV (1991) Anatomic evidence of nociceptive inputs to primary somatosensory cortex: relationship between spinothalamic terminals and thalamocortical cells in squirrel monkeys. J Comp Neurol 308:467–490
12. Graziano A, Jones EG (2004) Widespread thalamic terminations of fibers arising in the superficial medullary dorsal horn of monkeys and their relation to calbindin immunoreactivity. J Neurosci 24:248–256
13. Horn AC, Vahle-Hinz C, Bruggemann J et al. (1999) Responses of neurons in the lateral thalamus of the cat to stimulation of urinary bladder, colon, esophagus, and skin. Brain Res 851:164–174
14. Jones EG (1985) The Thalamus. Plenum, New York
15. Jones AK, Brown WD, Friston KJ et al. (1991) Cortical and subcortical localization of response to pain in man using positron emission tomography. Proc Biol Sci 244: 39–44
16. Kenshalo DR Jr, Giesler GJ Jr, Leonard RB et al. (1980) Responses of neurons in primate ventral posterior lateral nucleus to noxious stimuli. J Neurophysiol 43:1594–1614
17. Martin RJ, Apkarian AV, Hodge CJ Jr (1990) Ventrolateral and dorsolateral ascending spinal cord pathway influence on thalamic nociception in cat. J Neurophysiol 64:1400–1412
18. Ralston HJ, III (2003) Pain, the brain, and the (calbindin) stain. J Comp Neurol 459:329–333
19. Shi T, Apkarian AV (1995) Morphology of thalamocortical neurons projecting to the primary somatosensory cortex and their relationship to spinothalamic terminals in the squirrel monkey. J Comp Neurol 361:1–24
20. Shi T, Stevens RT, Tessier J et al. (1993) Spinothalamocortical inputs nonpreferentially innervate the superficial and deep cortical layers of SI. Neurosci Lett 160:209–213
21. Steriade M, Jones EG, Llinas RR (1990) Thalamic oscillations and signaling. Wiley Neuroscience, New York
22. Vahle-Hinz C, Detsch O (2002) What can in vivo electrophysiology in animal models tell us about mechanisms of anaesthesia? Br J Anaesth 89:123–142
23. Vos BP, Benoist JM, Gautron M et al. (2000) Changes in neuronal activities in the two ventral posterior medial thalamic nuclei in an experimental model of trigeminal pain in the rat by constriction of one infraorbital nerve. Somatosens Mot Res 17:109–122

N

Nociceptor Generator Potential

CARLOS BELMONTE

Instituto de Neurociencias de Alicante, University
Miguel Hernández-CSIC, San Juan de Alicante, Spain
carlos.belmonte@umh.es

Synonyms

Receptor potential; generator current

Definition

The local change in ▶ membrane potential caused by
the opening of ion channels in the peripheral terminals
of nociceptor neurons, when natural stimuli (mechanical, thermal, chemical) activate their transduction mechanisms.

Characteristics

Transduction of natural stimuli by the specialized membrane of sensory receptor cells leads ultimately to the opening and closing (gating) of ion channels and to the generation of local electrical signals. These were already described in early studies using invertebrate stretch receptor cells (Eyzaguirre and Kufler 1955) as well as in the receptor cells of specialized sensory organs in mammals, such as the cochlear hair cells, the olfactory neurons or the retinal photoreceptors, taking advantage of their accessibility to direct electrophysiological recording (for review see Gardner and Martin 2000). In all cases, the gating of ▶ transduction channels triggered by the stimulus caused charge transfer across the membrane and a gradual depolarization (or hyperpolarization) of an amplitude proportional to the intensity of the stimulus called the 'receptor or generator potential'.

The receptor endings of primary sensory neurons in mammals are not easily accessible to the conventional biophysical methods that were successfully applied to the cell soma. An indirect approach aimed at recording the small current flows associated with the opening of transduction channels in sensory endings was made in the middle of the 20th century using the pacinian corpuscle, a specialized mechanoreceptor that responds to very low mechanical forces and can be easily visualized and isolated from the mesentery of the cat. The pacinian corpuscle is formed by the nerve terminal of a large myelinated sensory axon surrounded by a number of concentric lamellae, which loses its myelin sheath and Schwann cells upon entering the corpuscle, running subsequently as a straight, bare nerve ending. In a series of classical studies (Gray and Sato 1953; Loewenstein 1961), the pacinian corpuscle isolated 'in vitro' was employed to record extracellularly the ▶ membrane potential changes associated with mechanical stimulation of the corpuscle surface, establishing that in the most distal part of the nerve terminal the stimulus

evoked a flow of generator current of an amplitude proportional to the magnitude of indentation (Fig. 1).
▶ Generator currents could summate temporally and propagate electrotonically (i.e. declining exponentially with distance) along the length of the axon. When the amplitude of the depolarization reaching the first node of Ranvier (located inside the corpuscle near to the point of entrance of the nerve) attained a critical level, an ▶ action potential was generated (Fig. 1). The conclusion of these and subsequent studies, was that the generator process in sensory receptor fibers takes place in a terminal portion of the nerve membrane that is not electrically excitable, i.e. cannot support a regenerative change in sodium conductance and that the process of transduction that leads to the generator potential is spatially separated from the point where propagated action potentials are produced. The firing frequency and the duration of the impulse discharge are proportional

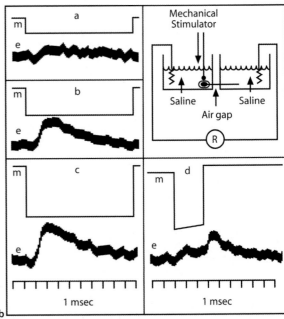

Nociceptor Generator Potential, Figure 1 (a) The pacinian corpuscle.
(b) Generator potentials recorded extracellularly in a pacinian corpuscle,
'in vitro'. a, b, and c, generator potentials (e) elicited by mechanical compressions of increasing magnitude shown in m. d. Short mechanical pulses elicit both "on" and "off" responses which sum. ((a) from Schmidt RF & Thews G, 1990, Physiologie des Menschen, 24. Auflage, Springer Verlag;
(b) after Gray JAB & Sato M, 1953, J Physiol 122:610–636)

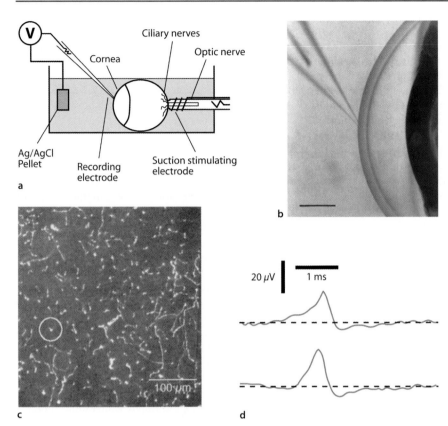

a

b

c

d

20 µV | 1 ms

Nociceptor Generator Potential, Figure 2 Recording of nerve terminal impulses in the guinea pig cornea. Schematic diagram of recording set-up (a) and photomicrograph (b) showing the location of the recording electrode. (c) confocal micrograph of nerve terminals in the cornea. (d) averages of spontaneously occurring nerve terminal impulses recorded from a mechano-nociceptor (upper trace) and a polymodal nociceptor (lower trace).

N

to the amplitude and duration of the generator potential (for details see Patton 1966; Gardner and Martin 2000). It has been speculated that the sequence of phenomena observed in the transduction process of mechanorecep-tor fibers is general to all mammalian sensory receptor endings, including nociceptive terminals, where the transduction channels opened by mechanical, thermal or chemical stimuli are thought to generate a local receptor or generator potential that will ultimately lead to impulse firing in the parent axon (Belmonte 1996). However, direct evidence for this extrapolation is still lacking, due to the difficulty of applying the intracellular or extracellular recording techniques used in other receptor classes to nociceptive nerve fibers intimately embedded in their surrounding tissues and with a diameter below 1 µ.

In recent years new technical approaches have offered indirect evidence of the presence of generator currents in nociceptive terminals. Extracellular activity of single ► nociceptive nerve endings was successfully recorded in the cornea of the eye (Fig. 2) using a large tip mi-croelectrode tightly applied against the corneal surface (Brock et al. 1998). Terminal sensory branches run be-tween corneal epithelium cells ending close to the most superficial epithelium layers; the high resistance seal formed by the electrode allowed the recording of the spontaneous and stimulus-evoked propagated impulse activity of the ending located immediately below the electrode tip. In these experiments, a depolarization preceding the propagated nerve terminal impulse, sug-gestive of a local generator current was occasionally observed in polymodal nociceptor endings (Brock et al. 1998). Likewise, in single nociceptive fibers of the rat skin, Sauer et al. (2004) using the 'threshold tracking technique' reported that heat and ► bradykinin stimu-lation of polymodal nociceptor endings was preceded by a reduction of threshold suggestive of a local depo-larization presumably corresponding to the generator potential.

Nevertheless, the location in nociceptors of the trans-formation site where generator currents give rise to propagated impulses when the depolarization exceeds threshold remains unknown. It has been suggested, based on morphological evidence that the patches of axonal membrane devoid of Schwann cell coating observed in the terminal portion of ► knee joint noci-ceptors correspond to the ► transduction sites where receptor potentials would be generated (Heppelmann et al. 1990) while action potentials occur at a more central point. However, in corneal polymodal nociceptor end-ings it has been shown that the most distant portion of the terminal possess sufficient density of ► tetrodotoxin-resistant sodium channels to sustain propagated action potentials (Brock et al. 1998), a characteristic that is not shared by cold-sensitive nerve fibers, whose pe-ripheral terminals seem to lack regenerative properties

(Brock et al. 2001). Thus, the possibility exists that in nociceptor terminals, the ion channels responsible for generator currents and those sustaining the production of propagated action potentials are not spatially segregated. This may have a functional significance in the profusely ramified nociceptor fibers. Action potentials originated at the peripheral endings by a direct action of the stimulus also propagate antidromically and invade terminals of the same parent axon that were not directly excited by the stimulus. A large proportion of nociceptor terminals contain vesicles filled with ▶ neuropeptides (CGRP, SP), that are released by the entrance of calcium ions driven by the invading antidromic action potential, thereby contributing to neurogenic inflammation.

References

1. Belmonte C (1996) Signal transduction in nociceptors: General principles. In: Belmonte C, Cervero F (eds) Neurobiology of nociceptors. Oxford University Press, Oxford, pp 243–257
2. Brock J, McLachlan EM, Belmonte C (1998) Tetrodotoxin-resistant impulses in single nerve terminals signalling pain. J Physiol 512:211–217
3. Brock JA, Pianova S, Belmonte C (2001) Differences between nerve terminal impulses of polymodal nociceptors and cold sensory receptors of the guinea-pig cornea. J Physiol 533:493–501
4. Eyzaguirre C, Kuffler SW (1955) Processes of excitation in the dendrites and in the soma of single isolated sensory nerve cells of the lobster and crayfish. J Gen Physiol 39:87–119
5. Gardner EP, Martin JH (2000) Coding of sensory information. In: Kandel E, Schwartz JH, Jessell TM (eds) Principles of Neural Sciences, 4th edn. McGraw-Hill, New York, pp 411–625
6. Gray JAB, Sato M (1953) Properties of the receptor potential in pacinian corpuscles. J Physiol 122:610–636
7. Heppelmann B, Messlinger K, Neiss WF, Schmidt RF (1990) Ultrastructural three-dimensional reconstruction of group III and group IV sensory nerve endings ("free nerve endings") in the knee joint capsule of the cat: evidence for multiple receptive sites. J Comp Neurol 292:103–16
8. Loewenstein WR (1959) The generation of electric activity in a nerve ending. Ann New York Acad Sc 81:367–387
9. Patton DH (1966) Receptor Mechanisms. In: Ruch TC and Patton HD (eds) Physiology and Biophysics. WB Saunders Co., Philadelphia and London, pp 95–112
10. Sauer SK, Weidner C, Averbeck B et al. (2004) Are generator potentials of rat cutaneous nociceptive terminals accessible to threshold tracking? J Neurophysiol (in press)

Nociceptor Inactivation

▶ Nociceptor, Adaptation

Nociceptor Sensitization

Definition

Process by which there is a decrease in nociceptor threshold and enhanced responses to suprathreshold stimuli. This phenomenon is an increment of the excitability of the nociceptor, due to a metabolic change induced by sensitizing agents such as pro-inflammatory mediators.

▶ Capsaicin Receptor
▶ Polymodal Nociceptors, Heat Transduction
▶ Thalamus, Clinical Pain, Human Imaging

Nociceptor(s)

Definition

Harmful stimuli activate the peripheral endings of primary afferent neurons, also called nociceptors. Their cell bodies lie in the dorsal root ganglia (DRG) or the trigeminal ganglia. Distinct classes of nociceptors encode discrete intensities and modalities of noxious stimuli. Receptor molecules that lend these specific properties to diverse classes of nociceptors and mediate transduction have been cloned. One important molecule is the vanilloid receptor TRPV1, which serves as a transducer of noxious thermal and chemical (e.g. protons) stimuli, and can be activated by capsaicin, the active ingredient of hot chili peppers. Conduction of nociceptive signals in nociceptors is mediated via activation of voltage-gated sodium channels. A family of nociceptor-specific tetrodotoxin (TTX)-resistant sodium channels modulates the excitability of primary afferents and likely mediates pathophysiological alterations thereof.

▶ Acute Pain Mechanisms
▶ Cancer Pain, Animal Models
▶ Cancer Pain Management, Nonopioid Analgesics
▶ COX-1 and COX-2 in Pain
▶ Cytokines, Effects on Nociceptors
▶ Descending Modulation and Persistent Pain
▶ Dorsal Root Ganglionectomy and Dorsal Rhizotomy
▶ Drugs Targeting Voltage-Gated Sodium and Calcium Channels
▶ Fibromyalgia, Mechanisms and Treatment
▶ Freezing Model of Cutaneous Hyperalgesia
▶ Functional Imaging of Cutaneous Pain
▶ Hypoalgesia, Assessment
▶ Mechanonociceptors
▶ Muscle Pain Model, Inflammatory Agents-Induced
▶ Nociceptor, Axonal Branching
▶ Nociceptor, Categorization
▶ Nociceptors, Cold Thermotransduction
▶ Nociceptors in the Dental Pulp
▶ NSAIDs, Mode of Action
▶ Opioids, Effects of Systemic Morphine on Evoked Pain
▶ Opioids in the Periphery and Analgesia
▶ Postherpetic Neuralgia, Pharmacological and Non-Pharmacological Treatment Options
▶ Postoperative Pain, Acute Pain Management, Principles
▶ Postoperative Pain, Acute Pain Team
▶ Somatic Pain
▶ Spinohypothalamic Tract, Anatomical Organization and Response Properties

Nociceptor, Adaptation

RICHARD A. MEYER, MATTHIAS RINGKAMP
Department of Neurosurgergy, School of Medicine,
Johns Hopkins University, Baltimore, MD, USA
rmeyer@jhmi.edu, platelet@jhmi.edu

Synonyms

Nociceptor Accommodation; Nociceptor Inactivation

Definition

The gradual decrease over time in the response of a nociceptor to a maintained noxious stimulus of fixed intensity.
Nociceptors Action Potentials and Post-Firing Excitability Changes

Characteristics

The response of nociceptors to a constant-temperature heat stimulus adapts with time. Unmyelinated nociceptors innervating the hairy skin of monkey can be separated into two classes based on the rate of adaptation to heat stimuli (Fig. 1). In response to a 53˚C stimulus, the discharge rate of quickly adapting C fibers is 20% of the peak response within 4s, whereas slowly adapting C fibers take more than 15 s to reach this level (Meyer and Campbell 1981). Myelinated fibers can also be separated into two classes based on their heat response: Type II fibers adapt quickly in a manner similar to quickly adapting C-fibers, whereas Type I fibers actually exhibit an increase in their response with time (Treede et al. 1998).

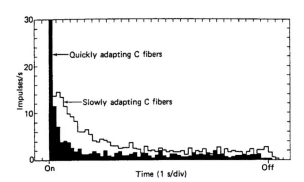

Nociceptor, Adaptation, Figure 1   Adaptation of response to heat (53˚C) in C-fiber nociceptor afferents in the monkey (From Meyer and Campbell 1981).

Nociceptors also exhibit a slowly adapting response to mechanical stimuli applied to their receptive field (Slugg et al. 2000). An exception to this rule exists for mechanically-insensitive nociceptors, which can develop a response to tonic pressure (Schmidt et al. 2000). The mechanisms underlying adaptation in nociceptors are not well understood, but calcium-dependent and -independent mechanisms appear to be involved.
▶ Nociceptors Action Potentials and Postfiring Excitability Changes

References

1. Meyer RA, Campbell JN (1981) Evidence for Two Distinct Classes of Unmyelinated Nociceptive Afferents in Monkey. Brain Res 224:149–152
2. Schmidt R, Schmelz M, Torebjörk HE et al. (2000) Mechano-Insensitive Nociceptors Encode Pain Evoked by Tonic Pressure to Human Skin. Neuroscience 98:793–800
3. Slugg RM, Meyer RA, Campbell JN (2000) Response of Cutaneous A- and C-Fiber Nociceptors in the Monkey to Controlled-Force Stimuli. J Neurophysiol 83:2179–2191
4. Treede R-D, Meyer RA, Campbell JN (1998) Myelinated Mechanically Insensitive Afferents from Monkey Hairy Skin: Heat-Response Properties. J Neurophysiol 80:1082–1093

Nociceptor, Axonal Branching

N

MARTIN SCHMELZ
Institute of Anaesthesiology, Operative Intensive Medicine and Pain Research, Faculty for Clinical Medicine Mannheim, University of Heidelberg, Mannheim, Germany
martin.schmelz@anaes.ma.uni-heidelberg.de

Synonyms

Axon reflex; neurogenic inflammation; Flare; Neurogenic Vasodilation; protein extravasation

Definition

Single nociceptive nerve fibers branch extensively in the periphery to form their receptive fields: branches can measure up to 9 cm in human skin. In addition, their terminal endings can also inhibit extensive branching in the micrometer range. Axonal branching is the structural basis for antidromic action potential propagation (axon reflex), leading to neurogenic inflammation.

Characteristics

Innervation Territories of Nociceptors

The receptive field of primary afferent nociceptors has been found to be very small in rodents. However, in humans, skin innervation territories measuring up to 9 cm in diameter have been found (Schmelz et al. 1997). Most of the available data on the structure of innervation territories and branching derive from skin, as they can more easily be analyzed as compared to deep somatic or visceral nociceptors. Extensive branching of skin nociceptors has also been found in monkey skin, with branching

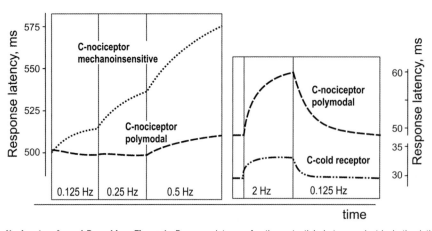

Nociceptor, Axonal Branching, Figure 1 Response latency of action potentials between electrical stimulation of the receptive endings in the skin and recording in the peripheral nerve (n. peroneaus) is shown. Left panel: Electrical stimulation at increasing frequency provokes increased response latency for different classes of afferent C-fibers (activity dependent slowing). The activity dependent slowing is most pronounced in mechano-insensitive C-nociceptors which slow down in conduction velocity even at low stimulatory frequencies of 0.125 or 0.25 Hz. The slowing of traditional mechano-responsive C-nociceptors ("polymodal") is far less pronounced and clearly separates between the two nociceptor classes (modified from Weidner et al. 1999). Right panel: At higher stimulation frequencies of 2 Hz polymodal nociceptors show a pronounced activity dependent slowing which clearly separates them from cold-sensitive C-fibers (C-cold receptor), which only slightly increase their response latency when stimulated at 2 Hz (modified from Serra et al. 1999).

points being rather proximal from the actual receptive field; interestingly, frequently unmyelinated branches of A delta fibers were found, which had a length of about 5 cm (Peng et al. 1999).

Axonal Properties of Different Nociceptor Classes

In human skin unmyelinated nociceptors fall into two basic classes: the majority of the fibers are mechano-heat sensitive polymodal nociceptors; however, about 20% are unresponsive to mechanical stimulation (Schmidt et al. 1995). These "silent" or "sleeping" nociceptors differ from conventional polymodal nociceptors in their receptive properties, their biophysical characteristics and their function. They have higher activation thresholds for heat and are not activated even by intense mechanical stimuli (Schmidt et al. 1995). Their innervation territories in the leg are larger (6 vs. 2 cm²), and conduction velocity is lower (0.8 vs. 1 m/s,) than in polymodal fibers (Schmidt et al. 1995). Most interestingly, their high transcutaneous electrical thresholds and their activity dependent hyperpolarization by far exceed the values observed in polymodal nociceptors. Although based on the axonal properties, analysis of activity dependent hyperpolarization allows classification of these two nociceptor classes (Weidner et al. 1999), and thus predicts sensory properties of their endings. Moreover, activity dependent hyperpolarization has also been shown to separate C-cold thermoreceptors from C-polymodal nociceptors (Fig. 1). It should be pointed out that this unexpected correlation between specific axonal properties and characteristics of sensory endings has a variety of implications. As mechanisms of activity-dependent hyperpolarization are currently being clarified on a molecular level, immunohistochemistry might in the future enable dif-

ferential staining and functional identification of axons. First clinical results confirm that this approach can be used to improve characterization of neuropathic axonal changes (Boettger et al. 2002).

Neurogenic Inflammation

Decades ago Thomas Lewis described the erythema arising in human skin in the surroundings of trauma as part of the "triple response" to noxious stimuli (Lewis et al. 1927). This "flare response" is dependent on the integrity of primary afferent nerves, but not on their central nervous connections. From his own findings and earlier work Lewis developed the concept of "axon reflex flare", i.e. the notion that "nocifensive" nerve fibers excited by a trauma send impulses not only into the central nervous system, but also via axon branches into the surrounding skin, where they trigger the release of a vasodilating substance from the nerve endings. Neuropeptides are now held responsible for the vasodilatation, which are produced by small dorsal root ganglion cells and transported in their thin axons to the central and peripheral nerve terminals. The main vasodilatory agent is probably CGRP which induces vasodilatation, but no plasmaextravasation (Brain 1996). The edema, caused by increased permeability of the endothelia for plasma proteins (neurogenic protein extravasation) can be attributed to the release of substance P. However, a variety of other neuropeptides like neurokinin A, neurokinin B, somatostatin, galanin, and recently, endomorphins have been also be found in primary afferent neurons. It should also be noted that in addition to the acute vascular effects, neuropeptides have important trophic functions and modulate the activity of local immune cells (Fig. 2).

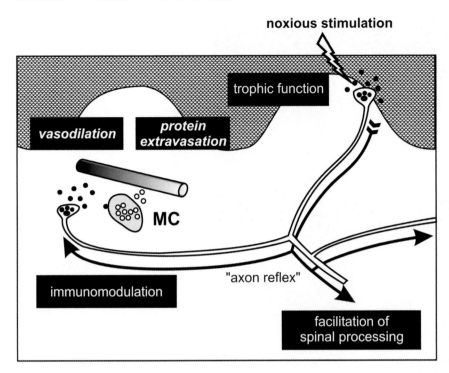

noxious stimulation

trophic function

vasodilation

protein extravasation

MC

immunomodulation

"axon reflex"

facilitation of spinal processing

Nociceptor, Axonal Branching, Figure 2 Schematical drawing of mechanisms involved in dermal neurogenic inflammation. Noxious stimulation of the skin (hatched area) results in generation of action potentials in nociceptors. The action potentials reach the arborisations of the axonal tree via the axon reflex (black arrows). By depolarization of the terminals, neuropeptides (black circles) are released. Key effects of neuropeptides are given in black squares. The involvement of mast cell mediators (MC, open circles) in vasodilation and protein extravasation in neurogenic inflammation is controversial.

Analysis of Neurogenic Inflammation

Chemical, thermal, and electrical stimulation has been widely used to elicit neurogenic inflammation, and direct evidence of neuropeptide release has been obtained using capsaicin as well as antidromic electrical nerve stimulation. In rodents, activation of polymodal nociceptors was sufficient to cause neurogenic inflammation (Gee et al. 1997). In contrast, mechano-insensitive, but heat- and chemosensitive C-nociceptors have been found responsible for the neurogenic vasodilation in pig skin (Gee et al. 1997; Lynn et al. 1996) and human (Sauerstein et al. 2000). The extent of the neurogenic erythema nicely matches the large cutaneous receptive fields of mechanoinsensitive nociceptors, and their high electrical thresholds also match the strong currents required to provoke neurogenic flare electrically. Thus, neurogenic inflammation in human differs from rodents, in which the neurogenic inflammation can be elicited by polymodal C nociceptors, and consists of a combination of vasodilation and protein extravasation (Sauerstein et al. 2000). In healthy volunteers no neurogenic protein extravasation could be induced (Sauerstein et al. 2000), but may develop under pathophysiological conditions (Weber et al. 2001).

Neurogenic Inflammation and Secondary Hyperalgesia

The areas of vasodilation and warming around a noxious stimulation site have been found to be similar to the areas of secondary mechanical hyperalgesia (punctate hyperalgesia) (Serra et al. 1998). However, recent results would suggest, that by blocking axonal action potential propagation by a local anesthetic, only the spread of axon

reflex vasodilation and warming can be blocked. In contrast, areas of punctate hyperalgesia developed symmetrically, even beyond a peripherally located "anesthetic strip" (Fig. 3).

Epidermal Axonal Branching

Under physiological conditions unmyelinated human nerve fibers entering the epidermis are found to be oriented straight up, and reach the outermost layers of viable skin without pronounced branching (Hilliges et al. 1995). Interestingly, in some human skin diseases extensive branching of epidermal nerve fibers has been described. Increased intradermal nerve fiber density has been found in patients with chronic pruritus. In addition, increased epidermal levels of neurotrophin 4 (NT4) have been found in patients with atopic dermatitis, and massively increased serum levels of NGF and SP have been found to correlate with the severity of the disease in such patients (Toyoda et al. 2002). Increased fiber density and higher local NGF concentrations were also found in patients with contact dermatitis. Most interestingly, intraepidermal sprouting has also been found as a physiological response to circular skin incision (Rajan et al. 2003): „collateral sprouting" from axons at the incision margins lead to centripedal reconstituting of skin innervation, probably due to higher local NGF concentrations in the denervated skin (Rajan et al. 2003). A similar mechanism might also explain findings in patients with diabetic neuropathy characterized by reduced epidermal innervation density, but higher degree of epidermal branching (Polydefkis et al. 2003). It will be of major interest in the future to assess the

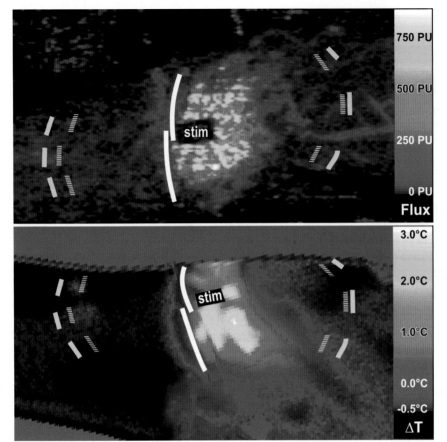

Nociceptor, Axonal Branching, Figure 3 Specimen of transcutaneous electrical stimulation (1 Hz, 50 mA, 0,5 ms; stimulation site ["stim"] is marked by a rectangle) provoking an area of increased superficial blood flow as assessed with a laser Doppler scanner (upper panel) and with an infrared thermocamera (lower panel). An anesthetic strip was induced by perfusing two intradermal microdialysis membranes (vertical white lines) with 2% lidocaine. The borders of hyperalgesia to punctate stimuli (grey lines) and to light stroking (dotted lines) are shown in the laser Doppler scan and the thermogram. (Modified from Klede et al. 2003).

effects of the local sprouting on the sensory function of the nociceptors. There is already evidence of increased epidermal nerve fiber sprouting in vulvodynia, and moreover, signs of nociceptor sensitization (Bohm-Starke et al. 2001). Taken together, these data would suggest that local inflammatory processes could initiate nociceptor sprouting and sensitization by increased NGF production.

References

1. Boettger MK, Till S, Chen MX (2002) Calcium-Activated Potassium Channel SK[1-] and IK[1-]Like Immunoreactivity in Injured Human Sensory Neurones and its Regulation by Neurotrophic Factors. Brain 125:252–263
2. Bohm-Starke N, Hilliges M, Brodda-Jansen G et al. (2001) Psychophysical Evidence of Nociceptor Sensitization in Vulvar Vestibulitis Syndrome. Pain 94:177–183
3. Brain SD (1996) Sensory Neuropeptides in the Skin, pp 229–244
4. Gee MD, Lynn B, Cotsell B (1997) The Relationship between Cutaneous C Fibre Type and Antidromic Vasodilatation in the Rabbit and the Rat. J Physiol 503:31–44
5. Hilliges M, Wang L, Johansson O (1995) Ultrastructural Evidence for Nerve Fibers Within All Vital Layers of the Human Epidermis. J Invest Dermatol: 134–137
6. Klede M, Handwerker HO, Schmelz M (2003) Central Origin of Secondary Mechanical Hyperalgesia. J Neurophysiol 90:353–359
7. Lewis T, Harris KE, Grant RT (1927) Observations Relating to the Influence of the Cutaneous Nerves on Various Reactions of the Cutaneous Vessels. Heart 14:1–17
8. Lynn B, Schutterle S, Pierau FK (1996) The Vasodilator Component of Neurogenic Inflammation is Caused by a Special Subclass of Heat-Sensitive Nociceptors in the Skin of the Pig. J Physiol 494:587–593
9. Peng YB, Ringkamp M, Campbell JN et al. (1999) Electrophysiological Assessment of the Cutaneous Arborization of Adelta-Fiber Nociceptors. J Neurophysiol 82:1164–1177
10. Polydefkis M, Griffin JW, McArthur J (2003) New Insights into Diabetic Polyneuropathy. JAMA 290:1371–376
11. Rajan B, Polydefkis M, Hauer P et al. (2003) Epidermal Reinnervation after Intracutaneous Axotomy in Man. J Comp Neurol 457:24–36
12. Sauerstein K, Klede M, Hilliges M et al. (2000) Electrically Evoked Neuropeptide Release and Neurogenic Inflammation Differ between Rat and Human Skin. J Physiol 529:803–810
13. Schmelz M, Schmidt R, Bickel A et al. (1997) Specific C-Receptors for Itch in Human Skin. J Neurosci 17:8003–8008
14. Schmidt R, Schmelz M, Forster C et al. (1995) Novel Classes of Responsive and Unresponsive C Nociceptors in Human Skin. J Neurosci 1995:333–341
15. Serra J, Campero M, Ochoa J (1998) Flare and Hyperalgesia after Intradermal Capsaicin Injection in Human Skin. J Neurophysiol 80:2801–2810
16. Serra J, Campero M, Ochoa J et al. (1999) Activity-Dependent Slowing of Conduction Differentiates Functional Subtypes of C Fibres Innervating Human Skin. J Physiol 515:799–811
17. Toyoda M, Nakamura M, Makino T et al. (2002) Nerve Growth Factor and Substance P are Useful Plasma Markers of Disease Activity in Atopic Dermatitis. Br J Dermatol 147:71–79
18. Weber M, Birklein F, Neundorfer B et al. (2001) Facilitated Neurogenic Inflammation in Complex Regional Pain Syndrome. Pain 91:251–257

19. Weidner C, Schmelz M, Schmidt R et al. (1999) Functional Attributes Discriminating Mechano-Insensitive and Mechano-Responsive C Nociceptors in Human Skin. J Neurosci 19:10184–10190

Nociceptor, Categorization

EDWARD PERL

Department of Cell and Molecular Physiology, School of Medicine, University of North Carolina, Chapel Hill, NC, USA

erp@med.unc.edu

Synonyms

Categorization of Nociceptors

Definition

Why categorize a mixed set of primary afferent neurons? As Lynn (1996) pointed out, classifying the components of a neuronal population into categories on the basis of shared features does more than one service. It facilitates communication by providing a shorthand to designate a subset with certain features. It also provides a way to deal with the large number of neurons in the mammalian nervous system that serves common functions. Moreover, appropriate classification of neurons can help facilitate concepts on development and the functional organization of nervous mechanisms.

Characteristics

Noxious and Nociceptor

Definition of certain classes of stimuli as noxious and creation of the term nociceptor (noci-receptor) were outgrowths of the dispute in the late 19th Century about the sensory nature of pain. Physicians and physiologists of those days generally accepted pain to be a sensation. On the other hand, philosophical critics of this idea argued that in contrast to accepted sensations, pain does not have a "well defined" physical or chemical stimulus (Perl 1996). Mechanical events, heat, cold, and chemical agents can all produce it. Charles Sherrington (1906), an eminent physiologist of the time, proposed an answer to this criticism with the logic that pain ordinarily results from tissue injury. Consequently, tissue damage represents a common denominator of natural stimuli for pain. He suggested that events producing disruption of tissue or representing a physical threat to its integrity could be labeled noxious regardless of their nature, thereby providing an encompassing definition for the stimuli evoking pain. In this concept, sense organs signaling the presence of noxious events were labeled noci-receptors (now shortened to nociceptors). Designation of stimuli as noxious creates its own problems. Tissues of the mammalian body are diverse with widely differing mechanical and thermal characteristics.

This means that quantitatively the intensity of an environmental or circumstantial event necessary to cause tissue damage varies over a substantial range. Compare mechanical durability of the cornea of the human eye to the skin on the sole of a human foot. Furthermore, subcutaneous tissues and organs are protected from many environmental changes and potential insults; their exposure to some conditions that are innocuous for the skin would lead to tissue injury and thereby should be considered noxious. Thus, the nature of noxious events and their signaling by sense organs must be considered in the context of tissue type and location.

Classification of Sense Organs as Nociceptors

A primary afferent neuron is appropriately considered to be a nociceptor if the intensity of the most effective "natural" stimulus that evokes conducted action potentials approaches or exceeds the noxious (damaging) level for the innervated tissue. This criterion implies that such sensory units respond weakly or not all to innocuous stimuli of any type. Since the nature and intensity of noxious stimuli will vary for different tissues, the responsive characteristics of nociceptors will differ from one tissue to another.

Observations demonstrating nociceptors to be distinctive categories of somatic sense organs provide evidence that more than one type innervate many tissues. How are these different types distinguished? Actually, nociceptor classification has evolved as information about them expands and the changing criteria sometimes have led to ambiguity. Given the view that the function of nociceptors is to transmit to the central nervous system information about events dangerous to the physical integrity of the tissue they innervate, a first order in their classification, and one commonly used, is the nature of effective stimuli or the events signaled.

Classification of Nociceptors by Effective Stimuli

Much information about nociceptors has come from study of the innervation of epithelial tissue, particularly the skin. Early in the documentation of cutaneous nociceptors as distinctive types of sense organs, it became evident that the skin is innervated by more than one type (Perl 1996). As already suggested, nociceptors can be distinguished and classified according to the nature of stimuli activating them. On this basis, several categories are demonstrable in mammalian skin (Perl 1996; Campbell and Meyer 1996). In terms of effective stimuli, the cornea, another epithelial tissue, is innervated by closely similar varieties (Belmonte and Gallar 1996). One kind of cutaneous nociceptor responds vigorously to strong mechanical stimulation, positively grading the frequency and number of impulses in proportion to stimulus intensity. Extreme temperatures (e.g., noxious heat, freezing) excite such mechanical nociceptors (high threshold mechanoreceptors) only after a delay. A second category of cutaneous nociceptor responds more globally, being promptly activated by heat, mechanical distortion and irritant chemicals including protons. The latter response pattern led to the designation of this class as polymodal nociceptors. A third kind, prominent in the innervation of glabrous skin, is excited by mechanical distortion and elevated skin temperature (mechanical-heat), but does not promptly respond to surface application of irritant chemicals or acid. A fourth type responds both to low skin temperatures and to noxious mechanical stimuli (mechanical-cold). In addition to these four categories, evidence exists for a class of primary afferents (labeled 'silent' nociceptors) that are only excited by mechanical stimuli when sensitized by local inflammation and for another category selectively excited by ▶ histamine (pruritus receptors).

Characterization by Conduction Velocity

Whereas the nature of effective stimuli represents an approach to classifying nociceptors that relates to function, it is not the only important criterion. Indications that peripheral stimuli evoke pain after distinctly different delays existed prior to documentation of nociceptors as a special set of peripheral sense organs. Transient application of a noxious mechanical or heat stimulus to distally located skin anecdotally and experimentally was noted to provoke a double pain response, one of short latency and a second delayed; these differences in latency can be attributed to differences in ▶ conduction velocity of peripheral nerve fibers responsible for the afferent messages. In addition to these distinctions of delay, "first" and "second" pain is reported to differ in quality of the sensation. This circumstantial evidence for conduction differences is consistent with findings that some categories of nociceptors have myelinated (A) and others unmyelinated (C) afferent fibers. Those with ▶ A fibers conduct much more rapidly (10–50×) than the ▶ C Fiber groups, and even though most A nociceptors have thinly thinly myelinated fibers (Aδ), a number from distal limb regions are in the medium myelinated range with Aβ (35–50 m/s) conduction velocities. A fiber and C fiber nociceptors also differ in other ways. For instance, several sets of C-fiber nociceptors express peptide mediators (e.g., substance P, CGRP) that are apparently absent in myelinated nociceptors. Furthermore, the central projections of A and C fiber nociceptors differ. These distinctions are consistent with certain differences in functions initiated by the A and C fiber categories.

Characterization by Tissue of Origin

Primary afferent neurons with responsive features of nociceptors innervate many mammalian tissues or organs, both somatic and visceral. In addition to skin and cornea these include teeth, skeletal muscle, tendon, joints, bone, urethra, ureter, urinary bladder, blood vessels, bronchi, heart, pleura and peritoneum, segments of the alimentary tract, meninges, and testis (Cervero 1996). These tissues differ substantially in physical and chemical attributes, differences that are reflected in part in the responsive and signaling features of innervating nociceptive fibers. The testis is innervated by nociceptors mimicking the broad activation of cutaneous polymodal nociceptors by being responsive to noxious mechanical, heat and chemical stimuli (Kumazawa 1996). In contractile tissues, unusually high tension is an effective excitant for part of the nociceptive innervation. Similarly, lowered pH (protons), by itself or in combination with anoxemia, activate or enhance the responsiveness of certain nociceptive afferents of skeletal muscle (Mense 1996). Circumstantial evidence suggests that subcutaneous tissues such as joints and muscle contain a number of primary afferent fibers that are unresponsive to mechanical or thermal stimuli until injury has induced inflammation and its chemical environment (Schaible and Schmidt 1996). The latter can be considered types of chemoreceptor. Thus, the classification of nociceptors must take into account the tissue innervated in addition to effective stimuli, and the diameter (conduction velocity) of the afferent fiber.

Characterization by Molecular Features

A presumption underlying hypotheses about differentiation and specialization of biological cells, in our case neurons, is that these processes are guided and controlled by the presence and expression of particular molecular entities. Relating factors associated with molecular expression to functionally important features of nociceptors is an ongoing effort and at present represents at most an emerging story with promise for future insights.

In one example, the heat responsiveness of polymodal nociceptors is attributed to a membrane receptor, ▶ TRPV1 (Caterina and Julius 2002). TRPV1 donates such reactivity when expressed in heterologous cells. TRPV1 is the endogenous receptor that is selectively activated by capsaicin, the substance that gives the sensation of heat upon ingestion of "hot" pepper. A structurally related membrane receptor, ▶ TRPV2, is predominantly expressed in different primary afferent neurons than TRPV1, and is proposed to provide a higher threshold heat response for a set of nociceptors different from the polymodal type. TRPV2 is neither excited by capsaicin nor acid (Caterina and Julius 2002). Other relationships between molecular features and categories of nociceptors include the immunocytochemical labeling of a subset of small diameter dorsal root ganglia (DRG) neurons and their processes for the peptides, ▶ substance P and ▶ CGRP. Both circumstantial and direct correlations indicate that at least some peptide-labeled elements are polymodal or mechanical-heat nociceptors (Lawson 1996; Lawson et al. 1997). The small substance P-containing neurons are mostly distinct from an isolectin IB4-binding population of presumed nociceptors (Lawson 1996). Thus, evidence for the common presence of TRPV1, TRPV2, or any other unique cellular constituent links the nociceptors

these differences worthy of further study. A tantalising possibility is that differences in electrophysiological properties between nociceptors and non-nociceptors, or even possibly between sub-classes of nociceptor, might provide a basis for novel analgesic drugs. Some work on ▶ sodium channel blockers is already published and this is likely to remain an active research field (Wood et al. 2004)

References

1. Blair NT, Bean BP (2002) Roles of Tetrodotoxin (TTX)-Sensitive Na$^+$ Current, TTX-Resistant Na$^+$ Current, and Ca^{2+} Current in the Action Potentials of Nociceptive Sensory Neurons. J Neurosci 22:10277–10290
2. Bostock H, Campero M, Serra J et al. (2003) Velocity Recovery Cycles of C Fibres Innervating Human Skin. J Physiol 553:649–663
3. Djouhri L, Fang X, Okuse K et al. (2003a) The TTX-Resistant Sodium Channel Nav1.8 (SNS/PN3): Expression and Correlation with Membrane Properties in Rat Nociceptive Primary Afferent Neurons. J Physiol 550:739–752
4. Djouhri L, Lawson SN (1999) Changes in Somatic Action Potential Shape in Guinea-Pig Nociceptive Primary Afferent Neurones during Inflammation *In Vivo*. J Physiol 520:565–576
5. Djouhri L, Newton R, Levinson SR et al. (2003b) Sensory and Electrophysiological Properties of Guinea-Pig Sensory Neurones Expressing Nav 1.7 (PN1) Na$^+$ Channel Alpha Subunit Protein. J Physiol 546:565–576
6. Fang X, Djouhri L, Black JA et al. (2002) The Presence and Role of the Tetrodotoxin-Resistant Sodium Channel Na(v)1.9 (NaN) in Nociceptive Primary Afferent Neurons. J Neurosci 22:7425–7433
7. Gee MD, Lynn B, Basile S et al. (1999) The Relationship between Axonal Spike Shape and Functional Modality in Cutaneous C-Fibres in the Pig and Rat. Neuroscience 90:509–518
8. Gee MD, Lynn B, Cotsell B (1996) Activity-Dependent Slowing of Conduction Velocity Provides a Method for Identifying Different Functional Classes of C-Fibre in the Rat Saphenous Nerve. Neuroscience 73:667–675
9. Grosskreutz J, Quasthoff S, Kuhn M et al. (1996) Capsaicin Blocks Tetrodotoxin-Resistant Sodium Potentials and Calcium Potentials in Unmyelinated C Fibres of Biopsied Human Sural Nerve *In Vitro*. Neurosci Lett 208:49–52
10. Lawson SN (2002) Phenotype and Function of Somatic Primary Afferent Nociceptive Neurones with C-, Adelta- or Aalpha/Beta-Fibres. Exp Physiol 87:239–244
11. Mayer C, Quasthoff S, Grafe P (1999) Confocal Imaging Reveals Activity-Dependent Intracellular Ca^{2+} Transients in Nociceptive Human C Fibres. Pain 81:317–322
12. Orstavik K, Weidner C, Schmidt R et al. (2003) Pathological C-Fibres in Patients with a Chronic Painful Condition. Brain 126:567–578
13. Serra J, Campero M, Bostock H et al. (2004) Two Types of C Nociceptors in Human Skin and their Behavior in Areas of Capsaicin-Induced Secondary Hyperalgesia. J Neurophysiol 91:2770–2781
14. Serra J, Campero M, Ochoa J et al. (1999) Activity-Dependent Slowing of Conduction Differentiates Functional Subtypes of C Fibres Innervating Human Skin [see comments]. J Physiol 515:799–811
15. Weidner C, Schmelz M, Schmidt R et al. (2002) Neural Signal Processing: The Underestimated Contribution of Peripheral Human C-Fibers. J Neurosci 22:6704–6712
16. Weidner C, Schmelz M, Schmidt, R et al. (1999) Functional Attributes Discriminating Mechano-Insensitive and Mechano-Responsive C Nociceptors in Human Skin. J Neurosci 19:10184–10190
17. Weidner C, Schmidt R, Schmelz M et al. (2003) Action Potential Conduction in the Terminal Arborisation of Nociceptive C-Fibre Afferents. J Physiol 547:931–940
18. Wood JN, Boorman JP, Okuse K et al. (2004) Voltage-Gated Sodium Channels and Pain Pathways. J Neurobiol 61:55–71

Nociceptors, Cold Thermotransduction

FÉLIX VIANA, ELVIRA DE LA PEÑA
Instituto de Neurociencias de Alicante, Universidad Miguel Hernández-CSIC, Alicante, Spain
felix.viana@umh.es, elvirap@umh.es

Synonyms

Cold Nociception; Noxious Cold Receptor; Cold Thermotransduction

Definition

A large fraction of nociceptors can be excited by application of cold temperatures to their peripheral endings. Most have the functional properties of C-type polymodal nociceptors. The molecular sensors involved in transducing strong cooling stimuli into an electrical signal are still unresolved; ▶ TRPA1 channels are contested candidates. Noxious and thermal signals are further processed in the brain to establish the intensity and quality of the sensation. Peripheral nerve injury can modify the process to give rise to ▶ cold allodynia or ▶ hyperalgesia.

Characteristics

Humans can feel a wide range of ambient temperatures. This capacity is fundamental for tactile recognition of objects and thermoregulation. Within the cold temperature range, the qualities of sensations evoked vary from pleasantly cool to extremely painful. The neutral zone, evoking no sensation upon temperature change of the skin ranges between 35°C and 31°C. Cutaneous temperatures of 30–15°C are generally perceived as cool to cold. Upon further temperature reduction, the perceptual qualities of the sensation change, becoming painful. The sensation of cold pain can have a burning, aching, prickling or stinging quality, depending on temperature and stimulus duration, possibly reflecting the activation of different classes of afferents. In contrast to the sharp threshold temperature for heat pain, the threshold for cold pain is less clearly defined and influenced by several factors such as rate of temperature change and stimulus area, indicating that mechanisms of temporal and spatial summation participate in encoding these sensations. Generally, the sensation turns painful only after a considerable delay, many seconds after cold application, which further complicates the definition of a threshold. Focal skin temperatures above approximately 43–45°C also evoke a ▶ paradoxical cold sensation in many individuals.

While significant advances in the cellular and molecular mechanisms responsible for temperature transduction by nerve terminals have taken place in recent years

N

(reviewed by Jordt et al. 2003; Patapoutian et al. 2003; Reid 2005), many important aspects of the function of ▶ cold thermoreceptors and nociceptors and how cold pain is encoded remain obscure. Thus, it is unknown which molecular and cellular factors determine the different temperature thresholds of individual sensory terminals. Also, the mechanisms involved in the development of pain by moderate cooling after nerve injury (▶ cold hyperalgesia) remain mysterious. These are important questions with implications in the treatment of disorders in which cold temperatures evoke pain.

The existence of separate, small, cold and warm cutaneous sensory spots has been known since the late 19th century. These findings lend support to von Frey's specificity theory of somesthesia, according to which sensory nerve fibers of the skin were sensitive to only one form of stimulation and acted as "labeled lines" for the transmission of information encoding a single perceptual quality. In contrast to the strict labeled line hypothesis, many studies also indicated that the perceptual quality of cold-evoked painful sensations is determined by the integrated activity of both nociceptive and non-nociceptive systems.

Psychophysical studies suggest that pure cooling and cold pain sensations result from the activation of different populations of receptors. In support of this view, humans show better detection ability in the innocuous cold compared to the noxious cold temperature range. Compression block of myelinated fiber conduction in cold-sensitive afferents shifts the pain threshold of cold stimulation towards higher temperatures, pointing to a convergent processing of thermal and nociceptive inputs (Yarnitsky and Ochoa 1990). The same occurs in certain diseases, including peripheral nerve lesions and neuropathic pain syndromes, which are often associated with cold hyperalgesia.

The anatomical substrates for these cold-sensitive spots are free nerve endings branching inside the superficial skin layers. Functional studies suggest that receptors sensing noxious cold may be located more deeply within the skin, some located along vein walls (Klement and Arndt 1992). The difference in location has important implications for interpreting experimental findings; the deeper location of nociceptive endings will result in a large discrepancy between the actual temperature of the receptor and the readings of the surface probe used to apply the cold stimulus. This lag in thermal readings will overestimate the apparent low temperature of activation of nociceptors to cold. As a matter of fact, temperature recordings inside the skin indicate that cold pain may be evoked with intracutaneous temperatures as high as 28°C (Klement and Arndt 1992).

Cold-Sensitive Fibers

Extending the psychophysical studies, single fiber recordings in various species, including primates, have identified a population of myelinated Aδ fibers excited by moderate decreases in the temperature of their receptive field. These fibers are insensitive to mechanical stimuli. They are the prototypical "low-threshold" cold thermoreceptors (Hensel 1981). At normal skin temperatures (33–34°C), cold thermoreceptors show a static ongoing discharge. On sudden cooling, they display a transient peak in firing that adapts to a new static level, often characterized by short bursts of impulses separated by silent intervals. Rewarming of the skin leads to silencing of the receptors. A mirror response is observed in warm receptors. Activation of these receptors is the probable mechanism responsible for the sensation of innocuous cold. In humans, microneurographic recordings confirmed the existence of cold thermoreceptors; the principal difference in primates was the lower conduction velocity and the regular pattern of discharge (Campero et al. 2001). ▶ Menthol, a natural substance found in leaves of certain plants, evokes cold sensations when applied at low doses to skin and mucosae. This effect is due to sensitization of cold thermoreceptors; they shift their threshold of activation to higher temperatures. However, other studies also show that topical application of high concentrations of menthol can sensitize nociceptors and evoke pain (Green 1992; Wasner et al. 2004).

Greater decreases in temperature recruit an additional population of receptors. Many of these high-threshold cold-sensitive fibers are also heat- and mechanosensitive and conduct slowly, which would classify them as C-type polymodal nociceptors. In humans, they are characterized by low and irregular firing rates (< 1 impulse/s) during cooling (Campero et al. 1996). Activation of these nociceptors is thought to underlie the sensation of cold pain. However, other fiber types also augment their discharge during strong cold stimuli, including high threshold cold receptors and a fraction of slowly adapting low threshold mechanoreceptors. Thus, it is still an open question as to the contribution of these various fibers to noxious cold sensations. Terminal stumps of damaged sensory fibers can be excited by moderate cooling stimuli. The majority are C-type and many are also menthol sensitive (Roza et al. 2006) Parallel input from primary sensory neurons carrying innocuous and noxious thermal information to the brain is suggested by the existence of anatomically and functionally distinct second-order neurons in lamina I of the spinal cord responsive to innocuous cooling, pure nociceptive stimuli or multimodal thermal and mechanical stimuli.

Cold Sensitive Neurons

To investigate the cellular mechanisms underlying cold sensing, many laboratories have turned to models that use primary sensory neurons maintained in culture (reviewed by Reid 2005). Activity in these cells can be monitored with calcium-sensitive fluorescent dyes (Fig. 1). Only a small fraction (10–15%) of sensory

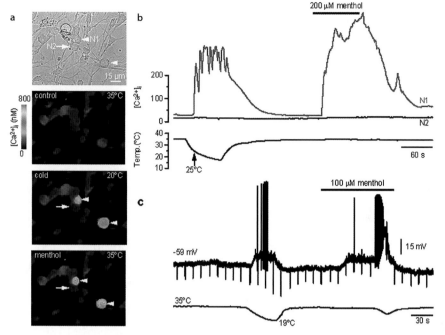

Nociceptors, Cold Thermotransduction, Figure 1 Identification and response characteristics of cold sensitive trigeminal neurons in culture. (a) A neuronal culture (1 day *in vitro*) obtained from the trigeminal ganglion showing the bright-field image (top) and (in descending order) the pseudocolor images of the fura-2 ratio intensity at 35°C, 20°C and 35°C in the presence of 200 μM menthol. Two of the neurons (marked with arrowheads) increased their resting calcium level during the cold stimulus, while the remaining cells did not change their calcium levels. (b) Intracellular calcium response to a cold ramp and 200 μM menthol application in the two neurons marked in (a). Only one of the cells responded to the stimuli. (c) Whole cell current clamp recordings of a cold sensitive neuron showing the potentiation of the cold response and the shift in temperature threshold by menthol.

neurons respond to application of cold stimuli with an elevation in their intracellular calcium concentration. Many of these cold sensitive neurons are also activated by cooling compounds like menthol (Fig. 1), suggesting that they are indeed cold thermoreceptors (Viana et al. 2002; McKemy et al. 2002; Reid et al. 2002). These studies further showed that cold sensitive neurons have distinct electrophysiological properties. A hallmark is their high excitability; they require minute excitatory currents to reach firing threshold. The increased excitability reflects the relative low expression of subthreshold voltage gated potassium currents in comparison with other sensory neurons. A high percentage of cold and menthol sensitive neurons are also excited by the algesic compound capsaicin, which can be interpreted as further evidence for the expression and role of ▶ TRPM8 channel s in polymodal nociceptive neurons (Viana et al. 2002; McKemy et al. 2002).

Molecular Sensors for Cold

Work in the 1970's attributed the activation of nerve terminals by cooling to the depolarization produced by inhibition of the Na^+/K^+ pump. However, the realization that individual terminals can be activated by variable low temperatures hinted at the existence of more specific mechanisms, such as membrane ion channels with distinct temperature thresholds of activation, as likely molecular sensors of innocuous and painful cold signals. In principle, excitation of nerve terminals by a cold temperature could involve opening of cation channels or closure of resting potassium channels (Fig. 2). In either case, the net result is a depolarizing generator potential and firing of action potentials by the terminal.

Following on the landmark identification of ▶ TRPV1, a cation channel activated by heat and capsaicin (Caterina et al. 1997), two research groups cloned two additional transient receptor potential (TRP) channels activated by decreases in temperature. These two ion channels, known as ▶ TRPM8 and ▶ TRPA1, are expressed in discrete, non-overlapping, subpopulations of primary sensory neurons (Story et al. 2003). So far, the best characterized channel in the molecular machinery for neuronal cold sensing is TRPM8. The data argue strongly for a primary role of TRPM8 in non-noxious cold detection. TRPM8 is a calcium permeable, voltage gated, nonselective cation channel that is activated by temperature and natural cooling compounds like menthol and eucalyptol (McKemy et al. 2002; Peier et al. 2002). TRPM8 is expressed selectively in a small population (10–15%) of primary sensory neurons of small diameter and most cold sensitive neurons are also excited by menthol. Many of the same neurons also express TRPM8 mRNA transcripts. Moreover, many cold sensitive neurons manifest a non-selective cation current with many biophysical and pharmacological properties consistent with the properties of TRPM8-dependent currents (reviewed by Reid 2005).

One important difference between native cold activated currents and cloned ▶ TRPM8 channels is the temperature threshold (de la Pena et al. 2005). Activation threshold of TRPM8 channels is around 25°C, a surprisingly low value. This is not a trivial issue for two reasons. First, it leaves unexplained the ability of many cold thermoreceptors to sense temperature decreases in the 33 to 26°C range. Second, the high threshold observed suggests that TRPM8 may also be a candidate for thermal nociception

N

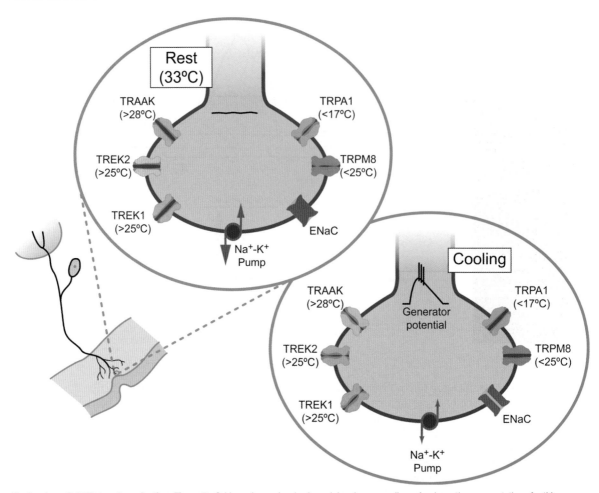

Nociceptors, Cold Thermotransduction, Figure 2 Cold sensing molecules in peripheral nerve endings. A schematic representation of a thin sensory fiber innervating the skin. The transduction of cold temperatures into an electrical signal takes place at free nerve endings. A free nerve ending with all the putative cold-sensing channels and their temperature thresholds. In the case of K^+ channels, closed by low temperature, the "threshold" value represents the lowest temperature at which the channels display significant activity. At normal skin temperatures, the terminal is kept hyperpolarized by the background activity of K^+ channels. Activity in the electrogenic Na^+-K^+ pump contributes to the hyperpolarization. Upon cooling, K^+ channels close and thermosensitive TRPs open, with a decrease in Na^+-K^+ pump activity, leading to a depolarizing receptor potential and spike firing.

as well. As already mentioned, this hypothesis is supported by some psychophysical studies in humans (Wasner et al. 2004; Green 1992). In turn, the discrepancy in thresholds may be explained by intrinsic modulation of TRPM8 channels by endogenous factors.

The identification of cold sensitive neurons that are insensitive to menthol points to additional cellular mechanisms in neuronal cold sensing (reviewed by Reid 2005). As a matter of fact, many high threshold cold sensitive neurons lack TRPM8 expression. The second cold sensitive TRP channel identified, ▶ TRPA1, is activated by much lower temperatures ($< 17°$C) than TRPM8 and has therefore been suggested to be important in the transduction of high threshold, painful, cold stimuli (Story et al. 2003). This channel is not activated by menthol but is potently activated by pungent compounds like cinnamaldehyde and isothiocyanates present in cinnamon oil, wasabi and mustard oil. However, other investigators have not been able to replicate

the cold sensitivity of TRPA1 channels (Jordt et al. 2004). Furthermore, the population of high threshold, menthol insensitive, cold activated neurons is not activated by mustard oil, which would suggest that their activation is not dependent upon TRPA1 activity (Babes et al. 2004). These findings make TRPA1 an uncertain candidate as a molecular sensor for noxious cold. In an interesting twist of events, recent studies suggest that TRPA1 channels are part of the mechanotransduction complex of vertebrate hair cells.

Cooling also activates ENaC channels, a member of the amiloride sensitive epithelial sodium channel family. However, a cold sensitive current matching the pharmacological profile of ENaC channels has not been documented in sensory neurons.

Alternatively, neuronal cold sensing may involve the closure of background potassium channels by cold (Fig. 2). TREK-1, TREK-2 and TRAAK, ▶ Two Pore Domain K+ Channels activated by fatty acids and mechanical stimuli, expressed in sensory neurons and with high sensitivity to temperature are good molecular candidates for this role (Kang et al. 2005; Maingret et al. 2000). The steep, rapid and gradual decrease in current flowing through these channels in a broad physiological temperature range (44–24°C) make them excellent candidates for thermal sensing in those terminals harboring them. In contrast to the direct temperature sensitivity of ▶ TRP channels, cell integrity is required for temperature sensitivity of these K^+ channels. Other background K^+ channels (i.e. TASK) are minimally affected by temperature. Experimental data implicating the closure of background potassium channels in cold transduction have been obtained in trigeminal and DRG neurons (Viana et al. 2002; Reid and Flonta 2001). However, the pharmacology or molecular nature of the conductance closed by cold temperature has not been addressed directly.

It is interesting that blockade of certain types of voltage-gated K^+ channels can render a population of sensory neurons cold sensitive. Experiments in trigeminal neurons showed that a slowly inactivating potassium current can act as a brake on excitability, reducing cold sensitivity (Viana et al. 2002). Neurons insensitive to cold and ▶ menthol could be transformed into cold sensitive neurons in the presence of low concentrations of 4-AP, a blocker for these channels.

It is important to emphasize that the various ionic mechanisms postulated in cold transduction are not mutually exclusive; if present in the same nerve terminal they could act synergistically to expand the dynamic range of temperature detection. Alternatively, activity of thermosensitive K^+ channels in those terminals with TRP channels opened by heat (i.e. TRPV2, TRPV3, TRPV4, TRPV1) would act as a brake on the excitatory actions of the latter.

Unfortunately, most recent data on thermosensitive ion channels have been obtained during *in vitro* animal studies, precluding a direct translation of these results to human physiology and pathophysiology. Much remains to be learnt about the differential expression pattern of the different thermosensitive channels and the functional properties of the sensory fibers expressing them. It is likely that other thermosensitive channels will be uncovered in the next few years, expanding the palette of putative molecular candidates for cold sensing.

In summary, psychophysical studies indicate that input from non-noxious thermal systems is essential for the thermal quality and the intensity of the pain sensation evoked by cold. Thermosensory afferent input normally inhibits cold evoked pain. At the molecular level, the diverse functional characteristics and broad range of temperature thresholds in the different afferent fibers suggests that each class of nerve terminal may operate with a combinatorial code of sensory receptors. The available evidence supports an important role for TRPM8 in sensing of innocuous cold temperatures in peripheral re-

ceptors (evidence reviewed by Reid, 2005). In addition, the participation of TRPM8 channels in certain forms of cold pain is a distinct possibility. Lacking genetic evidence (i.e. TRPM8-deficient mice) or specific pharmacological tools, this conclusion is not firm. The role of TRPA1 channels in the transduction of noxious cold pain is uncertain. Activity of background K^+ channels can certainly influence cold sensitivity, but their role as primary transducers has not been addressed directly. Not surprisingly, interest in the pharmacological profile of thermosensitive channels is very high. It is anticipated that modulators of these channels will provide new therapeutic options with which to treat certain forms of pain, including cold hyperalgesia and allodynia.

References

1. Campero M, Serra J, Bostock H et al. (2001) Slowly conducting afferents activated by innocuous low temperature in human skin. J Physiol 535:855–865
2. Campero M, Serra J, Ochoa JL (1996) C-polymodal nociceptors activated by noxious low temperature in human skin. J Physiol 497:565–572
3. Caterina MJ, Schumacher MA, Tominaga M et al. (1997) The capsaicin receptor: a heat-activated ion channel in the pain pathway. Nature 389:816–824
4. de la Pena E, Malkia A, Cabedo H et al. (2005) The contribution of TRPM8 channels to cold sensing in mammalian neurones. J Physiol 567:415–426
5. Green BG (1992) The sensory effects of l-menthol on human skin. Somatosens Mot Res 9:235–244
6. Hensel H (1981) Thermoreception and temperature regulation. Monogr Physiol Soc 38:1–321
7. Jordt SE, McKemy DD, Julius D (2003) Lessons from peppers and peppermint: the molecular logic of thermosensation. Curr Opin Neurobiol 13:487–492
8. Kang D, Choe C, Kim D (2005) Thermosensitivity of the two-pore domain K+ channels TREK-2 and TRAAK. J Physiol 564:103–116
9. Klement W, Arndt JO (1992) The role of nociceptors of cutaneous veins in the mediation of cold pain in man. J Physiol 449:73–83
10. Maingret F, Lauritzen I, Patel AJ et al. (2000) TREK-1 is a heat-activated background K(+) channel. EMBO J 19:2483–2491
11. McKemy DD, Neuhausser WM, Julius D (2002) Identification of a cold receptor reveals a general role for TRP channels in thermosensation. Nature 416:52–58
12. Patapoutian A, Peier AM, Story GM et al. (2003) ThermoTRP channels and beyond: mechanisms of temperature sensation. Nat Rev Neurosci 4:529–539
13. Peier AM, Moqrich A, Hergarden AC et al. (2002) A TRP channel that senses cold stimuli and menthol. Cell 108:705–715
14. Reid G (2005) ThermoTRP channels and cold sensing: what are they really up to Pflugers Arch 451:250–263
15. Reid G, Babes A, Pluteanu F (2002) A cold- and menthol-activated current in rat dorsal root ganglion neurones: properties and role in cold transduction. J Physiol 545:595–614
16. Roza C, Belmonte C, Viana F (2006) Cold sensitivity in axotomized fibers of experimental neuromas in mice. Pain 120:24–35
17. Story GM, Peier AM, Reeve AJ et al. (2003) ANKTM1, a TRP-like channel expressed in nociceptive neurons, is activated by cold temperatures. Cell 112:819–829
18. Viana F, de la Peña E, Belmonte C (2002) Specificity of cold thermotransduction is determined by differential ionic channel expression. Nat Neurosci 5:254–260
19. Wasner G, Schattschneider J, Binder A et al. (2004) Topical menthol–a human model for cold pain by activation and sensitization of C nociceptors. Brain 127:1159–1171
20. Yarnitsky D, Ochoa JL (1990) Release of cold-induced burning pain by block of cold-specific afferent input. Brain 113:893–902

N

Nociceptors, Immunocytochemistry

▶ Immunocytochemistry of Nociceptors

Nociceptors in the Dental Pulp

Matti V. O. Närhi
Department of Physiology, University of Kuopio,
Kuopio, Finland
matti.narhi@uku.fi

Synonyms

Intradental Nociceptors; Pulpal Nociceptors

Definition

▶ Nociceptors that are located inside the tooth in the
▶ dental pulp and in the ▶ dentinal tubules in the most inner layers of ▶ dentin. The intradental afferent innervation consists of both myelinated and unmyelinated nerve
fibers, which are mostly, if not exclusively, nociceptive.
The nerve fibers originate from the mandibular (lower
jaw) and maxillary (upper jaw) branches of the trigeminal nerve, and have their cell bodies in the ▶ trigeminal
ganglion.

Characteristics

Pulpal inflammation can be extremely painful. Also, the
intensity of the pain responses induced from teeth, e.g.
from exposed dentin, by external stimulation can reach
the maximum level of any pain score. The structure of
the intradental innervation gives a basis for such high
sensitivity. It should also be noted that pain is the predominant, if not the only, sensation that can be evoked
by activation of intradental nerves.

Structure of Intradental Innervation

The innervation of the dental pulp is exceptionally
rich (Fig. 1). Several hundred nerve fibers enter each
tooth (Byers 1984). Approximately 20–30% of them
are myelinated, mostly of smaller diameter, A–δ type,
although there are also some larger A–β type axons. A
great majority of the pulp nerve fibers are unmyelinated
(C-fibers). A small proportion, approximately 10%, of
the unmyelinated fibers are sympathetic efferents (see
Byers and Närhi 1999). Their activation causes vasoconstriction and consequently reduction in the pulpal
blood flow (Olgart 1996).
All intradental axons terminate as free nerve endings,
the C-fibers in the pulp proper and A-fibers both in the
pulp and a great number of them also in the ▶ predentin
and inner layers of dentin (Fig. 1.). The myelinated
nerve fibers branch abundantly and one axon may
have endings in more than a hundred dentinal tubules
(Byers 1984). The maximum distance that the fibers
penetrate into the tubules is approximately 100 – 150

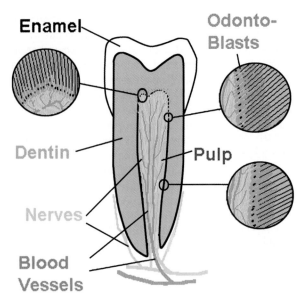

Nociceptors in the Dental Pulp, Figure 1 Schematic presentation of the
intradental innervation. A few branches from the alveolar nerve enter the
pulp through the apical foramen. These bundles extend further through
the root pulp and branch extensively, especially in the coronal pulp. The
terminal branches of the axons are free nerve endings, and are located
either in the pulp (especially the C-fibers) or in the tubules of the predentin
and inner layers of dentin (many of the A-fibers). See text for more details.

μm in the horns or tip of the coronal pulp. The pulp horns
are also the most densely innervated areas of the pulp. At
the pulp tip, approximately 50% of the tubules contain
nerve terminals, some of them even multiple endings
(Byers 1984). As there are 30000–40000 tubules/mm^2
of dentin (Brännström 1981), the density of the innervation of the pulp-dentin border at the tip of the coronal
pulp is exceptionally dense. However, there are fewer
nerve endings at the pulp-dentin border of the cervical
region, and yet exposed dentin in these areas can be
extremely sensitive, with innervation in the root being
especially sparse (Fig. 1) (Brännström 1981).

Function of Intradental Nociceptors

The similarity of the structure of the intradental innervation in human teeth to that in cats, dogs and monkeys
(Byers 1984) gives a morphological basis for studies,
where the function of intradental nerves in experimental
animals have been compared to the sensations evoked
by dental stimulation in man. Electrophysiological
recordings have revealed that A- and C-fibers of the
pulp are functionally different (Närhi 1985; Byers and
Närhi 1999). Comparison of those results to the sensory responses evoked by stimulation of human teeth
also indicated that activation of pulpal A- and C-fibers
may induce different types of pain sensations, namely
sharp and dull pain, respectively (Ahlquist et al. 1985;
Jyväsjärvi and Kniffki 1987). The intradental nerve
activity recordings in human teeth indicate that the
nerve function resembles that of experimental animals

(Edwall and Olgart 1976). The results of the single fiber recordings in cat and dog teeth also indicate that A-fibers are responsible for the sensitivity of dentin (Närhi 1985; Närhi et al. 1992), and that the intradental Aβ– and Aδ–fibers respond in a similar way to noxious dental stimulation (Närhi et al. 1992). Accordingly, they belong to the same functional group (Närhi et al. 1992 1996).

Pulpal A-fibers can be activated by a number of different stimuli applied at the tooth surface. Their responses are greatly enhanced if the dentin is exposed and the dentinal tubules are open (Närhi et al. 1992). Heat, cold, hypertonic solutions of various chemicals and desiccating air blasts, for example, applied to exposed dentin, evoke nerve responses with quite a similar pattern. The nerve firing starts immediately, or within a couple of seconds after the stimulus is applied, far before the stimuli, e.g. heat or cold, have reached the most inner layers of dentin and the pulp, where the nociceptors are located. So, the responses cannot be caused by a direct effect of the applied stimuli on the intradental nerve endings.

The stimuli, which induce pain from human teeth and activate the intradental nerves in experimental animals, are able to induce fluid flow in the dentinal tubules (Brännström 1981). Moreover, the fluid flow and the nerve responses induced by hydrostatic pressure are directly related (Vongsavan and Matthews 1994). Also, both the induction of the fluid flow, and the sensitivity of dentin are, to a great extent, dependent on the openness of the dentinal tubules (Brännström 1981; Närhi et al. 1992). Accordingly, the final stimulus for the nociceptors, which are responsible for the sensitivity of dentin (intradental A-fibers), seems to be the fluid flow in the tubules and, probably, the consequent mechanical deformation of the tissue and nerve endings in the pulp-dentin border (the so-called hydrodynamic mechanism of pulp nerve activation, Brännström 1981) (Fig. 2).

The hydrodynamic fluid flow is based on the strong capillary forces in the thin dentinal tubules (Brännström 1981). If dentinal fluid is extracted from the outer end of an open tubule by any stimulus, it is immediately replaced by a rapid outward fluid shift e.g. air-drying of dentine induces outward fluid flow and intense firing of the pulpal A-fibers (Närhi 1985). It also causes disruption of the tissues in the peripheral pulp (Brännström 1981). Thus, the capillary and hydrodynamic forces can considerably intensify the effect of the applied stimuli, and even a light stimulus such as an air blast can turn out to be noxious to the pulp.

The pulpal C-nociceptors are polymodal, and only activated if the external stimuli reach the pulp proper (Närhi 1985; Närhi et al. 1996). They do not respond to hydrodynamic stimulation. The C-fibers are activated by intense cold and heat applied to the tooth crown (Närhi et al. 1982; Jyväsjärvi and Kniffki 1987; Närhi et al. 1996). The response latencies are quite long, because the thermal stimuli have to reach the pulp where the nerve endings are located (Närhi 1985; Jyväsjärvi and Kniffki 1987; Närhi et al. 1996). The responses seem to be induced by a direct effect of heat and cold on the nerve endings. The C-nociceptors also respond to intense mechanical stimulation as well as to bradykinin, histamine and capsaicin applied to the exposed pulp (Närhi 1984; Närhi et al. 1992; Närhi et al. 1996).

Inflammation-Induced Changes in Pulpal Nociceptor Function

In healthy teeth the intradental nociceptors are well protected by the dental hard tissues and difficult to activate. Thus, pain is seldom induced from teeth during everyday activities. However, this is not the case when dentin with open tubules is exposed, because the effects of external stimuli are intensified by the hydrodynamic forces (Brännström 1981; Närhi et al. 1992). As in other tissue injuries, inflammation of the dental pulp can considerably sensitize the nociceptors (Brännström 1981;

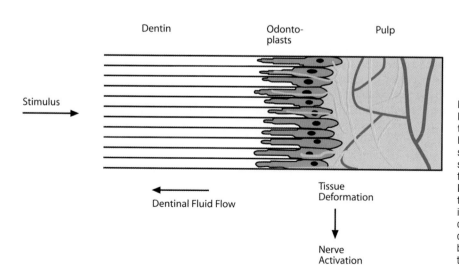

Nociceptors in the Dental Pulp, Figure 2 Activation of the intradental A-fibers by the hydrodynamic mechanism. Various stimuli applied to the exposed dentin surface are able to remove fluid from the outer ends of the dentinal tubules. Due to the high capillary force within the thin tubules the removed fluid is immediately replaced by a rapid outward fluid shift. This, in turn, distorts the tissue in the pulp-dentin border and, consequently, activates the nociceptors in the area.

Närhi et al. 1996). This may lead to extremely intense spontaneous pain (toothache), and exaggerated painful responses to external stimuli e.g. to hot or cold food or drinks. The change in pulpal nociceptor activity and sensitivity is caused by a number of different inflammatory mediators, which are released and/or synthesized in response to the tissue injury (Närhi et al. 1996; Byers and Närhi 1999).

Intradental A– and C-nociceptors are activated and sensitized by inflammatory mediators in the initial stages of inflammation, which include neurogenic reactions, e.g. ▶ axon reflexes (Närhi 1984; Närhi et al. 1992; Närhi et al. 1996; Olgart 1996). However, there are other longer-term neurogenic mechanisms which may contribute to the increased sensitivity (Byers and Närhi 1999). These include activation of silent pulpal nociceptors (Närhi et al. 1996; Byers and Närhi 1999), i.e. the proportion of pulpal A-fibers responding to dentinal stimulation is significantly higher in inflamed compared to normal teeth, and is especially profound among the slow-conducting Aδ fibers (Närhi et al. 1996). Moreover, the receptive fields of the single nerve fibers in inflamed teeth become expanded (Närhi et al. 1996). Both of these changes may be related to sprouting of the nociceptive nerve fibers (Kimberly and Byers 1988) and/or activation of normally unresponsive nerve terminals. These changes may contribute to the increased sensitivity of inflamed teeth.

In view of the dense innervation of the dental pulp, and the structural neural changes that can occur in inflamed teeth, it is clinically puzzling to find that pulpitis may frequently be almost or even completely asymptomatic. This can be partially due to central regulatory mechanisms, which may inhibit the impulse transmission in the trigeminal pain pathways (Sessle 2000). However, local mechanisms also seem to exist in the dental pulp itself, which may be important not only for the regulation of the inflammatory reactions, but also the sensitivity of the nociceptors (Närhi et al. 1996; Olgart 1996; Byers and Närhi 1999; Dionne et al. 2001). Endogenous opioids may inhibit the nerve activation and neuropeptide release from the nociceptive nerve endings. Also, somatostatin may have an inhibitory effect on the nociceptor activation. Furthermore, sympathetic nerve fibers seem to prevent the release of the neuropeptides, by virtue of their preterminal connections to the nociceptive nerve endings (Olgart 1996). Accordingly, a number of different central and peripheral regulatory mechanisms may be operating, and contribute to the great variability of the pain symptoms connected with pulpal inflammation.

References

1. Ahlquist ML, Franzen OG, Edwall LGA, Forss UG, Haegerstam GAT (1985) Quality of Pain Sensations Following Local Application of Algogenic Agents on the Exposed Human Tooth Pulp: A Psycho Physiological and Electrophysiological Study. In: Fields HL (ed) Advances in Pain Research and Therapy, vol 9. Raven Press, New York, pp 351–359

2. Beasley WL, Holland GR (1978) A Quantitative Analysis of the Innervation of the Pulp of Cat's Canine Tooth. J Comp Neurol 178:487–494
3. Brännstöm M (1981) Dentin and Pulp in Restorative Dentistry. Dental Therapeutics AB, Nacka, Sweden
4. Byers MR (1984) Dental Sensory Receptors. Int Rev Neurobiol 25:39–94
5. Byers MR, Närhi M (1999) Dental Injury Models: Experimental Tools for Understanding Neuroinflammatory Interactions and Polymodal Nociceptor Function. Crit Rev Oral Biol Med 10:4–39
6. Dionne RA, Lepinski AM, Jaber L, Gordon SM, Brahim JS, Hargreaves KM (2001) Analgesic Effects of Peripherally Administered Opioids in Clinical Models of Acute and Chronic Inflammation. Clin Pharmacol Ther 70:66–73
7. Edwall L, Olgart LM (1977) A New Technique for Recording of Intradental Sensory Nerve Activity in Man. Pain 3:121–126
8. Jyväsjärvi E, Kniffki K-D (1987) Cold Stimulation of Teeth: A Comparison between the Responses of Cat Intradental Aδ and C Fibres and Human Sensation. J Physiol 391:193–207
9. Kimberly CL, Byers MR (1988) Inflammation of Rat Molar Pulp and Periodontium Causes Increased Calcitonin Gene–Related Peptide and Axonal Sprouting. Anat Rec 222:289–300
10. Närhi MVO (1985) The Characteristics of Intradental Sensory Units and their Responses to Stimulation. J Dent Res 64:564–571
11. Närhi MVO (2001) Local Application of Morphine Inhibits the Intradental Nociceptor Responses to Mustard Oil but Not to Hydrodynamic Stimulation of Dentin. Society of Oral Physiology, Abstracts
12. Närhi M, Kontturi–Närhi V, Hirvonen T, Ngassapa D (1992) Neurophysiological Mechanisms of Dentin Hypersensitivity. Proc Finn Dent Soc 88:15–22
13. Närhi M, Yamamoto H, Ngassapa D (1996) Function of Intradental Nociceptors in Normal and Inflamed Teeth. In: Shimono M, Maeda T, Suda H and Takahashi K (eds) Dentin/pulp Complex. Quintessence Publ Co Tokyo, pp136–140
14. Olgart L (1996) Neurogenic Components of Pulp Inflammation. In: Shimono M, Maeda T, Suda H and Takahashi K (eds) Dentin/pulp Complex. Quintessence Publ Co Tokyo, pp 169–175
15. Sessle BJ (2000) Acute and Chronic Orofacial Pain: Brainstem Mechanisms of Nociceptive Transmission and Neuroplasticity and their Clinical Correlates. Crit Rev Oral Biol Med 11:57–91
16. Vongsavan N, Matthews B (1994) The Relationship between Fluid Flow in Dentine and the Discharge of Intradental Nerves. Archs Oral Biol 39 140S

Nociceptors in the Mucosa

▶ Nociceptors in the Orofacial Region (Skin/Mucosa)

Nociceptors in the Orofacial Region (Meningeal/Cerebrovascular)

KARL MESSLINGER
University of Erlangen-Nürnberg, Nürnberg, Germany
messlinger@physiologie1.uni-erlangen.de

Synonyms

Meningeal Afferents; Meningeal Nociceptors; Intracranial Nociceptors; Dural Receptors

Definition

Trigeminal afferents that respond to noxious (painful) stimulation of intracranial structures (cranial meninges and intracranial blood vessels). These afferents originate in the trigeminal ganglion and project centrally to the spinal trigeminal nucleus, and to some extent to the spinal dorsal horn of the first cervical segments. Activation of meningeal afferents produces the sensation of headache.

Characteristics

The afferent innervation of the meninges and intracranial blood vessels has long been associated with the generation of ▶ headaches. Intraoperative exploration of patients undergoing open head surgery has revealed that intracranial structures are differentially sensitive to various stimuli (Ray and Wolff 1940). Noxious mechanical, thermal or electrical stimulation of dural blood vessels and the main intracerebral arteries, but not other intracranial tissues, has been reported to be painful in these experiments. Since headache-like pain was the only sensation evoked from stimulation of these intracranial structures, meningeal afferents are generally attributed a nociceptive function. This concept has been confirmed by morphological findings. Afferent innervation of intracranial structures is restricted to Aδ and C fibres, which are known to terminate as ▶ non-corpuscular sensory endings. These nerve endings do not form distinct corpuscular end structures but disperse as small bundles of sensory fibres, partly encased by peripheral glia (Schwann

cells), along dural blood vessels and into the dural connective tissue (MeSSlinger et al. 1993; Fricke et al. 2001). Immunohistochemical preparations have shown that a considerable proportion of intracranial afferent fibres contain vasoactive neuropeptides, particularly ▶ calcitonin gene-related peptide (CGRP) (MeSSlinger et al. 1993). This vasodilatory neuropeptide is released from activated intracranial afferents, and has been suggested to be involved in the generation of ▶ migraine and other primary headaches (Edvinsson and Goadsby 1998). Experimentally, CGRP release from cranial dura mater can be quantitatively assessed *in vitro* and used as a measure for the activation of meningeal afferents by noxious stimuli. Using this method, it has been shown that not only classical noxious stimuli such as inflammatory mediators (Ebersberger et al. 1999); capsaicin, protons or heat, but also nitric oxide (NO) (Strecker et al. 2002) is able to release CGRP from rodent cranial dura. Another neuropeptide that has been identified immunohistochemically, in a smaller proportion of meningeal afferents, is substance P (MeSSlinger et al. 1993). Peripheral release of substance P is known to cause ▶ neurogenic inflammation, characterised by protein plasma extravasation, as well as other endothelial and perivascular changes. Neurogenic inflammation has been proposed to be a key factor in migraine pathophysiology (Moskowitz and Macfarlane 1993), but substance P was not found to be elevated during migraine attacks (Edvinsson and Goadsby 1998). In animal experiments, noxious stimulation of the meninges has failed to release detectable amounts of substance P in the periphery (Ebersberger et al. 1999), however, in

N

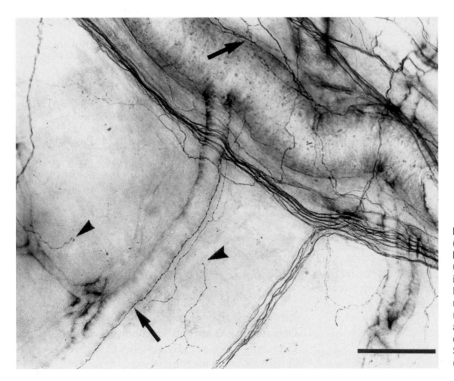

Nociceptors in the Orofacial Region (Meningeal/Cerebrovascular), Figure 1 Meningeal Afferents. CGRP immunoreactive nerve fibres in the rat dura mater encephali. Bundles and single immunopositive nerve fibres (arrows) run along the middle meningeal artery (MMA) and its branches, and terminate close to blood vessels (arrowheads). Scale bar 100 μm. Modified from (MeSSlinger et al. 1993).

the spinal trigeminal nucleus, increased substance P release during stimulation of rat dura mater with acidic solutions has been shown using a sensitive microprobe technique (Schaible et al. 1997). Therefore, substance P (and possibly CGRP), released from the central terminals of activated meningeal afferents, can be assumed to contribute to nociceptive transmission in the central trigeminal system.

Only a few direct electrophysiological recordings from intracranial afferents have been made in animal experiments. The teased fibre technique has been used to record from intracranial afferents running in the nasociliary nerve, which innervate fronto-medial parts of the supratentorial dura mater of the guinea pig (Bove and Moskowitz 1997). Another approach has been made in the rat to record with microelectrodes from the trigeminal ganglion, selecting neurons with dural receptive fields located around the middle meningeal artery or the large sinuses (Dostrovsky et al. 1991; Strassman et al. 1996). These studies are in accordance with the release studies mentioned above, and have shown afferent activation caused by noxious chemical stimuli (inflammatory mediators, capsaicin, and acidic buffer), heat and cold stimuli applied to the exposed dura mater, as well as mechanical stimulation of dural receptive fields. These studies also suggest that most, if not all, meningeal afferents can be regarded as ▶ polymodal nociceptors, which can be sensitized to mechanical stimuli through a cAMP mediated intracellular mechanism (Levy and Strassman 2002). There is evidence that most meningeal sensory endings express tetrodotoxin-resistant sodium channels, as has been reported frequently for visceral nociceptors (Strassman and Raymond 1999). In a new *in vitro* preparation of rat cranial dura, electrophysiological recordings from meningeal nerves are now made routinely in our laboratory. These experiments will provide additional insight into the response properties of meningeal afferents to stimuli such as nitric oxide and histamine, which are suggested to be key mediators in the generation of primary headaches.

Extracellular recordings from second-order neurones in the cat and the rat spinal trigeminal nucleus have shown that there is high convergence of afferent input from the meninges and orofacial region, most typically from the periorbital area (Davis and Dostrovsky 1988; Schepelmann et al. 1999). This observation has led investigators to assume that ▶ referred pain and hyperalgesia associated with headache may result from a ▶ central sensitization (Yamamura et al. 1999; Ellrich et al. 1999). The morphological and electrophysiological data taken from meningeal afferents suggest that intracranial pain (headache) may share more characteristics with visceral, rather than somatic, nociception and pain.

References

1. Bove GM, Moskowitz MA (1997) Primary Afferent Neurons Innervating Guinea Pig Dura. J Neurophysiol 77:299–308
2. Davis KD, Dostrovsky JO (1988) Responses of Feline Trigeminal Spinal Tract Nucleus Neurons to Stimulation of the Middle Meningeal Artery and Sagittal Sinus. J Neurophysiol 59:648–666
3. Dostrovsky JO, Davis KD, Kawakita K (1991) Central Mechanisms of Vascular Headaches. Can J Physiol Pharmacol 69:652–658
4. Ebersberger A, Averbeck B, Messlinger K, Reeh PW (1999) Release of Substance P, Calcitonin Gene-Related Peptide and Prostaglandin E$_2$ from Rat Dura Mater Encephali Following Electrical and Chemical Stimulation, *In Vitro*. Neuroscience 89:901–907
5. Edvinsson L, Goadsby PJ (1998) Neuropeptides in Headache. Eur J Neurol 5:329–341
6. Ellrich J, Andersen OK, Messlinger K, Arendt-Nielsen LA (1999) Convergence of Meningeal and Facial Afferents onto Trigeminal Brainstem Neurons: An Electrophysiological Study in Rat and Man. Pain 82:229–237
7. Fricke B, Andres KH, von Düring M (2001) Nerve Fibres Innervating the Cranial and Spinal Meninges: Morphology of Nerve Fiber Terminals and their Structural Integration. Microsc Res Technique 53:96–105
8. Levy D, Strassman AM (2002) Distinct Sensitizing Effects of the cAMP-PKA Second Messenger Cascade on Rat Dural Mechanonociceptors. J Physiol 538.2:483–493
9. Meßlinger K, Hanesch U, Baumgärtel M, Trost B, Schmidt RF (1993) Innervation of the Dura Mater Encephali of Cat and Rat: Ultrastructure and CGRP/SP-Like Immunoreactivity. Anat Embryol 188:219–237
10. Moskowitz MA, Macfarlane R (1993) Neurovascular and Molecular Mechanisms in Migraine Headaches. Cerebrovasc Brain Metab Rev 5:159–177
11. Ray BS, Wolff HG (1940) Experimental Studies on Headache: Pain Sensitive Structures of the Head and their Significance in Headache. Arch Surg 1:813–856
12. Schaible H-G, Ebersberger A, Peppel P, Beck U, Meßlinger K (1997) Release of Immunoreactive Substance P in the Trigeminal Brain Stem Nuclear Complex Evoked by Chemical Stimulation of the Nasal Mucosa and the Dura Mater Encephali - A Study with Antibody Microprobes. Neuroscience 76:273–284
13. Schepelmann K, Ebersberger A, Pawlak M, Oppmann M, Messlinger K (1999) Response Properties of Trigeminal Brain Stem Neurons with Input from Dura Mater Encephali in the Rat. Neuroscience 90:543–554
14. Strassman AM, Raymond SA, Burstein R (1996) Sensitization of Meningeal Sensory Neurons and the Origin of Headaches. Nature 384:560–564
15. Strassman AM, Raymond SA (1999) Electrophysiological Evidence for Tetrodotoxin-Resistant Sodium Channels in Slowly Conducting Dural Sensory Fibres. J Neurophysiol 81:413–424
16. Strecker T, Dux M, Messlinger K (2002) Nitric Oxide Releases Calcitonin Gene-Related Peptide from Rat Dura Mater Encephali Promoting Increases in Meningeal Blood Flow. J Vasc Res 39:489–496
17. Yamamura H, Malick A, Chamberlin NL, Burstein R (1999) Cardiovascular and Neuronal Responses to Head Stimulation Reflect Central Sensitization and Cutaneous Allodynia in a Rat Model of Migraine. J Neurophysiol 81:479–493

Nociceptors in the Orofacial Region (Skin/Mucosa)

BRIAN Y. COOPER
Department of Oral and Maxillofacial Surgery, University of Florida, Gainesville, FL, USA
bcooper@dental.ufl.edu

Synonyms

Polymodal nociceptor; High Threshold Mechanorecep-tor; mechanonociceptor; Mechanoheat Nociceptor; no-ciceptors in the skin; Nociceptors in the Mucosa

Definition

Nociceptors detect and encode stimuli with actual or potential tissue damaging properties. Many are also responsive to chemicals released from traumatized tissue, inflammatory and immune system cells. Noci-ceptors are notable among sensory afferents for their plasticity. Detection and encoding capacities undergo rapid quantitative and slower qualitative up regulatory adaptations (sensitization). These contribute to both peripheral and central nervous system changes, which mediate increased pain sensitivity following tissue or nervous system injury. These adaptations serve to pro-tect tissue from further damage and promote healing. Orofacial nociceptors supply a diverse set of tissues that include skin, muscle, bone and joints, but also highly specialized structures such as cornea, mucosa (oral and nasal) and teeth. Accordingly, some of the

anatomic and physiologic features are unique. The reader should examine the essays on corneal and tooth ▶ pulp nociceptors for further details.

Characteristics

Trigeminal nociceptors of skin and mucosa are a di-verse population of mechanical, thermal and chemically responsive afferents that detect and encode intense phys-ical, thermal and chemical events associated with actual or near tissue damage. The trigeminal root ganglion (TRG, gasserian ganglion, semilunar ganglion) contains cell bodies of orofacial skin and mucosal nociceptors. Trigeminal nociceptors are anatomically distinct from spinal nociceptors (derived from dorsal root ganglia), in that their central projections terminate in the brainstem rather than in the spinal cord. In other respects, they are very similar (Hu 2000; Sessle 2000). In addition to detection and encoding of noxious stimuli, nociceptors of the skin and mucosa are able to release neuropep-tides at both the peripheral and central processes. Peripherally, these peptides are involved in a variety of pro-inflammatory events (▶ plasma extravasation, mast cell degranulation, PLA$_2$ activation, healing),

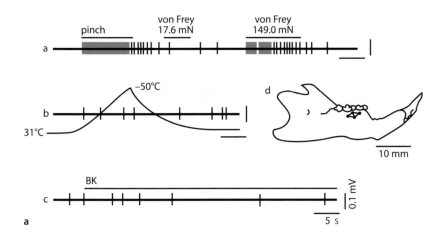

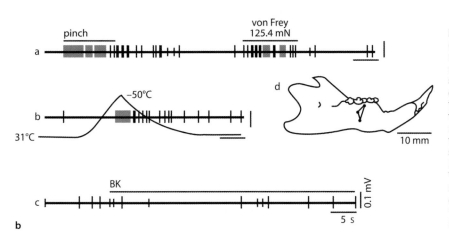

Nociceptors in the Orofacial Region (Skin/Mucosa), Figure 1 Mucosal nociceptors respond differentially to mechanical, chemical and thermal stimulation. (a) Brisk response of an Aδ HTM of the rat mucosa to mechanical stimulation. The fiber is less responsive to other modalities. (b) An Aδ MH responds to both mechanical and thermal stimuli. Reprinted from Neuroscience Letters 228, K. Toda, N. Ishii and Y. Nakamura, 'Characteristics of mucosal nociceptors in the rat oral cavity: an in vitro study', pp. 95-98, 1997 with permission from Elsevier. BK, bradykinin 0.1 uM.

while centrally they are released with primary neurotransmitters (e.g. glutamate) to modify the synaptic pain message at the first synapse (Cooper and Sessle 1993). The neuropeptides substance P and/or CGRP (calcitonin gene related peptide) are expressed in nociceptors; including, myelinated and unmyelinated nociceptors (Aδ and C class) that have been described in both facial and oral mucosa tissues (Aδ ▶ HTM, Aδ ▶ MH, Aδ PMN, C PMN) (see ▶ MH, ▶ HTM, ▶ PMN) (Cooper et al. 1991; Bongenhielm and Robinson 1996; Toda et al. 1997; Flores et al. 2001). Many nociceptors contain neither of these peptides. In the trigeminal ganglion, the small and medium sized cells represent the main populations of nociceptive neurons. The large neurons of the TRG may also contain nociceptive populations. Nociceptors are highly specialized to detect chemical agents associated with tissue trauma, and may sensitize following exposure to chemical algesics. Both peptidergic and non-peptidergic nociceptive afferents express cholinergic (▶ nAChr) (Liu et al. 1993; Carstens et al. 2000), ▶ purinergic (▶ P2X3 ; Eriksson et al. 1998, Xiang et al. 1998) or acid sensitive receptors and ▶ ion channels (▶ ASIC) (Ichikawa and Sugimoto 2002). These channels enable nociceptors to detect the presence of ATP, ACh or protons that are associated with tissue damage and inflammation. ATP and ACh are released from damaged cells, while high levels of protons may be associated with infection or ischemia due to compromise of the vascular supply. Many of these same populations express the ▶ capsaicin sensitive protein ▶ VR1 or the capsaicin insensitive ▶ VRL1 (TRPV1, TRPV2) (see ▶ VR1, ▶ VRL1, ▶ TRPV1, ▶ TRPV2), which transduce noxious heat stimuli and are critical to the development of heat sensitization (Ichikawa and Sugimoto 2000; Stenholm et al. 2002). Responses to cooling, ▶ bradykinin, ▶ PGE2 and histamine have also been described (Toda et al. 1997; Viana et al. 2002) (Fig. 1).

References

1. Bongenhielm U, Robinson PP (1996) Spontaneous and Mechanically Evoked Afferent Activity Originating from Myelinated Fibres in Ferret Inferior Alveolar Nerve Neuromas. Pain 67:399–406
2. Carstens E, Simons CT, Dessirier JM, Carstens MI, Jinks SL (2000) Role of Neuronal Nicotinic-Acetylcholine Receptors in the Activation of Neurons in Trigeminal Subnucleus Caudalis by Nicotine Delivered to the Oral Mucosa. Exp Brain Res 132:375–383
3. Cooper BY, Ahlquist ML, Friedman RM, Loughner BA, Heft MW (1991) Properties of High-Threshold Mechanoreceptors in the Gingival Mucosa I: Responses to Dynamic and Static Pressure. J Neurophysiol 66:1272–1279
4. Cooper, BY, Sessle BJ (1993) Physiology of Nociception in the Trigeminal System. In: Olesen J, Tfelt-Hansen P, Welch KMA (eds) The Headaches. Raven Press Ltd, New York, pp 87–92
5. Eriksson J, Bongenhielm U, Kidd E, Matthews B, Fried K (1998) Distribution of P2X3 Receptors in the Rat Trigeminal Ganglion after Inferior Alveolar Nerve Injury. Neurosci Lett 254:37–40
6. Flores CM, Leong AS, Dussor GO, Harding-Rose C, Hargreaves KM, Kilo S (2001) Capsaicin-Evoked CGRP Release from Rat Buccal Mucosa: Development of a Model System for Studying Trigeminal Mechanisms of Neurogenic Inflammation. Eur J Neurosci 14:1113–1120
7. Hu JW (2000) Neurophysiological Mechanism of Head Face and Neck Pain. In: Vernon H (ed) The cranio-cervical syndrome: mechanisms, assessment and treatment. Oxford, Boston, pp 31–48
8. Ichikawa H, Sugimoto T (2000) Vanilloid Receptor [1]-Like Receptor-Immunoreactive Primary Sensory Neurons in the Rat Trigeminal Nervous System. Neuroscience 101:719–725
9. Ichikawa H, Sugimoto T (2002) The Co-Expression of ASIC3 with Calcitonin Gene-Related Peptide and Parvalbumin in the Rat Trigeminal Ganglion. Brain Res 943:287–291
10. Liu L, Pugh W, Ma H, Simon SA (1993) Identification of Acetylcholine Receptors in Adult Rat Trigeminal Ganglion Neurons. Brain Res 617:37–42
11. Sessle BJ (2000) Acute and Chronic Craniofacial Pain: Brainstem Mechanisms of Nociceptive Transmission and Neuroplasticity, and their Clinical Correlates. Crit Rev Oral Biol Med 11:57–91
12. Stenholm E, Bongenhielm U, Ahlquist M, Fried K (2002) VRl- and VRL-l-Like Immunoreactivity in Normal and Injured Trigeminal Dental Primary Sensory Neurons of the Rat. Acta Odontol Scand 60:72–79
13. Toda K, Ishii N, Nakamura Y (1997) Characteristics of Mucosal Nociceptors in the Rat Oral Cavity: An *In Vitro* Study. Neurosci Lett 228:95–98
14. Viana F, de la Pena E, Belmonte C (2002) Specificity of Cold Thermotransduction is Determined by Differential Ionic Channel Expression. Nat Neurosci 5:254–260
15. Xiang Z, Bo X, Burnstock G (1998) Localization of ATP-Gated P2X Receptor Immunoreactivity in Rat Sensory and Sympathetic Ganglia. Neurosci Lett 256:105–108

Nociceptors in the Orofacial Region (Temporomandibular Joint and Masseter Muscle)

BRIAN E. CAIRNS
Faculty of Pharmaceutical Sciences, University of British Columbia, Vancouver, BC, Canada
brcairns@interchange.ubc.ca

Synonyms

Nociceptive Temporomandibular Joint Afferents; Nociceptive Masseter Muscle Afferents

Definition

Primary afferent fibers that innervate the ▶ temporomandibular joint (TMJ) and masticatory muscles, and are activated by noxious mechanical, chemical or thermal stimuli applied to these tissues. These afferent fibers transduce and convey information about potential or actual tissue injury from the orofacial region to the central nervous system.

Characteristics

TMJ Nociceptors

The TMJ is innervated by thinly myelinated and unmyelinated afferent fibers, with non-specialized endings, which contain clear and dense core vesicles. This suggests some of these afferent fibers release neuro-transmitters and neuropeptides, such as calcitonin gene related peptide (CGRP) and substance P, from their terminal endings (Kido et al. 1995). These small-diameter afferent fibers project, via the gasserian or trigeminal ganglion, to the trigeminal subnuclei interpolaris and caudalis (Casatti et al. 1999; Capra 1987; Widenfalk and Wiberg 1990), areas of the caudal brainstem which appear to be most important for the integration of nociceptive input from deep orofacial tissues. Electro-physiological studies have confirmed the projection of a subpopulation of TMJ afferent fibres with conduction velocities of less than 25 m/sec (Aδ and C fibres) to the caudal brainstem (Cairns et al. 2001 a,b). These fibres are activated by noxious mechanical and/or chemical stimuli and appear to function as nociceptors (Cairns et al. 2001 a,b).

TMJ afferent fibers, identified as mechanical nociceptors by their response to noxious protrusion or lateral movement of the TMJ, have been described (Cairns et al. 2001a; Loughner B et al. 1997). These fibers are not activated by innocuous jaw opening, but begin to discharge as lateral rotation of the jaw exceeds the normal range, and exhibit a progressively increased discharge with supra-normal rotation of the jaw. Some of these nociceptors also appear to encode rate of jaw rotation (Loughner B et al. 1997). The threshold of TMJ nociceptors to noxious mechanical rotation of the jaw is lower in females than males; however, this is apparently due to sex-related differences in the biome-chanical properties of the TMJ tissues (Loughner B et al. 1997).

TMJ nociceptors respond to injection of algogenic substances such as mustard oil, potassium chloride and ▶ glutamate into the TMJ, which also evokes a ▶ nociceptive reflex response in the jaw muscles (Cairns et al. 2001a; Cairns et al. 1998) The activity of TMJ nociceptors precedes, but has a markedly shorter duration, than reflex jaw muscle activity evoked by injection of glutamate into the TMJ. This finding has led to the speculation that a brief activation of TMJ nociceptors, by algogenic compounds such as glutamate, is sufficient to induce ▶ central sensitization, a period of prolonged increase in the excitability of trigeminal subnucleus caudalis neurons (Cairns et al. 2001a). Such a phenomenon may explain the diffuse referral pattern of TMJ pain, which may spread to include the masticatory and neck muscles, and why acute joint pain can sometimes significantly outlast the duration of nociceptive stimulation.

Sex-related differences in the chemical response characteristics of TMJ nociceptors have also been noted. The greatest response to algogenic compounds has been observed in small, mechanically sensitive afferent fibers with conduction velocities of less than 10 m/s, which suggests that these particular fibers function as polymodal nociceptors, i.e. nociceptors that respond

to more than one type of noxious stimulation. Sex-related differences in response to injection of glutamate into the TMJ have been best characterized. Injection of glutamate into the TMJ has been found to evoke significantly greater nociceptive reflex responses and discharge in polymodal nociceptors in females than in males (Cairns et al. 2001a) Such sex-related differences in TMJ nociceptor excitability may explain, in part, the increased prevalence of certain orofacial pain syndromes in women (Dao and LeResche 2000).

Algogenic compounds, such as mustard oil and glutamate, excite TMJ nociceptors in part through activation of peripheral NMDA and non-NMDA receptors (Cairns et al. 1998). This suggests that peripheral glutamate receptor antagonists may be of use in modifying the excitability of TMJ nociceptors under certain pathological conditions. In contrast, the peripheral endings of TMJ nociceptors are not excited by γ- ▶ aminobutyric acid (GABA), which is thought to depolarize the central endings of nociceptors (Cairns et al. 2001a). Indeed, the current evidence suggests that GABA may in fact decrease the excitability of TMJ nociceptors through activation of peripheral GABA$_A$ receptors (Cairns et al. 1999). This unexpected effect of GABA suggests that the activation of peripheral GABA$_A$ receptors may result in a local analgesia of the TMJ.

Masseter Muscle Nociceptors

Anatomical and electrophysiological studies have indicated that the ▶ masseter muscle is also innervated by thinly myelinated and unmyelinated trigeminal afferent fibers with non-specialized endings, which project to the trigeminal subnucleus interpolaris and caudalis (Cairns et al. 2002; Cairns et al. 2001b; Cairns et al. 2003; Capra and Wax 1989; Nishimori et al. 1986) These fibers are activated by noxious mechanical and/or chemical stimuli and appear to function as nociceptors (Cairns et al. 2002; Cairns et al. 2001b; Cairns et al. 2003).

About one-third of masseter muscle afferent fibers that project to subnucleus caudalis have mechanical thresholds that exceed the human pressure pain threshold (Cairns et al. 2003; Svensson et al. 2003). In uninjured masseter muscle, these nociceptors are predominantly Aδ fibers with conduction velocities of less than 10 m/sec (Cairns et al. 2002; Cairns et al. 2003). Most of these nociceptors exhibit slowly adapting responses to sustained noxious mechanical stimulation (Fig. 1). A significant sex-related difference in the mechanical threshold of these nociceptors has not been found.

Like TMJ nociceptors (see above), masseter muscle mechanical nociceptors also respond to the injection of algogenic substances such as ▶ hypertonic saline and glutamate, but not GABA, into their mechanoreceptive field (Cairns et al. 2002; Cairns et al. 2001; Cairns et al. 2003). The afferent discharge evoked by these algogenic substances is greatest in C fibers and in Aδ fibers with con-

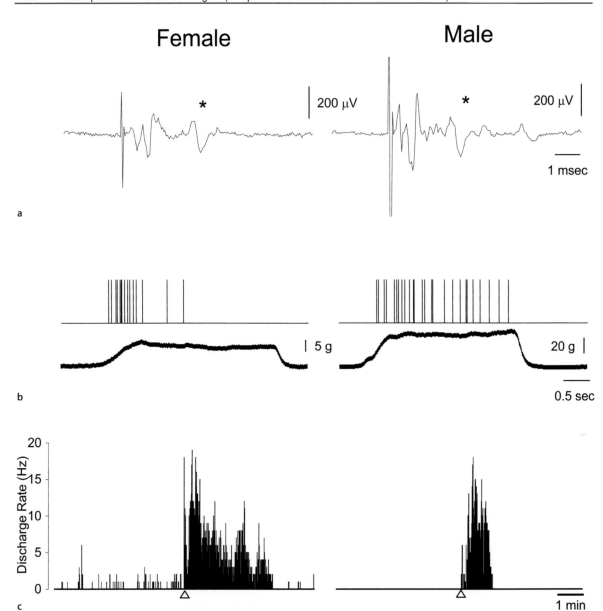

Nociceptors in the Orofacial Region (Temporomandibular Joint and Masseter Muscle), Figure 1 Examples of deep orofacial tissue nociceptor response characteristics. (a) The line drawing illustrates antidromic action potentials (*), evoked by electrical stimulation of the caudal brainstem, to confirm the central projection target of these masseter muscle Aδ nociceptors. (b) Sustained noxious mechanical stimulation of the masseter muscle with an electronic Von Frey hair (lower trace), resulted in a slowly adapting discharge (upper trace). (c) The peri-stimulus histograms illustrate the effect of injection of the algogenic substance glutamate into the masseter muscle. Note that glutamate-evoked nociceptor discharge was markedly greater in the female than in the male.

duction velocities of less than 10 m/s. Thus, these particular fibers appear to function as polymodal nociceptors. Glutamate consistently evokes significantly greater nociceptor discharges and pain responses in females than in males (Cairns et al. 2002; Cairns et al. 2001; Cairns et al. 2003) (see examples, Fig. 1). Thus, sex-related differences in masseter muscle nociceptor excitability appear to underlie, at least in part, the increased prevalence of masticatory muscle pain conditions suffered by women (Dao and LeResche 2000). Prolonged mechanical sensitization of the masseter muscle and its nociceptors has

also been demonstrated to occur after injection of glutamate into the masseter muscle, although there do not appear to be sex-related differences in this phenomenon (Cairns et al. 2002; Svensson et al. 2003).

Unlike TMJ nociceptors, current evidence suggests that glutamate-evoked afferent discharge in masseter nociceptors is predominantly mediated through activation of peripheral NMDA receptors (Cairns et al. 2003). Glutamate-induced mechanical sensitization is also mediated through activation of peripheral glutamate receptors (Cairns et al. 2002). Thus, peripheral NMDA receptor antagonists may prove to be particularly effective analgesics for the treatment of masticatory muscle pain.

Conclusion

The role of orofacial nociceptors is to transduce and convey information about the intensity and quality of orofacial pain. The characteristics of TMJ and masseter muscle nociceptors suggest that they may play a role not only in the development, but also in the maintenance of certain types of orofacial pain, and contribution to sex differences in TMJ and masticatory muscle pain.

References

1. Cairns BE, Sessle BJ, Hu JW (1998) Evidence that Excitatory Amino Acid Receptors within the Temporomandibular Joint Region are Involved in the Reflex Activation of the Jaw Muscles. J Neurosci 18:8056–8064
2. Cairns BE, Sessle BJ, Hu JW (1999) Activation of Peripheral GABAA Receptors Inhibits Temporomandibular Joint-Evoked Jaw Muscle Activity. J Neurophysiol 81:1966–1969
3. Cairns BE, Sessle BJ, Hu JW (2001a) Characteristics of Glutamate-Evoked Temporomandibular Joint Afferent Activity in the Rat. J Neurophysiol 85:2446–2454
4. Cairns BE, Hu JW, Arendt-Nielsen L, Sessle BJ, Svensson P (2001b) Sex-Related Differences in Human Pain Perception and Rat Afferent Discharge Evoked by Injection of Glutamate into the Masseter Muscle. J Neurophysiol 86:782–791
5. Cairns BE, Gambarota G, Svensson P, Arendt-Nielsen L, Berde CB (2002) Glutamate-Induced Sensitization of Rat Masseter Muscle Fibers. Neuroscience 109:389–399
6. Cairns BE, Svensson P, Wang K, Hupfeld S, Graven-Nielsen T, Sessle BJ, Berde CB, Arendt-Nielsen l (2003) Activation of Peripheral NMDA Receptors Contributes to Human Pain and Rat Afferent Discharges Evoked by Injection of Glutamate into the Masseter Muscle. J Neurophysiol 90:2098–2105
7. Capra NF (1987) Localization and Central Projections of Primary Afferent Neurons that Innervate the Temporomandibular Joint in Cats. Somatosens Res 4:201–213
8. Capra NF, Wax TD (1989) Distribution and Central Projections of Primary Afferent Neurons that Innervate the Masseter Muscle and Mandibular Periodontium: A Double-Label Study. J Comp Neurol 279:341–352
9. Casatti CA, Frigo L, Bauer JA (1999) Origin of Sensory and Autonomic Innervation of the Rat Temporomandibular Joint: A Retrograde Axonal Tracing Study with the Fluorescent Dye Fast Blue. J Dent Res 78:776–783
10. Dao TTT, LeResche L (2000) Gender Differences in Pain. J Orofac Pain 14:169–184
11. Dateoka Y, Shigenaga Y (1986) The Distribution of Muscle Primary Afferents from the Masseter Nerve to the Trigeminal Sensory Nuclei. Brain Res 372:375–381
12. Kido MA, Kiyoshima T, Ibuki T, Shimizu S, Kondo T, Terada Y, Tanaka T (1995) A Topographical and Ultrastructural Study of Sensory Trigeminal Nerve Endings in the Rat Temporomandibular Joint as Demonstrated by Anterograde Transport of Wheat Germ Agglutinin-Horseradish Peroxidase (WGA-HRP). J Dent Res 74:1353–1359
13. Loughner B, Miller J, Broumand V, Cooper B (1997) The Development of Strains, Forces and Nociceptor Activity in Retrodiscal Tissues of the Temporomandibular Joint of Male and Female Goats. Exp Brain Res 113:311–326
14. Nishimori T, Sera M, Suemune S, Yoshida A, Tsuru K, Tsuiki Y, Akisaka T, Okamoto T, Svensson P, Cairns BE, Wang K, Hu JW, Graven-Nielsen T, Arendt-Nielsen L, Sessle BJ (2003) Glutamate-Evoked Pain and Mechanical Allodynia in the Human Masseter Muscle. Pain 101:221–227
15. Widenfalk B, Wiberg M (1990) Origin of Sympathetic and Sensory Innervation of the Temporo-Mandibular Joint. A Retrograde Axonal Tracing Study in the Rat. Neurosci Lett 109:30–35

Nociceptors, Perireceptor Elements

▶ Perireceptor Elements

Nocifensive

Definition

Denoting a process or mechanism that acts to protect the body from injury.
▶ Nocifensive Behaviors of the Urinary Bladder
▶ Secondary Somatosensory Cortex (S2) and Insula, Effect on Pain Related Behavior in Animals and Humans

Nocifensive Behavior

Definition

Nocifensive behaviors are those that are evoked by stimuli that activate the nociceptive sensory apparatus. They are associated with protection against insult and injury typically in response to a noxious stimulus. Responses to noxious stimuli in animals may include behaviors resembling responses to pain in humans, such as limping, flinching, vocalization and reflexive withdrawal. Other specific pain-related responses in animals include tail and paw flicks, licking, and scratching. Responses to increased deep muscle and joint pain may include reduced exploration activity. In the viscera, nocifensive behaviors can be produced by hollow organ distension, ischemia, traction on the mesentery or stimulation of inflamed organs.
▶ Muscle Pain Model, Inflammatory Agents-Induced
▶ Nocifensive Behaviors (Muscle and Joint)
▶ Sensitization of Visceral Nociceptors

Nocifensive Behaviors Evoked by Myositis

▶ Muscle Pain Model, Inflammatory Agents-Induced

Nocifensive Behaviors, Gastrointestinal Tract

GERALD F. GEBHART

Department of Pharmacology, University of Pittsburgh, Pittsburgh, PA, USA

gf-gebhart@uiowa.edu

Synonyms

Pseudaffective; pseudoaffective; Gastrointestinal Tract, Nocifensive Behaviors

Definition

Nocifensor, a term introduced by Lewis (1936; see Lewis 1942; LaMotte 1992 for discussion), describes a system of "nerves" associated with local defense against injury. Nocifensive has since expanded as a term to describe behaviors associated with protection against insult and injury. Nocifensive behaviors are more complex than simple nociceptive flexor withdrawal reflexes, such as the tailflick reflex, and the term is particularly appropriate in the visceral realm, where stimuli considered to be adequate (e.g. hollow organ distension, ischemia, traction on the mesentery) are different from those Sherrington (1906) defined as adequate for activation of cutaneous nociceptors. The nocifensive behaviors produced by visceral stimulation are also considered pseudaffective (Sherrington 1906) (pseudoaffective), because responses to visceral stimulation are organized supraspinally.

Characteristics

Balloon distension of gastrointestinal tract organs has been widely employed in both human and non-human animal studies. Significantly, balloon distension of the esophagus, stomach or large bowel reproduces in humans the distribution of referred sensations, as well as the quality and intensity of discomfort and pain, arising from pathological visceral disorders (see Ness and Gebhart 1990 for review). In addition, balloon distension of hollow organs is a stimulus that is easy to control in terms of onset, duration and intensity, as opposed, for example, to a chemical or ischemic visceral stimulus. The nocifensive behaviors produced by balloon distension of hollow organs include changes in blood pressure, heart rate and respiration, and visceromotor reflexes (▶ visceromotor reflex/response). All of these responses are absent in spinally transected animals, but present following mid-collicular decerebration, thus revealing that they are responses integrated in the brainstem. All of these response measures are intensity-dependent and can be quantified as indices of visceral nociception.

Although balloon distension of hollow organs has been widely used, it wasn't until Ness parametrically characterized in the rat responses to colorectal distension that this model of visceral pain became widely accepted and widely used (Ness and Gebhart 1988). Similar parametric evaluation of responses to colorectal distension in the mouse (Kamp et al. 2003) and gastric distension in the rat (Ozaki et al. 2002) have since been described.

Colorectal Distension (CRD)

Balloons of different lengths and varying durations of distension have been reported in the literature. As Lewis (1942) noted, distension of hollow organs is most painful in humans when long, continuous segments of the gut are distended, which emphasizes the importance of ▶ spatial summation as an important consideration in CRD as a stimulus. Results using different length balloons in the rat are qualitatively similar, although greater intensities of stimulation are generally required with smaller balloons to produce quantitatively equivalent responses. The human literature (see Ness and Gebhart 1990 for citations and discussion) also established that constant pressure distension, rather than constant volume, was the appropriate stimulus. It should be appreciated that hollow organs throughout the viscera, and particularly within the gastrointestinal tract, accommodate as they fill. Thus, constant volume distension produces an inconstant intensity of stimulation as the organ musculature relaxes.

Balloon CRD produces contraction of the peritoneal musculature, representing what has been termed a visceromotor reflex. Among the responses to CRD, the visceromotor reflex recorded from the external oblique peritoneal musculature is perhaps the most reliable and experimentally least complicated measure to quantify. Indwelling arterial catheters to measure changes in blood pressure or heart rate produce equally robust and quantifiable measures of response to distension, but are more difficult to maintain than electromyographic electrodes sewn into the peritoneal musculature. Figure 1 illustrates graded visceromotor responses to increasing intensities of CRD in the mouse. The response threshold for CRD is typically between 20 mmHg and 25 mmHg in normal rat colon. In consideration of the response threshold for a subset of pelvic nerve afferent fibers that innervate the colon and spinal dorsal horn neuron responses to CRD, the intensity of CRD in the rat considered to be noxious is $\geq$ 30 mmHg. This interpretation is consistent with results from psychophysical studies in humans (e.g. Ness et al. 1990), in which increases in heart rate and blood pressure were produced by colon distension at intensities of distension less than reported as painful. Accordingly, quantification of pseudaffective responses to visceral stimulation requires interpretation with respect to the quality of the nocifensive behavior produced (e.g. visceromotor response). That is, changes in response measures may be apparent before a behavior is nocifensive, although thresholds for response are similar.

Clinical Use and Side Effects

NSAIDs are indicated in the treatment of:

- various pain states (e.g. headache, toothache and migraine), primarily pathophysiological pain involving nociceptors e.g. rheumatic pain and pain caused by bone metastases,
- defects of the ductus arteriosus Botalli (short circuit connection between arteria pulmonalis and aorta; non-closure after birth)
- fever (see ▶ NSAIDs and their indications)

Side effects of NSAIDs include:

- gastrointestinal disorders (e.g. dyspepsia), gastrointestinal erosion with bleeding, ulceration and perforation,
- kidney malfunctions with retention of sodium and water, hypertension
- inhibition of platelet aggregation,
- central nervous symptoms such as dizziness and headache,
- disturbance of uterine motility,
- skin reactions,
- triggering of asthma attacks in asthmatics. This side effect is a pseudo-allergic reaction where COX-inhibition increases the availability of substrates for lipoxygenase that are converted to broncho-constrictive leukotrienes (see ▶ NSAIDs, adverse effects and ▶ NSAID-Induced Lesions of the Gastrointestinal Tract).

Non-selective inhibitors of prostaglandin synthesis are contraindicated:

- in gastric and duodenal ulcer,
- in asthma,
- in bleeding disorders,
- during the last few weeks of pregnancy because of the danger of early sealing of the ductus Botalli.

Glucocorticoids increase the risk of gastrointestinal complications. Considerable caution is necessary when using NSAIDs in patients with severe liver and kidney damage and they should not be combined with coumatins. Owing to the limited experience obtained, these precautions and contraindications also apply to COX-2 selective inhibitors.

The following drug interactions are the most important that can occur when conventional NSAIDs are co-administered with other agents:

- the uricosuric effect of probenecid is reduced
- the diuretic effect of saluretics is weakened,
- the blood glucose lowering effect of oral antidiabetics is increased,
- the elimination of methotrexate is delayed and its toxicity is increased,
- the elimination of lithium ions is delayed,
- the anti-coagulation effect of coumatin derivatives is enhanced and
- the antihypertensive effect of ACE-inhibitors is reduced (see ▶ NSAIDs, pharmacokinetics).

Due to the short period of clinical use, the interaction profile of COX-2 selective inhibitors cannot be described at the present time.

Derivatives of Salicylic Acid

Salicylic acid for systemic use has been replaced by acetylsalicylic acid, amides of salicylic acid (salicylamide, ethenzamide, salacetamide), salsalate and diflunisal.

Acetylsalicylic Acid (Aspirin)

The esterification of the phenolic hydroxyl group in salicylic acid with acetic acid results not only in an agent with improved local tolerability, but also with greater antipyretic and anti-inflammatory activity and, in particular, more marked inhibitory effects on platelet aggregation (inhibition of thromboxane-A2 synthesis). Because of these qualities, acetylsalicylic acid is one of the most frequently used non-opioid analgesics and the most important inhibitor of platelet aggregation. Acetylsalicylic acid irreversibly inhibits both COX-1 and COX-2 by acetylating the enzymes. Since mature platelets lack a nucleus, they are unable to synthesize new enzyme. The anti-platelet effects of acetylsalicylic acid therefore persist throughout the lifetime of the platelet and the half-life of this effect is thus much longer than the elimination half-life of acetylsalicylic acid (15 min). Since new platelets are continuously launched into the circulation, the clinically relevant anti-platelet effect of aspirin lasts for up to 5 days. This is the reason why low doses of acetylsalicylic acid (ca. 100 mg per day) are sufficient in the prophylaxis of heart attacks.

After oral administration, acetylsalicylic acid is rapidly and almost completely absorbed, but in the intestinal mucosa it is partly deacetylated to salicylic acid, which also exhibits analgesic activity. The plasma half-life of acetylsalicylic acid is approximately 15 min, whereas that of salicylic acid at therapeutic dosages of acetylsalicylic acid is 2–3 h. Salicylic acid is eliminated more slowly when acetylsalicylic acid is administered at high dose rates because of saturation of the liver enzymes. The metabolites are mainly excreted via the kidney. The dosage of acetylsalicylic acid in the treatment of pain and fever is 1.5–3 g daily and in the prophylaxis of heart attacks 30–100 mg daily.

Side effects of acetylsalicylic acid administration include buzzing in the ears, loss of hearing, dizziness, nausea, vomiting and most importantly gastrointesti-

N

nal bleeding and gastrointestinal ulcerations including gastric perforation. The administration of acetylsalicylic acid in children with viral infections can, in rare cases, produce Reye's syndrome, involving liver damage, encephalopathy and a mortality rate exceeding 50%. Acute salicylate poisoning results in hyperventilation, marked sweating and irritability followed by respiratory paralysis, unconsciousness, hyperthermia and dehydration.

Derivatives of Acetic Acid

Indomethacin

Indomethacin is a strong inhibitor of both cyclooxygenase isoforms with a slight stronger effect in the case of COX-1. It is rapidly and almost completely absorbed from the gastrointestinal tract and has high plasma protein binding. The plasma half-life of indomethacin varies from 3 to 11 h due to intense enterohepatic cycling. Only about 15% of the substance is eliminated unchanged in the urine, the remainder being eliminated in urine and bile as inactive metabolites (O-demethylation, glucuronidation, N-deacylation). The daily oral dose of indomethacin is 50–150 mg (up to 200 mg).

Indomethacin treatment is associated with a high incidence (30%) of side effects typical for those seen with other NSAIDs (see above). Gastrointestinal side effects, in particular, are more frequently observed after indomethacin than after administration of other NSAIDs. The market share of indomethacin (approximately 5%) is therefore low as compared to that for other non-steroidal antirheumatic agents.

Diclofenac

Diclofenac is an exceedingly potent cyclooxygenase inhibitor slightly more efficacious against COX-2 than COX-1. Its absorption from the gastrointestinal tract varies according to the type of pharmaceutical formulation used. The oral bioavailability is only 30–80% due to a first-pass effect. Diclofenac is rapidly metabolised (hydroxylation and conjugation) and has a plasma half-life of 1.5 h. The metabolites are excreted renally and via the bile.

Epidemiological studies have demonstrated that diclofenac causes less serious gastrointestinal complications than indomethacin. However, a rise in plasma liver enzymes occurs more frequently with diclofenac than with other NSAIDs. The daily oral dose of diclofenac is 50–150 mg. Diclofenac is also available as eye-drops for the treatment of non-specific inflammation of the eye and for the local therapy of eye pain (see ► NSAIDs, pharmacokinetics).

Derivatives of Arylpropionic Acid

2-arylpropionic acid derivatives possess an asymmetrical carbon atom, giving rise to S- and R-enantiomers.

The S-enantiomer inhibits cyclooxygenases 2–3 orders of magnitude more potently than the corresponding R-enantiomer. This finding has led to the marketing of pure S-enantiomers (e.g. S-ibuprofen and S-ketoprofen) in some countries in addition to the racemates where the R-enantiomer is considered as "ballast". However, it is not yet proven whether 2-arylpropionic acids are better tolerated when given as S-enantiomer than as the racemate. Naproxen, for example, which is clinically available only as the S-enantiomer, does not cause less serious gastrointestinal side effects than, e.g. ibuprofen racemate.

Ibuprofen is the most thoroughly researched 2-arylpropionic acid. It is a relatively weak, nonselective inhibitor of COX. In epidemiological studies, ibuprofen compared to all other conventional NSAIDs, has the lowest relative risk of causing severe gastrointestinal side effects. Because of this, ibuprofen is the most frequently used OTC ("over the counter", sale available without prescription) analgesic. Ibuprofen is highly bound to plasma proteins and has a relatively short elimination half-life (approximately 2 h). It is mainly glucuronidated to inactive metabolites that are eliminated via the kidney. The typical single oral dose of ibuprofen as an OTC analgesic is 200–400 mg and 400–800 mg when used in anti-rheumatic therapy. The corresponding maximum daily doses are 1200 or 2400 mg, respectively but the dose in anti-rheumatic therapy in some countries can be as high as 3200 mg daily.

Other arylpropionic acids include naproxen, ketoprofen and flurbiprofen. They share most of the properties of ibuprofen. The daily oral dose of ketoprofen is 50–150 mg, 150–200 mg for flurbiprofen and 250–1000 mg for naproxen. Whereas the plasma elimination half-life of ketoprofen and flurbiprofen are similar to that of ibuprofen (1.5–2.5 h and 2.4–4 h, respectively), naproxen is eliminated much more slowly with a half-life of 13–15 h (see ► NSAIDs, pharmacokinetics).

Oxicams

Oxicams e.g. piroxicam, tenoxicam, meloxicam and lornoxicam are non-selective inhibitors of cyclooxygenases. Like diclofenac, meloxicam inhibits COX-2 slightly more potently than COX-1. This property can be exploited clinically with doses up to 7.5 mg per day, but at higher doses COX-1 inhibition becomes clinically relevant. Since the dose of meloxicam commonly used is 15 mg daily, this agent cannot be regarded as a COX-2 selective NSAID and considerable caution needs to be exercised when making comparisons between the actions of meloxicam and those of other conventional NSAIDs. The average daily dose in anti-rheumatic therapy is 20 mg for piroxicam and tenoxicam, 7.5–15 mg for meloxicam and 12–16 mg for lornoxicam. Some oxicams have long elimination half-lives (lornoxicam 3–5 h, meloxicam approximately 20 h, piroxicam approximately 40 h and tenoxicam approximately 70 h).

COX-2 Selective NSAIDs (COXIBs)

The development of the COXIBs has been based on the hypothesis that COX-1 is the physiological COX and COX-2 the pathophysiological isoenzyme. Inhibition of the pathophysiological COX-2 only is assumed to result in fewer side effects as compared to non-selective inhibition of both COX isoenzymes. Rofecoxib and celecoxib were the first substances approved that inhibit only COX-2 at therapeutic doses. Substances with higher COX-2-selectivity than rofecoxib and celecoxib have been recently approved or will shortly be approved (e.g. etoricoxib, parecoxib, lumiracoxib).

Unlike conventional NSAIDs, with the exception of lumiracoxib the "COXIBs" have no functional acidic group. The indications for these agents are in principle identical to those of the non-selective NSAIDs, although they have not yet received approval for the whole spectrum of indications of the conventional NSAIDs. Because they lack COX-1-inhibiting properties, COX-2-selective inhibitors show fewer side effects than conventional NSAIDs. However, they are not free of side effects because COX-2 has physiological functions that are blocked by the COX-2-inhibitors. The most frequently observed side effects are infections of the upper respiratory tract, diarrhoea, dyspepsia, abdominal discomfort and headache. Peripheral oedema is as frequent as with conventional NSAIDs. The frequency of gastrointestinal complications is approximately half that observed with conventional NSAIDs. The precise side effect profile of the selective COX-2-inhibitors, however, will only be known after several years of clinical use (see ▶ NSAID induced lesions of the gastrointestinal tract).

On September 30, 2004, MSD voluntarily withdrew rofecoxib from the market because of a colon cancer prevention study (APPROVe) suggesting that rofecoxib nearly doubled the rate of myocardial infarction and strokes as compared to placebo. Celecoxib, a less potent selective COX-2-inhibitor with a shorter half life showed a similar dose related problem in another colon cancer prevention trial (APC), but did not show an increased risk in an Alzheimer prevention trial (ADAPT) or in another colon cancer study (PreSAP). The reasons for these discrepancies are a matter of scientific debate (Tegeder, Geisslinger 2006). Many scientists favour a group effect of all coxibs, because the balance between two fatty acids, prostacyclin and thrombox-

ane A2 that control blood clotting and vasodilation may be disturbed after intake of selective COX-2-inhibitors. As a result of this possible imbalance, the risk for cardiovascular events may increase. However, there are also data suggesting that nonselective NSAIDs are also not safe with respect to thromboembolic events. In the aforementioned ADAPT trial, the nonselective NSAID naproxen significantly increased the risk of heart attacks and stroke (see ▶ NSAIDs, chemical structure and molecular mode of action; ▶ NSAIDs and their indications; ▶ NSAIDs, pharmacokinetics; ▶ NSAIDs, adverse effects; ▶ NSAIDs and cardio-vascular effects).

More than 20 years ago it was shown for the first time that chronic use of NSAIDs reduces the risk of colon cancer. The molecular mechanisms of the anti-carcinogenic effects of NSAIDs are still not fully understood. Predominantly, these effects have been suggested to be due to their COX-inhibiting activity. This notion is based on the observation that COX-2 is over-expressed in more than 80% of colon carcinomas and other cancer types and that an enhanced production of prostaglandins plays a crucial role in cell proliferation and angiogenesis. However, several *in vitro* and *in vivo* results cannot be explained by an enhanced COX-2 expression and PG-synthesis indicating that COX-2 independent mechanisms must also be involved. Until now five selective COX-2 inhibitors have been developed and partly introduced into clinical practice. Of these, only celecoxib has been approved by the FDA for adjuvant treatment of patients with familial adenomatous polyposis.

It has been shown that the antiproliferative effects of celecoxib are at least in part mediated through induction of a cell-cycle block (in G_1-phase) and apoptosis. These effects occurred in COX-2 expressing as well as in COX-2 deficient colon carcinoma cells (see ▶ NSAIDs, COX-independent actions and ▶ NSAIDs and cancer).

References

1. Fereira SH, Moncada S, Vane JR (1971) Indomethacin and aspirin abolish prostaglandin release from the spleen. Nat New Biol 231:237–239
2. Fu JY, Masferrer JL, Seibert K et al. (1990) The induction and suppression of prostaglandin H2 synthase (cyclooxygenase) in human monocytes. J Biol Chem 265:16737–16740
3. Tegeder I, Pfeilschifter J, Geisslinger G (2001) Cyclooxygenase-independent actions of cyclooxygenase inhibitors. FASEB J 15:2057–2072
4. Tegeder I, Geisslinger G (2006) Cardiovascular risk with cyclooxygenase inhibitors: general problem with substance specific differences? Naunyn-Schmiedeberg's Arch Pharmacol (373:1019)
5. Vane JR (1971) Inhibition of prostaglandin synthesis as a mechanism of action for aspirin-like drugs. Nat New Biol 231:232–235

N

NOP Receptor

Definition

The term NOP or ORL1 receptor (N for ▶ Nociceptin or ▶ orphanin-FQ N/OFQ) represents the G-protein coupled receptor that is closely related to MOP, DOP and KOP receptors, but responds to the peptide N/OFQ rather than any of the classical opioid drugs or peptides. It is expressed in many areas of the nervous system and has effects that may be analgesic or hyperalgesic depending on the anatomical region. The NOP receptor protein is produced by a single gene. When activated, the NOP receptor predominantly transduces cellular actions via inhibitory G-proteins. The electrophysiological consequences of NOP receptor activation are usually inhibitory.

▶ Opioid Electrophysiology in PAG

Noradrenaline

Definition

Noradrenaline is a catecholamine that acts as a neurotransmitter both centrally and peripherally by binding to adrenergic receptors. It is also known as norepinephrine.

▶ Descending Circuitry, Transmitters and Receptors

Noradrenergic

Definition

Neurons containing norepinephrine.

▶ Stimulation-Produced Analgesia

Noradrenergic and Serotonergic Inhibitory Pathways

Definition

Noradrenaline (acting via $\alpha 2$ receptors) and Serotonin (acting mainly via 5-HT$_1$ receptors) both exert inhibitory effects on nociception in the dorsal horn.

▶ Postoperative Pain, Transition from Parenteral to Oral Drugs

NOS

▶ Nitric Oxide Synthase

Noxious Cold Receptor

▶ Nociceptors, Cold Thermotransduction

Noxious Stimulus

A noxious stimulus is one that is painful and potentially damaging to normal tissues. Stimuli that are painful can be thermal, mechanical or chemical.

▶ Acute Pain Mechanisms
▶ Arthritis Model, Kaolin-Carrageenan Induced Arthritis (Knee)
▶ Descending Modulation and Persistent Pain
▶ Functional Imaging of Cutaneous Pain
▶ Gynecological Pain, Neural Mechanisms
▶ Human Thalamic Response to Experimental Pain (Neuroimaging)
▶ Metabotropic Glutamate Receptors in Spinal Nociceptive Processing
▶ Nociceptive Processing in the Amygdala, Neurophysiology and Neuropharmacology
▶ Polymodal Nociceptors, Heat Transduction
▶ Postoperative Pain, Acute Pain Management, Principles
▶ Postoperative Pain, Acute Pain Team
▶ Postoperative Pain, Pre-Emptive or Preventive Analgesia
▶ Psychological Aspects of Pain in Women
▶ Referred Muscle Pain, Assessment
▶ Somatic Pain
▶ Thalamic Nuclei Involved in Pain, Cat and Rat

Noxious Stimulus Intensity

Definition

The physical magnitude of a potentially injurious stimulus that is being applied to the body. This could be the amount of energy deposited from a mechanical or thermal stimulus, or a concentration of chemicals.

▶ Encoding of Noxious Information in the Spinal Cord

Noxious Stimulus Location

Definition

The body region that is being affected by a potentially injurious stimulus.

▶ Encoding of Noxious Information in the Spinal Cord

NPY

▶ Neuropeptide Y

NRS

▶ Numerical Rating Scale

NRSF

▶ Neuron Restrictive Silencer Factor

NSAID-Induced Lesions of the Gastrointestinal Tract

JOACHIM MÖSSNER

Medical Clinic and Policlinic II, University Clinical
Center Leipzig AöR, Leipzig, Germany
moej@medizin.uni-leipzig.de

Definition

Definition of gastrointestinal complications due to application of non-steroidal antiinflammatory drugs (▶ NSAIDs): ersosions, ulcers, bleeding erosions or bleeding ulcers, ulcer perforations. These lesions are mostly located in the stomach, less common in the upper duodenum. However, lesions are possible along the entire gastrointestinal tract, i.e. small gut and colon.

Characteristics

Pathogenesis of NSAID Induced Peptic Ulcers

Inhibition of prostaglandin synthesis in the stomach by NSAIDs seems to be the key pathogenetic factor. Prostaglandins of the E-type stimulate gastric blood circulation, mucus secretion and cell regeneration and inhibit acid secretion. Furthermore, NSAIDs exert direct side effects at the gastric mucosa besides this systemic effect. NSAIDs are weak acids. Within an acidic environment NSAIDs are not dissociated. As lipophilic substances they may penetrate the mucus and exert direct damaging effects.

Gastrointestinal Side Effects Due to Therapy with Non-Steroidal Anti-Inflammatory Drugs (NSAIDs)

Treatment with NSAIDs may cause life-threatening complications in the gastrointestinal tract such as bleeding or perforation. In many cases no symptoms precede. In a study by Sing et al. including 1,921 patients, 81% had no preceding symptoms (Sing et al. 1996). Very often complications affect rather old patients with co-morbidities. Thus, a rather high mortality may be a consequence. In patients on NSAIDs accessory risk factors increase the odds ratio of risk of peptic ulcer bleeding (Weil et al. 2000). In a case control study on 1,121 patients with bleeding ulcers, therapy with anti-coagulants increased the risk by 7.8, history of peptic ulcer by 3.8, heart insufficiency by 5.9, oral glucocorticosteroids by 3.1 and smoking by 1.6. The odds ratio increased multiplicatively when in addition to these risk factors NSAIDs were administered (Weil et al. 2000).

Primary Prophylaxis, Therapy, Secondary Prophylaxis of NSAID Induced Gastrointestinal Lesions

In primary prophylaxis of NSAID induced gastrointestinal lesions, one has to discuss the roles of coxibs, ▶ Helicobacter pylori eradication and prophylactic therapy with either misoprostol, histamine-2-receptor-antagonists (H2-blockers) or proton pump inhibitors (PPIs). In acute treatment of bleeding ulcers, endoscopic therapy is one of the most important mainstays. For treatment of NSAID induced gastrointestinal lesions, one has to compare the effectiveness of H2-blockers with that of misoprostol or PPIs. In secondary prophylaxis, H2-blockers have again to be compared with misoprostol, PPIs and H. pylori eradication. 15–20% of ulcers rebleed after successful endoscopic therapy. In primary prevention of NSAID induced gastrointestinal lesions one has to discuss the role of coxibes, -antagonists, and proton pump inhibitors (PPIs).

Intravenous omeprazole reduced this risk of recurrent bleeding after successful endoscopic treatment of bleeding peptic ulcers (Lau et al. 2000).

240 patients were randomly assigned to either placebo or omeprazole (80 mg bolus intravenously followed by 8 mg / h for 72 h). Thereafter, both groups received omeprazole 20 mg orally for 4 weeks. In the PPI group, 8 patients rebled (6.7%) within 30 days *versus* 27 (22.5%) (p< 0,001) in the placebo group. 5 patients died in the PPI group (4.2%) as compared to 12 (10%) in the placebo group. This difference did not reach statistical significance (p = 0.13).

In primary prevention of diclofenac associated ulcers and dyspepsia, omeprazole was compared with triple therapy in H. pylori positive patients (Labenz et al. 2002). Patients had no history of ulcer disease. Patients were on continuous NSAID therapy (diclofenac 2 × 50 mg / day). They received either French triple therapy for H. pylori eradication (PPI plus clarithromycin plus amoxicillin) followed by placebo or omeprazole or omeprazole alone or placebo alone. Ulcer incidence after 5 weeks was 1.2% *vs* 1.2% *vs* 0% *vs* 5.8% respectively. Thus, persistence of H. pylori gastritis and no inhibition of acid secretion were associated with an increased risk of ulcer development due to diclofenac therapy. In another study from China, H. pylori eradication decreased the risk of ulcer development when NSAID naive patients received long term NSAID therapy (Chan et al. 2002a).

N

A key question in prophylaxis is not only prevention of gastric or duodenal ulcers in patients on NSAID therapy but also prevention of serious ulcer complications such as bleeding or perforation. For misoprostol it has been clearly demonstrated that this substance reduces serious gastrointestinal complications in patients with rheumatoid arthritis receiving nonsteroidal anti-inflammatory drugs (Silverstein et al. 1995). 8,843 patients on NSAIDs were randomly assigned to either misoprostol (4×200 µg / day) versus placebo. 25 out of 4,404 patients on misoprostol developed ulcer complications as compared to 42 out of 4,439 in the placebo group (risk reduction around 40%; odds ratio 0.598 (95% CI, 0.364–0.982; P <0.049). However, 20% of patients on misoprostol terminated the therapy due to side effects such as severe diarrhea, as compared to 15% on placebo.

Therapy of NSAID Induced Peptic Ulcers

H2-antagonists, misoprostol and PPIs have been shown to be effective in healing gastric and duodenal ulcers. Omeprazole has been compared with the prostaglandin analogue misoprostol for ulcers associated with nonsteroidal anti-inflammatory drugs (Hawkey et al. 1998). Omeprazole was superior to misoprostol with regard to the percentage of healed ulcers after 4 weeks. A concomitant *H. pylori* gastritis favors the healing rates with a PPI. This effect could be due to endogenous prostaglandin synthesis induced by the gastritis and / or to the gastric acid buffering by ammonia produced by *H. pylori*.

When omeprazole was compared with ranitidine, the PPI therapy was significantly superior to the H2-receptor antagonist therapy in healing NSAID induced gastric or duodenal ulcers (Yeomans et al. 1998).

Secondary Prophylaxis of Gastrointestinal Complications Due to NSAIDs

The most efficient prophylaxis is certainly termination of any NSAID administration. However, this is not possible in many cases due to the underlying diseases. Further options are *H. pylori* eradication since an underlying *H. pylori* gastritis may increase the risk of NSAID induced lesions. Other options are administration of inhibitors of acid secretion such as PPIs or H2-blockers, treatment with misoprostol or switching from non-selective NSAIDs to coxibs. The choice of the most efficient prophylaxis can be based on the results of several controlled prospective studies but the reduction of risk by a switch to coxibs and additional acid inhibition by PPIs has not been studied.

H. pylori Eradication versus PPI

400 patients with a history of a bleeding ulcer due to NSAIDs or aspirin and concomitant *H. pylori* gastritis were randomly assigned to either *H. pylori* eradica-

tion or acid inhibition by omeprazole (20 mg per day). NSAID therapy (250 patients, naproxen 2×500 mg per day) or aspirin (150 patients, aspirin 80 mg per day) was continued for 6 months (Chan et al. 2001). The bleeding probability within 6 months in the aspirin group was 0.9% when omeprazole was used and 1.9% after *H. pylori* eradication. The difference was not statistically significant. Thus, *H. pylori* eradication is as efficient as inhibition of acid secretion when low dose aspirin is used. However, in the naproxen group, 18.8% rebled when *H. pylori* was eradicated as compared to 4.4% when omeprazole was used as prophylaxis. Thus, *H. pylori* eradication does not protect against ulcer recurrences when NSAID therapy is continued. In another study, patients with *H. pylori* gastritis who developed an ulcer complication under long-term therapy with aspirin (<325 mg per day) were enrolled (Lai et al. 2002). *H. pylori* was eradicated and after healing of the ulcers aspirin (100 mg per day) was continued. The PPI lansoprazole (30 mg per day) was compared to placebo for up to 12 months or until the occurrence of the next complication. 9 out of 61 (14.8%) patients developed an ulcer complication in the placebo group *versus* 1 out of 62 (1.2%) in the PPI group. 4 out of 10 patients had a re-infection by *H. pylori*, 2 out of 10 used further NSAIDs. Thus, in countries with a rather high risk of *H. pylori* re-infection or in cases of uncontrolled concomitant NSAID use, acid inhibition by PPIs seems to be more effective than *H. pylori* eradication alone when aspirin is continued. In a recent study from Hong Kong, patients who experienced ulcer bleeding after aspirin were switched to either clopidogrel (75 mg per day) or aspirin (80 mg per day) together with the pure enantiomer of omeprazole esomeprazole (2×20 mg per day). Both groups were *H. pylori* negative. 13 out of 161 rebled in the clopidogrel group *versus* 1 out of 159 in the aspirin plus esomeprazole group. Thus, a switch to clopidogrel does not offer any protection in contrast to efficient acid inhibition by esomeprazole (Chan et al. 2005).

Misoprostol versus PPI

When omeprazole was compared with misoprostol for ulcers associated with nonsteroidal anti-inflammatory drugs, misoprostol was slightly less effective than omeprazole in healing gastric and duodenal ulcers. In secondary prevention, omeprazole was superior. Furthermore, patients given omeprazole experienced fewer side effects (Hawkey et al. 1998).

Selective Cyclooxygenase-2 (COX-2) Inhibitors, So-called Coxibs, Solution of the Problem?

Coxibs do not inhibit aggregation of platelets. The gastrointestinal bleeding risk seems to be decreased. However, these drugs may increase the risk of cardiovascular diseases such as myocardial infarction

(Bombardier et al. 2000). Valdecoxib, given to patients undergoing coronary bypass surgery, was associated with an increased frequency of cerebro-vascular and renal complications (Ott et al. 2003). Patients receiving high doses of rofecoxib appear to die from sudden cardiac death more frequently than those that have not been exposed to cyclooxygenase inhibition (Graham et al. 2004). Similarly, a recent outcome study signalled more cardiac infarctions during long-term treatment with a Cox2 inhibitor (lumiracoxib), as compared to the naproxen treated control group (Farkouh et al. 2004). Nested case control studies (e.g. Hippisley-Cox et al, BMJ 2005) indicate, however, that a similar increase in risk of CV-events is seen with widely used non-selective inhibitors such as diclofenac or ibuprofen.

Conclusion

Theoretical, clinical and experimental evidence shows that effects of non-steroidal, anti-inflammatory drugs on the cardio-vascular system are of major clinical importance. The impact of these drugs on blood coagulation is well defined. Moreover, selective and non-selective NSAIDs increase blood pressure and lead to water and fluid retention, at least in some patients. The importance of the effect of selective Cox2 inhibitors on thrombosis, cardiac infarction and stroke is not completely clear. Nevertheless, these effective drugs should be used in patients at risk with caution and at low doses, for short periods of time.

References

1. Baigent C, Patrono C (2003) Selective Cyclooxygenase–2–Inhibitors, Aspirin, and Cardiovascular Disease: A Reappraisal. Arthritis Rheum 48:12–20
2. Bombardier C, Laine L, Reicin A, Shapiro D, Burgos-Vargas R, Davis B, Day R, Ferraz MB, Hawkey CJ, Hochberg MC, Kvien TK, Schnitzer TJ (2000) VIGOR Study Group. Comparison of Upper Gastrointestinal Toxicity of Rofecoxib and Naproxen in Patients with Rheumatoid Arthritis. VIGOR Study Group. N Engl J Med 343:1520–1528; pp following 1528
3. Brater DC (2002) Anti-Inflammatory Agents and Renal Function. Semin Arthritis Rheum 32:33–42
4. Brune K, Hinz B (2004) The Discovery and Development of Antiinflammatory Drugs. Arthritis Rheum 50:2391–2399
5. Cipollone F, Rocca B, Patrono C (2004) Cyclooxygenase–2 Expression and Inhibition in Atherothrombosis. Arterioscler Thromb Vasc Biol 24:246–255
6. Crofford LJ, Lipsky PE, Brooks P, Abramson SB, Simon LS, van de Putte LB (2000) Basic Biology and Clinical Application of Specific Cyclooxygenase–2 Inhibitors. Arthritis Rheum 43:4–13
7. Farkouh ME, Kirshner H, Harrington RA, Ruland S, Verheugt FW, Schnitzer TJ, Burmester GR, Mysler E, Hochberg MC, Doherty M, Ehrsam E, Gitton X, Krammer G, Mellein B, Gimona A, Matchaba P, Hawkey CJ, Chesebro JH (2004) TARGET Study Group. Comparison of Lumiracoxib with Naproxen and Ibuprofen, in the Therapeutic Arthritis Research and Gastrointestinal Event Trial (TARGET), Cardiovascular Outcomes: Randomised Controlled Trial. Lancet 364:675–684
8. FitzGerald GA (2002). The Choreography of Cyclooxygenases in the Kidney. J Clin Invest 110:33–34
9. Flower RJ (2003) The Development of COX2 Inhibitors. Nat Rev Drug Discov 2:179–191
10. Francois H, Coffman TM (2004) Prostanoids and Blood Pressure: Which Way is Up? J Clin Invest 114:757–759
11. Graham DJ, Campen D, Cheetham C, Hui R, Spence M, Ray WA (2004) Risk of Acute Cardiac Events among Patients Treated with Cyclooxygenase–2 elective and Non-Selective Nonsteroidal Antiinflammatory Drugs [Abstract 571]. The 20th International Conference on Pharmacoepidemiology & Therapeutic Risk Management, August 22–25, 2004. Bordeaux, France
12. Hara A, Yuhki K, Fujino T, Narumiya S, Ushikubi F (2003) Pathophysiological Roles of the Prostanoids in the Cardiovascular System: Studies Using Mice Deficient in Prostanoid Receptors. Nippon Yakurigaku Zasshi 122:384–390
13. Harris RC, Breyer MD (2001). Physiological Regulation of Cyclooxygenase–2 in the Kidney. Am J Physiol Renal Physiol 281:F1–11
14. Harris RC, Zhang MZ, Cheng HF (2004) Cyclooxygenase–2 and the Renal Renin-Angiotensin System. Acta Physiol Scand 181(4):543–547
15. Hawkey CJ (1999) COX2 Inhibitors. Lancet 353(9149):307–314
16. Hegi TR, Bombeli T, Seifert B, Baumann PC, Haller U, Zalunardo MP, Pasch T, Spahn DR (2004) Effect of Rofecoxib on Platelet Aggregation and Blood Loss in Gynaecological and Breast Surgery Compared with Diclofenac. Br J Anaesth 92:523–531
17. Hennan JK, Huang J, Barrett TD, Driscoll EM, Willens DE, Park AM, Crofford LJ, Lucchesi BR (2001) Effects of Selective Cyclooxygenase–2 Inhibition on Vascular Responses and Thrombosis in Canine Coronary Arteries. Circulation 104:820–825
18. Johnson AG (1997) NSAIDs and Increased Blood Pressure. What is the Clinical Significance? Drug Saf 17:277–289
19. Johnson DL, Hisel TM, Phillips BB (2003) Effect of Cyclooxygenase–2 inhibitors on Blood Pressure. Ann Pharmacother 37:442–446
20. Komhoff M, Grone HJ, Klein T, Seyberth HW, Nusing RM (1997) Localization of Cyclooxygenase–1 and –2 in Adult and Fetal Human Kidney: Implication for Renal Function. Am J Physiol 272:F460–468
21. Loftin CD, Trivedi DB, Tiano HF, Clark JA, Lee CA, Epstein JA, Morham SG, Breyer MD, Nguyen M, Hawkins BM, Goulet JL, Smithies O, Koller BH, Langenbach R (2001) Failure of Ductus Arteriosus Closure and Remodeling in Neonatal Mice Deficient in Cyclooxygenase–1 and Cyclooxygenase–2. Proc Natl Acad Sci USA 98:1059–1064
22. Malik KU, Sehic E (1990) Prostaglandins and the Release of the Adrenergic Transmitter. Ann N Y Acad Sci 604:222–236
23. McAdam BF, Catella-Lawson F, Mardini IA, Kapoor S, Lawson JA, FitzGerald GA (1999) Systemic Biosynthesis of Prostacyclin by Cyclooxygenase (COX)–2: The Human Pharmacology of a Selective Inhibitor of COX2. Proc Natl Acad Sci USA 96:272–277. Erratum in: Proc Natl Acad Sci USA 96:5890
24. Merritt JC, Bhatt DL (2004) The Efficacy and Safety of Perioperative Antiplatelet Therapy. J Thromb Thrombolysis 17:21–27
25. Narumiya S, Sugimoto Y, Ushikubi F (1999) Prostanoid Receptors: Structures, Properties, and Functions. Physiol Rev 79:1193–1226
26. Ott E, Nussmeier NA, Duke PC, Feneck RO, Alston RP, Snabes MC, Hubbard RC, Hsu PH, Saidman LJ, Mangano DT (2003) Multicenter Study of Perioperative Ischemia (McSPI) Research Group; Ischemia Research and Education Foundation (IREF) Investigators. Efficacy and Safety of the Cyclooxygenase–2 inhibitors Parecoxib and Valdecoxib in Patients Undergoing Coronary Artery Bypass Surgery. J Thorac Cardiovasc Surg 125:1481–1492
27. Pratico D, Tillmann C, Zhang ZB, Li H, FitzGerald GA (2001) Acceleration of Atherogenesis by COX1–Dependent Prostanoid Formation in Low Density Lipoprotein Receptor Knockout Mice. Proc Natl Acad Sci USA 98:3358–3363
28. Reuben SS, Connelly NR (2004). The Perioperative Use of Cyclooxygenase–2 Selective Nonsteroidal Antiinflammatory Drugs May Offer a Safer Alternative. Anesthesiology 100:748
29. Schwartz JI, Vandormael K, Malice MP, Kalyani RN, Lasseter KC, Holmes GB, Gertz BJ, Gottesdiener KM, Laurenzi M, Redfern KJ, Brune K (2002) Comparison of Rofecoxib, Celecoxib, and Naproxen on Renal Function in Elderly Subjects receiving a Normal-Salt Diet. Clin Pharmacol Ther 72:50–61

N

30. Simmons DL, Botting RM, Hla T (2004) Cyclooxygenase Isozymes: The Biology of Prostaglandin Synthesis and Inhibition. Pharmacol Rev 56:387–437
31. Ushikubi F, Sugimoto Y, Ichikawa A, Narumiya S (2000) Roles of Prostanoids Revealed from Studies Using Mice Lacking Specific Prostanoid Receptors. Jpn J Pharmacol 83:279–285
32. Wacker MJ, Tehrani RN, Smoot RL, Orr JA (2002) Thromboxane A(2) Mimetic Evokes a Bradycardia Mediated by Stimulation of Cardiac Vagal Afferent Nerves. Am J Physiol Heart Circ Physiol 282:H482–490
33. White WB, Kent J, Taylor A, Verburg KM, Lefkowith JB, Whelton A (2002) Effects of Celecoxib on Ambulatory Blood Pressure in Hypertensive Patients on ACE Inhibitors. Hypertension 39:929–934

NSAIDs and Coxibs

▶ Coxibs and Novel Compounds, Chemistry

NSAIDs and their Indications

RICHARD O. DAY, GARRY G. GRAHAM
Department of Physiology and Pharmacology, School of Medical Sciences and Department of Clinical Pharmacology, University of New South Wales, St Vincent's Hospital, Sydney, NSW, Australia
r.day@unsw.edu.au, ggraham@stvincents.com.au

Synonyms

Non-Steroidal Anti-Inflammatory Drugs and their indications; Antipyretic Analgesics; Aspirin-Like Drugs; simple analgesics; COX–2 selective inhibitors

Definitions

The term Non-Steroidal Anti-Inflammatory Drugs, NSAIDs, refers to a group of drugs whose major therapeutic activities are the suppression of pain (analgesia), reduced body temperature in fever (antipyresis) and decreased signs of inflammation (anti-inflammatory activity).

Characteristics

The NSAIDs can be separated into two major groups:

- non-selective NSAIDs, such as aspirin, ibuprofen and indomethacin, which also produce gastrointestinal damage, inhibit the aggregation of platelets, decrease kidney function in some patients and precipitate aspirin-induced asthma. The activity of these drugs is due to inhibition of two central enzymes involved in the synthesis of ▶ prostaglandins and related compounds. These central enzymes are cyclooxygenase–1 (COX–1) and COX–2.
- COX–2 selective inhibitors (coxibs or COX–1 sparing agents, CSIs) such as celecoxib, which have similar activities to the non-selective NSAIDs but have improved gastrointestinal tolerance, little or no effect

on platelets and, from present studies, no tendency to produce asthma. The COX-2 selective inhibitors tend to increase the incidence of heart attack and stroke although the incidence of these reactions is low and may not be significant at analgesic doses of all the COX-2 selective inhibitors.

In addition, there is the unique drug, paracetamol (acetaminophen), which has similar activities to the COX–2 selective inhibitors but has weaker anti-inflammatory activity.

History

Three well-known plant compounds, salicin, salicylaldehyde and methyl salicylate, are active analgesics, antipyretics and anti-inflammatory agents. All three owe their pharmacological activity to their metabolism to salicylate (Fig. 1). Salicin is the most well known because it is present in the bark of the willow tree, and in several other plants which were used in the treatment of pain and fever. The modern use of willow bark started in 1763, although it had been used in earlier times. Methyl salicylate is still widely used in liniments while salicylaldehyde has little modern use although, like salicin, it is still used in herbal preparations.

In the nineteenth century, salicin was superseded by synthetic salicylic acid and its salt, sodium salicylate (Fig. 1). In turn, the purely synthetic compound, aspirin, largely replaced salicylic acid and its salts. However, sodium salicylate continued to be used for many years in the treatment of rheumatic fever and, until recently, sodium and other salicylate salts were used as anti-inflammatory drugs for ▶ rheumatoid arthri-

NSAIDs and their Indications, Figure 1 Structures of the naturally occurring salicylate derivatives and the synthetic drug, aspirin. All compounds are metabolized to the pharmacologically active salicylate (the ionised form of salicylic acid). The effect of aspirin is due to the metabolite, salicylate, and also to the reaction in which a serine at the active site of both COX–1 and COX–2 is acetylated. The effect of aspirin is prolonged because of this covalent binding to COX–1 and COX–2, and also because the half life of salicylate is longer than that of aspirin.

tis. Salicylate is still of interest because it is an active metabolite of aspirin.

Mechanism of Action

The older, non-selective NSAIDs inhibit both COX–1 and COX–2 and, therefore, decrease the synthesis of all prostaglandins and related compounds, such as ► Thromboxane A2 and ► prostacyclin. The prostaglandins and related compounds are factors which can be synthesized widely throughout the body and produce a variety of physiological effects. For example, they potentiate the actions of painful mediators, such as bradykinin. Thus, by inhibiting the synthesis of prostaglandins, the non-selective NSAIDs are analgesic. Inhibition of the synthesis of prostaglandin also explains the antipyretic and anti-inflammatory actions of NSAIDs, as well as their common adverse effects (see below).

The discovery of two COX isoenzymes led to the development of the COX–2 selective inhibitors which retain the analgesic, antipyretic and anti-inflammatory activities, but have a much reduced risk of gastrointestinal toxicity, and do not inhibit platelet function or precipitate aspirin-induced asthma.

Both salicylate and paracetamol are poor inhibitors of COX–1 and COX–2 in broken cell preparations, but both drugs inhibit the production of prostaglandins by intact cells when the levels of the precursor, arachidonic acid, are low (Graham and Scott 2003). Consequently, it now appears that salicylate and paracetamol both produce their pharmacological effects by inhibition of prostaglandin synthesis. The pharmacological activities of paracetamol and salicylate are generally similar to those of the COX–2 selective inhibitors, but the actions of paracetamol and salicylate at a molecular level are not known.

The activity of aspirin is due, in part, to its metabolism to salicylate, but aspirin also inhibits both COX–1 and COX–2. In this regard, the acetyl group of aspirin is transferred to COX–1 and COX–2, the result being irreversible inhibition of both enzymes (Fig. 1). Although aspirin is rapidly hydrolyzed to salicylate *in vivo*, the irreversible inhibition of COX–1 leads to prolonged inhibition of platelet aggregation, an initial step in the coagulation of blood.

Clinical Uses of the NSAIDs

Pain

The NSAIDs are indicated for a wide variety of painful states affecting all organ systems and all ages of patients, and are particularly indicated when inflammation is a significant contributor to the painful state. Alone, they are not useful for severe, acute pain, for example pain of bone fractures, surgical procedures or myocardial infarction. In these cases, the opioids, such as morphine, are more effective analgesics. The opioids are very useful for the treatment of the pain of cancer, although they may be used with the NSAIDs for this indication. Although very effective analgesics, the opioids depress the function of the central nervous system and have well known addictive properties, actions which are not shown by the NSAIDs.

Musculoskeletal pain is the major indication for NSAIDs. Surveys have shown that 15–20% of individuals over the age of 65 years take NSAIDs regularly, and this is largely for musculoskeletal pain. ► Osteoarthritis has a prevalence of about 10% in western populations, and afflicts elderly people. Although osteoarthritis is not primarily an inflammatory disorder, NSAIDs are moderately effective at relieving pain and the muscle stiffness associated with osteoarthritis.

Paracetamol is a widely used analgesic and antipyretic drug, but without significant anti-inflammatory actions in usual doses in rheumatoid arthritis, although it does reduce swelling after oral surgery. Although the NSAIDs are, on average, somewhat more efficacious than paracetamol (Pincus et al. 2004), paracetamol is still recommended as first line treatment for osteoarthritis, not only because it is effective, but also because it is better tolerated than the NSAIDs. Inflammation is a relatively minor component of the pathophysiology of osteoarthritis, and this might explain the small advantage that NSAIDs demonstrate compared to paracetamol. Although little work has been done to evaluate the utility of combining NSAIDs with paracetamol, this practice has no obvious disadvantages and may control pain better than either drug alone. NSAIDs are also indicated for spinal pain, particularly lumbar and cervical mechanical origin pain, prevalent in middle to old age. So called 'soft tissue' rheumatic problems are common and include muscle strains and aches, tennis elbow, and many others. NSAIDs can be helpful if paracetamol is insufficient, along with physical and other non-pharmacological therapies. There is some controversy about whether continuous therapy with NSAIDs slow or increase the loss of cartilage from weight bearing joints in patients with osteoarthritis (Rashad et al. 1989). This issue remains to be resolved. Good pain relief has been achieved with NSAIDs in conditions of painful, often obstructed contraction, of smooth muscle. Examples are renal and biliary colic. This is because the smooth muscle contractions are dependent on prostaglandin synthesis. Again, NSAIDs outperform the opioids which have been traditionally used for these indications.

In a similar way, the pain associated with menstruation is dependent on prostaglandin synthesis and is therefore amenable to treatment with the non-selective NSAIDs. The COX–2 selective drugs relieve the pain of this condition and, because they have no significant anti-platelet effect, they do not increase menstruation related bleeding (Daniels et al. 2002).

A major, relatively new indication for the NSAIDs is perioperative pain. This has evolved with the availability of

N

the COX–2 selective inhibitors. In contrast to NSAIDs, including aspirin, the COX–2 selective inhibitors do not inhibit platelet aggregation so that blood clots normally. This property is particularly useful with the major shift to 'day only' surgery (Buvanendran et al. 2003). Renal function may, however, be decreased by NSAIDs after surgery (see below), and they should be used carefully in this situation.

Inflammation

Inflammatory rheumatic disorders exemplified by rheumatoid arthritis (RA) are an important indication for NSAIDs. Pain and stiffness especially in the morning are characteristic and debilitating. These symptoms are relieved by the non-selective NSAIDs or the COX–2 selective drugs, but there is no clear effect of either group on the progression of the condition to joint damage and loss of function. However, the NSAIDs have much to offer symptomatically to patients with rheumatoid arthritis. Consequently, the NSAIDs are very commonly used with the ▶ disease-modifying anti-rheumatic drugs (DMARDs). These are drugs which slow the progression of rheumatic arthritis in many patients. NSAIDs also have well defined roles in many other inflammatory, painful, arthritic states, including acute gout, ▶ ankylosing spondylitis and the arthritis often associated with psoriasis.

Migraine

The non-selective NSAIDs and the COX–2 selective inhibitors are good analgesics and, consequently, have an important place in the treatment of migraine (Goadsby et al. 2002). Their use soon after onset of an acute attack of migraine is most effective. Combination with an antiemetic is often required in order to suppress vomiting.

Other Clinical Uses

The non-selective NSAIDs have antithrombotic effects due to their inhibition of the formation of thromboxane A_2, a prostaglandin-like compound which leads to the aggregation of platelets and, therefore, the initiation of clotting of blood. Thromboxane A_2 is synthesized by a COX–1 dependent pathway in platelets and, therefore, all the non-selective NSAIDs have antithrombotic activity. Aspirin is, however, the preferred anti-platelet agent because of its long duration of action. As thromboxane A_2 is synthesized by a COX–1-dependent pathway, the COX–2 selective inhibitors do not have significant antithrombotic activity. This lack of antithrombotic activity may, however, be a cause for the major adverse reactions of these new NSAIDs, as is outlined below.

Adverse Effects

Gastrointestinal

Prostaglandins are cytoprotective in the stomach and small intestine. Thus, they are important in developing

mechanisms which protect the gastrointestinal tract from damage from the digestive enzymes and, in the stomach and duodenum, from the acidic contents. The non-selective NSAIDs commonly cause a variety of serious adverse reactions in the gastrointestinal tract, most importantly, perforations, ulceration and bleeding. Serious cases of gastrointestinal damage affect nearly 1% of chronic users of the older NSAIDs per year. Older, sicker patients, particularly those with previous peptic ulceration are most at risk.

Gastrointestinal tolerance is improved with ▶ enteric coating, co-prescription of antacids, ingestion with food, or rectal or parental routes of administration, but the risk of serious upper gastrointestinal bleeding remains. Another approach is to use the non-selective NSAIDs with prostaglandin analogues which are cytoprotective, or with drugs which decrease acid secretion by the stomach. A further approach is to use the COX–2 selective inhibitors or paracetamol. The COX–2 selective inhibitors were developed in order to decrease the gastrointestinal toxicity of the NSAIDs. This was successful and the use of the selective inhibitors, in preference to the non-selective NSAIDs, reduces the incidence of serious gastrointestinal damage (Silverstein et al. 2000).

A particular problem arises for patients who require long-term dosage with both low dose aspirin as an antithrombotic and a NSAID. It now appears that low doses of aspirin decrease the gastrointestinal sparing effects of the COX–2 selective inhibitors (Schmidt et al. 2004). Consequently, patients who require both an analgesic and low-dose aspirin are now often prescribed a non-selective NSAID and a cytoprotective drug, as well as aspirin (Barraclough et al. 2002).

Thrombosis

As discussed above, thromboxane A_2 is synthesized by a COX–1 dependent pathway in platelets, and therefore not affected by the COX–2 selective inhibitors. However, the selective COX–2 inhibitors may block the synthesis of prostacyclin, a vasodilator and antiplatelet factor which is largely synthesized through COX–2. Thus, there has been considerable concern that the selective COX–2 inhibitors may increase the incidence of ▶ thrombosis, causing myocardial infarction, for example. This concern has been confirmed by the withdrawal of one COX–2 selective inhibitor, rofecoxib, because of the increased occurrence of myocardial infarction during long term therapy (FitzGerald 2004). On the other hand, blood clotting often develops at atherosclerotic plaques in arteries. The development of atherosclerosis or reactions following thrombosis in the heart, in part, may be inflammatory processes, and the COX–2 selective inhibitors may usefully reduce this inflammation. Much research is presently directed at examining this possibility.

Renal Impairment and Hypertension

The NSAIDs and the COX–2 selective drugs both may precipitate renal failure. Risk factors include: age over 60, pre-existing renal impairment, dehydration, cirrhosis, congestive cardiac failure, salt restricted diets, or concomitant treatment with diuretics or inhibitors of angiotensin formation or action (Barraclough et al. 2002). The renal function of patients in these situations is considered to be more dependent on the function of prostaglandins than normal subjects and, therefore, inhibition of prostaglandin synthesis may produce marked depressant effects on renal function. Blood pressure may rise, in some cases quite substantially, during treatment with either the non-selective NSAIDs or the COX–2 selective agents (Barraclough et al. 2002; Whelton et al 2002). Consequently, it is now recommended that blood pressure should be monitored if dosage with the non-selective NSAIDs or the COX–2 selective drugs is commenced in patients taking antihypertensives, and the dosage of antihypertensives increased if blood pressure rises.

Asthma

Asthma is precipitated in up to 20% of asthmatics by aspirin and other non-selective NSAIDs. This reaction is produced by inhibition of COX–1 because asthma is not induced by the COX–2 selective inhibitors (West and Fernandez 2003). Paracetamol is also safer in aspirin-sensitive asthmatics, but does produce mild asthma in occasional patients (Jenkins 2000).

References

1. Barraclough DR, Bertouch JV, Brooks P et al. (2002) Considerations for the Safe Prescribing and Use of COX–2–Specific Inhibitors. Med J Aust 176:328–331
2. Buvanendran A, Kroin JS, Tuman KJ et al. (2003) Effects of Perioperative Administration of a Selective Cyclooxygenase–2–Inhibitor on Pain Management and Recovery of Function after Knee Replacement: A Randomized Controlled Trial. JAMA 290:2411–2418
3. Daniels SE, Talwalker S, Torri S et al. (2002) Valdecoxib, A Cyclooxygenase–2–Specific Inhibitor, is Effective in Treating Primary Dysmenorrhea. Obstet Gynecol 100:350–358
4. FitzGerald GA (2004) Coxibs and Cardiovascular Disease. N Engl J Med 351:1709–1711
5. Goadsby PJ, Lipton RB, Ferrari MD (2002) Migraine – Current Understanding and Treatment. N Engl J Med 346:257–270.
6. Graham GG, Scott KF (2003) Mechanisms of Action of Paracetamol and Related Analgesics. Inflammopharmacology 11:401–412
7. Jenkins C (2000) Recommending Analgesics for People with Asthma. Am J Therapeut 7:55–61
8. Pincus T, Koch G, Lei H et al. (2004) Patient Preference for Placebo, Acetaminophen (paracetamol) or Celecoxib Efficacy Studies (PACES): Two Randomised, Double Blind, Placebo Controlled, Crossover Clinical Trials in Patients with Knee or Hip Osteoarthritis. Ann Rheum Dis 63:931–939
9. Rashad S, Revell P, Hemingway A et al. (1989) Effect of Non-Steroidal Anti-Inflammatory Drugs on the Course of Osteoarthritis. Lancet 2:519–522
10. Schmidt H, Woodcock BG, Geisslinger G (2004) Benefit-Risk Assessment of Rofecoxib in the Treatment of Osteoarthritis. Drug Safety 27:185–196
11. Silverstein FE, Faich G, Goldstein JL et al. (2000) Gastrointestinal Toxicity with Celecoxib vs. Nonsteroidal Anti-Inflammatory Drugs for Osteoarthritis and Rheumatoid Arthritis: The Class Study: A Randomized Trial. JAMA 284:1247–1255
12. West PM, Fernandez C (2003) Safety of COX–2 Inhibitors in Asthma Patients with Aspirin Hypersensitivity. Ann Pharmacother 37:1497–1501
13. Whelton A, White WB, Bello AE et al. (2002) Effects of Celecoxib and Rofecoxib on Blood Pressure and Edema in Patients > 65 Years of Age with Systemic Hypertension and Osteoarthritis. Am J Cardiol 90:959–963

NSAIDs, Adverse Effects

IRMGARD TEGEDER
Center of Pharmacology, University Clinic Frankfurt, Frankfurt, Germany
tegeder@em.uni-frankfurt.de

Synonyms

NSAIDs; non-steroidal anti-inflammatory drugs; Non-Steroidal Anti-Rheumatic Drugs; cyclooxygenase inhibitors; NSAIDs, Side Effects

Definition

NSAIDs constitute a large group of chemically diverse substances that inhibit ▶ Cyclooxygenases activity and thereby prostaglandin synthesis. Traditional NSAIDs inhibit both COX-isoenzymes (COX-1 and COX-2). Novel NSAIDs ("coxibs") inhibit only COX-2. NSAIDs are mainly used as analgesics.

Characteristics

Overview

▶ Adverse effects of NSAIDs arise from the fact that it is impossible to inhibit exclusively the synthesis of ▶ prostaglandins that cause pain and inflammation. The inhibition of cyclooxygenases will always also affect the synthesis of prostaglandins and ▶ thromboxanes that are needed for physiological processes. In addition, COX inhibition may shift arachidonic acid metabolism to ▶ leukotriene synthesis because of the excess supply of substrate. This rule particularly applies to traditional NSAIDs that inhibit both COX-isoenzymes, but also holds true for COX-2 specific inhibitors.

COX-1 and COX-2 perform different tasks; this is allowed for by a different localization and regulation. COX-1 is expressed in all tissues and mainly produces prostaglandins and thromboxanes that are needed for the maintenance of physiological functions. COX-2 is not expressed in most healthy tissue but is upregulated after stimulation, which may be any kind of tissue damage. Hence, exclusively targeting COX-2 will not affect COX-1 derived physiological prostaglandins, and will therefore avoid many adverse effects that are typical for traditional NSAIDs. However, COX-2 is also constitutively expressed (see ▶ Constitutive Gene) in some tissues, so that COX-2 selective NSAIDs are not able to spare physiological prostaglandin production completely. In addition to common adverse effects, some substance specific side effects may occur, so the individual tolerability of NSAIDs may vary among patients.

Gastrointestinal Toxicity

Physiological prostaglandin E2 (PGE2) and prostacyclin (PGI2) in the stomach play an important role in the gastric defense mechanisms that protect the gastric epithelium from the acidic environment. PGE2 increases the production of gastric mucus, which builds a protective layer on the epithelium, while PGI2 maintains gastric blood flow. Inhibition of PG synthesis in the stomach causes serious adverse effects such as gastric erosions, bleeding, ulceration and perforation. A single dose of aspirin is sufficient to cause small erosions. The risk for serious GI toxicity increases considerably with long-term use of traditional NSAIDs and concomitant use of glucocorticoids.

Multiple clinical trials have demonstrated that COX-2 selective inhibitors cause less gastrointestinal toxicity than traditional NSAIDs. Particularly, serious side effects are reduced to the placebo level, suggesting that the physiological PG production in the stomach is mediated primarily by the COX-1 pathway. However, experimental studies have revealed that gastric damage only occurs if both COX-enzymes are inhibited collectively, but not with COX-1 or COX-2 inhibition alone. This indicates that COX-2 also is important for protection of the gastric mucosa (Halter et al. 2001). This idea is further supported by studies showing that COX-2 is ▶ upregulated in the stomach in the case of ulceration (Schmassmann et al. 1998) or other epithelial damage such as ▶ Helicobacter pylori infection (Seo et al. 2002), and contributes to the production of prostaglandins that are involved in healing processes such as PGJ2 (Gilroy et al. 1999). Hence, although COX-2 selective inhibitors are relatively safe for the healthy stomach, they may impair ulcer healing (Jones et al. 1999).

Renal Toxicity

COX-2 is constitutively expressed in the kidney and is highly regulated in response to alterations in intravascular volume (Harris et al. 1994). COX-2-derived PGs signal the release of ▶ renin from the renal ▶ juxtaglomerular apparatus, especially during volume depletion. PGs also maintain renal blood flow and regulate salt and water excretion.

COX-2 inhibition, both with traditional NSAIDs or selective COX-2 inhibitors, may transiently decrease urine sodium excretion in some subjects and induce mild to moderate elevation of blood pressure. Substance specific differences have been suggested. For example, rofecoxib users were at a significantly increased relative risk of new onset hypertension compared with patients taking celecoxib, nonspecific NSAIDs or no NSAID (Solomon et al. 2004). The risk for renal side effects is increased in patients with pre-existing renal or heart disease.

Platelet Aggregation and Cardiovascular System

Thrombocyte aggregation depends on thromboxane A2 (TXA2), which is produced by the COX-1 pathway in platelets. Hence, traditional NSAIDs inhibit platelet aggregation, and particularly aspirin, the irreversible unselective COX-inhibitor, causes a long-lasting prolongation of the bleeding time, which may increase the risk of bleeding e.g. during or after surgery. On the other hand, inhibition of thrombocyte aggregation may be the desired therapeutic effect of aspirin for patients with increased risk of thrombosis such as coronary heart disease, or it may be a welcome side-effect of traditional NSAIDs.

The activation of platelets by TXA2 is counterbalanced by vascular prostacyclin (PGI2) under physiological conditions. Systemic PGI2 is mainly produced through the COX-2 pathway (McAdam et al. 1999). Specific COX-2 inhibitors may therefore shift the balance between TXA2 and PGI2 towards TXA2 mediated thrombocyte aggregation. This may result in an increased risk of ▶ thrombotic events in predisposed patients. Recent large clinical trials have revealed an increased risk for thrombotic cardiovascular effects with rofecoxib and other COX-2 inhibitors. However, observational studies reported a similar risk with selective and unselective COX-inhibitors, suggesting that an imbalance between PGJ_2 and TXA_2 does not sufficiently explain the increased cardiovascular risk with these analgesics.

Bone Healing

PGs participate in inflammatory responses in the bone, increased ▶ osteoclast activity and subsequent bone resorption, and increased ▶ osteoblast activity and new bone formation.

Data from animal studies suggest that both non-specific and specific inhibitors of cyclooxygenases impair fracture healing. This is due to the inhibition of COX-2 (Zhang et al. 2002). Although these data raise concerns about the use of traditional NSAIDs and COX-2-specific inhibitors as anti-inflammatory or anti-analgesic drugs in patients undergoing bone repair, clinical reports have been inconclusive.

Aspirin Asthma

Inhibition of cyclooxygenase activity reduces arachidonic acid consumption for prostaglandin synthesis, and hence yields more substrate for leukotriene and endocannabinoid synthesis. While ▶ endocannabinoids may enhance the analgesic effects of certain NSAIDs (Ates et al. 2003), overproduction of cysteinyl leukotrienes may cause bronchial constriction and trigger asthma attacks in "aspirin-sensitive" patients (Szczeklik et al. 2001). Aspirin asthma has also been observed with other non-selective NSAIDs but not with COX-2 selective drugs. Similar mechanisms also account for the NSAID-evoked ▶ urticaria (Mastalerz et al. 2004).

Ototoxicity

A recent study suggested that salicylate induced tinnitus is mediated through an indirect activation of ▶ NMDA receptors in the cochlea, causing an increase of spontaneous auditory nerve activity. NMDA receptor activation is probably mediated by inhibition of prostaglandin synthesis (Guitton et al. 2003), and hence is not specific for salicylate. ▶ Tinnitus occurs at high plasma concentrations.

Pregnancy

COX-2-derived prostaglandins play a prominent role at all stages of female reproduction, from ovulation to implantation, ▶ decidualization and delivery. The regulation of prostaglandin release is mediated by transcriptional control of COX-2 and microsomal prostaglandin E synthase. Elevated uterine PGs or the enhanced sensitivity of the myometrium to PGs leads to contractions and labor. Hence, traditional NSAIDs as well as COX-2 inhibitors may prolong parturition, or may be used in the treatment of preterm labor (McWhorter et al. 2004).

In addition, prostaglandins regulate the transition to pulmonary respiration following birth that requires closure and remodeling of the ▶ ductus arteriosus. The maintenance of the ductus arteriosus in the open, or patent, state is dependent on prostaglandin synthesis, and the neonatal drop in prostaglandin E2 that triggers ductal closure is sensed through the EP4 receptor (Nguyen et al. 1997). Hence, NSAIDs may cause a premature DA closure if taken during late pregnancy, or may be used to induce DA closure in preterm infants.

References

1. Ates M, Hamza M, Seidel K et al. (2003) Intrathecally Applied Flurbiprofen Produces an Endocannabinoid-Dependent Antinociception in the Rat Formalin Test. Eur J Neurosci 17:597–604
2. Gilroy DW, Colville-Nash PR, Willis D et al. (1999) Inducible Cyclooxygenase may have Anti-Inflammatory Properties. Nat Med 5:698–701
3. Guitton MJ, Caston J, Ruel J et al. (2003) Salicylate Induces Tinnitus through Activation of Cochlear NMDA Receptors. J Neurosci 23:3944–3952
4. Halter F, Tarnawski AS, Schmassmann A et al. (2001) Cyclooxygenase-2 Implications on Maintenance of Gastric Mucosal Integrity and Ulcer Healing: Controversial Issues and Perspectives. Gut 49:443–453
5. Harris RC, McKanna JA, Akai Y et al. (1994) Cyclooxygenase-2 is Associated with the Macula Densa of Rat Kidney and Increases with Salt Restriction. J Clin Invest 94:2504–2510
6. Jones MK, Wang H, Peskar BM et al. (1999) Inhibition of Angiogenesis by Nonsteroidal Anti-Inflammatory Drugs: Insight into Mechanisms and Implications for Cancer Growth and Ulcer Healing. Nat Med 5:1418–1423
7. Mastalerz L, Setkowicz M, Sanak M et al. (2004) Hypersensitivity to Aspirin: Common Eicosanoid Alterations in Urticaria and Asthma. J Allergy Clin Immunol 113:771–775
8. McAdam BF, Catella-Lawson F, Mardini IA et al. (1999) Systemic Biosynthesis of Prostacyclin by Cyclooxygenase (COX)-2: the Human Pharmacology of a Selective Inhibitor of COX-2. Proc Natl Acad Sci USA 96:272–277
9. McWhorter J, Carlan SJ, Richichi K et al. (2004) Rofecoxib versus Magnesium Sulfate to Arrest Preterm Labor: A Randomized Trial. Obstet Gynecol 103:923–930
10. Nguyen M, Camenisch T, Snouwaert JN et al. (1997) The Prostaglandin Receptor EP4 Triggers Remodelling of the Cardiovascular System at Birth. Nature 390:78–81
11. Schmassmann A, Peskar BM, Stettler C et al. (1998) Effects of Inhibition of Prostaglandin Endoperoxide Synthase-2 in Chronic Gastro-Intestinal Ulcer Models in Rats. Br J Pharmacol 123:795–804
12. Seo JH, Kim H, Kim KH (2002) Cyclooxygenase-2 Expression by Transcription Factors in Helicobacter Pylori-Infected Gastric Epithelial Cells: Comparison between HP 99 and NCTC 11637. Ann NY Acad Sci 973:477–480
13. Solomon DH, Schneeweiss S, Levin R et al. (2004) Relationship between COX-2 Specific Inhibitors and Hypertension. Hypertension 44:140–145
14. Szczeklik A, Nizankowska E, Sanak M et al. (2001) Aspirin-Induced Rhinitis and Asthma. Curr Opin Allergy Clin Immunol 1:27–33
15. Weir MR, Sperling RS, Reicin A et al. (2003) Selective COX-2 Inhibition and Cardiovascular Effects: A Review of the Rofecoxib Development Program. Am Heart J 146:591–604
16. Zhang X, Schwarz EM, Young DA et al. (2002) Cyclooxygenase-2 Regulates Mesenchymal Cell Differentiation into the Osteoblast Lineage and is Critically Involved in Bone Repair. J Clin Invest 109:1405–1415

NSAIDs, Chemical Structure and Molecular Mode of Action

STEFAN A. LAUFER

Institute of Pharmacy, Eberhard-Karls University of Tuebingen, Tuebingen, Germany

stefan.laufer@uni-tuebingen.de

Definition

Structure and Metabolic Function of COX-1

COX-1 is a 70 kD enzyme, catalyzing the reaction of ▶ arachidonic acid to PGG2 (cyclooxygenase reaction) and consecutively PGG2 to PGH2 (peroxidase reaction) as outlined in Fig. 1.

There are distinct active sites for the ▶ Cyclooxygenases (COX) and the peroxidase reactions (Fig. 2).

Characteristics

Inhibitors of Cyclooxygenases

Different chemical classes can provide the structural features necessary to mimic arachidonic acid at the active site. The substrate, arachidonic acid is a C_{20} carboxylic acid with 4 isolated double bonds at positions 5, 8, 11 and 14. For the enzyme reaction, arachidonic acid must adapt to a "folded" conformation, allowing the oxygen to insert between C_9 and C_{11} and the ring closure between C_8 and C_{12} (Fig. 3).

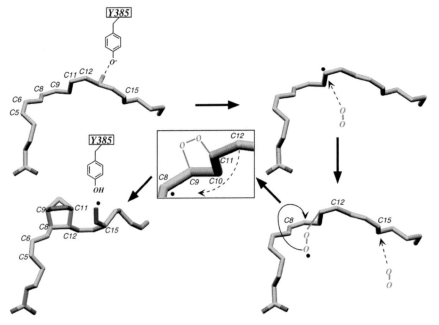

NSAIDs, Chemical Structure and Molecular Mode of Action, Figure 1 Reaction catalyzed by COX enzymes.

NSAIDs, Chemical Structure and Molecular Mode of Action, Figure 2 A ribbon representation of the Co^{3+}-oPGHS-1 monomer with AA bound in the COX channel. The EGF domain, MBD, and catalytic domain are shown in green, orange and blue, respectively; Co^{3+}-protoporphyrin IX is depicted in red, disulfide bonds (Cys36-Cys47, Cys37-Cys159, Cys4^1–Cys57, Cys59-Cys69, and Cys569-Cys575) in dark blue and side chain atoms for COX channel residues Arg120, Tyr355 and Tyr385 in magenta (from Malkowski et al. (2000)).

NSAIDs, Chemical Structure and Molecular Mode of Action, Figure 3 Mechanistic sequence for converting AA to PGG$_2$. Abstraction of the 13-proS hydrogen by the tyrosyl radical leads to the migration of the radical to C-11 on AA. The attack of molecular oxygen, coming from the base of the COX channel, occurs on the side interfacial to hydrogen abstraction. As the 11R-peroxyl radical swings over C-8 for an R-side attack on C-9 to form the endoperoxide bridge, C-12 is brought closer to C-8 *via* rotation about the C-10/C-11 bond, allowing the formation of the cyclopentane ring. The movement of C-12 also positions C-15 optimally for addition of a second molecule of oxygen, formation of PGG$_2$ and the migration of the radical back to Tyr385 (from Malkowski et al. (2000)).

To fix arachidonic acid in such a conformation, several interactions with the active site of the enzyme are necessary, e.g. ionic interaction (a salt bridge) between the carboxylic group and arginine 120, π-π interactions between the double bonds of arachidonic acid and aromatic amino acids and numerous hydrophobic interactions (Fig. 4).

All these structural features can be identified in many ► NSAID s. Most acidic NSAIDs are therefore believed to mimic arachidonic acid in its folded conformation at the active site of COX. Structure activity relationships follow these structural constrictions closely.

The activity against COX-1 clearly correlates with torsion angles around the π-electron systems and the overall lipophilicity of the molecule (Moser et al. 1990).

Two classes of compounds however have a distinctly different molecular mode of action,

- ASS acetylates Ser 530 irreversibly at the active site of the enzyme
- The oxicames are believed to interfere with the peroxidase active site, which also explains their structural difference.

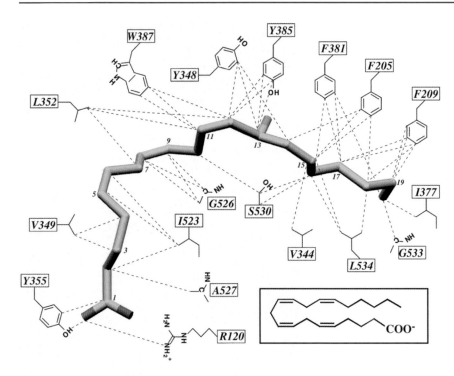

NSAIDs, Chemical Structure and Molecular Mode of Action, Figure 4 A schematic of interactions between AA and COX channel residues. Carbon atoms of AA are yellow, oxygen atoms red and the 13proS hydrogen blue. All dashed lines represent interactions within 4.0 A between the specific side chain atom of the protein and AA (from Malkowski et al. (2000)).

Most of the currently used NSAIDs, including diclofenac, ibuprofen, naproxen, piroxicam and indomethacin for instance, may produce full inhibition of both COX-1 and COX-2 with relatively poor selectivity under therapeutic conditions (Warner et al. 1999).

Acidic NSAIDs like diclofenac accumulate particularly in blood, liver, milt and bone marrow, but also in tissue with acidic extracellular pH values. Such tissues are mainly inflamed tissues such as gastric tissue and the manifolds of the kidney. In inflamed tissue, NSAIDs inhibit the pathological overproduction of prostaglandins. In contrast, neutral NSAIDs (paracetamol) and weakly acidic NSAIDs (metamizol) distribute themselves quickly and homogeneously in the organism. They also penetrate the blood-brain-barrier.

Fenamate Group

The core structure is 2-aminobenzoic acid (anthranilic acid). The 2-amino group is substituted with aromatic residues.

- flufenamic acid
- mefenamic acid
- meclofenamic acid
- nifluminic acid (core structure: 2-amino-pyridyl-3-carboxylic acid)

For topical application, the carboxylic acid group is esterified with diethyleneglycol

- etofenamate

Fenac Group

The core structure is 2-aminophenylacetic acid. The 2-amino group is substituted with aromatic residues.

- diclofenac
- felbinac (only used topically)

Heteroaryl Acetic Acid Group

- indomethacin
- acemetacine
- proglumetacine
- tolmetin (and its ring closed analog ketorolac)
- ionazolac

Profene Group

The core structure is 2-arylpropionic acid

- ibuprofen
- ketoprofen
- thiaprofen
- naproxen
- ketorolac (can be seen formally as a ring closed profene)

Oxicam Group

The core structure is 1,2-benzothiazine

- piroxicam
- tenoxicam
- lornoxicam
- droxicam

N

- cinoxicam
- sudoxicam
- meloxicam

Pyrazolone Group

The mode of action of the pyrazolones remains unclear. It is thought that they may not be involved in the inhibition of COX-1 or COX-2. The compounds of the pyrazol-3-on series at least are neutral molecules with no acidity. A central mode of action is suggested. They also act antispasmodically and are effective in visceral pain. In the past, pyrazolones were very frequently used nonsteroidal anti-inflammatory drugs. They show a high plasma protein binding and therefore have a high rate of interaction with other pharmaceuticals. Agranulocytosis is a rare but severe side effect.

The core structure is $3H$-pyrazol-3-on

- propyphenazone
- metamizol-Na
- phenazone

Pyrazolidindione

The core structure is pyrazolidin-3,5-dion

- phenylbutazone
- mofebutazone

COX-2 Selective Inhibitors

The isoform 2 of the COX enzyme catalyzes the identical reaction AA to PGG_2, the active site however is slightly different from COX-1 (Fig. 5).

Isoleucine 523 is replaced by valine 509, making the active site of COX-2 more "spacious". This difference can be used to generate COX-2 selective inhibitors, as this active site tolerates more bulky molecules. Celecoxib is capable of producing full inhibition of COX-1 and COX-2. However it shows a preferential selectivity toward COX-2 (>5 fold). The newer coxibs like rofecoxib strongly inhibit COX-2 with only weak activity against COX-1 (Warner et al. 1999).

A common pharmacophore cannot be identified, however vicinal diaryl systems (celecoxib, rofecoxib, valdecoxib) and sulfone or sulphonamide groups seem to be advantageous (Laufer et al. 2000). Lumiracoxib however is an excellent example of the fact that spatial demanding substituents (bulky groups) alone are sufficient to generate selectivity, even with a diclofenac-like pharmacophore.

Structural Features of Selective COX-2 Inhibitors

Sulfonamide structure

- celecoxib
- valdecoxib

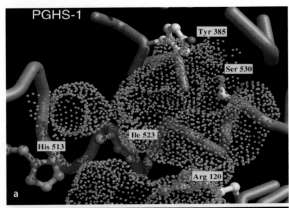
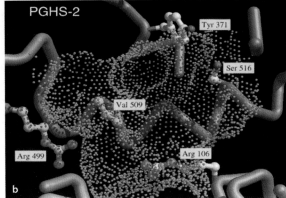

NSAIDs, Chemical Structure and Molecular Mode of Action, Figure 5 Comparison of the active site of COX-1 (PGHS-1) and COX-2 (PGHS-2) (from Wong et al. 1997).

Methylsulfone structure

- rofecoxib
- etoricoxib

Aryl acetic acid

- Lumiracoxib

Others:

- parecoxib (water soluble prodrug for parenteral application, rapidly metabolized to valdecoxib)

References

1. Moser P, Sallmann A, Wiesenberg L (1990) Synthesis and quantitative structure-activity relationships of diclofenac analogues. J Med Chem 33:2358–2368
2. Warner T; Giuliano F, Vojnovic I et al. (1999) Nonsteroid drug selectivities for cyclo-oxygenase-1 rather than cyclo-oxygenase 2 are associated with human gastrointestinal toxicity: A full in vitro analysis. Proc. Natl Acad Sci USA 96:7563–7568
3. Dannhardt G and Laufer S (2000) Structural approaches to explain the selectivity of COX-2 inhibitors: Is there a common pharmacophore? Current Medicinal Chemistry 7:1101–1112
4. Malkowski M; Ginell SL, Smith WL, Garavito RM (2000) The Productive Conformation of Arachidonic Acid Bound to Prostaglandin Synthase. Science 289:1933–1937
5. Wong E, Bayly E, Waterman HL et al. (1997) Conversion of prostaglandin G/H synthase-1 into an enzyme sensitive to PGHS-2-selective inhibitors by a double His$^{513}\rightarrow$Arg and Ile$^{523}\rightarrow$Val mutation. J Biol Chem 272:9280–9286

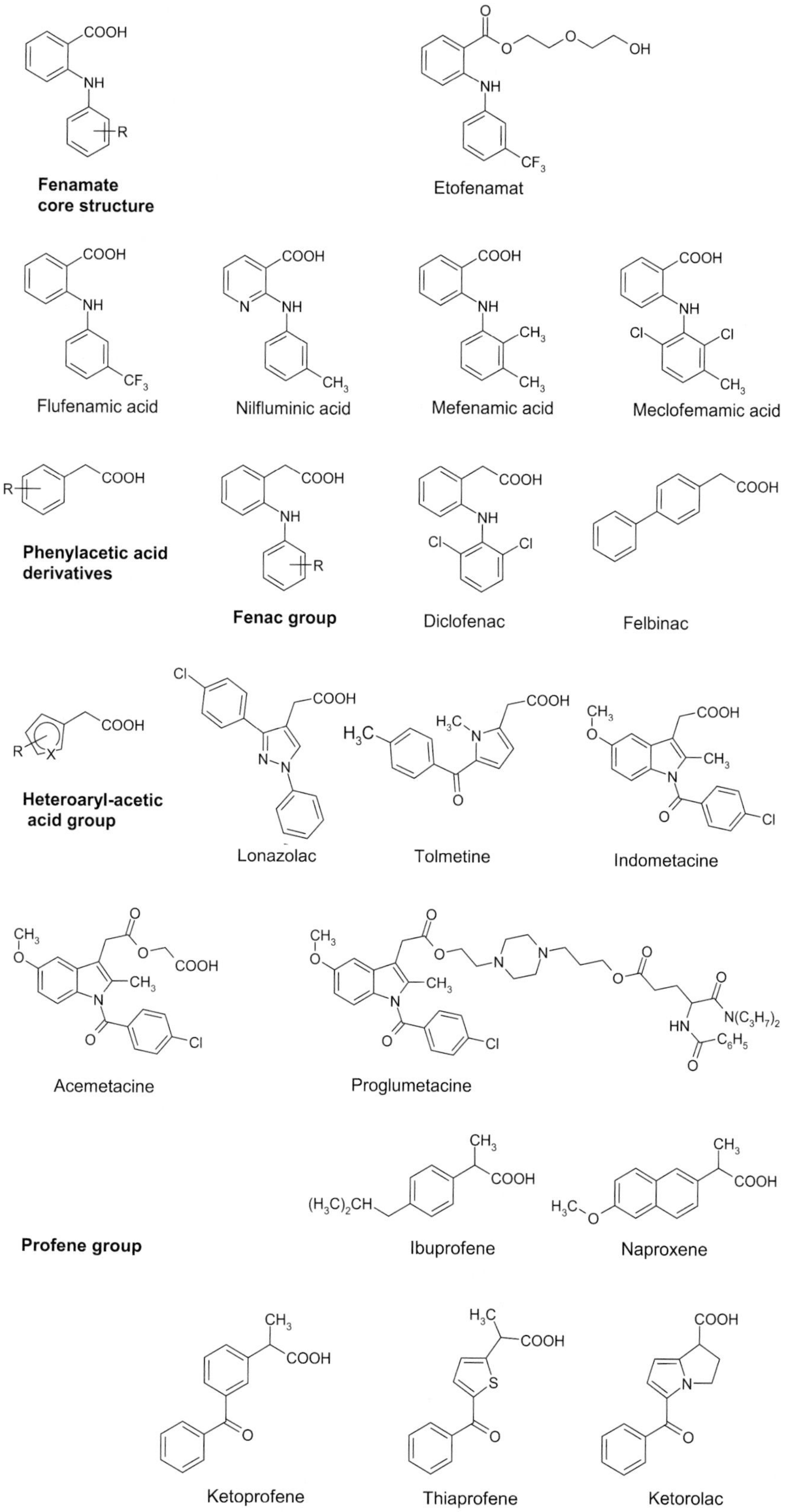

Fenamate core structure

Etofenamat

Flufenamic acid

Nilfluminic acid

Mefenamic acid

Meclofemamic acid

Phenylacetic acid derivatives

Fenac group

Diclofenac

Felbinac

Heteroaryl-acetic acid group

Lonazolac

Tolmetine

Indometacine

Acemetacine

Proglumetacine

Profene group

Ibuprofene

Naproxene

Ketoprofene

Thiaprofene

Ketorolac

NSAIDs, Chemical Structure and Molecular Mode of Action, Figure 6 Chemical structures of NSAIDs.

N

NSAIDs, COX-Independent Actions

ELLEN NIEDERBERGER, IRMGARD TEGEDER
Pharmacological Center Frankfurt, Clinical Center
Johann-Wolfgang Goethe University, Frankfurt,
Germany
e.niederberger@em.uni-frankfurt.de,
tegeder@em.uni-frankfurt.de

Synonyms

NSAIDs; non-steroidal anti-inflammatory drugs; COX;
cyclooxygenase; PGH-Synthase; Prostaglandin H Synthase

Definition

NSAIDs are among the most commonly used ▶ analgesics and anti-inflammatory drugs. The major mechanism of action is supposed to be the inhibition of
cyclooxygenase (COX) 1 and 2 enzymes, and thereby
prostaglandin synthesis. However, since aspirin was
reported to inhibit nuclear factor kappa B (NF-κB)
activation (Kopp and Ghosh 1994), it is increasingly
recognized that certain NSAIDs have various biological
effects that are independent of cyclooxygenase activity and prostaglandin synthesis, and may account, at
least in part, for their analgesic, anti-inflammatory and
antiproliferative effects. These effects mainly occur at
drug concentrations beyond the IC_{50} (▶ IC50 value) for
COX-inhibition, and therefore probably occur primarily at high concentrations. Various mechanisms have
been shown to be involved (Tegeder et al. 2001) and are
summarized in this essay. A schematic overview over
these mechanisms is shown in figure 1.

Characteristics

Effects on Transcription Factors

Nuclear Factor Kappa B (NF-κB)

NF-κB is an important mediator of the cellular response to a variety of extracellular stress stimuli. As
homodimers and heterodimers, Rel/NF-κB proteins
bind to DNA target sites and regulate gene transcription
of pro-inflammatory mediators and proteins that are
involved in cell death or survival. Various NSAIDs
including salicylates, sulindac, ibuprofen and R- and
S-flurbiprofen, inhibit NF-κB activation. While aspirin,
ibuprofen and sulindac also inhibit COX-activity, R-
flurbiprofen and salicylic acid are inactive in this regard,
and therefore do not cause typical NSAID-evoked side
effects that are due to COX-inhibition. Indomethacin,
ketoprofen and ketorolac do not inhibit NF-κB. Hence,
in contrast to COX-inhibition, NF-κB inhibition is not
a "class-effect" The COX–2 selective inhibitors rofecoxib and celecoxib have different effects on NF-κB.
While rofecoxib inhibits its activation in RAW 264.7
macrophages (Niederberger et al. 2003), celecoxib

further increases LPS-induced NF-κB-activation. The
latter effect of celecoxib results in a loss of its anti-
inflammatory efficacy at high doses in an experimental
inflammatory model in rats (Niederberger et al. 2003),
suggesting that effects on NF-κB are important for the
anti-inflammatory efficacy of some COX-inhibitors.
As a stress signalling molecule, NF-κB is also involved
in the regulation of cell death and survival, either as
being essential for the induction of ▶ apoptosis or
more commonly as an inhibitor of apoptosis. Whether
NF-κB promotes or inhibits apoptosis appears to depend on the cell type and the type of inducer. NF-κB
is persistently active in numerous human cancer cells.
This is suggested to contribute to increased resistance
towards chemo– or radiotherapy. NSAIDs that inhibit
NF-κB may eliminate this resistance mechanism and
thereby re-increase cancer cell sensitivity towards
apoptosis inducing treatments. Hence, inhibition of
NF-κB in tumour cells may contribute to the observed
anti-tumour activity of various NSAIDs including S-
and R-Flurbiprofen (Wechter et al. 1997), celecoxib
(Grosch et al. 2001), sulindac and aspirin (Thun et al.
1991).

AP–1

The transcription factor AP–1 is a homo- or heterodimer
of Jun, Fos and Fra oncogenes. AP–1 is activated by various stimuli including UV-irradiation, growth factors and
inflammatory cytokines. Some of the genes known to
be regulated by AP–1 are involved in the immune and
inflammatory responses or tumour formation and progression. AP–1 regulated genes partially overlap with
genes that are regulated by NF-κB. Inhibition of AP–1
has been shown for aspirin, sodium salicylate, piroxicam, R-flurbiprofen and the selective COX–2 inhibitors
celecoxib and NS398 in various cell types. However, it
is not presently known to what extent effects on AP–1
contribute to the anti-inflammatory or anti-proliferative
effects of NSAIDs, because different AP–1 homo- and
heterodimers may have either stimulating or inhibiting
effects on gene transcription (Grosch et al. 2003), and
the number of genes that are regulated by AP–1 is high.
Therefore, the result of NSAID-induced AP–1 inhibition may greatly vary.

Effects on Cellular Kinases

Inhibitor Kappa B Kinase Complex (IKK)

In most cells NF-κB exists in the cytoplasm in an
inactive complex bound to inhibitor IκB proteins. NF-
κB is activated upon phosphorylation and subsequent
proteasome-mediated proteolysis of IκB. The key regulatory step in this pathway is the activation of an IκB
kinase (IKK) complex. IKK consists of two catalytic
subunits, IKKα and IKKβ, and a regulatory subunit
(IKKγ) that regulates binding of activators. Liberated
NF-κB translocates from the cytoplasm to the nucleus
where it binds to the κB-sites of target genes and reg-

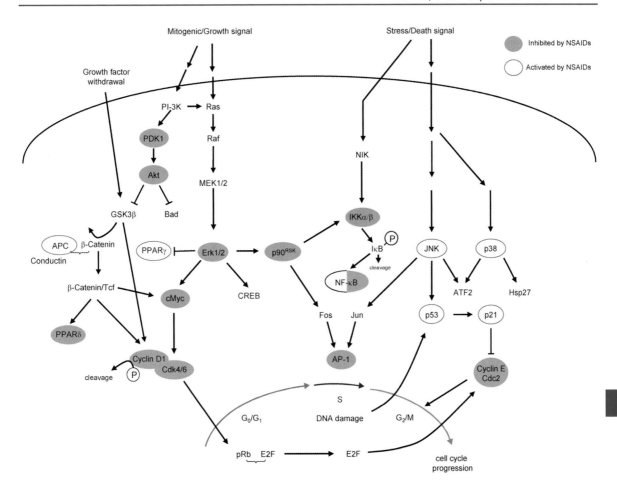

NSAIDs, COX-Independent Actions, Figure 1, Systematic overview of COX-independent NSAIDs effects. → activation or induction; ⊣ inhibition ⬤ inhibited by NSAIDs; ◯ activated by NSAIDs Abbreviations: Akt/PKB, protein kinase B; APC adenomatous polyposis coli tumor suppressor gene; AP-1 activator protein-1; Cdk, cyclin dependent kinase; CREB, cAMP response element binding protein; Erk, extracellular signal regulated kinase; GSK3β, glycogen synthase kinase 3 beta; Hsp, heat shock protein; IKK, I-kappa kinase; JNK, Jun N-terminal kinase; MAPK, mitogen activated kinase; MEK/MKK, mitogen-activated protein kinase kinase; NIK, nuclear factor-kappaB inducing kinase; NF-κB, nuclear factor kappa B; PDK, phosphoinositol-dependent kinase; PI-3K, phosphatidylinositol-3-kinase; PKC, protein kinase C; PPAR, peroxisome proliferator activated receptor; pRb, retinoblastoma protein; p90RSK, ribosomal S6 kinase; Tcf, T cell factor.

ulates their transcription. Various NSAIDs including aspirin, sodium salicylate and sulindac inhibit the ATP binding to IKKβ, and thereby its catalytic activity (Yin et al. 1998). However, the IKK inhibitory potency of these NSAIDs is low, and the specificity of aspirin-induced IKK, and thereby NF-κB inhibition, has been doubted.

Mitogen Activated Protein (MAP)-Kinase Cascade

MAP-kinases (MAPK) play a central role in the differentiation and proliferation of several cell types, and can be activated by various extracellular stimuli. AP–1 is one downstream target of the MAP-kinase family members including extracellular signal regulated kinases (Erk-1 and -2; p42/p44 MAPK), c-Jun N-terminal kinases (JNK1-3) and p38 MAPK. Erk activation has been implicated in growth promotion and cell survival, whereas JNK and p38 MAPK activation are associated with stress responses and apoptosis. Recent results have shown that the effect of NSAIDs on MAP-kinases

largely depends on the cellular context. In cancer cells, the ability of NSAIDs to modulate MAPK activities may play an important role in the cytotoxicity and induction of apoptosis.

Aspirin and sodium salicylate were shown to inhibit activation of Erk-1 and -2 under certain circumstances. Inhibition of angiogenesis by COX–2 selective and unselective NSAIDs has been shown to be mediated through inhibition of Erk-2 activity and interference with its nuclear translocation in vascular endothelial cells (Tsujii et al. 1998). p38 MAPK was reported to be activated by sodium salicylate in human fibroblasts leading to induction of apoptosis. TNFα-induced JNK activation was also inhibited by salicylate in human fibroblasts. Oppositely, in HT-29 colon cancer and COS-1 cells, salicylate treatment resulted in activation of JNK.

Protein Kinase B (PKB/Akt)

The protein kinase B (PKB/Akt) promotes cell proliferation and survival, thereby contributing to cancer progression. Activation of Akt occurs by translocation of the kinase to the cell membrane and phosphorylation through phospho-inositide-dependent kinase 1 (PDK1). The COX–2 selective inhibitor celecoxib has been shown to induce apoptosis in prostate carcinoma (Hsu et al. 2000), hepatocarcinoma and colon carcinoma cells by inhibiting the phosphorylation of PKB/Akt, thereby blocking its anti-apoptotic activity. The effects of celecoxib on Akt depended in part on the inhibition of PDK1. Inhibition of PKB/Akt by celecoxib has also been observed in vascular smooth muscle cells leading to inhibition of neointima formation after ballon injury. Similarly, sulindac has been described to inhibit Akt-phosphorylation in lung adenocarcinoma cells. Aspirin has been shown to either activate or inhibit Akt-activation, dependent on the cell type.

Effects on Cell Cycle Proteins

The progression through the various phases of the cell cycle is regulated by cyclins and cyclin-dependent kinases (Cdks). The function of cyclins is primarily controlled by changes in cyclin transcription, while Cdks are regulated by phosphorylation. The activity of the Cdk/cyclin complex is inhibited by p21 and p27. Sodium salicylate inhibits the proliferation of vascular smooth muscle cells through up-regulation of these cell cycle inhibitors. This is probably caused by salicylate-induced up-regulation of p53, which is the primary regulator of p21 transcription. Similar to salicylates, sulindac, sulindac sulfide and celecoxib inhibited the proliferation of colon carcinoma cells and caused them to accumulate in the G_0/G_1 phase. This effect was attributed to inhibition of cyclin-dependent kinases and/or up-regulation of p27 and p21.

Modulation of the Activity of Nuclear Receptor Family Members

Activation of Peroxisome Proliferator Activated Receptor (PPAR)

PPARs α, δ and γ are nuclear hormone receptors that control the transcription of genes involved in energy metabolism, cell differentiation, apoptosis and inflammation. PPARs bind to sequence-specific DNA response elements as a heterodimer with the retinoic acid receptor (RXR). PPARγ is highly expressed in adipose tissue, and plays an important role in the regulation of genes involved in lipid utilization and storage, adipocyte differentiation, insulin action and inflammation. Indomethacin binds to PPARγ and induces the differentiation of mesenchymal stem cells into adipocytes ► in vitro. Some other NSAIDs including ibuprofen, fenoprofen and flufenamic acid also bind and activate PPARγ. However, they are less potent than indomethacin.

In addition to the role in adipogenesis and inflammation, PPARγ is highly expressed in normal large intestine and in breast, colon and prostate cancer. PPARγ-agonists such as troglitazone and 15deoxy-PGJ$_2$ were able to induce differentiation and apoptosis in tumour cells, suggesting that PPARγ suppresses tumour cell proliferation. Indomethacin was shown to reduce the colonogenic activity of prostate cancer cells and increased the antiproliferative effect of 5–fluorouracil in colon cancer cells. This effect was supposed to be mediated through activation of PPARγ.

PPARδ is a nuclear transcription factor that is activated by prostacyclin. Inhibition of COX-activity with aspirin or other NSAIDs causes inhibition of PPARδ, which has been identified as one of the downstream targets of the WNT-β-catenin pathway (He et al. 1999). This pathway plays a crucial role in embryonic development and carcinogenesis. PPARδ expression is normally controlled by the APC tumour suppressor. However, during colon carcinogenesis, APC function is almost always lost, leading to a dysfunction of β-catenin and uncontrolled PPARδ expression. This is considered as a crucial initiating step in tumour transformation. The suppression of PPARδ activity by various NSAIDs, including aspirin and sulindac, can compensate for the loss of APC or β-catenin dysfunction and thereby reduce colon carcinogenesis. Hence, the inhibition of PPARδ activity may contribute to the chemopreventive effects of some NSAIDs.

Other Targets

Intracellular Carbonic Anhydrase

Carbonic anhydrases play an important role in the extracellular acidification. Several studies suggest a possible involvement of these enzymes in tumour progression resulting from the acidic extracellular pH. Celecoxib and valdecoxib inhibit carbonic anhydrases. This effect is supposed to depend on their sulfonamide structure, and is therefore not shared by rofecoxib or etoricoxib.

Acid Sensing Ion Channels (ASICs)

H^+-gated currents mediated by acid sensing ion channels (ASICs) are involved in acidosis which occurs under inflammatory conditions and in tumours. Various NSAIDs including aspirin, salicylic acid, flurbiprofen, ibuprofen and diclofenac are inhibitors of these H^+-gated channels, thereby inhibiting acid induced pain reaction and inflammatory responses.

Ca^{2+}-Release

Treatment with some COX–2 inhibitors increased intracellular calcium levels in osteoblasts, PC–12 and HUVEC cells. This effect might be mediated by a block of endoplasmatic reticulum Ca^{2+}-ATPases, and may increase the risk of cardiovascular events in predisposed patients.

References

1. Grosch S, Tegeder I, Niederberger E et al. (2001) COX–2 Independent Induction of Cell Cycle Arrest and Apoptosis in Colon Cancer Cells by the Selective COX–2 Inhibitor Celecoxib. FASEB J 15:2742–2744

2. Grosch S, Tegeder I, Schilling K et al. (2003) Activation of c-Jun-N-terminal-Kinase is Crucial for the Induction of a Cell Cycle Arrest in Human Colon Carcinoma Cells caused by Flurbiprofen Enantiomers. FASEB J 17:1316–1318

3. He TC, Chan TA, Vogelstein B et al. (1999) PPARdelta is an APC-Regulated Target of Nonsteroidal Anti-Inflammatory Drugs. Cell 99:335–345

4. Hsu AL, Ching TT, Wang DS et al. (2000) The Cyclooxygenase-2 Inhibitor Celecoxib Induces Apoptosis by Blocking Akt Activation in Human Prostate Cancer Cells Independently of Bcl-2. J Biol Chem 275:11397–11403

5. Kopp E, Ghosh S (1994) Inhibition of NF-Kappa B by Sodium Salicylate and Aspirin. Science 265:956–959

6. Niederberger E, Tegeder I, Schafer C et al. (2003) Opposite Effects of Rofecoxib on Nuclear Factor-kappa B and Activating Protein-1 Activation. J Pharmacol Exp Ther 304:1153–1160

7. Tegeder I, Pfeilschifter J, Geisslinger G (2001) Cyclooxygenase-Independent Actions of Cyclooxygenase Inhibitors. FASEB J 15:2057–2072

8. Thun MJ, Namboodiri MM, Heath CW Jr (1991) Aspirin Use and Reduced Risk of Fatal Colon Cancer. N Engl J Med 325:1593–1596

9. Tsujii M, Kawano S, Tsuji S et al. (1998) Cyclooxygenase Regulates Angiogenesis Induced by Colon Cancer Cells. Cell 93:705–716

10. Wechter WJ, Kantoci D, Murray ED Jr et al. (1997) R-Flurbiprofen Chemoprevention and Treatment of Intestinal Adenomas in the APC(Min)/+ Mouse Model: Implications for Prophylaxis and Treatment of Colon Cancer. Cancer Res 57:4316–4324

11. Yin MJ, Yamamoto Y, Gaynor RB (1998) The Anti-Inflammatory Agents Aspirin and Salicylate Inhibit the Activity of I(kappa)B Kinase-Beta. Nature 396:77–80

NSAIDs, Mode of Action

MARIA BURIAN

Pharmacological Center Frankfurt, Clinical Center Johann-Wolfgang Goethe University, Frankfurt, Germany

burian@em.uni-frankfurt.de

Synonyms

NSAIDs; non-steroidal anti-inflammatory drugs; Aspirin-Like Drugs; Non-Selective COX-Inhibitors; cyclooxygenase; COX; Prostaglandin H Synthase; PGHS

Definition

Non-steroidal anti-inflammatory drugs (NSAIDs) are among the most widely prescribed and used drugs for the management of pain, especially of pain in inflammatory conditions. Despite the wide use of NSAIDs over the last century, little was known on the mode of actions of these drugs for a long time. Initially, the principle mode of the antinociceptive action of NSAIDs was related to their anti-inflammatory activity, and attributed to the inhibition of the production of prostaglandins at the peripheral site of inflammation (peripheral mode of action) (Vane 1971). The traditional belief in the exclusively peripheral action of NSAIDs, however, has been challenged by the growing evidence showing the dissociation between the anti-inflammatory and antinociceptive effects of NSAIDs (McCormack and Brune 1991). This is the basis for the hypothesis of additional antinociceptive mechanisms existing with NSAIDs, where the inhibition of prostaglandin synthesis in CNS appears to be universally applicable for all NSAIDs (central mode of action).

While inhibiting prostanoid synthesis, NSAIDs do not typically elevate the normal pain threshold, but mainly normalize the increased pain threshold observed in ▶ inflammatory pain (▶ hyperalgesia), so that their antinociceptive effect should rather be defined as anti-hyperalgesic instead of analgesic.

Characteristics

Prostanoid Synthesis

Despite the diverse chemical structure of aspirin-like drugs, all NSAIDs bear a common pharmacological property of inhibiting the formation of prostanoids. Prostanoids are formed by most cells and act as lipid mediators. They are synthesized from membrane-released arachidonic acid mobilized by phospholipases (PLA$_2$) when cells are activated by mechanical trauma, cytokines, growth factors, etc. (Fig. 1). Conversion of arachidonic acid to prostanoid end-products occurs by cyclooxygenases (COX), an enzyme also known as prostaglandin H synthase (PGHS), at two different sites of the enzyme. It is initially cyclized and oxidized to the endoperoxide PGG$_2$ at the cyclooxygenase site of the COX. This product is then reduced to a second endoperoxide, PGH$_2$, at the peroxidase site of the COX enzyme. Subsequent formation of prostaglandin end-products from PGH$_2$ depends on the presence of the specific synthase enzymes that produce functionally important prostanoids PGD$_2$, PGE$_2$, PGF$_{2\alpha}$, PGI$_2$ (prostacyclin) and TXA$_2$ (thromboxane), which mediate their effects through the specific receptors: PGD$_2$ (DP$_1$, DP$_2$ receptors), PGE$_2$ (EP$_1$, EP$_2$, EP$_3$, EP$_4$ receptors), PGF$_{2\alpha}$ (FP receptor), PGI$_2$ (IP receptors) and TXA$_2$ (TP$_\alpha$ and TP$_\beta$ receptors).

Inhibition of Cyclooxygenases by NSAIDs

NSAIDs inhibit the formation of prostanoids by several different effects on COX, including irreversible inactivation of COX (e.g. aspirin) or reversible competitive inhibition (e.g. ibuprofen). COX is represented by two isoforms, COX-1 and COX-2, which are membrane-associated enzymes with a 63% amino acid sequence similarity. The identification of two isoforms of COX in the early 1990s offered a simple and attractive hypothesis: COX-1, being found in almost all cells, is the constitutive "house-keeping" enzyme responsible for production of basal "beneficial" PGs, which are vital for protecting the stomach through mucus production or maintenance of renal blood flow. In contrast, COX-2, in which expression is low or undetectable in most cells but increased dramatically in a variety of pathological

N

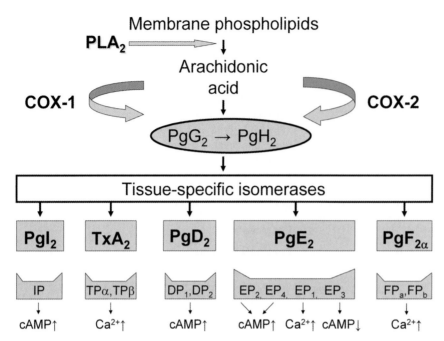

NSAIDs, Mode of Action, Figure 1 Prostanoids are synthesized from membrane-released arachidonic acid mobilized by phospholipases (PLA_2). Conversion of arachidonic acid to prostanoid end-products occurs by COX-1 and COX-2 at two different sites of the enzyme. It is initially cyclized and oxidized to the endoperoxide PGG_2 at the cyclooxygenase site of the COX and then reduced to a second endoperoxide, PGH_2 at the peroxidase site of the COX enzyme. Tissue-specific isomerases catalyze subsequent formation of prostaglandin end-products including PGD_2, PGE_2, $PGF_{2\alpha}$, PGI_2 (prostacyclin) and TXA_2 (thromboxane). These prostanoids exert their effects by acting through the specific receptors: PGD_2 (DP_1, DP_2 receptors), PGE_2 (EP_1, EP_2, EP_3, EP_4 receptors), $PGF_{2\alpha}$ (FP receptor), PGI_2 (IP receptors) and TXA_2 (TP_α and TP_β receptors). The "relaxant" receptors IP, DP_1, EP_2 and EP_4 signal through Gs-mediated increases in intracellular cyclic adenosine monophosphate (cAMP). The "contractile" receptors EP_1, FP and TP signal through Gq-mediated increases in intracellular calcium. The EP_3 receptor is regarded as an "inhibitory" receptor that couples to Gi and decrease cAMP formation.

conditions, is the inducible enzyme responsible for "pathological" production of prostanoids in different conditions ranging from inflammation to cancer.

NSAIDs are non-selective inhibitors of COX (both COX-1 and COX-2). Initially, the favourable anti-inflammatory, anti-nociceptive and antipyretic effects of NSAIDs were solely attributed to the inhibition of COX-2, while the concomitant inhibition of COX-1 was supposed to lead to adverse reactions of the drugs (gastrointestinal and renal toxicities). With time, especially along with the introduction/gaining experience of selective COX-2 inhibitors (e.g. celecoxib, rofecoxib, etc.), this concept turned out to be more complicated than initially thought, indicating that both COX-1 and COX-2 have physiological and pathological roles, so that the inhibition of both isoforms may be responsible for favourable and unfavourable pharmacological effects of NSAIDs.

Cyclooxygenases and Prostanoids at the Peripheral Site

In injured tissue, COX-2 is the predominant isoform expressed and a main source of prostanoids during inflammation. The significant induction of COX-2 is found in activated polymorponuclear leucocytes, phagocytosing mononuclear cells and fibroblasts, which are abundantly present at the site of inflammation. However, COX-1 is also involved in the modulation of the

inflammatory response, and is mainly increased in circulating monocytes and stimulated mast cells at the early inflammatory phase. Thus, both COX isoforms are involved in the inflammatory reaction in the periphery, and may contribute to the generation and maintenance of inflammatory pain. The earliest prostanoid response is dependent on COX-1, but COX-2 becomes a major source of prostanoids along with the progression of inflammation. NSAIDs-mediated inhibition of COX-1 and COX-2 at the site of inflammation results in the attenuation of peripheral ▶ sensitization associated with inflammatory pain (Fig. 2).

Cyclooxygenase and Prostanoids in CNS

In contrast to the periphery, in the CNS both COX-1 and COX-2 are expressed constitutively (Beiche et al. 1996). These isoforms are present in neurons and non-neuronal elements of the spinal cord and brain (Maihofner et al. 2000). The peripheral inflammatory reactions associated with tissue injury result in the release of pro-inflammatory cytokines, such as IL-1β, which may enhance the up-regulation of COX-2 in the CNS (Samad et al. 2001). This up-regulation is paralleled to the substantial elevation of prostanoids in the cerebrospinal fluid and typical nociceptive behaviour of the animals in experimental pain models. Therefore, COX-2 appears to be mainly responsible

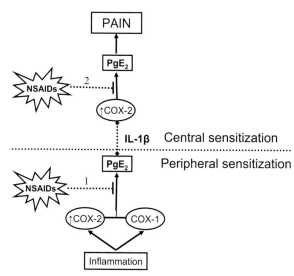

NSAIDs, Mode of Action, Figure 2 The inhibition of prostaglandin synthesis by NSAIDs takes place at both the site of peripheral inflammation (1) and at the spinal level (2), indicating that peripheral and central mechanisms may be responsible for their antinociceptive action. NSAIDs-mediated inhibition of COX-1 and COX-2 at the peripheral site results in the attenuation of peripheral sensitization, whereas inhibition of the up-regulated COX-2 in CNS leads to the attenuation of central hyperalgesia. Peripheral and central hyperalgesia are hallmarks of inflammatory pain.

for the central processing of pain after peripheral inflammation. COX-1, however, can also become the source of spinal prostaglandins in response to peripheral inflammation under specific conditions, as has been particularly demonstrated in COX-2 deficient knockout mice. NSAIDs-mediated inhibition of COX-1 and COX-2 in CNS results in the attenuation of central sensitization associated with inflammatory pain (Fig. 2).

Mechanisms of Prostaglandin-Mediated Hyperalgesia

Prostaglandins are potent sensitizing agents, which are able to modulate multiple sites along the nociceptive pathway enhancing transduction (peripheral sensitization), as well as transmission (central sensitization), of the nociceptive information (Woolf 1983).

Peripheral Sensitization

Direct and indirect mechanisms of the peripheral sensitizing action of prostanoids have been suggested. The direct effects are mediated by their action upon prostaglandin receptors and modulation of ion channels in ▶ nociceptors. The indirect effects are produced through enhancing the sensitivity of nociceptors to noxious agents, including heat and bradykinin. Both direct and indirect sensitizing effects of prostanoids lead to the enhanced transduction of the nociceptive information and manifest as peripheral hyperalgesia. NSAIDs-mediated inhibition of prostanoid synthesis in the periphery results in the attenuation of peripheral hyperalgesia associated with inflammatory pain (peripheral ▶ antihyperalgesic effect).

Central Sensitization

The sensitizing effects of prostanoids in CNS are mediated by their action on presynaptic and postsynaptic membranes of the primary afferent synapse in the dorsal horn of the spinal cord. Acting via prostanoid receptors located on the presynaptic membrane, prostanoids may cause the enhancement of nociception via facilitation of the spinal release of the excitatory neurotransmitter ▶ glutamate and neuropeptides (▶ substance-P and/or ▶ calcitonin gene-related peptide). At the postsynaptic level, prostanoids can directly activate deep dorsal horn neurons and/or block the inhibitory glycinergic neurotransmission onto dorsal horn neurons. All this leads to the enhanced transmission of the nociceptive activity to the brain, and manifests as central hyperalgesia. NSAIDs-mediated inhibition of prostanoid synthesis in CNS results in the attenuation of central hyperalgesia associated with inflammatory pain (central antihyperalgesic effect).

Central and Peripheral Antihyperalgesic Effects of NSAIDs

From the pharmacological point of view, the contribution of the central versus peripheral mechanisms to the overall antihyperalgesic effects of NSAIDs depends on:

- the site of drug delivery (e.g. systemic, local-peripheral, epidural, spinal intracerebro-ventricular);
- uptake and distribution from the site of drug delivery, as determined by factors including the drug's physical and chemical properties, specific transport mechanisms, local and systemic blood flow, and tissue barriers to drug permeation, such as the blood-brain barrier.

One of the accepted approaches to prove that NSAIDs act upon CNS to alleviate pain is an assessment of their antinociceptive activity, following a direct application of NSAIDs to spinal or supraspinal structures. This approach has gained its particular importance in behavioural animal studies. The intrathecal delivery of various NSAIDs has been shown to be effective in the reduction of behavioural hyperalgesia in several animal models of acute, short-term and long-term inflammatory pain (Brune et al. 1991). The antihyperalgesic effects have been observed with doses that are significantly lower than those needed to produce the similar degree of antinociception by systemic administration. Clinical relevance of the central antinociceptive mechanisms of the antinociceptive action of NSAIDs has been demonstrated in patients with intractable pain due to various types of cancer conditions. In these patients, intrathecal administration of small doses of lysine-acetylsalicylate (equivalent to acetylsalicylic acid 500 µg/kg) has been shown to bring rapid and prolonged pain relief (Pellerin et al. 1987).

The evidence for a clinically relevant peripheral antinociceptive action has been obtained with locally applied NSAIDs, where the effective antinociceptive effect of NSAIDs versus placebo has been established with intra-articular and topical applications of NSAIDs (Romsing et al. 2000).

The contribution of central versus peripheral mechanisms to the total antihyperalgesic effect of NSAIDs has been studied in the human experimental pain model of "freeze lesion". The experimental hyperalgesia in this model was produced by short-lasting freezing of volunteer's skin. The relative contribution of the central component of orally administered diclofenac has accounted for approximately 40% of the total antihyperalgesic efficacy of the drug (Burian et al. 2003).

Conclusion

NSAIDs are potent antinociceptive agents, whose efficacy in reducing pain is widely recognized in various pain conditions, including post-surgical pain and persistent pain states, such as arthritis and cancer. Although NSAIDs have long been used in clinical practice, the mechanism of their antihyperalgesic action remains controversial. It appears that the inhibition of prostaglandin synthesis by NSAIDs takes place both at the site of peripheral inflammation and at the spinal level, indicating that peripheral and central mechanisms are responsible for their antinociceptive action. The contribution of peripheral and central COX-dependent mechanisms to the overall antinociceptive action of NSAIDs is individual for each drug, and is dependent on the site of drug delivery, as well as pharmacokinetic characteristics of the drug determining its penetration to the sites of action (e.g. peripheral and spinal COX).

References

1. Beiche F, Scheuerer S, Brune K et al. (1996) Up-Regulation of Cyclooxygenase-2 mRNA in the Rat Spinal Cord following Peripheral Inflammation. FEBS Lett 390:165–169
2. Brune K, Beck WS, Geisslinger G et al. (1991) Aspirin-Like Drugs may Block Pain Independently of Prostaglandin Synthesis Inhibition. Experientia 47:257–261
3. Burian M, Tegeder I, Seegel M et al. (2003) Peripheral and Central Antihyperalgesic Effects of Diclofenac in a Model of Human Inflammatory Pain. Clin Pharmacol Ther 74:113–120
4. Maihofner C, Tegeder I, Euchenhofer C et al. (2000) Localization and Regulation of Cyclooxygenase-1 and -2 and Neuronal Nitric Oxide Synthase in Mouse Spinal Cord. Neuroscience 101:1093–1108
5. McCormack K, Brune K (1991) Dissociation between the Antinociceptive and Anti-Inflammatory Effects of the Non-Steroidal Anti-Inflammatory Drugs. A Survey of their Analgesic Efficacy. Drugs 41:533–457
6. Pellerin M, Hardy F, Abergel A et al. (1987) Chronic Refractory Pain in Cancer Patients. Value of the Spinal Injection of Lysine Acetylsalicylate. 60 Cases. Presse Med 16:1465–1468
7. Romsing J, Moiniche S, Ostergaard D et al. (2000) Local Infiltration with NSAIDs for Postoperative Analgesia: Evidence for a Peripheral Analgesic Action. Acta Anaesthesiol Scand 44:672–683
8. Samad TA, Moore KA, Sapirstein A et al. (2001) Interleukin-1beta-Mediated Induction of Cox-2 in the CNS Contributes to Inflammatory Pain Hypersensitivity. Nature 410:471–475
9. Vane JR (1971) Inhibition of Prostaglandin Synthesis as a Mechanism of Action for Aspirin-Like Drugs. Nat New Biol 231:232–235
10. Woolf CJ (1983) Evidence for a Central Component of Post-Injury Pain Hypersensitivity. Nature 306:686–688

NSAIDs, Pharmacogenetics

CARSTEN SKARKE
Institute of Clinical Pharmacology, pharmazentrum frankfurt/ZAFES, Institute of Clinical Pharmacology, Johann-Wolfgang Goethe University, Frankfurt, Germany
skarke@em.uni-frankfurt.de

Synonyms

Inherited Variability of Drug Response; Pharmacogenetics of NSAIDs

Definition

Pharmacogenetics seeks to explore how genetic variants influence the pharmacokinetic and pharmacodynamic properties of a given drug, by determining how mutations in the genes that encode drug metabolizing enzymes, drug targets and drug transporters influence drug response.

Characteristics

Nonsteroidal anti-inflammatory drugs (NSAID) block the formation of prostaglandins by inhibiting the rate-limiting cyclooxygenase (COX) enzymes, COX–1 and COX–2, also known as prostaglandin H_2 synthases (PGHS1 and PGHS2). Since prostaglandins participate in mediating the inflammatory response, the pharmacological activity of NSAIDs consists mainly of antinociceptive, anti-inflammatory and antipyretic properties. Variations of this pharmacological activity can arise as a basic principle from mutations in proteins, which (i) influence the bioavailability of a drug, (ii) vary the binding affinity to the drug target, or (iii) modify drug elimination. Since NSAIDs possess a high solubility and high permeability (Yazdanian et al. 2004), and were not found to be a substrate of drug efflux transporters, it is unlikely that the disposition varies on a genetic basis. Far more expected are mutations in the cyclooxygenase enzymes as drug targets and the metabolizing enzymes as determinants of drug elimination. The majority of such mutations are ► single nucleotide polymorphisms (SNP), which consist of an exchange of one nucleotide often, but not always, leading to an alteration in the amino-acid sequence of the resulting protein, provided that the SNP is located within the coding region of the ► gene.

Polymorphisms in the Cyclooxygenase-1 Gene

The COX–1 gene is located on ► chromosome 9 and consists of 11 exons. Several SNPs have been described (Halushka et al. 2003), of which so far only some single nucleotide polymorphisms have drawn attention regarding a possible functional consequence leading to a decreased enzyme function or binding affinity. This was based on a computerized evaluation of the likelihood that a resulting amino acid exchange would lead to a phenotypic alteration (Ulrich et al. 2002). The SNPs 22C>T (arginine to tryptophan at position 8, R8W) and 50>T (proline to leucine at position 17, P17L) in ▶ exon 2 and the SNPs 688G>A (glycine to serine at position 230, G230S) and 709C>A (leucine to methionine at position 237, L237M) in exon 7 were considered as first-line candidates. Using human platelets as a system to study COX–1 activity, ▶ heterozygous carriers of the SNP 50C>T were determined to show a significantly greater inhibition of prostaglandin H_2 production after aspirin exposure than carriers of the CC50 ▶ genotype. The possible mechanism for the increased sensitivity to aspirin was seen in a decrease of COX–1-enzyme levels. Since the 50C>T was found in complete ▶ linkage disequilibrium with -842A>G, a mutation in the COX–1 promoter, this SNP may also account for the functional impact, possibly because ▶ gene transcription is repressed (Halushka et al. 2003). However, with an allele frequency of 18% in Caucasians, a multitude of patients would be affected, but the overall contribution of these SNPs in explaining the interindividual variability of the pharmacological response to NSAIDs still remains to be determined.

Polymorphisms in the Cyclooxygenase-2 Gene

For the COX–2 gene on chromosome 1, a substantial number of SNPs was described for the promoter and the ten exons. However, so far, only the polymorphism -765G>C in the promoter was linked to a significantly lower promoter activity for carriers of the -765C- ▶ allele, displaying decreased plasma levels of the C-reactive protein in patients with coronary heart surgery (Papafili et al. 2002). How this polymorphism may eventually interfere with NSAID-induced effects still remains unclear, but because carriers of the CC-765 genotype presented with a more severe course of aspirin-induced asthma, reflected by an increased consummation of oral corticosteroids (Szczeklik et al. 2004), a possible relevance is under consideration.

Polymorphisms in Metabolizing Enzyme Genes

Many NSAIDs are hepatically metabolized by the cytochrome P450 (CYP) system. Diclofenac, ibuprofen, flurbiprofen, naproxen, piroxicam, tenoxicam, meloxicam, mefenamic acid and celecoxib are listed as substrates for one of the most important isoforms, CYP2C9. Polymorphisms in the CYP2C9 gene are recognized to account for variable NSAID pharmacokinetics. Among numerous mutations, the alleles CYP2C9*2 (Cys144, Ile359, Asp360) and CYP2C9*3 (Arg144, Leu359, Asp360) are of particular importance in the Caucasian population, due to the reduced intrinsic

metabolic activity combined with a high allele frequency of 8–14% and 4–16%, respectively. For flurbiprofen, which is exclusively metabolized by CYP2C9, most of the pharmacokinetic variability could be explained by the CYP2C9 genotype, with most pronounced effects in carriers of the CYP2C9*3-allele (Lee et al. 2003). That the CYP2C9*3-allele is mostly responsible for the interindividual variability was also seen when the oral clearance of celecoxib was reduced more than two-fold in ▶ homozygous carriers of the CYP2C9*3 allele as compared to the non-mutated volunteers, while no significant influence was determined for the CYP2C9*2 allele (Kirchheiner et al. 2003). In the presence of nonfunctional CYP2C9-alleles, other cytochrome isoforms (CYP3A4) might compensate by increasing their contribution. This might be the reason why no evidence was seen that CYP2C9 mutations were a determinant for the diclofenac-induced hepatotoxicity (Aithal et al. 2000). Significant pharmacokinetic differences were also seen for racemic and S-(+)-ibuprofen between carriers of one or two CYP2C9*3 alleles and non-mutated alleles (Kirchheiner et al. 2002), while the CYP2C9*2 variant only displayed a compromised metabolic activity when found in combination with the CYP2C8*3 (K139, R399) mutation (Garcia-Martin et al. 2004). In fact, the two alleles CYP2C9*2 and CYP2C8*3 were shown to be in linkage disequilibrium (Yasar et al. 2002). Further information about CYP450 alleles is available at http://www.imm.ki.se/CYPalleles/.

The metabolism of NSAIDs further involves glucuronidation by uridine 5t'-diphosphoglucose glucuronosyl transferase (UGT) enzymes. Since most NSAIDs first undergo CYP450-mediated transformation to inactive metabolites, it is rather unlikely that UGT-alleles with a compromised catalytic activity cause a change in drug response due to drug accumulation. However, this perception may be challenged by rofecoxib, which after UGT2B15-mediated glucuronidation with minor contribution of UGT2B7 and UGT1A9 (Zhang et al. 2003), and deglucuronidation in the lower gastrointestinal tract, may cycle enterohepatically and reappear again in the plasma as rofecoxib. This explains the observed second maximum concentration peak in the concentration-time curves (Baillie et al. 2001), and serves as an example that mutations rendering the UGT less metabolically active could gain clinical importance in special circumstances. The current nomenclature can be accessed at http://som.flinders.edu.au/FUSA/ClinPharm/UGT/allele_table.html.

Substrates of the N-acetyltransferase 2 (NAT2) show three different acetylation phenotypes depending on the possession of two non-mutated alleles (fast), two mutated alleles (slow) or one non-mutated allele combined with a mutated allele (intermediate). The current knowledge that alleles are associated with a compromised catalytic function can be retrieved from

N

http://www.louisville.edu/medschool/pharmacology/ NAT.html. NAT2 plays an important role in the detoxification of sulfasalazine metabolites; hence accumulation in slow acetylator genotypes was associated with the onset of adverse reactions such as infectious mononucleosis-like syndrome (Ohtani et al. 2003), acute pancreatitis (Tanigawara et al. 2002), discoid (Sabbagh et al. 1997) or systemic lupus erythematosus (Gunnarsson et al. 1997). Metamizol (dipyrone) also qualifies as an NAT2-substrate, but differences in drug response according to the acetylation ► phenotype have not yet been reported. The distribution of the polymorphic alleles in the NAT2 gene is an example of the relevance of the ethnic background, since frequency of genotypes associated with fast or intermediate acetylation ranges from approx. 40% in the European population to approx. 90% in the Japanese.

Impact of Non-Functional Alleles on Drug-Drug-Interaction

A patient genotyped as a compound carrier of non-functional CYP2C9*2/*3 alleles presented with normal INR values after therapeutic warfarin dosing. However, when a concomitant analgesic therapy was introduced with celecoxib, the INR rapidly increased (>10) with extensive ecchymosis (Malhi et al. 2004). The impaired warfarin-metabolizing capacity of the CYP2C9*2/*3 alleles had no clinically significant effect on the INR, but when these CYP2C9*2/*3 alleles were challenged by the second substrate celecoxib, which in addition exhibits a high affinity for CYP2C9, the metabolizing rate of (S)-warfarin via CYP2C9 rapidly decreased, while the metabolism of the 2–5 × less potent (R)-warfarin by CYP 1A2 and 2C19 was not affected. This observation should represent a possible mechanism for how a drug interaction may be elicited in the drug metabolizing system. However, in this particular observation this has to be further elucidated, since the warfarin-celecoxib interaction was not seen in healthy volunteers (Karim et al. 2000).

Celecoxib was shown to inhibit the CYP2D6-mediated metabolism of metoprolol in healthy volunteers, with a more pronounced rise in the plasma concentration-time profile in carriers of two functional alleles as compared to one allele. Such an effect is not anticipated with two mutated alleles leading to a minimum of CYP2D6 catalytic function (poor metabolizer). (Werner et al. 2003). Although little information is available of such induced drug interactions, further research may elucidate more, since over 40 drugs are listed as CYP2D6 substrates (see http://medicine.iupui.edu/flockhart/table.htm).

Aspirin-Induced Asthma

Patients with aspirin-induced asthma represent about 10% of all asthma-diseased adults. Inhibition of COX–1 leads to an excess supply of substrate for lipoxygenases which causes a surplus of bronchoconstrictory leukotrienes, of which cysteinyl-leukotrienes (Cys-LT)

were determined as major mediators. The formation of Cys-LTs is regulated by the leukotriene (LT) C4-synthase gene, where a polymorphism in the promoter (-444A>C) was significantly more frequent in aspirin-induced asthma patients (Sanak et al. 1997; Sanak et al. 2000). However, since a relation of this polymorphism to disease severity or aspirin intolerance was not seen in a large cohort of asthma patients and healthy controls, the functional consequence of the C-444 genotype remains to be determined.

Conclusion

So far, little is known about the impact of pharmacogenetics on the therapeutic effect of NSAIDs. There is evidence that polymorphisms in the major drug metabolizing enzyme cytochrome P450 2C9 lead to a modified pharmacokinetic profile of its substrates, of which diclofenac, ibuprofen, naproxen and celecoxib are the most important ones. Polymorphisms in the drug targets COX–1 and COX–2 might alter drug response, but due to the preliminary character of such data, it is still too early to estimate the clinical relevance.

References

1. Aithal GP, Day CP, Leathart JB et al. (2000) Relationship of Polymorphism in CYP2C9 to Genetic Susceptibility to Diclofenac-Induced Hepatitis. Pharmacogenetics 10:511–518
2. Baillie TA, Halpin RA, Matuszewski BK et al. (2001) Mechanistic Studies on the Reversible Metabolism of Rofecoxib to 5-Hydroxyrofecoxib in the Rat: Evidence for Transient Ring Opening of a Substituted 2-Furanone Derivative using Stable Isotope-Labeling Techniques. Drug Metab Dispos 29:1614–1628
3. Garcia-Martin E, Martinez C, Tabares B et al. (2004) Interindividual Variability in Ibuprofen Pharmacokinetics is Related to Interaction of Cytochrome P450 2C8 and 2C9 Amino Acid Polymorphisms. Clin Pharmacol Ther 76:119–127
4. Gunnarsson I, Kanerud L, Pettersson E et al. (1997) Predisposing Factors in Sulphasalazine-Induced Systemic Lupus Erythematosus. Br J Rheumatol 36:1089–1094
5. Halushka MK, Walker LP, Halushka PV (2003) Genetic Variation in Cyclooxygenase 1: Effects on Response to Aspirin. Clin Pharmacol Ther 73:122–130
6. Karim A, Tolbert D, Piergies A et al. (2000) Celecoxib does not Significantly Alter the Pharmacokinetics or Hypoprothrombinemic Effect of Warfarin in Healthy Subjects. J Clin Pharmacol 40:655–663
7. Kirchheiner J, Meineke I, Freytag G et al. (2002) Enantiospecific Effects of Cytochrome P450 2C9 Amino Acid Variants on Ibuprofen Pharmacokinetics and on the Inhibition of Cyclooxygenases 1 and 2. Clin Pharmacol Ther 72:62–75
8. Kirchheiner J, Stormer E, Meisel C et al. (2003) Influence of CYP2C9 Genetic Polymorphisms on Pharmacokinetics of Celecoxib and its Metabolites. Pharmacogenetics 13:473–480
9. Lee CR, Pieper JA, Frye RF et al. (2003) Differences in Flurbiprofen Pharmacokinetics between CYP2C9*1/*1, *1/*2, and *1/*3 Genotypes. Eur J Clin Pharmacol 58:791–794
10. Malhi H, Atac B, Daly AK et al. (2004) Warfarin and Celecoxib Interaction in the Setting of Cytochrome P450 (CYP2C9) Polymorphism with Bleeding Complication. Postgrad Med J 80:107–109
11. Ohtani, T., A. Hiroi, M. Sakurane and F. Furukawa (2003) Slow Acetylator Genotypes as a Possible Risk Factor for Infectious Mononucleosis-Like Syndrome Induced by Salazosulfapyridine. Br J Dermatol 148:1035–1039
12. Papafili A, Hill MR, Brull DJ et al. (2002) Common Promoter Variant in Cyclooxygenase-2 Represses Gene Expression: Ev-

idence of Role in Acute-Phase Inflammatory Response. Arterioscler Thromb Vasc Biol 22:1631–1636

13. Sabbagh N, Delaporte E, Marez D et al. 1997) NAT2 Genotyping and Efficacy of Sulfasalazine in Patients with Chronic Discoid Lupus Erythematosus. Pharmacogenetics 7:131–135
14. Sanak M, Pierzchalska M, Bazan-Socha S et al. (2000) Enhanced Expression of the Leukotriene C(4) Synthase due to Overactive Transcription of an Allelic Variant Associated with Aspirin-Intolerant Asthma. Am J Respir Cell Mol Biol 23:290–296
15. Sanak M, Simon HU, Szczeklik A (1997) Leukotriene C4 Synthase Promoter Polymorphism and Risk of Aspirin-Induced Asthma. Lancet 350:1599–1600
16. Szczeklik W, Sanak M, Szczeklik A (2004) Functional Effects and Gender Association of COX–2 Gene Polymorphism G-765C in Bronchial Asthma. J Allergy Clin Immunol 114:248–253
17. Tanigawara Y, Kita T, Aoyama N et al. (2002) N-acetyltransferase 2 Genotype-Related Sulfapyridine Acetylation and its Adverse Events. Biol Pharm Bull 25:1058–1062
18. Ulrich CM, Bigler J, Sibert J et al. (2002) Cyclooxygenase-1 (COX1) Polymorphisms in African-American and Caucasian Populations. Hum Mutat 20:409–410
19. Werner U, Werner D, Rau T et al. (2003) Celecoxib Inhibits Metabolism of Cytochrome P450 2D6 Substrate Metoprolol in Humans. Clin Pharmacol Ther 74:130–137
20. Yasar U, Lundgren S, Eliasson E et al. (2002) Linkage between the CYP2C8 and CYP2C9 Genetic Polymorphisms. Biochem Biophys Res Commun 299:25–28
21. Yazdanian M, Briggs K, Jankovsky C et al. 2004) The "High Solubility" Definition of the Current FDA Guidance on Biopharmaceutical Classification System may be too Strict for Acidic Drugs. Pharm Res 21:293–299
22. Zhang JY, Zhan J, Cook CS et al. (2003) Involvement of Human UGT2B7 and 2B15 in Rofecoxib Metabolism. Drug Metab Dispos 31:652–658

NSAIDs, Pharmacokinetics

BRUNO OERTEL, JÖRN LÖTSCH
Institute for Clinical Pharmacology, Pharmaceutical Center Frankfurt, Johann Wolfgang Goethe University, Frankfurt, Germany
j.loetsch@em.uni-frankfurt.de

Synonyms

Plasma Concentration Versus Time Profiles; Pharmacokinetics of the NSAIDs

Definition

The pharmacokinetics describes the journey of a drug molecule through the body. The journey includes its release from the drug product, its ▶ absorption into the body system, for some substances its bio-activation via ▶ metabolism, the ▶ distribution to its site of action and back into the blood, and its ▶ elimination from the body either via transformation into inactive metabolites, which are then excreted, or direct excretion of the active entity. The goal of pharmacokinetics is to describe the time course of the drug concentrations in the organism in order to derive dosing regimens that provide most effective clinical drug actions with least side effects.

Characteristics

NSAIDs are mainly administered orally. Formulations for intravenous, intramuscular, topical, rectal or intraocular administration are also available for some NSAIDs. The pharmacokinetics of the NSAIDs is best described by the LADME model, which describes the Liberation, Absorption, Distribution, Metabolism and Elimination of a drug. The concentration versus time profiles of the drug depends on these five processes.

The ▶ liberation of the active ingredient from a pharmaceutical product is mainly the result of the galenic engineering (tablet coating, tablet disintegration, particle size, etc.). Enteric- and sustained release-coatings are often used with NSAIDs to reduce their gastrointestinal toxicity. While the effectiveness of the coating for reduction of the toxicity is doubted, its influence on the absorption of the drug due to delayed release is clear. Once freed from the pharmaceutical formulation, the absorption of a drug is mainly defined by its physicochemical properties. Most of the NSAIDs are carbonic acids, or at least have an acidic function in their molecular structure. They pass the gastrointestinal wall by a passive ▶ diffusion process and are rapidly and extensively absorbed from the stomach and proximal small intestine, with peak plasma concentrations generally occurring within 2–3 h post-administration, or within 30 min in the case of fast release formulations. However, although absorption is extensive, some NSAIDs (e.g. diclofenac) have a low ▶ bioavailability because they are subject to a considerable ▶ First-Pass Metabolism that takes place in the intestinal wall and in the liver. Most NSAIDs are metabolised by ▶ phase-1 metabolic reactions such as oxidation, hydroxylation, demethylation, deacetylation, and hepatic conjunctions (▶ phase–2 metabolic reactions such as glucuronidation and sulphation), or both, with subsequent excretion into urine or bile. In addition, acetyl salicylic acid is deacetylated directly in the blood. The lower the bioavailability is, the fewer molecules reach the circulation and are available for transport to their site of action. Once the molecules of the NSAIDs have reached the blood, they are extensively bound to plasma proteins, especially to albumin. Their ▶ volume of distribution (Vd) is usually small, mainly between 0.1 and 0.3 l/kg body weight, which approximates plasma volume. After excretion into the bile, several NSAIDs undergo an ▶ enterohepatic recirculation. That is, they are re-absorbed from the intestine after cleavage of the phase–2-conjugates (i.e. glucuronides or sulphates) by intestinal human or bacterial glucuronidases or sulfatases. Depending on the elimination process (metabolism or excretion via the kidney or the bile), NSAIDs differ in their speed of elimination, which is usually numerically characterized by the ▶ elimination half-life values ($t_{1/2}$). The half-life of the NSAIDs can vary within and between individuals due to organ damage (i.e. kidney or liver

N

failure) or due to genetic polymorphisms of the enzymes involved in the metabolism of the NSAIDs. For example, some NSAIDs are metabolised via cytochrome P450 2C9 (CYP2C9), for which mutations resulting in a less-functional or non-functional enzyme have been described. Furthermore, pharmacokinetic drug-drug interactions can occur that results in inhibition of enzymes or of transporters involved in the elimination of the NSAIDs, with the consequence of altered, often decreased, rates of elimination, and thus increased half-lives of the NSAIDs (Davies and Skjodt 2000).

In the following, the pharmacokinetic properties will be described in more detail for the particular class of NSAIDs.

Salicylic Acid Derivatives

The salicylic acid derivatives are rapidly and completely absorbed after oral administration. The reduced bioavailability and very short elimination half-life of acetyl salicylic acid is the result of an extensive first-pass metabolism by hydrolysis of acetyl salicylic acid to salicylic acid and acetic acid (Fig. 1), which takes place while passing the gastrointestinal mucosa, in the liver and in the blood. Due to the irreversible acetylation of the amino acid serine at position 530 of the COX-1 protein in platelets, the half-life of the anti-thrombotic effect of acetyl salicylic acid is much longer than the half-life of acetyl salicylic acid in plasma. Thus, a clinically relevant aggregation of platelets will only be re-established after enough new platelets have been produced, which is several days after administration of acetyl salicylic acid, at a time when the drug has already completely been eliminated from plasma for some days.

Salicylic acid is an active metabolite of acetyl salicylic acid. It has a longer elimination half-life than acetyl salicylic acid. During treatment with high or repetitive doses of salicylic acid or diflunisal, the elimination half-life can increase due to saturation of liver enzymes involved in the metabolism (non-linear kinetic). Salicylic acid and its metabolites are excreted via the kidney. The renal elimination rate of salicylic acid is influenced by the urinary pH. Therefore, acidifying agents (e.g. ammonium chloride) decrease its excretion, while alkalinising agents such as sodium bicarbonate increase the urinary excretion. Salicylates can displace the anticonvulsants phenytoin and valproic acid from their plasma protein binding sites, and prevents the elimination of

valproic acid due to inhibition of its main metabolic pathway, the β-oxidation. To prevent intoxication due to increased free plasma levels, combination of the drugs should be avoided (Brouwers and de Smet 1994; Needs and Brooks 1985).

In contrast to other salicylic acid derivatives, sulfasalazine and its active metabolite 5-aminosalicylic acid are only poorly absorbed, and therefore remain mainly within the gastrointestinal tract. Sulfasalazine and salsalat are prodrugs, and are mainly used for the treatment of ulcerative colitis and Crohnt's disease. While salsalat is an ester of two salicylic acid molecules, which is rapidly absorbed and then hydrolysed, the anti-inflammatory effect of sulfasalazine is probably attributed to its metabolite 5-aminosalicylic acid.

Arylpropionic Acids

Chirality results when three-dimensional repositioning produces different forms (enantiomers) of the same molecule. A chiral drug exists as a pair of molecules that are each other's mirror image, called S-enantiomer and R-enantiomer. The most common example of chirality is a sp^3-hybridised tetrahydral carbon atom, to which 4 different atoms are attached (Fig. 2). Such a sp^3-hybridised tetrahedral chiral carbon atom is the common structural feature of the arylpropionic acids, and is located within their propionic acid side chain. Most of the arylpropionic acids are marketed as racemats, i.e. as mixtures of both enantiomers. In addition, pure S-enantiomers are available for ibuprofen and ketoprofen. Naproxen is available and clinically used only as S-enantiomer. This is because the S-enantiomers have been shown to possess almost the whole pharmacologic activity. However, more recent studies have also demonstrated some pharmacologic effects of the R-enantiomers.

Enantiomers of arylpropionic acids have different physical properties such as water solubility and differ in their pharmacokinetics. For example, a stereoselectivity, i.e., a different pharmacokinetic behaviour of the S- and R-enantiomers of ibuprofen and flurbiprofen has been reported (Davies and Skjodt 2000). Some arylpropionic

Aspirin (ASA)   Salicylic acid   Acetic acid

NSAIDs, Pharmacokinetics, Figure 1 Hydrolysis of acetyl salicylic acid.

Diclofenac   **4′-Hydroxy-Diclofenac**

NSAIDs, Pharmacokinetics, Figure 2 Chirality of the arylpropionic acids.

NSAIDs, Pharmacokinetics, Table 1 Pharmacokinetics of the salicylic acid derivates

Drug	F [%]	PB [%]	t_{Max} [h]	Vd [L/kg]	CL [L/h/kg]	$t_{1/2}$ [h]	Active Metabolites	Remarks
Salicylic acid (SA)	100	80–90	0.5–2	0.17	4.2	2–3 (–30)	No	Dose-dependent half-life due to saturation of liver enzymes involved in the metabolism
Aspirin (ASA)	68	85–95	0.4–0.5	0.15	0.6–3.6	14–20 min	Salicylic acid (SA)	Hydrolysis through non-specific esterases while passing the gut wall, in plasma and liver
Diflunisal	100	99.8	2–3	0.10	0.0066	5–20	No	Dose-dependent half-life due to saturation of liver enzymes involved in the metabolism
Sulfasalazine (Prodrug)	<15	>99.3	3–12	NR	1	4–11	5-Aminosalicylic acid (F = 10–30%, t_{Max} 10 h)	Bacteria mediated splitting in anti-inflammatory active 5-Aminosalicylic acid and sulfapyridine. Half-life dependent on slow or fast acetylation by polymorphic enzyme
Salsalate (Prodrug)	100	NR	1.5	NR	NR	1.1(–16)	Salicylic acid (SA)	Rapid esterase hydrolysis in two molecules of salicylic acid in the small intestine and plasma

F: oral bioavailability, PB: binding to plasma proteins, t_{Max}: time from administration until maximum plasma concentrations are reached, Vd/F: volume of distribution, divided by bioavailability (because data from systemic administration that are needed to calculate the true Vd are usually not available, and the volumes are derived from data after oral drug administration, and have therefore been corrected for bioavailability), CL. Drug clearance, describing the speed of its elimination from the body, $t_{1/2}$: half-life in plasma

NSAIDs, Pharmacokinetics, Table 2 Pharmacokinetics of the arylpropionic acid derivates

Drug	F [%]	PB [%]	t_{Max} [h]	Vd [L/kg]	CL [L/h/kg]	$t_{1/2}$ [h]	Active Metabolites	Remarks
Ibuprofen (Rac/S) *	100	98–99	1–2	0.15	0.045	1.5–3	No	Unidirectional inversion to S-(+)-enantiomer with an inversion-rate R:S=50-80%. Metabolising enzymes (Phase 1): CYP2C9. Dose-dependent binding to plasma proteins
Flurbiprofen (Rac) *	100	>99	1.5	0.1	0.018	3–6	No	Unidirectional inversion to S-(+)-enantiomer. Inversion-rate R:S=0-5%
Ketoprofen (Rac/S) *	81-84	98.7	0.5-3	0.11	0.072	2–4	No	Unidirectional inversion to S-(+)-enantiomer. Inversion-rate R:S 10%
Naproxen (S) *	100	>99	2–4	0.10–0.16	0.0042	12–15	No	Dose-dependent binding to plasma proteins
Tiaprofenic acid (Rac) *	100	98	NR	0.4–1	0.036–0.084	3-6	No	Negligible R to S conversion upon oral administration
Fenoprofen (Rac) *	NR	>99	2	0.08–0.11	NR	1.5–3	NR	

* available as racemate and/or single S-(+)-enatiomer

F: oral bioavailability, PB: binding to plasma proteins, t_{Max}: time from administration until maximum plasma concentrations are reached, Vd/F: volume of distribution, divided by bioavailability (because data from systemic administration that are needed to calculate the true Vd are usually not available, and the volumes are derived from data after oral drug administration, and have therefore been corrected for bioavailability), CL. Drug clearance, describing the speed of its elimination from the body, $t_{1/2}$: half-life in plasma

acids undergo a unidirectional inversion of the inactive R-enantiomer to the active S- enantiomer (Fig. 3). The extent of the inversion is variable from drug to drug and is most substantial for R-(-)-ibuprofen, while it is negligible for R-(-)-flurbiprofen (Table 2) (Geisslinger et al. 1994).

Diclofenac   **Lumiracoxib**

NSAIDs, Pharmacokinetics, Figure 3 Unidirectional inversion of the arylpropionic acids.

The arylpropionic acids get fast and near complete absorption. They have no extensive first-pass metabolism and their elimination is, with the exception of naproxen, quite fast. Ibuprofen and naproxen bind in a concentration-dependent manner to plasma proteins. There is an increase in the unbound fraction of the drug at doses greater than 600 mg and 500 mg, respectively, resulting in an increased ► clearance and reduced area under curve (AUC) of the total-drug. A decreased clearance of S-(+)-ibuprofen is reported in carriers of certain genetic polymorphisms, which results in a CYP2C9 enzyme with decreased or absent functionality (see ► NSAIDs, Pharmacogenetics).

Heteroaryl Acetic Acids

Diclofenac, aceclofenac, ketorolac and lumiracoxib are heteroaryl acetic acids. They are fast and nearly completely absorbed. Due to an extensive first pass metabolism, diclofenac has a decreased systemic availability. The primary metabolite of diclofenac, 4'-hydroxy-diclofenac (Fig. 4), is produced by the genetically polymorphic CYP2C9. The amount of 4'-hydroxy-diclofenac excreted in urine and bile accounts

for 30% and 10–20%, respectively, of an oral dose of diclofenac (van der Marel et al. 2004). Data from experiments in laboratory animals suggest that 4'-hydroxy-diclofenac has 30% of the anti-inflammatory and antipyretic activity of diclofenac. Aceclofenac, an ester of diclofenac, appears to inhibit both COX isoforms through conversion into diclofenac and its metabolite 4'-hydroxy-diclofenac (Hinz et al. 2003). Ketorolac is a chiral NSAID and is marketed as a racemic mixture of the S-(-)- and the R-(+)-enantiomeric isoforms. The S-(-)-form possesses the analgesic and ulcerogenic activity. There is no evidence for an inversion of R-(+)-ketorolac to S-(-)-ketorolac in man, but the pharmacokinetics of ketorolac shows enantioselectivity. The S-(-)-form has a two times shorter plasma half-life and greater clearance in adults than the R-(+)-Form, and the elimination half-life of S-(-)-ketorolac seems to be further increased in children (Kauffman et al. 1999; Mroszczak et al. 1996). While the other heteroaryl acetic acids are classical NSAIDs, lumiracoxib is a selective inhibitor of COX–2. Its molecular structure is very similar to that of diclofenac (Fig. 5) and very different from the other COX–2 selective agents (diarylheterocycles). This difference is reflected in the pharmacokinetic properties of lumiracoxib, which are more similar to those of the classical acidic NSAIDs than to the diarylheterocycles.

Diarylheterocycles

The diarylheterocycles (celecoxib, rofecoxib, etoricoxib, and oxaprozin) have a higher selectivity to the COX–2 isoform compared to the classical NSAIDs. With the exception of oxaprozin, the diarylheterocycles do not possess an acidic function in their molecule. They are very lipophilic and poorly water-soluble. Since absorption of the drug molecules requires their

NSAIDs, Pharmacokinetics, Figure 4 Primary metabolite of diclofenac.

NSAIDs, Pharmacokinetics, Table 3 Pharmacokinetics of the Heteroaryl acetic acids

Drug	F [%]	PB [%]	t_{Max} [h]	Vd [L/kg]	CL [L/h/kg]	$t_{1/2}$ [h]	Active Metabolites	Remarks
Diclofenac	30–80	>99	0.37–89	0.1–0.2	0.26–0.45	1.1–1.7	4't-Hydroxy-Diclofenac (30% activity of diclofenac in animal models)	Extensive first-pass metabolism Metabolising enzymes (Phase 1): CYP2C9, CYP3A4, CYP3A5 Prodrug of diclofenac: Aceclofenac
Tolmetin	100	99-	0.5–1	0.1	NR	2 (5)	No	Biphasic elimination with a rapid phase ($t_{1/2} = 2$ h), followed by a slow phase ($t_{1/2} = 5$ h)
Ketorolac (Rac)	80–100	>99	0.3–1	0.1–0.3	0.03	2.1–2.9(S) 3.3–6.7[®]	No	S-(-)-Ketorolac is the active enantiomer Stereoselective metabolism with increased clearance for the active S-(-)-enantiomer
Lumiracoxib	66–80.8	>98	1-4	7.3–10.7 (L)	NR	3-6	4'-Hydroxy-Lumiracoxib (Potency and selectivity is similar to Lumiracoxib)	Metabolising enzymes (Phase 1): CYP2C9

F: oral bioavailability, PB: binding to plasma proteins, t_{Max}: time from administration until maximum plasma concentrations are reached, Vd/F: volume of distribution, divided by bioavailability (because data from systemic administration that are needed to calculate the true Vd are usually not available, and the volumes are derived from data after oral drug administration, and have therefore been corrected for bioavailability), CL. Drug clearance, describing the speed of its elimination from the body, $t_{1/2}$: half-life in plasma

NSAIDs, Pharmacokinetics, Table 4 Pharmacokinetics of the Diarylheterocycles

Drug	F [%]	PB [%]	t_{Max} [h]	Vd [L]	CL [L/h]	$t_{1/2}$ [h]	Active Metabolites	Remarks
Celecoxib	NR (22–40 in dogs)	>97	2–3	339–571	23.7–27.8	8–12	No	Metabolising enzymes (Phase 1): CYP2C9, CYP3A4
Rofecoxib	92–93	85	2–4	86–91	7.2–8.5	10–17	No	Metabolism: Cytosolic Reduction
Valdecoxib	83	>98	3	54.5	6	8-11	Yes (10% of the Valdecoxib dose with decreased anti-inflammatory activity)	Prodrug of Valdecoxib: Parecoxib (i.v.) Metabolising enzymes (Phase 1): CYP2C9, CYP3A4, Non-CYP450
Etoricoxib	100	NR	0.5–1.5	82–156	4.92–8.04	18.9–30.9	NR	-
Oxaprozin	95	99	2.4–3.1	0.16–0.24 (L/kg)	0.15–0.3 (L/h/kg)	41.4–54.9	No	-

F: oral bioavailability, PB: binding to plasma proteins, t_{Max}: time from administration until maximum plasma concentrations are reached, Vd/F: volume of distribution, divided by bioavailability (because data from systemic administration that are needed to calculate the true Vd are usually not available, and the volumes are derived from data after oral drug administration, and have therefore been corrected for bioavailability), CL. Drug clearance, describing the speed of its elimination from the body, $t_{1/2}$: half-life in plasma

dissolution in fluids, special formulations have had to be developed to enhance their water solubility, and thus to ensure their absorption. Compared to the classical NSAIDs, diarylheterocycles show very different pharmacokinetics, particularly the volume of distribution, the plasma clearance and the elimination half-life (Ahuja et al. 2003; Alsalameh et al. 2003).

Enolic Acids

Members of the enolic acids family (piroxicam, meloxicam, tenoxicam, lornoxicam) are weakly acidic by virtue of the enolic 4-hydroxy substituent (Fig. 6). They are well absorbed and extensively bound to plasma proteins. Due to this plasma protein binding, their apparent volumes of distribution are small. They are

NSAIDs, Pharmacokinetics, Table 5   Pharmacokinetics of the Enolic acids

Drug	F [%]	PB [%]	t Max [h]	Vd [L/kg]	CL [L/h/kg]	t 1/2 [h]	Active Metabolites	Remarks
Piroxicam	NR (100)	99	2–3	0.1–0.2	0.002–0.003	30–70	No	Prodrugs of piroxicam: Ampiroxicam, droxicam, pivoxicam
Meloxicam	100	>99.5	3–9	0.1–0.2	0.0066	20	No	Metabolising enzymes (Phase 1): CYP2C9
Tenoxicam	100	>98.5	2	0.15	0.001–0.002	49–81	No	Metabolising enzymes (Phase 1): CYP2C9
Isoxicam	100	98	10	0.1–0.2	0.3 (L/h)	30–50	No	Increased $t_{1/2}$ for about 10% of a population, eventually due to polymorphic enzyme
Lornoxicam	NR	99.7	0.5–2.5	0.1–0.2	1.5–3.4 (L/h)	3–5	NR	Metabolising enzymes (Phase 1): CYP2C9
Azapropa-zone	60-100	>99.5	3–6	8.4–15.4 (L)	0.48-0.73 (L/h)	11.5–17.1	NR	-
Phenyl-butazone	90	>98	NR	0.02-0.15	0.09 (L/h)	29–175	Oxyphen-butazone γ-Hydroxy-phenyl-butazone	Dose-dependent half-life
Oxyphen-butazone	NR	97–98	NR	0.15	NR	27–64	NR	-

F: oral bioavailability, PB: binding to plasma proteins, t_{Max}: time from administration until maximum plasma concentrations are reached, Vd/F: volume of distribution, divided by bioavailability (because data from systemic administration that are needed to calculated the true Vd are usually not available and the volumes are derived from data after oral drug administration and have therefore be corrected for bioavailability), CL. Drug clearance, describing the speed of its elimination from the body, $t_{1/2}$: half-life in plasma

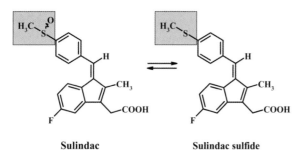

Sulindac   **Sulindac sulfide**

NSAIDs, Pharmacokinetics, Figure 5   Structural similarity of lumiracoxib to classical NSAIDs.

(R)-Enantiomer | **(S)-Enantiomer**

NSAIDs, Pharmacokinetics, Figure 6   Acidic nature of piroxicam.

mainly eliminated by hepatic metabolism (Olkkola et al. 1994). The polymorphic CYP2C9 provides the major catabolic pathway for tenoxicam and meloxicam, and are therefore candidates for an altered pharmacokinetic due to genetic polymorphisms (see ▶ NSAIDs, Pharmacogenetics). The elimination is usually slow. The elimination half-lives of the oxicams are long, with the exception of lornoxicam. Therefore, the oxicams have a tendency to accumulate in patients.

Phenylbutazone and oxyphenbutazone tend to accumulate due to the slow metabolism and renal elimination. In addition, they have a high potential to interact with other drugs, particularly with oral anticoagulants, anticonvulsants and oral antihyperglycaemic agents, by either inhibiting metabolic pathways or by displacement from plasma protein binding sites (Brouwers and de Smet 1994).

Indole and Indene Acetic Acids

Indomethacin, its prodrug acemetacin, sulindac and etodolac are all accounted to the indole and indene acetic acids. Their bioavailability is high and their binding to plasma proteins after absorption is extensive. They undergo extensive enterohepatic circulation, which results in a prolonged elimination half-life compared to the other NSAIDs because the already eliminated drug is re-absorbed. About 60% of an oral dose of indomethacine is excreted in the urine, while about 40% is excreted in the faeces after biliary secretion (Helleberg 1981).

Nursing Home Residents

Definition

Chronic pain is more frequent in nursing home residents than in a community sample. Uncontrolled pain is a frequent cause of admission to nursing homes.
▶ Psychological Treatment of Pain in Older Populations

Nutraceuticals

SCOTT MASTERS
Caloundra Spinal and Sports Medicine Centre,
Caloundra, QLD, Australia
scotty1@ozemail.com.au

Synonyms

Glucosamine; chondroitin; Avocado-Soybean-Unsaponifiables

Definition

▶ Nutraceuticals are loosely defined as foods with a health benefit. They are naturally occurring substances that can be used as drugs in order to treat specific symptoms, or to modify disease processes. In the field of osteoarthritis, four nutraceuticals have been recognised and studied: ▶ glucosamine, ▶ chondroitin, glycosaminoglycan polysulfuric acid, and ▶ Avocado-Soybean-Unsaponifiables (ASU).

Glucosamine is a hexosamine sugar that is a component of almost all human tissues. It is one of the two molecules that form the repeating units of certain glycosaminoglycans, which in turn form the matrix of all connective tissues (Deal and Moskowitz 1999). Glycosaminoglycans, and therefore glucosamine, form a large component of articular cartilage, which is the tissue that is primarily damaged in osteoarthritis.

Chondroitin sulphate is the principal glycosaminoglycan found in articular cartilage. It is composed of a long unbranched polysaccharide chain, with a repeating disaccharide structure of N-acetyl galactosamine and glucuronic acid (Deal and Moskowitz 1999). Chondroitin sulphate is a strongly charged polyanion, which endows cartilage with water-binding properties. Functionally, this allows the cartilage matrix to absorb compression forces, and thereby protect the underlying bone from damage.

Glycosaminoglycan polysulfuric acid is an extract from bovine cartilage and bone marrow, which contains a variety of glycosaminoglycans, including chondroitin and chondroitin sulphate (Pavelka et al. 1995; Pavelka et al. 2000).

ASUs are unsaponifiable fractions of one-third avocado oil and two-thirds soybean oil (Maheu et al. 1998; Blotman et al. 1997; Appleboom et al. 2001).

Characteristics

Mechanism

Glucosamine has been shown to reach the articular cartilage after oral, intra-muscular and intravenous administration (Deal and Moskowitz 1999; McAlindon et al. 2000; Pavelka et al. 2003). It is preferentially incorporated by human chondrocytes into GAGS (Deal and Moskowitz 1999; Pavelka et al. 2003), and stimulates the synthesis of proteoglycans (Deal and Moskowitz 1999; McAlindon et al. 2000; Pavelka et al. 2003; Reginster et al. 2001).

Glucosamine and chondroitin sulphate have been shown to have anti-inflammatory effects (Deal and Moskowitz 1999; Pavelka et al. 2003; Reginster et al. 2001), positive effects on cartilage metabolism *in vitro*, and anti-arthritic effects in animal models (Deal and Moskowitz 1999; McAlindon et al. 2000; Towheed et al. 2002). These results suggest possible structure-modifying and disease-modifying roles for glucosamine and chondroitin in osteoarthritis.

In laboratory studies, glycosaminoglycan polysulfuric acid has been found to stimulate cartilage metabolism, and to inhibit the catabolic effects of interleukin-1 (Pavelka et al. 1995; Pavelka et al. 2000).

ASUs have also shown some anti-osteoarthritis properties both *in vitro* and *in vivo* (Maheu et al. 1998; Blotman et al. 1997; Appleboom et al. 2001).

Application

Nutraceuticals have been promoted for the treatment of osteoarthritis, on the grounds that they are natural substances that might promote healing or impede further deterioration of damaged cartilage.

Nutraceuticals are mainly taken by the oral route, as a tablet capsule or powder, and are also available as a cream. Although the majority of trials have focused on osteoarthritis of the knee, nutraceuticals are marketed for relief in a wide variety of conditions e.g. arthritis pain, fibromyalgia, and joint swelling.

Efficacy

One pragmatic (Deal and Moskowitz 1999) and four systematic reviews (McAlindon et al. 2000; Towheed et al. 2002; Richy et al. 2003; Leeb et al. 2000) in the last five years on the use of glucosamine and chondroitin in osteoarthritis reached similar conclusions. A number of randomised controlled trials showed benefits from these agents greater than that of placebo, in terms of reduction of pain and increased function. Others showed equivalent or better efficacy than treatment with ▶ non-steroidal anti-inflammatory drugs (NSAIDs). However, the reviews offer caution regarding the methodological problems associated with many of the studies, and advise that the treatment effects are probably exaggerated.

Important points raised by these reviews include:

N

- The ▶ effect-sizes in the larger and better quality studies are smaller than those of other studies.
- Many trials suffer from inadequate blinding and absence of intention-to-treat analysis of results.
- Publication bias may apply, in that studies with statistically significant and positive results are more likely to be published than studies with negative results.
- Manufacturer support was prevalent in many of the early trials.

These problems are not unique to trials of nutraceuticals, for they have also been noted in trials of drugs for osteoarthritis. Nevertheless, they constitute grounds for caution when interpreting or stating the results of trials. A further factor is that all of the early trials with positive results were of European origin. Later studies, conducted in the USA and in England, have found glucosamine to be no more effective than placebo for the relief of pain (Rindone et al. 2000; Hughes and Carr 2002).

Less contentious is the effect of glucosamine on the prevention of disease progression. Two randomised controlled trials have assessed the long-term effects of glucosamine sulphate on knee osteoarthritis (Pavelka et al. 2003; Reginster et al. 2001). Both studies compared the effects of placebo with that of 1500 mg glucosamine sulphate daily for three years. In both studies, patients treated with glucosamine showed greater reductions in pain, and greater improvements in function, as measured by the Western Ontario and McMaster Universities osteoarthritis index (WOMAC). Both studies also demonstrated significantly less loss of joint space width in those patients treated with glucosamine. The second study (Pavelka et al. 2003) showed that the ▶ NNT for preventing clinically substantial loss of joint space was 11.

For glycosaminoglycan polysulfuric acid the evidence has not been favourable. For the relief of pain it is no more effective than placebo (Pavelka et al. 1995). It does not protect against loss of joint space (Pavelka et al. 2000). Three studies of ASUs found greater reductions in pain and greater improvements in function than those following treatment with placebo ((Maheu et al. 1998; Blotman et al. 1997; Appleboom et al. 2001). These agents also had significant effects in reducing the need of patients to use NSAIDs.

Safety

No major toxicity problems have emerged with the use of these nutraceuticals. In particular, glucosamine has been shown to be safe in the two trials with three-year follow-up (Pavelka et al. 2003; Reginster et al. 2001). Side effects were similar to those of placebo, and no specifically adverse effects were uncovered.

Some chondroitin preparations are derived from bovine cartilage. Due to the recent European epidemic of bovine spongioform encephalopathy (BSE) and its transmission to humans (resulting in variant Creutzfeldt-Jakob disease), all bovine derived products are being re-evaluated for potential transmission risks. On the List of Tissues with Suspected Infectivity (World Health Organisation), bovine cartilage is listed as Category IV (no detectable infectivity). Most other commercially available chondroitin products are derived from shark cartilage.

Conclusions

The evidence for the use of nutraceuticals in the treatment of OA of the knee is growing. However, doubts remain about their effect-size when compared with placebo; and the efficacy of these agents has not been compared with other regimens of long-term treatment of osteoarthritis. It is still not evident if they are a cost–effective substitute for treatment with NSAIDs or exercise; or if they are a worthwhile addition to such treatment. Nor has their efficacy been determined for osteoarthritis of joints other than those studied to date, or for other painful conditions.

References

1. Appleboom T, Scheuermans J, Verbrugger G, Henroitin Y, Reginster JY (2001) Symptoms Modifying Effect of Avocado/Soybean Unsaponifiables (ASU) in Knee Osteoarthritis. A Double Blind, Prospective, Placebo-Controlled Study. Scand J Rheumatol 30:242–247
2. Blotman F, Maheu E, Wulwik A, Caspard H, Lopez A (1997) Efficacy and Safety of Avocado/Soybean Unsaponifiables in the Treatment of Symptomatic Osteoarthritis of the Knee and Hip. A Prospective, Multicenter, Three-Month, Randomized, Double-Blind, Placebo-Controlled Trial. Rev Rhum (Engl Ed) 64:825–834
3. Deal CL, Moskowitz RW (1999) Nutraceuticals as Therapeutic Agents in Osteoarthritis. The Role of Glucosamine, Chondroitin Sulfate, and Collagen Hydrolysate. Rheum Disc Clin N Am 25:379–395
4. Hughes R, Carr A (2002) A Randomised, Double-Blind, Placebo-Controlled Trial of Glucosamine Sulphate as an Analgesic in Osteoarthritis of the Knee. Rheumatology 41:279–284
5. Leeb B, Schweitzer H, Mantag, Smolen JS (2000) A Metaanalysis of Chondroitin Sulfate in the Treatment of Osteoarthritis. J Rheumatol 27:205–211
6. Maheu E, Mazieres B, Valat JP, Loyau G, Le Loet X, Bourgeois P, Grouin JM, Rozenberg S (1998) Symptomatic Efficacy of ASU in the Treatment of Osteoarthritis of the Knee and Hip. Arthritis Rheum 41:81–91
7. McAlindon DM, LaValley MP, Gulin JP, Felson DT (2000) Glucosamine and Chondroitin for Treatment of Osteoarthritis. JAMA 283:1469–1475
8. Pavelka K, Gatterova J, Gollarova V, Urbanova Z, Sedlackova M, Altman RD (2000) A 5-Year Randomised Controlled, Double-Blind Study of Glycosaminoglycan Polysulfuric Acid Complex (Rumalon®) as a Structure Modifying Therapy in Osteoarthritis of the Hip and Knee. Osteoarthritis Cartilage 8:335–342

ship of the pain complaint to the presence of pathology is often unclear in women with chronic pelvic pain. Given the difficulties of applying the IASP pelvic pain definition to clinical research, several medical societies have recently taken a lead in revising the definition of chronic pelvic pain. The International Continence Society has defined "pelvic pain syndrome" as the occurrence of persistent or recurrent episodic pelvic pain associated with symptoms suggestive of lower urinary tract, sexual, bowel or gynecological dysfunction in the absence of proven infection or other obvious pathology (Abrams 2002). The European Association of Urology has suggested to extend this definition by considering two subgroups based on the presence or absence of well-defined conditions that produce pain (Fall 2004). The American College of Obstetricians and Gynecologists has proposed the following definition: chronic pelvic pain is non-cyclic pelvic pain of 6 or more months duration that localizes to the anatomic pelvis, anterior abdominal wall at or below the umbilicus, the lumbosacral back or the buttocks and is of sufficient severity to cause functional disability or lead to medical care. A lack of physical findings does not negate the significance of a patient's pain, and normal examination results do not preclude the possibility of finding pelvic pathology (ACOG 2004).

Some chronic gynecological pain syndromes present with very specific clinical characteristics. ▶ Interstitial cystitis is a chronic pelvic pain syndrome characterized by urinary frequency, urgency and pelvic pain. Women are 10 times more frequently affected than men. Clemons et al. (2002) found that 38% of women presenting with chronic pelvic pain and undergoing laparoscopic evaluation are ultimately diagnosed with interstitial cystitis. Certain chronic gynecological pain syndromes are related to specific phases of the menstrual cycle. ▶ Premenstrual syndrome (ACOG 2000) and ▶ dysmenorrhea are cyclic gynecological pain syndromes associated with gonadal hormonal changes during the menstrual cycle. In the majority of chronic pelvic pain patients no specific pathology can be identified that might account for the pain complaint. However, it is important to keep in mind that chronic pelvic pain can be a typical symptom of certain pelvic diseases and it is imperative to work-up patients appropriately. In women who undergo a ▶ laparoscopy to evaluate chronic pelvic pain, the prevalence of endometriosis is about 33% (Howard 1993). Chronic pelvic pain and pelvic adhesions are well-known sequelae of ▶ pelvic inflammatory disease (PID ▶ Chronic Pelvic Pain, Pelvic Inflammatory Disease and Adhesion). Chronic pelvic pain occurs in up to 36% of women who have suffered from PID and in up to 67% after three or more episodes of PID (Safrin et al. 1992).

In addition to gynecological pain syndromes characterized by pain localized to the pelvic cavity, gynecological pain syndromes localized to the urogenital floor have been described. Specific terms have been coined for these conditions; however, similar to the definitions of chronic pelvic pain, many of these definitions are currently being revised. Chronic perineal pain is referred to as ▶ pudendal neuralgia, if electrophysiological evaluation confirms impairment of the ▶ pudendal nerve (Bensignor et al. 1993). Vulvar pain occurring in the absence of an underlying recognizable disease has become an increasingly common clinical problem and is referred to as ▶ vulvodynia. Two subgroups are recognized (Moyal-Barracco and Lynch 2004), generalized vulvodynia and localized vulvodynia, including pain localized to the vulvar vestibule – ▶ vestibulodynia (vulvar vestibulitis) and to the clitoris – ▶ clitorodynia (clitoral pain) (Gordon 2002). ▶ Dyspareunia is defined as "recurring genital pain associated with sexual activity". The most common form of superficial dyspareunia in pre-menopausal women is provoked vestibulodynia (Harlow et al. 2001). Vaginismus (see ▶ dyspareunia and vaginismus) is defined as recurrent or persistent involuntary ▶ Muscle Spasm of the outer third of the vagina interfering with ▶ sexual intercourse. Like women with dyspareunia, these patients have difficulty with and pain during vaginal penetration activities.

Epidemiology of Chronic Gynecological Pain Syndromes

Epidemiological studies of chronic gynecological pain syndromes are difficult, due to the lack of agreed upon definitions, as discussed above. Epidemiological data from the USA showed that 14.7% of women in their reproductive ages reported chronic pelvic pain (Mathias et al. 1996). Extrapolating to the total female population suggested an estimated 9.2 million chronic pelvic pain sufferers in the United States alone. Analysis of a large primary care database from the United Kingdom demonstrated that the annual prevalence rate of chronic pelvic pain (see ▶ epidemiology of chronic pelvic pain) in women is 38 / 1000, which is comparable to the prevalence rate of asthma (Zondervan et al. 1999a). Diagnoses related to the urinary or gastrointestinal tracts were more common than gynecologic causes (Zondervan et al. 1999b). Populations at risk of having chronic pelvic pain seem to be women with a history of pelvic inflammatory disease, endometriosis, interstitial cystitis, irritable bowel syndrome, obstetric history, previous abdominopelvic surgery, musculoskeletal disorders and physical and sexual abuse (Abrams et al. 2002).

A survey of ▶ Sexual Dysfunctions, analyzing data from the National Health and Social Life Survey, reported that 16% of women between the ages of 18 and

O

59 years living in households throughout the United States experience pain during sex (Laumann et al. 1999). When these data were analyzed by age group, the highest number of women reporting pain during sex was in the 18–29 years age group. The location and etiology of pain was not analyzed in this study. Approximately 15% of pre-menopausal women suffer from vulvar vestibulitis (provoked vestibulodynia), the most common form of superficial dyspareunia (Harlow et al. 2001; Goetsch 1991).

Neurobiology of Gynecological Pain

Over the last 20 years the basic neurobiology of the pelvis, despite the complexity of this region of the body, has come to be a reasonably well-developed discipline (Berkley 2001; Burnett and Wesselmann 1999). In general, the pelvis and the pelvic floor are innervated by both divisions of the autonomic nervous system, the sympathetic and ▶ parasympathetic divisions, as well as by the somatic and sensory nervous systems. In a broad anatomical view, dual projections from the thoracolumbar and sacral segments of the spinal cord carry out this innervation, converging primarily into discrete peripheral neuronal plexuses before distributing nerve fibers throughout the pelvis (Fig. 1). Interactive neuronal pathways routing from higher origins in the brain through the spinal cord add to the complexity of neuronal regulation in the pelvis.

The inferior hypogastric plexus is considered to be the major neuronal integrative center, innervating multiple pelvic organs, including the genital and reproductive tract structures, the urinary bladder, proximal urethra, distal ureter, rectum and internal anal sphincter. The inferior hypogastric plexus receives sympathetic and parasympathetic input. Sympathetic nerves originate in the thoracolumbar segments of the spinal cord (T10-L1) and condense into the ▶ superior hypogastric plexus. Nerve fibers project from the superior hypogastric plexus as paired hypogastric plexuses destined for the inferior hypogastric plexuses. Parasympathetic preganglionic efferents arise from sacral spinal cord segments S2-S4 and fuse as the pelvic splanchnic nerve before entering the inferior hypogastric plexus. Parasympathetic afferents have cell bodies located in the S2-S4 dorsal root ganglia and course also within the pelvic splanchnic nerve. In addition to its parasympathetic efferent and afferent component, the pelvic splanchnic nerve also receives postganglionic axons from the caudal sympathetic chain ganglia. Somatic efferent and afferent innervation to the pelvis is supplied through the sacral nerve roots (S2-S4) and their ramifications. The sacral nerve roots emerge from the spinal cord forming the sacral plexus, from which the pudendal nerve diverges (S2-S3). Traditionally it was thought that ascending pathways for visceral and other types

of pain were mainly the spinothalamic and spinoreticular tracts. However, three previously undescribed pathways that carry visceral nociceptive information have been discovered, the dorsal column pathway, the spino(trigemino)-parabrachio-amygdaloid pathway and the spino-hypothalamic pathway (Cervero and Laird 1999). Specifically the dorsal column pathways play a key role in the processing of pelvic pain and neurosurgeons have successfully used punctate midline myelotomy to relieve pelvic pain due to cancer (Willis and Westlund 2001).

The gynecological pain syndromes belong to the category of visceral pain syndromes (Wesselmann 1999a). Research in animal models of visceral pain has shown that several kinds of sensory receptors exist in most internal organs and that different pain states are mediated by different neurophysiological mechanisms (Cervero and Jänig 1992). Acute visceral pain is triggered by the activation of high threshold visceral afferents and by the high frequency bursts that these stimuli evoke in intensity coding afferent fibers, which are afferents with a range of responsiveness in the innocuous and noxious ranges. Prolonged forms of visceral stimulation result in sensitization of high-threshold receptors and activation of previously unresponsive afferent fibers, ▶ silent nociceptors (Häbler et al. 1988). This increased afferent activity enhances the excitability of central neurons and leads to the development of persistent pain states. There are two components of visceral pain: "true visceral pain" – deep visceral pain arising from inside the body and "▶ visceral referred pain" – pain that is referred to segmentally related somatic and also other visceral structures. Referred visceral-somatic pain mechanisms have been demonstrated to occur within minutes after uterine inflammation in an animal model of pelvic pain (Wesselmann and Lai 1997). ▶ Secondary hyperalgesia ▶ (referred hyperalgesia) usually develops at the referred site (Giamberardino and Vecchiet 1994). When examining and treating a woman with chronic gynecological pain it is important to consider both aspects of the pain syndrome (true and referred pain) including the pain deep in the pelvic cavity and pain referred to somatic structures (lower back and legs) and other visceral organs. The mechanisms of referred viscero-visceral pain (see ▶ visceral referred pain) might explain the substantial overlap observed between chronic pelvic pain and other abdominal symptoms (Abrams et al. 2002). Considering the concept of referred visceral pain will allow the physician to look at the global picture of visceral dysfunction, rather than "chasing" one aspect of the visceral pain syndrome out of context.

There is increasing evidence derived from studies in rodents that gynecological pain perception is subject to dynamic processes including ▶ cross-system

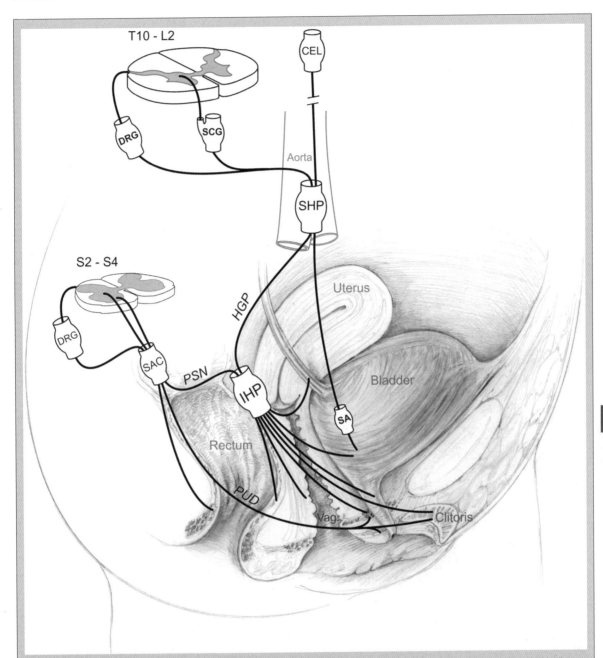

Obstetric and Gynecological Pain, Figure 1 Schematic drawing showing the innervation of the pelvic area in females. Although this diagram attempts to show the innervation in humans, much of the anatomical information is derived from animal data . CEL, celiac plexus; DRG, dorsal root ganglion; HGP, hypogastric plexus; IHP, inferior hypogastric plexus; PSN, pelvic splanchnic nerve; PUD, pudendal nerve; SA, short adrenergic projections; SAC, sacral plexus; SCG, sympathetic chain ganglion; SHP, superior hypogastric plexus; Vag., Vagina (From Wesselmann et al. 1997; with permission of the International Association for the Study of Pain).

► viscero-visceral and viscero-somatic convergence, wide-spread divergence and convergence of information flow throughout the CNS, ► central sensitization and hormonal modulation (Berkeley 2001). This dynamic view allows the explanation of some of the puzzling and confusing aspects of chronic gynecological pain syndromes, including poor correlation of pathology and pain intensity, referred pain phenomena and co-existenceof gynecological pain with painful conditions associated with different systems.

Chronic Gynecological Pain and Psychological Aspects

There is a growing literature focusing on the role of abusive experiences in gynecological pain syndromes including ► physical abuse and ► sexual abuse during childhood and adulthood. These studies are often difficult to compare due to the lack of uniformly agreed upon definitions of sexual and physical abuse. In addition many studies are flawed by the lack of appropriate control groups utilizing pain patients, small sample sizes and samples with significant self-selection factors. In contrast to retrospective studies based on recall, which have documented a relationship between abusive experiences and chronic gynecological pain syndromes, a recent prospective study of childhood sexual and physical abuse found no association with adult pain symptoms (Raphael et al. 2001). Clearly, further research into the complex interactions between abuse in child and adulthood and chronic gynecological pain syndromes is urgently needed, in order to address these complex psychosocial factors appropriately when treating women with chronic gynecological pain syndromes. Gynecological pain syndromes can have a significant impact on sexual functioning ► (Gynecological Pain and Sexual Functioning) and this impact might be modulated by the etiology, duration and location of pain, previous sexual function and psychosocial as well as partner related factors (Berman et al. 2003; Weijmar Schultz et al. 2003). While there are anecdotal reports that women with chronic pelvic pain are more psychologically impaired and difficult to manage, a recent study did not confirm this impression. When compared to pain controls, women with chronic pelvic pain did not score higher on a measure of depressive symptoms, did not report more pain-related disability and did not exhibit unique or different coping strategies (Heinberg et al. 2004).

Gynecological Pain: Assessment and Treatment

Chronic pelvic pain is often thought to be primarily of gynecological origin. However, it is important to realize that all other structures in the pelvic cavity including the urinary tract, the lower gastrointestinal tract and the pelvic blood vessels have to be included in the differential diagnosis. Musculoskeletal, neurological and psychiatric etiologies have to be considered. Thus the differential diagnosis is complicated and a thorough work-up is necessary. Since history and physical examination often do not allow the identification of an etiology for the chronic pain syndrome, laparoscopy has been the routine tool in the investigation of chronic pelvic pain for diagnostic confirmation, histological documentation and patient reassurance (Howard 1993). Endometriosis and adhesions (► Chronic Pelvic Pain, Pelvic Inflammatory Disease and Adhesions) are the most common findings; however, the extent of pelvic pathology is often not correlated to the intensity of the pelvic pain complaint. ► Laparoscopic Pain Mapping is a diagnostic laparoscopy under local anesthesia, with or without conscious sedation, aimed at identifying sources or

generators of pain in women with chronic pelvic pain. A ► superior hypogastric plexus block applied at the time of laparoscopic pain mapping may improve the predictability of the efficacy of presacral neurectomy (Steege 1998). However, prospective randomized studies will be necessary to determine whether this novel technique of laparoscopic pain mapping improves outcomes in patients with chronic pelvic pain leading to more specific medical and surgical treatments.

Treatment for chronic gynecological pain is directed towards symptomatic pain management and includes a wide range of approaches (see review in Wesselmann 2001). The absence of standardized and validated treatment protocols for chronic gynecological pain syndromes continues to frustrate patients and physicians. Physicians need to be aware that patient outcomes in chronic pelvic pain are influenced by the quality of the doctor-patient interaction (► Chronic Gynaecological Pain, Doctor-Patient Interaction) (Selfe et al. 1998). Traditionally surgical approaches towards the treatment of chronic gynecological pain syndromes have been very common. However, since it has been realized that there is not a linear correlation between the intensity of pelvic pain and pelvic pathology (if any), indications for surgery have been limited to women where pelvic pathology that might account for the pain complaint has been clearly identified. Despite the fact that it is a very common chronic pain syndrome, very little is known about effective pharmacological treatment for chronic gynecological pain. Further research on the pathophysiological mechanisms and controlled clinical trials are desperately needed to design improved pharmacological treatment strategies. Despite these limitations and need for improvement, currently available pharmacological treatment strategies, which have mainly been evaluated for other chronic pain syndromes, can be successfully applied to women with chronic gynecological pain, including NSAIDs, ► antidepressant drugs, ► Anticonvulsant (Agent), local anesthetic antiarrhythmics and ► opioids. Nerve blocks employed for chronic gynecological pain syndromes include ► superior hypogastric plexus blocks for pain in the pelvic cavity and ► pudendal nerve blocks for perineal pain syndromes. A typical characteristic of chronic pelvic pain is that patients not only present with deep pelvic pain, but also with referred pain to somatic structures. ► Physical Therapy and ► trigger point injections have been reported to be successful in the relief of ► myofascial pain associated with chronic gynecological pain syndromes (Weiss 2001). Neurosurgical approaches include presacral neurectomy for gynecological pain syndromes in the pelvic cavity, surgical decompression of the ► pudendal nerve in intractable pudendal neuralgias and limited midline myelotomy for the relief of malig-

laboratory studies allow closer control of the noxious stimulus and extraneous variables. However, laboratory studies are also limited by ethical constraints, and the degree to which they can simulate the environment of the chronic pain sufferer.

Acknowledging the limitations of laboratory studies, Linton and Gotestam (1985) reported inducing learned pain responses in healthy individuals with no existing learned pain responses. Over fifteen trials they verbally reinforced (with praise) the pain reports of subjects in the presence of a noxious stimulus (a blood pressure cuff which was inflated to a painful level). In their first experiment they found that pain reports could be operantly conditioned to increase and decrease, relative to a control condition, even though the intensity of the cuff pressure was kept stable across trials. In their second experiment the experimenters found that, with verbal reinforcement for reports of increased pain, the pain reports of subjects were maintained and increased even when the intensity of the noxious stimulus decreased. In contrast, for those in the control condition who were not given verbal reinforcement for reports of increased pain, subjects' pain reports decreased as the intensity of the painful stimulus decreased.

Schmidt et al. (1989) argued that instead of providing support for the reinforcement hypothesis, Linton and Gotestam's findings could have been interpreted as evidence of augmentation and amplification of sensations. However, this is unlikely, since Linton and Gotestam (1985) found that the pain reports of subjects could be positively reinforced up and down in the presence of a stable noxious stimulus.

Lousberg et al. (1996) reported a replication study based on Linton and Gotestam's (1985) paradigm, but using brief electric shocks as the noxious stimulus with a sample of healthy volunteers. In addition to pain ratings, Lousberg et al. also used psychophysiological measures of skin conductance response and skin conductance level. The results replicated those found previously by Linton and Gotestam, with the experimental group reporting significantly increased pain levels, relative to the control group. Interestingly, the experimenters also found a similar effect in skin conductance responses, although not on skin conductance levels. Thus, Lousberg et al's results revealed an effect of verbal conditioning not only on pain ratings but on a physiological measure as well.

Interestingly, Lousberg (1994) reported failure at an attempted replication of their results. Lousberg et al. (1996) also reported failure in an attempt to 'down condition' (train reductions in pain reporting). They considered that these findings may have been due to modified 'punishing responses' (expressions of surprise that pain was lower) for lower pain ratings in the experimental group during 'up-conditioning'. However, the variable findings clearly called for further investigation.

Flor et al. (2002) replicated Linton and Gotestam's earlier findings with a sample of chronic pain patients and normal, matched control subjects. Like Lousberg et al. (1996) they used an aversive electrical stimulus, but also recorded EEG, EOG, heart rate, skin conductance and muscle tension levels. Flor et al. used a similar reinforcement paradigm to that described by Linton and Gotestam, but the reinforcer in this case was a 'smiley' face on a computer screen whose mouth could be modified (up for positive feedback and down for negative feedback). Flor et al. also provided (or withdrew) tokens that could be exchanged for small amounts of money as additional sources of reinforcement. Flor et al. also examined reinforcement for increased and decreased pain reports. Their results showed that both patient and normal groups responded according to the reinforcement contingencies, in both directions (increased and decreased pain). Interestingly, Flor et al. also found that extinction of both the (previously reinforced) increased verbal pain reports and associated cortical responses (measured N150-component of somatosensory evoked potentials) took longer in the patient group. The patient group also displayed prolonged elevated electromyogram levels in this task, relative to the normal controls. Flor et al. concluded that their data provided support for the operant conditioning of pain responses, and indicated that chronic back pain patients are more easily influenced by reinforcement contingencies than healthy controls.

In a similar vein to these earlier studies, Chambers et al. (2002) demonstrated that the interactions of mothers with their daughters, but not sons, could also modulate (up and down) the experience of pain in children subjected to cold-pressor pain in the laboratory. Importantly, Chambers et al. demonstrated this effect with observed facial activity as a non-verbal pain measure and not just self-reported pain ratings.

Recently, Jolliffe and Nicholas (2004) also replicated Linton and Gotestam's original findings. They used a similar paradigm, but a larger sample size and tests for the influence of other possible confounding factors, such as awareness of the response-reinforcement contingencies, heightened somatic awareness, anxiety, gender and locus of control. None of these variables was found to influence the results that supported those reported by the earlier researchers.

Taken together, these studies provide general support for the thesis that pain reports can be operantly conditioned and this effect can be reflected in measures of skin conductance responses, facial activity and cortical responses as well. These studies also support Fordyce's original contention that pain responses (or behaviours) could be, to some extent, independent of any noxious stimulus. The treatment implications are that those interacting with chronic pain patients should be alert to the possibility that their responses to reports of pain by patients could well act to reinforce

O

and maintain such behaviours, and may complicate the clinical presentation and assessment/management of such cases.

References

1. Cairns D, Pasino JA Comparison of Verbal Reinforcement and Feedback in the Operant Treatment of Disability due to Chronic Low Back Pain. Behav Ther 197 8:621–630
2. Chambers CT, Craig KD, Bennett SM (2002) The Impact of Maternal Behavior on Children's Pain Experiences: An Experimental Analysis. J Pediatr Psychol 27:293–301
3. Flor H, Knost B, Birbaumer N (2002) The Role of Operant Conditioning in Chronic Pain: An Experimental Investigation. Pain 95:111–118
4. Fordyce WE (1976) Behavioural Methods for Chronic Pain and Illness. Mosby, St. Louis
5. Gil KM, Ross SL, Keefe FJ (1988) Behavioral Treatment of Chronic Pain: Four Pain Management Protocols. In: France RD, Krishnan KRR (eds) Chronic Pain. American Psychiatric Press, Washington, pp 376–413
6. Jolliffe CD, Nicholas MK (2004) Verbally Reinforcing Pain Reports: An Experimental Test of the Operant Model of Chronic Pain. Pain 107:167–175
7. Keefe FJ, Block AR (1982) Development of an Observation Method for Assessing Pain Behavior in Chronic Low Back Pain Patients. Behav Ther 13:363–375
8. Latimer PR (1982) External Contingency Management for Chronic Pain: Critical Review of Evidence. Am J Psychiatry 139:1308–1312
9. Linton SJ, Gotestam KG (1985) Controlling Pain Reports through Operant Conditioning: A Laboratory Demonstration. Percep Motor Skills 60:427–437
10. Lousberg R (1994) Chronic Pain: Multiaxial Diagnostics and Behavioral Mechanisms. PhD thesis. Universitaire Pers Maastricht, Maastricht
11. Lousberg R, Groenman NH, Schmidt AJM et al. (1996) Operant Conditioning of the Pain Experience. Percep Motor Skills 83:883–900
12. Morley S, Eccleston C, Williams (1999) A Systematic Review and Meta Analysis of Randomised Control Trials of Cognitive Behavioural Therapy for Chronic Pain in Adults, Excluding Headache. Pain 80:1–13
13. Pavlov IP (1927) Conditioned Reflexes. Trans. GV Anrep. Oxford University Press
14. Schmidt AJM, Gierlings REH, Peters ML (1989) Environmental and Interoceptive Influences on Chronic Low Back Pain Behaviour. Pain 38:137–143
15. White B, Sanders SH (1986) The Influence of Patient's Pain Intensity Ratings of Antecedent Reinforcement of Pain Talk or Well Talk. J Behav Ther Exp Psychiatry 17:155–159

Operant Process

Operant Treatment

Operant Treatment of Chronic Pain

HERTA FLOR
Department of Clinical and Cognitive Neuroscience at the University of Heidelberg, Central Institute of Mental Health, Mannheim, Germany
flor@zi-mannheim.de

Synonyms

Behavioral Treatment; Operant-Behavioral Treatment

Definition

The operant treatment of pain is based on Fordyce's operant conditioning model of pain, and involves behavioral exercises to reduce pain behaviors and to increase healthy behaviors in many areas of life, including medication reduction.

Characteristics

The operant conditioning formulation proposed by Fordyce (1976, 1988) has substantially contributed to our understanding of chronic pain and has had a significant impact on treatment and rehabilitation. The operant model of chronic pain is presented in the essay ▶ operant perspective on pain. This article will focus on operant treatment. Based on the assumption that pain behaviors have been positively reinforced and health behaviors have not been adequately reinforced, extinguished or punished, the operant approach focuses on the restructuring of pain-incompatible behaviors, and the reduction of pain behaviors such as lack of physical activity, guarding and bracing, excessive use of medication, and emphasizes the responses of the patients' significant others to pain. Three areas of intervention are primarily addressed: (1) modification of the response of significant others to the patient's pain-related and health-related behaviors; (2) decrease of observable pain behaviors and increase of activity levels of the patient in areas such as activities at home, work-related behaviors, social and leisure time behaviors (including social skills training), and interaction with significant others and health care providers; and (3) modification of medication-intake and other illness-related behaviors.

In the original studies, the operant treatment was usually conducted in an inpatient setting because of greater control of the environment and the contingencies of reinforcement. More recently, operant treatments have also been used in outpatient settings. They have the advantage that the home is a more natural environment than the hospital, the patient can practice in his or her own home environment, and it is easier to involve significant others in treatment. Thus, outpatient treatment gains should be more readily maintained. It is, moreover, more cost-effective, especially if it is delivered in a group setting.

Opiates - Pharmacology of Pain

FRANK PORRECA

Departments of Pharmacology and Anesthesiology,
University of Arizona, Health Sciences Center,
Tucson, AZ, USA
frankp@u.arizona.edu

Introduction

The efficacy of the opioid alkaloids, morphine and codeine, as well as that of their derivatives, as analgesics in conditions of acute pain is well established in clinical practice. Morphine, the major opiate alkaloid, is the prototypic analgesic and serves as the reference standard against which the analgesic activity of pain treatments are measured in clinical and preclinical paradigms. Opiate analgesics are routinely used in post-operative pain and in the treatment of many painful conditions of short and medium term duration and are gaining acceptance in the treatment of some chronic pain states as well. A complicating factor in the use of opioids to manage chronic pain conditions is the decrease in analgesic activity observed over time, at least in some patients, indicative of the phenomenon of analgesic ▶ tolerance. Opioids exert their antinociceptive activity through peripheral, spinal and supraspinal sites and adaptations induced by opioids at these multiple levels of the neuraxis may be contributing factors in the expression of tolerance. There is evidence to indicate that long-term opioid exposure may result in activation of pain facilitatory systems from medullary sites that oppose the analgesic actions of these compounds. The engagement of descending pain facilitatory mechanisms can paradoxically result in the expression of a hyperalgesic state, which can act as a "physiological antagonist" of analgesia, in essence manifesting as "antinociceptive tolerance." The chapters included in this section discuss many different aspects of opioid mediated action and the neurophysiological adaptations that can contribute to the effects of these compounds over time.

Opioid Receptors and Endogenous Opioids

The discovery of a receptor selective for opioids was reported almost simultaneously by three different groups in 1973 (Pert and Snyder 1973a; Pert and Snyder 1973b; Simon 1973) and precipitated an increased interest in the field of pain research. This discovery was rapidly followed by the identification and characterization of endogenous ligands for this receptor. Almost immediately thereafter, the pentapeptide ▶ enkephalins (Hughes et al. 1975; Kosterlitz and Hughes 1975), the ▶ endorphins (Cox et al. 1975) and ▶ dynorphin (Goldstein et al. 1979) were described.

Concurrently, behavioral studies and experiments performed with isolated tissue preparations revealed the existence of three subtypes of the ▶ opioid receptor, identified as mu, kappa and delta (Lord et al. 1977; Martin et al. 1976; Waterfield et al. 1978); this was later confirmed through cloning techniques (Zaki et al. 1996). Although different subtypes have not been cloned, it is possible for example that post-transcriptional events may occur to produce these subtypes (Zaki et al. 1996). The production of antibodies to these receptors allowed for anatomical location (Arvidson et al. 1995; Kalyuzhny et al. 1996; Mansour et al. 1994, 1995) and this led to localization of these receptors in pain pathways including the central and peripheral terminations of sensory fibers and in ascending pain transmission pathways as well as in descending pain modulatory systems. Collectively, these findings suggested that opioids may exert their antinociceptive activity through several mechanisms, providing their overall analgesic actions through anatomical synergy. These discoveries also provided strong evidence for the existence of an ▶ endogenous pain control system, with implications for the understanding of tolerance, dependence and withdrawal.

The Distributions of the Opioid Receptors Are Consistent with Pain Pathways

Spinal Sites of Action

The distribution and anatomical localization of the opioid receptors have been extensively explored through immunohistochemistry, autoradiography, radioligand binding and *in situ* hybridization of message for the receptors (Bzdega et al. 1993; Mansour et al. 1995). The distribution of opioid receptors is consistent with known pathways related to the processing of nociceptive signals. The opioid receptors are predominant in the outer laminae of the spinal dorsal horn, with a less extensive distribution in lamina V and around the central canal and are sparse within the intermediate laminae (Besse et al. 1991; Quirion et al. 1983). These sites are consistent with the distribution of the terminals of nociceptors from the periphery and viscera. Studies employing a variety of techniques established that a substantial proportion of the opioid receptors found in the outer laminae reside on the terminals of primary afferent nociceptive C-fibers and that message for the opioid receptors is found principally in nociceptive C- and A-delta dorsal root ganglia (DRG) neurons (Arvidsson et al. 1995; Besse et al. 1991; Ji et al. 1995). This distribution is consistent with a role in the regulation of nociceptive inputs without altering innocuous sensory signals. Accordingly, it was found that activation of mu-opioid receptors predictably inhibited Ca^{++} channels of small diameter nociceptors and not of

O

large diameter myelinated A-beta cells and suggested that mu-receptor activation selectively inhibits the activity of C-fibers (Taddese et al. 1995). Approximately 20–30% of spinal opioid receptors reside on either interneurons or on cell bodies of second order neurons that transmit nociceptive inputs to supraspinal sites that process nociceptive signals (Besse et al. 1991).

The presence of opioid receptors in the spinal cord suggests a direct spinal antinociceptive action of opioids. The direct spinal application of morphine or of enkephalins into the spinal space produced dose dependent, ► naloxone reversible antinociception to noxious thermal stimuli (Yaksh et al. 1977a). Mid-thoracic spinalization reduced the potency of systemic, but not of spinal, morphine against a noxious evoked spinal reflex (Advokat 1989). The iontophoretic application of morphine into the outer laminae of the dorsal horns of the spinal cord also attenuated the responses of dorsal horn units to noxious stimuli (Duggan et al. 1976). These observations supported the hypothesis that opioids may act directly at spinal sites to modulate nociceptive spinal reflexes and nociceptive inputs and the spinal administration of morphine has now become routine medical practice in the treatment of pain.

Supraspinal Sites of Action

The microinjection of opioids into the cerebral ventricles has been shown to produce dose dependent antinociception in several species, including mice and rats, suggesting a supraspinal modulation of nociceptive inputs (Erspamer et al. 1989; Jiang et al. 1990; Miaskowski et al. 1991; Porreca et al. 1984). Autoradiographic studies have demonstrated that there are significant levels of opioid receptor mRNA in many cortical, diencephalic and brainstem regions in addition to spinal loci (Mansour et al. 1994; Mansour et al. 1995). In particular, significant expression of message for opioid receptors was found in the periaqueductal gray (PAG) and the rostral ventromedial medulla (RVM), regions that are critical to expression of supraspinal antinociceptive manipulations (Basbaum et al. 1978; Basbaum and Fields 1978; Fields and Anderson 1978). The microinjection of morphine into the PAG produced dose dependent, naloxone reversible antinociception to peripheral noxious stimuli (Lewis and Gebhart 1977; Yaksh et al. 1976). Moreover, PAG sites that were responsive to morphine also produced antinociception in response to electrical stimulation (Lewis and Gebhart 1977; Yeung et al. 1977). The microinjection of morphine into the PAG attenuated the activity of projection neurons in the dorsal horn in response to peripheral nociceptive stimuli (Bennett and Mayer 1979). The RVM is recognized as a critical region with respect to nociceptive processing and modulation, re-

ceiving inputs from the spinal dorsal horn and from rostral sites as well (Fields and Basbaum 1999; Fields and Heinricher 1985; Fields et al. 1983). Electrophysiological studies on the responses of RVM neurons to noxious thermal stimulation have identified the existence of ► on-cells and ► off-cells (Fields 1992; Fields and Basbaum 1999; Heinricher et al. 2003). The off-cells are tonically active and pause in firing immediately before the animal withdraws from the noxious thermal stimulus, whereas the on-cells accelerate firing immediately before the nociceptive reflex occurs. An additional class, the "neutral" cells were initially characterized by the absence of response to noxious thermal stimulation. It is now generally understood that the activity of the off-cells correlates with inhibition of nociceptive input and nocifensive responses and these neurons may be the source of descending inhibition of nociceptive inputs (Fields 1992; Fields and Basbaum 1999; Heinricher et al. 2003). In contrast, the response characteristics of the on-cells suggest that these neurons are the source of descending facilitation of nociception (Fields 1992; Fields and Basbaum 1999; Heinricher et al. 2003; McNally 1999;). Accordingly, manipulations that facilitate responses to nociceptive stimuli also increase on-cell activity (Fields and Basbaum 1999; Fields 2000; Heinricher and Roychowdhury 1997; Heinricher et al. 2003;). For example, prolonged delivery of a noxious thermal stimulus produced increased on-cell activity along with a facilitation of nociceptive reflexes (Morgan and Fields 1994). Moreover, inactivation of RVM neuronal activity with lidocaine blocked the facilitated withdrawal response (Morgan and Fields 1994). It is now generally accepted that a spino-bulbo-spinal loop may be important to the development and maintenance of exaggerated pain behaviors produced by persistent noxious stimuli (Heinricher et al. 2003; Ossipov et al. 2001; Suzuki et al. 2002; Suzuki et al. 2004). Morphine microinjection or electrical stimulation in the RVM has produced naloxone sensitive antinociception by activating spinopetal mechanisms (Kiefel et al. 1993; McGowan and Hammond 1993; Rossi et al. 1993). Studies employing retrograde tracing methods demonstrated the existence of opioid expressing neurons that project from the RVM to the spinal cord to provide a descending inhibition of nociceptive inputs (Kalyuzhny et al. 1996). It was also proposed that opioids exert indirect effects on RVM projection neurons and have both direct and indirect effects on bulbospinal neurons (Kalyuzhny et al. 1996).

Synergistic Actions at Spinal / Supraspinal Sites

An important aspect of morphine-mediated antinociception is the existence of a synergistic interaction between morphine given spinally and supraspinally. The administration of a 1:1 fixed ratio of morphine administered intrathecally and into the cerebral ventricles produced an approximate 30-fold increase in potency when evaluated in the tail-flick test and a 45-fold increase in the hot plate test compared to supraspinal morphine alone (Yeung and Rudy 1980). Isobolographic analyses employing several dose ratios demonstrated a hyperbolic function with a strong degree of curvature and it was concluded that potentiation would occur at all possible combinations of spinal and supraspinal levels of morphine after systemic injection (Miyamoto et al. 1991; Roerig and Fujimoto 1988; Yeung and Rudy 1980). Situations where the antinociceptive effect of morphine was diminished corresponded with a loss of spinal / supraspinal synergy. For example, repeated exposure to systemic morphine abolished the synergistic antinociceptive effect of morphine given into the PAG and spinally (Siuciak and Advokat 1989). Similarly, rats with peripheral nerve injury demonstrate a loss of spinal morphine potency along with a loss of the spinal / supraspinal synergy (Bian et al. 1999). Restoration of the spinal site of morphine activity with an NMDA antagonist restored supraspinal-spinal synergy and increased the potency of systemically given morphine in animals with nerve injury (Bian et al. 1999).

Paradoxical Opioid Induced Hyperalgesia

A number of clinical reports exist that show that opioid administration can paradoxically elicit abnormally heightened pain sensations. Long-term spinal morphine provoked hyperesthesias and allodynia that were unrelated to the original pain complaint in cancer patients (Ali 1986; Arner et al. 1988; De Conno et al. 1991). The spinal infusion of sufentanil in a patient with neuropathic pain secondary to arachnoiditis and laminectomy evoked hyperesthesias in the lower extremities (Devulder 1997). This abnormal pain state was described as being qualitatively different from the original complaint and included the back, abdomen and both legs. Cancer patients who received high doses of intrathecal morphine by bolus injections also reported paradoxical intense pain within 0.5 hour of the injections (Stillman et al. 1987).
Animal studies have clearly demonstrated that opioid administration may produce an abnormal, paradoxical hyperalgesic state (Gardell et al. 2002b; Mao et al. 1994; Mayer et al. 1995a; Vanderah et al. 2000; Vanderah et al. 2001b). The repeated daily injection of spinal or systemic morphine produced enhanced responses of the tail or hind paw to noxious thermal stimuli within 8 days (Mayer et al. 1995b; Trujillo and

Akil 1994). The continuous exposure to opioids produced behavioral signs of exaggerated pain and importantly, such pain occurred while the opioid was continuously present in the system (Gardell et al. 2002b; Vanderah et al. 2000; Vanderah et al. 2001b). The continuous spinal infusion of [D-Ala^2,N-Me-Phe^4,Gly-ol^5]enkephalin (DAMGO) delivered through an osmotic minipump or of morphine administered by subcutaneous pellets produced antinociceptive tolerance to spinal DAMGO or morphine (Vanderah et al. 2000). These animals expressed tactile and thermal hypersensitivities (Vanderah et al. 2000; Vanderah et al. 2001b) while the opioids were still being administered (Vanderah et al. 2000; Vanderah et al. 2001b) and changes did not result from changes in metabolism or metabolites since blood levels of opiates were constant over the period of infusion (Ossipov, Stiller and Porreca, unpublished observations).
This paradoxical hyperalgesia and the neurobiological adaptations which underlie this state may play an important role in the requirement for increased levels of opioids to maintain a constant degree of antinociception, perhaps reflecting the expression of antinociceptive tolerance (Gardell et al. 2002b; Vanderah et al. 2000; Vanderah et al. 2001a; Vanderah et al. 2001b). Clinically, the need for increasing doses of opioids in cases of chronic pain, at least in some patients, is well documented and can present a major obstacle to providing adequate pain relief over a long period of time (Cherney and Portenoy 1999; Foley 1993; Foley 1995). In spite of much intensive research, however, the mechanisms that underlie the development of tolerance to the analgesic effects of opioids remain largely unknown. Many studies have focused on changes occurring at the cellular level in order to gain an appreciation of the mechanisms that drive the development of antinociceptive tolerance (e.g. Childers 1991; Sabbe and Yaksh 1990). Although alterations in subcellular processes appear potentially to contribute to the phenomenon of tolerance, the present level of understanding of such processes is insufficient to allow for the direct correlation of intracellular changes with those occurring at the level of the neuronal circuits mediating antinociception or analgesia. Nevertheless, opioid induced up-regulation of peptidic neuromodulators such as cholecystokinin (CCK) or dynorphin may supply endogenous physiological antagonists to endogenous or exogenous opioid activity. These changes may be related to the activation of descending facilitation of nociception. Consequently, pain may be considered as a physiological antagonist of analgesia and increased states of pain require increased levels of pain relieving opiate, resulting in "opiate tolerance" (Vanderah et al. 2001a).

O

Opioid Induced Paradoxical Pain Is Promoted by Descending Facilitation from the RVM

As noted above, the on-cells of the RVM are an important source of descending pain facilitatory projections. The microinjection of CCK into the RVM has enhanced nociceptive input and attenuated the morphine induced reduction of on-cell responses to nociception, suggesting that these neurons may be activated by CCK (Heinricher and McGaraughty 1996). The microinjection of lidocaine into the RVM of rats with persistent exposure to morphine produced a reversible block of both tactile and thermal hyperesthesias and abolished antinociceptive tolerance to morphine (Vanderah et al. 2001b). Prolonged morphine exposure elicited a 5-fold increase in basal CCK in the RVM (Xie et al. 2005). The microinjection of CCK into the RVM produced tactile and thermal hyperesthesias whereas a CCK_2 antagonist in the RVM abolished opioid induced hyperesthesias (Xie et al. 2005). Moreover, the microinjection of a CCK_2 antagonist into RVM or lesions of the dorsolateral funiculus abolished both behavioral signs of enhanced pain and antinociceptive tolerance in response to persistent morphine exposure (Xie et al. 2005).

Spinal Dynorphin and Opioid Induced Paradoxical Pain

Considerable evidence has demonstrated that enhanced expression of spinal dynorphin is pronociceptive and promotes facilitated pain states. A single spinal injection of dynorphin has produced long lasting tactile allodynia in rats and mice (Laughlin et al. 1997; Vanderah et al. 1996). Elevations in spinal dynorphin content are also seen in animals with prolonged, constant exposure to opioids either systemically or spinally (Gardell et al. 2002b; Vanderah et al. 2001a; Vanderah et al. 2001b). Spinal infusion of DAMGO elicited enhanced responses to tactile and noxious thermal stimuli and also caused an elevation in dynorphin content in the lumbar cord (Vanderah et al. 2000). The spinal injection of antiserum to dynorphin blocked enhanced responses in the DAMGO-treated rats and unmasked the antinociceptive action of the DAMGO that was still infused (Vanderah et al. 2000). Furthermore, dynorphin antiserum blocked the rightward displacement of the dose-effect curve for spinal morphine in DAMGO infused rats, indicating a blockade of antinociceptive tolerance (Vanderah et al. 2000). Bilateral lesions of the DLF, which were shown to block abnormal pain and tolerance to the antinociceptive effect of morphine, also prevented the up-regulation of spinal dynorphin (Gardell et al. 2003). Thus, manipulations that block opioid induced pain, in this case due to spinal infusion of opioid, also block the behavioral manifestation of antinociceptive tolerance. The data show that sustained opioid administration leads to elevated spinal dynorphin content, which in turn promotes an abnormal pain state and increases the requirement for opioid dose in order to produce a comparable antinociceptive effect to that in animals without increased nociception, resulting in an apparent manifestation of antinociceptive tolerance.

The precise mechanisms through which increased spinal dynorphin expression promotes pain and consequently the manifestation of opioid tolerance remain to be elucidated but appear to be related to an enhanced release of transmitters from primary afferent terminals. Dynorphin produced a dose dependent release of glutamate and aspartate elicited by exogenous dynorphin in the hippocampus and spinal cord (Faden 1992; Skilling et al. 1992). More recently, the capsaicin stimulated release of calcitonin gene related peptide (CGRP) was potentiated by dynorphin $A_{(2-13)}$, a non-opioid fragment, in spinal cord sections *in vitro* (Claude et al. 1999; Gardell et al. 2002a; Gardell et al. 2003). In addition, dynorphin also facilitated capsaicin evoked substance P release from trigeminal nuclear slices and this effect was abolished by MK-801, but not by opioid antagonists (Arcaya et al. 1999). Most recently, it was demonstrated that persistent exposure to morphine pellets implanted subcutaneously produced enhanced capsaicin evoked release of CGRP from spinal tissue (Gardell et al. 2002b; Gardell et al. 2003). This enhanced, evoked release was blocked by the addition of antiserum to dynorphin in the perfusion medium. Moreover, the disruption of descending facilitation from supraspinal sites by selective ablation of RVM neurons that express the mu-opioid receptor or by surgical lesions of the DLF prevented opioid induced abnormal pain, spinal dynorphin upregulation and enhanced capsaicin evoked release of CGRP (Gardell et al. 2002b; Gardell et al. 2003). Finally, enhanced capsaicin evoked release of CGRP was also blocked by the NMDA antagonist MK-801 (Gardell et al. 2002b; Gardell et al. 2003). More recently, the introduction of NMDA, dynorphin $A_{(1-17)}$ or dynorphin $A_{(2-17)}$ into the lumbar spinal cord through a microdialysis catheter elicited a prolonged release of prostaglandin E2 and of excitatory amino acids (Koetzner et al. 2004). These observations provide a mechanism through which pathologically elevated levels of spinal dynorphin may promote enhanced pain (Koetzner et al. 2004).

Summary

The opioid analgesics have been employed throughout our history for the treatment and control of pain. The opioids, exemplified by the prototype morphine, represent the most efficacious means of controlling pain at the present time. The analgesic activity of opioids is mediated through activity at spinal and supraspinal sites. Opioids may act directly at the spinal level to block incoming nociceptive inputs. Alternatively, opioids may activate supraspinal sites that activate descending pain inhibitory systems to block the transmission of nociceptive signals to supraspinal structures. Paradoxically, the very same substances that are so efficacious against pain may actually cause an abnormal pain phenomenon themselves by eliciting the activation of endogenous pronociceptive systems. Persistent exposure to the opioids causes an increase in the presence of the pronociceptive neurotransmitter CCK, which acts as an endogenous modulator of antinociceptive activity. One means through which this is achieved is through the activation of a descending facilitation from the RVM. These findings reveal the complex neurobiological adaptations that result from opioid administration and raise questions as to the optimal use of opioids for the management of pain in humans, as well as suggesting alternative approaches to improve the use of this class of compounds for the management of chronic pain states.

References

1. Advokat C (1989) Tolerance to the antinociceptive effect of morphine in spinally transected rats. Behav Neurosci 103:1091–1098
2. Ali NM (1986) Hyperalgesic response in a patient receiving high concentrations of spinal morphine. Anesthesiology 65:449
3. Arcaya JL, Cano G, Gomez G et al. (1999) Dynorphin A increases substance P release from trigeminal primary afferent C-fibers. Eur J Pharmacol 366:27–34
4. Arner S, Rawal N, Gustafsson LL (1988) Clinical experience of long-term treatment with epidural and intrathecal opioids –a nationwide survey. Acta Anaesthesiol Scand 32:253–259
5. Arvidsson U, Dado RJ, Riedl M et al. (1995) delta-Opioid receptor immunoreactivity:distribution in brainstem and spinal cord, and relationship to biogenic amines and enkephalin. J Neurosci 15:1215–1235
6. Basbaum AI, Fields HL (1978) Endogenous pain control mechanisms: review and hypothesis. Ann Neurol 4:451–462
7. Basbaum AI, Clanton CH, Fields HL (1978) Three bulbospinal pathways from the rostral medulla of the cat: an autoradiographic study of pain modulating systems. J Comp Neurol 178:209–224
8. Bennett GJ, Mayer DJ (1979) Inhibition of spinal cord interneurons by narcotic microinjection and focal electrical stimulation in the periaqueductal central gray matter. Brain Res 172:243–257
9. Besse D, Lombard MC, Besson JM (1991) Autoradiographic distribution of mu, delta and kappa opioid binding sites in the superficial dorsal horn, over the rostrocaudal axis of the rat spinal cord. Brain Res 548:287–291
10. Bian D, Ossipov MH, Ibrahim M et al. (1999) Loss of antiallodynic and antinociceptive spinal / supraspinal morphine synergy in nerve-injured rats: restoration by MK-801 or dynorphin antiserum. Brain Res 831:55–63
11. Bzdega T, Chin H, Kim H et al. (1993) Regional expression and chromosomal localization of the delta opiate receptor gene. Proc Natl Acad Sci USA 90:9305–9309
12. Cherney NI, Portenoy RK (1999) Practical issues in the management of cancer pain. In:Wall PD, Melzack R (eds) Textbook of Pain. Churchill Livingstone, Edinburgh, pp 1479–1522
13. Childers SR (1991) Opioid receptor-coupled second messenger systems. Life Sci 48:1991–2003
14. Claude P, Gracia N, Wagner L et al. (1999) Effect of dynorphin on ICGRP release from capsaicin-sensitive fibers. Abstracts of the 9th World Congress on Pain 9:262
15. Cox BM, Opheim KE, Teschemacher H et al. (1975) A peptide-like substance from pituitary that acts like morphine. 2. Purification and properties. Life Sci 16:1777–1782
16. De Conno F, Caraceni A, Martini C et al. (1991) Hyperalgesia and myoclonus with intrathecal infusion of high-dose morphine. Pain 47:337–339
17. Devulder J (1997) Hyperalgesia induced by high-dose intrathecal sufentanil in neuropathic pain. J Neurosurg Anesthesiol 9:146–148
18. Duggan AW, Davies J, Hall JG (1976) Effects of opiate agonists and antagonists on central neurons of the cat. J Pharmacol Exp Ther 196:107–120
19. Erspamer V, Melchiorri P, Falconieri-Erspamer G et al. (1989) Deltorphins:a family of naturally occurring peptides with high affinity and selectivity for delta opioid binding sites. Proc Natl Acad Sci USA 86:5188–5192
20. Faden AI (1992) Dynorphin increases extracellular levels of excitatory amino acids in the brain through a non-opioid mechanism. J Neurosci 12:425–429
21. Fernandes M, Kluwe S, Coper H (1977) The development of tolerance to morphine in the rat. Psychopharmacology 54:197–201
22. Fields HL (1992) Is there a facilitating component to central pain modulation? APS Journal 1:71–78
23. Fields HL (2000) Pain modulation: expectation, opioid analgesia and virtual pain. Prog Brain Res 122:245–253
24. Fields HL, Anderson SD (1978) Evidence that raphe-spinal neurons mediate opiate and midbrain stimulation-produced analgesias. Pain 5:333–349
25. Fields HL, Basbaum AI (1999) Central nervous system mechanisms of pain modulation. In: Wall PD, Melzack R (eds) Textbook of Pain. Churchill Livingstone, Edinburgh, pp 309–329
26. Fields HL, Heinricher MM (1985) Anatomy and physiology of a nociceptive modulatory system. Philos Trans R Soc Lond B Biol Sci 308:361–374
27. Fields HL, Bry J, Hentall I et al. (1983) The activity of neurons in the rostral medulla of the rat during withdrawal from noxious heat. J Neurosci 3:2545–2552
28. Foley KM (1993) Opioids. Neurol Clin 11:503–522
29. Foley KM (1995) Misconceptions and controversies regarding the use of opioids in cancer pain. Anticancer Drugs 6:4–13
30. Gardell LR, Burgess SE, Dogrul A et al. (2002a) Pronociceptive effects of spinal dynorphin promote cannabinoid-induced pain and antinociceptive tolerance. Pain 98:79–88
31. Gardell LR, Wang R, Burgess SE et al. (2002b) Sustained morphine exposure induces a spinal dynorphin-dependent enhancement of excitatory transmitter release from primary afferent fibers. J Neurosci 22:6747–6755
32. Gardell LR, Vanderah TW, Gardell SE et al. (2003) Enhanced evoked excitatory transmitter release in experimental neuropathy requires descending facilitation. J Neurosci 23:8370–8379
33. Goldstein A, Tachibana S, Lowney LI et al. (1979) Dynorphin-(1–13), an extraordinarily potent opioid peptide. Proc Natl Acad Sci USA 76:6666–6670
34. Heinricher MM, McGaraughty S (1996) CCK modulates the antinociceptive actions of opioids by an action within the rostral ventromedial medulla: a combined electrophysiological and behavioral study. In: Abstracts of the 8th World Congress on Pain, Vancouver. IASP Press, Seattle, p 472
35. Heinricher MM, Roychowdhury SM (1997) Reflex-related activation of putative pain facilitating neurons in rostral ventromedial medulla requires excitatory amino acid transmission. Neuroscience 78:1159–1165

O

36. Heinricher MM, Pertovaara A, Ossipov MH (2003) Descending modulation after injury. In: Dostrovsky DO, Carr DB, Koltzenburg M (eds) Proceedings of the 10th World Congress on Pain. IASP Press, Seattle, pp 251–260

37. Hughes J, Smith T, Morgan B et al. (1975) Purification and properties of enkephalin –the possible endogenous ligand for the morphine receptor. Life Sci 16:1753–1758

38. Ji RR, Zhang Q, Law PY et al. (1995) Expression of mu-, delta-, and kappa-opioid receptor-like immunoreactivities in rat dorsal root ganglia after carrageenan-induced inflammation. J Neurosci 15:8156–8166

39. Jiang Q, Mosberg HI, Porreca F (1990) Antinociceptive effects of [D-Ala2]deltorphin II, a highly selective delta agonist in vivo. Life Sci 47:PL43–47

40. Kalyuzhny AE, Arvidsson U, Wu W et al. (1996) mu-Opioid and delta-opioid receptors are expressed in brainstem antinociceptive circuits: studies using immunocytochemistry and retrograde tract-tracing. J Neurosci 16:6490–6503

41. Kiefel JM, Rossi GC, Bodnar RJ (1993) Medullary mu and delta opioid receptors modulate mesencephalic morphine analgesia in rats. Brain Res 624:151–161

42. Koetzner L, Hua XY, Lai J et al. (2004) Nonopioid actions of intrathecal dynorphin evoke spinal excitatory amino acid and prostaglandin E2 release mediated by cyclooxygenase-1 and -2. J Neurosci 24:1451–1458

43. Kosterlitz HW, Hughes J (1975) Some thoughts on the significance of enkephalin, the endogenous ligand. Life Sci 17:91–96

44. Laughlin TM, Vanderah TW, Lashbrook J et al. (1997) Spinally administered dynorphin A produces long-lasting allodynia: involvement of NMDA but not opioid receptors. Pain 72:253–260

45. Lewis VA, Gebhart GF (1977) Morphine-induced and stimulation-produced analgesias at coincident periaqueductal central gray loci: evaluation of analgesic congruence, tolerance, and cross-tolerance. Exp Neurol 57:934–955

46. Lord JA, Waterfield AA, Hughes J et al. (1977) Endogenous opioid peptides: multiple agonists and receptors. Nature 267:495–499

47. Mansour A, Fox CA, Burke S et al. (1994) Mu, delta, and kappa opioid receptor mRNA expression in the rat CNS: an in situ hybridization study. J Comp Neurol 350:412–438

48. Mansour A, Fox CA, Akil H et al. (1995) Opioid-receptor mRNA expression in the rat CNS: anatomical and functional implications. Trends Neurosci 18:22–29

49. Mao J, Price DD, Mayer DJ (1994) Thermal hyperalgesia in association with the development of morphine tolerance in rats:roles of excitatory amino acid receptors and protein kinase C. J Neurosci 14:2301–2312

50. Martin WR, Eades CG, Thompson JA et al. (1976) The effects of morphine- and nalorphine- like drugs in the nondependent and morphine-dependent chronic spinal dog. J Pharmacol Exp Ther 197:517–532

51. Mayer DJ, Mao J, Price DD (1995a) The development of morphine tolerance and dependence is associated with translocation of protein kinase C. Pain 61:365–374

52. Mayer DJ, Mao J, Price DD (1995b) The development of morphine tolerance and dependence is associated with translocation of protein kinase C. Pain 61:365–374

53. McGowan MK, Hammond DL (1993) Antinociception produced by microinjection of L-glutamate into the ventromedial medulla of the rat: mediation by spinal GABAA receptors. Brain Res 620:86–96

54. McNally GP (1999) Pain facilitatory circuits in the mammalian central nervous system: their behavioral significance and role in morphine analgesic tolerance. Neurosci Biobehav Rev 23:1059–1078

55. Miaskowski C, Taiwo YO, Levine JD (1991) Contribution of supraspinal mu- and delta-opioid receptors to antinociception in the rat. Eur J Pharmacol 205:247–252

56. Miyamoto Y, Morita N, Kitabata Y et al. (1991) Antinociceptive synergism between supraspinal and spinal sites after subcuta-neous morphine evidenced by CNS morphine content. Brain Res 552:136–140

57. Morgan MM, Fields HL (1994) Pronounced changes in the activity of nociceptive modulatory neurons in the rostral ventromedial medulla in response to prolonged thermal noxious stimuli. J Neurophysiol 72:1161–1170

58. Ossipov MH, Lai J, Malan TP Jr et al. (2001) Tonic descending facilitation as a mechanism of neuropathic pain. In: Hansson PT, Fields HL, Hill RG et al. (eds) Neuropathic Pain: Pathophysiology and Treatment. IASP Press, Seattle, pp 107–124

59. Pert CB, Snyder SH (1973a) Opiate receptor: demonstration in nervous tissue. Science 179:1011–1014

60. Pert CB, Snyder SH (1973b) Properties of opiate-receptor binding in rat brain. Proc Natl Acad Sci USA 70:2243–2247

61. Porreca F, Mosberg HI, Hurst R et al. (1984) Roles of mu, delta and kappa opioid receptors in spinal and supraspinal mediation of gastrointestinal transit effects and hot-plate analgesia in the mouse. J Pharmacol Exp Ther 230:341–348

62. Quirion R, Zajac JM, Morgat JL et al. (1983) Autoradiographic distribution of mu and delta opiate receptors in rat brain using highly selective ligands. Life Sci 33 Suppl 1:227–230

63. Roerig SC, Fujimoto JM (1988) Morphine antinociception in different strains of mice: relationship of supraspinal-spinal multiplicative interaction to tolerance. J Pharmacol Exp Ther 247:603–608

64. Rossi GC, Pasternak GW, Bodnar RJ (1993) Synergistic brainstem interactions for morphine analgesia. Brain Res 624:171–180

65. Sabbe MB, Yaksh TL (1990) Pharmacology of spinal opioids. J Pain Symptom Manage 5:191–203

66. Simon EJ (1973) In search of the opiate receptor. Am J Med Sci 266:160–168

67. Siuciak JA, Advokat C (1989) The synergistic effect of concurrent spinal and supraspinal opiate agonisms is reduced by both nociceptive and morphine pretreatment. Pharmacol Biochem Behav 34:265–273

68. Skilling SR, Sun X, Kurtz HJ et al. (1992) Selective potentiation of NMDA-induced activity and release of excitatory amino acids by dynorphin: possible roles in paralysis and neurotoxicity. Brain Res 575:272–278

69. Stillman MJ, Moulin DE, Foley KM (1987) Paradoxical pain following high-dose spinal morphine. Pain 4

70. Suzuki R, Morcuende S, Webber M et al. (2002) Superficial NK1-expressing neurons control spinal excitability through activation of descending pathways. Nat Neurosci 5:1319–1326

71. Suzuki R, Rahman W, Hunt SP et al. (2004) Descending facilitatory control of mechanically evoked responses is enhanced in deep dorsal horn neurones following peripheral nerve injury. Brain Res 1019:68–76

72. Taddese A, Nah SY, McCleskey EW (1995) Selective opioid inhibition of small nociceptive neurons. Science 270:1366–1369

73. Trujillo KA, Akil H (1994) Inhibition of opiate tolerance by non-competitive N-methyl-D-aspartate receptor antagonists. Brain Res 633:178–188

74. Vanderah TW, Laughlin T, Lashbrook JM et al. (1996) Single intrathecal injections of dynorphin A or des-Tyr-dynorphins produce long-lasting allodynia in rats: blockade by MK-801 but not naloxone. Pain 68:275–281

75. Vanderah TW, Gardell LR, Burgess SE et al. (2000) Dynorphin promotes abnormal pain and spinal opioid antinociceptive tolerance. J Neurosci 20:7074–7079

76. Vanderah TW, Ossipov MH, Lai J et al. (2001a) Mechanisms of opioid-induced pain and antinociceptive tolerance:descending facilitation and spinal dynorphin. Pain 92:5–9

77. Vanderah TW, Suenaga NM, Ossipov MH et al. (2001b) Tonic descending facilitation from the rostral ventromedial medulla mediates opioid-induced abnormal pain and antinociceptive tolerance. J Neurosci 21:279–286

78. Waterfield AA, Lord JA, Hughes J et al. (1978) Differences in the inhibitory effects of normorphine and opioid peptides on the responses of the vasa deferentia of two strains of mice. Eur J Pharmacol 47

79. Xie JY, Herman DS, Stiller CO et al. (2005) Cholecystokinin in the rostral ventromedial medulla mediates opioid-induced hyperalgesia and antinociceptive tolerance. J Neurosci 25:409–416

80. Yaksh TL, Yeung JC, Rudy TA (1976) Systematic examination in the rat of brain sites sensitive to the direct application of morphine: observation of differential effects within the periaqueductal gray. Brain Res 114:83–103

81. Yaksh TL, Huang SP, Rudy TA (1977a) The direct and specific opiate-like effect of met5-enkephalin and analogues on the spinal cord. Neuroscience 2:593–596

82. Yaksh TL, Kohl RL, Rudy TA (1977b) Induction of tolerance and withdrawal in rats receiving morphine in the spinal subarachnoid space. Eur J Pharmacol 42:275–284

83. Yeung JC, Rudy TA (1980) Multiplicative interaction between narcotic agonisms expressed at spinal and supraspinal sites of antinociceptive action as revealed by concurrent intrathecal and intracerebroventricular injections of morphine. J Pharmacol Exp Ther 215:633–642

84. Yeung JC, Yaksh TL, Rudy TA (1977) Concurrent mapping of brain sites for sensitivity to the direct application of morphine and focal electrical stimulation in the production of antinociception in the rat. Pain 4:23–40

85. Zaki PA, Bilsky EJ, Vanderah TW et al. (1996) Opioid receptor types and subtypes:the delta receptor as a model. Annu Rev Pharmacol Toxicol 36:379–401

gion of the central nervous system under consideration. In general, MOP and KOP receptors develop early in rodents and humans and the δ receptor appears later. In the human fetus, μ and κ opioid receptors appear at the start of the second trimester and mature through prenatal life. ▶ Delta opioid receptors (DOP) are generally absent prenatally in the human, although they can be transiently expressed. In the rat and other non-primate species, results are comparable: early appearance of MOP and KOP opioid receptors that peak between one and two weeks after birth, at which time the numbers decrease until adult levels are reached shortly thereafter. DOP receptors are first detected at the end of the first week after birth and are not likely to be fully functional until even later. In all cases, receptor affinity remains unchanged with age. Peptide development in general is also early and regionally specific, although the endomorphins mature relatively late (figure 1). Met-enkephalin-, dynorphin- and β-endorphin-like proteins can be detected by day 11.5 in the rat embryo, preceding the maturation of the recep-

tors, although in some regions opioids appear at the end of the first postnatal week.

Pharmacokinetics of Morphine

Morphine kinetics differ with both age and with body weight. In the adult, the major active metabolites of morphine are morphine-3-glucuronide (M3G) and morphine-6-glucuronide (M6G). M3G may have anti-opioid properties whereas M6G has analgesic effects (Christrup 1997). In the infant, M3G is the major metabolite. Although neither M3G nor M6G readily cross the blood brain barrier in the adult, whether they do or not in the infant is not known. Steady state morphine levels require 24–48 h of treatment for morphine, and at least 5 days of treatment for the metabolites (Saarenmaa et al. 2000). At six months of age, the full body clearance rate for morphine is about 80% of that of the adult (Bouwmeester et al. 2004). Metabolite clearance likewise increases with age. Thus, morphine doses in the infant must, out of necessity, be lower for

O

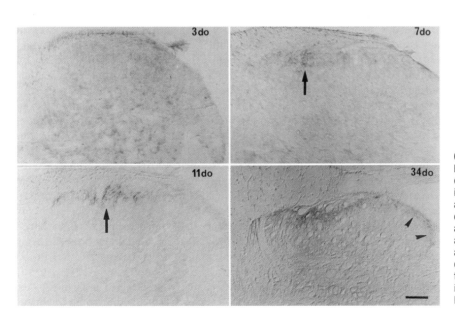

Opiates During Development, Figure 1 Maturation of endomorphin-2-like immunoreactivity in the lumbar dorsal horn of the rat at 4 different ages. Note the absence of staining at 3 days and the light and limited distribution of staining at 7 and 11 days (arrows). Staining at 34 days of age is more widely distributed in the lateral aspects of the dorsal horn (arrowheads). Bar is 100 μm. From Barr and Zadina, Neuroreport, 1999.

the premature infant or neonate than the older infant. Like morphine, fentanyl clearance is slower in the infant than in the older child and adult.

Development of Analgesia

In animal models (mostly rodent), the infant is generally more responsive to noxious stimuli (e.g. more likely to experience "pain") than the older animal, and is differentially responsive to opiate-induced analgesia. Although it is not known for certain why the infant is more sensitive to injury, the organization of the nervous system is clearly different in the infant than the adult (Fitzgerald 1991). ▶ Receptive fields of the infant, human or rodent, are larger and more diffuse. The afferent input of noxious stimulation in the infant is by ▶ A-fibers rather than ▶ C Fiber and the A fibers terminate in lamina 2 of the spinal cord ▶ dorsal horn. In the rat, these inappropriately targeted fibers retract and are replaced by C-fibers over the first three weeks of life. Further, inhibitory processes are not mature in the infant. Descending inhibitory processes engaged by opiates develop late in the infant rat, around the end of the second week of life, due to the late growth of functional descending bulbospinal projections. Diffuse noxious inhibitory processes within the spinal cord, where injury to one limb reduces nociception in a heterotopic region, also do not appear until sometime in the third week of life. Thus, in the absence of multiple inhibitory processes, the infant is unable to dampen the effects of injury (Fitzgerald 1991).

Opiates, despite the immaturity of the opioid peptides and receptors, are quite effective analgesics in the infant. This has been demonstrated numerous times in many paradigms. Morphine and fentanyl are the most effective treatments for pain in human neonates undergoing invasive medical treatment and postoperative care. Infants treated aggressively with opiates during and after surgery show decreased morbidity and mortality (Anand and Hickey 1987; Anand et al. 1987). Nonetheless, little detail is known of the best opiate, dose, dosing regimen, and match of opiate to type of pain. Issues of gestational age, body weight, and criticalness of illness only add to these complications (van Lingen et al. 2002).

The immaturity of the blood brain barrier may also contribute to the differential effectiveness of the opiate in the infant, by allowing more opiate to enter the central nervous system. There may also be yet undefined pharmacodynamic factors that account for this increased sensitivity. However, in the infant even more than the adult, the effectiveness of particular opiates is dependent on the type of nociceptive test and the intensity of the noxious stimulus. Intense thermal stimuli are less amenable to relief by morphine in the newborn rat pup, whereas analgesia to lower the intensity of mechanical noxious stimuli occurs quite early. The complexity is well illustrated by data showing that the relative analgesic effectiveness of buprenorphine, fentanyl and morphine in the infant compared to the adult is dependent on the type

of analgesic test. Morphine is most effective in the infant in thermal tests, but buprenorphine is most effective in tests of pain that are models for inflammatory insult (McLaughlin and Dewey 1994).

Moreover, there is regional specificity to the actions of the opiates. For example, due to the lack of descending inhibition, brain administration is less effective than spinal administration in the infant rat, although that is dependent on the type of analgesic test. In rats, administration of opiates in a manner that targets the spinal cord is quite effective as an analgesic (Barr et al. 1992; Marsh et al. 1999). In human children, these procedures are not common, but the clinical literature suggests that they are effective (e.g. Collins et al. 1995).

In both the adult and the infant, there are untoward side-effects that affect treatment. One of these is respiratory depression, a well-known effect of opiates. Initially part of the reluctance to treat infants was out of concern for these actions. Although still a concern, infants are not likely to be more sensitive to the respiratory effects of opiates than are adults. Two other concerns are dependence and ▶ tolerance that occur with repeated exposure.

Dependence

As in the adult, opiates such as morphine produce ▶ physical dependence. The human infant can become dependent due to medical treatment with opiates or by passive exposure through placental transfer, if the mother uses heroin or other opiates. When therapeutic opiate treatment is discontinued or when the opiate dependent mother gives birth, the infant shows a clear withdrawal syndrome that consists of increased irritability, disruption of sleep/wake states, incessant crying, and other physical signs. This is termed the "narcotic abstinence syndrome". As might be expected, higher doses and longer exposure increase risk for this syndrome.

In the rodent, withdrawal exists quite early, even in utero. In the infant rat, withdrawal is clearly different from withdrawal in the adult rat, and is characterized by increased separation-induced ultrasonic vocalizations (crying), increased activity and a unique set of behaviors not normally seen in pups not in withdrawal. The dysphoric state induced by opiate withdrawal occurs later, around the second week of life in the infant rat. Autonomic signs are minimal. In the adult, ▶ NMDA glutamate receptor antagonists, when given concomitantly with morphine, reduce withdrawal; but in the infant that treatment is ineffective (Zhu and Barr 2001). In contrast, AMPA blockers or ▶ nitric oxide inhibitors reduce dependence in the infant as they do in the adult. Thus, it is likely that the fundamental mechanisms mediating the chronic effects of opiates differ in the neonate.

Treatment with opiates is the preferred initial therapy for narcotic abstinence syndrome, and the only treatment for which there is evidence of efficacy. Morphine and methadone are currently the most commonly prescribed opioids to treat infant withdrawal, but which is more effective has not been determined. Clinically, there are no accepted or proven non-opioid treatments for the withdrawal syndrome. Barbiturate, benzodiazepines, and other sedatives are ineffective. The preclinical data suggest that NMDA antagonists, effective in the adult, are not likely to work in the human infant.

Tolerance

Tolerance also occurs to chronic opiate use in both human and animal infants. The tolerance is substantially less than that seen in the adult for reasons that are not understood. There are differences in intracellular signaling mechanisms that are age dependent that might account for this; as for dependence, tolerance to morphine in the infant is not NMDA receptor mediated.

Summary

Opioid receptors and peptides mature early during development but in a complex manner. Opiates are effective well-characterized drugs for the treatment of pain in the premature and full term infant. Regardless of the philosophical debate as to whether or not the infant can experience "pain", opiate treatment reduces morbidity and mortality in the infant patient. Opiates tend to be cleared more slowly in the premature or newborn full-term infant, and issues of the unique developmental effects of metabolites remain unaddressed. Whether or not different opiates are differentially effective for different painful procedures is not known. As in the adult, there are problems with iatrically induced tolerance and dependence, and with dependence in infants born of opiate using mothers. The most effective treatments are opiate based.

References

1. Anand KJ, Hickey PR (1987) Pain and its Effects in the Human Neonate and Fetus. N Engl J Med 317:1321–1329
2. Anand KJ, Sippell WG, Aynsley-Green A (1987) Randomised Trial of Fentanyl Anaesthesia in Preterm Babies Undergoing Surgery: Effects on the Stress Response. Lancet 1:62–66
3. Anand KJS, Craig KD (1996) New Perspectives on the Definition of Pain. Pain 67:3–6
4. Barr GA, Miya DY, Paredes W (1992) Analgesic Effects of Intraventricular and Intrathecal Injection of Morphine and Ketocyclazocine in the Infant Rat. Brain Res 584:83–91
5. Barr GA, Zadina JE (1999) Maturation of endomorphin-2 in the dorsal horn of the medulla and spinal cord of the rat. Neuroreport 10:3857–60
6. Bouwmeester NJ, Anderson BJ, Tibboel D et al. (2004) Developmental Pharmacokinetics of Morphine and its Metabolites in Neonates, Infants and Young Children. Br J Anaesth 92:208–217
7. Christrup LL (1997) Morphine Metabolites. Acta Anaesthesiol Scand 41:116–122
8. Collins JJ, Grier HE, Kinney HC et al. (1995) Control of Severe Pain in Children with Terminal Malignancy. J Pediatr 126:653–657
9. Derbyshire SW (2001) Fetal Pain: An Infantile Debate. Bioethics 15: 77–84.
10. Fitzgerald M (1991) Development of Pain Mechanisms. Brit Med Bull 47:667–675
11. Lingen RA van, Simons SH, Anderson BJ et al. (2002) The Effects of Analgesia in the Vulnerable Infant during the Perinatal Period. Clin Perinatol 29:511–534
12. Marsh D, Dickenson A, Hatch D et al. (1999) Epidural Opioid Analgesia in Infant Rats I: Mechanical and Heat Responses. Pain 82:23–32
13. McLaughlin CR, Dewey WL (1994) A Comparison of the Antinociceptive Effects of Opioid Agonists in Neonatal and Adult Rats in Phasic and Tonic Nociceptive Tests. Pharmacol Biochem Behav 49:1017–1023
14. Saarenmaa E, Neuvonen PJ, Rosenberg P et al. (2000) Morphine Clearance and Effects in Newborn Infants in Relation to Gestational Age. Clin Pharmacol Ther 68:160–166
15. Snyder SH, Pasternak GW (2003) Historical Review: Opioid Receptors. Trends Pharmacol Sci 24:198–205
16. Zhu H, Barr GA (2001) Opiate Withdrawal during Development: Are NMDA Receptors Indispensable? Trends Pharmacol Sci 22:404–408

Opiates, Rostral Ventromedial Medulla and Descending Control

MARY M. HEINRICHER
Department of Neurological Surgery, Oregon Health Science University, Portland, OR, USA
heinricm@ohsu.edu

Definition

The recognition that supraspinal structures can exert control over sensory processing at the level of the spinal cord has a long history. However, the realization that descending controls have a specific role in the regulation of spinal pain processing achieved prominence in 1969, with the demonstration of analgesia during electrical stimulation of the midbrain periaqueductal gray (PAG) (Reynolds 1969). This phenomenon came to be called "stimulation-produced analgesia" (SPA). Subsequent intensive investigations of SPA led to the definition of a central pain modulatory network, now known to span the neuraxis, with critical links in the PAG and ▶ rostral ventromedial medulla (RVM) (Fields and Basbaum 1999). Non-selective activation of the RVM was shown to inhibit behavioral responses to noxious stimuli, and this antinociception is in large part due to interference with nociceptive processing at the level of the spinal cord. Moreover, further investigation has now demonstrated that the RVM exerts bidirectional control over nociception. The best current evidence, as described below, is that different physiologically defined populations of RVM neurons mediate antinociceptive and pronociceptive effects of RVM manipulation.

The anatomical substrate for spinal modulation of nociception from the RVM is a large projection from this region to the dorsal horn. The projection travels through the dorsolateral funiculus, and terminates at all levels of the spinal cord, in laminae known to be involved in nociception. The specifics of how the RVM projection interfaces with nociceptive circuitry at the level of the dorsal horn to alter nociception remain unresolved. A major input to the RVM is the PAG, which channels input from higher structures, including hypothalamus and amygdala, to the RVM.

The delineation of this brainstem pain modulating system has thus been a major breakthrough in defining pain modulation as a separable function of the nervous system, and in showing that the influence of psychological variables on pain could have an understandable neural basis.

Characteristics

Interest in the PAG/RVM descending modulatory network was heightened when it became apparent that this system was also an important substrate for opioid analgesia. The RVM, and especially the PAG, are rich in opioid receptors and opioid peptides. The RVM is required for the full analgesic action of systemically administered morphine, and focal application of morphine or mu-opioid agonists within the RVM is sufficient to produce potent behavioral analgesia (Yaksh et al. 1988). The neural basis of mu-opioid analgesia within the RVM has been studied in depth. There is now clear evidence that the antinociceptive effects of mu-opioid agonists within the RVM require activation of a class of RVM neurons termed "▸ off-cells (RVM)" (Fig. 1), which exert a net inhibitory effect on nociception (Heinricher et al. 1994). The proximal event in opioid activation of

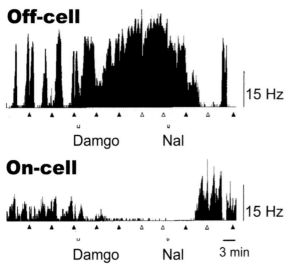

Off-cell

15 Hz

Damgo   Nal

On-cell

15 Hz

Damgo   Nal   3 min

Opiates, Rostral Ventromedial Medulla and Descending Control, Figure 1 Focal application of the mu-opioid agonist DAMGO within the RVM activates an off-cell whilst inhibiting an on-cell recorded simultaneously on the same electrode. Ratemeter records show firing rate in 1 s bins, with tail flick trials performed at 5min intervals (indicated by triangles below the trace). DAMGO was infused following a baseline period, and resulted in activation of the off-cell and suppression of on-cell firing. Inhibition of the tail flick reflex ("analgesia") is indicated by open triangles at 15 and 20 min after DAMGO. Changes in cell activity and antinociception were reversed by systemic administration of naloxone (1 mg/kg). Adapted with permission from Heinricher et al. (1994) Disinhibition of off-cells and antinociception produced by an opioid action within the rostral ventromedial medulla. Neuroscience 63:279–288.

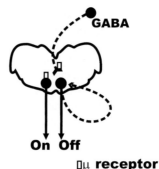

Opiates, Rostral Ventromedial Medulla and Descending Control, Figure 2 Off-cell activation is triggered by presynaptic inhibition of a GABAergic input originating from outside of the RVM, and reinforced by an excitatory input (mediated by an NMDA receptor, not shown). The excitatory link could be within the RVM (i.e. mutual excitation among off-cells) or via extra-RVM pathways. Parallel inhibition of on-cells by the opioid likely contributes to antinociception, although under normal conditions on-cell inhibition is not sufficient to produce antinociception. Mu-opioid receptors are thus located both presynaptically (on inhibitory inputs to off-cells) and post-synaptically (on on-cells).

the off-cells is disinhibition. That is, the direct effect of mu-opioid agonists is to inhibit a GABAergic input to the off-cells. This disinhibition in turn leads to a positive feedback process, resulting in further off-cell activation and behavioral antinociception (Fig. 2) (Heinricher et al. 2001; Heinricher and Tortorici 1994; Pan et al. 1990). In addition to the indirect activation of off-cells, mu-opioid agonists inhibit another class of neurons in RVM, termed "▸ on-cells (RVM)" (Fig. 1). It was originally thought that on-cells served as inhibitory interneurons within the RVM. However, on-cells are known to project to the dorsal horn, and the recent demonstration that blocking the reflex-related activity of on-cells does not disinhibit off-cells, argues very strongly that on-cells are not inhibitory interneurons. Rather, they are now thought to constitute a descending influence that is in parallel with the antinociceptive output of the off-cells (Fig. 2). Given that suppression of on-cell discharge is not by itself sufficient to produce measurable behavioral antinociception (Heinricher et al. 1999), it is unlikely that on-cells exert a potent tonic effect on nociception under normal conditions. However, direct opioid inhibition of on-cells may assume an important role in inflammatory or other abnormal pain states, in which these neurons are very likely to contribute to hyperalgesia.

A third class of RVM neurons - " ▸ neutral cells (RVM)" - do not respond to noxious stimulation or to opioid application. Their role in pain modulation is unknown. It is likely that neutral cells comprise a heterogeneous group that includes the serotonergic neurons in this region. The idea that RVM serotonergic neurons do not respond to opioids has presented something of an enigma, since pharmacological studies point to descending serotonergic projections as central to descending pain modulation, including opioid analgesia. One possible way to reconcile the behavioral and physiological observations is to propose that the serotonergic outflow enables or "gates" other descending influences that are directly inhibitory or facilitatory.

Delta Opioid Actions in the RVM

Insight into the role of the delta opioid receptor in the RVM remains at an early stage, at least in comparison to our understanding of the mu receptor (Heinricher and Fields 2003). Delta receptors are found in the RVM, although there is some disagreement as to whether they are localized to cell bodies or exclusively to axon terminals. Direct microinjection of delta opioid receptor agonists, especially delta2 agonists, within the RVM produces a modest hypoalgesia in behavioral tests. Given the presence of delta receptors and evidence for a behavioral effect of delta agonists in the RVM, it is somewhat surprising that *in vitro* electrophysiological studies have found no evidence for delta receptor effects on RVM neurons. *In vivo*, identified on- and off-cells exhibit only modest changes in response patterns after microinjection of the delta2 agonist deltorphin. Although subtle compared to the effects of mu agonists within the RVM, these alterations in neuronal firing are consistent with the relatively small behavioral change produced by delta agonists in this region.

Kappa Opioid Actions in the RVM

The role of the kappa receptor within the RVM is at present somewhat controversial. Focal application of kappa agonists within the RVM has been reported to produce potent analgesia by one group (Ackley et al. 2001), while other investigators find that kappa compounds have no effect by themselves on nociception, but interfere with the analgesic actions of mu-opioids (that is, that they have an "anti-analgesic" effect) (Pan 1998). While the sex of the subjects may account for some of the discrepant results, it does not appear to be a complete explanation.

As with the behavioral analyses, electrophysiological findings are also controversial. Only *in vitro* studies have been reported to date. Pan and colleagues found that mu and kappa receptors are expressed by separate populations of RVM neurons (referred to as ► secondary cells (RVM) and ► primary cells (RVM), respectively). They therefore proposed that the behavioral anti-analgesic effect of kappa agonists given by microinjection in the RVM could be explained by kappa inhibition of off-cells, the inhibitory output neurons of the RVM (Pan 1998). However, it is not known whether off-cells respond to kappa agonists, as this has not been tested *in vivo*. Moreover, recent work in the RVM slice by Marinelli et al. (Marinelli et al. 2002) showed that mu- and kappa-opioid receptor types are commonly co-expressed by spinally projecting RVM neurons, with

only a small subset demonstrating kappa responses in the absence of mu responses. Other workers have shown that kappa agonists act presynaptically within the RVM (Ackley et al. 2001).

Physiological Recruitment of Opioids within the RVM

What is the physiological role of opioids within the RVM? Opioid receptor antagonists, microinjected into the RVM, do not alter nociceptive responses, indicating that endogenous opioids do not maintain an ongoing tone under normal conditions. Endogenous opioid-mediated effects are likely to be important in stress-induced analgesia, although relatively few studies have focused specifically on the RVM. Interestingly, enhanced delta activity is thought to contribute to the well-documented increase in the analgesic potency of opioids in inflammatory pain states. Hurley and Hammond (2001) suggest a novel interaction of mu- and delta-receptor mediated effects within the RVM following inflammation.

Among the other neurotransmitters and neuropeptides known to influence opioid-sensitive pain modulating circuits within the RVM are ► acetylcholine, ► serotonin, neurotensin, norepinephrine, ► cholecystokinin and ► orphanin FQ/nociceptin. Understanding the many inputs to the RVM, and how these systems are recruited and modified to interact with opioid actions under physiological and pathophysiological conditions, remain important areas for future work.

References

1. Ackley MA, Hurley RW, Virnich DE et al. (2001) A Cellular Mechanism for the Antinociceptive Effect of a Kappa Opioid Receptor Agonist. Pain 91:377–388
2. Fields HL, Basbaum AI, Heinricher MM (2005) Central nervous system mechanisms of pain modulation. In: McMahon S and Koltzenburg M (eds) Wall PD, Melzack's Textbook of Pain, 5th edn. Elsevier, London, pp 125–142
3. Heinricher MM, Fields HL (2003) The Delta Opioid Receptor and Brain Pain-Modulating Circuits. In: Chang KJ, Porreca F, Woods J (eds) The Delta Receptor: Molecular and Effect of Delta Opioid Compounds. Marcel Dekker, New York, pp 467–480
4. Heinricher MM, McGaraughty S, Farr DA (1999) The Role of Excitatory Amino Acid Transmission within the Rostral Ventromedial Medulla in the Antinociceptive Actions of Systemically Administered Morphine. Pain 81:57–65
5. Heinricher MM, Morgan MM, Tortorici V et al. (1994) Disinhibition of Off-Cells and Antinociception Produced by an Opioid Action within the Rostral Ventromedial Medulla. Neuroscience 63:279–288
6. Heinricher MM, Schouten JC, Jobst EE (2001) Activation of Brainstem N-methyl-D-aspartate Receptors is required for the Analgesic Actions of Morphine given Systemically. Pain 92:129–138.
7. Heinricher MM, Tortorici V (1994) Interference with GABA Transmission in the Rostral Ventromedial Medulla: Disinhibition of Off-Cells as a Central Mechanism in Nociceptive Modulation. Neuroscience 63:533–546
8. Hurley RW, Hammond DL (2001) Contribution of Endogenous Enkephalins to the Enhanced Analgesic Effects of Supraspinal Mu-opioid Receptor Agonists after Inflammatory Injury. J Neurosci 21:2536–2545

O

9. Marinelli S, Vaughan CW, Schnell SA et al. (2002) Rostral Ventromedial Medulla Neurons that Project to the Spinal Cord Express Multiple Opioid Receptor Phenotypes. J Neurosci 22:10847–10855
10. Pan ZZ (1998) μ-Opposing Actions of the Kappa-Opioid Receptor. Trends Pharmacol Sci 19:94–98
11. Pan ZZ, Williams JT, Osborne PB (1990) Opioid Actions on Single Nucleus Raphe Magnus Neurons from Rat and Guinea-Pig *In Vitro*. J Physiol 427:519–532
12. Reynolds DV (1969) Surgery in the Rat during Electrical Analgesia Induced by Focal Brain Stimulation. Science 154:444–445
13. Yaksh TL, Al-Rodhan NRF, Jensen TS (1988) Sites of Action of Opiates in Production of Analgesia. Prog Brain Res 77:371–394

Opioid

Definition

A class of drugs with a molecular structure similar to opium. All opiates have analgesic effects and other effects, some of them adverse. Examples of opiates include morphine, codeine and fentanyl. Opioid is a generic term that refers to all molecules, either natural or synthetic, either small molecule or peptide, which exert morphine-like pharmacological actions. The predominant pharmacologic property of therapeutic interest is analgesia, the selective relief of pain. Other pharmacologic actions include sedation, respiratory depression, decreased gastrointestinal motility, nausea, and vomiting. Opioids exert their actions through a family of seven-transmembrane, G_i/G_o-coupled receptors, traditionally identified as μ, κ, and δ (a.k.a. MOR, KOR, and DOR). Morphine is the prototypical μ opioid agonist.

▶ Analgesia During Labor and Delivery
▶ Cancer Pain Management, Cancer-Related Breakthrough Pain, Therapy
▶ Cancer Pain Management, Principles of Opioid Therapy, Dosing Guidelines
▶ Cancer Pain Management, Principles of Opioid Therapy, Drug Selection
▶ Cytokine Modulation of Opioid Action
▶ Deep Brain Stimulation
▶ Forebrain Modulation of the Periaqueductal Gray
▶ Hot Plate Test (Assay)
▶ Opioids, Clinical Opioid Tolerance
▶ Opioid Peptide Co-Localization and Release
▶ Opioid Receptor Localization
▶ Pain Treatment, Implantable Pumps for Drug Delivery
▶ Postoperative Pain, Acute Pain Management, Principles
▶ Postoperative Pain, Opioids
▶ Postoperative Pain, Postamputation Pain, Treatment and Prevention

Opioid Adverse Effects

Definition

Unwanted and unpleasant effects of opioid drugs when used in pain management.
▶ Cancer Pain Management, Principles of Opioid Therapy, Drug Selection

Opioid Analgesia

Definition

Pain-inhibitory effects of opioid drugs such as morphine or opioid-receptor agonist drugs.
▶ Opioid Analgesia, Strain Differences
▶ Psychological Aspects of Pain in Women

Opioid Analgesia and Sex Differences

▶ Sex Differences in Opioid Analgesia

Opioid Analgesia, Strain Differences

JEFFREY S. MOGIL
Department of Psychology, McGill University, Montreal, QC, Canada
jeffrey.mogil@mcgill.ca

Synonyms

Opioid analgesia; Genotypic Influences on Opioid Analgesia; Genetic Factors Contributing to Opioid Analgesia

Definition

The efficacy of the pain-inhibitory neural circuitry activated by opioid compounds differs among individuals. The contribution of inherited genetic factors to such interindividual variability in responses to drugs (i.e. ▶ pharmacogenetics) is most easily studied by comparing subpopulations of a species, especially ▶ inbred strains. Robust strain differences in the magnitude and neurochemical mediation of opioid analgesia have been observed in both mice and rats. The genes underlying these strain differences are starting to be identified, and appear to play similar roles in analgesic variability in humans.

Characteristics

Morphine at standard doses exhibits a wide range of clinical efficacies against postoperative and chronic pain. A human twin study revealed that morphine inhibition of experimental pain is likely to be ▶ heritable (Liston et al. 1981), and successful selective breeding has demonstrated the heritability of opioid analgesia in mice (see Mogil et al. 1996b). The identification of genes (and their common DNA sequence variants, or ▶ alleles) underlying the variable pharmacodynamic and pharmacokinetic properties of opioid analgesics would allow individualized treatment of pain, to maximize efficacy and minimize side effects in each patient.

Differential sensitivity of laboratory mouse and rat populations to opioid drugs has long been noted (see Mogil 1999). The genetic contribution to such variability can be assessed using inbred strains, in which repeated brother–sister matings have eliminated genetic ▶ heterozygosity, rendering each individual virtually isogenic to (i.e. a clone of) all others of that strain. By comparing multiple strains tested simultaneously, genetic components (differences between strain means) and environmental components (within–strain error) of analgesic variability can be partitioned. Large "strain surveys" of opioid analgesia have been performed in the mouse (Wilson et al. 2003) and rat (Morgan et al. 1999). Robust differences in half–maximal analgesic doses ($AD_{50}s$) were noted; in one study of morphine ranged almost 4–fold among 12 inbred strains (see Fig. 1). Strain differences can be observed regardless of the route of opioid administration. The magnitude of strain differences has been shown to depend on opioid efficacy and stimulus intensity (Morgan et al. 1999). Genotype-dependence of analgesia is not limited to exogenous opioids; with strain differences also being documented for stress–induced analgesia and non–opioid drug analgesia (see Mogil 1999). In the few studies that have ever looked, pharmacokinetic considerations do not appear to explain these strain differences (e.g. Mas et al. 2000). In addition to analgesic magnitude, the physiological processing of analgesia also appears to be strain-dependent. For example, forced swims in 15°C water produce opioid-mediated (naloxone-sensitive) analgesia in male DBA/2J mice, but non-opioid-mediated analgesia in male C57BL/6J mice (Mogil and Belknap 1997). Similarly, analgesia from the κ–opioid agonist, U50,488, is reversed by the N–methyl-D-aspartate receptor antagonist, MK–801, in male mice of a number of strains, but not in C3HeB/FeJ mice (unpublished data). Elegant pharmacological studies have shown that heroin analgesia is predominantly mediated by μ receptors in three inbred strains, by κ receptors in two others, and by δ receptors in yet another (Rady et al. 1998). Such qualitative differences among strains suggest differential neural circuit organization, as has been demonstrated for coeruleospinal projections (Clark and Proudfit 1992).

Dose-Response Curves

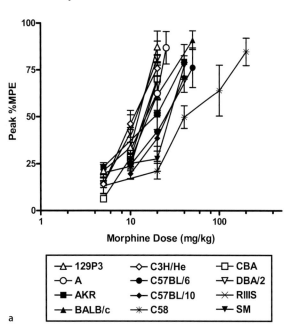

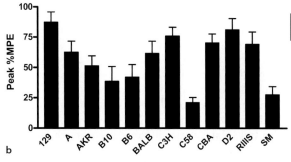

20 mg/kg Morphine

Opioid Analgesia, Strain Differences, Figure 1 Genotype-dependent sensitivity to systemic morphine analgesia in 12 inbred mouse strains (all "J" substrains; from Wilson et al. 2003). All mice were tested for baseline sensitivity on the 49°C hot water tail-withdrawal assay, administered 5–200 mg/kg (i.p.) morphine sulfate, and retested 15, 30 and 60 min. post-injection. Symbols in (a) represent mean ± S.E.M. peak (over the 60 min. time course) percentage of the maximum possible effect (%MPE) at each dose. Associated $AD_{50}s$ range from 10.5 mg/kg (129P3) to 38.5 mg/kg (C58). The 12 strains appear to group into three clusters: a sensitive group (open symbols), a resistant group (closed symbols and cross), and the very resistant C58 strain (asterisk). The peak %MPE at one dose common to all strains, 20 mg/kg, is shown in (b).

The strongest predictor of strain-dependent morphine AD_{50} is the baseline sensitivity to the noxious stimulus being inhibited by morphine. Generally speaking, strains sensitive to nociception are resistant to analgesia, and strains resistant to nociception are sensitive to analgesia (Mogil et al. 1996a). This might imply that the underlying genetic contribution is to ▶ opioid tone and/or related to ▶ fractional receptor occupancy of opioid receptors (Elmer et al. 1998). The phenomenon is not limited to morphine anal-

Opioid Analgesia, Strain Differences, Table 1   QTLs for morphine inhibition of hot-plate nociception in DBA/2 and C57BL/6 mice.

Chrom.	Loc. [a]	LOD [b]	Candidate Gene/Protein [c]	Reference
1	10 cM	4.7†	Oprk1, κ–opioid receptor (6 cM)	Mogil et al. unpublished data
9*	20 cM	5.2†	—	—
9*	42 cM	4.5	Htr1b, serotonin–1B receptor (46 cM)	Hain et al. 1999 J. Pharmacol. Exp. Ther. 291:444–449
10*	9 cM	7.5	Oprm, μ–opioid receptor (8 cM)	Belknap et al. 1995 Life Sci. 57:PL117–PL124

[a]Location in centiMorgans (cM; approximately 1 million base pairs) from the proximal end of the chromosome of the peak statistical evidence for genetic linkage. The 95% confidence intervals in this type of study are generally very large, however
[b]Logarithm of the odds (LOD) score for linkage of morphine analgesia to the defined genomic region. The conservative threshold for "significant" linkage is LOD = 4.3
[c]Gene and the protein it codes that may underlie the QTL, supported by evidence presented in the cited reference. The gene's chromosomal location in cM is given in parentheses
*The existence of these QTLs was independently replicated in a different laboratory using different progenitor strains (A/J and SM/J) (Mizuo et al. 2000, *International Narcotics Research Conference*, Seattle)
†Significant linkage in female mice only; no evidence for linkage whatsoever was obtained in male mice

gesia, however, having also been demonstrated for clonidine, epibatidine, U50,488, and the cannabinoid agonist, WIN55–212,2 (Wilson et al. 2003). In fact, these five analgesics show a high degree of genetic correlation with each other, suggestive of the existence of "master" genes responsible for variability in both nociception and analgesia across a wide range of compounds (Wilson et al. 2003).

When male and female subjects have been tested simultaneously for opioid analgesia, a strong interaction between genotype and sex has been noted (see Mogil 2003). Sex differences (see ► Gender and Pain) can be demonstrated in some genotypes but not others, and even the direction of the sex difference may depend on the subject's genotype. The converse is, of course, also true: some strain differences are much larger in one sex than the other.

Different physiological effects of a drug may have independent genetic bases. For example, in a study comparing the sensitivity of three inbred strains on six behavioral effects of morphine (analgesia, hyperlocomotion, hypothermia, muscular rigidity, antidiuresis and constipation), almost every possible rank-ordering of strain was observed (Belknap et al. 1989). With respect to analgesia specifically, strains sensitive to morphine inhibition of thermal nociception on the tail-withdrawal or hot-plate tests, are *not* necessarily the same strains sensitive to morphine inhibition of chemical nociception on the formalin or abdominal constriction tests (Mogil et al. 1996a; Elmer et al. 1998). The dependence of analgesia pharmacogenetics on the type of pain being inhibited is a generalizable phenomenon, also applicable to clonidine (Wilson et al. 2003) and pregabalin (manuscript submitted).

Of opioid analgesics, only morphine and U50,488 have been subjected to ► quantitative trait locus (QTL) mapping, a technique allowing the broad localization of trait variability genes to chromosomal regions as the first step towards their identification. Once the genes underlying the QTLs are identified, one can search for the DNA sequence variants (e.g. ► single-nucleotide polymorphisms) responsible for the strain difference. Although it is not necessarily true that murine polymorphisms will be preserved in humans, there is some reason to expect that similar genes will be trait-relevant and genetically variable in both rodents and humans. For morphine inhibition of thermal (hot plate) nociception, using the sensitive DBA/2 and resistant C57BL/6 strains (see Fig. 1) as parental genotypes, four significant QTLs have been uncovered, that together account for two–thirds of the additive genetic variance and one-quarter of the overall trait variance (Bergeson et al. 2001). These QTLs, and the genes likely underlying each QTL, are shown in Table 1. As can be seen, in two cases the QTLs are sex-specific. A female–specific QTL was also uncovered for U50,488 inhibition of hot water tail–withdrawal nociception (Mogil et al. 2003). This QTL, on distal mouse chromosome 8, was determined by convergent mouse mutant and pharmacological data to be *Mc1r*, encoding the melanocortin-1 receptor (Mogil et al. 2003).

Success in identifying genes responsible for mouse or rat strain differences will be of purely academic interest unless those same genes are shown to be relevant to human individual differences. Thus, more attention is being paid to "translational" genetic strategies. If a particular gene is postulated to be important for a trait, and that gene has known sequence variants in humans, an association or ► allele dosage study can be performed. The possible roles of the human *OPRM* (μ-opioid receptor) and *OPRD* (δ–opioid receptor) genes are currently being investigated. Following the determination that the mouse *Mc1r* gene affected κ-opioid analgesia in female mice, the human *MC1R* gene (also responsible for red hair and fair skin) was found to affect pentazocine inhibition of experimental pain in human women (Mogil et al. 2003). Findings such as these may revolutionize pain treatment, by allowing more effective usage of existing compounds, identifying new molecular targets for drug development, and facilitating the regulatory approval of new drugs based on the ability to identify likely "responders."

References

1. Belknap JK, Noordewier B, Lamé M (1989) Genetic Dissociation of Multiple Morphine Effects among C57BL/6J, DBA/2J and C3H/HeJ Inbred Mouse Strains. Physiol Behav 46:69–74
2. Bergeson SE, Helms ML, O'Toole LA, Jarvis MW, Hain HS, Mogil JS, Belknap JK (2001) Quantitative Trait Loci Influencing Morphine Antinociception in Four Mapping Populations. Mamm Genome 12:546–553
3. Chesler EJ, Ritchie J, Kokajeff A et al. (2003) Genotype-dependence of gabapentin and pregabalin sensitivity: the pharmacogenetic mediation of analgesia is specific to the type of pain being inhibited. Pain 106:325–35
4. Clark FM, Proudfit HK (1992) Anatomical Evidence for Genetic Differences in the Innervation of the Rat Spinal Cord by Nora-drenergic Locus Coeruleus Neurons. Brain Res 591:44–53
5. Elmer GI, Pieper JO, Negus SS, Woods JH (1998) Genetic Variance in Nociception and its Relationship to the Potency of Morphine-Induced Analgesia in Thermal and Chemical Tests. Pain 75:129–140
6. Liston EH, Simpson JH, Jarvik LF, Guthrie D (1981) Morphine and Experimental Pain in Identical Twins. Prog Clin Biol Res 69:105–116
7. Mas M, Sabater E, Olaso MJ, Horga JF, Faura CC (2000) Genetic Variability in Morphine Sensitivity and Tolerance between Different Strains of Rats. Brain Res 866:109–115
8. Mogil JS (1999) The Genetic Mediation of Individual Differences in Sensitivity to Pain and its Inhibition. Proc Natl Acad Sci USA 96:7744–7751
9. Mogil JS (2004) The Interaction between Sex and Genotype in the Mediation of Pain and Pain Inhibition. Pain Med 1:197–205
10. Mogil JS, Belknap JK (1997) Sex and Genotype Determine the Selective Activation of Neurochemically-Distinct Mechanisms of Swim Stress-Induced Analgesia. Pharmacol Biochem Behav 56:61–66
11. Mogil JS, Kest B, Sadowski B, Belknap JK (1996a) Differential Genetic Mediation of Sensitivity to Morphine in Genetic Models of Opiate Antinociception: Influence of Nociceptive Assay. J. Pharmacol. Exp Ther 276:532–544
12. Mogil JS, Sternberg WF, Marek P, Sadowski B, Belknap JK, Liebeskind JC (1996b) The Genetics of Pain and Pain Inhibition. Proc Natl Acad Sci USA 93:3048–3055
13. Mogil JS, Wilson SG, Chesler EJ, Rankin AL, Nemmani KVS, Lariviere WR, Groce MK, Wallace MR, Kaplan L, Staud R, Ness TJ, Glover TL, Stankova M, Mayorov A, Hruby VJ, Grisel JE, Fillingim RB (2003) The Melanocortin–1 Receptor Gene Mediates Female-Specific Mechanisms of Analgesia in Mice and Humans. Proc Natl Acad Sci USA 100:4867–4872
14. Morgan D, Cook CD, Picker MJ (1999) Sensitivity to the Discriminative Stimulus and Antinociceptive Effects of μ-Opioids: Role of Strain of Rat, Stimulus Intensity, and Intrinsic Efficacy at the μ-Opioid Receptor. J Pharmacol Exp Ther 289:965–975
15. Rady JJ, Elmer GI, Fujimoto JM (1998) Opioid Receptor Selectivity of Heroin Given Intracerebroventricularly Differs in Six Strains of Inbred Mice. J Pharmacol Exp Ther 288:438–445
16. Wilson SG, Smith SB, Chesler EJ, Melton KA, Haas JJ, Mitton BA, Strasburg K, Hubert L, Rodriguez-Zas SL, Mogil JS (2003) The Heritability of Antinociception: Common Pharmacogenetic Mediation of Five Neurochemically-Distinct Analgesics. J Pharmacol Exp Ther 304:547–559

Opioid Analgesic

Definition

Opioid analgesics are pharmacologic agents whose mechanism of action involves interaction with receptors for endogenous opioids. Opioid receptors located in the central nervous system, with their endogenous ligands, including enkephalin, β-endorphin, and dynorphin, form part of an endogenous system modulating nociception.

▶ Cancer Pain Management, Opioid Side Effects, Uncommon Side Effects

Opioid Analgesic Actions Outside the Central Nervous System

▶ Opioids in the Periphery and Analgesia

Opioid Antagonists

Definition

Naloxone is generally recognized as the classical opioid antagonist drug, which possesses affinity but lacks efficacy for opioid receptors. At sufficient doses, naloxone will block mu, delta and kappa opioid receptors, although low doses are reportedly more selective for mu opioid receptors. Naltrexone and β-chlornaltrexamine are other examples of non-selective opioid antagonist drugs. Newer drugs possess greater selectivity for one or another opioid receptor subtypes. For instance, β-funaltrexamine and CTOP are selective mu opioid antagonists, naltrindole and naltriben are selective delta opioid antagonists, and norbinaltorphimine is a selective kappa opioid antagonist.

▶ Nitrous Oxide Antinociception and Opioid Receptors

Opioid Dose Titration

Definition

The clinical practice of increasing opioid dosage to achieve analgesia without unwanted adverse effects.

▶ Cancer Pain Management, Principles of Opioid Therapy, Drug Selection

Opioid Electrophysiology in PAG

MacDonald J. Christie, P.B. Osborne
Pain Management Research Institute and Kolling
Institute, University of Sydney, Sydney, NSW,
Australia
macc@med.usyd.edu.au

Synonyms

Periaqueductal grey; periaqueductal gray; central grey;
Central Gray/Central Grey; opiate

Definition

The midbrain periaqueductal grey (PAG) is one of the
major brain targets for the analgesic actions of opioid
drugs and endogenously released opioids. The PAG contributes to a descending inhibitory neural network. When
PAG output neurons are activated, nociceptive neurotransmission at the level of the dorsal horn of the spinal
cord is inhibited. Opioids are thought to produce analgesia in the PAG by a disinhibitory mechanism via direct
inhibition of GABAergic neurotransmission impinging
on descending output neurons.

Characteristics

The PAG, as the name suggests, is a cell dense region surrounding the cerebral aqueduct extending from the third
ventricle to the pontine division of the fourth ventricle.
Anatomical, physiological and behavioural studies all
indicate that the PAG is organized into distinct functional
columns that extend along the rostrocaudal axis. The different functional columns are considered to be involved
in the expression of distinct patterns of autonomic and
behavioural responses (Bandler and Shipley 1994).
All of the major types of opioid receptor, μ– (▶ MOP),
δ– (▶ DOP) and κ– (▶ KOP) and N/OFQ (▶ NOP) receptors, are expressed abundantly in PAG (Mansour et
al. 1995). The first three of these are considered to mediate antinociceptive actions in PAG, with the μ–receptor
mediating the analgesic actions of most clinically useful
opioids. The N/OFQ receptor is closely related to μ–,
δ– and κ–receptors, but is not activated by classical
opioid agonists. Activation of the N/OFQ receptor in
PAG functionally antagonizes the effects of morphine.
Endogenous opioids derived from each of the major pro-hormone precursors are also richly expressed
within the PAG (Fallon and Leslie 1986). These include pro-opiomelanocortin (POMC), which produces
▶ β–endorphin from nerve terminals of hypothalamic
neurons, proenkephalin from intrinsic neurons and projections from several brain regions, and pro-dynorphin
also from intrinsic neurons and projections from several
brain regions.
Direct microinjection of opioid receptor agonists into
the PAG produces analgesia in experimental animals.
Agonists for each receptor type have antinociceptive

actions when microinjected into PAG (Ossipov et
al. 1995). However, μ–receptor agonists are more efficacious than δ– or κ–agonists. Microinjected opioids
produce antinociception more effectively in the ventrolateral PAG, particularly in the most caudal area, than in
lateral or dorsal columns (Jansen and Yaksh 1985). Electrical stimulation of the PAG in experimental animals
and humans also produces analgesia that can be reversed
by opioid receptor antagonists such as naloxone, but
only when stimulation is located in the ventrolateral
area. This implies that electrical stimulation of ventrolateral PAG releases endogenous opioids. Stimulation
of other areas of the PAG can also produce antinociception, but the effects are generally not reversed by opioid
antagonists (see Bandler and Shipley 1994).
The mechanisms by which opioids modulate electrical
excitability in PAG are summarized in Figure 1. These
mechanisms provide a general explanation for the analgesic actions of μ– and κ–opioid agonists in PAG, as well
as the anti-opioid actions of N/OFQ.

Postsynaptic Actions of Opioids in PAG

Opioid receptors, where expressed on the somatic membrane, inhibit electrical excitability of PAG neurons (see
Williams et al. 2001 for review). Inhibition occurs via
actions that are typical of the subfamily of inhibitory
G-protein coupled receptors, to which all of the opioid
receptors belong. Opioid agonists activate inhibitory G-
proteins (predominantly Gi) to simultaneously reduce
currents through voltage-gated calcium channels, and
enhance currents through inwardly rectifying potassium
channels in PAG neurons. Both actions inhibit neuronal
excitability. The principal calcium channels inhibited
by opioids are the N– and ▶ P/Q channels, which play
a major role in regulation of membrane excitability as
well as neurotransmitter release. The potassium channel is probably a ▶ GIRK subtype that hyperpolarizes
the membrane to reduce excitability. Opioid agonists
also inhibit adenylyl cyclase in PAG. While this has
little effect on excitability under basal conditions, it
reduces currents through a protein kinase A dependent,
non-selective cation channel that is activated when
adenylyl cyclase and hence cAMP levels are elevated
in the neuron. The latter mechanism of opioid action is
also inhibitory.
Opioids display the actions described above only in a
subpopulation of neurons in PAG. Actions mediated by
μ–receptors have been observed in brain slices and isolated neurons from rat PAG. Although μ–agonists act
on approximately 30% of all lateral and ventrolateral
PAG neurons, only 14% of those in the ventrolateral PAG
that project to the rostral ventromedial medulla are sensitive to μ-agonists (Osborne et al. 1996). This observation supports the proposal (see Williams et al. 2001) that
μ–opioids act predominantly on GABAergic interneurons in PAG, and not on neurons that form part of the descending projection to the rostral ventromedial medulla.

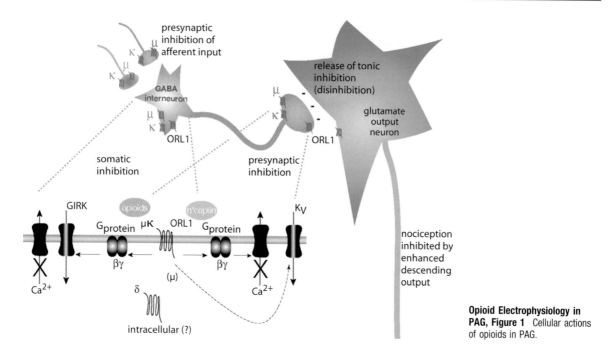

Opioid Electrophysiology in PAG, Figure 1 Cellular actions of opioids in PAG.

However, it should be noted that in the same study, 56% of descending projection neurons in the lateral PAG were sensitive to μ–agonists, so the interpretation may only be true for the ventrolateral PAG which mediates opioid antinociception.

Almost all PAG neurons of the rat are inhibited via the same mechanisms described above by the ORL1 agonist, N/OFQ. By contrast, no electrophysiological effects of κ– or δ–receptor agonists were observed in rat PAG, although both receptors are expressed in the region. Failure of δ–receptors to affect membrane currents is probably due to their largely intracellular localisation (Commons 2003). Density of κ–receptors in rat PAG might not be sufficiently high to produce robust cellular physiological effects in rats. In mouse PAG, opioids act on μ–, δ– and κ–receptors in about 80%, 20%, and 20% of PAG neurons, respectively (Vaughan et al. 2003). It should be noted that κ– and δ–receptor agonists produce physiological effects including antinociception when microinjected into rat PAG, although these are generally weaker than μ-receptor actions. Failure to detect actions on membrane currents or synaptic transmission (see below) may, therefore, indicate that these cellular measures are not sufficiently sensitive to detect small effects on large populations of cells, or during specific physiological conditions such as stress, which induces translocation of δ–receptors to the surface membrane in PAG (Commons 2003).

Presynaptic Actions of Opioids in PAG

Opioid receptors are also abundantly expressed on nerve terminals in PAG (Commons 2003). Opioids acting on μ-receptors presynaptically inhibit both GABAergic and glutamatergic synapses impinging on all PAG neurons, and the maximum inhibition is similar for both types of synapse (Vaughan et al. 1997b). Inhibition is due to a reduction in probability of transmitter release that reduces both electrically-evoked and spontaneous synaptic transmission in both terminal types. However, the intracellular mechanisms of opioid action differ between GABAergic and glutamatergic synapses. In glutamatergic synapses, the mechanisms coupling opioid receptors to reduced probability of quantal release of glutamate have not been resolved, with the exception of some dependence on inhibition of voltage-gated calcium channels under conditions of exaggerated calcium entry into the nerve terminal. In GABAergic nerve terminals, presynaptic inhibition is mediated by activation of a voltage-gated potassium channel, (Kv) and that inhibition can be prevented by the Kv blockers, 4–aminopyridine and α–dendrotoxin (Vaughan et al. 1997b). The mechanism that couples opioid receptors to the Kv channel involves activation of phospholipase A$_2$ that mobilizes arachidonic acid, followed by formation of its metabolites via 12–lipoxygenase. Inhibitors of 5–lipoxygenase and cyclooxygenase potentiate presynaptic inhibition by opioids in PAG, presumably by shunting metabolism of arachidonic acid through the 5–lipoxygenase pathway. This process could provide one of the mechanisms of non-steroidal analgesia in the central nervous system. In addition to this mechanism, μ–opioids inhibit GABAergic synapses in PAG via inhibition of voltage-gated calcium channels, under conditions of exaggerated calcium entry into the nerve terminal (CW Vaughan, unpublished observations).

Opioids acting on κ– and δ–receptors do not produce presynaptic inhibition in rat PAG, and ORL1 agonists inhibit synaptic transmission in about 50% of recordings (Vaughan et al. 1997a). In mouse PAG, μ–opioids inhibit GABAergic synapses in all neurons, while κ–receptor agonists do so in about 50% of neurons, and δ–agonists are without effect.

Functional Consequences of Cellular Actions of Opioids in PAG

Although opioids inhibit both inhibitory (GABAergic) and excitatory (glutamatergic) synapses, the dominant action is probably on GABAergic synapses, because there is a large GABAergic tone in PAG (Chieng and Christie 1994). This would explain observations (e.g. Behbehani et al. 1990) that μ–opioids produce excitatory actions on PAG neurons under recording conditions that enhance GABAergic tone. Opioids also inhibit the soma of very few neurons in ventrolateral PAG that descend to the rostral ventromedial medulla, suggesting that the major effect of opioids is to disinhibit these output neurons. Disinhibition of descending output from the PAG *in vivo* is known to produce antinociception, so this is presumably the mechanism of action of μ–opioids to produce analgesia in PAG. However, the actions of μ–opioids on glutamatergic synapses, as well as descending projection neurons in the lateral PAG, still require explanation.

Stimulation of ORL1 receptors inhibits GABAergic and glutamatergic synapses in some PAG neurons, and might be expected to produce antinociception (Vaughan et al. 1997a). However, these receptors are also located on the cell bodies of all PAG neurons, including output neurons. Thus, any disinhibition produced presynaptically on output neurons would be expected to be blocked by the direct somatic inhibitory actions of N/OFQ on output neurons. This organisation of receptors would predict that ORL receptor stimulation in PAG would be expected to block the antinociceptive actions of opioids, which has been observed in microinjection studies (Morgan et al. 1997).

All of the major opioid receptor types are expressed in PAG neurons. The membrane actions are summarized below. Opioids couple to inhibition of voltage-gated calcium channels and activation of potassium channels via Gi-protein βγ–subunits in the membrane of PAG neurons and nerve terminals, although different potassium channels are involved in the soma (GIRK) and nerve terminal (Kv). Opioids inhibit both soma and nerve terminal excitability of intrinsic (presumably GABAergic) neurons, but not neurons that project the rostral ventromedial medulla. This disinhibits these output neurons to produce antinociception. The exception is the ORL1 receptor, which directly inhibits the output neurons to block opioid antinociception.

References

1. Bandler R, Shipley MT (1994) Columnar Organization in the Midbrain Periaqueductal Gray: Modules for Emotional Expression? Trends Neurosci 17:379–389
2. Behbehani MM, Jiang M, Chandler SD (1990) The Effect of [Met]enkephalin on the Periaqueductal Gray Neurons of the Rat: An *In Vitro* Study. Neuroscience 38:373–80
3. Chieng B, Christie MJ (1994) Inhibition by Opioids Acting on mu-Receptors of GABAergic and Glutamatergic Postsynaptic Potentials in Single Rat Periaqueductal Gray Neurones *In Vitro*. Br J Pharmacol 113:303–9
4. Commons KG (2003) Translocation of Presynaptic Delta Opioid Receptors in the Ventrolateral Periaqueductal Gray after Swim Stress. J Comp Neurol 464:197–2003
5. Fallon JH, Leslie FM (1986) Distribution of Dynorphin and Enkephalin Peptides in the Rat Brain. J Comp Neurol 249:293–336
6. Jensen TS, Yaksh TL (1986) Comparison of Antinociceptive Action of Morphine in the Periaqueductal Gray, Medial and Paramedial Medulla in Rat. Brain Res 36:99–113
7. Mansour A, Fox CA, Akil H, Watson SJ (1995) Opioid-Receptor mRNA Expression in the Rat CNS: Anatomical and Functional Implications. Trends Neurosci 18:22–9
8. Morgan MM, Grisel JE, Robbins CS, Grandy DK (1997) Antinociception Mediated by the Periaqueductal Gray is Attenuated by Orphanin FQ. Neuroreport 8:3431–4
9. Osborne PB, Vaughan CW, Wilson HI, Christie MJ (1996) Opioid Inhibition of Rat Periaqueductal Gray Neurones with Identified Projections to Rostral Ventromedial Medulla *In Vitro* . J Physiol 490:383–9
10. Ossipov MH, Kovelowski CJ, Nichols ML, Hruby VJ, Porreca F (1995) Characterization of Supraspinal Antinociceptive Actions of Opioid Delta Agonists in the Rat. Pain 62:287–93
11. Vaughan CW, Ingram SL, Christie MJ (1997a) Actions of the ORL1 Receptor Ligand Nociception on Membrane Properties of Rat Periaqueductal Gray Neurons *In Vitro*. J Neurosc 17:996–1003
12. Vaughan CW, Ingram SL, Connor MA, Christie MJ (1997b) How Opioids Inhibit GABA-Mediated Neurotransmission. Nature 390:611–614
13. Vaughan CW, Bagley EE, Drew GM, Schuller A, Pintar JE, Hack SP, Christie MJ (2003) Cellular Actions of Opioids on Periaqueductal Gray Neurons from C57B16/J Mice and Mutant Mice Lacking MOR-1. Br J Pharmacol 139:362–367
14. Williams JT, Christie MJ, Manzoni O (2001) Cellular and Synaptic Adaptations Mediating Opioid Dependence. Physiol Rev 81:299–343

Opioid Hyperexcitability

Definition

Opioid hyperexcitability is a syndrome that includes whole body hyperalgesia and allodynia, abdominal muscle spasms and symmetrical jerking of legs; methadone is preferred.

▶ Postoperative Pain, Opioids

Opioid Hypoalgesia

▶ Opioids, Effects of Systemic Morphine on Evoked Pain

Opioid-Induced Analgesia

Definition

Analgesia produced by administration of opioids.
▶ Forebrain Modulation of the Periaqueductal Gray

Opioid-Induced Bowel Dysfunction

▶ Cancer Pain Management, Gastrointestinal Dysfunction as Opioid Side Effects

Opioid-Induced Neurotoxicity

Definition

A syndrome of neuropsychiatric consequences of opioid administration. The features of OIN include cognitive impairment, severe sedation, hallucinosis, delirium, myoclonus, seizures, hyperalgesia, and allodynia.
▶ Cancer Pain Management, Opioid Side Effects, Cognitive Dysfunction

Opioid-Induced Release of CCK

CARL-OLAV STILLER
Division of Clinical Pharmacology and Department of Medicine, Karolinska University Hospital, Stockholm, Sweden
carl-olav.stiller@ki.se

Synonyms

Neuronal Release; increased extracellular levels; release of CCK

Definition

Cholecystokinin (CCK) was first identified as a gastrointestinal hormone, contracting the gallbladder and stimulating the secretion of the exocrine pancreas (Jorpes and Mutt 1966). CCK (or gastrin-like immunoreactivity) was demonstrated in the CNS (Vanderhaeghen et al 1975). The predominant form of CCK in gastrointestinal tissue is CCK-33, whereas the predominant form in the CNS is the sulphated CCK-8 (Rehfeld 1978).

"Release of CCK" refers to neuronal release. However, a direct measurement of synaptic release of CCK in nervous tissue has so far not been possible. Instead, information on release has to be obtained by indirect measures. This assay is based on *in vivo* microdialysis (▶ In vivo CCK release by microdialysis), *in vitro* release (▶ In vitro CCK release) and receptor ▶ binding studies. Studies of the behavioral effects of

CCK-antagonists in combination with opioids are not addressed here.

Characteristics

In Vitro Release Studies

The effect of opioids on CCK-like immunoreactivity (CCK-LI) release *in vitro* may seem confusing, since not only inhibition (Table 1), but also potentiation (Table 2) or a biphasic effect (Table 3) on potassium induced release have been reported.

Even though an opioid induced inhibition of potassium induced release of CCK in tissue sections may seem to be a good indicator for the drug effect *in vivo*, it has to be kept in mind that potassium stimulation induces a depolarization of both inhibitory and excitatory neurons. Thus, the interpretation of inhibited potassium induced release by opioids is difficult.

In Vivo Release Studies

With regard to clinical relevance, an *in vivo* situation, preferably using awake animals, may seem more appropriate. Furthermore, studies on the effect of opioids on CCK release should focus on the basal non-stimulated release.

Systemic administration of morphine, at doses ranging from 2.5 mg/kg to 10 mg/kg, have been demonstrated to induce an increased outflow of CCK-LI in the frontal cortex (Becker et al. 1999), the nucleus accumbens (Hamilton et al. 2000), and the dorsal horn of the spinal cord in the rat *in vivo* (de Araujo Lucas et al. 1998; Gustafsson et al. 1999).

Opioid Receptors Mediating CCK – LI Release

In order to determine which opioid receptor mediates CCK-LI release *in vivo*, the effect of different opioid antagonists on morphine induced release has been studied (Table 4).

δ–opioid antagonists blocked the CCK-LI release of morphine, and δ–opioid agonists mimicked the CCK-LI releasing effect of morphine. A delta mediated inhibition of CCK-LI release is also supported by some *in vitro* experiments (Table 2).

With regard to the effect of μ–opioid receptor activation on CCK-LI release, this opioid receptor does not seem to induce CCK-LI release. The *in vitro* data indicate an inhibitory effect on the potassium evoked release (Table 1). We could not demonstrate an increased non-stimulated CCK-LI level in the dorsal horn *in vivo* during local (1 μM in the microdialysis perfusion medium) or systemic (1 mg/kg s.c.) administration of the selective μ–opioid receptor agonist DAMGO (Gustafsson et al. 2001). However, since the basal CCK-LI level in the microdialysate was close to the detection limit of the RIA, the possibility of μ–opioid receptor mediated inhibition of CCK-release should not be excluded.

Opioid-Induced Release of CCK, Table 1 Opioid induced inhibition of potassium induced release of CCK-LI *in vitro*

Region (species)	Opioid agonist	Agonist concentration in perfusate [M]	Effect reversed by antagonist	Reference
Hypothalamus (cat/rat)	Non selective: Morphine	10^{-11}–10^{-8}+10^{-5}	Non selective: Naloxone	(Micevych et al. 1982, 1984, 1985)
	δ–opioid agonist: DADL	10^{-12}–10^{-10}	Non selective: Naloxone	
Substantia nigra (rat)	µ–opioid agonist:			(Benoliel et al. 1992)
	DAGO	10^{-5}	Non selective: Naloxone	
	Morphiceptin (PL017)	10^{-5}	Non selective: Naloxone	
Dorsal lumbar spinal cord (rat)	µ–opioid agonist: DAGO	10^{-8}–10^{-5}	Non selective: Naloxone	(Benoliel et al. 1994)

Opioid-Induced Release of CCK, Table 2 Opioid induced potentiation of potassium induced release of CCK-LI *in vitro*

Region (species)	Opioid agonist	Agonist concentration in perfusate [M]	Effect reversed by antagonist	Reference
Substantia nigra (rat)	δ–agonist:			(Benoliel et al. 1992)
	D-Pen2, D-Pen5–enkephalin	5×10^{-5}		
	Tyr-D-Thr-Gly-Phe-Leu-Thr (DTLET)	3×10^{-6}	δ-antagonist: ICI-154129	
Dorsal lumbar spinal cord (rat)	Non-selective: Morphine	10^{-5}		(Benoliel et al. 1991)

Opioid-Induced Release of CCK, Table 3 Biphasic effect of opioids on potassium induced release of CCK-LI *in vitro*

Region (species)	Opioid agonist	Agonist concentration for inhibition [M]	Agonist concentration for excitation [M]	Antagonist for reversal of effect	Reference
Dorsal lumbar spinal cord (rat)	δ–agonist: DTLET	10^{-8}–3×10^{-6}	10^{-5}	δ-antagonist: Naltrindole ICI 154129	(Benoliel et al. 1991, 1994)
	Non-selective: Morphine	10^{-8}–10^{-7}	10^{-5}	Inhibition: Naloxone Excitation: Naltrindole ICI 154129	

Opioid-Induced Release of CCK, Table 4 Reversal of opioid induced *in vivo* release of CCK-LI by opioid antagonists

Region (species)	Opioid agonist (dose)	Effect reversed by antagonist	Effect not affected by	Reference
Frontal cortex (rat)	Non-selective: Morphine (10 mg/kg i.p)	Non-selective: Naloxone (1.5 mg /kg i.p.) (10 µM)	µ–antagonist: CTOP (10 µM)	(Becker et al. 1999)
		δ–antagonist: Naltrindole:10µM	κ–antagonist: nor-BNI:10 µM	
		δ2–antagonist: Naltriben:10 µM	δ1–antagonist: BNTX:10 µM	
	δ2–agonist: [D-Ala2] deltorphin II (1 µM)	δ2–antagonist: Naltriben:10 µM		
Dorsal lumbar spinal cord (rat)	Non-selective: Morphine (5 mg/kg s.c.)	Non-selective: Naloxone: 2 mg/kg s.c. ; 10 µM	µ–antagonist: CTOP:10 µM	(Gustafsson et al. 1999, 2001)
		δ–antagonist: Naltrindole:10 µM	κ–antagonist: nor-BNI:10 µM	
	δ–agonist: BW373U86 (1 mg/kg s.c.)	δ–antagonist: Naltrindole; 10 µM		
	δ2–agonist: [D-Ala2] deltorphin II (1 µM)			

An indirect indication of δ–opioid receptor mediated release of CCK is also provided by a receptor binding study with a selective CCK-B radioligand (Ruiz-Gayo et al. 1992). Following an intracerebroventricular (ICV) injection of the δ–opioid receptor agonist BUBUC, but not the μ–opioid receptor agonist DAMGO, the specific binding of the CCK-B radioligand decreased. According to the author's interpretation, an endogenous release of CCK competes with the radioligand for the receptor and decreases the specific binding.

The combined experimental evidence indicates that agonist activation of δ–opioid receptors, probably of the δ₂–opioid receptor subtype, induces release of CCK. A decrease of CCK-release by opioids is only reported in conditions of potassium stimulation.

Mechanisms of Opioid-Induced Release of CCK-LI

The exact mechanisms responsible for the opioid induced release of CCK-LI have not been determined so far. The morphine-induced release of CCK-LI is calcium dependent, indicating a neuronal origin. Furthermore, we have demonstrated that an influx of calcium at presynaptic terminals, through voltage-dependent calcium channels (VDCCs) of the L– and N–type, is essential for morphine-induced release of CCK-LI in the dorsal horn (Gustafsson et al. 1999).

Since opioid-receptor activation normally induces inhibition of neuronal activity and reduces transmitter release, a disinhibition of local inhibitory neurons (i.e. GABA-neurons), a mechanism which has been demonstrated in the periaqueductal gray *in vivo* (Stiller et al. 1996), could be an alternative. However, no evidence for this mechanism in the dorsal horn has been provided so far. Furthermore, we could not demonstrate that perfusion of the dialysis probe with the GABA-A antagonist bicuculline (100 μM in the perfusion medium) increased the extracellular levels of CCK-LI in the spinal cord (Gustafsson 2001). An opioid mediated disinhibition of other inhibitory neurotransmitters (e.g. glycine) could still be an option.

However, opioid receptor activation may not only mediate an inhibition, but also excitation (for review see Crain and Shen 1990). If δ–opioid receptors are present in CCK-containing nerve cells in the dorsal horn, a direct activation of δ–opioid receptors should release CCK-LI in this region. Such a mechanism should be insensitive to the sodium channel blocking agent tetrodotoxin (TTX). However, TTX inhibited the morphine induced CCK-LI release (Gustafsson et al. 1999), suggesting that a local propagation of action potentials in the dorsal horn seems to be a prerequisite for the opioid induced release of CCK. It is possible that the opioid induced CCK-LI release involves several neurons.

An opioid induced release of excitatory amino acids, which in turn stimulate the release of CCK, is indicated by the observation that administration of NMDA or AMPA antagonists prevents the morphine-induced release of CCK-LI in the dorsal horn (Gustafsson 2001). In addition, spinal morphine (100 μM in the perfusion fluid) induced a several fold increase of the extracellular glutamate concentration in the dorsal horn *in vivo* (Gustafsson 2001).

References

1. Becker C, Hamon M, Cesselin F, Benoliel JJ (1999) Delta(2)-Opioid Receptor Mediation of Morphine-Induced CCK Release in the Frontal Cortex of the Freely Moving Rat. Synapse 34:47–54
2. Benoliel JJ, Bourgoin S, Mauborgne A, Legrand JC, Hamon M, Cesselin F (1991) Differential Inhibitory/Stimulatory Modulation of Spinal CCK Release by mu and delta Opioid Agonists, and Selective Blockade of mu-Dependent Inhibition by Kappa Receptor Stimulation. Neurosci Lett 124:204–207
3. Benoliel JJ, Collin E, Mauborgne A, Bourgoin S, Legrand JC, Hamon M, Cesselin F (1994) Mu and delta Opioid Receptors Mediate Opposite Modulations by Morphine of the Spinal Release of Cholecystokinin-Like Material. Brain Res 653:81–91
4. Benoliel JJ, Mauborgne A, Bourgoin S, Legrand JC, Hamon M, Cesselin F (1992) Opioid Control of the In Vitro Release of Cholecystokinin-Like Material from the Rat Substantia Nigra. J Neurochem 58:916–922
5. Crain SM, Shen KF (1990) Opioids Can Evoke Direct Receptor-Mediated Excitatory Effects on Sensory Neurons. Trends Pharmacol Sci 11:77–81
6. de Araujo Lucas G, Alster P, Brodin E, Wiesenfeld-Hallin Z (1998) Differential Release of Cholecystokinin by Morphine in Rat Spinal Cord. Neurosci Lett 245:13–16
7. Gustafsson H (2001), Opioid-Induced Cholecystokinin Release in the CNS-Neurochemical Mechanisms and Effects of Sciatic Nerve Lesion; PhD thesis, Karolinska Institutet; ISBN 91–628–4440–7
8. Gustafsson H, Afrah A, Brodin E, Stiller CO (1999) Pharmacological Characterization of Morphine-Induced In Vivo Release of Cholecystokinin in Rat Dorsal Horn: Effects of Ion Channel Blockers. J Neurochem 73:1145–1154
9. Gustafsson H, Afrah AW, Stiller CO (2001) Morphine-Induced In Vivo Release of Spinal Cholecystokinin is Mediated by delta-Opioid Receptors-Effect of Peripheral Axotomy. J Neurochem 78:55–63
10. Hamilton ME, Redondo JL, Freeman AS (2000) Overflow of Dopamine and Cholecystokinin in Rat Nucleus Accumbens in Response to Acute Drug Administration. Synapse 38:238–242
11. Jorpes E, Mutt V (1966) Cholecystokinin and pancreozymin, one single hormone? Acta Physiol Scand 66:196–202
12. Micevych PE, Yaksh TL, Go VL (1982) Opiate-Mediated Inhibition of the Release of Cholecystokinin and Substance P, but not Neurotensin from Cat Hypothalamic Slices. Brain Res 250:283–289
13. Micevych PE, Yaksh TL, Go VL (1984) Studies on the Opiate Receptor-Mediated Inhibition of K⁺–Stimulated Cholecystokinin and Substance P Release from Cat Hypothalamus In Vitro. Brain Res 290:87–94
14. Micevych PE, Yaksh TL, Go VW, Finkelstein JA (1985) Effect of Opiates on the Release of Cholecystokinin from In Vitro Hypothalamus and Frontal Cortex of Zucker Lean (Fa/-) and Obese (fa/fa) Rats. Brain Res 337:382–385
15. Rehfeld JF (1978) Localisation of gastrins to neuro- and adenohypophysis. Nature 271:771–773
16. Ruiz-Gayo M, Durieux C, Fournié-Zaluski MC, Roques BP (1992) Stimulation of delta-Opioid Receptors Reduces the In Vivo Binding of the Cholecystokinin (CCK)-B-Selective Agonist [3H]pBC 264: Evidence for a Physiological Regulation of CCKergic Systems by Endogenous Enkephalins. J Neurochem 59:1805–1811
17. Stiller CO, Bergquist J, Beck O, Ekman R, Brodin E (1996) Local Administration of Morphine Decreases the Extracellular Level of GABA in the Periaqueductal Gray Matter of Freely Moving Rats. Neurosci Lett 209:165–168

O

18. Vanderhaeghen JJ, Signeau JC, Gepts W (1975) New peptide in the vertebrate CNS reacting with antigastrin antibodies. Nature 257:604–605

Opioid Modulation by Cytokines

▶ Cytokine Modulation of Opioid Action

Opioid Modulation of Nociceptive Afferents In Vivo

DAVID C. YEOMANS[1], ALEXANDER TZABAZIS[2]

[1]Department of Anesthesia, Stanford University, Stanford, CA, USA

[2]Department of Anesthesia, University of Erlangen, Erlangen, Germany

dcyeomans@stanford.edu, tzabazis@web.de

Synonyms

Opioid therapy for primary afferents; first order sensory neurons

Definition

Modulation of primary afferents by endogenous or exogenous opioids. Primary afferents are sensory neurons with one peripheral process innervating a peripheral tissue area (▶ receptive field), and one central process that enters the dorsal horn of the spinal cord via a dorsal root. The cell bodies of primary afferents are located in the ▶ dorsal root ganglia (DRG) or trigeminal ganglia (TG). Opioid targets are either receptors on pre- or postsynaptic membranes of central terminals in the dorsal horn, and/or peripheral opioid receptors on nociceptive endings in the innervated tissue. Modulation can be achieved by systemic or local application of drugs (agonists or antagonists) or gene therapy (de novo or altered expression of an "antinociceptive" gene or knockdown of a "pronociceptive" gene).

Characteristics

Physiology of the spinal and peripheral opioid system

In 1976, Yaksh and Rudy discovered that spinally administered opioids could produce analgesia. Due to reduced side effects, this new route of administration for opioids became the gold standard for relief of severe pain. Antinociceptive effects of spinally applied opioids are predominantly mediated by pre- and/or postsynaptic μ-opioid receptors, ▶ δ-opioid receptors and ▶ κ-opioid receptors, mainly in laminae 1 and 2 (Rexed) of the dorsal horn of the spinal cord. Methionine (met-) and leucine (leu)-enkephalin, ▶ Beta(β)-Endorphin, ▶ dynorphin, α-neoendorphin and ▶ endomorphin I and II are all endogenous opioids with different affinities for the different opioid receptor subtypes. The preferential endogenous ligand for μ-opioid receptors are β-endorphin and endomorphin I and II. Enkephalins favour δ-, and dynorphins have the highest affinity for κ-opioid receptors. However, one should keep in mind that receptor affinity depends on the type of fragment that is released by the enzymatic cleavage from the precursor, which again depends on the tissue where this process has taken place (Zaki et al. 1996; Wall and Melzack 1999).

Opioid receptors can also be found on peripheral nociceptive endings (Fields et al. 1980). These receptors are upregulated by peripheral inflammation, which enhances the potency of endogenous and exogenous opioids. The appearance of opioid receptors within minutes to hours after onset of inflammation suggests their preexistence, although they cannot be readily detected in uninjured tissue. A possible explanation for this sudden availability of opioid receptors on nociceptive terminals, might be an unblocking of the perineurium at a very early stage of inflammation within 12 hours (Antonijevic et al. 1995), and/or at a later time point by sprouting of the terminals.

Studies in knockout mice reveal different contributions of opioid receptors and endogenous opioids in mediating nociceptive behaviour (Table 1) (Kieffer and Gaveriaux-Ruff 2002). Activation of the μ-opioid receptor induces both desirable analgesic effects, as well as undesirable effects of exogenous opioids like respiratory depression and constipation, making this receptor a difficult but widely used therapeutic target for systemic drug treatment.

Opioid receptors are ▶ Type-II Receptors, i.e. their action is carried forward by a second messenger G-protein. Stimulation of presynaptic μ– and δ2–receptors is associated with a reduction in calcium influx (Ca^{2+}) leading to a hyperpolarization of the terminal, and a reduced release of neurotransmitters such as ▶ glutamate, and ▶ neuropeptides such as ▶ substance P. Activated postsynaptic opioid receptors stabilize membrane potentials by enhancing the outward flow of potassium (K^+), and decreasing the amplitude of excitatory postsynaptic potentials.

Intrathecally administered pertussis toxin (PTX) produces thermal hyperalgesia and allodynia in mice (Womer et al. 1997) by inactivation of the inhibitory G_i and G_0 proteins that are involved in the intracellular signalling process. This disinhibition leads to a predominance of excitation, ▶ wind-up, and reduces the analgesic potency of many μ-agonists, like morphine and DAMGO. Antinociception mediated by mixed μ-agonists/antagonists like buprenorphine, however, is less affected. The effectiveness of buprenorphine as opposed to other exogenous μ-agonists, even after intrathecal PTX, indicates that the mechanism of action of buprenorphine does not entirely depend on PTX-sensitive, intracellular signalling pathways,

Opioid Modulation of Nociceptive Afferents In Vivo, Table 1   Changes in nociception as observed in different knockout mice (Kieffer and Gaveriaux-Ruff 2002)

Pain/ hyperalgesia	MOR-/-	DOR-/-	KOR-/-	β end-	Penk-	Pdyn-
thermal	↑	↔	↔	↔	↑	↑
mechanical	↔	↔	↔	n/a	n/a	↔
chemical	↓	n/a	↑	n/a	↓	↔
inflammatory	shorter duration of hyperalgesia	n/a	n/a	n/a	n/a	n/a
neuropathic	n/a	n/a	n/a	n/a	n/a	shorter duration of hyperalgesia

Abbreviations: MOR, μ-opioid receptor; DOR, δ-opioid receptor; KOR, κ-opioid receptor; βend, β-endorphin; Penk, preproenkephalin; Pdyn, predynorphin.

which might explain its special role in the treatment of ► neuropathic pain (McCormack et al. 1998).

Modulation of central projections

As with endogenous opioids, intrathecally applied exogenous opioids also have different affinities for different opioid receptors (Table 2). Whereas κ-agonists do not attenuate either Aδ–or C–thermonociceptor-mediated responses, μ–, δ1– and δ2–opioid agonists are effective on both. DPDPE (δ1–selective agonist) showed parallel dose-response curves for Aδ– and C–mediated antinociception, indicating similar mechanisms of action. On the other hand, μ-agonists (DAMGO and morphine) and a δ2–selective agonist (DSLET) produced non-parallel dose-response curves, indicating that the mechanisms by which these drugs act are different for the two types of nociception. Specifically, μ– and δ2–agonists seem to act presynaptically on C-fiber afferent terminals, but they attenuate responses to Aδ–mediated nociception on dorsal horn neurones, i.e. postsynaptically (Lu et al. 1997). It has recently been shown (Jones et al. 2003) that knockdown of μ-opioid receptors in primary afferents, by way of a recombinant herpes vector, attenuates the potency of μ-receptor-selective agonists for C–, but not for Aδ–fibers. These findings support the observations of Lu et al., as herpes viruses usually do not jump synapses, i.e. they act on primary afferents only

Opioid Modulation of Nociceptive Afferents In Vivo, Table 2 Antinociceptive potency of exogenous opioids on Aδ- and C-fiber mediated behavior in the paw withdrawal test. Parallel dose-response curves indicate similar mechanisms of action, which allows comparison of potencies on Aδ- and C-mediated analgesia

Substance	A δ	C	dose-response curves
Morphine (μ-agonist)	++*	++*	non-parallel
DAMGO (μ-agonist)	+++*	+++*	non-parallel
DPDPE (δ1–agonist)	+*	++*	parallel
DSLET (δ2-agonist)	+*	+*	non-parallel
U50488 (κ–agonist)	0	0	-

* indicates reversibility by μ-, δ1– and δ2–antagonists, respectively

(Lu et al. 1997). Consistent with these results are the observations of Taddese et al., that activation of the μ-opioid receptor inhibited presynaptic calcium channels preferentially on small nociceptors, but had minimal effects on larger nociceptors, whereas ► somatostatin had the opposite effects (Taddese et al. 1995). Several groups (Wilson et al. 1999; Bras et al. 2001; Wilson and Yeomans 2002; Glorioso et al. 2003) have used herpes virus-based vectors for delivery of transgenes to the nervous system. The natural properties of the herpes simplex virus to enter dorsal root ganglia via peripheral infection, and to become latent there, allows a phenotypic alteration of the first cell in the pathway of nociception. Pain therapy, based on this technology, should minimize adverse side effects of opioids like constipation or respiratory depression. Delivery of a transgene-encoding opioid peptide precursor (human preproenkephalin) leads to synthesis of enkephalin peptides in sensory neurons in mice (Figure 1) (Wilson et al. 1999). Baseline withdrawal latencies to noxious radiant heat were similar in animals infected with proenkephalin-encoding and control viruses. However, after sensitization of C-fibers with ► capsaicin and Aδ-fibers with ► dimethylsulfoxide (DMSO), thermal hyperalgesia was reduced or eliminated in mice infected with proenkephalin-encoding virus for at least 7 weeks.

Modulation of nociceptive terminals

Peripheral localized administration of endogenous and exogenous opioids have been shown to mediate antinociception in models of inflammatory and neuropathic pain (Stein et al. 2003). For example, intra-articular application of morphine during knee surgery, with a dose that does not lead to systemic effects, produced a significant, naloxone-reversible and long lasting analgesic effect (Stein 1995).

Similarly, after infection of primary afferents with a viral vector encoding for preproenkephalin A (HSVLatEnk1), the majority of met-enkephalin-like material accumulated at the proximal side of the ligatured sciatic nerve, while much less was seen in ligatured L4–L5 roots (Bras et al. 2001). In HSVLatEnk1–infected animals

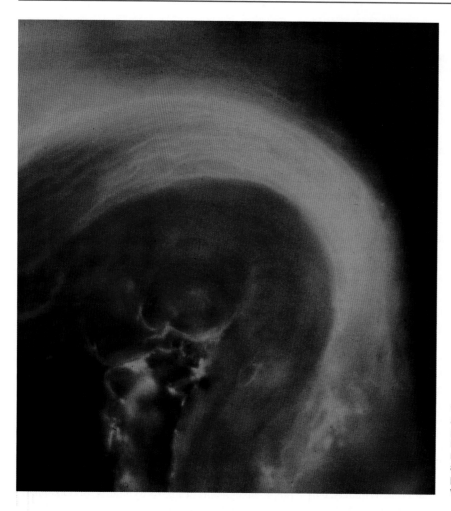

Opioid Modulation of Nociceptive Afferents In Vivo, Figure 1 Human pro-enkephalin immunofluroescence in primary afferent fibers of mouse dorsal root 6 weeks after application of a human preproenkephalin-encoding herpes vector to the skin.

without sciatic nerve ligation, subcutaneous microdialysis showed significantly higher basal levels of met-enkephalin-like material in the interstitial fluid of the hindpaw, indicating that overexpressed peptides have reached a releasable compartment. Electrical stimulation of the sciatic nerve revealed an approximately three-fold higher overflow of met-enkephalin-like material in HSVLatEnk1–infected rats as compared to control rats. These data suggest that overexpression of antinociceptive genes like preproenkephalin in primary afferents leads to a combined analgesic effect, i.e. effects on nociceptive terminals and central projections. Expression and release of opioid peptides are also very likely to be induced by hormones (e.g. corticotropin-releasing hormone, CRH) and cytokines (Interleukin 1, IL–1) in ► immune cells (B and T lymphocytes, macrophages, and monocytes) (Stein et al. 2003). The released endogenous opioids from immune cells can interact with peripheral receptors on nociceptive terminals. As many painful conditions are accompanied or sustained by inflammatory processes, inducing overexpression of endogenous opioids in immune cells could provide a promising therapeutic approach to the treatment of pain.

References

1. Antonijevic I, Mousa SA, Schäfer M, Stein C (1995) Perineurial Defect and Peripheral Opioid Analgesia in Inflammation. J Neurosci 15:165–172
2. Bras J-MA, Becker C, Bourgoin S, Lombard M-C, Cesselin F, Hamon N, Pohl M (2001) Met-Enkephalin is Preferentially Transported into the Peripheral Processes of Primary Afferent Fibres in Both Control and HSV1–Driven Proenkephalin A Overexpressing Rats. Neurosci 103:1073–1083
3. Fields HL, Emson PC, Leigh BK, Gilbert RFT, Iversen LL (1980) Multiple Opiate Receptor Sites on Primary Afferent Fibers. Nature 284:351–353
4. Glorioso JC, Mata M, Fink DJ (2003) Exploiting the Neurotherapeutic Potential of Peptides: Targeted Delivery using HSV Vectors. Expert Opin Biol Ther 3:1233–1239
5. Jones TL, Sweitzer SM, Wilson SP, Yeomans DC (2003) Afferent Fiber-Selective Shift in Opiate Potency following Targeted Opioid Receptor Knockdown. Pain 106:365–371
6. Kieffer BL, Gaveriaux-Ruff C (2002) Exploring the Opioid System by Gene Knockout. Prog Neurobiol 66:285–306
7. Lu Y, Pirec V, Yeomans DC (1997) Differential Antinociceptive Effects of Spinal Opioids on Foot Withdrawal Responses Evoked by C Fibre or A Delta Nociceptor Activation. Br J Pharmacol 121:1210–1216
8. McCormack K, Prather P, Chapleo C (1998) Some New Insights into the Effects of Opioids in Phasic and Tonic Nociceptive Tests. Pain 78:79–98
9. Stein C (1995) The Control of Pain in Peripheral Tissue by Opioids. N Eng J Med 332:1685–1690

Opioid Peptides from the Amphibian Skin, Table 2 Affinity and selectivity for mu and delta opioid receptors, biological activities on guinea pig ileum (GPI) and mouse vas deferens (MVD) preparations and analgesic potency of dermorphins and deltorphins

Compounds	K_i, nM (mean ± S.E.)			IC_{50}, nM (mean ± S.E.)		Analgesia
	µ-system	δ-system	µ / δ	GPI	MVD	AD_{50} nmol/rat
Morphine	11±1.5	500±48	22×10^{-3}	150±18.5	1215±115	8.7±1.1
Dermorphin						
dermorphin	0.6±0.02	929±41	6.1×10^{-4}	1.29±0.11	16.5±1.3	0.035±0.01
[Hyp^6]derm	0.7±0.03	1200±131	5.8×10^{-4}	1.6±0.12	18.1±2.9	
[Lys^7]derm	0.09±0.008	1105±185	8.1×10^{-5}	1.15±0.13	13.6±1.5	0.026±0.009
[Lys^7-OH]derm	5.7 ±0.51	1150±172	4.9×10^{-3}	3.82±0.45	56.3±7.8	
[Trp^4,Asn^5]derm	0.9±0.052	480±45	1.9×10^{-3}	5.00±0.52	73.7±9.1	0.43±0.04
[Trp^4,Asn^7]derm	0.32±0.026	690±57	4.6×10^{-4}	0.58±0.06	6.6±0.9	2.086±0.31
Deltorphin						
D-Ala^2-delt I	1985±224	0.78±0.08	2545	1239±203	0.18±0.02	15±3.0
D-Ala^2-delt II	2222±233	1.03±1.09	2157	2500±170	0.37±0.03	54±6.0
D-Ala^2,Gly^4-delt	13.5±2.1	3.26± 0.7	4.14	22±3	2.62±0.32	2.5±0.3
D-Met^2-delt	693±37	1.18±0.21	587	1476±185	0.97±0.05	20±5.0
D-Leu^2-delt	>10000	>10000	-	> 5000	2480±378	
D-Leu^2-delt(1–10)	-	-	-	1684±403	37.0±3.9	
D-Ile^2-delt	1021±57	24±3	42.6	4200±475	7.0±0.9	6.7±1.0
D-alle^2-delt	452±68	54±65	8.4	3200±307	70±8.2	9.8±1.2

K_i, equilibrium inhibition constant of the competing ligand; mu-opioid receptors have been labeled with [^{3}H]DAMGO, 0.5 nM; delta opioid receptors have been labeled with [^{3}H]deltorphin I, 0.3 nM; µ/δ represents selectivity for the mu receptors *versus* delta receptors.

and Phe^3 aromatic rings in definite orientations best suited for delta receptor docking (Negri and Giannini 2003).

Dermorphin affinity for mu opioid receptors and its opioid potency in guinea pig ileum preparations (GPI) (see ▶ GPI (guinea pig ileum) and MVD (mouse vas deferns)) are 20 and 100 times higher respectively than those of morphine. Among other dermorphins, [Lys7]dermorphin shows an affinity and selectivity for mu opiate receptors 6 times higher than dermorphin and 100 times higher than morphine (Table 2). Like mu opiate agonists, dermorphins produce antinociception but also catalepsy, respiratory depression, constipation, tolerance and dependence, albeit to a lower degree than morphine. Dermorphin induced antinociception takes place at supraspinal and spinal levels. Owing to its low CNS permeability and bioavailability, the analgesic potency of dermorphin is about 250 times higher than that of morphine after icv injection but comparable to that of morphine after sc injection. [Lys7]dermorphin and some synthetic analogs bearing a hydrophilic group (a basic amino acid or a glycosyl residue) at the C-terminal end of the molecule enter the CNS in 7 to 10 times

higher amounts than dermorphin, suggesting facilitated transport across the blood brain barrier by a carrier or endocytosis. The amphibian opioid with the highest analgesic potency and efficacy is [Lys7]dermorphin (AD_{50} 30 pmol/rat by the intracerebroventricular route (icv), 0.22 µmol/kg by the subcutaneous route (sc)). The ratio of antinociceptive to respiratory depressant ED_{50} doses was 17 times lower for [Lys7]dermorphin than for morphine. Indeed, [Lys7]dermorphin, in the range of analgesic doses (36–120 pmol, icv, 0.12–4.7 µmol/kg, sc) significantly increases respiratory frequency and minute volume of rats breathing air or hypoxic inspirates. The early onset ventilatory stimulation produced by [Lys7]dermorphin and ascribed to the intact peptide is mediated by serotonergic descending excitatory pathways that stimulate neurons of the brainstem respiratory network (Negri et al. 1998). In rats and mice, central or peripheral administration of the dermorphin-like peptides induces a significantly slower development of tolerance to the antinociceptive effect than with morphine. Withdrawal symptoms precipitated by naloxone are less intense in peptide dependent than in morphine dependent rats (Negri et al. 2000).

The discovery of deltorphins provided the tools for the functional characterization of the delta opiate system. While D-Ala^2-deltorphins have delta binding affinity similar to D-Met^2-deltorphin, they consistently have the highest delta opiate selectivity (Table 2). The rank order of selectivity ($K_i\delta / K_i\mu$) is D-Ala^2-deltorphin I = D-Ala^2-deltorphin II > D-Met^2-deltorphin >> D-Ile^2-deltorphin >>D-Leu^2-deltorphin heptadecapeptide or its N-terminal decapeptide fragment. Both D-Met^2-deltorphin and D-Ala^2-deltorphins are highly resistant to enzyme degradation. D-Ala^2-deltorphins I and II cross the blood-brain barrier *in vivo* and *in vitro* (Fiori et al. 1997). Recently, D-Ala^2-deltorphin II was identified as a transport substrate of organic anion transporting polypeptides (Oatp/OATP), a family of polyspecific membrane transporters, strongly expressed in the rat and human blood-brain barrier (Negri and Giannini 2003).

In mice, D-Ala^2-deltorphin II by the icv route (EC$_{50}$ = 2.1 nmol/mouse) is half as potent as morphine and the analgesic effect is antagonized by the delta selective antagonist, naltrindole. Repeated injection of D-Ala2-deltorphin II induces tolerance to the antinociceptive effect. Isobolographic analysis shows that the supraspinal antinociception induced by the delta opioid agonist DPDPE and the spinal antinociception induced by D-Ala^2-deltorphin II are synergistic in many nociceptive tests, suggesting that the compounds act on distinct delta opiate receptors (Kovolevski et al. 1999). In rats, intrathecal injections of D-Ala^2-deltorphin II (from 0.6 nmol/rat) produce a naltrindole reversible antinociception, by inhibiting the nociceptive neurons in the superficial and deeper dorsal horn of the medulla. Conversely, when injected icv in rats, D-Ala2-deltorphin II was a weak partial agonist (> 30 nmol/rat) and induces fleeting naloxone sensitive antinociception. Both D-Ala2-deltorphin I and D-Met2-deltorphin at doses between 6.5 and 52 nmol/rat induce a naloxone sensitive analgesia. Data suggest that the delta agonists play a predominantly modulatory role in antinociception rather than a primary role. In mice and in rats, the intensity of delta opiate analgesia depends on coactivation of mu opiate receptors by endogenous or exogenous opiates. Deltorphin induced analgesia is weaker in homozygote mice with a disrupted mu opiate receptor gene than in wild type mice.

Injections of the deltorphins into the rat brain ventricles, ventral tegmental area and nucleus accumbens at doses 10–100 times lower than those inducing analgesia (0.06 to 3.8 nmol/rat) invariably increase locomotor activity and induce stereotyped behavior. Deltorphin induced motor activity is antagonized by the delta selective antagonist, naltrindole. Repeated icv injections of D-Ala^2-deltorphin II in naive rats induce tolerance to the stimulant effects. High doses (10-50 nmol/rat) of all the D-Met^2-deltorphin analogs and His^4-substituted D-Ala^2-deltorphins induce non-opioid motor dysfunc-

tion that is completely blocked by the non-competitive NMDA antagonist, dextrorphan. Because the deltorphin peptides do not induce dependence, and because they stimulate respiratory activity and leave the rate of transit through the small intestine unchanged (Negri et al. 2000; Negri and Giannini 2003), they are excellent candidates as drugs to relieve acute or chronic pain in humans.

References

1. Barra D, Mignogna G, Simmaco M et al. (1994) [D-Leu^2]Deltorphin, a 17 amino acid opioid peptide from the skin of the Brazilian hylid frog, *Phyllomedusa burmeisteri*. Peptides 15:199–202
2. Broccardo M, Erspamer V, Falconieri-Erspamer G et al. (1981) Pharmacological data on dermorphins, a new class of potent opioid peptides from amphibian skin. Br J Pharmacol 73:625–31
3. Erspamer V (1994) Bioactive secretions of the Amphibian integument. In: Heatwole H (ed) Amphibian Biology. Surrey Beatty & Son, Chipping Norton, pp 178–350
4. Erspamer V, Melchiorri P, Falconieri-Erspamer G et al. (1989) Deltorphins: a family of naturally occurring peptide with high affinity and selectivity for delta-opioid binding sites. Proc Natl Acad Sci USA 86:5188–92
5. Fiori A, Cardelli P, Negri L et al. (1997) Deltorphin transport across the blood-brain barrier. Proc Natl Acad Sci USA 94:9469–74
6. Kovolevski CJ, Bian D, Ruby H et al. (1999) Selective opioid delta agonists elicit antinociceptive supraspinal/ spinal synergy in the rat. Brain Res 843:12–17
7. Kreil G, Barra D, Simmaco M et al. (1989) Deltorphin, a novel amphibian skin peptide with high selectivity and affinity for delta-opioid receptors. Eur J Pharmacol 162:123–8
8. Montecucchi PC, De Castiglione R, Erspamer V (1981) Identification of dermorphin and Hyp-dermorphin in skin extract of the Brazilian frog Phyllomedusa rohdeii. Int J Peptide Prot Res 17:316–21
9. Negri L and Giannini E (2003) Deltorphins. In: Chang KJ, Porreca F, Woods JH (eds) The delta receptors, molecule and effects of delta opioid compounds. Marcel Dekker Book Chapters, pp 175–189
10. Negri L, Falconieri-Erspamer G, Severini C et al. (1992) Dermorphin related peptides from the skin of Phyllomedusa bicolor and their amidated analogs activate two mu-opioid receptor subtypes which modulate antinociception and catalepsy, in the rat. Proc Natl Acad Sci USA 89:7203–7
11. Negri L, Lattanzi R, Tabacco F et al. (1998) Respiratory and cardiovascular effects of the mu-opioid receptor agonist [Lys^7]dermorphin in awake rats. Br J Pharmacol 124:345–55
12. Negri L, Melchiorri P, Lattanzi R (2000) Pharmacology of Amphibian opiate peptides. Peptides 21:1639–47
13. Wechselberger C, Severini C, Kreil G et al. (1998) A new opioid peptide predicted from clone cDNAs from skin of Pachymedusa dacnicolor and Agalychinis annae. FEBS Lett 429:41–3

Opioid Pseudo-Pharmacological Ceiling Dose

Definition

The results of adverse effects on dose titration of pure opioid agonists.

▶ Cancer Pain Management, Principles of Opioid Therapy, Drug Selection

Opioid Receptor Localization

CATHERINE ABBADIE[1], GAVRIL W. PASTERNAK[2]
[1]Department of Pharmacology, Merck Research
Laboratories, Rahway, NJ, USA
[2]Laboratory of Molecular Neuropharmacology,
Memorial Sloan-Kettering Cancer Center, New York,
NY, USA
catherine_abbadie@merck.com, pasterng@mskcc.org

Definition

Opioids have long played a major role in pharmacology, representing one of the oldest classes of clinically important pharmaceuticals (Pasternak 1993; Reisine and Pasternak 1996). Opioid receptor binding to brain membranes was first demonstrated in 1973, and represents one of the earliest neurotransmitter receptors localized within the central nervous system using autoradiographic techniques. Presently, three distinct classes of opioid receptors have been identified. All three classes of opioid receptors are members of the ▶ G-protein-coupled receptor family, and have the typical seven transmembrane domains seen with this large family of membrane receptors. Opioids bind to the extracellular face of the receptor and activate intracellular G-proteins. The opioid receptors are almost exclusively inhibitory, activating primarily G_o and G_i. The three opioid receptor classes are structurally homologous, but each is encoded by a separate gene.

Early autoradiographic studies of the brain, defining the regional distribution of opioid receptors, used a variety of radioligands that we now know are not very selective. Although these initial studies firmly established the presence of opioid binding sites in brain regions known to be important in mediating opioid actions, it is almost certain that they were labeling more than one class of binding site. With the cloning of the receptors (for review see Pasternak 2001; Kieffer and Gaveriaux-Ruff 2002; Wei and Loh 2002), it is now possible to selectively localize them at the mRNA level using in situ hybridization, and at the protein level immunohistochemically.

Mu Receptors

Morphine and most clinical opioid analgesics act though the mu- ▶ opiate receptors, making these receptors particularly important. However, this class of receptor is complex, with over a dozen different splice variants of the mu receptor having been cloned. While these may provide potential insights into early pharmacological studies implying different mu receptor subtypes for morphine analgesia versus respiratory depression or constipation, it complicates the interpretation their distributions.

Delta Receptors

Delta receptors were first proposed shortly after the discovery of the enkephalins, their endogenous ligand. The development of highly selective, stable delta compounds has greatly facilitated studies of the pharmacology of this receptor, and the cloning of the DOR–1 has enabled studies of this receptor at the molecular level. Delta opioids produce analgesia, but with far less respiratory depression and constipation. There is strong pharmacological evidence for delta receptor subtypes, but functional splice variants have not yet been reported.

Kappa₁ Receptors

Kappa receptors were initially suggested from classical *in vivo* pharmacological studies long before the identification of its endogenous ligand, dynorphin A. The synthesis of highly selective ligands has helped to define the kappa₁ receptor, both biochemically and pharmacologically. Kappa₁ receptors can produce analgesia, but through mechanisms distinct from those of the other receptor classes. However, the clinical use of kappa receptor ligands has been limited by their psychotomimetic side-effects.

A kappa receptor with the appropriate pharmacological profile has been cloned, KOR–1, and it has high homology with the other opiate receptors. In addition to the nervous system, kappa₁ receptors are also present in other tissues, particularly immune cells.

Other Kappa Receptors

Several other kappa receptor classes have been proposed. U50,488H is a potent, and highly selective, kappa₁ receptor agonist. Kappa₂ receptors, initially defined by their insensitivity to traditional mu, delta and kappa₁ opioids, display a unique binding profile and may correspond to dimers of KOR–1 and DOR–1 receptors. Kappa₃ receptors represent another class of U50,488H–insensitive receptors totally distinct from any other class.

Opioid-Receptor-Like (ORL–1) Receptor

A fourth member of the opiate receptor family has been cloned that is highly selective for the peptide orphanin FQ/nociceptin (▶ OFQ/N). The pharmacology of OFQ/N is complex, with actions depending upon both dose and route. Despite the similarity of the cloned receptor with other members of the opioid receptor family, OFQ/N shows no appreciable affinity for traditional opioid receptors and opioids bind very poorly to the ORL–1 receptor. However, the ORL–1 receptor will dimerize with MOR–1, yielding a complex with a profoundly different binding profile, in which traditional mu opioids potently compete with OFQ/N and vice versa.

Conclusion

The opioid system is comprised of three major classes of receptors, with each being encoded by a different gene, as well as the ORL–1 receptor. Furthermore, the gene encoding MOR–1 generates a large number of variants, many of which bind morphine and related mu opioids

O

with high affinity. Their close structural and ligand binding characteristics make it difficult to localize a single variant.

Characteristics

The first attempt to look at opioid distribution in the brain used autoradiographic approaches. These early studies defining their distributions used various opioid ligands, and quickly established the presence of opioid binding sites in brain regions presumed to be important in mediating opioid actions. However, as our understanding of opioid receptors has expanded, it has become apparent that opioids act through a family of receptors, as described earlier. Equally important, many of the ligands initially thought to be "selective" are now known not to be, complicating the interpretation of these earlier studies.

Following the cloning of the opioid receptors, their distributions within the brain were evaluated using in situ hybridization and immunohistochemistry. Unlike traditional receptor autoradiography, the selectivity of both techniques is excellent. In situ hybridization labels mRNA and identifies the cell bodies responsible for synthesizing the receptors. However, the receptors themselves are often transported long distances along axons. Thus, it is also important to localize with subcellular resolution the receptors at protein level. The epitopes identified from the cloned receptors has provided unique, and very selective, tools for immunohistochemistry. However, even some of antisera do not distinguish among some of the splice variants. Thus, even now, localization studies must be interpreted cautiously, taking into account the possibility that a specific epitope might be contained within more than one variant.

A complete description of the distribution of opioid receptors is beyond the scope of this entry. Detailed descriptions of the mRNA of MOR–1 have been published, (Mansour et al. 1994), as have the distributions of the peptides (Ding et al. 1996), DOR–1 (Arvidsson et al. 1995a) and KOR–1 (Arvidsson et al. 1995b). The descriptions below refer primarily to opioid receptor localization in relationship to pain pathways and are based primarily upon studies with rodents, although the distributions in human tissues are quite similar (Fig. 1).

Peripheral Opioid Receptors

Mu, delta and kappa opioid receptors have been identified in rat and human ▶ nerve terminals in the skin (for review see Stein et al. 2001). These fibers are the peripheral terminals of neuronal cell bodies that are localized in the ▶ dorsal root ganglia (DRG). Within the DRG, approximately 50% of all neurons express MOR 1, whereas only 20% express DOR–1 or KOR–1. MOR–1 and KOR–1 are found almost exclusively in small diameter myelinated (Aδ fibers) and unmyelinated (C fibers) axons, whereas DOR–1 is also found in large diameter fibers (Aαβ fibers). Opioid receptors are synthesized in the DRG and then transported to the nerve endings, both in the periphery and centrally in the ▶ spinal cord, via axonal transport. In inflammatory states, all three types of receptors have been shown to be upregulated, facilitating peripheral-mediated opioid analgesia.

It has been suggested that opioid receptors are also located on sympathetic post-ganglionic terminals, and that they contribute to opioid antinociception. However, direct attempts to localize opioid receptors in sympathetic ganglia have failed. Additionally, chemical sympathectomy with 6-hydroxydopamine does not modify opioid receptor expression in the dorsal root ganglia, nor does it change the analgesic effect of either mu, delta or kappa agonists in an inflammatory model of pain. Immune cells have also been shown to express opioid receptors; however, their role in mediating analgesia remains unclear.

Spinal Cord

In the spinal dorsal horn, expression of mu, delta and kappa opioid receptors is intense in the superficial laminae (laminae I–II), where nociceptive Aδ and C fibers terminate. Opioid receptors are located presynaptically on axons from the DRG neurons, as well as post-synaptically on cell bodies that can be visualized by in situ hybridization, and immunohistochemically. In deeper laminae of the dorsal horn, and in the ventral horn, mu and kappa opioid receptor expression is weaker, whereas delta receptors are found throughout the dorsal and ventral horns including motoneurons. Two splice variants of the mu opioid receptor, MOR–1C and MOR–1D, are expressed almost exclusively in unmyelinated axons in the superficial laminae of the spinal cord (Abbadie et al. 2001). Furthermore, confocal studies indicate that neurons in the dorsal horn express either MOR–1 or MOR–1C, but rarely both.

In pain pathways, ascending projections originating from the deep laminae terminate in different areas than projections originating from lamina I (Gauriau and Bernard 2002). Deep laminae neurons project to caudal reticular areas, including the lateral reticular nucleus, the subnucleus reticularis dorsalis, and the gigantocellular lateral paragigantocellular reticular nuclei. Lamina I neurons project to the thalamus, including the ventral posterolateral nucleus, ventral posteromedial, posterior nuclear group and triangular posterior nuclei (Willis and Westlund 1997). Lamina I neurons also project to the lateral parabrachial area.

The distribution of opioid receptors in the spinal trigeminal nucleus is similar to the distribution in the spinal cord.

Brainstem

Moderate expression of MOR–1 is observed in regions of the pons and medulla, particularly those involved in

MOR1   DOR1   KOR1

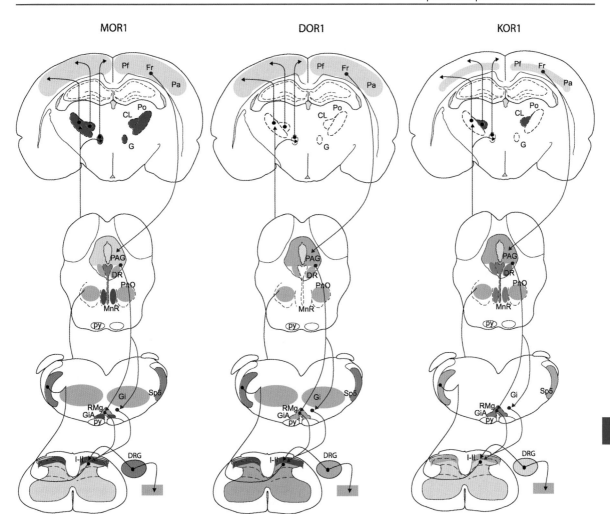

Opioid Receptor Localization, Figure 1 Opioid receptor distribution in relationship with pain pathways. These schematics represent the ascending (arrows on the left side) and descending (arrows on the right side) pain pathways. Distributions of MOR-1, DOR-1 and KOR-1, based on *in situ* hybridization and immunohistochemistry studies are indicated by the blue shading. Nociceptive information is transmitted from the periphery to the spinal cord. Pain perception mainly depends upon the activation of the spinothalamic tract. Neurons in the spinal cord project to thalamic nuclei, which in turn project to subcortical and cortical areas, particularly those within the limbic system. Nociceptive information is also transmitted by the spino-parabrachial tract (not represented in this schematic) which projects to the amygdala and hypothalamus. There are also spino-limbic pathways that contribute to different aspects of pain (emotional, autonomic) by influencing different cortical areas. These ascending pain sensory pathways are subject to modulatory control by descending modulatory circuits. These circuits originate in the limbic forebrain, and via brainstem connections, control the transmission of pain signals at their first central relay in the spinal cord. These modulatory circuits mediate the action of morphine and their action is mediated by the release of endogenous opioid peptides. Abbreviations, I-II, superficial laminae of the spinal cord; CL, centrolateral thalamic nucleus; DR, dorsal raphe nucleus; DRG, dorsal root ganglia; Fr, frontal cortex; G, gelatinosus nucleus; Gi, gigantocellular reticular nucleus; GiA, gigantocellular reticular nucleus part alpha; MnR, median raphe nucleus; Pa, parietal cortex; PAG, periaqueductal grey; Pf, prefrontal cortex; PnO, pontine reticular nucleus; Po, posterior thalamic nuclear group; py, pyramidal tract; RMg, raphe magnus nucleus; Sp5, spinal trigeminal nucleus. Schematics are modified from (Paxinos and Watson 1997).

mediating analgesia such as the raphe magnus, intermediate reticular, gigantocellular reticular and lateral paragigantocellular nuclei. Opioids also act on regions of the brainstem to activate descending pain inhibitory systems, which consist of descending serotoninergic and noradrenergic neurons (Basbaum and Fields 1984). Indeed microinjections of morphine into the lateral paragigantocellular nucleus, raphe magnus nucleus and periaqueductal grey induce profound analgesic effects. The periaqueductal grey, medial and dorsal raphe nuclei also contain moderate MOR–1, but intense KOR–1 labeling.

Intense expression of MOR–1 is also seen in the nucleus of the solitary tract, ambiguus nucleus and parabrachial nucleus. These brainstem structures mediate the respiratory and cardiovascular side effects of opioids. Neurons in the lateral parabrachial area project to the extended amygdala, the hypothalamus, the periaqueductal grey matter, and the ventrolateral medulla and have been implicated in emotional and autonomic aspects of pain

(Willis and Westlund 1997; Gauriau and Bernard 2002). DOR–1 expression is low or absent in all hindbrain and midbrain structures such as the periaqueductal grey, raphe nucleus or parabrachial nucleus.

Midbrain and Forebrain

MOR–1 expression has been demonstrated in the thalamic nuclei involved in the transmission of nociceptive information, including the centrolateral, ventrolateral and ventromedial thalamic nuclei and posterior thalamic nuclear group. Only the centrolateral and geniculate nuclei express KOR. Little or no expression of DOR–1 is observed in the rodent thalamus. In the hypothalamus, one splice variant of MOR–1 is found in various nuclei, whereas MOR–1 distribution is limited (Abbadie et al. 2000).

In the ▶ cerebral cortex, MOR–1 is weakly expressed in layers II–IV, while DOR–1 expression is moderate to intense in layers II, III, V and VI, and KOR–1 is only found in layer VI.

Conclusion

Overall, there is an excellent correlation between the localization of opioid receptors and pain pathways. Opioid receptors are distributed at various sites from nerve endings in the skin, to the cerebral cortex and various nuclei located along nociceptive pathways, such as the dorsal raphe or the lateral parabrachial nucleus.

References

1. Abbadie C, Pan YX, Pasternak GW (2000) Differential Distribution in Rat Brain of mu-Opioid Receptor Carboxy Terminal Splice Variants MOR-1C-Like and MOR-1-Like Immunoreactivity: Evidence for Region-Specific Processing. J Comp Neurol 419:244–256
2. Abbadie C, Pasternak GW, Aicher SA (2001) Presynaptic Localization of the Carboxy-Terminus Epitopes of the mu-Opioid Receptor Splice Variants MOR-1C and MOR-1D in the Superficial Laminae of the Rat Spinal Cord. Neuroscience 106:833–842
3. Arvidsson U, Dado RJ, Riedl M, Lee JH, Law PY, Loh HH, Elde R, Wessendorf MW (1995a) delta-Opioid Receptor Immunoreactivity: Distribution in Brainstem and Spinal Cord, and Relationship to Biogenic Amines and Enkephalin. J Neurosci 15:1215–1235
4. Arvidsson U, Riedl M, Chakrabarti S, Vulchanova L, Lee JH, Nakano AH, Lin X, Loh HH, Law PY, Wessendorf MW, et al. (1995b) The kappa-Opioid Receptor is Primarily Postsynaptic: Combined Immunohistochemical Localization of the Receptor and Endogenous Opioids. Proc Natl Acad Sci USA 92:5062û5066
5. Basbaum AI, Fields HL (1984) Endogenous Pain Control Systems: Brainstem Spinal Pathways and Endorphin Circuitry. Annu Rev Neurosci 7:309–338
6. Ding YQ, Kaneko T, Nomura S, Mizuno N (1996) Immunohistochemical Localization of mu-Opioid Receptors in the Central Nervous System of the Rat. J Comp Neurol 367:375–402
7. Gauriau C, Bernard JF (2002) Pain Pathways and Parabrachial Circuits in the Rat. Exp Physiol 87:251–258
8. Kieffer BL, Gaveriaux-Ruff C (2002) Exploring the Opioid System by Gene Knockout. Prog Neurobiol 66:285–306
9. Mansour A, Fox CA, Burke S, Meng F, Thompson RC, Akil H, Watson SJ (1994) Mu, delta, and kappa Opioid Receptor mRNA Expression in the Rat CNS: An In Situ Hybridization Study. J Comp Neurol 350:412–438
10. Pasternak GW (1993) Pharmacological Mechanisms of Opioid Analgesics. Clin Neuropharmacol 16:1–18
11. Pasternak GW (2001) Insights into mu-Opioid Pharmacology: The Role of mu-Opioid Receptor Subtypes. Life Sci 68:2213–2219
12. Paxinos G, Watson C (1997) The Rat Brain in Stereotaxic Coordinates. Academic Press, San Diego, CA
13. Reisine T, Pasternak GW (1996) Opioid Analgesics and Antagonists. In: Hardman JG, Limbird LE (eds) Goodman and Gilman's: The Pharmacological Basis of Therapeutics. McGraw-Hill, New York, pp 521–556
14. Stein C, Machelska H, Schafer M (2001) Peripheral Analgesic and Anti-Inflammatory Effects of Opioids. Z Rheumatol 60:416–424
15. Wei LN, Loh HH (2002) Regulation of Opioid Receptor Expression. Curr Opin Pharmacol 2:69–75
16. Willis WD, Westlund KN (1997) Neuroanatomy of the Pain System and of the Pathways that Modulate Pain. J Clin Neurophysiol 14:2–31

Opioid Receptor Trafficking in Pain States

CATHERINE M. CAHILL[1], ANNE MORINVILLE[2], ALAIN BEAUDET[2]
[1]Queen's University, Kingston, ON, Canada
[2]Montreal Neurological Institute, McGill University, Montreal, QC, Canada
cahillc@post.queensu.ca, annemorinville@yahoo.ca, abeaudet@frsq.gouv.gc.ca

Synonyms

Trafficking; opioid receptor targeting; opioid receptor recruitment; opioid receptor sorting; opioid receptor redistribution

Definition

Receptor ▶ trafficking is the constitutive or regulated movement of a receptor protein within the cell, whether between sub-cellular compartments, or towards or away from plasma membranes. The presence of opioid receptors (OR) at the cell surface is essential for regulating opioid signal transduction and subsequent cellular functions. Following agonist activation, receptor ▶ internalization plays an important role in cellular responsiveness, by depleting the cell surface of receptors and contributing to the processes of receptor ▶ desensitization and re-sensitization. Likewise, receptor insertion in plasma membranes through recycling of internalized receptors, and/or targeting of reserve receptors from intracellular stores, is critical for controlling the number of plasma membrane receptors accessible for stimulation, and thereby for regulating various neuronal responses including pain transmission.

Characteristics

Background

Three genes have been identified to encode for three opioid receptors (OR): ▶ mu (μ), ▶ delta (δ), and ▶ kappa

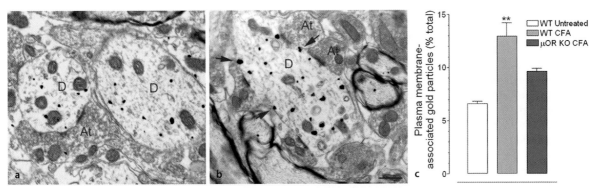

Opioid Receptor Trafficking in Pain States, Figure 1 Trafficking of δOR to neuronal plasma membranes of postsynaptic neurons in the dorsal spinal cord following induction of peripheral inflammation. Electron microscopic distribution of δOR in dendrites from the ipsilateral dorsal spinal cord of sham-injected (a) versus CFA-injected (b) rats. Silver-intensified immunogold labeling of δOR demonstrates a predominantly intracellular localization of the receptor in both conditions. However, the number of gold particles is higher over the plasma membrane of dendrites in CFA-treated than in sham-injected animals (arrows). (c) Quantitative analysis of the subcellular distribution of immunoreactive δOR in dendrites from the lumbar spinal cord of untreated wild-type (WT), CFA-treated WT, and μOR knock-out (KO) mice. Data are expressed as the percentage of dendrite-associated gold particles present on plasma membranes. Note that the percentage of membrane-associated δOR is significantly higher in CFA-injected than in sham-treated WT mice, and that this effect is absent in CFA-treated μOR KO mice. D, dendrite; At, axon terminal. Scale bar = 0.4 μm.

(κ). All OR inhibit the transmission of pain and are located on peripheral and central branches of somatic and visceral sensory afferents, as well as at various locations within the central nervous system including the spinal cord, midbrain, and cerebral cortex. Within the last few decades, great advances have been made in our understanding of the physiological and pharmacological properties of OR, as well as of their implication in mechanisms of acute and chronic pain. By comparison, much less is known about the mechanisms of OR intraneuronal trafficking, specifically, the physiological function or maladaptive processes that are linked to these trafficking events (for reviews see Roth et al. 1998; von Zastrow et al. 2003).

The first documentation of OR trafficking in models of persistent and chronic pain was generated by studies on axonal transport in peripheral sensory afferents. Thus, autoradiographic and immunohistochemical studies have demonstrated that induction of inflammatory pain via local injection of chemical irritants, antigens, or cytokines resulted in an increase in the synthesis and expression of OR in the cell bodies of sensory afferent neurons (► dorsal root ganglia, DRG). This increased expression led, in turn, to enhanced axonal transport of OR in the sciatic nerve, and hence to an increase in their density in the inflamed tissue (Hassan et al. 1993; Ji et al. 1995). Ligation of the nerve following induction of tissue inflammation resulted in an accumulation of all three OR in the sciatic nerve, both proximal and distal to site of ligation, indicating both antero- and ► retrograde transport of multiple OR. This enhanced transport was postulated to underlie the augmented antinociceptive potency of OR agonists following either spinal or local administration of opiates in models of inflammation (Antonijevic et al. 1995; Cahill et al. 2003). Similarly, μOR were found to be up-regulated in DRG

► ipsilateral to the site of nerve injury in a model of neuropathic pain (Truong et al. 2003). In this latter study, the OR protein was trafficked to axonal endbulbs of Cajal just proximal to the site of nerve injury, within aberrantly regenerating small axons in the epineurial sheath, and in residual small axons distal to the nerve constriction. These changes resulted in an increase in anti-allodynic and anti-hyperalgesic effects of locally or peripherally applied opioid agonists, suggesting that the accumulation of μOR to sites of neuromas, and concomitant disruption of the blood–nerve barrier, provided a means for enhanced agonist access to the receptors (Antonijevic et al. 1995).

Cell Trafficking of δOR in Chronic Pain

We postulated that, likewise, changes in receptor trafficking might underlie the enhanced antinociceptive potency of δOR agonists administered intrathecally in rodents with unilateral hind paw inflammation (Hylden et al. 1991; Qiu et al. 2000). To test this hypothesis, we used electron microscopic immunocytochemistry to quantify the ultrastructural distribution of δOR in neurons of the dorsal spinal cord of rats and mice, subjected, or not, to peripheral inflammation via intraplantar injection of Complete Freund's Adjuvant (CFA). In non-treated animals, the bulk of δOR immunoreactivity was associated with neuronal cell bodies and ► dendrites, in conformity with in situ hybridization and radioligand binding data (Cahill et al. 2001a). Within these structures, only a small proportion of immunoreactive receptors were found on the plasma membrane, the majority being associated with intracellular vesicular stores (Cahill et al. 2001a; Cheng et al. 1997). By contrast, 72h after CFA injection, the proportion of δOR associated with plasma membranes was significantly increased in both species within dendrites from lam-

0

inae III–V of the dorsal horn ipsilateral to the side of inflammation, compared to both untreated controls and to the ▶ contralateral spinal cord (Cahill et al. 2003; Morinville et al. 2004a). This change in sub-cellular compartmentalization was positively correlated with an augmented antinociceptive effect of δOR agonists following spinal administration (Cahill et al. 2003). The increase in δOR plasma membrane density was partly due to recruitment of reserve receptors from intracellular reserve stores, since it was accompanied by a statistical decrease in the mean distance separating intracellular receptors from the closest plasma membrane.

A similar increase in the targeting of δOR to neuronal plasma membranes had previously been documented by us in rats and mice subjected to sustained treatment with morphine for 48h (Cahill et al. 2001b; Morinville et al. 2003). Similar to the results obtained in CFA-treated mice, this increase in δOR targeting was not accompanied by corresponding augmentations in either δOR mRNA, protein expression, or [^{125}I]–deltorphin binding levels, suggesting that it was not due to enhanced receptor production, but solely to increased recruitment to the surface (Morinville et al. 2004b). Most importantly, this targeting effect of morphine was the result of a selective stimulation of μOR, as it was no longer observed in μOR-KO mice (Morinville et al. 2003).

To determine whether the CFA-induced targeting of δOR to dendritic membranes was also due to stimulation of μOR, we repeated the CFA experiments in transgenic μOR knock-out animals. The CFA-induced recruitment of δOR to neuronal plasma membranes was totally abolished in these animals, suggesting that it was dependent on the activation of μOR through pain-induced release of endogenous μOR-acting peptides (Morinville et al. 2004a).

Functional Significance

In summary, alterations in the sub-cellular distribution of OR, as the result of either acute or chronic stimulation, or of adaptive changes in response to injury, can have dramatic pathophysiological consequences on pain transmission. In the case of δOR, the increase in cell surface receptor density induced by the chronic inflammatory pain process has major pharmacological implications in allowing for increased therapeutic efficacy of analgesic drugs selective for the δOR. In other pain model systems, OR have been demonstrated to be involved in activity-dependent synaptic plasticity, a process known to be fundamental to the development of chronic pain states (Woolf & Salter 2000). Studying phenomena of receptor trafficking and internalization will hopefully provide another venue that allows either better diagnostic, or alternative novel, strategies for the treatment of chronic pain syndromes.

References

1. Antonijevic I, Mousa SA, Schafer M., Stein C (1995) Perineurial Defect and Peripheral Opioid Analgesia in Inflammation. J Neurosci 15:165–172
2. Cahill CM, McClellan KA, Morinville A, Hoffert C, Hubatsch D, O'Donnell D, Beaudet A (2001a) Immunocytochemical Distribution of delta Opioid Receptors in Rat Brain: Antigen-Specific Sub-Cellular Compartmentalization. J CompNeurol 440:65–84
3. Cahill CM, Morinville A, Hoffert C, Hubatsch D, O'Donnell D, Beaudet A (2003) Up-Regulation and Trafficking of δOR in a Model of Chronic Inflammatory Pain; Positive Correlation with Enhanced D-[Ala2]deltorphin-Induced Antinociception. Pain 101:199–208
4. Cahill CM, Morinville A, Lee M-C, Vincent JP, Beaudet A (2001b) Targeting of delta Opioid Receptor to the Plasma Membrane following Chronic Morphine Treatment. J Neurosci 21:7598–7607
5. Cheng PY, Liu-Chen LY, Pickel VM (1997) Dual Ultrastructural Immunocytochemical Labeling of mu and delta Opioid Receptors in the Superficial Layers of the Rat Cervical Spinal Cord. Brain Res 778:367–380
6. Hassan AH, Ableitner A, Stein C, Herz A (1993) Inflammation of the Rat Paw Enhances Axonal Transport of Opioid Receptors in the Sciatic Nerve and Increases their Density in the Inflamed Tissue. Neuroscience 55:185–195
7. Hylden JL, Thomas DA, Iadarola MJ, Nahin RL, Dubner R (1991). Spinal Opioid Analgesic Effects are Enhanced in a Model of Unilateral Inflammation/Hyperalgesia: Possible Involvement of Noradrenergic Mechanisms. Eur J Pharmacol 194:135–143
8. Ji RR, Zhang Q, Law PY, Loh HH, Elde R, Hökfelt T (1995) Expression of mu-, delta-, and kappa-Opioid Receptor-Like Immunoreactivities in Rat Dorsal Root Ganglia after Carrageenan-Induced Inflammation. J Neurosci 15:8156–8166
9. Morinville A, Cahill CM, Esdaile MJ, Aibak H, Collier B, Kieffer BL, Beaudet A (2003) Regulation of delta Opioid Receptor Trafficking through mu-Opioid Receptor Stimulation: Evidence from mu-Opioid Receptor Knock-Out Mice. J Neurosci 23:4888–4898
10. Morinville A, Cahill CM, Kieffer B, Collier B, Beaudet A (2004) Mu Opioid Receptor Knockout Prevents Changes in delta-Opioid Receptor Trafficking Induced by Chronic Inflammatory Pain. Pain 109:266–273
11. Morinville A, Cahill CM, Aibak H et al. (2004b) Morphine-induced changes in delta opioid receptor trafficking are linked to somatosensory processing in the rat spinal cord. J Neurosci 24:5549–5559
12. Qiu C, Sora I, Ren K, Uhl G, Dubner R (2000) Enhanced delta-Opioid Receptor-Mediated Antinociception in mu-Opioid Receptor-Deficient Mice. Eur J Pharmacol 387:163–169
13. Roth BL, Willins DL, Kroeze WK (1998) G Protein-Coupled Receptor (GPCR) Trafficking in the Central Nervous System: Relevance for Drugs of Abuse. Drug Alcohol Depend 51:73–85
14. Truong W, Cheng C, Xu QG, Li XQ, Zochodne DW (2003) Mu Opioid Receptors and Analgesia at the Site of a Peripheral Nerve Injury. Ann Neurol 53:366–375
15. von Zastrow M, Svingos A, Haberstock-Debic H, Evans C (2003) Regulated Endocytosis of Opioid Receptors: Cellular Mechanisms and Proposed Roles in Physiological Adaptation to Opiate Drugs. Curr Opin Neurobiol 13:348–353
16. Woolf, C.J., Salter, M.W. (2000). Neuronal Plasticity: Increasing the Gain in Pain. Science 288:1765–1769

Opioid Receptors

GAVRIL W. PASTERNAK

Department of Neurology, Memorial Sloan-Kettering Cancer Center, New York, NY, USA

pasterng@mskcc.org

Synonyms

Opiate Receptors; MOR–1; DOR–1; KOR–1

Definition

Opioid receptors are proteins located on the surface of cells that bind opiate and opioid peptide drugs selectively and with high affinity.

Characteristics

Opioids act by interacting with specific recognition sites on the surface of the cell termed receptors. The concept of opiate receptors goes back over fifty years. The first opioids, morphine and codeine, were isolated from opium over a hundred years ago, which was followed by the synthesis of thousands of derivatives in an effort to dissociate analgesia from side-effects. The rigid structure activity relationships of these compounds led to the suggestion of very specific binding sites. Indeed, these structure-activity relationships led to models of the binding pocket decades before the receptors were cloned. The classification of these receptors became more complex with the observations of the interactions between nalorphine and morphine. Differing only by the substitution of the N-methyl group by an N-allyl group, the two drugs were quite distinct pharmacologically. Whereas morphine is an effective analgesic, nalorphine was one of the first antagonists. However, if given at sufficiently high doses, nalorphine was also able to elicit analgesia, leading Martin to propose two subtypes of opioid receptors. He suggested that nalorphine was an antagonist at the M, or morphine receptor, and an agonist at the N, or nalorphine, receptor. Martin extended this classification based upon detailed pharmacological observations *in vivo*, to propose specific receptors for morphine (mu) and for ketocyclazocine (kappa) (Martin et al. 1976). The subsequent discovery of the endogenous opioid peptides (Table 1), led Kosterlitz and co-workers to propose an ► enkephalin-selective receptor, termed delta (Lord et al. 1977) (► delta opioid receptor). Goldstein and colleagues then identified

dynorphin A as the endogenous ligand for the kappa receptor (► kappa opioid receptor). Pharmacological studies have suggested these three major families of receptors, as well as subtypes (Table 2).

Opiate Receptor Binding Sites

The initial concept of opioid receptors, and the suggestion of receptor classes, had been inferred by classical pharmacological studies. Receptor binding studies provided the verification of these sites at the biochemical level. Opioid binding sites within the nervous system were first reported in 1973 using mu ligands (Snyder and Pasternak 2003). In these initial studies, the receptors were labeled by incubating brain membranes with radiolabeled opioids of high specific activity, and washing away the unbound drug. Specificity of the labeled sites was established by demonstrating that only active opioids completed the binding. A number of studies then explored the nature of the binding, demonstrating its protein nature, and differences in the binding of agonists and antagonists. As the kappa and delta classes of opioid receptors were described and suitable radioligands became available, they, too, were verified in binding studies.

During the course of these studies exploring the binding of a variety of opioids, evidence surfaced for subpopulations of sites, starting with mu receptors (Wolozin and Pasternak 1981; Pasternak and Snyder 1975). Early binding studies identified a very high affinity binding component, which was subsequently found to be uniquely sensitive to the antagonists naloxonazine and naloxazone. Under conditions *in vivo*, in which this high affinity binding site was blocked, naloxonazine was able to antagonize selected mu actions, such as supraspinal analgesia, but not others, such as respiratory depression or the inhibition of gastrointestinal transit. The mu binding and mu actions sensitive to naloxonazine were termed mu_1, and those mu sites and functions that were insensitive were termed mu_2 (Wolozin and Pasternak 1981). The complexity of

Opioid Receptors, Table 1 Selected Opioid Peptides

Opioid Peptide	Amino Acid Sequence
[Leu^5]enkephalin	**Tyr –Gly –Gly –Phe –Leu**
[Met^5]enkephalin	**Tyr –Gly –Gly –Phe–Met**
Dynorphin A	**Tyr –Gly –Gly –Phe –Leu**–Arg–Arg–Ile–Arg––Pro–Lys-Leu-Lys-Trp-Asp-Asn–Gln
Dynorphin B	**Tyr –Gly –Gly –Phe –Leu**–Arg–Arg–Gln–Phe–Lys–Val–Val–Thr
α–Neoendorphin	**Tyr –Gly –Gly –Phe –Leu**–Arg–Lys–Tyr–Pro–Lys
β$_h$–Endorphin	**Tyr –Gly –Gly –Phe –Met**–Thr–Ser–Glu-Lys-Ser-Gln-Thr-Pro-Leu-Val-Thr-Leu-Phe-Lys-Asn-Ala-Ile-Ile-Lys-Asn-Ala-Tyr-Lys-Lys-Gly-Glu
Endomorphin–1	Tyr–Pro–Trp–Phe-NH$_2$
Endomorphin–2	Tyr–Pro–Phe–Phe-NH$_2$

Opioid Receptors, Table 2 Pharmacological classification of opioid receptors and their actions

Receptor	Clone	Actions
Mu	MOR–1	Sedation
Mu$_1$		Supraspinal and peripheral analgesia
		Prolactin release; Feeding
Mu$_2$		Spinal Analgesia; Respiratory depression,
		Inhibition of gastrointestinal transit,
		Guinea pig ileum bioassay; Feeding
Kappa		
Kappa$_1$	KOR–1	Analgesia; Dysphoria; Diuresis; Feeding
Kappa$_2$	(KOR–1/DOR–1 dimer)	Unknown
Kappa$_3$		Analgesia
Delta	DOR–1	Mouse vas deferens bioassay, feeding
Delta$_1$		Supraspinal analgesia
Delta$_2$		Spinal &supraspinal analgesia

Some actions assigned to general families have not yet been correlated with a specific subtype. Some pharmacologically defined subtypes have not been correlated with specific clones.

mu subtypes increased with studies of the morphine metabolite morphine–6β–glucuronide, a highly selective mu opioid with a pharmacology distinct from that of morphine (Pasternak 2001b).

The suggestion of receptor subtypes was not limited to mu receptors. Using selective delta ligands, investigators also demonstrated differences suggesting the existence of delta receptor subtypes (Mattia et al. 1991). Kappa receptor subtypes were proposed by several groups. These distinctions were based in a large part upon the kappa-selective drug U50,488H. First, the kappa receptors were separated into U50,488H-sensitive and insensitive sites (Zukin et al. 1988) The U50,488H sensitive sites were designated as kappa$_1$. These kappa$_1$ receptors were further subdivided by their sensitivity towards several endogenous opioids, α–neoendorphin and dynorphin B (Clark et al. 1989). Dynorphin A is the endogenous ligand for kappa$_1$, and competes at all kappa$_1$ sites with high affinity. In contrast, there are subpopulations of kappa$_1$ binding sites that are sensitive to dynorphin B and α–neoendorphin and those that are not. Two subdivisions of the U50,488H insensitive sites have also been suggested. The kappa$_2$ receptors were defined by the benzomorphan ethylketocyclazocine, while the kappa$_3$ receptor was defined in both binding studies and pharmacologically using the novel opioid nalox-

one benzoylhydrazone. Similar conclusions came from detailed computer modeling (Rothman et al. 1992)

Molecular Biology of Opioid Receptors

The various opioid receptor classes were initially defined pharmacologically and in receptor binding assays. It took almost twenty years for the receptors to be cloned (Uhl et al. 1994). The delta receptor (▶ DOR-1) was the first one to be cloned (Evans et al. 1992; Kieffer et al. 1992), followed quickly by mu (▶ MOR–1) and kappa$_1$ (▶ KOR–1) receptors. All the opioid receptors are traditional G protein coupled receptors, with seven transmembrane domains, an extracellular amino (N) terminus and an intracellular carboxy (C) terminus (Fig. 1). The three clones predicted very similar proteins, particularly within the transmembrane domains. DOR–1 and KOR–1 are comprised of three exons that encode the full protein, with the first encoding the NH$_2$–terminus through the first transmembrane domain, the second encoding the next three transmembrane domains, and the third encoding the last three transmembrane domains and the COOH-terminus. MOR–1 is similar in that there are three exons that encode the NH$_2$–terminus, all seven transmembrane domains and most of the intracellular COOH-terminus. However, it differs from the others in that there are twelve additional amino acids at the tip of the COOH-terminus encoded by exon 4. The binding pocket is within the membrane and is comprised of the seven transmembrane domains of the receptor. When expressed, each receptor showed the anticipated selectivity in receptor binding assays, and sensitivity

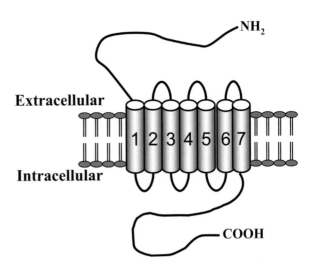

Opioid Receptors, Figure 1 Schematic of the opioid receptors. Like traditional G-protein coupled receptors, the opioid receptors have seven transmembrane (TM) domains. DOR–1 and KOR–1 both have three exons that encode the receptor protein. The first TM is encoded by the first translated exon, the next three TM by the second and the last three TM by the third translated exon. Although MOR–1 has this same exon structure from the extracellular N-terminus through to the seven TM regions, MOR–1 has an additional exon that encodes the terminal 12 amino acids in the C-terminus. The structure of this region is more complex with the MOR–1 variants.

Mouse MOR-1 3'-Splice variants

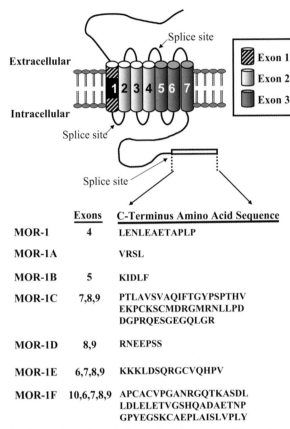

	Exons	C-Terminus Amino Acid Sequence
MOR-1	4	LENLEAETAPLP
MOR-1A		VRSL
MOR-1B	5	KIDLF
MOR-1C	7,8,9	PTLAVSVAQIFTGYPSPTHV EKPCKSCMDRGMRNLLPD DGPRQESGEGQLGR
MOR-1D	8,9	RNEEPSS
MOR-1E	6,7,8,9	KKKLDSQRGCVQHPV
MOR-1F	10,6,7,8,9	APCACVPGANRGQTKASDL LDLELETVGSHQADAETNP GPYEGSKCAEPLAISLVPLY

Opioid Receptors, Figure 2 Schematic of the mouse MOR–1 variants. MOR–1 undergoes alternative splicing at the C-terminus inside the cell. The exons responsible for encoding the terminal amino acids and its sequence are presented.

in functional assays when looking at their ability to activate G-proteins.

Pharmacological studies strongly implied the existence of subtypes of the receptors. With regards to mu receptors, this concept is supported with the isolation of a number of different splice variants of MOR–1 in mice, rats and humans (Pasternak 2001a). Many of the variants generate full length receptors that differ only in the tip of the intracellar C-terminus. As noted above, in MOR–1 the terminal 12 amino acids are encoded by exon 4. These other variants have alternative exons instead of exon 4 that encode sequences of different lengths and amino acid composition (Fig. 2). All the variants contain the same first three exons that encode transmembrane domains that define the binding pocket. Thus, it is not surprising that they all show high affinity and selectivity for mu opioids. However, functional studies have shown differences in the sensitivity of these variants to different opioid ligands. Thus, the concept of multiple ► Mu(μ)-Opioid Receptor has been confirmed at the molecular level, although the relation-

ship between these variants and the pharmacologically defined subtypes is still not certain.

The situation is less clear with the delta receptor subtypes. Although DOR–1 undergoes splicing, no functional splice variants have been uncovered. KOR–1 corresponds to the kappa$_1$ subtype. Again, despite the presence of alternative splicing, there are no additional functional KOR–1 variants. There is evidence to suggest that kappa$_2$ receptors are generated by a dimer of KOR–1/DOR–1. The kappa$_3$ receptors are the least understood of all the pharmacologically defined variants. Antisense mapping studies have suggested an association with the receptor for orphanin FQ/nociceptin, but the two receptors are clearly not identical.

Functional Studies

The overall pharmacology of these agents is quite complex (Reisine and Pasternak 1996). Highly selective agonists and antagonists are available for these drugs, permitting the evaluation of the actions of individual classes of opioid receptors. All the opioid receptor classes, and even all the proposed subtypes, have been implicated in analgesia, with many involved with other actions as well. With mu opioids, these actions include respiratory depression, sedation and the inhibition of gastrointestinal transit. The actions of the kappa and delta drugs are less well studied clinically.

Analgesia results from the activation of opioid receptors in the brain, spinal cord or periphery. However, the simultaneous activation of more than one site, such as when the drugs are given systemically, leads to more profound responses due to synergistic interactions among the sites. This was first demonstrated between the brain and the spinal cord, and has been extended to peripheral sites as well. Chronic administration of opioids leads to a progressive decline in activity, or ► tolerance. Drugs within the same class show cross tolerance, but agents from different classes do not. ► Dependence is also seen with chronic administration. Unlike ► addiction, which implies drug-seeking behaviors, dependence is a physiological response to the chronic administration of the agents and is observed with all subjects.

Correlating these opioid actions with the cloned receptors has been a major goal. Shortly after the initial cloning of MOR–1, antisense approaches demonstrated the importance of the MOR–1 gene in morphine analgesia. This was further confirmed using knockout models (► knockout mice). Several different animal models were generated that were deficient in MOR–1. All the animal models revealed the absence of morphine analgesia as well as other morphine effects. However, one of these animal models was quite unusual. Despite the disruption of exon 1, additional mRNA transcripts from the MOR–1 gene continued to be made. Furthermore, although morphine was inactive in this animal model at the highest doses tested, some mu opioids, such as morphine-6β-glucuronide and heroin, retained their

O

analgesic potential despite the inactivity of morphine. This provides further evidence supporting the existence of pharmacologically distinct mu receptor subtypes. Knockout models have also been evaluated for delta (DOR–1) and kappa₁ (KOR–1) receptors. The loss of the receptors in both cases led to the loss of activity of their respective classes of drugs. Together, these experiments confirm the importance of each of these receptors in the analgesic actions of the drugs involved.

Conclusion

The concept of opiate receptors goes back many years. Initial studies, based upon traditional pharmacological approaches, implied the existence of several families of receptors and subtypes which have now been confirmed with the cloning of these receptors. The concept of subtypes of mu receptors is supported by the identification of splice variants of MOR–1.

- ▶ Opioids in the Periphery and Analgesia
- ▶ Opioids in the Spinal Cord and Modulation of Ascending Pathways (N. gracilis)
- ▶ Postoperative Pain, Opioids

References

1. Clark JA, Liu L, Price M, Hersh B, Edelson M, Pasternak GW (1989) Kappa opiate receptor multiplicity: Evidence for two U50,488–sensitive kappa₁ subtypes and a novel kappa₃ subtype. J Pharmacol Exp Ther 251:461–468
2. Evans CJ, Keith DE, Jr, Morrison H, Magendzo K, Edwards RH (1992) Cloning of a delta opioid receptor by functional expression. Science 258:1952–1955
3. Kieffer BL, Befort K, Gaveriaux-Ruff C, Hirth CG (1992) The δ-opioid receptor: Isolation of a cDNA by expression cloning and pharmacological characterization. Proc Natl Acad Sci USA 89:12048–12052
4. Lord JAH, Waterfield AA, Hughes J, Kosterlitz HW (1977) Endogenous opioid peptides: multiple agonists and receptors. Nature 267:495499
5. Martin WR, Eades CG, Thompson JA, Huppler RE, Gilbert PE (1976) The effects of morphine and nalorphine-like drugs in the nondependent and morphine-dependent chronic spinal dog. J Pharmacol Exp Ther 197:517–532
6. Mattia A, Vanderah T, Mosberg HI, Porreca F (1991) Lack of antinociceptive cross tolerance between [D-Pen²,D-Pen⁵]enkephalin and [D-Ala²]deltorphin II in mice: evidence for delta receptor subtypes. J Pharmacol Exp Ther 258:583–587
7. Pasternak GW (2001a) Incomplete cross tolerance and multiple mu opioid peptide receptors. Trends Pharmacol Sci 22:67–70
8. Pasternak GW (2001b) Insights into mu opioid pharmacology - The role of mu opioid receptor subtypes. Life Sci 68:2213–2219
9. Pasternak GW, Snyder SH (1975) Identification of a novel high affinity opiate receptor binding in rat brain. Nature 253:563–565
10. Reisine T, Pasternak GW (1996) Opioid analgesics and antagonists. In: Hardman JG, Limbird LE (eds) Goodman & Gilman's the Pharmacological Basis of Therapeutics. McGraw-Hill, New York, pp 521–556
11. Rothman RB, Bykov V, Xue BG, Xu H, De Costa BR, Jacobson AE, Rice KC, Kleinman JE, Brady LS (1992) Interaction of opioid peptides and other drugs with multiple kappa receptors in rat and human brain. Evidence for species differences. Peptides 13:977–987
12. Snyder SH and Pasternak GW (2003) Historical review: Opioid receptors. Trends Pharmacol Sci 24:198–205.
13. Uhl GR, Childers S, Pasternak GW (1994) An opiate-receptor gene family reunion. Trends Neurosci 17:89–93
14. Wolozin BL and Pasternak GW (1981) Classification of multiple morphine and enkephalin binding sites in the central nervous system. Proc Natl Acad Sci USA 78:6181–6185
15. Zukin RS, Eghbali M, Olive D, Unterwald E, Tempel A (1988) Characterization and visualization of rat and guinea pig brain kappa opioid receptors: Evidence for kappa₁ and kappa₂ opioid receptors. Proc Natl Acad Sci USA 85:4061–4065

Opioid Receptors at Postsynaptic Sites

ANDREW J. TODD
Spinal Cord Group, Institute of Biomedical and Life Sciences, University of Glasgow, Glasgow, UK
a.todd@bio.gla.ac.uk

Synonyms

Postsynaptic Opioid Receptors

Definition

Postsynaptic opioid receptors are those that are located on the cell bodies and dendrites of neurons, rather than on their axon terminals. Opioids administered to the spinal cord can produce analgesia, and part of this effect is mediated by opioid receptors on the terminals of ▶ nociceptive primary afferents. Activation of these receptors reduces the release of excitatory neurotransmitter from the nociceptive afferents, and this is referred to as a presynaptic action. However, opioid receptors are also present on certain neurons in the spinal cord (post-synaptic opioid receptors), and these are thought to contribute to opioid analgesia.

Characteristics

Anatomical Distribution of Opioid Receptors in the Spinal Cord

The distribution of opioid receptors in the spinal cord was initially investigated by using ▶ radio-ligand binding. Numerous studies were carried out with this method, and these showed that the highest concentration of receptors was in the superficial part of the dorsal horn (▶ Rexed's laminae I and II). Transection of dorsal roots led to a substantial reduction of this opioid binding, presumably due to loss of presynaptic receptors on primary afferent terminals. However, significant binding was still seen in the superficial dorsal horn after rhizotomy, and this was thought to result from the presence of opioid receptors on spinal cord neurons. The cloning of μ, δ and κ opioid receptors meant that antibodies could be raised against them and used to investigate their distribution in the spinal cord by means of ▶ immunocytochemistry (Arvidsson et al. 1995a; Arvidsson et al. 1995b; Kemp et al. 1996; Harris and Drake 2001; Spike et al. 2002). With this approach, all 3 receptors have been found to be concentrated in laminae I and II of the dorsal horn, which matches the results obtained with radio-ligand binding. Immunocytochemical studies have shown that μ and κ receptors are present on both dorsal horn neurons (postsynaptic opioid receptors) and primary afferents (presynaptic receptors) (Arvidsson et al. 1995b; Kemp et al. 1996; Harris and Drake 2001; Spike et al. 2002), while δ receptors in the dorsal horn appear to be restricted to the terminals of primary afferents (Arvidsson et al. 1995b). Relatively little is known about postsynaptic κ opioid receptors, except that they have been seen on a few neuronal cell bodies in laminae I and II (Harris and Drake 2001). In contrast, several studies have demonstrated μ opioid receptors on dorsal horn neurons. Since μ opioid receptors play a fundamental role in opioid analgesia and more is known about their distribution, they will be the main focus of this article. Most of the studies on μ opioid receptors have been carried out with an antibody raised against the first identified form of the protein (MOR1), and these have shown that numerous immunoreactive cells are present in the superficial part of the dorsal horn (Arvidsson et al. 1995b; Kemp et al. 1996; Spike et al. 2002) (Fig. 1). MOR[1]-immunoreactivity is present on small neurons that are generally located in lamina II, where they make up approximately 10% of the neuronal population (Spike et al. 2002). As very few ▶ projection neurons are seen in this lamina, it is likely that the cells with MOR1 are interneurons, with axons that terminate locally in the spinal cord. Lamina II contains both excitatory (▶ glutamatergic) and inhibitory (▶ GABAergic) interneurons. The great majority of cells with MOR1 do not contain GABA (Kemp et al. 1996), and it is therefore likely that most of them are excitatory interneurons. The responses of MOR[1]-expressing neurons in lamina II have been investigated by examining activation of the immediate early gene ▶ c-fos after different forms of noxious stimulation (Spike et al. 2002). It was found that although approximately 15% of these cells up-regulated *c-fos* in response to noxious thermal stimulation, very few did so following mechanical or chemical noxious stimuli. This suggests that at least some of the MOR[1]-expressing neurons in lamina II of the spinal dorsal horn may be selectively activated by noxious thermal stimuli.

Although most immunocytochemical studies have used antibodies raised against MOR1, it is now known that there are several other ▶ splice variants of the μ opioid receptor and two of these, known as MOR1C and MOR1D, have been found in the spinal cord (Abbadie et al. 2000). Like MOR1 itself, these splice variants were both present at highest concentrations in the superficial laminae; however, significant amounts of MOR1C were also observed near the central canal. MOR1C (like MOR1) was found on cell bodies in lamina II, and was also present on primary afferents. In contrast, MOR1D-immunoreactivity was seen on neurons in lamina I, but not on primary afferents (Abbadie et al. 2000). Lamina I contains many projection neurons, and this therefore raises the possibility that some of these might express MOR1D, which would allow a direct inhibitory action of μ opioid agonists on the output cells of the dorsal horn.

In situ hybridisation histochemistry has also been used to investigate the locations of cells that express the 3 opioid receptors (Maekawa et al. 1994; Mansour et al. 1994; Schafer et al. 1994); however, the results with this approach have been inconsistent. Thus, one study reported

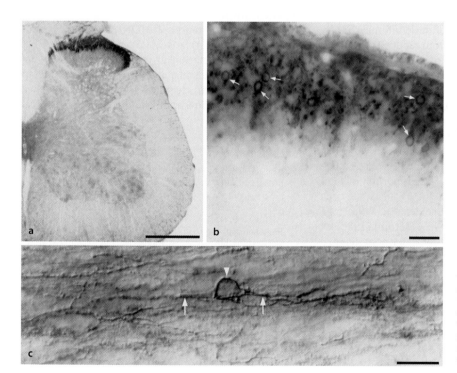

Opioid Receptors at Postsynaptic Sites, Figure 1 The appearance of MOR1 in the rat spinal cord revealed with immunocytochemistry. (a) In a transverse section of the spinal cord, MOR[1]-immunoreactivity is seen to be highly concentrated in the upper part of the dorsal horn (laminae I and II). (b) At higher magnification it is possible to see several MOR[1]-immunoreactive cell bodies (some of which are marked with arrows). (c) This image shows part of a longitudinal (parasagittal) section through the spinal cord. The cell body (arrowhead) and dendrites (arrows) of a MOR[1]-immunoreactive neuron can be seen. Scale bars: a = 500 μm; b, c = 20 μm. (Reprinted from Neuroscience, 75, Kemp et al. The μ-opioid receptor (MOR-1) is mainly restricted to neurons that do not contain GABA or glycine in the superficial dorsal horn of the rat spinal cord, pp 1231–1238, Copyright (1996), with permission from Elsevier).

that neurons with mRNA for the μ receptor are present throughout the dorsal horn, with the highest levels in the superficial laminae (Maekawa et al. 1994), while another found that they were present in the deeper laminae of the dorsal horn with few in the superficial part (Mansour et al. 1994). Neurons with mRNA for the κ receptor have been seen concentrated in the superficial laminae (Schafer et al. 1994), throughout the spinal grey matter (Maekawa et al. 1994), and in the deeper parts of the dorsal horn but not the superficial part (Mansour et al. 1994). The reasons for these discrepancies are unknown.

Responses of Dorsal Horn Neurons to Drugs that Act on the μ Opioid Receptor

The actions of opioid agonists on neurons in the superficial dorsal horn have been studied *in vitro* in slices of spinal cord and brainstem. Yoshimura and North (1983) demonstrated that ▶ opioid peptides could hyperpolarise many neurons in lamina II of the spinal cord, and that this effect was mediated by an increase in K^+ conductance. Subsequent studies have shown that this involves μ (rather than δ) opioid receptors (Jeftinija 1988; Grudt and Williams 1994; Schneider et al. 1998), which is consistent with anatomical observations that μ, but not δ, receptors are present on dorsal horn neurons. Hyperpolarisation resulting from activation of μ opioid receptors will have an inhibitory effect on these neurons. This, taken together with the fact that many of the lamina II cells with MOR1 are excitatory (Kemp et al. 1996), and that at least some respond to noxious stimuli (Spike et al. 2002), has led to the suggestion that excitatory interneurons with μ opioid receptors in lamina II normally play a role in conveying nociceptive information to projection cells in other laminae of the dorsal horn. Inhibition of these interneurons by μ opioid agonists would therefore reduce the input to projection neurons following noxious stimuli, and this would result in analgesia (reduced perception of pain). Although the hyperpolarising effect of μ opioid agonists on lamina II neurons appears at first sight to be compatible with the results of anatomical studies, there are certain discrepancies. Firstly, while only 10% of lamina II neurons are MOR[1]-immunoreactive (Spike et al. 2002), effects of μ agonists are seen on a much higher proportion of neurons. The proportion of lamina II neurons hyperpolarised by μ agonists has been variously estimated as 39% (Schneider et al. 1998), 50% (Yoshimura and North 1983) or 75% (Jeftinija 1988) for the rat spinal cord, 60% for hamster spinal cord (Schneider et al. 1998), and 86–90% for the trigeminal nucleus of rat and guinea pig (Grudt and Williams 1994). While sampling bias in recording experiments may contribute to this effect, it is unlikely to explain such a dramatic difference. It is possible that MOR1C is present on some neurons that are not MOR[1]-immunoreactive, and this could increase the proportion of cells with functional μ opioid receptors. Secondly, a "post-synaptic" action of

μ agonists has been reported on many cells in deeper laminae of the dorsal horn, in areas where radio-ligand binding and immunocytochemistry both suggest that there are low levels of opioid receptors.

Internalisation of MOR1 as a Means of Studying its Activation

Activation of receptors on the surface of neurons sometimes causes them to leave the plasma membrane and enter the cytoplasm on small membrane-bound vesicles (endosomes). Since internalised receptors can be identified with immunocytochemistry, this phenomenon can be used to investigate various aspects of receptor activation, for example dose-response relationships and time-course. It has been found that various μ-selective agonists cause internalisation of MOR1 on lamina II neurons, although morphine did not produce this effect (Trafton et al. 2000). The doses of μ agonists that were needed to cause MOR1 internalisation were similar to those that have been shown to produce hyperpolarisation of lamina II neurons (Grudt and Williams 1994), and also to doses that produced analgesia in behavioural tests (Trafton et al. 2000). Although this does not prove that postsynaptic actions of μ opioid drugs contribute to spinal opioid analgesia, they are compatible with this suggestion. Interestingly, noxious stimulation did not evoke MOR1 internalisation, either in normal animals or in those with a chronic inflammation (Trafton et al. 2000). This suggests that although postsynaptic μ opioid receptors may be involved in analgesia produced by the administration of opioid drugs, endogenous opioid peptides that act on μ receptors are not released in sufficient amounts to activate this system following noxious stimulation. It has recently been shown that direct electrical stimulation of the dorsal horn *in vitro* can cause internalisation of MOR1 in lamina II neurons (Song and Marvizon 2003), which suggests that in some circumstances neurons in the dorsal horn are able to release sufficient quantities of opioid peptides to activate postsynaptic receptors. It remains to be shown whether this occurs under physiological or pathological conditions.

References

1. Abbadie C, Pan Y, Drake CT et al. (2000) Comparative Immuno-histochemical Distributions of Carboxy Terminus Epitopes from the μ-Opioid Receptor Splice Variants MOR-1D, MOR-1 and MOR-1C in the Mouse and Rat CNS. Neuroscience 100:141–153
2. Arvidsson U, Dado RJ, Riedl M et al. (1995a) δ-Opioid Receptor Immunoreactivity: Distribution in Brainstem and Spinal Cord, and Relationship to Biogenic Amines and Enkephalin. J Neurosci 15:1215–1235
3. Arvidsson U, Riedl M, Chakrabarti S et al. (1995b) Distribution and Targeting of a μ-Opioid Receptor (MOR1) in Brain and Spinal Cord. J Neurosci 15:3328–3341
4. Grudt TJ, Williams JT (1994) μ-Opioid Agonists Inhibit Spinal Trigeminal Substantia Gelatinosa Neurons in Guinea Pig and Rat. J Neurosci 14:1646–1654
5. Harris JA, Drake CT (2001) Kappa Opioid Receptor Density is Consistent along the Rostrocaudal Axis of the Female Rat Spinal Cord. Brain Res 905:236–239

6. Jeftinija S (1988) Enkephalins Modulate Excitatory Synaptic Transmission in the Superficial Dorsal Horn by Acting at μ-Opioid Receptor Sites. Brain Res 460:260–268
7. Kemp T, Spike RC, Watt C et al. (1996) The μ-Opioid Receptor (MOR1) is Mainly Restricted to Neurons that do not Contain GABA or Glycine in the Superficial Dorsal Horn of the Rat Spinal Cord. Neuroscience 75:1231–1238
8. Maekawa K, Minami M, Yabuuchi K et al. (1994) *In Situ* Hybridization Study of μ- and κ-Opioid Receptor mRNAs in the Rat Spinal Cord and Dorsal Root Ganglia. Neurosci Lett 168:97–100
9. Mansour A, Fox CA, Burke S et al (1994) Mu, Delta, and Kappa Opioid Receptor mRNA Expression in the Rat CNS: an *In Situ* Hybridization Study. J Comp Neurol 350:412–438
10. Schafer MK, Bette M, Romeo H et al. (1994) Localization of κ-Opioid Receptor mRNA in Neuronal Subpopulations of Rat Sensory Ganglia and Spinal Cord. Neurosci Lett 167:137–140
11. Schneider SP, Eckert WA III, Light AR (1998) Opioid-Activated Postsynaptic, Inward Rectifying Potassium Currents in Whole Cell Recordings in Substantia Gelatinosa Neurons. J Neurophysiol 80:2954–2962
12. Song B, Marvizon JC (2003) Dorsal Horn Neurons Firing at High Frequency, but not Primary Afferents, Release Opioid Peptides that Produce μ-Opioid Receptor Internalization in the Rat Spinal Cord. J Neurosci 23:9171–9184
13. Spike RC, Puskar Z, Sakamoto H et al. (2002) MOR-[1]-Immunoreactive Neurons in the Dorsal Horn of the Rat Spinal Cord: Evidence for Nonsynaptic Innervation by Substance P-Containing Primary Afferents and for Selective Activation by Noxious Thermal Stimuli. Eur J Neurosci 15:1306–1316
14. Trafton JA, Abbadie C, Marek K et al. (2000) Postsynaptic Signaling via the μ-Opioid Receptor: Responses of Dorsal Horn Neurons to Exogenous Opioids and Noxious Stimulation. J Neurosci 20:8578–8584
15. Yoshimura M, North RA (1983) Substantia Gelatinosa Neurones Hyperpolarized *In Vitro* by Enkephalin. Nature 305:529–530

Opioid Responsiveness

Definition

Opioid responsiveness is the probability that adequate analgesia without intolerable and unmanageable side effects can be obtained during opioid dose titration.

▶ Cancer Pain Management, Principles of Opioid Therapy, Drug Selection
▶ Opioid Rotation
▶ Opioid Rotation in Cancer Pain Management

Opioid Responsiveness in Cancer Pain Management

SEBASTIANO MERCADANTE
La Maddalena Cancer Pain Relief & Palliative Care Unit Center, Palermo, Italy
terapiadeldolore@la-maddalena.it

Definition

The degree of analgesia obtained following dose escalation to an endpoint determined by either analgesia or intolerable adverse effects. It is a continuum of response rather than a quantal, yes or no, phenomenon, consistent with the inter-individual variability that characterizes opioid analgesia, and the occurrence of dose-dependent effects.

Characteristics

Chronic opioid therapy has been recognized as standard management for cancer pain. Analgesia can be achieved with different opioid dosages in individuals, as there is effectively no ceiling to their analgesic effect. However, the proportion of adverse effects that the patient can tolerate may limit this process. Several factors can interfere with an appropriate analgesic opioid response. The unpredictable individual response in terms of analgesia and toxicity depends on patient-related factors, drug-selective effects, and pain-related factors (Portenoy et al. 1990). The need for opioid escalation may indicate an abrupt change in the underlying disease, or reveal a previously unknown complication, indicating a change in the relation between dose and response. Primary tumors may have different evolutions in terms of distant metastases and then pain mechanisms, and can also modify the opioid response through the intervention of some metabolic factors, like cytokines. Several studies have indicated that increases in opioid doses during a chronic morphine treatment were related to a progression of disease, generating an increase in pain (Collin et al. 1993), supporting the view that development of ▶ tolerance to opioids is unlikely to be the driving force for loss of analgesia in patients who have alternative reasons for increasing pain. On the other hand, a reduced potency of the analgesic effects of opioids following its repeated administration may occur, reflecting the development of tolerance. Tolerance to analgesic and non-analgesic effects commonly occur, although other factors may be operant that allow the patient to tolerate higher doses of opioids (Portenoy 1995). Opioid response may also be drug-selective, a possibility suggested by the remarkable variability of individual patients and their response to different drugs. Different receptorial attitudes may explain these differences among opioids, in terms of ▶ efficacy. Moreover, asymmetric tolerance among opioids exists.

The pain mechanism may influence the opioid response. ▶ Neuropathic pain is considered to be less responsive to opioid treatment in comparison to ▶ nociceptive pain. Recent evidence suggests that hyperalgesia consequent to nerve injury and tolerance, both involve the ▶ N-methyl-D-aspartate (NMDA)-receptor and share part of intracellular events producing a state of neural hyperexcitation (Mao et al. 1995). Neuropathic pain has been shown to require higher doses of opioids to achieve acceptable analgesia, which is often accompanied by greater toxicity and rapid tolerance. Opioid-related side effects are often associated with neuropathic cancer pain syndromes. The clinical characteristics of neuropathic pain do not predict responses to opioids. Indeed,

O

patients with neuropathic pain did not show a particular disadvantage compared to those exhibiting nociceptive pain, unless associated with neurological impairment (Mercadante et al. 1999). Thus, neuropathic pain can still be responsive to analgesic treatment and does not result in an inherent resistance to opioids (Portenoy et al. 1990; Bruera et al. 1995; Mercadante et al. 1992). The temporal pattern of pain may also limit the opioid response. ▶ Breakthrough pain, episodic pain that interrupts basal analgesia, is commonly associated with a poor prognosis (Portenoy and Hagen 1990). The difficulty in the treatment consists in the temporal pattern of this kind of pain, involving almost the same site of basal pain. ▶ Breakthrough pain may be spontaneous, occurring without an identifiable precipitating event, and precipitant factors, volitional and non-volitional, have been identified in more than 50% of patients. The most well known form of breakthrough pain is incident pain, due to movement and commonly caused by bone metastases. The difficulty with incident pain is not a lack of response to systemic opioids, but rather that the doses required to control the incident pain produce unacceptable adverse effects when the patient is at rest or pain spontaneously stops (Mercadante et al. 2002).

Absorption, metabolism, and elimination may alter the opioid responsiveness. For example, patients with a gastrointestinal tract that is not functioning normally because of a mucosal damage or bowel resection may have a reduction in absorption of drugs, therefore requiring an increase in opioid dosage. Morphine metabolites are involved in various ways in determining the complex effects of morphine, both favourable and adverse, and may complicate the clinical use of morphine in the treatment of cancer pain. While morphine-6-glucuronide (M6G) binds the opioid receptors exerting a relevant analgesic activity, the principal morphine metabolite morphine-3-glucuronide (M3G), has been shown to functionally antagonize the analgesic effects of morphine, possibly contributing to the development of tolerance. Such metabolites are hydrophilic substances eliminated by the kidney. The accumulation of toxic metabolites during chronic morphine therapy can reduce the opioid response, leading to severe and intolerable adverse effects, even in patients with apparently normal renal function (Mercadante and Portenoy 2001).

Strategies to Improve the Opioid Response

Considering the importance of opioids in the management of chronic pain, countermeasures should be taken to limit the interference with opioid responsiveness. The countermeasures begin with a comprehensive evaluation of the causes that can contribute to worsening pain or altered pain perception, including recurrent disease, psychological distress, and the history of previous opioid use. These approaches may produce either a leftward shift of the analgesia curve or a rightward shift of the toxicity curve (Portenoy 1996).

One approach to the patient with pain that is poorly responsive to opioids is the co-administration of adjuvants, such as antidepressants and anticonvulsants. Antidepressants may improve depression, enhance sleep and provide decreases in perception of pain. The analgesic effect of tricyclics is not directly related to antidepressant activity. The analgesic ▶ efficacy of the tricyclic antidepressants has been established in many painful disorders with a neuropathic mechanism (Portenoy 1996). These substances are commonly used, although no scientific evidence exists of their advantages when added to opioids for cancer pain. Combination with opioids may introduce further risks of toxicity. Anti-inflammatory drugs have some opioid sparing effect, and may allow the lowering of opioid doses, reducing the risk of toxicity.

Another strategy to address poor opioid response is the aggressive management of adverse effects. This approach may open the therapeutic window and allow higher and more effective opioid doses. Different symptomatic drugs have been used, although few studies could demonstrate the validity of this approach (Cherny et al. 2002).

Alternately, the poor opioid response could be managed targeting analgesic tolerance and attempt to reduce or prevent it. Agents that block the activity of NMDA-receptors may provide new tools for the treatment of poorly responsive pain syndromes, particularly neuropathic ones. There are clinical reports about the use of ketamine, although this drug is hard to manage due to its excitatory adverse effects and should be used by skilled people (Mercadante and Portenoy 2001).

The treatment of breakthrough pain is challenging for physicians. A rescue dose of an opioid can provide a means to treat breakthrough pain in patients already stabilized on a baseline opioid regimen. Most opioids administered by oral route, including morphine, oxycodone and hydromorphone, have a relatively slow onset of effect (about 30–45 minutes), and the pain onset may be so rapid that an oral dose may not provide sufficiently prompt relief, even if taken as needed. Subcutaneous or intravenous administration is timely and an effective route of administration. Oral transmucosal dosing is a noninvasive approach to the rapid onset of analgesia. Fentanyl, incorporated in a hard matrix on a handle, is rapidly absorbed and has been shown to have an onset of pain relief similar to intravenous morphine, i.e. within 10 minutes. Titration of the rescue dose should be attempted in an individual way to identify the most appropriate dose, as no relationship between basal dose and rescue dose has been found in studies with transmucosal fentanyl (Mercadante et al. 2002).

Most patients receive morphine as the first drug for their pain conditions. The ratio of metabolites to the parent compound is less during parenteral administration than oral administration. In some situations, this difference in the production of metabolites could account for the occurrence of fewer adverse effects during parenteral morphine administration. Thus, ▶ switching from oral administration to a continuous parenteral administration, both subcutaneously or intravenously may reduce the metabolite-morphine relationship and decrease the toxicity due to accumulation of the metabolites. Adverse effects may also be reduced in intensity with the use of the spinal route, although the administration of local anesthetics with an opioid may provide additional analgesia, and permit the recapture of patients unresponsive to spinal morphine administered alone. Epidural clonidine in combination with morphine has demonstrated some benefit in neuropathic pain conditions (Mercadante 1999). Many simple procedures of regional anesthesia may be helpful in some selected cases.

As opioids have differential effects on selective subsets of opioid receptors in the central nervous system, and cross tolerance between opioids is incomplete, a shift from one opioid to another is a useful option when the side effect-analgesic relationship is inconvenient. This pharmacological approach is named opioid rotation or switching. To restore a more advantageous analgesia-toxicity relationship, sequential trials of different opioids have been suggested. The degree of cross-tolerance may change as opioid doses are escalated, and care must be taken in applying an equianalgesic dose table to patients on high doses of opioids (Bruera et al. 1996).

Finally, cancer pain is a complex experience, which involves personality, learning, and situational components. Although difficult to assess, psychological status plays an important role in the experience of cancer pain and may influence the need for opioid escalation. The degree of psychological distress has been reported as a major negative prognostic factor for opioid responsiveness. It is possible to attain better analgesia following the introduction of psychological interventions or psychotropic medication.

References

1. Bruera E, Schoeller T, Wenk R, MacEachern T, Marcellino S, Hanson J, Suarez-Almazor M (1995) A Prospective Multicenter Assessment of the Edmonton Staging System for Cancer Pain. J Pain Symptom Manage 10:348–355
2. Bruera E, Pereira J, Watanabe S, Belzile M, Kuehn N, Hanson J (1996) Opioid Rotation in Patients with Cancer Pain: A Retrospective Comparison of Dose Ratios Between Methadone, Hydromorphone, and Morphine. Cancer 78:852–857
3. Cherny N, Ripamonti C, Pereira J et al. (2001) Strategies to Manage the Adverse Effects of Oral Morphine: An Evidence-Based Report. J Clin Oncol 19:2542–2554
4. Collin E, Poulain P, Gauvain-Piquard A, Petit G, Pichard-Leandri E (1993) Is Disease Progression the Major Factor in Morphine "Tolerance" in Cancer Pain Treatment? Pain 55:319–326
5. Mao J, Price D, Mayer DJ (1995) Experimental Mononeuropathy Reduces the Antinociceptive Effects of Morphine: Implications for Common Intracellular Mechanisms Involved in Morphine Tolerance and Neuropathic Pain. Pain 61:353–364
6. Mercadante S, Maddaloni S, Roccella S, Salvaggio L (1992) Predictive Factors in Advanced Cancer Pain Treated only by Analgesics. Pain 50:51–155
7. Mercadante S (1999) Problems of Long-Term Spinal Opioid Treatment in Advanced Cancer Patients. Pain 79:1–13
8. Mercadante S, Portenoy RK (2001) Opioid poorly responsive cancer pain. Part 3. Clinical strategies to improve opioid responsiveness. J Pain Symptom Manage 21:338–354
9. Mercadante S, Radbruch L, Caraceni A et al. (2002) Episodic (Breakthrough) Pain. Cancer 94:832–839
10. Portenoy RK, Hagen NA (1990) Breakthrough Pain: Definition, Prevalence, and Characteristics. Pain 41:273–281
11. Portenoy RK, Foley KM, Inturrisi CE (1990) The Nature of Opioid Responsiveness and its Implications for Neuropathic Pain: New Hypotheses Derived from Studies of Opioid Infusions. Pain 43:273–286
12. Portenoy RK (1995) Tolerance to Opioid Analgesics: Clinical Aspects. Cancer Surveys 21:49–65
13. Portenoy RK (1996) Adjuvant Analgesic Agents. Hematol Oncol Clin North Am 10:103–119

Opioid Rotation

CHARLES E. INTURRISI
Department of Pharmacology, Weill Medical College of Cornell University and The Pain and Palliative Care Service, Memorial Sloan-Kettering Cancer Center, New York, NY, USA
ceintur@med.cornell.edu

Definition

▶ Opioid rotation refers to the substitution or switching from one opioid to another to achieve a more favorable therapeutic outcome.

Characteristics

The individualization of the dose of an opioid is essential for the appropriate and successful management of pain with these drugs (Inturrisi 2002). When gradual ▶ dose titration is limited by adverse effects, opioid rotation is one of the alternative therapeutic strategies that should be employed (Indelicato and Portenoy 2002). This approach is based on clinical observations that the interindividual response to opioids varies widely, and that the switch to an alternative opioid often results in an "opening in the therapeutic window" by reducing limiting adverse effects (Pereira et al. 2001; Indelicato and Portenoy 2002; Inturrisi 2002). Unfortunately, while there is general agreement about the utility of opioid rotation, the factors underlying interindividual variation cannot yet be readily identified in most patients, and therefore no consensus has been reached on the steps that should be used in converting the dose from one opioid to the alternative (Ripamonti et al. 1998; Mercadante 1999; Pereira et al. 2001; Indelicato and Portenoy 2002). However, a rational pharmacological approach begins with the recognition that opioid rotation requires knowledge of the ▶ relative potency relationship between the two opioids involved in the therapeutic situation. Relative potency refers to the ratio of doses of two drugs required to produce the same level of effect (▶ Equianalgesic Dose) (Houde et

O

al. 1965). As defined, it can only be obtained from dose-response data. The most reliable data is obtained from randomized, double blind, crossover studies, where the dose-response curves are generated and comparisons are made in the equianalgesic effect range to reduce errors associated with extrapolation (Houde et al. 1965). An equianalgesic dose table provides evidence based values for estimates of the relative potency of different opioids administered by commonly used routes of administration (for example, see Table 1). Importantly, the table simplifies comparisons, by relating the potency of each opioid to that of a 10 mg intramuscular dose of morphine. Nevertheless, an equianalgesic dose table does not provide all of the essential information needed for dose conversion in individual patients. The table (Table 1) presents the mean estimate of relative potency, but not the confidence limits which define the range of values where the estimate will fall 95 percent of the time. If the confidence limits are wide, as they are for the estimates used to construct the table (Houde et al. 1965), then any ratio number derived from the table and used as the sole means of calculating the equianalgesic dose for opioid rotation will be subject to this variation. The table (Table 1) was originally intended as the starting point for the estimation of the conversion dose ratio, with the consideration of indi-

vidual patient factors and clinical experience to guide the final dose selection. Some of the factors affecting opioid response, and therefore the equianalgesic dose, are intrinsic to the patient and some are intrinsic to the drug. For example, with repetitive dosing the opioid will accumulate until steady-state is reached. Opioids with a short ► elimination half-life will reach steady-state sooner than those with a longer elimination half-life (Inturrisi 2002). Even at an apparent steady-state, the analgesic responses vary widely among cancer patients. Estimates of the concentration of methadone required to produce 50% pain relief at steady-state vary nearly 10 fold (Inturrisi et al. 1990). For some opioids, including morphine, active metabolites can accumulate with repetitive dosing, and their contribution to the therapeutic and adverse effects of these opioids remains controversial (Penson et al. 2000; Skarke et al. 2003). Some opioids have nonopioid effects that can influence opioid responses. Methadone has NMDA receptor antagonist activity in animal studies that are not seen with morphine or hydromorphone. NMDA receptor antagonists prevent or reverse opioid tolerance, and are antihyperalgesic in models of injury-induced pain (Davis and Inturrisi 1999). Factors intrinsic to the patient that can influence ► opioid responsiveness include the mechanism and intensity of the patient's

Opioid Rotation, Table 1   Opioid Analgesics used for Severe Pain

Name	Equianalgesic im Dose [a]	Starting Oral Dose Range (mg) [a]	Comments	Precautions
morphine	10	30	Standard of comparison for opioid analgesics. Several sustained-release dosage forms	lower doses for aged patients; impaired ventilation; bronchial asthma; increased intracranial pressure; liver failure
hydromorphone	1.5	4–8	Slightly shorter acting. HP im dosage form for tolerant patients	like morphine
oxycodone	10	15–30	Immediate- release and sustained-release dosage forms.	like morphine
methadone	10	10	good oral potency; long plasma half-life	like morphine; may accumulate with repetitive dosing causing excessive sedation
levorphanol	2	2–4	like methadone	like methadone
fentanyl	0.1	–	Transdermal preparation. See package insert for equianalgesic dosing	Transdermal creates skin reservoir of drug-12–hour delay in onset and offset. Fever increases absorption
meperidine	75	not recommended	slightly shorter acting; used orally for less severe pain	normeperidine (toxic metabolite) accumulates with repetitive dosing causing CNS excitation; not for patients with impaired renal function or receiving monoamine oxidase inhibitors

For these equianalgesic im doses (also see comments) the time of peak analgesia in nontolerant patients ranges from one-half to one hour and the duration from four to six hours. The peak analgesic effect is delayed and the duration prolonged after oral administration.
[a]These doses are recommended starting doses from which the optimal dose for each patient is determined by titration and the maximal dose limited by adverse effects. For single IV bolus doses use half the im dose.
Im, intramuscular; po, oral
Adapted from, Table 1, Inturrisi, C.E., Clin. J. Pain, 18 (2002) S3–S13

pain. It is generally recognized that pain generated by injury to the nervous system, i.e. neuropathic pain, is often less responsive to opioids (Portenoy et al. 1990). Advanced age and decreased renal function can increase opioid responsiveness, while the development of opioid tolerance decreases the response to opioids (Inturrisi 2002). Current information is not sufficient to assure us that any one of these factors equally affect the response to each opioid in the table, and therefore can be ignored while calculating a ratio. Thus, it is generally accepted that tolerance does not appear to develop at the same rate to all opioids (Pasternak 2001). Indeed, this concept of ▶ incomplete cross tolerance among opioids provides one of the rationales for opioid rotation, but also needs to be accounted for in the calculation of the rotation dose. Many of the pharmacokinetic and pharmacodymamic factors outlined above can be expected to make a significant contribution to the response seen after multiple dosing with the alternate drug rather than after a single dose. A systemic review of estimates of the ▶ equianalgesic dose ratios reported in studies that utilized chronic opioid administration was conducted by Pereira et al. (2001). This review identified many of the issues discussed above, and also noted that the equianalgesic dose ratio may change according to the direction of the opioid switch. This complication is neither well appreciated nor has it been systematically evaluated.

Given these caveats, two principles that clearly emerge are that the rotation dose should be some fraction of the equianalgesic dose calculated from Table 1, and that some form of ▶ dose titration is required to provide a margin of safety (Ripamonti et al. 1998; Mercadante 1999; Pereira et al. 2001; Indelicato and Portenoy 2002). The overarching consideration in selecting a dosing schedule for opioid rotation is first to limit the risk of overdose as one opioid is discontinued and the substitute is introduced. The dose of the new opioid is calculated from the equianalgesic dose table (Table 1). This estimated dose is then reduced by 25 to 50% for opioids other than methadone (Indelicato and Portenoy 2002; Inturrisi 2002). For methadone, the estimated dose is reduced by 75 to 90% (Indelicato and Portenoy 2002). This estimated dose may also be adjusted based on the medical condition of the patient and the severity of the pain (Indelicato and Portenoy 2002). Ripamonti (Ripamonti et al. 1998) observed that in cancer patients the estimated equianalgesic dose ratio of morphine to methadone increased as a function of the prior morphine dose, so that no single dose ratio was appropriate for both opioid-naïve patients and patients who were receiving short or longer duration morphine therapy at the time they were switched to methadone. The data indicate that those patients who were receiving the highest doses of morphine were relatively more sensitive to the analgesic effects of methadone than predicted by the dose ratio derived from the table.

Therefore, patients with prior morphine experience require a greater reduction in the estimated methadone dose than relatively morphine-naïve patients. It is not known whether this variability in the estimated dose ratio between morphine and methadone is unidirectional, or if it should also be considered when switching from methadone to morphine. Recognition of the complexity of estimating the equianalgesic dose has led several investigators to conduct both prospective and retrospective studies aimed at better defining the equianalgesic dose ratios. Thus, from retrospective studies in palliative care patients, the ratio of morphine to hydromorphone was estimated to be approximately 5 to 1 (Pereira et al. 2001). However, this ratio (morphine to hydromorphone) was only approximately 3.5 to 1 when patients were shifted from hydromorphone to morphine (Pereira et al. 2001) This led to the suggestion that the values in Table 1 should be modified to reflect these estimates (Pereira et al. 2001). This change in the relative potency estimates could decrease or eliminate the need to reduce the dose calculated from the table in the manner described above. Whether this provides a safer and more convenient approach remains to be verified. Nevertheless, anyone planning to use opioid rotation should carefully consider these approaches (Ripamonti et al. 1998; Mercadante 1999; Pereira et al. 2001).

The ▶ dosing regimen to be employed should also reflect the understanding that the estimated dose is just that, a starting dose from which the optimal dose for that patient will be achieved by careful dose titration up or down. Alternatively, the dose can be fixed and the ▶ dosing interval adjusted to optimize the response. Usually some combination of these two approaches provides the necessary flexibility. Where both opioids have relatively short ▶ elimination half lives (e.g. morphine and hydromorphone), the final estimated dose of the new opioid can be substituted for current opioid, provision made for a rescue dose (usually 5 to 15% of the total daily dose) and titration with the new opioid begun (Indelicato and Portenoy 2002). Often the new opioid is administered on a fixed interval schedule as was the previous opioid (Indelicato and Portenoy 2002). An important exception to this approach are the opioids with relatively long elimination half lives (see Inturrisi 2002). The most important of these is methadone, whose half-life is much longer than that of morphine and subject to significant interindividual variation (Inturrisi 2002). Early studies employed a patient-controlled dosage regimen of oral methadone, which fixed the dose of methadone but allowed the dosing interval to be determined by the duration of the patient's pain relief after methadone (Sawe et al. 1981). This "▶ as needed dosage regimen during the titration phase of rotation to methadone is still advocated" (Foley and Houde 1998). More recent versions of the fixed dose with an "as needed" interval approach for methadone rotation have been described (Morley et al. 1993; Mercadante 1999).

O

Others have proposed that the switch from morphine to methadone be more gradual, over 3 to 4 days, and that a portion of the morphine dose (1/3) be substituted with methadone each day (Bruera et al. 1995; Ripamonti et al. 1998). These approaches also incorporate our current understanding of the need to further reduce the dose of methadone from the estimate obtained using the unmodified table (Table 1) (Morley et al. 1993; Bruera et al. 1995; Mercadante 1999) and they take into account the complex relationship discussed above between prior morphine experience and the response to methadone (Ripamonti et al. 1998).

This discussion has focused on the rotation of opioids by the oral route of administration because most of the studies have employed this route.

However, some data are available on opioid rotation that involves the transdermal and the parenteral routes (Mercadante 1999; Pereira et al. 2001; Indelicato and Portenoy 2002).

Given the current limitations in our knowledge of dose conversion strategies, additional controlled studies of opioid rotation are essential so that more specific guidelines for opioid rotation can be developed, and this useful method of optimizing pain relief can be both improved and simplified.

References

1. Bruera E, Watanabe S, Fainsinger RL, Spachynski K, Suarez-Almazor M, Inturrisi C (1995) Custom-Made Capsules and Suppositories of Methadone for Patients on High-Dose Opioids for Cancer Pain. Pain 62: 141–146
2. Davis AM, Inturrisi CE (1999) d-Methadone Blocks Morphine Tolerance and N-methyl-D-aspartate-induced Hyperalgesia. J Pharmacol Exp Ther 289: 1048–1053
3. Foley KM, Houde RW (1998) Methadone in Cancer Pain Management: Individualize Dose and Titrate to Effect. J Clin Oncol 16: 3213–3215
4. Houde RW, Wallenstein SL, Beaver WT (1965) Clinical Measurement of Pain. In: deStevens G (ed) Analgesics. Academic Press, Inc., New York, pp 75–122
5. Indelicato RA, Portenoy RK (2002) Opioid Rotation in the Management of Refractory Cancer Pain. J Clin Oncol 20: 348–352
6. Inturrisi CE (2002) Clinical Pharmacology of Opioids for Pain. Clin J Pain 18: S3–S13
7. Inturrisi CE, Portenoy RK, Max MB, Colburn WA, Foley KM (1990) Pharmacokinetic-Pharmacodynamic Relationships of Methadone Infusions in Patients with Cancer Pain. Clin Pharmacol Ther 47: 565–577
8. Mercadante S (1999) Opioid Rotation for Cancer Pain: Rationale and Clinical Aspects. Cancer 86: 1856–1866
9. Morley JS, Watt JW, Wells JC, Miles JB, Finnegan MJ, Leng G (1993) Methadone in Pain Uncontrolled by Morphine. Lancet 342: 1243
10. Pasternak GW (2001) Incomplete Cross Tolerance and Multiple mu Opioid Peptide Receptors. Trends Pharmacol Sci 22: 67–70
11. Penson RT, Joel SP, Bakhshi K, Clark SJ, Langford RM, Slevin ML (2000) Randomized Placebo-Controlled Trial of the Activity of the Morphine Glucuronides. Clin Pharmacol Ther 68: 667–676
12. Pereira J, Lawlor P, Vigano A, Dorgan M, Bruera E (2001) Equianalgesic Dose Ratios for Opioids. A Critical Review and Proposals for Long-Term Dosing. J Pain Symptom Manage 22: 672–687
13. Portenoy RK, Foley KM, Inturrisi CE (1990) The Nature of Opioid Responsiveness and its Implications for Neuropathic Pain: New Hypotheses Derived from Studies of Opioid Infusions. Pain 43: 273–286
14. Ripamonti C, Groff L, Brunelli C, Polastri D, Stavrakis A, De Conno F (1998) Switching from Morphine to Oral Methadone in Treating Cancer Pain: What is the Equianalgesic Dose Ratio? J Clin Oncol 16: 3216–3221
15. Sawe J, Hansen J, Ginman C, Hartvig P, Jakobsson PA, Nilsson MI, Rane A, Anggard E (1981) Patient-Controlled Dose Regimen of Methadone for Chronic Cancer Pain. Br Med J (Clin Res Ed) 282: 771–773
16. Skarke C, Darimont J, Schmidt H, Geisslinger G, Lotsch J (2003) Analgesic Effects of Morphine and Morphine-6-glucuronide in a Transcutaneous Electrical Pain Model in Healthy Volunteers. Clin Pharmacol Ther 73: 107–121

Opioid Rotation in Cancer Pain Management

ROSE-ANNE INDELICATO, RUSSELL K. PORTENOY
Department of Pain and Palliative Care, Beth Israel Medical Center, New York, NY, USA
rportenoy@chpnet.org

Definition

Converting from one opioid to an alternative opioid with the goal of achieving a more favorable balance between analgesia and side effects.

Characteristics

Chronic opioid therapy remains the cornerstone of treatment for moderate to severe cancer pain. Optimization of therapy relies on individualization of opioid dosing. This process involves gradual dose titration until adequate analgesia or the development of unmanageable side effects has been reached. ▶ Opioid responsiveness refers to the likelihood that a favorable balance between pain relief and side effects can be achieved during dose titration (Portenoy 2000). Poor responsiveness can be due to a number of factors, including co-morbid medical conditions that predispose to toxicity, pain pathophysiology associated with limited analgesic response, and pharmacological effects such as active metabolite accumulation associated with dehydration or renal insufficiency (Portenoy 1999; Mercadante and Portenoy 2001a; Mercadante and Portenoy 2001b).

The management of a patient who experiences a poor response to an opioid drug begins with a comprehensive pain assessment, including physical examination. Based on this assessment, the clinician may implement one of the following strategies (Indelicato and Portenoy 2002):

- More aggressive therapy for side effects.
- Administration of a co-analgesic (non-opioid or ▶ adjuvant analgesic) with the goal of reducing the systemic opioid requirement.
- Intraspinal therapy to reduce the systemic opioid requirement.

- Nonpharmacological interventions, such as transcutaneous nerve stimulation (TENS), neural blockade, cognitive approaches, or complementary therapies to reduce systemic opioid requirement.
- Opioid rotation to a different opioid with the hope of a more favorable balance between analgesia and side effects.

Opioid rotation is based on the variability of response to different opioids. As a result of this variation, a switch to an alternative drug may produce a better balance between analgesia and side effects (Galer et al. 1992, Cherny et al. 1995; Bruera et al. 1996a).

To reduce the risk of overdosing or underdosing as one opioid is discontinued and another is started, the clinician must have a working knowledge of the ▶ equianalgesic dose table. This dosing table provides evidence-based values for the relative potencies among different opioid drugs and routes of administration. These values were established from well-controlled single-dose assays conducted in cancer populations with limited exposure to opioid analgesics (Houde et al. 1966). The standard to which all relative potencies are compared is defined as morphine 10 mg parenterally. The equianalgesic table offers a broad guide for dose selection when switching from one opioid to another. The clinician must first calculate the total daily dosage of the current opioid, including the fixed schedule dosing and the supplemental doses taken as needed for breakthrough pain.

In many cases, the calculated dose of the new opioid must be reduced to minimize the risk of overdosage (Derby et al. 1998, Anderson et al. 2001). The usual starting point for dose reduction from the calculated equianalgesic dose is 25–50%. The following guidelines should be followed when converting from one opioid analgesic to another (Indelicato and Portenoy 2002):

a) Calculate the equianalgesic dose of the new opioid based on the equianalgesic table.
b) If switching to any opioid other than methadone or fentanyl, decrease the equianalgesic dose by 25–50%.
c) If switching to methadone, reduce the dose by 75–90%.
d) If switching to transdermal fentanyl (Duragesic®), do not reduce the equianalgesic dose.
e) Consider further changes in the adjusted equianalgesic dose based on medical condition and pain:
    If the patient is elderly or has significant cardiopulmonary, hepatic or renal disease, consider further dose reduction.
    If the patient has severe pain, consider a lesser dosage reduction or forego any dose reduction.
f) Calculate a rescue dose as 5–15% of the total daily opioid dose and administer at an appropriate interval.
g) Reassess and titrate the new opioid as needed.

This reduction is justified by:

- The potential for incomplete cross-tolerance between opioid drugs (potentially leading to effects, including side effects that would be greater than expected when a switch to a new analgesic is implemented).
- The interindividual variability in the relative potencies among opioids (ratios listed on the equianalgesic table may be more or less than the ratio that would be found if a single dose study was done in the individual patient).
- The need for dosage adjustment for conditions that increase opioid risk (including advanced age and medical co-morbidities).
- The possible difference in relative potencies in single dose assays compared to repeated dose assays.

There are exceptions to the dosage reductions previously mentioned. The first is a conversion to a transdermal fentanyl system (TFS). When this formulation was developed, conversion guidelines were created that incorporated a safety factor, precluding the need for additional dose reduction in most patients.

The second exception occurs with a conversion to methadone. A larger dosage reduction in the calculated equianalgesic dose (75–90%) is supported by data that demonstrate a much higher potency than expected when switching to methadone from another pure mu agonist, such as morphine (Ripamonti et al. 1998; Bruera et al. 1996b; Shimoyama et al. 1997). These data suggest that the potency of methadone following a switch from another mu agonist is dependent on the dose of the prior drug (Bruera et al. 1996b; Shimoyama et al. 1997); a dose of 500 mg or more of morphine requires a larger dose reduction (90%) than a smaller dose. This greater-than-expected potency is thought to be related to the d-isomer which represents 50% of the commercially available racemic mixture in the United States. This isomer blocks the N-methyl-D-aspartate (NMDA) receptor, and in turn may produce analgesic effects and partially reverse opioid tolerance (Elliot et al. 1994; Hagen and Wasylenko 1999).

Conversion Example

Mr. J was a 64-year-old man with a history of prostate cancer and metastases to the thoracic spine. His back pain had been well controlled with modified-release oxycodone 80 mg every 12 h and oxycodone 5 mg, 1–2 tablets every 4 h as needed for breakthrough pain. He usually took 4 tablets per day. He developed an increase in the intensity of his back pain. Physical exam and MRI ruled out spinal cord compression. He had no other medical co-morbidities. His dosage of oxycodone was initially increased to 80 mg every 12 h and his oxycodone dose was increased to 4–5 tablets per dose, which he took twice daily. This change improved pain relief, but he developed sedation and dizziness. The plan was to switch to oral morphine.

O

1. Calculate the 24 h total of oxycodone:

   (modified-release oxycodone 80 mg × 2) + (oxycodone 20 mg × 2)

   160 mg + 40 mg = 200 mg of oxycodone/day

2. Convert to the oral morphine equivalent using the equianalgesic table:

   oxycodone 20 mg = morphine 30 mg

   oxycodone 200 mg = morphine 300 mg

3. Decrease the morphine dosage by 25%:

   morphine 300 mg × 25% = 75 mg

   morphine 300 mg–75 mg = 225 mg

4. Convert the 24 h total to a fixed schedule:

   morphine 225 mg/24 h = modified-release morphine 120 mg every 12 h. The dosage has been rounded up given the tablet dosage size available.

5. Calculate a rescue dose. The rescue dose may be calculated as a dose that is 5–15% of the total daily dose:

   morphine 240 mg/d × 5% = 12 mg; morphine 240 mg/d × 10% = 24 mg; and morphine 240 mg/d × 15% = 36 mg

   A rescue dose of 30 mg every 4 h as needed is reasonable.

References

1. Anderson R, Saiers JH, Abram S et al. (2001) Accuracy in Equianalgesic Dosing: Conversion Dilemmas. J Pain Symptom Manage 21:397–406
2. Bruera EB, Pereira J, Watanabe S et al. (1996a) Systemic Opioid Therapy for Chronic Cancer Pain: Practical Guidelines for Converting Drugs and Routes. Cancer 78:852–857
3. Bruera EB, Pereira J, Watanabe S et al. (1996b) Opioid Rotation in Patients with Cancer Pain. Cancer 78:852–857
4. Cherny NI, Chang V, Frager G et al. (1995) Opioid Pharmacotherapy in the Management of Cancer Pain: A Survey of Strategies used by Pain Physicians for the Selection of Analgesic Drugs and Routes of Administration. Cancer 76:1288–1293
5. Derby S, Chin J, Portenoy RK (1998) Systemic Opioid Therapy for Chronic Cancer Pain: Practical Guidelines for Converting Drugs and Routes of Administration. CNS Drugs 9:99–109
6. Elliot K, Hynanski A, Inturrisi CE (1994) Dextromethorphan Attenuates and Reverses Analgesic Tolerance to Morphine. Pain 59:361–368
7. Galer BS, Coyle N, Pasternak GW et al. (1992) Individual Variability in the Response to Different Opioids: Report of Five Cases. Pain 49:87–91
8. Hagen NA, Wasylenko E (1999) Methadone: Outpatient Titration and Monitoring Strategies in Cancer Patients. J Pain Symptom Manage 18:369–375
9. Houde RW, Wallenstein SL, Beaver WT (1966) Evaluation of Analgesics in Patients with Cancer Pain. In: Lasagna L (ed) International Encyclopedia of Pharmacology and Therapeutics. Pergamon Press, Oxford, pp 59–98
10. Indelicato RA, Portenoy, RK (2002) Opioid Rotation in the Management of Refractory Cancer Pain. J Clin Oncol 20:348–352
11. Mercadante S, Portenoy RK (2001a) Opioid Poorly Responsive Cancer Pain. Part 3: Clinical Strategies to Improve Opioid Responsiveness. J Pain Symptom Manage 21:338–354
12. Mercadante S, Portenoy RK (2001b) Opioid Poorly-Responsive Cancer Pain. Part 1: Clinical Considerations. J Pain Symptom Manage 21:144–150
13. Portenoy RK (2000) Contemporary Diagnosis and Management of Pain in Oncologic and AIDS Patients, 3rd edn. Handbooks in Health Care Company, Newtown, PA
14. Portenoy RK (1999) Managing Cancer Pain Poorly Responsive to Systemic Opioid Therapy. Oncology 13:25–29
15. Ripamonti C, Groff L, Brunelli C et al. (1998) Switching from Morphine to Oral Methadone in Treating Cancer Pain: What is the Equianalgesic Ratio? J Clin Oncol 16:3216–3221
16. Shimoyama N, Shimoyama M, Megumi S et al. (1997) D-Methadone is Antinociceptive in Rat Formalin Test. J Pharmacol Exp Ther 283:648–652

Opioid Switch

Definition

Clinical practice of changing from one opioid to another, s. also Opioid Rotation.
▶ Cancer Pain Management, Principles of Opioid Therapy, Drug Selection

Opioid Therapy in Cancer Pain Management, Route of Administration

LUKAS RADBRUCH
Department of Palliative Medicine, University of Aachen, Aachen, Germany
lradbruch@ukaachen.de

Synonyms

Application route; delivery route

Definition

Before they can effect their analgesic activity, opioids must be transferred to their sites of action, usually the opioid receptors in the dorsal horn of the spinal cord or brain. The route of administration is the method by which the opioid enters the body. By altering the pharmacokinetics of the opioid, the route also influences the effects (or pharmacodynamics). The course of analgesia is different for oral, subcutaneous or intrathecal application (Table 1). The side effect profile may be different for different application routes. Preference for a given application route in an individual patient may influence the choice of the opioid.

Characteristics

Oral Administration

The administration of opioids "by the mouth" is one of the major recommendations of the World Health Organization (1996). The oral route as the first-line approach has been confirmed by other cancer pain guidelines (Agency for Health Care Policy and Research, US Department of Health and Human Services 1994; Hanks et al. 2001). The approach is easy and comfortable and finds high acceptance with the patients. No technical

nurse) to suspect problematic drug-taking or a history of drug abuse should alert the patient's palliative care team, thus beginning the assessment and management process (Lundberg and Passik 1997), which includes use of empathic and truthful communication. This approach entails starting the assessment interview with broad questions about the role of drugs (e.g. nicotine, caffeine) in the patient's life, and gradually becoming more specific in focus to include illicit drugs. Third, the development of clear treatment goals is essential for the management of drug abuse. The distress of coping with a life-threatening illness and the availability of prescription drugs for symptom control can make complete abstinence an unrealistic goal (Passik and Portenoy 1998). Rather, a harm reduction approach should be employed. A written agreement between the team and patient helps to provide structure to the treatment plan, establishes clear expectations, and outlines the consequences of aberrant drug-taking, and the inclusion of spot urine toxicology screens and pill counts in the agreement can be useful in maximizing compliance. Fourth, the team should consider using longer acting drugs (e.g. transdermal fentanyl patch or modified-release opioids). The longer duration and slow onset may help reduce aberrant drug-taking behaviors when compared to the rapid onset and increased frequency of dosage associated with short-acting drugs. Fifth, the team should make plans to reassess frequently the adequacy of pain and symptom control. Finally, the team should involve family members and friends in the treatment to help bolster social support and functioning. Becoming familiar with the family may help the team identify family members who are themselves drug abusers, and who may potentially divert the patient's medications and contribute to the patient's non-compliance.

Managing addiction problems in patients with cancer is labor intensive and time-consuming. Clinicians must recognize that virtually any centrally acting drug, and any route of administration, can potentially be abused. The problem does not lie in the drugs themselves. The effective management of patients with pain who engage in aberrant drug-taking behavior necessitates a comprehensive approach, and provides a practical means to manage risk, treat pain effectively and assure patient safety.

References

1. Groerer J, Brodsky M (1992) The Incidence of Illicit Drug Use in the United States, 1962–1989. Brit J Addiction 87:1345
2. Lundberg JC, Passik SD (1997) Alcohol and Cancer: A Review for Psycho-Oncologists. Psycho-Oncology 6:253–266
3. Passik SD, Portenoy RK (1998) Substance Abuse Issues in Palliative Care. In: Berger AM, Portenoy RK, Weissman DE (eds) Principles and Practice of Supportive Oncology. Lippincott Raven Publishers, Philadelphia, pp 513–530
4. Portenoy RK (1994) Opioid Tolerance and Efficacy: Basic Research and Clinical Observations. In: Gebhardt G, Hammond D, Jensen T (eds) Proceedings of the VII World Congress on Pain.

Progress in pain research and management, vol 2. IASP Press, Seattle, p 595
5. Rinaldi RC, Steindler EM, Wilford BB et al. (1988) Clarification and Standardization of Substance Abuse Terminology. JAMA 259:555

Opioid Tolerance

▶ Opioids, Clinical Opioid Tolerance

Opioid Tolerance and Glutamate Homeostasis

▶ Glutamate Homeostasis and Opioid Tolerance

Opioid Tone

Definition

A hypothesis whereby endogenous opioid peptides are released in a tonic manner, in the absence of any evoking stimulus. The presumed effect of opioid tone would be to produce a constant state of analgesia, as the opioids bind to and activate opioid receptors. The sometimes observed hyperalgesic effect of the opioid antagonist, naloxone, has been attributed to opioid tone.

▶ Opioid Analgesia, Strain Differences

Opioids and Bladder Pain/Function

DAGMAR WESTERLING, KARL-ERIK ANDERSSON
Departments of Clinical Pharmacology, Anesthesiology and Intensive Care, Lund University Hospital, Lund, Sweden
Dagmar.westerling@skane.se,
karl-erik.andersson@klinfarm.lu.se

Definitions

Opioids are ligands (agonists and antagonists) at opioid receptors (κ, δ and μ, or OR 1–3). Opioid receptors are mainly located on primary afferents in the dorsal horn and in several supraspinal centres of importance for micturition control, such as the periaqueductal grey. There are also opioid receptors on primary afferents in peripheral tissues, including the bladder.

Bladder pain may be evoked from distension, inflammation and/or physical damage (surgery, bladder stone, tumour growth etc). Bladder pain is a type of ▶ Visceral Nociception and Pain. Opioid receptor agonists may be effective in the treatment of some types of bladder pain Bladder function comprises collection, storage and emission of urine. The bladder and urethra constitute a functional unit, which is under spinal and supraspinal nervous control.

Administration of analgesic doses of opioid agonists may cause pain relief but also urinary retention due to a dose dependent depression of micturition reflexes, by actions at local, spinal and/or supraspinal sites.

Characteristics

Bladder Function

Anatomy

The lower urinary tract consists of the ▶ urinary bladder and the urethra. The bladder can be divided into two main components: the bladder body, which is located above the ureteral orifices, and the base, consisting of the trigone, urethrovesical junction, deep detrusor and the anterior bladder wall (Fig. 1). The bladder is a hollow smooth muscle organ, lined by a mucous membrane, and covered on its outer aspect partly by peritoneal serosa and partly by fascia. Its muscular wall is formed of smooth muscle cells, which comprise the detrusor muscle. The detrusor is structurally and functionally different from e.g. trigonal and urethral smooth muscle. The urethra contains both smooth and striated muscles, the latter forming the external urethral sphincter (rhabdosphincter).

Innervation of the Urinary Bladder

The urinary bladder receives sympathetic, parasympathetic, sensory and somatic-motor innervation via the hypogastric, the pelvic and the pudendal nerves (Morrison et al. 2002) (Fig. 2) The smooth muscle layers of the bladder wall receive autonomic (mainly sympathetic but also parasympathetic fibres) and afferent innervation. The striated muscle of the external sphincter is under voluntary somato-motor control. There is a considerable overlap in the source of the innervation. Primary afferent nerves from the bladder have their cell bodies in

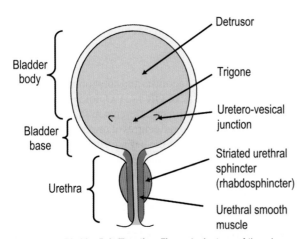

Opioids and Bladder Pain/Function, Figure 1 Anatomy of the urinary bladder. The bladder can be divided into two main components: the bladder body, which is located above the ureteral orifices, and the base, consisting of the trigone, urethrovesical junction, and the detrusor.

the dorsal root ganglia of the thoracolumbar and sacral spinal cord. From the dorsal root ganglia, sensory nerve cell bodies project both to the bladder, where information is received, and to the spinal cord, where the efferent pathways originate, and where the ▶ primary afferents of the urinary bladder connect to the spinothalamic tracts.

The primary afferents are myelineated (Aδ) and thin unmyelineated (C) fibres, with nerve endings in the lamina propria and in the smooth muscle layers of the bladder and urethra. Retrograde tracing studies have shown that most of the sensory innervation of the bladder and urethra originates in the thoracolumbar region and travels via the pelvic nerve. In addition, some afferents originating in ganglia at the thoracolumbar level of the sympathetic outflow project via the hypogastric nerve. The sensory nerves of the striated muscle in the rhabdosphincter travel in the pudendal nerve to the sacral region of the spinal cord. Sacral sensory nerve terminals are uniformly distributed to all areas of the detrusor and urethra, whereas lumbar sensory nerve endings are most frequent in the trigone, and scarce in the bladder body. In the urinary bladder of both humans and animals, sensory nerves have been identified suburothelially as well as in the detrusor muscle. Suburothelially, they form a nerve plexus, which lies immediately beneath the epithelial lining. Some terminals may even be located within the basal parts of the urothelium. This suburothelial plexus is relatively sparse in the dome of the bladder, but becomes progressively denser near the bladder neck, and it is particularly prominent in the trigone.

The hypogastric and pelvic pathways are implicated, not only in the sensations associated with normal bladder filling, but also with bladder pain. The pelvic and pudendal pathways are also concerned with the sensation that micturition is imminent, and with thermal sensations from the urethra. The incoming information controls the activity in the parasympathetic, sympathetic and somatic efferent nerves to the lower urinary tract. Under normal conditions there is little ongoing activity in the primary afferent nerves corresponding to little or no conscious sensations from the empty and slowly filling urinary bladder.

Physiology, Initiation of Micturition

Bladder pressure increases very modestly during normal collection and storage of urine. When bladder pressure reaches an individual level of around 25–35 cm H_2O, there is an urge to void. Under normal conditions this is a non-painful sensation. The smooth muscle of the detrusor contracts and urine is passed if the bladder neck, internal and external sphincters are relaxed at the same time. All of this requires a complex combination of nervous stimulation and inhibition (Fig. 3)

Myogenic activity, distension of the detrusor, and signals from the urothelium may initiate voiding (Ander-

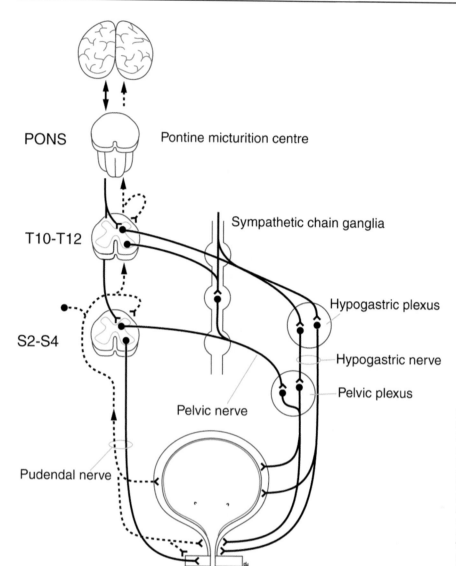

Opioids and Bladder Pain/Function, Figure 2 Innervation of the urinary bladder. The urinary bladder receives efferent sympathetic (hypogastric nerve), parasympathetic (pelvic nerve), and somatic-motor (pudendal nerve) innervation. Afferent (sensory) information is conveyed via the hypogastric, pelvic and the pudendal nerves. In the figure, only afferent pathways in the pudendal nerve have been indicated (dotted line).

sson 2002). The normal stimulus for initiating micturition is distension of the bladder, activating mechanoreceptors in the bladder wall. A high level of activity can be recorded in small myelinated afferent nerves (Aδ), which reach the lumbosacral spinal cord via the dorsal root ganglia. These Aδ afferents connect to a spinobulbospinal reflex consisting of an ascending limb from the lumbosacral spinal cord, an integration centre in the rostral brain stem, which is known as the pontine micturition centre (PMC), and a descending limb from the PMC back to the parasympathetic nucleus in the lumbosacral spinal cord. In the foetus and neonate, afferent information is conveyed by small unmyelinated (C-fibre) vesical afferents, which have a high mechanical threshold. Activity in these fibres is suppressed during development ("silent C-fibres"), but may be activated when the long reflex is damaged, as in spinal cord injuries, or by inflammation of the bladder mucosa, for example.

Extracellular adenosine triphosphate (ATP) has been found to mediate excitation of small-diameter sensory neurons via P2X$_3$ receptors, and it has been shown that bladder distension causes release of ATP from the urothelium. In turn, ATP can activate P2X$_3$ receptors on suburothelial afferent nerve terminals to evoke a neural discharge. However, it is not only ATP, but also a cascade of inhibitory and stimulatory transmitters/mediators that are most probably involved in the transduction mechanisms underlying the activation of afferent fibres during bladder filling. The urothelium may serve as a mechanosensor which, by producing NO, ATP and other mediators, can control the activity in afferent nerves, and thereby the initiation of the micturition reflex. The ► firing of suburothelial afferent nerves, and the threshold for bladder activation, may be modified by both inhibitory (e.g. NO) and stimulatory (e.g. ATP, tachykinins, prostanoids) mediators.

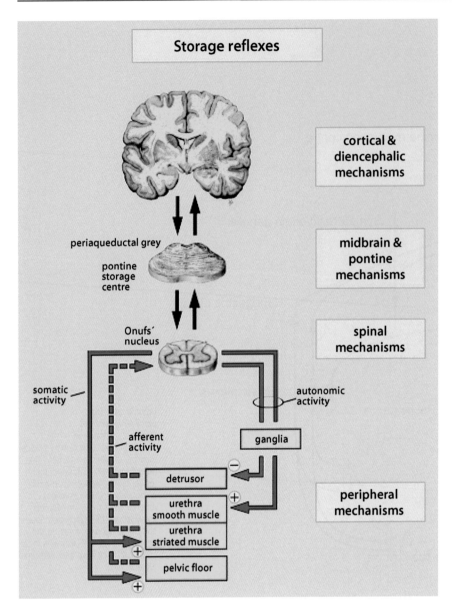

Storage reflexes

cortical & diencephalic mechanisms

midbrain & pontine mechanisms

spinal mechanisms

peripheral mechanisms

periaqueductal grey

pontine storage centre

Onufs' nucleus

somatic activity

autonomic activity

afferent activity

ganglia

detrusor

urethra smooth muscle

urethra striated muscle

pelvic floor

Opioids and Bladder Pain/Function, Figure 3a Normal function and physiology of the urinary bladder. During urine storage, there is continuous and increasing afferent activity (interrupted green line) from the bladder. There is no spinal parasympathetic outflow (red line -) that can contract the bladder. The sympathetic outflow to urethral smooth muscle, and the somatic outflow to urethral and pelvic floor striated muscles (continuous green lines +) keep the outflow region closed.

These mechanisms can be involved in the generation of bladder overactivity, causing urge, frequency and incontinence, but also in bladder pain.

Pathophysiology: Effect of Inflammation and Distension

If micturition is prevented and bladder pressure increases above 25–35 cm H_2O, the sensation of bladder fullness becomes more and more unpleasant, and most subjects describe this as painful (Ness et al. 1998). The pressure in the bladder, although painful, is not even near pressure levels that potentially might be harmful to the tissues. Pain arising from the bladder is usually reported from the lower abdomen above the symphysis, but may also be referred to the inner thigh, groin and knees.

Inflammation of the bladder may be caused by infections (acute bacterial or viral cystitis) or there may be no identifiable causing agent (e.g. ▶ interstitial cystitis). Exposure to chemicals (poisoning, cytostatics etc) and radiation may also lead to inflammation. Bladder inflammation causes distress, severe pain and micturition disturbances with an increase in voiding frequency and a decrease in micturition volume. The bladder lamina propria is invaded by inflammatory cells, and there is edema and extravasation of plasma proteins.

Inflammation of the bladder causes increased firing in the afferent nerve fibres "silent" under normal conditions, which leads to increased sensitivity in the dorsal horn. This is due to activation of several receptors/systems, including N-Methyl D-Aspartate (NMDA) receptors, nitric oxide (NO), Nerve Growth

A replication-incompetent recombinant HSV vector, deleted for the essential immediate early HSV gene ICP4, has also been demonstrated to provide a pain-relieving effect in rodent models. Despite being unable to replicate in epithelial cells, the PE-expressing replication-incompetent HSV vector injected subcutaneously establishes a "latent" state in DRG (Goss et al. 2001), and reduces spontaneous pain behavior during the delayed phase in the formalin test of inflammatory pain (10 minutes to 1 hour after injection of formalin) without affecting the acute pain score. This effect is reversed by intrathecal administration of naltrexone (Goss et al. 2001). The analgesic effect was limited to the injected limb; formalin testing of the limb contralateral to the injection reveals no analgesic effect on that side (unpublished observation).

The vector-mediated analgesic effect of the PE-expressing vector persists for several weeks before waning. Animals tested four weeks after vector inoculation have shown no significant reduction in pain related behavior during the delayed phase of the formalin test (Goss et al. 2001), but animals re-inoculated with the vector four weeks after the initial inoculation, and then tested with formalin injection at 5 weeks, show a substantial and significant return of the antinociceptive effect (Goss et al. 2001).

In the spinal nerve ligation model of neuropathic pain, subcutaneous inoculation of the PE-expressing HSV vector into the foot one week after spinal nerve ligation produces an antiallodynic effect that lasts for several weeks before waning (Hao et al. 2003). Reinoculation of the vector 6 weeks after the initial inoculation re-establishes the antiallodynic effect; the magnitude of the effect produced by the reinoculation is at least as great as that produced by the initial injection, and persists for a longer time after the reinoculation than the effect produced by the initial inoculation . Intraperitoneal naloxone reverses the antiallodynic effect.

The effect of the PE-expressing HSV vector-mediated antiallodynic effect in neuropathic pain is continuous throughout the day. Animals tested repeatedly at different times through the day show a similar elevation in threshold at all times tested (Hao et al. 2003). Intraperitoneal morphine produces a greater antiallodynic effect than the vector alone, but inoculation of the maximum dose of morphine produces an antiallodynic effect that persists for only 1 to 2 hours before waning. The effect of vector-mediated enkephalin (acting predominantly at δ opioid receptors) and morphine (acting predominantly at MOR) is additive. The ED_{50} of morphine was shifted from 1.8 μg/kg in animals with neuropathic pain from spinal nerve ligation, treated with PBS or inoculated with a control vector expressing *lac*Z, to 0.15 μg/kg in animals injected with the PE-expressing vector one week after spinal nerve ligation. Twice daily inoculation of morphine (10 mg/kg IP) in spinal nerve ligated animals, results in the development of tolerance by one week; be-

yond that time, continued twice-daily administration of morphine has no antiallodynic effect. Animals inoculated with the PE-expressing vector one week after spinal nerve ligation continue to demonstrate the antiallodynic effect of the vector, despite the induction of tolerance to morphine (Hao et al. 2003).

In a rodent model of pain resulting from cancer in bone, created by implantation of NTCT 2472 cells into the distal femur, subcutaneous inoculation of the PE-expressing replication incompetent HSV vector into the plantar surface of the foot, one week after tumor injection, produces a significant reduction in ambulatory pain score compared to control vector-inoculated tumor-bearing animals. This effect is reversed by intrathecal naltrexone (Goss et al. 2002).

The experimental evidence demonstrates that replication incompetent HSV vectors can be used to target delivery of genes with analgesic potential to neurons of the DRG, resulting in the local spinal release of analgesic substances to produce focal analgesic effects. The efficacy of this intervention in different models, which recapitulate essential features of the several subtypes of chronic pain, sets the stage for further development in two directions. The same approach may be used to express other molecules that might be anticipated to have significant analgesic effects at the spinal level, such as other inhibitory neurotransmitters, anti-inflammatory cytokines, or neurotrophic factors that produce analgesic effects in specific types of chronic pain . The second direction will be to determine whether HSV-mediated gene transfer will prove effective in the treatment of pain in patients. Replication-incompetent HSV vectors are appropriate for human use, and a proposal for a phase I human trial to examine the safety and tolerability of subcutaneous inoculation of an HSV vector deleted for the IE genes ICP4, ICP22, ICP27 and ICP41, and expressing human PE under the control of the HCMV IEp, was presented to the Recombinant Advisory Committee at the NIH in June 2002, and is now under review by the U.S. Food and Drug Administration.

References

1. Antunes Bras JM, Epstein AL, Bourgoin S, Hamon M, Cesselin F, Pohl M (1998) Herpes Simplex Virus 1–Mediated Transfer of Preproenkephalin A in Rat Dorsal Root Ganglia. J Neurochem 70:1299–1303
2. Braz J, Beaufour C, Coutaux A, Epstein AL, Cesselin F, Hamon M, Pohl M (2001) Therapeutic Efficacy in Experimental Polyarthritis of Viral-Driven Enkephalin Overproduction in Sensory Neurons. J Neurosci 21:7881–7888
3. DeLuca NA, McCarthy AM, Schaffer PA (1985) Isolation and Characterization of Deletion Mutants of Herpes Simplex Virus Type 1 in the Gene Encoding Immediate-Early Regulatory Protein ICP4. J Virol 56:558–570
4. Finegold AA, Mannes AJ, Iadarola MJ (1999) A Paracrine Paradigm for *In Vivo* Gene Therapy in the Central Nervous System: Treatment of Chronic Pain. Hum Gene Ther 10:1251–1257
5. Fink DJ, Glorioso JC (1997) Engineering Herpes Simplex Virus Vectors for Gene Transfer to Neurons. Nat Med 3:357–359
6. Goss JR, Harley CF, Mata M, O'Malley ME, Goins WF, Hu X-P, Glorioso JC, Fink DJ (2002) Herpes Vector-Mediated Expression

of Proenkephalin Reduces Pain-Related Behavior in a Model of Bone Cancer Pain. Ann Neurol 52:662–665

7. Goss JR, Mata M, Goins WF, Wu HH, Glorioso JC, Fink DJ (2001) Antinociceptive Effect of a Genomic Herpes Simplex Virus-Based Vector Expressing Human Proenkephalin in Rat Dorsal Root Ganglion. Gene Ther 8:551–556

8. Hao S, Mata M, Goins W, Glorioso JC, Fink DJ (2003) Transgene-Mediated Enkephalin Release Enhances the Effect of Morphine and Evades Tolerance to Produce a Sustained Antiallodynic Effect. Pain 102:135–142

9. Kim SH, Chung JM (1992) An Experimental Model for Peripheral Neuropathy Produced by Segmental Spinal Nerve Ligation in the Rat. Pain 50:355–363

10. Krisky DM, Wolfe D, Goins WF, Marconi PC, Ramakrishnan R, Mata M, Rouse RJ, Fink DJ, Glorioso JC (1998) Deletion of Multiple Immediate-Early Genes from Herpes Simplex Virus Reduces Cytotoxicity and Permits Long-Term Gene Expression in Neurons. Gene Ther 5:1593–1603

11. Sah DW, Ossipo MH, Porreca F (2003) Neurotrophic Factors as Novel Therapeutics for Neuropathic Pain. Nat Rev Drug Discov 2:460–472

12. Wilson SP, Yeomans DC, Bender MA, Lu Y, Goins WF, Glorioso JC (1999) Antihyperalgesic Effects of Infection with a Preproenkephalin-Encoding Herpes Virus. Proc Natl Acad Sci USA 96:3211–3216

13. Wu N, Watkins SC, Schaffer PA, DeLuca NA (1996) Prolonged Gene Expression and Cell Survival after Infection by a Herpes Simplex Virus Mutant Defective in the Immediate-Early Genes Encoding ICP4, ICP27 and ICP22. J Virol 70:6358–6368

14. Xu Y, Gu Y, Xu GY, Wu P, Li GW, Huang LY (2003) Adeno-Associated Viral Transfer of Opioid Receptor Gene to Primary Sensory Neurons: A Strategy to Increase Opioid Antinociception. Proc Natl Acad Sci USA 100:6204–6209

Opioids and Inflammatory Pain

C. ZÖLLNER, M. SCHÄFER
Clinic for Anesthesiology and Operative Intensive Medicine, Charité-University Clinical Center Berlin, Campus Benjamin Franklin, Berlin, Germany
zoellner@zop-admin.ukbf.fu-berlin.de,
mischaefer@zop-admin.ukbf.fu-berlin.de

Synonyms

Opioids and Opioid Receptor Function in Inflammation; Inflammatory Pain and Opioids

Definition

In addition to the traditional belief that opioids elicit antinociception via opioid receptors within the central nervous system, recent research has shown that they also elicit antinociception via opioid receptors located on peripheral nerve terminals of sensory neurons. Such antinociceptive effects in the periphery are particularly prominent under painful inflammatory conditions.

Characteristics

Peripheral Opioid Receptors and Inflammation

Pain can be relieved by systemic administration of opioids acting on specific opioid receptors (OR) within the central nervous system. However, substantial side-effects such as sedation, nausea, vomiting, respiratory

depression or respiratory arrest can occur following i.v. opioid administration. In animal experiments, it was shown that local application of μ-opioid receptor (MOR) agonists into inflamed tissue elicited a pronounced antinociceptive effect (Stein et al. 1988). These results suggest that MOR agonists have a peripheral site of action within inflamed tissue. All three opioid receptor types (μ, δ and κ) are present on peripheral sensory neurons and are functionally involved in analgesia. As already known from the central side of action, peripheral OR increase potassium currents and decrease calcium currents in the cell bodies of sensory neurons. These effects can diminish the neuronal firing of peripheral sensory neurons (Woolf and Salter 2000). In addition, opioids can activate inhibitory G-proteins ($G_{i/o}$) which lead to a decrease in the second messenger adenylate cyclase (cAMP) content. Saturation and competition experiments indicate that the pharmacological characteristics of these peripheral OR are very similar to those in the brain.

In primary sensory neurons, the neuronal cell body is located in the ► dorsal root ganglion (DRG) (Fig. 1). OR have been found on small-to-medium-diameter neuronal cell bodies within the DRG, and on central as well as peripheral nerve terminals of primary afferent neurons (Mousa et al. 2001). Peripheral analgesic effects of opioids are greatly enhanced within inflamed tissue. Following the induction of inflammation, MOR mRNA increases within the lumbar spinal cord (Maekawa et al. 1996). In addition, the ► axonal transport of MOR from DRG to the peripheral nerve terminals is increased (Hassan et al. 1993). This was demonstrated for various neuroreceptors, including MOR in peripheral nerves (Laduron and Castel 1990). This increase is reduced by ligation of the sciatic nerve, indicating that inflammation enhances the peripherally directed axonal transport of MOR (Hassan et al. 1993). In addition, the number of peripheral sensory nerve terminals is increased in inflamed tissue, a phenomenon known as sprouting (Stein 1995). It might be that inflammation can also disrupt the perineurium, which is a normally a rather impermeable barrier. This allows opioid agonists easier access to peripheral MOR. In conclusion, OR are present in the periphery and mediate potent analgesic effects after peripheral opioid application. An inflammatory process can result in a profound increase in the density of MOR in the DRG, an increase in the axonal transport of MOR to the periphery, and in the enhanced sprouting of MOR$^+$ peripheral sensory nerve terminals. This might explain why locally applied opioids are more effective within inflamed compared to non-inflamed tissue.

Inflammation and Exogenous Opioids

Quantification of MOR binding sites by ligand-binding experiments confirmed an increase in MOR within the DRG during inflammation. Together with immunohistochemistry experiments, it was shown that this increase

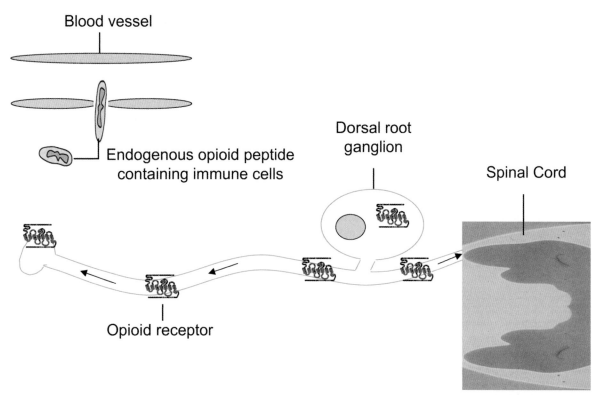

Opioids and Inflammatory Pain, Figure 1   Primary afferent sensory neuron with its cell body (DRG). Opioid receptors are synthesized in the cell body of the DRG and transported towards its central (right) and peripheral (left) terminals. Under inflammatory conditions, immune cells migrate into the tissue. Exogenous (e.g. stressful stimuli) or endogenous (e.g. corticotropin-releasing-hormone, Interleukin 1) stimuli release opioid peptides from monocytic cells or lymphocytes. The endogenous ligands for opioid receptors reduce the excitability of the primary afferent neuron.

in MOR binding sites of DRG was due to an increase in both the number of MOR⁺ neurons and the density of MOR⁺ staining per neuron (Mousa et al. 2001). The affinity of certain opioid agonists (e.g. ▶ DAMGO, ▶ Buprenorphine) to MOR remained unchanged during inflammation. However, in a ▶ G protein coupling assay, it was shown that the alteration in the density of MOR in the DRG and the periphery during inflammation could lead to an increase in the number of ▶ G proteins activated (Zöllner et al. 2003). Interestingly, these changes did not occur either at spinal, supraspinal (e.g. hypothalamus) or at contralateral DRG regions. Subsequent to the MOR up-regulation in DRG, more OR are axonally transported towards the peripheral nerve endings. With a certain delay, an up-regulation in MOR can also be seen within inflamed subcutaneous tissue. In addition, neuronal OR in the inflamed paw might undergo changes owing to the specific milieu of inflamed tissue (e.g. low pH), which could contribute to an increase in opioid efficacy (Selley et al. 1993). These adaptive changes underscore the important differences in MOR binding and signalling between normal and inflamed tissue.

Inflammation and Endogenous Opioid Peptides

The natural ligands for OR are opioid peptides. So far, five different peptides have been described in

the neuroendocrine and central nervous system: β-endorphin (βEND), enkephalin (ENK), dynorphin (DYN), ▶ endomorphine 1 and endomorphine 2. The endogenous opioid peptides are released from vesicles in a calcium dependent way. In inflammatory conditions, opioid peptide-containing immune cells migrate from the circulation to the inflamed site (Fig. 1). Upon certain exogenous stressful stimuli (e.g. cold water swim stress or postoperative pain), these cells can locally release opioid peptides that subsequently bind to OR on sensory neurons, where they can increase the nociceptive thresholds of peripheral sensory neurons in inflamed tissue. The analgesic effects of endogenous opioid peptides can be blocked by antibodies against opioid peptides and by immunosuppression, suggesting involvement of the immune system in inflammatory pain control (Machelska et al. 2002). It has been shown that opioid-containing cells are predominantly granulocytes during early and monocytes or macrophages during later stages of inflammation (Rittner et al. 2001). The endogenous opioid-mediated analgesia increases in parallel with the ▶ immune cell recruitment and the degree of inflammation. Other endogenous stimuli have been identified to trigger opioid secretion from immune cells. For instance, Corticotropin-releasing hormone (CRH) stimulates the release of opioid peptides from immune cells that subsequently activate OR on sensory nerve endings (Schäfer et al. 1997). These results indicate that the activation of the endogenous opioid production and release from immune cells might be a new approach to the development of peripherally acting analgesics.

Peripheral Opioids and Clinical Implications

Since the first demonstration of the analgesic efficacy of ▶ Intra-Articular Morphine (Stein et al. 1991), many clinical studies have confirmed that application of peripheral opioids in patients with acute and chronic arthritic pain resulted in significant pain reduction. These effects were shown to be dose-dependent and reversible by naloxone, indicating a specific effect at OR. In addition, the intraarticular application of naloxone after knee arthroscopy increased pain in the presence of endogenous opioid peptides within synovial tissue. These studies in humans have shown that a stressful stimulus (e.g. surgery) leads to a tonic release of endogenous opioids to reduce inflammatory pain by activating intraarticular OR (Oliveira et al. 1999). These findings suggest that opioids are released from immune cells in inflamed tissue and can activate peripheral OR to attenuate clinically important pain. It was shown that these endogenous opioids do not interfere with exogenous morphine and do not produce ▶ tolerance to exogenous morphine at peripheral OR (Stein et al. 1996). In addition, local opioid analgesia was shown in patients with dental surgery (Likar et al. 1998) and acute visceral pain (Rorarius et al. 1999). In summary, peripheral opioids significantly reduce pain in patients with acute and chronic inflammatory diseases. In comparison to central acting opioids, the peripheral administration of morphine did not show any side-effects like respiratory depression, sedation or nausea.

References

1. Hassan AH, Ableitner A, Stein C et al. (1993) Inflammation of the Rat Paw Enhances Axonal Transport of Opioid Receptors in the Sciatic Nerve and Increases their Density in the Inflamed Tissue. Neuroscience 55:185–195
2. Laduron PM, Castel MN (1990) Axonal Transport of Receptors. A Major Criterion for Presynaptic Localization. Ann NY Acad Sci 604:462–469
3. Likar R, Sittl R, Gragger K et al. (1998) Peripheral Morphine Analgesia in Dental Surgery. Pain 76:145–150
4. Machelska H, Mousa SA, Brack A et al. (2002) Opioid Control of Inflammatory Pain Regulated by Intercellular Adhesion Molecule-1. J Neurosci 22:5588–5596
5. Maekawa K, Minami M, Masuda T et al. (1996) Expression of mu- and kappa-, but not delta-, Opioid Receptor mRNA is Enhanced in the Spinal Dorsal Horn of the Arthritic Rats. Pain 64:365–371
6. Mousa SA, Zhang Q, Sitte N et al. (2001) Beta-Endorphin-Containing Memory Cells and μ-Opioid Receptors Undergo Transport to Peripheral Inflamed Tissue. J Neuroimmunol 115:778
7. Oliveira L, Paiva AC, Vriend G (1999) A Low Resolution Model for the Interaction of G Proteins with G Protein-Coupled Receptors. Protein Eng 12:1087–1095
8. Rittner H, Brack A, Machelska H et al. (2001) Opioid Peptide-Expressing Leukocytes: Identification, Recruitment, and Simultaneously Increasing Inhibition of Inflammatory Pain. Anesthesiology 95:505–508
9. Rorarius M, Suominen P, Baer G et al. (1999) Peripherally Administered Sufentanil Inhibits Pain Perception after Postpartum Tubal Ligation. Pain 79:83–88
10. Schäfer M, Mousa SA, Stein C (1997) Corticotropin-Releasing Factor in Antinociception and Inflammation. Eur J Pharmacol 323:1–10
11. Selley DE, Breivogel CS, Childers SR (1993) Modification of G Protein-Coupled Functions by Low-pH Pretreatment of Membranes from NG108-15 Cells: Increase in Opioid Agonist Efficacy by Decreased Inactivation of G Proteins. Mol Pharmacol 44:731–741
12. Stein C (1995) The Control of Pain in Peripheral Tissue by Opioids. N Engl J Med 332:1685–1690
13. Stein C, Comisel K, Haimerl E et al. (1991) Analgesic Effect of Intraarticular Morphine after Arthroscopic Knee Surgery. N Engl J Med 325:1123–1126
14. Stein C, Millan MJ, Shippenberg TS et al. (1988) Peripheral Effect of Fentanyl upon Nociception in Inflamed Tissue of the Rat. Neurosci Lett 84:225–228
15. Stein C, Pfluger M, Yassouridis A et al. (1996) No Tolerance to Peripheral Morphine Analgesia in Presence of Opioid Expression in Inflamed Synovia. J Clin Invest 98:793–799
16. Woolf CJ, Salter MW (2000) Neuronal Plasticity: Increasing the Gain in Pain. Science 288:1765–1769
17. Zöllner C, Shaqura M, Bopaiah CP et al. (2003) Painful Inflammation Induced Increase in μ-Opioid Receptor Binding and G-Protein Coupling in Primary Afferent Neurons. Mol Pharmacol 64:202–210

Opioids and Muscle Pain

KATHLEEN A. SLUKA
Physical Therapy and Rehabilitation Science Graduate Program, University of Iowa, Iowa City, IA, USA
kathleen-sluka@uiowa.edu

Synonyms

Musculoskeletal pain; Morphine and Muscle Pain

Definition

Muscle pain is pain that originates in muscle tissue and results in an increased sensitivity of the muscle to noxious stimuli. This pain can be a result of tissue injury, inflammation, exercise, or ischemia. Opioids are a class of compounds utilized to treat pain that activate opioid receptors. There are 3 types of opioid receptors, μ, δ, and κ, which are located peripherally and throughout the central nervous system.

Characteristics

Muscle pain is characterized as a deep aching pain, and is associated with increased pain to deep pressure applied over the muscle, as well as ▶ referred pain to areas remote from the site of injury. Clinically, ▶ fibromyalgia, ▶ myofascial pain, ▶ myositis and ▶ strain are common forms of pain associated with tissue injury and/or pain in the muscle.

Animal models of muscle pain include inflammatory, induced by injection of carrageenan into the muscle tissue, and non-inflammatory, induced by repeated injections of acid into the muscle (Kehl et al. 2000; Sluka et al. 2001). These models of muscle pain result in ▶ secondary hyperalgesia to mechanical (von Frey filaments) and heat stimuli. Further, ▶ primary hyperalgesia, as measured by a decrease in grip force, is present following carrageenan inflammation of the muscle (Kehl et al. 2000). The primary and secondary hyperalgesia associated with carrageenan muscle inflammation, is reversed by systemic administration of the opioid agonists morphine and levorphanol (Kehl et al. 2001; Radhakrishnan et al. 2003). In the non-inflammatory model of muscle pain, produced by repeated intramuscular acid injections, systemic morphine and intrathecal μ– and δ– opioid agonists reverse the secondary mechanical hyperalgesia (Sluka et al. 2002). Thus, these data show that animal models of muscle pain are responsive to μ- and δ- opioid activation at receptors that could be located peripherally, spinally or supraspinally.

In humans, muscle pain can be produced by infusion of hypertonic saline into the muscle, direct electrical stimulation of the muscle, or eccentric contraction of the muscle (▶ DOMS). The pain associated with intramuscular hypertonic saline infusion is reversed by epidural injection of the opioid agonist, fentanyl (50 or 100 μg) (Eichenberger et al. 2003), suggesting a role for spinal opioid receptors in pain reduction. The pain associated with DOMS is reduced by activation of peripheral opioid receptors with morphine–6–β–glucuronide (M6Gl; a major metabolite of morphine that does not cross blood brain barrier) (Tegeder et al. 2003), but not by systemic administration of several opioid agonists (Barlas et al. 2000), suggesting a role for peripheral opioid receptors. The pain from electrical stimulation of the muscle is inhibited by the systemic administration of the opioid agonist, remifentanil. Remifentanil produces a greater inhibition of pain induced by electrical stimulation of the muscle when compared to the inhibition of pain from electrical stimulation of the skin, suggesting that muscle pain is more sensitive to opioids than cutaneous pain (Curatolo et al. 2000). Thus, there is evidence that in human subjects muscle pain is responsive to opioid agonists, and these effects could be as a result of activation of receptors located peripherally, spinally or supraspinally.

The use of opioids in the treatment of clinical muscle pain, either acute or chronic, is not common. However, there are a few studies, done predominately with patients with fibromyalgia or acute muscle sprain, which suggest treatment of muscle pain with opioids is effective. Mild to moderate pain resulting from acute muscle strain of the low back or soft tissue injury is effectively treated with a mild opioid (Tylenol with codeine), reducing pain by approximately 50% (Brown et al. 1986; Muncie et al. 1986). However, when compared to treatment with an anti-inflammatory, there was an equivalent reduction and more side effects with the opioid (Brown et al. 1986). In patients with fibromyalgia, a more chronic pain condition, systemic administration of opioid agonists reduced spontaneous pain, as measured by a visual analogue scale (Biasi et al. 1998) and ▶ temporal summation (Price et al. 2002). Spinal administration (epidural) of opioid agonists also reduces spontaneous pain, tenderness, and lower limb fatigue (Bengtsson et al. 1989). Thus, clinically, the use of opioid treatment for muscle pain conditions is supported by results from basic science, experimental muscle pain models, and clinical studies using people with muscle sprain and fibromyalgia. However, a number of muscle pain conditions, such as myositis and myofascial pain, have not been investigated to date regarding the effectiveness of either short term or long-term opioid treatment.

References

1. Barlas P, Craig JA, Robinson J, Walsh DM, Baxter GD, Allen JM (2000) Managing Delayed-Onset Muscle Soreness: Lack of Effect of Selected Oral Systemic Analgesics. Arch Phys Med Rehabil 81:966–972
2. Bengtsson M, Bengtsson A, Jorfeldt L (1989) Diagnostic Epidural Opioid Blockade in Primary Fibromyalgia at Rest and During Exercise. Pain 39:171–180
3. Biasi G, Manca S, Manganelli S, Marcolongo R (1998) Tramadol in the Fibromyalgia Syndrome: A Controlled Clinical Trial versus Placebo. Int J Clin Pharmacol Res. 18:13–19
4. Brown FL Jr, Bodison S, Dixon J, Davis W, Nowoslawski J (1986) Comparison of Diflunisal and Acetaminophen with Codeine in the Treatment of Initial or Recurrent Acute Low Back Strain. Clin Ther 9 Suppl C 52–58
5. Curatolo M, Petersen-Felix S, Gerber A, Arendt-Nielsen L (2000) Remifentanil Inhibits Muscular more than Cutaneous Pain in Humans. Br J Anaesthesia 85:529–532
6. Eichenberger U, Giani C, Petersen-Felix S, Graven-Nielsen T, Arendt-Nielsen L, Curatolo M (2003) Lumbar Epidural Fentanyl: Segmental Spread and Effect on Temporal Summation and Muscle Pain. Br J Anaesthesia 90:467–473
7. Kehl LJ, Trempe TM, Hargreaves KM (2000) A New Animal Model for Assessing Mechanisms and Management of Muscle Hyperalgesia. Pain 85:333–343
8. Muncie HL Jr, King DE, DeForge B (1986) Treatment of Mild to Moderate Pain of Acute Soft Tissue Injury: Diflunisal vs. Acetaminophen with Codeine. J Fam Pract 23:125–127
9. Price DD, Staud R, Robinson ME, Mauderli AP, Cannon R, Vierck CJ (2002) Enhanced Temporal Summation of Second Pain and its Central Modulation in Fibromyalgia Patients. Pain. 99:49–59
10. Radhakrishnan R, Bement M, Skyba D, Kehl L, and Sluka K (2004) Models of muscle pain: Carrageenan model and acidic saline model. In: Enna SJ, Williams M, Ferkany J, Kenakin T, Porsolt R, and Sullivan J (eds) Current Protocols in Pharmacology. John Wiley & Sons, Hoboken, NJ, pp 5.35.1–5.35.28
11. Sluka KA, Kalra A, Moore SA (2001) Unilateral Intramuscular Injections of Acidic Saline Produce a Bilateral, Long-Lasting Hyperalgesia. Muscle Nerve 24:37–46
12. Sluka KA, Rohlwing JJ, Bussey RA, Eikenberry SA, Wilken JM (2002) Chronic Muscle Pain Induced by Repeated Acid Injection is Reversed by Spinally Administered μ and δ- but not κ, Opioid Receptor Agonists. J Pharmacol Exp Ther 302:1146–1150
13. Tegeder I, Meier S, Burian M, Schmidt H, Geisslinger G, Lotsch J (2003) Peripheral Opioid Analgesia in Experimental Human Pain Models. Brain 126:1092–1102

O

Opioids and Nucleus Gracilis

▶ Opioids in the Spinal Cord and Modulation of Ascending Pathways (N. gracilis)

Opioids and Opioid Receptor Function in Inflammation

▶ Opioids and Inflammatory Pain

Opioids and Reflexes

CLAIRE D. ADVOKAT
Department of Psychology, Louisiana State University,
Baton Rouge, LA, USA
cadvoka@lsu.edu

Synonyms

Spinal nociceptive tail flick withdrawal reflex; Hindlimb Flexor Reflex; Reflexes and Opioids

Definitions

The tail flick (TF) withdrawal reflex is a spinally mediated standard measure of pain sensitivity. In the most common procedure, a beam of high intensity light is focused on the tail, and the response time is automatically measured and defined as the interval between the onset of the thermal stimulus and the abrupt flick of the tail. Typically, several determinations are made, and the mean score is taken as the response latency. Increases in latency are interpreted to indicate an antinociceptive, i.e. analgesic, response. To reduce tissue damage, animals not responding after a predetermined cut-off score are assigned the maximum score.

The hindlimb flexor reflex is a spinally mediated withdrawal response of the hindlimb. Typically, flexor reflexes are elicited by electrical stimulation of the hindpaw. The reflex has 2 components; a short latency component that appears within 20 – 100 msec and is elicited by low threshold, non-nociceptive stimulation, and a longer latency component that appears at about 150 – 450 msec, in response to high threshold, nociceptive, C-fiber stimulation (>6.8 + 0.2 mA).

Characteristics

Modern views of opiate action in the central nervous system (CNS) originated with the classic experiments of Wikler and colleagues, who demonstrated that systemically- administered opiates could suppress polysynaptic spinal nociceptive responses, such as the hindlimb flexor reflex and the tail withdrawal reflex, after ▶ spinal transection (Wikler 1950; Advokat and Burton 1987). While this showed that opiates could act directly at the level of the spinal cord, the doses required in the spinal animal were larger than the doses needed in the intact animal, to produce the same effect. This observation led to the hypothesis that opiate analgesia was not only due to a direct action of the drug in the brain and the spinal cord, but was also mediated by an additional, indirect, effect of opiates in the brain, which increased descending supraspinal inhibition of spinal nociceptive reflexes (Advokat 1988).

This view was supported by studies of the analgesic effect of morphine, administered concomitantly into the ▶ intrathecal space and the third cerebral ventricle (Yeung and Rudy 1980) or the ▶ periaqueductal gray (Siuciak and Advokat 1989a) of rats. Concurrent morphine administration to these sites had a ▶ synergistic effect on spinal antinociception, measured with the tail flick or ▶ hot plate assay. The total amount of morphine concurrently administered to the brain and spinal cord, necessary to produce an ED_{50} in these studies, was substantially less than the amount required separately at each site to produce the same effect. Furthermore, the total amount administered concomitantly to both sites was similar to the total concentration at these sites, which produced the same effect after systemic morphine administration (Advokat 1988). This confirmed that morphine-induced analgesia depended on a combined action at both spinal and supraspinal sites, but it did not indicate the nature of that interaction.

Some insight into this process was provided by studies in which morphine was administered intrathecally to the spinal cord of acute (1 day) spinally transected rats (Siuciak and Advokat 1989b). In this situation, the antinociceptive effect on spinal reflexes was considerably more potent than in the intact animal (Fig. 1a). These data demonstrated that the analgesic effect of spinal morphine at the spinal level was increased by either spinal transection or by supraspinally-administered morphine. The interpretation of this phenomenon was that spinal transection and intracerebral morphine administration produced the same effect on spinal opiate analgesia, because they eliminated (spinal transection) or suppressed (supraspinal morphine administration) an inhibitory action exerted by descending pathways on opiate-induced spinal antinociception.

The fact that systemically administered morphine was *less* potent in the acute spinal, compared to the intact animal, appeared to conflict with this hypothesis. However, it was subsequently shown that the amount of morphine reaching the spinal cord after acute spinalization was less than the concentration obtained at the same doses in intact rats (Advokat and Gulati 1991), demonstrating that the apparent decrease in potency of systemically-administered morphine might have been due to a disruption in the distribution of the drug to the CNS.

Several implications follow from these findings. First, they suggest that mechanisms responsible for descending control of spinal reflexes, *per se,* may be different

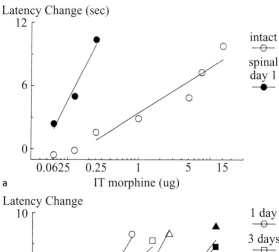

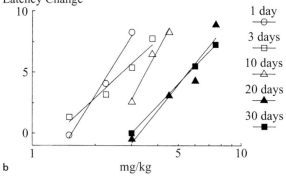

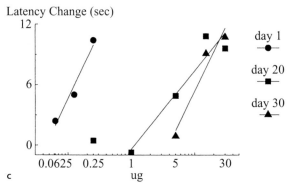

Opioids and Reflexes, Figure 1 (a) Dose-response functions to intrathecal (IT) morphine in Intact (open circles) and Acute Spinal rats (filled circles) on the tail flick test. The data show that, 24 hours after spinal transection, the antinociceptive effect of spinally administered morphine is profoundly increased (Siuciak and Advokat 1989b). (b) Dose-response functions to subcutaneous morphine in Intact rats and in rats spinally transected for either 3, 10, 20 or 30 days. The data show a gradual decline in the antinociceptive effect of systemic morphine within a month after spinal transection (Advokat and Burton 1987). (c) Dose-response functions to intrathecal morphine in rats that were spinally transected either 1 day, 20 or 30 days previously. The data show a gradual decline in the antinociceptive effect of intrathecal morphine within a month after spinal transection (Siuciak and Advokat 1989b).

from those which mediate descending control of the effects of opiates on those same reflexes. A corollary of this proposition is that supraspinal mechanisms may also mediate the development of tolerance to opiate inhibition of spinal reflexes. That is, repeated administration of morphine may not only produce tolerance locally, at supraspinal and spinal sites, chronic opi-

ate exposure may also reduce the inhibitory effect of morphine acting through descending pathways. This hypothesis would be consistent with the observation that tolerance to systemic morphine administration does not necessarily confer tolerance to the effect of morphine at the level of the spinal cord (Siuciak and Advokat 1989a; Siuciak and Advokat 1989b; Advokat et al. 1987; Advokat 1989). Second, there is no reason to assume that opiates would be unique in producing effects at the spinal cord by a combination of direct and indirect mechanisms. The spinal action of other pharmacological agents, or endogenous neurotransmitters that are involved in the control of spinal reflex function, may also be supraspinally modulated (Advokat 1993). Such influences may be relevant to mechanisms responsible for ▶ neuropathic pain states that can occur after trauma or damage to the central nervous system (Wolf and Advokat 1995). Third, descending modulation may not only be inhibitory, but may also facilitate the effect of drugs on spinal reflexes. Fourth, supraspinal modulation may not be limited to nociceptive reflexes, but may also be exerted on a variety of other spinal reflexes. Finally, the effects observed after an acute spinal transection might not be permanent, and could conceivably change over time as a result of neurophysiological adaptations, such as neuronal degeneration or receptor alterations, following spinal transection.

The possibility that the effects of an acute spinal transection might be modified over time, led to the development of the chronic spinal preparation as a model of ▶ spinal cord injury (SCI). SCI, produced by trauma to, or disease of, the nervous system, frequently leads to both ▶ spasticity and chronic pain in a majority of patients. Although the spinalized rat does not 'perceive' the nociceptive stimulus applied below the lesion, the reflex withdrawal of both the tail and the hindlimb is preserved, providing a model for evaluating reflex function in chronic spinal animals.

Initial studies of morphine-induced antinociception in this preparation, showed that during the first month following spinal transection, there was a gradual decrease in potency of the antinociceptive effect of morphine, whether administered systemically (Fig. 1b) (Advokat and Burton 1987) or directly onto the spinal cord (Fig. 1c) (Siuciak and Advokat 1989b). These results are consistent with other evidence from animal models and clinical observations, that the effect of opiate drugs is at least attenuated in neuropathic pain states produced by damage to the nervous system.

As with SCI in humans, a permanent and stable spastic response of the hindlimbs was also observed, developing in chronic spinal rats during the first few weeks following transection (Duke and Advokat 2000). This permitted the simultaneous assessment of the effect of antinociceptive and antispastic agents in the same, *in vivo*, unanesthetized animals. By concurrent electrophysiological measurement of the hindlimb flexion response, and recording of the nociceptive tail flick reflex in the same animals, the antispastic, as well as antinociceptive effect, of morphine was evaluated in this model (Advokat and Duke 1999). The results (Fig. 2) showed first, that, while the analgesic effect of systemic morphine was reduced in chronic spinal rats, the same doses were still effective against hindlimb spasticity. The hyperreactive hindlimb flexion reflex was decreased by 50% at doses that produced no change in the nociceptive response of the tail to a noxious thermal stimulus, in the same animals. This demonstrated a separation between the dose-response functions of the two behaviors, indicating that the antispastic action occurs at a dose that does not produce an analgesic effect.

Second, the data in Figure 2 also show that, at the highest dose (8 mg/kg), there was a significant reversal of the effect of morphine on both behaviors. While this dose was large enough to produce an antinociceptive effect, it also *increased* the flexion response to more than 200% of baseline. That is, morphine simultaneously decreased the reaction to a normally painful stimulus, and increased the spastic response to a nonpainful stimulus. This may be an example of the clinical phenomenon of "opioid-related" ▶ myoclonus that has been reported in cancer patients, which was "highly" associated with nerve dysfunction due to spinal cord lesions.

The observation that a single drug can modulate nociception and spasticity in the chronic spinal rat is not limited to morphine, but is relevant to the action of other pharmacological agents used in treating pain and

spasticity in SCI. Studies with the antispastic agent baclofen have also shown a separation between the antinociceptive action of low doses and an antispastic, muscle-relaxant, effect of higher doses, in chronic spinal rats (Advokat et al. 1999). The usefulness of the chronic spinal rat has also been demonstrated in recent studies of the ▶ Alpha(α) 2-Adrenergic Agonist, clonidine, on spinal reflex function (Advokat 2002).

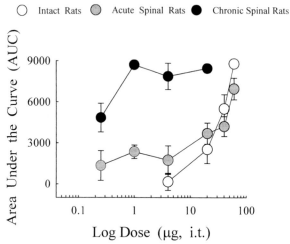

Opioids and Reflexes, Figure 3 Dose-response functions to intrathecal clonidine on the tail flick test, in Intact (open circles), Acute Spinal (shaded circles) and Chronic Spinal rats (solid circles). The data represent the mean ± S.E.M. of the area under the time-effect curve (at 30, 60 and 90 minutes) for separate groups of rats (n = 3 to 6) tested after administration of the indicated doses of clonidine. There was a significant dose-dependent effect of clonidine within each of the three experimental conditions. Clonidine-induced antinociception in Intact rats was the same as that in Acute Spinal rats, but was greatly increased in Chronic Spinal rats (Advokat 2002).

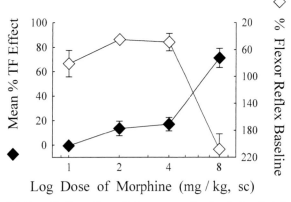

Opioids and Reflexes, Figure 2 Dose-response functions for the effect of subcutaneous morphine on the tail flick withdrawal reflex (left axis, filled symbols) and the flexor withdrawal reflex (right axis, open symbols) of chronic spinal rats. Separate groups of spinally transected rats were tested at each dose; both tests were administered to each animal. The data show a separation in the effect of morphine on these two measures. At low doses of 1 to 4 mg/kg, there is minimal antinociception and a maximum antispastic effect. At the highest, 8 mg/kg dose, antinociception is maximum while the antispastic action is reversed, and a profound hyperreactive response is elicited (Advokat and Duke 1999).

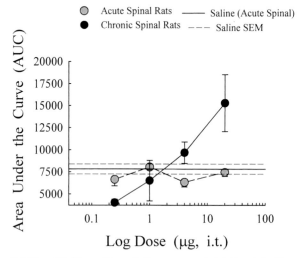

Opioids and Reflexes, Figure 4 Dose-response to intrathecal clonidine on the flexor reflex of Acute Spinal (shaded circles) and Chronic Spinal rats (solid circles). The data were obtained from the same animals whose tail flick test results are summarized in Fig. 3. There was no difference among the doses in Acute Spinal rats and no group differed from the saline condition. However, the same doses produced a significant dose-dependent effect in Chronic Spinal rats (Advokat 2002).

projections not only to the spinal dorsal horns, but also to the ventral and intermediolateral gray matter. Thus, opiate administration has direct sensory, motor and autonomic effects. For example, modulation of sympathetic outflow affects thermoregulation, which can influence nociceptive reactions to thermal stimulation (Tjolsen and Hole 1992). Parasympathetic modulation includes opiate actions within the vagal projection system of the brain stem (e.g. nucleus solitarius), and vagal activation can exert inhibitory influences on nociception (Ammons et al. 1983). Other brain stem effects involve modulation of defensive motor actions associated with nociception (e.g. fight or flight behaviors associated with rage or fear) (Braez 1994). Similarly, vocalizations related or unrelated to pain are suppressed via influences within the periaqueductal gray and associated structures (Cooper and Vierck 1986). In general, opiate influences on the brain stem are inhibitory for behavioral output and physiological reactions but excitation can result, depending on the dose and site of pharmacological application.

In addition to specific effects on nociceptive reactions, regulation of arousal by brain stem projection systems is susceptible to opiate modulation. Patterns of cortical EEG activity are modified by opiate actions within the brain stem and rostrally (Matejcek et al. 1988), and a generalized behavioral suppression results from therapeutic doses of morphine, particularly for primates (Vierck et al. 1984). Low doses of systemic morphine are sedative, promoting sleep and aiding recuperation from painful injuries. These effects on arousal can appear to represent analgesia by suppression of attention, particularly when high doses of morphine are administered.

Cerebral projection of nociception is susceptible to modulation via opiate agonist application to the thalamus and somatosensory cortex, and these effects are diverse (Wamsley 1983). For example, opiate receptor distribution in the medial thalamus is particularly high, and opiate receptors are present in cingulate, insular and prefrontal cortical regions. Opiate modulation at these sites is consistent with observations that systemic morphine reduces affective (emotional) and motivational responses to pain (Beecher 1957). Opiate actions within limbic projection systems (e.g. the septal area, amygdaloid nuclei and hypothalamus) are likely to be responsible for rewarding effects of opiates such as euphoria (Koob 1992). Also, nociceptive activation of the limbic system accesses brain stem systems of descending modulation, to influence autonomic and hormonal responses integral to diverse ► homeostatic adaptations to nociceptive input. Systemic morphine actions on limbic system processing include influences on the hypothalamic-pituitary-adrenal axis, and modulation of hypothalamic output of numerous hormonal releasing factors and of pituitary hormonal secretion (Wood and Iyengar 1988). Relevance of these actions to a comprehensive regulation of behavioral and physiological reactions to pain is indicated by demonstrations of extensive nociceptive projections to the limbic system. The multiple actions of opiate agonists make apparent some important considerations concerning experimental evaluation of systemic morphine's effects relevant's to control over clinical pain. Reflex tests are relatively insensitive and do not reveal numerous cerebral actions of morphine on pain sensations and reactions. Also, observation of responses to phasic input from myelinated nociceptors is not useful. Evaluation of responses to C nociceptor input appears to be necessary, and is especially informative if ► temporal summation (windup) of pain is produced. Attenuation of central sensitization produced by prolonged C nociceptor input is likely to be an important component of the clinical utility of systemic agonists (Price et al. 1985). Also, tests of responses to stimulation of inflamed tissue have revealed low-dose effects of systemic morphine on behavioral tests that are otherwise insensitive (Stein et al. 1989), indicating that peripheral actions constitute an important component of the effectiveness of systemic morphine for certain forms of clinical pain. In contrast, systemic morphine is relatively ineffective for control of chronic pain that can result from lesions within the central nervous system that interrupt nociceptive input to sites that contain opiate receptors (Arner and Meyerson 1988). Thus, morphine modulates nociceptive transmission to and within the central nervous system, but is less effective for attenuation of abnormal "spontaneous" activity that can result from deafferentation of pain transmission systems.

References

1. Ammons W, Blair R, Foremen R (1983) Vagal Afferent Inhibition of Primate Thoracic Spinothalamic Neurons. J Neurophysiol 50:926–940
2. Arner S, Meyerson BA (1988) Lack of Analgesic Effect of Opioids on Neuropathic and Idiopathic Forms of Pain. Pain 33:11–23
3. Beecher HK (1957) Measurement of Pain; Prototype for the Quantitative Study of Subjective Sensations. Pharmacoll Rev 9:59–209
4. Braez J (1994) Neuroanatomy and Neurotransmitter Regulation of Defensive Behaviors and Related Emotions in Mammals. Braz J Med Biol Res 27:811–829
5. Cooper BY, Vierck CJ Jr (1986) Vocalizations as Measures of Pain in Monkeys. Pain 26:393–408
6. Cooper BY, Vierck CJ Jr, Yeomans DC (1986) Selective Reduction of Second Pain Sensations by Systemic Morphine in Humans. Pain 24:93–116
7. Dickenson AH, Sullivan AF (1986) Electrophysiological Studies on the Effects of Intrathecal Morphine on Nociceptive Neurones in the Rat Dorsal Horn. Pain 24:211–222
8. Gebhart G (1982) Opiate and Opioid Peptide Effects on Brain Stem Neurons: Relevance to Nociception and Antinociceptive Mechanisms. Pain 12:93–140
9. Jurna I, Heinz G (1979) Differential Effects of Morphine and Opioid Analgesics on A and C Fibre-Evoked Activity in Ascending Axons of the Rat Spinal Cord. Brain Res 171:573–576
10. Koob G (1992) Drugs of Abuse: Anatomy, Pharmacology and Function of Reward Pathways. Trends Pharmacol Sci 13:177–184

11. Matejcek M, Pokorny R, Ferber G et al. (1988) Effect of Morphine on the Electroencephalogram and other Physiological and Behavioral Parameters. Neuropsychobiology 19:202–211
12. Price DD, Von der Gruen A, Miller J et al. (1985) A Psychophysical Analysis of Morphine Analgesia. Pain 22:261–269
13. Stein C, Millan MJ, Shippenberg TS et al. (1989) Peripheral Opioid Receptors Mediating Antinociception in Inflammation. Evidence for Involvement of *Mu*, *Delta* and *Kappa* Receptors. J Pharmacol Exp Therap 248:1269–1275
14. Tjolsen A, Hole K (1992) The Effect of Morphine on Core and Skin Temperature in Rats. Neuroreport 3:512–514
15. Vierck CJ, Acosta-Rua A, Nelligan R et al. (2002) Low Dose Systemic Morphine Attenuates Operant Escape but Facilitates Innate Reflex Responses to Thermal Stimulation. J Pain 3:309–319
16. Vierck CJ Jr, Cooper BY, Cohen RH et al. (1984) Effects of Systemic Morphine on Monkeys and Man: Generalized Suppression of Behavior and Preferential Inhibition of Pain Elicited by Unmyelinated Nociceptors. In: von Euler C, Franzen O, Lindblom U et al. (eds) Somatosensory Mechanisms. MacMillan Press, London, pp 309–323
17. Wamsley J (1983) Opioid Receptors: Autoradiography. Pharmacological Reviews 35:69–83
18. Wood PL, Iyengar S (1988) Central actions of Opiates and Opioid Peptides. In: Pasternak GW (ed) The Humana Press, pp 307–356
19. Woolfe G, MacDonald AD (1944) The Evaluation of the Analgesic Action of Pethidine Hydrochloride (Demorol). J Pharmacol ExpTher 80:300–307
20. Yeomans DC, Proudfit HK (1996) Nociceptive Responses to High and Low Rates of Noxious Cutaneous Heating are Mediated by Different Nociceptors in the Rat: electrophysiological. Pain 68:141–150
21. Yeomans DC, Cooper BY, Vierck CJ Jr (1995) Comparisons of Dose-Dependent Effects of Systemic Morphine on Flexion Reflex Components and Operant Avoidance Responses of Awake Non-Human Primates. Brain Res 670:297–302
22. Zieglgänsberger W, Bayerl H (1976) The Mechanism of Inhibition of Neuronal Activity by Opiates in the Spinal Cord of Cat. Brain Res 115:111–128

Opioids in Geriatric Application

PERRY G. FINE
Pain Management and Research Center, University of Utah, Salt Lake City, UT, USA
fine@aros.net

Definition

By convention, geriatric patients are those 65 years of age and older. This age group represents the fastest growing segment of the total population of developed nations. Physiologically, older patients differ significantly from those in younger age groups in a variety of ways. The physiologic changes of aging, along with acute and chronic pathologic conditions and altered drug disposition frequently lead to increased pain-producing problems, this is in addition to changing sensory perception and the ability to communicate or cope with distress, and these normal and pathologic changes influence drug disposition. The rate of aging is influenced by genetic and environmental factors, so the trajectory of changes is different from person to person. Neverthe-

less, with the passage of time, senescence is inevitable, and aging is marked by several common traits:
Rates of gene transcription, lipofuscin and extracellular matrix cross-linking, and protein oxidation are altered, among other biochemical and tissue changes.
Physiologic capacity diminishes.
Adaptive processes to physiologic stress (e.g. increases in cardiac output; thermo-regulation; GI transit rate) are blunted.
Susceptibility and vulnerability to diseases are increased.
There is an accelerating rise in mortality with advancing age after maturation occurs.
These factors must be taken into account when assessing older patients with significant pain. Decisions about goals of therapy, when and how to prescribe opioid ▶ analgesics, and what effects to anticipate will be strongly influenced by these circumstances. They are oftentimes considerably different than the types of concerns relevant to younger patients;

Characteristics

Pain Prevalence, Etiology and Features

Persistent and recurrent episodic pains are highly prevalent in older patients. About 5% of older Americans reportedly take prescription analgesics for most of a given year (Cooner and Amorosi 1997). Causes of pain in older patients are often from multiple etiologies. Most commonly, these include skeletal diseases such as osteoarthritis and degenerative spinal disorders, and ▶ neuropathic pain syndromes such as ▶ post-herpetic neuralgia and painful ▶ diabetic polyneuropathy. Also, pain-producing cardiovascular ailments and malignancies gain prevalence, adding to the overall burden of aging.
Surveys over the last several years have shown that serious pain is a frequent finding among both community dwelling and institutionalized older individuals, and it is largely under-treated in most settings except hospice, where comfort is a focus of care (Helme and Gibson 1999). Between 45–80% of nursing home residents are reported to have moderate to severe pain on a regular basis that is not adequately treated.
Although the adverse consequences of pain in older persons are not necessarily unique, they are oftentimes amplified, due to coexisting problems, including cognitive impairment, balance disturbances, deconditioning, sensory impairments, and other co-morbidities. As a result, the ill effects of pain, such as mood disorders (especially depression), social isolation, poor sleep, gait disturbance and inability to perform self-care and routine activities of daily living (ADLs) are compounded. The use of multiple medications for concurrent disease and symptom management creates an additional confound in the management of pain in geriatrics. Drug-drug and drug-disease interactions are, as a result, a far

more significant concern in this group of patients. The consequences of drug-related adverse effects, such as falls, confusion, or ▶ obstipation can have much graver consequences than in younger patients. Overall, however, as a pharmacological class, the risks associated with opioid analgesics are considerably less compared to other commonly prescribed drugs in older patients (Doucet et al. 1996).

Aging and Opioid Pharmacology

Consistent with current theories of aging, the great individual variability observed in older persons is more likely to be the result of "tightly controlled but individually different cell and tissue-specific patterns of gene expression", rather than age-specific genetic instability (Arking 2001). Each patient's history, environmental exposure, and genetic makeup contributes to a unique pattern of organ function (or dysfunction) and subjective response to therapy (Barja 1998). Evidence suggests that sensitivity to drugs that act in the central nervous system, best demonstrated in studies of opioid analgesics, increases with age (Rooke et al. 2002). Age has long been known to be an independent predictor of response to opioids (Belleville et al. 1971). In decile groupings, after the age of forty, there appears to be a linear age-related increase in responsiveness to fixed morphine doses with regard to pain intensity differences in post-operative patients. This correlates with changes in drug absorption, distribution, metabolism and clearance, all of which are influenced by body composition changes (e.g. muscle:fat), reduced serum protein levels, cardiac output and organ perfusion (Fine 2004). Notwithstanding the multiple pharmacokinetic (▶ pharmacokinetics) alterations that influence opioid blood levels over time, the cause of increased sensitivity to opioids appears to be mostly a function of reduced central nervous system resilience (Guay et al. 2002). In addition, it has been postulated that increased sensitivity to the effects of opioids, both therapeutic and toxic, are related to the high prevalence of subclinical malnutrition in community and institutional dwelling geriatric patients. In the few studies that have specifically evaluated pharmacodynamic (▶ pharmacodynamics) effects of analgesic drugs in older patients, the rate of drug delivery, rather than the absolute dose of drug over time, influences both analgesia and adverse effects, including the most feared risk of life-threatening respiratory depression (Aburun et al. 2002). Opioids have been shown to affect immune system responses and neuro-endocrine function. A systematic review of the literature did not reveal any conclusive age-specific, or age-related, effects of pain or opioids on human immune functioning (Page 2003). However, this is an area that requires further study, since patients are being treated for more protracted periods of time with opioids, and overall life expectancy is increasing. The potential for chronic opioid therapy to

reduce testosterone levels in males requires ongoing assessment, in addition to a risk-benefit analysis, in terms of pain treatment, hormone depletion and hormone replacement.

Indications and Guidelines

Opioid analgesics are most effectively used to achieve positive therapeutic goals when they are incorporated into a comprehensive non-pharmacologic, pharmacologic, behavioral and functional improvement (rehabilitative) pain management plan of care (Fine 2004) (see also ▶ non-pharmacologic pain management). The American Geriatrics Society has recently produced a clinical guideline based upon a systematic review of the literature, which outlines principles for analgesic use in older patients (Fine 2001). Key points with regard to opioids include:

- All older patients with functional impairment or diminished quality of life as a result of persistent pain are candidates for pharmacologic therapy.
- There is no role for ▶ placebos in the management of pain. Their use is unethical.
- The least toxic means of achieving pain relief should be used. When systemic medications are indicated, non-invasive routes should be considered first.
- Opioid analgesic drugs may help relieve moderate to severe pain, especially ▶ nociceptive pain. (As an update, though, it should be noted that recent studies have demonstrated the efficacy of opioids in the management of various neuropathic pain conditions (Rowbotham et al. 2003).
- Opioids for episodic (non-continuous) pain should be prescribed as needed, rather than around the clock.
- Long-acting or sustained-release analgesic preparations should be used for continuous pain;
- ▶ Breakthrough pain should be identified and treated by the use of fast-onset, short-acting preparations.
- Constipation and opioid-related gastrointestinal symptoms should be prevented. Assessment of bowel function should be an initial and ongoing process during every follow-up visit for patients receiving analgesics.
- Non-opioid pain-modulating medications may be appropriate for some patients with neuropathic pain and some other chronic pain conditions.
- Patients taking analgesic medications should be monitored closely:
- Patients should be reevaluated frequently for drug efficacy and side effects during initiation, titration, or any change in dose of analgesic medications.
- Patients should be reevaluated regularly for drug efficacy and side effects throughout long-term analgesic drug maintenance.
- Patients on long-term opioid therapy should be evaluated periodically for inappropriate or dangerous drug-use patterns.

O

- Clinical endpoints should be decreased pain, increased function and improvements in mood and sleep, not decreased drug dose.

Non Self-Reporting Patients

One of the more significant challenges in geriatric care is the management of symptoms in patients who are unable to provide an adequate history or narrative of their complaints. Most typically, these are patients suffering from severe cognitive impairments with associated verbal loss from advanced dementing illnesses (e.g. Alzheimers Disease, multi-infarct dementia). In these cases, it is incumbent upon practitioners to anticipate and appreciate the myriad co-existing conditions that typically cause pain in this population, and to develop the skills necessary to recognize symptoms, assess them, and sufficiently treat and monitor outcomes of therapy in patients who cannot self-report. Behavioral disturbances can be, and oftentimes are, mistaken as part and parcel of the dementing illness, rather than a manifestation of pain. Changes in usual behaviors, alterations in eating/sleeping/interpersonal response patterns, vocalizations, and various forms of agitation have been shown to be associated with pain perception that is modifiable by both pharmacologic and non-pharmacologic means. The decision to initiate and titrate opioid therapy must be based upon a high index of suspicion, combined with a failure to provide comfort through other means. An "N of 1" trial of opioid analgesics may be the best means of testing the hypothesis that a non self-reporting patient is experiencing pain. This approach has been shown to be effective at distinguishing analgesic- from non-analgesic-responsive behaviors, while significantly decreasing inappropriate use of psychotropic drugs that may only mask symptoms (Kovach et al. 1999). By sorting out causality in this way, and actively treating their pain, an important contribution to the maintenance of these vulnerable patients' dignity, and basic humanistic care, can be made.

References

1. Aburun F, Monsel S, Langeron O, Coriat P, Riou B (2002). Postoperative Titration of Intravenous Morphine in the Elderly Patient. Anesthesiology 96:17–23
2. AGS Panel on Persistent Pain in Older Persons (2002) The Management of Persistent Pain in Older Persons. J Am Geriatr Soc 50: S205–S224
3. Arking R (2001) The Biology of Aging: What Is It and When It Will Become Useful. Infertility and Reproductive Medicine Clinics of North America 12:469–487
4. Barja G (1998) Mitochondrial Free Radical Production and Aging in Mammals and Birds. Ann NY Acad Sci 854:224–238
5. Belleville JW, Forrest WH, Miller E et al. (1971) Influence of Age on Pain Relief from Analgesics: A Study of Postoperative Patients. JAMA 217:1835–1841
6. Cooner E, Amorosi S (1997) The Study of Pain in Older Americans. Louis Harris and Associates, New York
7. Doucet J, Chassagne P, Trivalle C et al. (1996) Drug-Drug Interactions Related to Hospital Admissions in Older Adults: A Prospective Study of 1000 Patients. J Am Geriatr Soc 44:944–948
8. Fine PG (2001) Opioid Analgesics in Older People. In: Ferrell BA (ed) Clinics in Geriatric Medicine: Pain Management in the Elderly. WB Saunders Company, Philadelphia, pp 479–485
9. Fine PG (2004) Pharmacological Management of Persistent Pain in Older Patients. Clin J Pain 20:220–226
10. Guay DRP, Lackner TE, Hanlon JT (2002) Pharmacologic Management. In: Weiner DK, Herr K, Rudy TE (eds) Persistent Pain in Older Adults. Springer, New York, pp 160–187
11. Helme RD, Gibson SJ (1999) Pain in Older People. In: Crombie IK, Croft PR, Linton SJ, et al. eds. Epidemiology of Pain. Seattle, IASP Press, pp 103–312
12. Kovach CR, Weissman DE, Griffie J et al. (1999). Assessment and Treatment of Discomfort for People with Late-Stage Dementia. J Pain Symptom Manage 18:412–419
13. Page GG (2003) The immune-suppressive effects of pain. Adv Exp Med Biol 521:117–25.
14. Rooke GA, Reeves JG, Rosow C (2002) Anesthesiology and Geriatric Medicine: Mutual Needs and Opportunities. Anesthesiology 96:2–4
15. Rowbotham MC, Twilling L, Davies MS, Reisner L, Taylor K, Mohr D (2003) Oral Opioid Therapy for Chronic Peripheral and Central Neuropathic Pain. New Engl J Med 348:1223–1232

Opioids in Sympathetically Maintained Pain

▶ Opioids in the Management of Complex Regional Pain Syndrome

Opioids in the Management of Complex Regional Pain Syndrome

SRINIVASA N. RAJA, SHEFALI AGARWAL
Department of Anesthesiology and Critical Care Medicine, Johns Hopkins University School of Medicine, Baltimore, MD, USA
sraja@jhmi.edu

Synonyms

Opioids in Sympathetically Maintained Pain

Definition

The role of opioids in the management of chronic non-cancer pain states has been a topic of considerable debate. Physicians' concerns about the use of opioids for pain states other than that resulting from cancer, e.g. neuropathic pain, include the risk of addiction, tolerance to the opioid effect, and lack of efficacy. The belief that nociceptive pain responds to opioids, while neuropathic pain is resistant to opioids, stems from the report by Arner and Meyerson (1988). These investigators compared the effectiveness of infusions of opioid and placebo in a mixed group of forty eight patients with neuropathic, nociceptive and idiopathic pain. Twelve patients in this group had neuropathic pain; four of these twelve patients had combined neuropathic and nociceptive pain. Only one of the eight patients with neuropathic pain alone, and one in the combined neuropathic/nociceptive group, responded positively to the opioid infusion test. These observations were in contrast with the reduction in pain in all of the 15 subjects with nociceptive pain after opioid infusions. This report has been controversial and criticized for an inherent selection bias in the study design (neuropathic pain patients were being treated with narcotics analgesics in moderately high doses prior to study) and for its small sample size. More recent clinical studies suggest that neuropathic pain is not resistant to opioids; however, the drug doses required to attenuate neuropathic pain may be higher than that required to relieve nociceptive pain.

Characteristics

Effect of Opioids in CRPS

A neuropathic pain state that is characterized by ongoing pain, allodynia (pain to normally innocuous stimuli), and significant limitation of function is Complex Regional Pain Syndrome (types I and II, formerly known as Reflex Sympathetic Dystrophy and Causalgia, respectively). The pathophysiology of this disease is uncertain, and hence therapies are aimed at symptomatic relief and functional rehabilitation. Opioids are often used in the management of patients with CRPS to alleviate the ongoing pain when more conservative therapies fail, and to help the patient participate in active physical therapy treatments.

Various therapeutic approaches have been proposed to alleviate the pain in patients with CRPS, but there is paucity of controlled clinical trials that have evaluated the beneficial effects of opioid therapies in patients with CRPS. Although the published literature is limited, growing clinical experience along with clinical re-evaluation of issues related to safety, efficacy and addiction or abuse, shows that some patients can achieve analgesia and improved function and quality of life without the occurrence of intolerable side effects. Since there are no controlled trials of opioid effects in a population of patients with CRPS, we will review the available data from studies of patients with neuropathic pain (a subset of patients in some of these studies have been diagnosed to have CRPS).

Effects of Opioids in Other Neuropathic Pain States

Initial proof of the principle of the effectiveness of opioids on neuropathic pain was achieved using brief intravenous (I.V.) infusion studies (Rowbotham et al. 1991), comparing the effects of I.V. infusions of morphine, lidocaine and placebo in 19 patients with post herpetic neuralgia, using a double blind, crossover design. A 33% decline in pain intensity was observed after morphine (0.3 mg/kg) infusion, compared to a 13% reduction with placebo. Pain relief ratings were also higher during the morphine sessions than lidocaine or placebo sessions.

Several subsequent studies have confirmed the beneficial role of opioids in the treatment of various neuropathic pain states. In a double blind crossover trial, the infusion of the opioid fentanyl was more effective in reducing the intensity of neuropathic pain, compared to the active placebo, diazepam, and the inert placebo, saline (Dellemijn and Vanneste 1997). Two recent additional randomized, controlled, crossover studies have reported beneficial effects of intravenous opioids on central pain and post-amputation pains (Attal et al. 2002, Wu et al. 2002). All four trials described above report a mean pain relief of 30–55% with opioids in the group of patients studied, but significant individual variations were observed. In contrast, the placebo response varied from an increase in pain of 5% to a 25% decrease in pain.

Infusion studies help demonstrate that opioids are likely to provide analgesia in patients with neuropathic pain. However, they may not predict whether therapy with oral opioids is likely to be similarly beneficial. A number of controlled trials published during the last five years have provided evidence for a beneficial effect of oral opioids in chronic neuropathic pain. In a crossover trial, the effects on pain of twice daily controlled release oxycodone treatment were studied in 50 patients with postherpetic neuralgia (Watson and Babul 1998). Subjects began with either placebo or 10 mg oxycodone twice a day and titrated to 60 mg per day. A significant decrease in overall pain intensity and pain relief was observed in the oxycodone treatment period as compared to the placebo period. Fifty eight percent of patients experienced at least moderate pain relief with oxycodone as compared to 18% with placebo. In addition, disability scores were lower during treatment with oxycodone. A similar decrease in pain and greater pain relief compared to placebo was observed in a multi-center, randomized, placebo-controlled trial in patients with distal symmetric diabetic neuropathy, treated with the weak opioid agonist tramadol (Harati et al. 1998, Raja et al. 2002), compared with the change in pain intensity and pain relief with opioids and tricyclic antidepressants in patients with postherpetic neuralgia. They observed similar reductions in pain intensity with both drugs, but patients reported greater satisfaction with the opioid therapy as compared to the therapy with tricyclic antidepressants (50% vs. 34%). Rowbotham et al. (2003) compared treatment with low (0.15 mg) – and high – strength (0.75 mg) capsules of levorphanol in a heterogenous group of patients with peripheral or central neuropathic pain states. They reported a greater reduction in intensity with higher doses of opioids

O

than with lower doses. The mean dose of levorphanol in the high strength group was 8.9 mg/day, approximately equivalent to 135–270 mg of oral morphine and 90–135 mg of oxycodone. A double blind placebo controlled trial in neuropathic patients who were being treated with spinal cord stimulators, however, failed to demonstrate a significant effect of morphine on pain at lower doses, between 60 and 90 mg/day (Harke et al. 2001).

In summary, several studies have demonstrated that oral therapy with opioids can result in a reduction in neuropathic pain intensity. Studies also indicate that therapy with opioids can be associated with side effects, and the risk-benefit ratio needs to be evaluated carefully. More careful studies need to be conducted in future, to examine if patients with CRPS are likely to benefit from therapy with opioids similar to that observed in patients with other neuropathic pain states.

References

1. Arner S, Meyerson BA (1988) Lack of Analgesic Effect of Opioids on Neuropathic and Idiopathic Forms of Pain. Pain 33:11–23
2. Attal N, Guirimand F, Brasseur L, Gaude V, Chauvin M, Bouhassira D (2002) Effects of IV Morphine in Central Pain – A Randomized Placebo-Controlled Study. Neurology 58:554–563
3. Dellemijn PL, Vanneste JA (1997) Randomised Double-Blind Active-Placebo-Controlled Crossover Trial of Intravenous Fentanyl in Neuropathic Pain. Lancet 349:753–758
4. Harati Y, Gooch C, Swenson M, Edelman S, Greene D, Raskin P, Donofrio P, Cornblath D, Sachdeo R, Siu CO, Kamin M (1998) Double-Blind Randomized Trial of Tramadol for the Treatment of the Pain of Diabetic Neuropathy. Neurology 50:1842–1846
5. Harke H, Gretenkort P, Ladleif HU, Rahman S, Harke O (2001) The Response of Neuropathic Pain and Pain in Complex Regional Pain Syndrome I to Carbamazepine and Sustained-Release Morphine in Patients Pretreated with Spinal Cord Stimulation: A Double-Blinded Randomized Study. Anesth Analg 92:488–495
6. Raja SN, Haythornthwaite JA, Pappagallo M, Clark MR, Travison TG, Sabeen S, Royall RM, Max MB (2002) Opioids versus Antidepressants in Postherpetic Neuralgia: A Randomized, Placebo-Controlled Trial. Neurology 59:1015–1021
7. Rowbotham MC, Reisner-Keller LA, Fields HL (1991) Both Intravenous Lidocaine and Morphine Reduce the Pain of Postherpetic Neuralgia. Neurology 41:1024–1028
8. Rowbotham MC, Twilling L, Davies PS, Reisner L, Taylor K, Mohr D (2003) Oral Opioid Therapy for Chronic Peripheral and Central Neuropathic Pain. N Engl J Med 348:1223–1232
9. Watson CP, Babul N (1998) Efficacy of Oxycodone in Neuropathic Pain: A Randomized Trial in Postherpetic Neuralgia. Neurology 50:1837–1841
10. Wu CL, Tella P, Staats PS, Vaslav R, Kazim DA, Wesselmann U, Raja SN (2002) Analgesic Effects of Intravenous Lidocaine and Morphine on Post-Amputation Pain: A Randomized Double-Blind, Active-Placebo-Controlled, Crossover Trial. Anesthesiology 96:841–848

Opioids in the Modulation of Ascending Pathways

▶ Opioids in the Spinal Cord and Modulation of Ascending Pathways (N. gracilis)

Opioids in the Periphery and Analgesia

CHRISTOPH STEIN
Department of Anaesthesiology and Intensive Care Medicine, Campus Benjamin Franklin, Charité University Medicine Berlin, Berlin, Germany
christoph.stein@charite.de

Synonyms

Peripheral Opioid Analgesia; Peripheral Mechanisms of Opioid Analgesia; Opioid Analgesic Actions Outside the Central Nervous System

Definition

Opioid analgesia produced outside the central nervous system by interaction of endogenous or exogenous opioids with opioid receptors on peripheral sensory neurons.

Characteristics

Opioids can produce potent analgesia by activating opioid receptors outside the central nervous system, thus avoiding centrally mediated unwanted effects. Peripheral opioid receptors are localized on ▶ primary afferent neurons. The cell bodies of these neurons in dorsal root ganglia express mu-, delta- and kappa-opioid receptor mRNAs and proteins (reviewed in Stein et al. 2001; Stein et al. 2003). ▶ Opioid receptors are intraaxonally transported into the neuronal processes (Hassan et al. 1993), and are detectable on peripheral sensory nerve terminals in animals (Stein et al. 1990) and in humans (Stein et al. 1996). Co-localization studies have confirmed the presence of opioid receptors on ▶ C and A Fibers, on transient receptor potential vanilloid subtype-1 (TRPV-1) carrying visceral fibers, and on neurons expressing isolectin B4, ▶ substance P and/or ▶ calcitonin-gene-related peptide, consistent with the phenotype of ▶ nociceptors (reviewed in Stein et al. 2003). Sympathetic neurons and immune cells can also express opioid receptors but their functional role in pain control is unclear (reviewed in Stein et al. 2001). The binding characteristics (affinity) of peripheral and central opioid receptors are similar (Hassan et al. 1993; Zöllner et al. 2003).

Opioid Receptor Signaling in Primary Afferent Neurons

All three types of opioid receptors mediate the inhibition of high-voltage activated calcium currents in cultured primary afferent neurons. These effects are transduced by G-proteins (G_i and/or G_o). In addition, opioids – via inhibition of adenylyl cyclase – suppress tetrodotoxin-resistant sodium- and nonselective cation currents stimulated by inflammatory agents (Stein et al. 2001), which may account for the notable efficacy of peripheral opioids in inflammatory and ▶ neuropathic pain (Stein 1993; Stein et al. 2003). Consistent with their

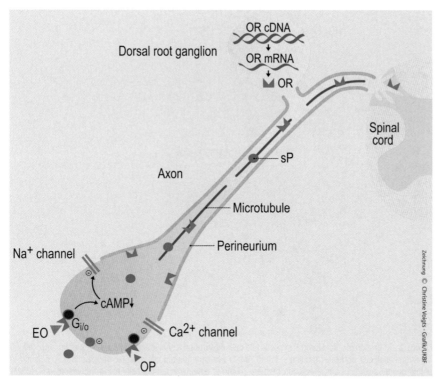

Opioids in the Periphery and Analgesia, Figure 1 Opioid receptor transport and signaling in primary afferent neurons. Opioid receptors (OR) and neuropeptides (e.g. substance P [sP]) are synthesized in the dorsal root ganglion, and transported along intraaxonal microtubules into central and peripheral processes of the primary afferent neuron. At the terminals OR are incorporated into the neuronal membrane and become functional receptors. Upon activation by exogenous (EO) or endogenous opioids (opioid peptides [OP]) OR couple to inhibitory G-proteins ($G_{i/o}$). This leads to direct or indirect (via decrease of cyclic adenosine monophosphate [cAMP]), suppression (-) of Ca^{++} and/or Na^+ currents, respectively, and to subsequent attenuation of sP release. The permeability of the perineurium is increased within inflamed tissue (from Stein et al. 2003).

O

effects on ion channels, opioids attenuate the excitability of peripheral nociceptor terminals, the propagation of action potentials, the release of excitatory proinflammatory neuropeptides (substance P, calcitonin gene-related peptide) from peripheral sensory nerve endings, and vasodilatation evoked by stimulation of C-fibers (Stein et al. 2001). All of these mechanisms result in analgesia and/or anti-inflammatory actions (Fig. 1).

Peripheral Opioid Receptors and Tissue Injury

Peripheral opioid analgesic effects are augmented under conditions of tissue injury such as ► inflammation, neuropathy, or bone damage (Kalso et al. 2002; Stein 1993; Stein et al. 2001). One underlying mechanism is an increased number ("upregulation") of peripheral opioid receptors. In dorsal root ganglia, the synthesis and expression of opioid receptors can be increased by peripheral tissue inflammation (Zöllner et al. 2003; Pühler et al. 2004). Subsequently, the axonal transport of opioid receptors is greatly enhanced (Hassan et al. 1993), leading to their upregulation and to enhanced agonist efficacy at peripheral nerve terminals. In addition, the specific milieu (low pH, prostanoid release) of inflamed tissue can increase opioid agonist efficacy by enhanced G-protein coupling and by increased neuronal cyclic adenosine monophosphate levels. Inflammation

also leads to an increase in the number of sensory nerve terminals ("sprouting") and disrupts the perineurial barrier, thus facilitating the access of opioid agonists to their receptors (Stein et al. 2003). Clinical studies have indicated that the perineural application of opioid agonists along uninjured nerves (e.g. axillary plexus) does not reliably produce analgesic effects, supporting the notion that inflammation promotes accessibility and/or efficient coupling of opioid receptors in primary afferent neurons (Stein et al. 2003). The secretion of endogenous opioid ligands within inflamed tissue (Rittner et al. 2005; Mousa et al. 2004) may produce additive/synergistic interactions at peripheral opioid receptors. In some models, peripheral opioid analgesia is resistant to development of ► tolerance, and clinical studies suggest a lack of cross-tolerance between peripheral exogenous and endogenous opioids in synovial inflammation (Stein et al. 2003).

Endogenous Ligands of Peripheral Opioid Receptors

Three families of ► opioid peptides are well characterized, the endorphins, enkephalins and dynorphins. They bind to all three opioid receptors. Each family derives from a distinct gene and the respective precursors proopiomelanocortin (POMC), proenkephalin and prodynorphin. The most extensively examined source

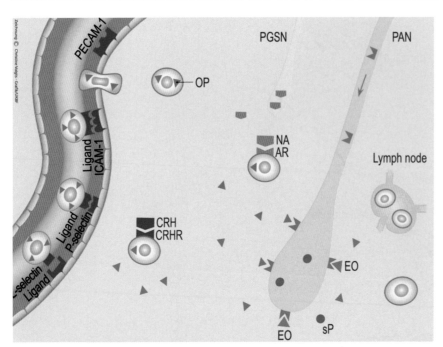

Opioids in the Periphery and Analgesia, Figure 2 Migration of opioid-producing cells and opioid secretion within inflamed tissue. P-selectin, intercellular adhesion molecule-1 (ICAM-1) and platelet-endothelial cell adhesion molecule-1 (PECAM-1) are upregulated on vascular endothelium. L-selectin is coexpressed by immune cells producing opioid peptides (OP). L- and P-selectin mediate rolling of opioid-containing cells along the vessel wall. ICAM-1 mediates their firm adhesion and diapedesis. Adhesion molecules interact with their respective ligands. In response to stress or releasing agents (corticotropin-releasing hormone [CRH], sympathetic neuron-derived noradrenaline [NA], interleukin-1β [IL-1]), the cells secrete OP. CRH, NA and IL-1 elicit OP release by activating CRH receptors (CRHR), adrenergic receptors (AR) and IL-1 receptors (IL-1R), respectively. OP or exogenous opioids (EO) bind to opioid receptors on primary afferent neurons leading to analgesia (Fig. 1). Afterwards immune cells, depleted of the opioids, migrate to regional lymph nodes.

of opioids interacting with peripheral opioid receptors are immune cells (Rittner et al. 2005). Transcripts and peptides derived from POMC and proenkephalin, as well as the prohormone convertases PC1/3 and PC2, necessary for their posttranslational processing, were detected in such cells (Smith 2003; Mousa et al. 2004). The expression of immune-derived opioids is stimulated by viruses, endotoxins, cytokines, corticotropin releasing hormone (CRH) and adrenergic agonists (Smith 2003). POMC mRNA, β-endorphin, met-enkephalin and dynorphin are found in circulating cells and lymph nodes in conditions of painful inflammation. These peptides are upregulated in lymphocytes, monocytes/macrophages and granulocytes within injured tissue (Cabot et al. 1997; Rittner et al. 2005). Circulating opioid-containing leukocytes migrate to injured tissue directed by ▶ Adhesion Molecules and chemokines (Brack et al. 2004). In inflamed tissue, β-endorphin-containing leukocytes co-express L-selectin, and opioid cells, vascular P-selectin; ICAM-1 and PECAM-1 are simultaneously upregulated. Blocking selectins or ICAM-1 reduces the number of opioid cells and intrinsic analgesia (Machelska et al. 1998; Rittner et al. 2005) (Fig. 2).

The release of opioids from immunocytes can be stimulated by environmental stress, sympathetic neuron-derived noradrenaline, interleukin-1β (IL-1) or CRH (Schäfer et al. 1994; Schäfer et al. 1996; Stein et al. 1993; Rittner at al. 2005) (Fig. 2). This release is receptor-specific and calcium-dependent, and it is mimicked by elevated extracellular potassium, consistent with a regulated secretory pathway, as in neurons and endocrine cells (Cabot et al. 1997). *In vivo*, the secreted opioid peptides bind to opioid receptors on sensory neurons and elicit analgesia within injured tissue (Stein et al. 1993; Schäfer et al. 1994; Schäfer et al. 1996). The efficacy of this pain inhibition is proportional to the number of opioid-producing immunocytes (Rittner et al. 2001). CRH-, IL-1 and stress-induced analgesia can be extinguished by immunosuppression (Schäfer et al. 1994; Stein et al. 1990), and by blocking the extravasation of opioid-containing leukocytes (Machelska et al. 1998). In patients undergoing knee surgery, opioid cells accumulate in the inflamed synovium and attenuate postoperative pain (Stein et al. 1993). Apparently, these immune-derived opioids do not induce cross-tolerance to locally administered morphine (Stein et al. 1996).

Preclinical Studies on Peripheral Opioid Analgesics

This basic research has stimulated the development of novel opioid ligands acting exclusively in the periphery without central side-effects. A common approach is the use of hydrophilic compounds with minimal capability to cross the blood-brain-barrier. Among the first compounds were the mu-agonist loperamide (originally known as an antidiarrheal drug) and the kappa-agonist asimadoline. Peripheral restriction was also achieved with newly developed arylacetamide and peptidic kappa-agonists (Stein et al. 2003). While earlier attempts to demonstrate peripheral opioid analgesia in normal tissue failed, they were more successful in models of pathological pain (Stein 1993; Stein et al. 2003). In inflammation of the rat paw, the local injection of low, systemically inactive doses of mu-, delta- and kappa-agonists produced analgesia that was dose-dependent, stereospecific and reversible by selective antagonists. Some agonists produced both peripheral analgesic and anti-inflammatory effects (Stein et al. 2001). Possible underlying mechanisms of the latter include a reduced release of proinflammatory neuropeptides or cytokines, and a diminished expression of adhesion molecules. Potent antinociception was also shown in models of nerve damage and of visceral, thermal and bone pain (Stein et al. 2003).

Clinical Studies on Peripheral Opioid Analgesics

Controlled studies have demonstrated significant analgesic effects following the local application of opioids at sites of injury (Kalso et al. 2002; Stein et al. 2001). The intraarticular administration of the mu-agonist morphine is the best examined clinical application (Kalso et al. 2002). After knee surgery, it dose-dependently reduces pain scores and/or supplemental analgesic consumption by a peripheral mechanism of action and without side-effects (Kalso et al. 2002; Stein et al. 2001). Intraarticular morphine is active in the presence of opioid-containing inflammatory cells (Stein et al. 1996) and in chronic rheumatoid and osteoarthritis. Its effect is similar to a standard intraarticular local anesthetic or steroid injection and is long lasting (up to 7 days), possibly due to morphine's anti-inflammatory activity. Other trials showed efficacy of local opioid injections in bone pain, dental pain, corneal abrasions and visceral pain (Stein et al. 2003). Several studies found no peripheral effects of opioids. The majority of those trials examined the injection of agonists into the non-inflamed environment along nerve trunks (Stein et al. 2003). This suggests that intraaxonal opioid receptors may be „in transit", and not available as functional receptors at the membrane. Novel peripherally restricted opioids have recently entered human trials, including a kappa-agonist that markedly reduced visceral pain in patients with chronic pancreatitis without severe side-effects (Stein et al. 2003). Beyond the absence of central side-effects, such novel compounds may offer advantages such as anti-inflammatory effects, lack of

tolerance, lack of constipation, lack of gastrointestinal, hepatic, renal and thromboembolic complications (typically associated with ▶ NSAIDs, Survey), and efficacy in neuropathic pain (Stein et al. 2003).

References

1. Brack A, Rittner HL, Machelska H et al. (2004) Control of inflammatory pain by chemokine-mediated recruitment of opioid-containing polymorphonuclear cells. Pain 112:229–238
2. Cabot PJ, Carter L, Gaiddon C et al. (1997) Immune Cell-Derived β-Endorphin: Production, Release and Control of Inflammatory Pain in Rats. J Clin Invest 100:142–148
3. Hassan AHS, Ableitner A, Stein C et al. (1993) Inflammation of the Rat Paw Enhances Axonal Transport of Opioid Receptors in the Sciatic Nerve and Increases their Density in the Inflamed Tissue. Neuroscience 55:185–195
4. Kalso E, Smith L, McQuay HJ et al. (2002) No Pain, No Gain: Clinical Excellence and Scientific Rigour – Lessons Learned from IA Morphine. Pain 98:269–275
5. Machelska H, Cabot PJ, Mousa SA et al. (1998) Pain Control in Inflammation Governed by Selectins. Nat Med 4:1425–1428
6. Mousa SA, Shakibaei M, Sitte N et al. (2004) Subcellular pathways of beta-endorphin synthesis, processing and release from immunocytes in inflammatory pain. Endocrinology 145:1331–1341
7. Pühler W, Zöllner C, Brack A et al. (2004) Rapid upregulation of mu opioid receptor mRNA in dorsal root ganglia in response to peripheral inflammation depends on neuronal conduction. Neuroscience 129:473–479
8. Rittner HL, Brack A, Machelska H et al. (2001) Opioid Peptide-Expressing Leukocytes: Identification, Recruitment, and Simultaneously Increasing Inhibition of Inflammatory Pain. Anesthesiology 95:500–508
9. Rittner HL, Machelska H, Stein C (2005) Leukocytes in the regulation of pain and analgesia. J Leukoc Biol 78:1215–1222
10. Schäfer M, Carter L, Stein C (1994) Interleukin-1β and Corticotropin-Releasing-Factor Inhibit Pain by Releasing Opioids from Immune Cells in Inflamed Tissue. Proc Natl Acad Sci USA 91:4219–4223
11. Schäfer M, Mousa SA, Zhang Q et al. (1996) Expression of Corticotropin-Releasing Factor in Inflamed Tissue is required for Intrinsic Peripheral Opioid Analgesia. Proc Natl Acad Sci USA 93:6096–6100
12. Smith EM (2003) Opioid Peptides in Immune Cells. Adv Exp Med Biol 521:51–68
13. Stein C (1993) Peripheral Mechanisms of Opioid Analgesia. Anesth Analg 76:182–191
14. Stein C, Hassan AHS, Lehrberger K et al. (1993) Local Analgesic Effect of Endogenous Opioid Peptides. Lancet 342:321–324
15. Stein C, Hassan AHS, Przewlocki R et al. (1990) Opioids from Immunocytes Interact with Receptors on Sensory Nerves to Inhibit Nociception in Inflammation. Proc Natl Acad Sci USA 87:5935–5939
16. Stein C, Machelska H, Schäfer M (2001) Peripheral Analgesic and Anti-Inflammatory Effects of Opioids. Z Rheumatol 60:416–424
17. Stein C, Pflüger M, Yassouridis A, Hoelzl J et al. (1996) No Tolerance to Peripheral Morphine Analgesia in Presence of Opioid Expression in Inflamed Synovia. J Clin Invest 98:793–799
18. Stein C, Schäfer M, Machelska H (2003) Attacking Pain at its Source: New Perspectives on Opioids. Nat Med 9:1003–1008
19. Zöllner C, Shaqura MA, Bopaiah CP et al. (2003) Painful Inflammation-Induced Increase in mu-Opioid Receptor Binding and G-Protein Coupling in Primary Afferent Neurons. Mol Pharmacol 64:202–210

O

Opioids in the Spinal Cord and Central Sensitization

ANTHONY H. DICKENSON
Department of Pharmacology, University College
London, London, UK
anthony.dickenson@ucl.ac.uk

Definition

Activation of the N-methyl-D-apartate (▶ NMDA) receptor causes a major excitatory drive in the dorsal horn of the spinal cord where ▶ wind-up and associated ▶ central sensitization is induced. Once the NMDA receptor is activated, inhibitory controls may be compromised, simply since greater levels of excitability will require greater inhibitory controls. Combinations of NMDA antagonists plus opioids therefore predictably synergise to produce marked inhibitory effects.

Characteristics

Some of the very first studies on glutamate as a transmitter involved the spinal cord. The NMDA receptor has become an increasingly important target site for potential analgesics, as evidence accumulates for a role of the receptor in the enhancement of spinal processing of painful messages and in many long term events in the brain, including ▶ long-term potentiation and excitotoxic cell death. However, this important role of the receptor in a number of CNS functions can lead to problems in terms of side-effects.

There is now little doubt that glutamate seen in primary afferent terminals in laminae I, III and IV of the dorsal horn is a releasable transmitter. In the case of C-fibres, glutamate may coexist with peptides such as substance P and CGRP, which would make it highly likely that a noxious stimulus releases both peptides and excitatory amino-acids from the afferent nociceptive fibres (Battaglia and Rustioni 1988). Large A fibres, terminating in deeper laminae, have glutamate, yet do not normally contain peptides. Thus, glutamate is involved in the transmission of both high and low threshold information from afferents into the spinal cord. In addition to a key role in transmission from afferent fibres, there is further evidence that transmission, at least from trigemino- and spinothalamic tract cells, also involves glutamate (Dickenson 1997).

Although a number of studies have demonstrated that glutamate is released from both low and high threshold afferents, electrophysiological studies would indicate that, in general, only noxious events, at least under normal conditions, activate the NMDA receptor. It could be suggested that peptides may allow the differentiation between large A-fibre and C fibre inputs, since only C-fibre stimulation will elicit peptide release. Consequently, C-fibre induced release of excitatory peptides may provide the required depolarization to remove the

Mg^{++} block of the receptor and allow NMDA receptor activation (Dickenson 1997).

Wind-Up

Wind-up is the term given to a short-term increase in excitability of spinal neurones. When a constant C-fibre stimulus is delivered, the response of deep dorsal horn neurone increases rapidly after the first few stimuli, and then decays slowly after cessation of the stimulus. If a train of stimuli are given, at frequencies of about 0.5 Hz and above, the responses of the neurone to the first few stimuli remains constant. However, as the stimulus continues, there is a rapid incremental increase in firing of the neurone, and cumulative long slow depolarization such as those mediated by peptides including substance P seen with intracellular recordings, associated with increased action potentials. The neurone firing can increase by up to 20-fold the initial rate. Although wind-up is only induced by C-fibre stimulation, once the process has occurred, all responses of the neurones are enhanced and a post-discharge, firing following the C-fibre latency band, is evoked. Thus, noxious stimuli, applied at sufficient intensities, can enhance spinal excitatory events by mechanisms that are restricted to the spinal cord. Wind-up, in normal animals, is only produced by stimulation at C-fibre, and possibly also A-delta, stimulation, but not by low-intensity stimuli (Dickenson 1997). With regard to the functional significance of wind-up, it has been shown that high frequency C-fibre stimulation results in a marked and prolonged increase in the ▶ flexion withdrawal reflex, recorded from motoneurones in spinal rats. It is evident that a number of physiological inputs, causing repeated C-fibre activity, should activate the NMDA receptor, if the intensity and area of stimulus is sufficient. This has turned out to be the case, and there is evidence for involvement of the NMDA receptor in inflammatory pain, neuropathic pain, allodynia and ischaemic pain, and all processes in which the receptor alters the normal relationship between stimulus and response (Dickenson 1997; Price 1994). In these persistent pain states the NMDA receptor is vital both in establishing the augmented pain state, and in maintaining this state. Higher frequency stimulation of afferents can lead to NMDA-dependent ▶ long-term potentiation in the spinal cord, where the enhanced responses now last for hours (Ikeda et al. 2003; Rygh et al. 2000). This pivotal role of the NMDA receptor in the plasticity of the pain signalling system makes it an attractive target for development of new analgesics.

The NMDA receptor is of course not restricted to spinal pain pathways, and it is not surprising that NMDA receptor antagonists, such as the channel blocker ketamine and competitive antagonists, are associated with a range of adverse effects. In volunteers and patients, key roles of the receptor have been shown in states of capsaicin induced central hypersensitivity and after nerve injury response (Dickenson 1997; Price 1994). The increased excitability leads not simply to increased pain ratings, but may well also increase the area of pain as has been seen in animal studies. However, the clinical use of NMDA receptor antagonists has been fraught by the simple fact that as therapeutic levels are attained, side-effects are on the verge of unacceptable. One possible approach to avoid the side-effects associated with global block of NMDA receptors is to target a particular receptor type by its subunit makeup. This was justified by animal studies that demonstrated that NR2B selective antagonists may have clinical utility for the treatment of pain conditions with a reduced side-effect profile compared to existing NMDA receptor antagonists (Boyce et al. 2001).

NMDA Receptor Interactions with Opioids

Accumulating evidence indicates plasticity in opioid controls. The degree of effectiveness of morphine analgesia is subject to modulation by other transmitter systems in the spinal cord, and by pathological changes induced by peripheral nerve injury. In neuropathic pain states, a number of explanations can be given for this reduction in opioid actions. A potential marked loss of pre-synaptic opioid receptors as a result of nerve section can occur, although this appears not to be a factor in less severe nerve injuries. Possibly, more importantly, an up-regulation of the "anti-opioid peptide" ► cholecystokinin, after damage to peripheral nerve, could also contribute to the reduced morphine analgesia. In reality, a combination of factors is likely to be the cause of the particular problems that arise in the control of neuropathic pains with opioid drugs (Dickenson and Suzuki 2002). The CNS operates by a balance between excitation and inhibition. Thus, the profound excitations produced by NMDA receptor involvement in pain related responses of spinal cord neurones can further shift the balance in favour of excitation. The enhanced levels of firing will then lead to a reduced effectiveness of a given dose of an opioid. Reductions in opioid controls can be overcome by dose-escalation if excessive side-effects do not intervene, and one approach could be spinal delivery where high local levels can be achieved.

An approach that could be considered would be to use a combination of an NMDA antagonist with an opioid such as morphine. The dual actions of these pharmacological agents could be beneficial. The fact that NMDA receptor antagonists are effectively anti-hyperalgesic agents, reducing the hyperexcitability, means that the addition of an analgesic such as an opioid would enable the baseline response to also be inhibited. Interestingly, some opioids such as methadone, pethidine and ketobemidone appear to have both mu opioid receptor actions and weaker, but potentially functionally relevant, NMDA receptor blocking actions (Ebert et al. 1995). This additional action of these opioids, non-competitive NMDA antagonism, has been revealed by

both binding and electrophysiological approaches, but it remains unclear as to whether the non-opioid component of their actions contributes at all to their *in vivo* profile (Carpenter et al. 2000).

The spinal actions of opioids and their mechanisms of analgesia involve: 1) reduced transmitter release (e.g. glutamate and peptides) from nociceptive C-fibres (75 % of spinal opioid receptors are pre-synaptic) so that spinal neurones are less excited by incoming painful messages, and 2) post-synaptic inhibitions of neurones conveying information from the spinal cord to the brain (Dickenson and Suzuki 2002). From electrophysiogical studies, a moderate dose of morphine, or indeed, any opioid, will initially profoundly inhibit neuronal activity evoked by C-fibre stimulation, delaying or abolishing activity indicative of pre-synaptic inhibition of transmitter release. However, as the stimulation continues, as wind-up is induced, the neuronal excitations produced by post-synaptic NMDA receptor activation breaks through the opioid inhibitions so that at moderate doses, opioids can only delay the onset of wind-up without inhibiting the process itself (Chapman and Dickenson 1992). Higher doses of opioid, presumably activating post-synaptic receptors as well, will abolish responses.

At supraspinal sites, opiate actions are becoming increasingly well understood but exact mechanisms are still elusive. Morphine can act to alter descending pathways from the brain to the cord which involve noradrenaline and serotonin, and these pathways then act to reduce spinal nociceptive activity. Actions of opioids on descending systems may be of particular relevance to pain states where supraspinal facilitatory pathways are superimposed on spinal hypersensitivity (Porreca et al. 2002; Suzuki et al. 2002).

Marked inhibitions can be produced through synergism between the combination of low threshold doses of morphine with low doses of NMDA receptor antagonists (Chapman and Dickenson 1992) using neuronal measures. In a model of neuropathic pain using behaviour against which morphine fails to be antinociceptive, the combined application of an NMDA antagonist, in this case MK-801, with morphine, restored the ability of morphine to inhibit the response (Yamamoto and Yaksh 1992). A human study on the flexion reflex in volunteers confirmed this idea, but indicated that the combination of ketamine and morphine had actions that rely on the type of afferent input (Bossard et al. 2002). These studies suggest that in the absence of NMDA receptor antagonists devoid of side-effects, the co-administration of a low dose of an NMDA antagonist with a low-dose of an opioid may deliver a good pain control with minor side-effects. However, there are some other important issues. Neurones in lamina I of the spinal cord have projections to ► parabrachial/PAG areas, whereas many deep cells project in the ► spinothalamic tract (Todd 2002). NMDA-dependent wind-up is clear and obvious

0

in deep cells and almost absent in lamina I cells, although both neuronal types support LTP when high-frequency stimuli are given (Dickenson 1997; Ikeda et al. 2003; Rygh et al. 2000). This suggests that in pain states other than those activated by very high frequency stimuli, spinothalamic inputs will be potentiated through wind-up like mechanisms, whereas inputs to emotional areas will not. This may then lead to dissociation between the emotional and sensory -discriminative aspects of pain. However, opioids have identical dose-response curves for ▶ Laminae I and V Neurones which would agree well with their ability to modulate both components of the sensation. As a consequence, the opioid-NMDA interaction will only be on lamina V activity, so that the sensory responses to pain could be expected to be altered more than the emotional aspects by a combination. However, an added complexity regarding lamina V, is that once LTP is induced morphine, at doses that completely suppress LTP, does not alter the underlying process. Thus, reversal of the opioid inhibition is only to the post-LTP response level (Rygh et al. 2000). Therefore, complex interactions of opioids with spinal mechanisms of hyperexcitability are likely, but further exploration of this area could lead to useful clinical advances.

References

1. Battaglia G, Rustioni A (1988) Coexistence of Glutamate and Substance P in Dorsal Root Ganglion Cells of the Rat and Monkey. J Comp Neurol 277:302–312
2. Bossard AE, Guirimand F, Fletcher D et al. (2002) Interaction of a Combination of Morphine and Ketamine on the Nociceptive Flexion Reflex in Human Volunteers. Pain 98:47–57
3. Boyce S, Wyatt A, Webb J et al. (1999) Selective NMDA NR2B Antagonists Induce Antinociception without Motor Dysfunction: Correlation with Restricted Localisation of NR2B Subunit in Dorsal Horn. Neuropharmacology 38:611–623
4. Carpenter K, Chapman V, Dickenson AH (2000) Neuronal Inhibitory Effects of Methadone are Predominantly Opioid Receptor Mediated in the Rat Spinal Cord In Vivo. Eur J Pain 4:19–26
5. Chapman V, Dickenson AH (1992) The Combination of NMDA Antagonism and Morphine Produces Profound Antinociception in the Rat Dorsal Horn. Brain Res 573:321–323
6. Dickenson AH (1997) Mechanisms of Central Hypersensitivity: Excitatory Amino Acid Mechanisms and their Control. In: Dickenson AH, Besson JM (eds) The Pharmacology of Pain. Springer Berlin Heidelberg New York, pp 167–196
7. Dickenson AH, Suzuki R (1999) Function and Dysfunction of Opioid Receptors in the Spinal Cord. In: Kalso E, McQuay HJ, Wiesenfeld-Hallen Z (eds) Opioid Sensitivity of Chronic Non-cancer Pain, Progress in Pain Research and Management, vol 14. IASP Press, Seattle, pp 1–28
8. Ebert B, Andersen S, Krogsgaard-Larsen P (1995) Ketobemidone, Methadone and Pethidine are Non-Competitive N-methyl-d-aspartate Antagonists in the Rat Cortex and Spinal Cord. Neurosci Letts 187:165–168
9. Ikeda H, Heinke B, Ruscheweyh R et al. (2003) Synaptic Plasticity in Spinal Lamina I Projection Neurons that Mediate Hyperalgesia. Science 299:1237–1240
10. Price DD, Mao J, Mayer DJ (1994) Central Neural Mechanisms of Normal and Abnormal Pain States. In: Fields H et al. (eds) Pharmacological Approaches to the Treatment of Chronic Pain: New Concepts and Critical Issues. Progress in pain research and management, vol 1. IASP Press, Seattle, pp 61–84
11. Porreca F, Ossipov M, Gebhart G (2002) Chronic Pain and Medullary Descending Facilitation. Trends Neurosci 25:319–325
12. Rygh L, Green M, Athauda N et al. (2000) The Effect of Spinal Morphine following Long-Term Potentiation of Wide Dynamic Range Neurones in the Rat. Anesthesiology 92:140–146
13. Suzuki R, Morcuende S, Webber S et al. (2002) Superficial NK1 Expressing Neurons Control Spinal Excitability through Activation of Descending Pathways. Nat Neurosci 5:1319–1326
14. Todd AJ (2002) Anatomy of Primary Afferents and Projection Neurones in the Rat Spinal Dorsal Horn with Particular Emphasis on Substance P and the Neurokinin 1 Receptor. Exp Physiol 87:245–249
15. Yamamoto T, Yaksh TL (1992) Studies on the Spinal Interaction of Morphine and the NMDA Antagonist MK-801 on the Hyperesthesia Observed in a Rat Model of Sciatic Mononeuropathy Neurosci Lett 1992:135:67–70

Opioids in the Spinal Cord and Modulation of Ascending Pathways (N. gracilis)

RIE SUZUKI, ANTHONY H. DICKENSON
Department of Pharmacology, University College London, London, UK
ucklrsu@ucl.ac.uk, anthony.dickenson@ucl.ac.uk

Synonyms

Opioids in the Modulation of Ascending Pathways; Opioids and Nucleus Gracilis

Definition

Spinally applied opioids have been shown to produce powerful ▶ antinociception behaviourally, both in acute pain models (tail flick, hot plate, von Frey) as well as in more chronic pain states (for review see Dickenson and Suzuki 1999). These actions are mediated through the activation of ▶ opioid receptors, which are found in abundance in the ▶ superficial dorsal horn of the spinal cord, the periphery and at various supraspinal sites, such as the nucleus gracilis (NG), parabrachial area (PB), periaqueductal gray (PAG), rostroventral medulla (RVM) and thalamus.

Characteristics

The NG is an area in the brainstem that receives afferent input from direct projections of myelinated and unmyelinated primary afferent fibres, as well as second-order projections from ▶ postsynaptic dorsal column (PSDC) neurones of the spinal cord (lamina III–V) (Willis and Coggeshall 2004). A large proportion of NG neurones project to the contralateral thalamus via the medial lemniscus, although a smaller population has axons terminating within the ▶ dorsal column nuclei, and hence appear to be interneurones. Substantial evidence exists for a role of dorsal column nuclei in the processing of visceral nociceptive input (Willis et al. 1999). This structure is of particular interest since it has been involved in various pathological conditions (Miki et al. 2000; Miki et al. 2002; Schwark and Ilyinsky 2001). The observation that ipsilateral lesions of the dorsal column or microinjection of lidocaine into the NG suppresses ► tactile allodynia (but not ► thermal hyperalgesia) (Sun et al. 2001), led studies to speculate that the NG may be implicated in mediating tactile hypersensitivity following peripheral nerve injury. In parallel with these findings, plasticity in NG neurones has been reported after tissue and nerve injury, which include electrophysiological and neuro-chemical alterations (Al-Chaer et al. 1997; Ma and Bisby 1998; Miki et al. 1998; Suzuki and Dickenson 2002). Clinically, a limited midline myelotomy at T8-10 level has been shown to relieve cancer pain in patients (for refs see Willis et al. 1999).

To study how activity in the NG can be modulated by spinal opioids, *in vivo* electrophysiological approaches were employed to record the responses of deep dorsal horn neurones after peripheral nerve injury. Spinal application of morphine was shown to selectively modulate noxious cutaneous input to the NG (Suzuki and Dickenson 2002). Morphine attenuated the noxious Aδ- and C-fibre evoked responses of NG neurones, as well as responses evoked by mechanical punctate and heat stimuli. In contrast, the innocuous brush-evoked responses and Aβ-fibre evoked activity remained relatively unaltered, in keeping with the proposed specific action of morphine on noxious inputs. Remarkably, responses evoked by mechanical punctate stimuli (von Freys of 2 and 9 grams) were dramatically attenuated by morphine administration in nerve injured animals, an effect that was not observed in sham control animals. These von Frey filaments are normally innocuous when applied to the rat hindpaw; however, after nerve injury, rats show aversive behaviours to the stimulus, a sign indicative of mechanical allodynia. The finding that neuronal responses evoked by normally innocuous stimuli are robustly inhibited by morphine after neuropathy is interesting, since this suggests an alteration in spinal opioid control, particularly on low threshold signalling systems. Whilst the efficacy of opioids in acute pain conditions is well established, the issue of opioid sensitivity in chronic neuropathic pain remains a much debated subject (Rowbotham 2001). Although previous behavioural studies have demonstrated a general lack of effect of intrathecally-administered morphine after neuropathy, morphine administered via the systemic route was shown to reverse tactile hypersensitivity (Bian et al. 1995; Lee et al. 1995), suggesting that these actions may be mediated through the supraspinal activation of opioid receptors, and subsequent activation of descending modulatory systems (Bian et al. 1995). Interestingly, the neuronal counterpart of this activity, as assessed by innocuous von Frey evoked activity recorded in NG neurones, is sensitive to intrathecal morphine treatment, and shows robust inhibition after nerve injury (Suzuki and Dickenson 2002).

The exact mechanism by which spinal morphine inhibits NG neuronal activity remains unclear; however several possibilities exist. One possibility is that spinal morphine, directly or indirectly, inhibits the PSDC pathway that originates from lamina III–V of the dorsal horn. The PSDC pathway projects via the dorsal funiculus and dorsolateral funiculus to the dorsal column nuclei, and the conduction velocities of their axons indicate they are small to medium-sized myelinated fibres (Willis and Coggeshall 2004). Dendrites of PSDC neurones have been shown to extend to lamina I and II, allowing them to receive monosynaptic input from small diameter fibres. Morphine applied spinally can, therefore, modulate the activity of PSDC neurones, through presynaptic inhibition of neurotransmitter release from nociceptive afferents. Alternatively, C-fibres can send collaterals through to the dorsal column from the lumbar segment. In this case, morphine may dampen excitability in these collateral fibres running to the GN via hyperpolarisation of the nerve terminals of small diameter fibres. The finding that low intensity mechanical evoked responses of NG neurones are selectively attenuated by spinal morphine after nerve injury, possibly suggests an acquired *de novo* opioid sensitivity of Aβ-fibres (through a phenotypic switch).

Another electrophysiological study investigating the role of the PSDC pathway in visceral nociceptive processing demonstrated that morphine administration into the sacral cord robustly suppressed the responses of NG neurones to colorectal distension (CRD), but not to noxious cutaneous stimuli (Al-Chaer et al. 1996), suggesting that the latter responses are largely conveyed by the ascending collaterals of primary afferent fibres. Recordings were also made in PSDC neurones and morphine was similarly effective in reducing the responses of PSDC neurones to CRD and also to noxious cutaneous stimuli.

Thus, the NG represents an important area of the brainstem that is involved in the relay of nociceptive visceral and somatic inputs to the VPL nucleus of the thalamus. Input to the NG is mediated through direct projections of primary afferent fibres, and indirectly through the PSDC system which originates from laminae III–V of the spinal cord. Furthermore, these inputs are sensitive to spinally administered opioids and can be modulated by agents such as morphine. Since the NG has been implicated in tactile hypersensitivity that accompanies pathological conditions such as neuropathy, the fact that spinal morphine can modulate the activity of these neurones may have important clinical implications, particularly in the treatment of static allodynia.

References

1. Al-Chaer E, Westlund K, Willis W (1997) Sensitization of Postsynaptic Dorsal Column Neuronal Responses by Colon Inflammation. Neuroreport 8:3267–3273
2. Al-Chaer E, Lawand N, Westlund K et al. (1996) Pelvic Visceral Input into the Nucleus Gracilis is Largely Mediated by the

Postsynaptic Dorsal Column Pathway. J Neurophysiol 76:2675–2690

3. Bian D, Nichols ML, Ossipov MH et al. (1995) Characterization of the Antiallodynic Efficacy of Morphine in a Model of Neuropathic Pain in Rats. Neuroreport 6:1981–1984
4. Dickenson A, Suzuki R (1999) Function and Dysfunction of Opioid Receptors in the Spinal Cord. In: Kalso E, McQuay H, Wiesenfeld-Hallin Z (eds) Opioid Sensitivity of Chronic Noncancer Pain. Progress in Pain Research and Management. IASP Press, Seattle, pp 17–44
5. Lee YW, Chaplan SR, Yaksh TL (1995) Systemic and Supraspinal, but not Spinal, Opiates Suppress Allodynia in a Rat Neuropathic Pain Model. Neurosci Lett 199:111–114
6. Ma W, Bisby MA (1998) Partial and Complete Sciatic Nerve Injuries Induce Similar Increases of Neuropeptide Y and Vasoactive Intestinal Peptide Immunoreactivities in Primary Sensory Neurons and their Central Projections. Neuroscience 86:1217–1234
7. Miki K, Iwata K, Tsuboi Y et al. (1998) Responses of Dorsal Column Nuclei Neurons in Rats with Experimental Mononeuropathy. Pain 76:407–415
8. Miki K, Iwata K, Tsuboi Y et al. (2000) Dorsal Column Thalamic Pathway is Involved in Thalamic Hyperexcitability following Peripheral Nerve Injury: A Lesion Study in Rats with Experimental Mononeuropathy. Pain 85:263–271
9. Miki K, Zhou Q-Q, Guo W et al. (2002) Changes in Gene Expression and Neuronal Phenotype in Brain Stem Pain Modulatory Circuitry after Inflammation. J Neurophysiol 87:750–760
10. Rowbotham M (2001) Efficacy of Opioids in Neuropathic Pain. In: Hansson P, Fields H, Hill R et al. (eds) Neuropathic Pain: Pathophysiology and Treatment. IASP Press, Seattle, pp 203–213
11. Schwark H, Ilyinsky O (2001) Inflammatory Pain Reduces Correlated Activity in the Dorsal Column Nuclei. Brain Res 889:295–302
12. Sun H, Ren K, Zhong C et al. (2001) Nerve Injury-Induced Tactile Allodynia is Mediated via Ascending Spinal Dorsal Column Projections. Pain 90:105–111
13. Suzuki R, Dickenson A (2002) Nerve Injury-Induced Changes in Opioid Modulation of Wide Dynamic Range Dorsal Column Nuclei Neurones. Neuroscience 111:215–228
14. Willis W, Coggeshall R (2004) Sensory Pathways in the Dorsal Funiculus. In: Willis W and, Coggeshall R Sensory Mechanisms of the Spinal Cord. Kluwer Academics/Plenum Press, New York, pp 597–664
15. Willis W, Al-Chaer E, Quast M et al. (1999) A Visceral Pain Pathway in the Dorsal Column of the Spinal Cord. Proc Natl Acad Sci USA 96:7675–7679

Opioids, Kappa Receptors and Visceral Pain

PIERRE J. M. RIVIÈRE
Ferring Research Institute, San Diego, CA, USA
pierre.riviere@ferring.com

Synonyms

κ-opioid receptors; kappa receptors and visceral pain; kappa-opioid receptors; KOR

Definitions

κ– (kappa) opioid receptors are a subtype of opioid receptors. They are differentiated from other opioid receptors subtypes (mu and delta) by distinct gene, protein, tissue expression pattern, functional properties and side effect profile. Kappa-opioid receptor agonists are particularly effective analgesics in visceral pain models.

Characteristics

Kappa-Opioid Receptors, Pharmacological Subtypes and Cloned Receptor

Pharmacological studies have long established the existence of κ– (kappa) opioid receptors that are functionally differentiated from μ– (mu) and δ– (delta) opioid receptor subtypes (Martin et al. 1976). Radioligand studies have also provided evidence of heterogeneity of kappa binding sites in brain membrane preparations, characterizing two main binding sites termed κ_1 and κ_2, each of them being further subdivided into high (κ_{1a}–, κ_{2a}–) and low affinity (κ_{1b}–, κ_{2b}–) binding sites (Rothman et al. 1990). However, only one kappa-opioid receptor (KOR1) has so far been cloned in human and rodents (Simonin et al. 1995). Its pharmacology is virtually identical to the previously characterized κ_1–receptor. KOR1 is a seven transmembrane domains (7TM) receptor, coupled to G-proteins (G-protein coupled receptors, GPCR) and negatively coupled to adenylate cyclase.

Kappa-Agonists

Most of the kappa-agonists available so far have been optimized at the κ_1–binding site or the cloned KOR1. Thus, they are all κ_1-selective, with agonist potencies in the nanomolar range (typically 0.1 to 10 nM). Prototypic representatives of this class of compounds include both organic (U50,488, enadoline/CI–977, asimadoline/EMD61753, ADL 10–010, ADL 10–0116) and peptidic molecules (FE 200665 and FE 200666) (Binder et al. 2001; Rivière et al. 1999). U50,488 and enadoline are brain-penetrating compounds (Rivière et al. 1999), while the others have various degrees of peripheral selectivity, ranging from moderate (asimadoline) (Rivière et al. 1999), ADL 10–0101, ADL 10–0116 (Murphy et al. 2000) to high (FE 200665, FE 200666) (Rivière et al. 1999).

Opioid Receptors and Pain Pathways

Opioid receptors are expressed on nerves involved in pain transmission (ascending sensory pathways) and modulation (descending inhibitory pathways) in the periphery, the spinal cord and the brain. Opioid receptors are mainly present on peptide-rich C-fibers of primary sensory afferents, where they prevent the activation and sensitization of these fibers and inhibit the release of pain transmitters. Upon activation by selective agonists, each opioid receptor subtype elicits different degrees of analgesia that varies greatly relative to the experimental conditions including: receptor subtype selectivity of the pharmacological agent, somatic vs. visceral pain, supra-spinal vs. spinal or peripheral site of action, and acute vs. inflammatory or chronic pain.

Analgesic Effects of Kappa-Agonists in Visceral Pain Models

Kappa-agonists are particularly potent analgesics after systemic administration in a wide variety of visceral pain models (Burton and Gebhart 1998; Su et al. 2002).

The antinociceptive effects of kappa-agonists in visceral pain are consistent across a multitude of experimental conditions, irrespective of species (rats or mice), targeted visceral organs (duodenum, colon, bladder, vagina, uterus or peritoneum), nature of noxious stimuli (distension or chemical irritant), nature of measured endpoint (cardiovascular, visceromotor or electrophysiological responses, anesthetized or conscious animals, basal or inflammatory pain and chemical nature of kappa-agonists (organic molecules or peptides). Experimental visceral inflammation decreases pain thresholds, increases pain response and enhances the analgesic potency of kappa-agonists (Burton and Gebhart 1998; Langlois et al. 1994; Langlois et al. 1997; Sengupta et al. 1999). Peritoneal irritation-induced pain is also associated with gastrointestinal transit inhibition (Friese et al. 1997; Riviere et al. 1993; Riviere et a. 1994). In these conditions, blockade by kappa-agonists of peritoneal irritation-induced pain results in a reversal of intestinal ileus. The ability of kappa-agonists to reverse peritoneal irritation-induced ileus is correlated with their antinociceptive potency in this model (Friese et al. 1997). These data suggest that kappa-agonists might be appropriate to treat post operative pain associated with ileus.

Involvement of Peripheral κ_1–Receptors in Kappa-Agonists Induced Visceral Analgesia in Intact Animals

In visceral pain models using intact animals, kappa-agonists are active at relatively low doses (typically 0.010 to 0.5 mg/kg, systemic route), and the rank order for analgesic potencies (Rivière et al. 1999; Burton and Gebhart 1998; Friese et al. 1997b) is consistent with that for agonist activity at the cloned KOR1. In these conditions, the analgesic effects of kappa-agonists are generally blocked by opioid antagonists (Burton and Gebhart 1998; Diop et al. 1994a; Diop et al. 1994b; Friese et al. 1997a; Langlois et al. 1994; Langlois et al. 1997), validating the involvement of opioid receptors, likely κ_1, considering the selectivity of the agonists for κ_1–receptors. Furthermore, in these models, the effects of kappa-agonists are generally blocked by peripherally restricted opioid antagonists, and/or peripherally restricted kappa-agonists are also equally effective compared to brain penetrating compounds in these models (Rivière et al. 1999; Burton and Gebhart 1998; Friese et al. 1997b; Sandner-Kiesling et al. 2002), suggesting that the κ_1–receptors involved in mediating kappa-agonist responses are located in the periphery.

Involvement of Non-Opioid Blockade of Sodium Currents in Kappa-Agonists Direct Effects on Visceral Sensory Input

Kappa-agonists have a direct inhibitory effect on visceral sensory input in the periphery. They inhibit the firing of decentralized pelvic afferents activated by colorectal distension (CRD) (Joshi et al. 2000; Sengupta et al. 1996; Sengupta et al. 1999; Su et al. 1997; Su et

al. 2002). These effects require higher doses than those needed in visceral pain models using intact animals (about 10–fold higher doses, typically 5 to 10 mg/kg, arterial administration) (Joshi et al. 2000; Sengupta et al. 1996; Sengupta et al. 1999; Su et al. 1997; Su et al. 2002). The inhibitory activity on pelvic afferents is not correlated with the rank order of potency at the cloned KOR1. The response to kappa-agonists cannot be completely antagonized by high doses of non-selective opioid antagonists or selective kappa antagonists (Sengupta et al. 1996; Su et al. 1997). KOR1 antisense oligodeoxynucleotide pretreatment does not alter the response to kappa-agonists (Joshi et al. 2000) and different enantiomers of U50,488, despite marked differences in agonist activity at κ_1–receptors; they are all equally potent and effective in inhibiting the firing of pelvic afferents (Su et al. 2002). Taken together, these data indicate the involvement of a non-opioid mechanism in the response to kappa-agonists in decentralized pelvic afferents. Whole cell patch-clamp experiments performed on rat colonic sensory neurons have established that organic, but not peptidic, kappa-agonists, when used at micromolar concentrations (i.e. about a 1,000–fold higher concentration than those for kappa-agonists activity), have non-opioid sodium channel blocking properties (Joshi et al. 2003).

Clinical Data on Kappa-Agonists in Visceral Pain

Very limited clinical information is available regarding kappa-agonists in visceral pain. Fedotozine was the first compound with kappa-agonist activity to be evaluated for visceral pain in a clinical setting. The compound was superior to placebo in reducing abdominal pain and bloating in non-ulcer dyspepsia (Fraitag et al. 1994) and irritable bowel syndrome (IBS) (Dapoigny et al. 1995). It also increased pain perception thresholds to colonic distension in IBS patients (Delvaux et al. 1999). Fedotozine is an atypical kappa-agonist, being a mixed kappa/mu ligand (Allescher et al. 1991), with high affinity for the κ_{1a}–binding site (Lai et al. 1994), and relatively low affinity for the cloned KOR1 (Lai et al. 1994).

More recently, a pilot study reported that the kappa-agonist, ADL 10-0101, was effective in reducing pain in patients suffering from chronic pancreatitis (Eisenach et al. 2003). ADL 10–0101 is a classical κ_1/KOR[1-]selective agonist combined with peripheral selectivity. The analgesic response appeared to be robust and was not associated with the CNS side-effects of brain penetrating kappa-agonists, suggesting that the compound did not reach the brain, and therefore supporting the hypothesis that its effects were mediated in the periphery. The onset of analgesia was immediate, reaching a plateau within 60 min, and remaining at maximal levels for the duration of the monitoring period (4 hours). During this time interval, the plasma levels of the compound are estimated to have ranged from high nanomolar (first hour, during and after administration) to intermediate/low nanomolar levels (~ 100 nM or less, 3rd and 4th hours). The plasma levels, at least during the last two hours of the study, when visceral analgesia was still maximal, were probably too low to elicit a non-specific sodium channel blockade, but were perfectly suitable to activate κ_1–receptors. Despite these preliminary and encouraging results, more definitive clinical proof of the concept for the therapeutic relevance of peripheral κ_1–receptors in visceral pain is still needed.

Side Effect Profile of Kappa–Agonists

The development and use of kappa-agonists has been limited by their side effects, which include primarily sedation and dysphoria (Rivière and Junien 2000). Unlike mu-agonists, kappa-agonists do not inhibit intestinal transit, induce euphoria, addiction or respiratory depression (Rivière and Junien 2000).

Kappa-Agonists, Targeted Clinical Profile for Visceral Pain

Since the unwanted side effects of kappa-agonists (sedation, dysphoria) are restricted to kappa receptors located in the CNS, i.e. beyond the blood brain barrier, and because the targeted kappa–receptors in visceral pain are located in the periphery, kappa-agonists with high peripheral selectivity are expected to be efficacious and safe for the treatment of visceral pain. Therapeutic indications for peripherally restricted kappa-agonists may include abdominal surgery associated with postoperative pain and ileus, pancreatitis pain, dysmennorhea, labor pain and irritable bowel syndrome.

References

1. Allescher HD, Ahmad S, Classen M, Daniel EE (1991) Interaction of Trimebutine and Jo-1196 (Fedotozine) with Opioid Receptors in the Canine Ileum. J Pharmacol Exp Ther 257:836–842
2. Binder W, Machelska H, Mousa S, Schmitt T, Riviere PJ, Junien JL, Stein C, Schafer M (2001) Analgesic and Anti-Inflammatory Effects of Two Novel Kappa-Opioid Peptides. Anesthesiology 94:1034–1044
3. Burton MB, Gebhart GF (1998) Effects of Kappa-Opioid Receptor Agonists on Responses to Colorectal Distension in Rats With and Without Acute Colonic Inflammation. J Pharmacol Exp Ther 285:707–715
4. Dapoigny M, Abitbol JL, Fraitag B (1995) Efficacy of Peripheral Kappa Agonist Fedotozine versus Placebo in Treatment of Irritable Bowel Syndrome. A Multicenter Dose-Response Study. Dig Dis Sci 40:2244–2249
5. Delvaux M, Louvel D, Lagier E, Scherrer B, Abitbol JL, Frexinos J (1999) The Kappa Agonist Fedotozine Relieves Hypersensitivity to Colonic Distention in Patients with Irritable Bowel Syndrome. Gastroenterology 116:38–45
6. Diop L, Riviere PJ, Pascaud X, Dassaud M, Junien JL (1994a) Role of Vagal Afferents in the Antinociception Produced by Morphine and U–50,488H in the Colonic Pain Reflex in Rats. Eur J Pharmacol 257:181–187
7. Diop L, Riviere PJ, Pascaud X, Junien JL (1994b) Peripheral Kappa-Opioid Receptors Mediate the Antinociceptive Effect of Fedotozine on the Duodenal Pain Reflex in Rat. Eur J Pharmacol 271:65–71
8. Eisenach JC, Carpenter R, Curry R (2003). Analgesia from a Peripherally Active Kappa-Opioid Receptor Agonist in Patients with Chronic Pancreatitis. Pain 101:89–95
9. Fraitag B, Homerin M, Hecketsweiler P (1994) Double-Blind Dose-Response Multicenter Comparison of Fedotozine and Placebo in Treatment of Nonulcer Dyspepsia. Dig Dis Sci 39:1072–1077
10. Friese N, Diop L, Lambert C, Riviere PJ, Dahl SG (1997a) Antinociceptive Effects of Morphine and U-50,488H on Vaginal Distension in the Anesthetized Rat. Life Sci 61:1559–1570
11. Friese N, Chevalier E, Angel F, Pascaud X, Junien JL, Dahl SG, Riviere PJ (1997b) Reversal by Kappa-Agonists of Peritoneal Irritation-Induced Ileus and Visceral Pain in Rats. Life Sci 60:625–634
12. Joshi SK, Lamb K, Bielefeldt K, Gebhart GF (2003) Arylacetamide Kappa-Opioid Receptor Agonists Produce a Tonic- and Use-Dependent Block of Tetrodotoxin-Sensitive and -Resistant Sodium Currents in Colon Sensory Neurons. J Pharmacol Exp Ther 307:367–372
13. Joshi SK, Su X, Porreca F, Gebhart GF (2000) Kappa-Opioid Receptor Agonists Modulate Visceral Nociception at a Novel, Peripheral Site of Action. J Neurosci 20:5874–5879
14. Kamp EH, Jones RC, III, Tillman SR, Gebhart GF (2003) Quantitative Assessment and Characterization of Visceral Nociception and Hyperalgesia in Mice. Am J Physiol Gastrointest Liver Physiol 284:G434–G444
15. Lai J, Ma SW, Zhu RH, Rothman RB, Lentes KU, Porreca F (1994) Pharmacological Characterization of the Cloned Kappa-Opioid Receptor as a Kappa 1b Subtype. Neuroreport 5:2161–2164
16. Langlois A, Diop L, Friese N, Pascaud X, Junien JL, Dahl SG, Riviere PJ (1997) Fedotozine Blocks Hypersensitive Visceral Pain in Conscious Rats: Action at Peripheral Kappa-Opioid Receptors. Eur J Pharmacol 324:211–217
17. Langlois A, Diop L, Riviere PJ, Pascaud X, Junien JL (1994) Effect of Fedotozine on the Cardiovascular Pain Reflex Induced by Distension of the Irritated Colon in the Anesthetized Rat. Eur J Pharmacol 271:245–251
18. Martin WR, Eades CG, Thompson JA, Huppler RE, Gilbert PE (1976) The Effects of Morphine- and Nalorphine-Like Drugs in the Nondependent and Morphine-Dependent Chronic Spinal Dog. J Pharmacol Exp Ther 197:517–532
19. Murphy DM, Koblisch M, Gauntner EK, Little PJ, Gottshall SL, Garver DD, DeHaven-Hudkins DL (2000) A Screening Process for In Vivo Assessment of Blood-Brain Barrier Penetration for Kappa (k) Opioid Receptor Agonists. Drug Metabolism Reviews 32[S2], 179, Abstract
20. Rivière PJM, Junien JL (2000) Opioid Receptors, Targets for New Gastrointestinal Drug Development. In: Gaginella TS, Guglietta A (eds) Drug Development, Molecular Targets for GI Diseases. Humana Press, Totowa, NJ, pp 203–238
21. Riviere PJ, Pascaud X, Chevalier E, Le Gallou B, Junien JL (1993) Fedotozine Reverses Ileus Induced by Surgery or Peritonitis: Action at Peripheral Kappa-Opioid Receptors. Gastroenterology 104:724–731
22. Riviere PJ, Pascaud X, Chevalier E, Junien JL (1994) Fedotozine Reversal of Peritoneal-Irritation-Induced Ileus in Rats: Possible Peripheral Action on Sensory Afferents. J Pharmacol Exp Ther 270:846–850
23. Rivière PJM, Vanderah TW, Porreca F, Houghton R, Schteingart C, Trojnar J, Junien JL (1999) Novel Peripheral Peptidic Kappa-Agonists. Acta Neurobiologiae Experimentalis 59[3], 186, Abstract
24. Rothman RB, Bykov V, De Costa BR, Jacobson AE, Rice KC, Brady LS (1990) Interaction of Endogenous Opioid Peptides and Other Drugs with Four Kappa-Opioid Binding Sites in Guinea Pig Brain. Peptides 11:311–331
25. Sandner-Kiesling A, Pan HL, Chen SR, James RL, DeHaven-Hudkins DL, Dewan DM, Eisenach JC (2002) Effect of Kappa-Opioid Agonists on Visceral Nociception Induced by Uterine Cervical Distension in Rats. Pain 96:13–22
26. Sengupta JN, Snider A, Su X, Gebhart GF (1999) Effects of Kappa-Opioids in the Inflamed Rat Colon. Pain 79:175–185

27. Sengupta JN, Su X, Gebhart GF (1996) Kappa, but not mu or delta, Opioids Attenuate Responses to Distention of Afferent Fibers Innervating the Rat Colon. Gastroenterology 111:968–980
28. Simonin F, Gaveriaux-Ruff C, Befort K, Matthes H, Lannes B, Micheletti G, Mattei MG, Charron G, Bloch B, Kieffer B (1995) Kappa-Opioid Receptor in Humans: cDNA and Genomic Cloning, Chromosomal Assignment, Functional Expression, Pharmacology, and Expression Pattern in the Central Nervous System. Proc Natl Acad Sci USA 92:7006–7010
29. Su X, Joshi SK, Kardos S, Gebhart GF (2002) Sodium Channel Blocking Actions of the Kappa-Opioid Receptor Agonist U50,488 Contribute to its Visceral Antinociceptive Effects. J Neurophysiol 87:1271–1279
30. Su X, Sengupta JN, Gebhart GF (1997) Effects of Opioids on Mechanosensitive Pelvic Nerve Afferent Fibers Innervating the Urinary Bladder of the Rat. J Neurophysiol 77:1566–1580

Oral Opioids

KOK KHOR
Department of Pain Management, Prince of Wales Hospital, Randwick, NSW, Australia
kekhor@bigpond.com

Synonyms

Narcotics, Major Analgesics

Definition

Opioids are drugs chemically related to morphine. They are strong analgesics, used to relieve moderate to severe chronic pain when ► paracetamol and ► NSAIDs, Survey (NSAIDs) are not effective or limited by adverse reactions.

Characteristics

Historical Background

In the form of opium, opioids have been used for centuries to provide relief from pain. In the modern era, the active agents of opium have been isolated, and related compounds have been synthesised in an effort to produce drugs with different potencies and duration of action (Table 1).

Application

Opioids are routinely used to provide relief of pain during and immediately after surgical procedures. They are used to relieve persistent pain in patients with cancer.

They are used to provide relief of severe pain following acute injury. In these applications, there is little or no controversy. Indeed, the use of opioids for these conditions could be regarded as a hallmark of conventional medical practice.

More contentious is the use of opioids for ► chronic pain not caused by cancer, and for which there appears to be no other effective treatment. The vast majority of patients in this state suffer from musculoskeletal pain. In the 1950s, medical opinion considered that the risk of addiction far outweighed the benefits of long-term therapy with opioids, but in 1986 Portenoy and Foley (Portenoy and Foley 1986) reported that opioids could be used effectively and safely for non-cancer pain. Nevertheless, their use has remained controversial. Concerns persist about efficacy, adverse effects, development of tolerance, addiction, drug diversion, and scrutiny of provider prescription by governmental health agencies (Portenoy 1996; Fanciullo and Cobb 2001).

Routes of Administration

Opioids can be administered by a variety of routes. Continuous or intermittent, subcutaneous, intramuscular, or intravenous injections are typically used for postoperative pain, or the pain of acute injury. Intrathecal or epidural routes can be used for postoperative pain and for cancer pain, or other chronic pain. Some preparations are available for rectal, sublingual, intranasal, and transdermal administration. Preparations for oral use are available for patients who are able to swallow, and who can obtain adequate analgesia by this route of administration.

Adverse Effects

Common adverse effects leading to cessation of therapy include constipation, somnolence, confusion, nausea and dizziness (Roth et al. 2000; Caldwell et al. 1999; Peloso et al. 2000). Stable dosing of opioids without concurrent use of other centrally acting drugs generally does not lead to cognitive and psychomotor impairment. Good management of pain often leads to improvement in cognitive function (Fanciullo and Cobb 2001).

With chronic opioid dosing, physical dependence does develop, but patients are often stigmatised by being inaccurately labelled "addicted" (Portenoy 1996). Ad-

Oral Opioids, Table 1 Opioids commonly used in Pain Medicine

Natural Opium Derivatives	Semisynthetic Derivatives	Synthetic Compounds
morphine	diacetylmorphine (heroin)	methadone
codeine	dihydromorphinone	meperidine (pethidine)
	dihydrohydroxymorphinone	fentanyl
	buprenorphine	
	oxycodone	

diction, however, is rare when opioids are used to treat pain, if patients have no prior history of opioid abuse (Portenoy 1996). Whereas addiction is characterised by drug-seeking behaviour, patients with chronic pain seek relief.

A confounding issue is that some individuals feign pain in order to obtain drugs that they subsequently sell-on to addicts. This is perhaps the leading problem currently concerning the use of opioids for chronic pain, for there is no reliable method for detecting fraudulent individuals who obtain opioids for diversion (Portenoy 1996). It is, therefore, imperative that physicians make a valid diagnosis before prescribing opioids, and be alert to potential abuse.

Efficacy

For postoperative pain, cancer pain, and the pain of acute injury, the efficacy of opioids is not questioned. Their obvious and virtually universal effectiveness obviates the need for randomised controlled trials. The only issues in these arenas are securing an optimum dose, which may be very high in some cases, and combating side-effects that may arise.

In the context of chronic musculoskeletal pain, opioids have not been uniformly successful in relieving pain and improving function. Nevertheless, a subpopulation of patients is able to achieve sustained pain-relief without substantial toxicity, functional deterioration or aberrant behaviours (Portenoy 1996; Fanciullo and Cobb 2001; Graziotti and Goucke 1997). The opioid doses required are generally low, and stabilize during long-term administration, suggesting that tolerance is rarely the "driving force" for dose escalation or diminishing efficacy (Roth et al. 2000; Arkinstall et al. 1995; Jamison et al. 1998). A significant number of patients (30–50%) will cease therapy early because of intolerance to adverse events or ineffectiveness (Roth et al. 2000; Caldwell et al. 1999; Moulin et al. 1996). Some will achieve relief when different opioids are used.

Osteoarthritis

Codeine and oxycodone are significantly more effective than placebo (Roth et al. 2000; Caldwell et al. 1999; Peloso et al. 2000) when used for osteoarthritis. Analgesia is accompanied by an improvement in physical function and sleep (Roth et al. 2000; Caldwell et al. 1999; Peloso et al. 2000; Fleischman et al. 1999). After an initial titration period, analgesia is maintained long-term (up to 18 months) (Roth et al. 2000). However, typical opioid related side-effects complicate treatment, and account for a number of patients ceasing therapy (Roth et al. 2000; Caldwell et al. 1999). Since they act by a different mechanism, opioids are synergistic with NSAIDs, and can be used to spare increases in NSAID dose, and thereby avoid seriously adverse effects of NSAIDs (Caldwell et al. 1999).

Low Back Pain

Two trials, although not a third, showed codeine, morphine, and methadone to be more effective than placebo for the relief of pain (Arkinstall et al. 1995; Moulin et al. 1996; Maier et al. 2002). Others have shown that opioids achieve significantly better relief of pain than usual care (Haythornthwaite et al. 1998) or NSAIDs (Jamison et al. 1998).

The degree of relief, however, was only modest. Opioids do not abolish pain. Furthermore, although some have found improvement in function and mood (Arkinstall et al. 1995), others found no improvement in these outcome measures (Moulin et al. 1996). ► Multidisciplinary treatment may be required to accomplish reductions in disability and suffering related to chronic pain (Haythornthwaite et al. 1998).

Management Strategies

Numerous guidelines (Portenoy 1996; Fanciullo and Cobb 2001; Graziotti and Goucke 1997) are available for physicians to identify those patients who might benefit from the long-term use of opioids, to achieve optimal outcomes.

The patient should have objective evidence of organic pathology causing pain, and be psychologically stable, with appropriate mood and behaviour; be reliable; be in a stable social environment; have health-support systems and no prior history of substance abuse (Graziotti and Goucke 1997). Alerting features include unsanctioned dose escalations, continued use despite severe side-effects, manipulative behaviour to obtain more drugs (and from multiple prescribers), hoarding, and diversion of drugs (Portenoy 1996; Graziotti and Goucke 1997). An opioid contract can be used to inform the patient of risks of addiction, tolerance, dependence, and to set limits of opioid use and reasons for discontinuation of therapy (Portenoy 1996; Fanciullo and Cobb 2001).

Only one doctor who has an established therapeutic relationship with the patient should prescribe the opioid and assess the outcome of therapy. Failure to reach predetermined goals is an indication to cease prescribing (Graziotti and Goucke 1997).

Sustained release (morphine, oxycodone) or long acting (methadone) preparations are the drugs of choice because of single or twice-daily dosing and stable blood concentration. Immediate release preparations may be used for dose finding before commencement of sustained release agents, and are useful for breakthrough pain. Intramuscular pethidine is not suitable for chronic use because of its short half life, increased risk of dependence, and potential for central excitatory effects. Codeine is unsuitable because of its short duration of action (Graziotti and Goucke 1997).

A trial of oral opioids can be conducted over four to six weeks, with clearly defined goals and endpoints. A low dose of a sustained-release morphine or oxycodone is started twice-daily, with the outcome assessed after one to two weeks. Patients with fluctuating pain conditions require a variable dosing regimen, with immediate release morphine or oxycodone every 4 hours. Improvement in analgesia should be the minimal requirement, and patients should show improved function. Persistence with opioid therapy is contraindicated if the patient fails to achieve at least partial analgesia at a moderate dose, or if the dose rapidly escalates in opioid-naïve patients within a month of starting treatment. At the end of the trial period, if expected outcomes have not been achieved, the drug dose is tapered over a few days and ceased. Patients who are prescribed opioids on an ongoing basis should be reviewed monthly by the prescribing physician, with a detailed review by a pain management centre undertaken annually, at which analgesic efficacy, level of function, and aberrant behaviour, can be assessed (Graziotti and Goucke 1997).

References

1. Arkinstall W, Sandler A, Goughnour B et al. (1995) Efficacy of Controlled-Release Codeine in Chronic Non-Malignant Pain: A Randomized, Placebo-Controlled Clinical Trial. Pain 62:169–178
2. Caldwell JR, Hale ME, Boyd RE et al. (1999) Treatment of Osteoarthritis Pain with Controlled Release Oxycodone or Fixed Combination Oxycodone Plus Acetaminophen Added to Non-Steroidal Anti-Inflammatory Drugs: A Double-Blind, Randomized, Multicenter, Placebo Controlled Trial. J Rheumatol 26:862–869
3. Fanciullo G, Cobb J (2001) The Use of Opioids for Chronic Non-Cancer Pain. Int J Pain Med & Pall Care 1:49–55
4. Fleischman RM, Kamin M, Olson WH et al. (1999) Safety and Efficacy of Tramadol for the Signs and Symptoms of Osteoarthritis. Arthr Rheum 42:S144
5. Graziotti PJ, Goucke CR (1997) The Use of Oral Opioids in Patients with Chronic Non-Cancer Pain. MJA 167:30–34
6. Haythornthwaite JA, Menefee LA, Quatrano-Piacentini BA et al. (1998) Outcome of Chronic Opioid Therapy for Non-Cancer Pain. J Pain Symptom Manage 15:185–194
7. Jamison RN, Raymond SA, Slawsby EA et al. (1998) Opioid Therapy for Chronic Non-Cancer Back Pain. Spine 23:2591–2600
8. Maier C, Hildebrandt J, Klinger R et al. (2002) Morphine Responsiveness, Efficacy and Tolerability in Patients with Chronic Non-Tumor Associated Pain - Results of a Double-Blind Placebo-Controlled Trial (MONTAS). Pain 97:223–233
9. Moulin DE, Lezzi A, Amireh R et al. (1996) Randomised Trial of Oral Morphine for Chronic Non-Cancer Pain. Lancet 347:143–147
10. Peloso PM Bellamy N, Bensen W et al. (2000) Double-Blind Randomized Placebo Control Trial of Controlled Release Codeine in the Treatment of Osteoarthritis of the Hip or Knee. J Rheumatol 27:764–771
11. Portenoy RK (1996) Opioid Therapy for Chronic Non-Malignant Pain: A Review of the Critical Issues. J Pain Symptom Manage 11:203–217
12. Portenoy R, Foley K (1986) Chronic Use of Opioid Analgesics in Non-Malignant Pain: Report of 38 Cases. Pain 25:171–186
13. Roth SH, Fleishmann RM, Burch FX et al. (2000) Around-the-Clock, Controlled-Release Oxycodone Therapy for Osteoarthritis-Related Pain. Arch Intern Med 160:853–860

Ordinary Cramp

Definition

The term „ordinary" usually includes conditions most frequently referred to as muscle cramps in normal or pathologic conditions, characterized by high-frequency, high-amplitude discharge of potentials on the EMG recordings.

▶ Muscular Cramps

Ordinary Headache

▶ Headache, Episodic Tension Type

Ordine®-morphine-hydrochloride

▶ Postoperative Pain, Morphine

Organ or Body Part Dysfunction

▶ Impairment, Pain-Related

Orofacial Pain, Movement Disorders

PETER SVENSSON
Department of Clinical Oral Physiology, University of Aarhus, Aarhus, Denmark
psvensson@odont.au.dk

Synonyms

Temporomandibular disorders; Mandibular Dysfunction; Muscle Hyperactivity; bruxism; Tremor; oral dystonia, dyskinesia

Definition

Perturbations of normal jaw functions that are either likely to cause pain in orofacial tissues or are the consequences of pain, i.e. a broad and unspecific term that covers a variety of pathophysiological mechanisms and clinical conditions.

Orofacial Pain

Barry J. Sessle[1, 2],
Jonathan O. Dostrovsky[2]
[1]Faculty of Dentistry, University of Toronto,
Toronto, ON, Canada
[2]Department of Physiology, Faculty of Medicine,
University of Toronto, Toronto, ON, Canada
barry.sessle@utoronto.ca,
j.dostrovsky@utoronto.ca

Although pain arising from the craniofacial region shares many features with the pain originating in other body regions, there are several pain conditions that are unique to this region. One of the best known and most prevalent is toothache, which results primarily from activation of nociceptors in the tooth pulp or dentine. A description of the clinical features, pathophysiology and management of dental pain is provided in the essay ► dental pain, etiology, pathogenesis and management. Two other well-known conditions unique to the trigeminal system are trigeminal neuralgia and temporomandibular disorders (TMD) and these are described in the essays ► trigeminal neuralgia, etiology, pathogenesis and management ► temporomandibular joint disorders and ► orofacial pain, movement disorders. Although postherpetic neuralgia can occur outside the orofacial region, facial tissues are often affected; its features are discussed in ► postherpetic neuralgia, etiology, pathogenesis and management. In addition to these well-described pain states, there are several other conditions that are more difficult to classify, diagnose and manage. The best examples of these poorly defined conditions are atypical facial pain and burning mouth syndrome (BMS), which are described in the essay ► atypical facial pain, etiology, pathogenesis and management. The problem of classification and taxonomy of orofacial pain is discussed in the essay ► orofacial pain, taxonomy/classification. The relationships and interactions of pain with sleep and with oral movement disorders (e.g. tremor, dystonia and dyskinesia) and parafunctions such as bruxism are discussed in the essays ► orofacial pain, sleep disturbance and ► orofacial pain, movement disorders. Headaches are of course also very common in the orofacial region and originate primarily as a result of activity in nociceptive afferents innervating the intracerebral vessels and meninges. The clinical features and underlying mechanisms of headaches are covered in ► migraine, pathophysiology and ► non-migraine headaches.

The Scope of Orofacial Pain

In addition to the wide range of pain conditions manifested in the orofacial area, epidemiological studies (e.g. LeResche 2001; Lipton et al. 1993) have revealed the very high prevalence of orofacial pain. Fortunately, some of the chronic conditions that are extremely painful or bothersome (e.g. trigeminal neuralgia, postherpetic neuralgia) are relatively uncommon (see ► trigeminal neuralgia, etiology, pathogenesis and management ► postherpetic neuralgia, etiology, pathogenesis and management). However, conditions such as TMD, BMS, headaches and toothaches are quite common and collectively have a prevalence of 10–15% or more in different populations (see ► temporomandibular joint disorders ► atypical facial pain, etiology, pathogenesis and management ► dental pain, etiology, pathogenesis and management ► migraine, pathophysiology and ► non-migraine headaches). Translated into worldwide figures, this means that at any one time TMD for example affects half a billion persons around the world! Studies in humans have drawn attention to the female predominance and to the importance of psychosocial influences as predisposing or modulating influences in many of these conditions, especially those that are chronic in nature and to the enormous economic as well as social costs of orofacial pain (Feinmann and Newton-John 2004; LeResche 2001; Sessle 2000). For example, changes in mental state (e.g. pain affect, depression) and sleep are frequent accompaniments of pain, as noted in the essays ► orofacial pain, sleep disturbance and ► temporomandibular joint disorders and there is evidence that in some situations pain may be the cause of these changes, in other cases the consequence. Also, the annual health care costs plus lost productivity, compensation, etc for pain are in the order of $120B in the USA alone (see ► Pain in the Workplace, Compensation and Disability Management). By conservative estimates, orofacial pain including headache would represent a third of these costs and so the cost to the US economy of orofacial pain each year is approximately $40B! Added to this economic burden is the personal suffering and disrupted quality of life of the orofacial pain patient and their interactions with family and friends. As pointed out in the various essays cited above, there have been some important advances in our knowledge of the clinical features and possible underlying mechanisms, although much remains to be learned and adequate therapy is still lacking in many cases.

Aetiology and Pathogenesis of Orofacial Pain Conditions

The aetiology and underlying processes of most acute pain conditions occurring in the face and mouth are now reasonably well understood, although there are still several points requiring clarification, as outlined in ► nociceptive processing in the brainstem. We now know for example that trauma, dental caries or infection are the most common causes of acute pain from the tooth, as pointed out in ▶ dental pain, etiology, pathogenesis and management, although the precise mechanisms and factors involved in the activation or sensitization of pulpal or dentinal afferents are not fully resolved (see ▶ nociceptors in the dental pulp). However, the biological processes giving rise to chronic orofacial pain are still poorly understood and it is clear from several essays on this topic that the aetiology of most of the chronic pain conditions expressed in the orofacial region is unclear and that their pathogenesis is still unresolved. This has impacted upon their diagnosis and management and even upon the classification schemes used to describe these conditions (see below and also ▶ orofacial pain, taxonomy/classification). The predisposing or risk factors related to each of these conditions are also poorly understood and this is exemplified by our limited ability to explain the female predominance in most of these chronic pain conditions. Nonetheless, with the recent emphasis on the need for a scientific underpinning and for an evidence basis for diagnostic and management approaches advocated for orofacial pain, some long-held beliefs are being laid to rest. For example, the past emphasis on occlusal factors, including sleep bruxism, as being of prime aetiological importance in TMD and related conditions, has not held up to scientific scrutiny, as the essays ▶ temporomandibular joint disorders and ▶ orofacial pain, sleep disturbance, and recent systematic reviews (e.g. Forssell and Kalso 2004) have pointed out. But we clearly have a long way to go to identify the aetiological mechanisms and risk factors predisposing to most of the chronic orofacial pain states. There is in particular a need for longitudinal population based studies to help define the factors that have been implicated for most conditions (e.g. gender, genetic, age, comorbidity, trauma).

There is also a need for a greater emphasis on the development of animal models to help improve our understanding of the aetiology and pathogenesis of these conditions. Many of the current concepts on orofacial pain mechanisms draw largely upon findings from spinal models of chronic pain. Given the uniqueness of some of the orofacial pain conditions (e.g. trigeminal neuralgia, BMS), there is a need to apply and test these concepts within the framework of the trigeminal system by developing chronic orofacial pain models. Recent approaches that show much promise for improving our understanding of inflammatory or neuropathic orofacial pain conditions include the use of inflammatory irritants or complete Freund's adjuvant in inducing musculoskeletal pain (e.g. Dubner and Ren 2004; Henry 2004; Ren and Dubner 1999; Woda and Pionchon 2000) and of trigeminal nerve damage in evoking nociceptive pain (Iwata et al. 2004; Woda and Pionchon 2000). From the limited trigeminal studies to date (see below) and from analogous studies in animal models of pain in the spinal system (see ▶ animal models and experimental tests to study nociception and pain and ▶ peripheral neuropathic pain), the mechanisms that appear to be involved in the pathogenesis of these chronic orofacial pain states include ectopic impulses generated in damaged afferent fibres, peripheral sensitization of afferent fibres, central sensitization of central nociceptive neurones, changes in segmental and descending inhibitory and facilitatory influences on nociceptive transmission and phenotypic changes in afferent fibres and central nociceptive neurones, including enhanced sympathetic modulation of afferent fibres and central sprouting of afferent fibres (see ▶ nociceptive processing in the brainstem). It has been suggested for instance that abnormal firing of trigeminal primary afferents leading to changes in central nociceptive pathways may be important in trigeminal neuralgia and neuropathic orofacial pain conditions (e.g. Devor et al. 2002; Iwata et al. 2004). Also, findings from inflammatory trigeminal models have led to suggestions (Hargreaves 2001; Sessle 1999; Sessle 2000) that both peripheral sensitization and central sensitisation may explain the allodynia, hyperalgesia, diffuse and often referred pain and limitations of jaw movements that are characteristic of TMD (see ▶ orofacial pain, movement disorders and ▶ temporomandibular joint disorders) or several types of toothache including the "hot" tooth (see ▶ dental pain, etiology, pathogenesis and management). The animal models and correlated human studies also draw attention to the close interplay between pain and other CNS functions, such as sleep, anxiety and depression (see ▶ orofacial pain, sleep disturbance) and between sensory and motor systems in the expression of acute or chronic orofacial pain (see ▶ orofacial pain, movement disorders). While Svensson (see essay ▶ orofacial pain, movement disorders) also notes that a pain adaptation may apply in TMD, future research of this model needs to explain the cause of the pain and address the long-term motor consequences of chronic pain.

Classification and Diagnostic Approaches and Issues

There is clearly a need for a practical, comprehensive and unified classification system for the variety of pain conditions that occur in the orofacial region. Zakrzewska (2004) has noted that classification schemes need to be valid, reliable, comprehensive, flexible and generalizable, but this is certainly not the case for orofacial pain. As revealed in ▶ orofacial pain, taxonomy/classification, several classification schemes for orofacial pain have been developed, but there is disagreement or inconsistency between them on a number of points. There has recently been a move towards a mechanisms based classification, but application of such a scheme to orofacial pain or indeed pain elsewhere in the body is stymied by a lack of clear definition of the specific mechanisms applicable to the development and maintenance of each of these conditions, especially many of the neuropathic pain states (see ▶ peripheral neuropathic pain and ▶ neuropathic pain of central origin).

Also related to the classification issues are the difficulties associated with differential diagnosis of orofacial pain conditions. While some orofacial pain states are reasonably well defined and readily discernable (e.g. trigeminal neuralgia, postherpetic neuralgia see ▶ trigeminal neuralgia, etiology, pathogenesis and management; ▶ postherpetic neuralgia, etiology, pathogenesis and management), many are complicated by vague or varying symptomatology, referral of pain, depression and concomitant pain elsewhere in the body (e.g. some toothaches, TMD; see ▶ dental pain, etiology, pathogenesis and management and ▶ temporomandibular joint disorders) or are diagnosed by exclusion (e.g. atypical facial pain, see ▶ atypical facial pain, etiology, pathogenesis and management). As a consequence of these features, it is not uncommon for a condition to be misdiagnosed and inappropriate therapy instituted (Truelove 2004; Vickers et al. 1998; also see below).

There are also available a multitude of diagnostic and assessment approaches that have been developed for orofacial pain (see ▶ dental pain, etiology, pathogenesis and management ▶ atypical facial pain, etiology, pathogenesis and management ▶ temporomandibular joint disorders ▶ orofacial pain, movement disorders). Clinical examination procedures, radiographic scans and common sensory assessment techniques (e.g. tooth pulp vitality tests) have long been mainstays of clinical diagnostic approaches. Over the past 2–3 decades, there have been substantive improvements in a number of these approaches that have been specifically developed for chronic as well as acute orofacial pains. While many of these particular approaches are not part of standard clinical practice, they have found extensive application in experimental or clinical studies of these conditions, and include pressure pain or tolerance thresholds, visual analogue scales, McGill pain questionnaire, quantitative sensory testing (QST), and magnetic resonance imaging (e.g. Bushnell 2001; Eliav et al. 2004; Essick 2004; Jaaskelainen 2004; Svensson et al. 2004). Although some of the orofacial pain states have reliable and validated diagnostic approaches, e.g. the research diagnostic criteria for TMD (see ▶ temporomandibular joint disorders), there are not yet any 'gold standards' for diagnosis of most of the conditions (Eliav et al. 2004; Essick 2004; Goulet 2001; Jaaskelainen 2004; Svensson et al. 2004). Clearly there is room for further development and standardization and validation of assessment and diagnostic techniques for orofacial pain.

Management Approaches and Issues

Some orofacial pain conditions, especially those that are chronic in nature, are often dealt with by medical specialists, but the dentist is the front line clinician for most orofacial pain conditions. Indeed dentists have been at the forefront in developing therapeutic procedures to control pain, a prime example being the introduction of gas anesthesia 160 years ago by dentists. Through these and subsequent developments, nearly all acute orofacial pain and procedural pain can be readily controlled and managed by general anesthetics, local anesthetics, analgesic drugs, etc. A case in point is the variety of management approaches available to the clinician for acute toothache (see ▶ dental pain, etiology, pathogenesis and management). Similarly, for the chronic orofacial pain conditions, a multitude of approaches are available and several so-called alternative medicine approaches (e.g. acupuncture, herbal remedies) have additionally become widely available over the past 2 decades. The essays on ▶ temporomandibular joint disorders; ▶ atypical facial pain, etiology, pathogenesis and management; ▶ trigeminal neuralgia, etiology, pathogenesis and management; ▶ postherpetic neuralgia, etiology, pathogenesis and management as well as recent extensive reviews (e.g. Forssell and Kalso 2004; Stohler and Zarb 1999; Truelove 2004; Watson 2004; Widmer 2001) have noted that while some of these techniques have proven efficacy for certain orofacial pain conditions (e.g. trigeminal neuralgia, postherpetic neuralgia), the efficacy of most management approaches currently in use has not been validated or fully tested for their specificity and sensitivity. Indeed, several common management strategies have a limited scientific underpinning and so in a sense it could be argued that some conditions are often overtreated or have inappropriate treatment rendered. One example is the case of occlusal adjustments for TMD. Another is the not uncommon misdiagnosis of cases of atypical facial pain or trigeminal neuralgia where as a consequence the therapy instituted may be inappropriate and may be associated with an exacerbation of the pain and suffering of the patient (e.g. Truelove 2004; Vickers et al. 1998) (see ▶ atypical facial pain, etiology, pathogenesis and management).

Such considerations emphasize the need for well-designed cohort studies, randomized controlled trials (RCTs) etc to test the efficacy, validity, specificity, sensitivity and reliability of a number of management and diagnostic strategies currently in use for pain in the face and mouth, as well as the need for an increased focus on enhancing pain educational programmes for health professionals and students who will be called upon to care for patients with orofacial pain (Attanasio 2002; Sessle 2003; Widmer 2001).

Concluding Remarks

The challenges ahead in clarifying the mechanisms underlying the aetiology and pathogenesis of orofacial pain offer the reward of better diagnostic and management approaches than currently exist. Management approaches for many of these conditions are relatively ineffective or unproven (e.g. BMS) or are varied in view of the so-called multifactorial nature of the condition (e.g. TMD). Nonetheless, emerging technologies in imaging, sensory testing (e.g. QST), biological markers and molecular biology hold out promise of improved therapeutic approaches for these conditions.
► Psychiatric Aspects of Pain and Dentistry

References

1. Attanasio R (2002) The study of temporomandibular disorders and orofacial pain from the perspective of the predoctoral dental curriculum. J Orofac Pain 16:176–180
2. Bushnell MC (2001) Perception and behavioral modulation of pain. In: Lund JP, Lavigne GJ, Dubner R, Sessle BJ (eds) Orofacial Pain. From Basic Science to Clinical Management. Quintessence, Chicago, pp 107–114
3. Devor M, Amir R, Rappaport ZH (2002) Pathophysiology of trigeminal neuralgia: the ignition hypothesis. Clin J Pain 18:4–13
4. Dubner R, Ren K (2004) Brainstem mechanisms of persistent pain following injury. J Orofac Pain 18:299–305
5. Eliav E, Gracely RH, Nahlieli O, Benoliel R (2004) Quantitative sensory testing in trigeminal nerve damage assessment. J Orofac Pain 18:339–344
6. Essick GK (2004) Psychophysical assessment of patients with posttraumatic neuropathic trigeminal pain. J Orofac Pain 18:345–354
7. Feinmann C, Newton–John T (2004) Psychiatric and psychological management consideration associated with nerve damage and neuropathic trigeminal pain. J Orofac Pain 18:360–365
8. Forssell H, Kalso E (2004) Application of principles of evidence–based medicine to occlusal treatment for temporomandibular disorders: Are there lessons to be learned? J Orofac Pain 18:9–22
9. Goulet J–P (2001) The path to diagnosis. In: Lund JP, Lavigne GJ, Dubner R et al. (eds) Orofacial Pain. From Basic Science to Clinical Management. Quintessence, Chicago, pp 167–182
10. Hargreaves KM (2001) Neurochemical factors in injury and inflammation of orofacial tissues. In: Lund JP, Lavigne GJ, Dubner R et al. (eds) Orofacial Pain. From Basic Science to Clinical Management. Quintessence, Chicago, pp 59–66
11. Henry JL (2004) Future basic science directions into mechanisms of neuropathic pain. J Orofac Pain 18:306–310
12. Iwata K, Tsuboi Y, Shima A et al. (2004) Central neuronal changes after nerve injury: neuroplastic influences of injury and aging. J Orofac Pain 18:293–298
13. Jaaskelainen SK (2004) The utility of clinical neurophysiological and quantitative sensory testing for trigeminal neuropathy. J Orofac Pain 18:355–359
14. LeResche L (2001) Epidemiology of orofacial pain. In: Lund JP, Lavigne GJ, Dubner R et al. (eds) Orofacial Pain. From Basic Science to Clinical Management. Quintessence, Chicago, pp 15–25
15. Lipton JA, Ship JA, Larach-Robinson D (1993) Estimated prevalence and distribution of reported orofacial pain in the United States. J Am Dent Assoc 124:115–121
16. Ren K, Dubner R (1999) Central nervous system plasticity and persistent pain. J Orofac Pain 13:155–163
17. Sessle BJ (1999) The neural basis of temporomandibular joint and masticatory muscle pain. J Orofac Pain 13:238–245
18. Sessle BJ (2000) Acute and chronic craniofacial pain: brainstem mechanisms of nociceptive transmission and neuroplasticity, and their clinical correlates. Crit Rev Oral Biol Med 11:57–91
19. Sessle BJ (2003) Outgoing president's address: Issues and Initiatives in pain education, communication, and research. In: Proceedings of the 10th World Congress on Pain. IASP Press, Seattle, pp 3–12
20. Stohler CS, Zarb GA (1999) On the management of temporomandibular disorders: a plea for a low-tech, high-prudence therapeutic approach. J Orofac Pain 13:255–261
21. Svensson P, Baad-Hansen L, Thygesen T et al. (2004) Overview on tools and methods to assess neuropathic trigeminal pain. J Orofac Pain 18:332–338
22. Truelove E (2004) Management issues of neuropathic trigeminal pain from a dental perspective. J Orofac Pain 18:374–380
23. Vickers ER, Cousins MJ, Walker S et al. (1998) Analysis of 50 patients with atypical odontalgia. A preliminary report on pharmacological procedures for diagnosis and treatment. Oral Surg Oral Med Oral Pathol Oral Radiol Endod 85:24–32.
24. Watson CPN (2004) Management issues of neuropathic trigeminal pain from a medical perspective. J Orofac Pain 18:366–373
25. Widmer CG (2001) Current beliefs and educational guidelines. In: Lund JP, Lavigne GJ, Dubner R et al. (eds) Orofacial Pain. From Basic Science to Clinical Management. Quintessence, Chicago, pp 27–36
26. Woda A, Pionchon P (2000) A unified concept of idiopathic orofacial pain: pathophysiologic features. J Orofac Pain 14:196–212
27. Zakrzewska JM (2004) Classification issues related to neuropathic trigeminal pain. J Orofac Pain 18:325–331

0

Characteristics

Normal jaw-motor functions involve fast, precise, highly coordinated and pain-free movement of the mandible during chewing, swallowing, speech, yawning etc. Deviation from normal jaw movements can be recognized as altered range of motion, irregular movements, postural changes and eventually noises such as clicking or grating sounds from the temporomandibular joint (TMJ). There has been a longstanding "chicken or egg" debate in the dental community, whether changes in jaw-motor function will cause pain or pain will cause changes in jaw-motor function. However, syntheses of recent experimental and clinical studies have provided a better description of the relationship between different types of orofacial pain complaints and jaw-motor function.

Temporomandibular Disorders (TMD)

TMD pains are considered a cluster of related pain conditions in the masticatory muscles, TMJ and associated structures, i.e. a form of orofacial musculoskeletal pain. The chewing pattern in patients with TMD pains differ in several characteristic ways compared to control subjects (Stohler 1999). For example, the movements of the mandible are smaller and tend to be more irregular, and the average and maximum opening velocity are slower. In accordance, it has been shown that TMD pain patients have a significantly longer duration of the chewing cycle. Furthermore, the jaw-closing muscles (masseter, temporalis) are significantly less activated during the agonist phase (jaw-closing), but significantly increased during the antagonist phase (jaw-opening) in TMD pain patients. The maximal voluntary ▶ occlusal force and electromyographic (EMG) activity are also reduced, and the endurance time at submaximal contractions is significantly shorter when compared with control subjects (Svensson and Graven-Nielsen 2001). With the mandible in its rest or ▶ postural position (normally 2–3 mm distance between the teeth), increased EMG activity, frequently referred to as muscle hyperactivity, has sometimes been reported in the jaw-closing muscles of TMD pain patients when compared to control subjects. However, firm conclusions have not been reached due to confounding factors in the studies, such as EMG cross-talk from facial muscles, inadequate control groups and prevalence of bruxism (see later). Recently, very small (1–2 μV) EMG increases have been found in well-controlled studies, although the diagnostic and pathophysiological significance of this finding remains unclear. It has also been reported that TMD pain patients may have abnormalities in mandibular kinaesthesia, which could influence the rest position of the mandible, and possibly underlie the common perception in TMD pain patients that the teeth do not fit together properly.

Traditionally, the interaction between pain and jaw-motor function has been explained by the vicious cycle concept, where muscle hyperactivity leads to pain and pain reinforces the muscle hyperactivity (Travell et al. 1942). The dental version of the vicious cycle was thought to be initiated by misalignment of the teeth (malocclusion), leading to changes in postural activity and chewing patterns. However, this stereotyped relation between pain and jaw-motor function was challenged in a series of critical papers (Lund et al. 1991). Furthermore, it was pointed out that comparable findings with slower movements and less EMG activity in the agonist phase, and more EMG activity in the antagonist phase, could also be observed during other dynamic motor tasks like gait and other repetitive movements in various musculoskeletal pain conditions (Graven-Nielsen et al. 2000). Analyses of the literature led to the formulation of the pain-adaptation model,

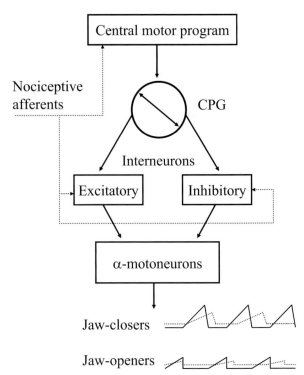

Orofacial Pain, Movement Disorders, Figure 1 Highly schematic presentation of the pain-adaptation model modified after Lund et al. 1991. Thin nociceptive afferents (dotted lines) from orofacial tissues influence both the central motor program and the central pattern generator (CPG) and networks with excitatory and inhibitory interneurons in the brainstem. There is a shift in the normal drive to the alpha-motoneuron pool so that the jaw-closing muscles are less activated (dotted line) during pain in their agonist phase and more activated in their antagonist phase. The same is true for the jaw-opening muscles. The consequences of this reorganization of the motor function are slower and smaller jaw movements.

which strongly contrasts with the vicious cycle model (Lund et al. 1991) (Fig. 1). The pain-adaptation model predicts that the consequences of orofacial nociceptive inputs to premotoneurons in the brainstem during agonist function are a facilitation of inhibitory pathways to the alpha-motor neurons, and during antagonist function a facilitation of excitatory pathways. The essential prerequisite for the model is a collection of premotorneurons, constituting the ▶ central pattern generator in the brainstem and groups of inhibitory and excitatory interneurons. The pain-adaptation model explains many of the jaw-motor consequences of TMD pain, but does not provide any explanation for the origin of the pain. Nevertheless, the pain-adaptation model has made it clear that no causal link between changes in jaw-motor function (mandibular dysfunction) and pain can be derived from cross-sectional clinical studies, because pain in itself has a significant influence on jaw-motor function. Johansson and Sojka (1991) presented an alternative model to explain muscle tension and spread of muscle pain, which integrates the gamma-motoneuron system and, most recently the sympathetic nervous system in the pathophysiological mechanisms. Further research will be necessary to test the hypotheses and pivotal parts of these different models.

Human experimental pain studies have nevertheless helped to clarify the interaction between orofacial pain and jaw-motor function. It has been shown that painful injections of e.g. hypertonic saline into the human masseter muscle, causes a reduction of the agonist EMG burst during empty open-close jaw-movements and during gum-chewing (Lund et al. 1991; Svensson et al. 1996). Experimental masseter pain also reduces the maximum displacement of the mandible in the lateral and vertical axes, and slows down the maximum velocity during jaw-opening and jaw-closing. Thus, experimental muscle pain studies have consistently shown a decrease in agonist EMG activity in the range of 10–15%, a small increase in the antagonist EMG activity and modest reductions in maximum displacements. These findings are in accordance with other experimental pain studies and recording of muscle activity during gait and repetitive shoulder movements in humans (Graven-Nielsen et al. 2000). In relation to the postural EMG activity, a small, but significant, increase in the EMG activity of the jaw-closing muscles, both during hypertonic saline-evoked pain and during the imagination of pain, has been demonstrated (Stohler 1999). Furthermore, ▶ experimental jaw muscle pain is associated with a short (<30–60 s) increase in EMG activity recorded with either intramuscular wire or surface EMG electrodes (Svensson and Graven-Nielsen 2001). Generally, the magnitude of these increases in human EMG activity is comparatively small in the jaw-closing muscles and relatively short-lived, which does not seem to justify the term muscle hyperactivity.

The experimental findings in humans are furthermore supported by observations in animal preparations of mastication. In decerebrated rabbits with cortically-driven mastication, noxious pressure applied to the zygoma or intramuscular injection of hypertonic saline causes a significant reduction in the agonist EMG burst, significant increases in the duration of the masticatory cycle, and significantly smaller amplitudes (Westberg et al. 1997). Thus, dynamic jaw-motor function seems to be reflexly changed by nociceptive activity. The relatively small EMG changes in the human jaw-closing muscles with the mandible at rest contrast with the significant EMG increases (300–400%) observed in animal studies using intramuscular EMG electrodes to record nocifensive reflex jaw responses following noxious stimulation of TMJ or muscle tissue (e.g. Hu et al. 1993; Cairns et al. 1998). The evidence of facilitation of EMG activity in both jaw-closing and jaw-opening muscles of rats and cats, following injection of various algesic substances into the deep craniofacial tissues, indicates that nociceptive afferents supplying these tissues activate excitatory pathways projecting to the alpha-motoneuron pools of the jaw-opening and jaw-closing muscles (Sessle 2000). The co-contraction of the jaw-opening and jaw-closing muscles may serve as a "splinting" effect and reduce jaw movements (Sessle 2000), in accordance with the pain adaptation model (Lund et al. 1991), although the finding that noxious stimulation induces co-activation of these muscles at rest may not be entirely consistent with this model.

However, animal and human studies could differ in some aspects. For example, human pain studies are performed in conscious human beings, and the influence of higher-order brain centers cannot be excluded. The finding that chewing sometimes increases the perceived intensity of pain also suggests that higher-order brain centers could contribute to pain-induced changes in chewing. Furthermore, human studies are performed with a food bolus in the mouth, whereas many of the animal studies have usually involved empty open-close jaw-movements. The motor programs related to such different types of jaw-movements could also be differentially influenced by pain. Nevertheless, the human experimental and animal studies are in general agreement with each other, and in general, support the pain-adaptation model.

In summary, the sensory-motor integration in patients with TMD pain seems to apply to the pain-adaptation model. Several human experimental pain studies and animal trials substantiate this hypothesis. However, there are still important issues that will need to be explained. For example, the pain-adaptation model cannot explain the origin of pain. Moreover, the long-term consequences of an adapted jaw-motor function to a chronic painful input is unknown, and there might be conditions where the jaw muscles are not "allowed" to adapt, e.g. when the same load or work is required.

Bruxism and Oral Parafunctions

Bruxism is considered an involuntary activity of the jaw muscles, which is characterized in subjects who are awake by jaw clenching and sometimes tooth gnashing and grinding (Lavigne et al. 2003). In sleep bruxism, both jaw clenching and tooth grinding are observed. The jaw muscle activity can be classified as either rhythmic (phasic), sustained (tonic) or a mixture of both types (Lavigne et al. 2003). It is estimated that about 8% of the adult population are sleep bruxers, but as many as 60% will demonstrate some form of rhythmic masticatory muscle activity. Thus, sleep bruxism can be viewed as an exaggerated normal behavior, which in some cases can be associated with significant destruction of the teeth. A point of discussion has been if sleep bruxism is related to TMD pain. About 20–30% of sleep bruxers report jaw muscle pain, which could either be due to a kind of localized post-exercise muscle soreness, or alternatively, a generalized muscle pain condition like fibromyalgia. However, several studies have now found that patients with the most jaw muscle EMG activity during sleep are actually those with the fewest muscle symptoms. One consideration is that protective mechanisms in painful conditions will also prevent the overuse of muscles during sleep.

Human experimental studies have nevertheless clearly shown that sustained voluntary EMG activity (grinding or clenching) of a certain intensity and duration can lead to symptoms both in jaw muscles and TMJs (e.g. Arima et al. 1999); however, the level of pain is rather low and short-lived in accordance with the notion that jaw muscles are extremely fatigue-resistant. The current view is, therefore, that bruxism and other parafunctional jaw activities are only modest risk factors for the development or maintenance of TMD pain.

Tremor, Orofacial Dystonia and Dyskinesia

The human mandible trembles at about 3–8 Hz when it is in its rest position with the jaw muscles relaxed, although the amplitude of this movement is too low to be detected visually (Jaberzedah et al. 2003). There is evidence that the mandible in the rest position is under a "pulsatile control", where fluctuating activity in central neural pulse generators activate both the jaw-opening and jaw-closing alpha-motoneurons. Recently, it was shown that hypertonic saline-evoked pain in the masseter muscle caused a reduction in the power of the resting jaw tremor (Jaberzadeh et al. 2003). This indicates that jaw muscle pain is capable of tonically modulating the amplitude of the outputs from the central "pulsatile control" generators that drive the alternating activation of antagonistic muscles, which produce jaw tremor at rest and during jaw movements.

For completeness, neurological conditions such as oral dyskinesia and dystonia will also be briefly mentioned, since they can be associated with orofacial pain complaints. Mandibular dyskinesia is involuntary, often continuous, repetitive movements of the tongue, lips, cheeks and jaw (Clark and Takeuchi 1995), and can be linked to withdrawal of neuroleptics (tardive dyskinesia). Orofacial dystonia is also involuntary, intermittent and momentarily sustained contraction of the orofacial or jaw muscles, which are normally only present during wakefulness. The pathophysiology may involve disorders of the central motor pathways and in particular the basal ganglia. Pain in these conditions is traditionally thought to be due to excessive muscle contractions.

In summary, movement disorders and orofacial pain covers a wide range of clinical conditions with different pathophysiological mechanisms and manifestations.

References

1. Arima T, Svensson P, Arendt-Nielsen L (1999) Experimental Grinding in Healthy Subjects: A Model for Post-Exercise Jaw Muscle Soreness. J Orofac Pain 13:104–114
2. Cairns BE, Sessle BJ, Hu JW (1998) Evidence that Excitatory Amino Acid Receptors within the Temporomandibular Joint Region are Involved in the Reflex Activation of the Jaw Muscles. J Neurosci 18:8056–8064
3. Clark GT, Takeuchi H (1995) Temporomandibular Dysfunction, Chronic Orofacial Pain and Oral Motor Disorders in the 21st Century. Calif Dent Assoc J 23:41–50
4. Graven-Nielsen T, Svensson P, Arendt-Nielsen L (2000) Effect of Muscle Pain on Motor Control: A Human Experimental Approach. Adv Physiother 2:26–38
5. Hu JW, Yu X-M, Vernon H, Sessle BJ (1993) Excitatory Effects on Neck and Jaw Muscle Activity of Inflammatory Irritant Applied to Cervical Paraspinal Tissues. Pain 55:243–250
6. Jaberzadeh S, Svensson P, Nordstrom MA, Miles TS (2003) Differential Modulation of Tremor and Pulsatile Control of Human Jaw and Finger by Experimental Muscle Pain. Exp Brain Res 150:520–524
7. Johansson H, Sojka P (1991) Pathophysiological Mechanisms Involved in Genesis and Spread of Muscular Tension in Occupational Muscle Pain. Med Hypotheses 135:196–203
8. Lavigne GJ, Kato T, Kolta A, Sessle BJ (2003) Neurobiological Mechanisms Involved in Sleep Bruxism. Crit Rev Oral Biol Med 14:30–46
9. Lund JP, Donga R, Widmer CG, Stohler CS (1991) The Pain-Adaptation Model: A Discussion of the Relationship between Chronic Musculoskeletal Pain and Motor Activity. Can J Physiol Pharmacol 69:683–694
10. Sessle BJ (2000) Acute and Chronic Craniofacial Pain: Brainstem Mechanisms of Nociceptive Transmission and Neuroplasticity, and their Clinical Correlates. Crit Rev Oral Biol Med 11:57–91
11. Stohler CS (1999) Craniofacial Pain and Motor Function: Pathogenesis, Clinical Correlates, and Implications. Crit Rev Oral Biol Med 10:504–518
12. Svensson P, Arendt-Nielsen L, Houe L (1996) Sensory-Motor Interactions of Human Experimental Unilateral Jaw Muscle Pain: A Quantitative Analysis. Pain 64:241–249
13. Svensson P, Graven-Nielsen T (2001) Craniofacial Muscle Pain: Review of Mechanisms and Clinical Manifestations. J Orofac Pain 15:117–145
14. Travell J Rinzler S Herman M (1942) Pain and Disability of the Shoulder and Arm. Treatment by Intramuscular Infiltration with Procaine Hydrochloride. J Am Med Assoc 120:417–422
15. Westberg K-G, Clavelou P, Schwartz G, Lund JP (1997) Effects of Chemical Stimulation of Masseter Muscle Nociceptors on Trigeminal Motoneuron and Interneuron Activities during Fictive Mastication in the Rabbit. Pain 73:295–308

Orofacial Pain, Sleep Disturbance

Giles J. Lavigne
Facultés de Médecine Dentaire et de Médecine, Université de Montréal, Montréal, QC, Canada
gilles.lavigne@umontreal.ca

Synonyms

Sleep Disturbance; Poor Sleep Quality

Definition

Chronic pain is a major cause of ► sleep disturbances and complaints. Its major influence is to increase the magnitude and/or the frequency of arousal and ► awakening in sleep. A day with intense pain could be followed by sleep of poor quality, and poor sleep may be followed by more pain on the next day.

Characteristics

Sleep is a physiological state usually characterized by isolation from the environment, except when an unpleasant, potentially harmful or life-threatening event occurs. During sleep, sensory perception is attenuated to prevent sleep disruption by non-relevant input in order to promote sleep consolidation. The perception of pain in sleep should rather be termed nociception, since sleep is associated with an altered state of consciousness. The presence of pain during wakefulness, as well as the intrusion of pain in the sleeping period, are potentially associated with fatigue and lower sleep quality (e.g. complaints of non-restorative sleep), daytime sleepiness and risk of accidents, low memory performance, etc. Although the influence of chronic orofacial muscle and/or temporomandibular joint pain on sleep does not differ from that of pain in other parts of the body, the impact of trigeminal neuralgia or neuropathy on sleep is unknown.

Epidemiology and Risk Factors

It is well known that ≈2/3 of chronic orofacial pain patients report poor sleep quality (Dao et al. 1994; Morin et al. 1998; Riley III et al. 2001; Yatani et al. 2002). The exacerbation of poor sleep in chronic pain patients could be associated with several risk factors:

1. Anxiety, catastrophising, depression, etc.
2. Alcohol, caffeine, nicotine and medications known to disturb sleep (e.g. cardio-active drugs, analgesics)
3. Sleep disorders such as insomnia, sleep apnea, periodic limb movement in sleep

Chronic pain patients frequently experience insomnia with an odds ratio of 1.5–2.0 (Moldofsky 2001). Risk factors in chronic orofacial muscle pain (e.g. myofascial pain alone or with temporomandibular arthralgia) include a history of trauma, jaw clenching habit, somatization and female gender (Huang et al. 2002). However, the link between orofacial pain and tooth grinding during sleep, termed sleep bruxism, is much less clear: only 1 sleep bruxism patient in 5 shows such a relation in the presence of objective sleep measures carried out in the laboratory. Sleep related headache and occasional temporomandibular joint lock or sounds are not uncommon. Sleep complaints with generalized pain sensitivity are not specific to the orofacial pain population, since they are found in the presence of other symptoms such as bowel complaints and frequent headaches that occur with chronic fatigue syndrome, fibromyalgia and temporomandibular disorders (Aaron et al. 2000; Moldofsky 2001).

Interaction Between Pain and Sleep

In most cases, a new pain episode will precede complaints of poor sleep (Morin et al. 1998; Riley III et al. 2001). By contrast, when chronic pain sets in (e.g. burn pain after a few days, fibromyalgia) a vicious circle is reported: a day with high pain is followed by a night of poor sleep, and sleep of poor quality is followed by reports of higher pain the next day (Raymond et al. 2001). However, this interaction only explains a low percentage of the variability in pain and sleep complaints; other influences such as physical and/or psychological disabilities, fatigue, depression and the risk factors mentioned above also have to be factored into the equation (Nicassio et al. 2002; McCracken and Iverson 2002).

Sleep Architecture and Pain

A normal sleep period is characterized by alternated ► sleep stages (light St 1&2 to deep St 3&4 to Rapid Eye Movement (REM) sleep) that occur 3–5 times in a normal sleep period of 7–9 hours. We usually spend approximately 50–65% of a night in St 1&2, 20–25% in St 3&4, and 10–20% in REM sleep. The roles of sleep are to recover from fatigue, maintain cognitive function (e.g. memory consolidation and performance, concentration) and help overall biological regeneration. Sleep disruption (e.g. fragmentation) that interferes with sleep continuity is reported to induce some complaints of fatigue and poor cognitive performance the next day. Interestingly, recent findings have suggested that when sleep is restricted to 4 and 6 hours per day for 14 days, subjects showed deficits in cognitive performance (Van Dongen et al. 2003). The impact of chronic pain on cognitive function (e.g. memory, concentration, fatigue, driving ability) during wakefulness, and the benefit of a nap (e.g. <20 min with mainly light sleep vs. 60–90 min nap that allows the occurrence of deep and REM sleep) or pain medications, need to be investigated (Brousseau et al. 2003).

The duration of sleep stages in most chronic pain patients is normal, although some disruption in the microstructure of sleep has been found, e.g. sleep transition (termed sleep stage shift), frequent and long arousals termed awakenings (see Table 1). The quality of deep sleep (St 3&4) of chronic pain patients was initially described to be perturbed, due to the intrusion of so-called fast Alpha waves (as estimated on the electroencephalographic (► EEG) sleep traces; see also Glossary for definition), but this concept has been revisited. It is currently suggested that the sleep of chronic pain patients is under the influence of a EEG "protective" mechanism termed ► cyclic alternating pattern (CAP) (Moldofsky 2001). CAP is a natural rhythm in sleep in which every 20–60 seconds there is a brief arousal (named a ► micro-arousal), which allows the individual to adjust his/her body temperature, heart and respiratory rate to the environment. This physiological activity is like a "sentinel" that protects and/or prepares the body for a rapid awakening in the presence of a threatening situation. In the presence of sleep disruptive influences (e.g. sound, sleep apnea, periodic limb movement and pain), arousal or CAP rate per hour of sleep could be increased.

Sleep is also a state normally associated with a reduction in heart rate variability, due to a change in the balance of components of the autonomic nervous system. In light and deep sleep, a parasympathetic dominance "slows down" the cardiac activity, while during the awake or REM sleep state there is a cardiac-

O

Orofacial Pain, Sleep Disturbance, Table 1

Sleep changes that could be produced by pain (low to moderate level of evidence)
Lower sleep efficacy (% time asleep over total time in bed: usually >85%)
Longer duration of light sleep (stage 1)
Lower duration of deep sleep (Stages 3&4)
Lower density of slow wave EEG activity usually associated with un-refreshing sleep
Higher density of K complexes in EEG activity
More frequent sleep stage shift (transition from deep sleep to light sleep) and unstable deep sleep
Presence of more than 15 micro-arousals/hr (3–10 sec EEG changes with heart rate increase and possible rise in muscle tone) in young adults; more than 29/hr of sleep in older adults
In the presence of an usual number of micro-arousals/hr of sleep, a rise in sympathetic-cardiac activity, a high CAP rate and Alpha EEG intrusions in deep sleep (St 3&4)
High rate of awakening in sleep (e.g. >4/hr sleep)

sympathetic dominance, characterized by a higher cardiac activity/variability. The absence of a reduction in cardiac activity during light or deep sleep may cause un-refreshing or non-restorative sleep. This suggestion is supported by findings showing that fibromyalgia and insomniac patients maintain a high sympathetic cardiac activity (Martínez-Lavín et al. 1998; Moldofsky 2001; Brousseau et al. 2003). The specificity of this hypothesis to explain poor sleep in pain patients needs to be demonstrated in the absence of anxiety, which is highly prevalent in fibromyalgia and insomnia.

Experimental Pain and Sleep Fragmentation Models

During sleep, in comparison to the waking state, most sensory stimulation needs to be more intense to evoke a physiological response such as micro-arousal, awakening or a behavioural reaction during awakening. An auditory alarm needs to be over 65 dB to waken a sleeping subject, although sound in the range of 40 dB is known to cause sleep perturbations. In an experimental setting, sleep can be disrupted in two ways: ► Sleep fragmentation or deprivation. Sleep fragmentation is a brief intrusion in sleep that causes a transitional change in the sleep process (sleep stage shift, micro-arousal or awakening without a conscious response from the subject). Sleep deprivation is either a total prevention of sleep or is limited to a specific sleep stage (e.g. St 3&4). To be able to induce sleep deprivation, the subject has to be monitored with polysomnography recordings. When sleep onset becomes apparent (e.g. drowsiness to sleep St 1), a verbal command or a sensory stimulation is applied to maintain wakefulness. Both fragmentation and deprivation have potential consequences for functioning the next day (e.g. fatigue, sleepiness, boredom, irritability, poor memory performance) that could influence pain reports or clinician assessment of pain. For research purposes, the effects of three sensory pain modalities on sleep have been investigated: thermal (heat-cold thermode, laser heat),

mechanical (finger-joint pressure) and chemical (hypertonic saline or other algesic substance injection) (Drewes et al. 1997; Lavigne et al. 2000; Lavigne et al. 2004). Electric shock has also been used to test nociceptive - polysynaptic flexion reflex latency and amplitude (Sandrini et al. 2001). The use of these models, have confirmed that pain perception during sleep, similar to other sensory stimulations during sleep, is lower. However, it remains to be proven that the use of the three sensory modalities or the flexion reflex mimic clinical pain. It appears that the duration of the stimulation needs to be long enough (over 60 sec) to trigger a response that is similar to that observed in a situation associated with awakening in sleep, e.g.: "I was suddenly woken up by a toothache". The validation of such models in the study of sleep and pain interaction is in progress.

Management

Sleep and pain interactions can be managed with classical approaches (see Table 2), (Brousseau et al. 2003). First, educate the patient about sleep "hygiene" to identify bad life habits that could exacerbate the problem (e.g. late day exercise, late meal, alcohol, poor sleep schedule, TV or computer in bedroom). In the presence of musculoskeletal pain-related problems, physical management (e.g. physical therapy, osteopathy, massage or fasciatherapy) could be beneficial. Light exercise is also recognized as being beneficial. However, an assessment needs to be made of the advantage and risk of a daytime nap; too long a nap could disrupt the circadian rhythm and induce prolonged sleep inertia/low cognitive functioning in the hours after the nap.

Second, if the presence of a sleep disorder is in doubt, it is strongly recommended that consultation with a sleep medicine physician be arranged, in order to rule out sleep disorders that create health risks (e.g. sleep apnea patients have a moderate to high risk of vehicle accident

Orofacial Pain, Sleep Disturbance, Table 2

Management guidelines for sleep and pain interaction (most have low level of evidence)
Sleep hygiene – life style
Bedroom should be an oasis, good mattress, etc
Avoid caffeine, nicotine and alcoholic products in evening
Relaxation (e. g. abdominal breathing, imagery, hot bath-hydrotherapy)
Use a regular sleep schedule as much as possible
Avoid heavy meals in the evening
Daytime nap should be in the afternoon and no more than 20 min
Light exercise program may be beneficial; avoid intense exercise late in the day
Physical therapy – massage
Sleep disorders diagnosis
Respiratory: sleep apnea &hypoapnea, upper airway resistance, snoring
Movement: periodic limb movement, sleep bruxism, abnormal swallowing, Parkinson-related activity, REM behaviour disorder, etc
Circadian – sleep cycle related: insomnia, hypersomnia, sleep-wake schedule shift, drug or alcohol abuse, narcolepsia, etc
Medication
Analgesics, AINS (Anti-inflammatory non-steroidal analgesics): morphine (risk of sleep disruption), gabapentin, pregabalin
Muscle relaxants: cyclobenzaprine (1/2 co) or clonazepan (low dose, not every evening) in early evening to prevent morning sleepiness and risk of vehicle accident
Sleep facilitators: zaleplon, (triazolam), temazepam, zopiclone, zolpidem and gabapentin at low dose (empirical basis so far)
Antidepressants: amitriptyline (low dose), trazodone, nefazodone and mirtazapine
Others: Valerian, Lavender, Kava, Cannabis: Additive effect possible (Consult: www.nccam.nih.gov)

and hypertension with a shorter life expectancy) or exacerbate poor sleep (e.g. periodic limb movement, nightmare, upper airway resistance).

Third, some medication (analgesics, muscle relaxants, sleep facilitators) could be used on a short-term basis to improve sleep and reduce pain. Opioid effects on sleep need to be further characterized, since some evidence suggests a disruption of the so-called restorative deep sleep (also termed slow wave activity sleep). In the presence of a severe sleep and pain problem, antidepressants could improve sleep and assist in the management of concomitant psychological conditions (e.g. anxiety, depression), but caution is suggested, since there is limited evidence bearing on their use for this purpose. Psychological support may also be considered in some cases to improve relaxation, life style or manage concomitant conditions.

References

1. Aaron LA, Burke MM, Buchwald D (2000) Overlapping Conditions Among Patients with Chronic Fatigue Syndrome, Fibromyalgia, and Temporomandibular Disorder. Arch Intern Med 160:221–227
2. Brousseau M, Manzini C, Thie NMR, Lavigne GJ (2003) Understanding and Managing the Interaction Between Sleep and Pain: An Update for the Dentist. J Can Dent Assoc 69:437–442
3. Dao TTT, Lavigne GJ, Feine JS, Lund JP, Goulet J-P (1994) Quality of Life and Pain in Myofascial Pain Patients and Bruxers. J Dent Res 73:2047
4. Drewes AM, Nielsen KM, Arendt-Nielsen L, Birket-Smith L, Hansen LM (1997) The Effect of Cutaneous and Deep Pain on the Electroencephalogram During Sleep - An Experimental Study. Sleep 20:623–640
5. Huang GJ, Leresche L, Critchlow CW, Martin MD, Drangholt MT (2002) Risk Factors for Diagnostic Subgroups of Painful Temporomandibular Disorders (TMD). J Dent Res 81:284–288
6. Lavigne GJ, Zucconi M, Castronovo C, Manzini C, Marchettini P, Smirne S (2000) Sleep Arousal Response to Experimental Thermal Stimulation During Sleep in Human Subjects Free of Pain and Sleep Problems. Pain 84:283–290
7. Lavigne GJ, Brousseau M, Kato T, Mayer P, Manzini C, Guitard F, Montplaisir JY (2004) Experimental pain perception remains equally active over all sleep stages. Pain 110:646-655
8. Martínez-Lavín M, Hermosillo AG, Rosas M, Soto M-E (1998) Circadian Studies of Autonomic Nervous Balance in Patients with Fibromyalgia: A Heart Rate Variability Analysis. Arthri Rheum 41:1966–1971
9. McCracken LM, Iverson GL (2002) Disrupted Sleep Patterns and Daily Functioning in Patients with Chronic Pain. Pain Res Manage 7:75–79
10. Moldofsky H (2001) Sleep and Pain: Clinical Review. Sleep Med Rev 5:387–398
11. Morin CM, Gibson D, Wade J (1998) Self-Reported Sleep and Mood Disturbance in Chronic Pain Patients. Clin J Pain 14:311–314
12. Nicassio PM, Moxham EG, Schuman CE, Gervirtz RN (2002) The Contribution of Pain, Reported Sleep Quality, and Depressive Symptoms to Fatigue in Fibromyalgia. Pain 100:271–279
13. Raymond I, Nielsen TA, Lavigne GJ, Manzini C, Choinière M (2001) Quality of Sleep and its Daily Relationship to Pain Intensity in Hospitalized Adult Burn Patients. Pain 92:381–388
14. Riley III JL, Benson MB, Gremillion HA, Myers CD, Robinson ME, Smith CL, Waxenberg LB (2001) Sleep Disturbances in

Orofacial Pain Patients: Pain-Related or Emotional Distress? J Craniomandib Pract 19:106–113

15. Sandrini G, Milanov I, Rossi B, Murri L, Alfonsi E, Moglia A, Nappi G (2001) Effects of Sleep on Spinal Nociceptive Reflexes in Humans. Sleep 24:13–17

16. Van Dongen HP, Maislin G, Mullington JM, Dinges DF (2003) The Cumulative Cost of Additional Wakefulness: Dose-Response Effects on Neurobehavioral Functions and Sleep Physiology from Chronic Sleep Restriction and Total Sleep Deprivation. Sleep 26:117–126

17. Yatani H, Studts J, Cordova M, Carlson CR, Okeson JP (2002) Comparison of Sleep Quality and Clinical and Psychological Characteristics in Patients with Temporomandibular Disorders. J Orofac Pain 16:221–228

Orofacial Pain, Taxonomy/Classification

ANTOON F. C. DE LAAT

Department of Oral/Maxillofacial Surgery, Catholic University of Leuven, Leuven, Belgium
antoon.delaat@med.kuleuven.ac.be

Synonyms

Diagnostic subdivisions; Taxonomy, Orofacial Pain

Definition

The development and establishment of widely accepted definitions, and a classification system for the different orofacial pain conditions.

Characteristics

Composing and validating a classification is a continuously ongoing process, driven by new scientific data or better insights into pathophysiological processes. Ideally, a classification should be complete, and all the syndromes described should have clear exclusion and inclusion criteria. Unfortunately, this system of "complete truth" does not exist and will probably never be reached. Although this may sound frustrating, it provides, however, the necessary flexibility (also in regard of syndromes or definitions under debate) to convince as many users as possible to share a common language. One of the first classification schemes for orofacial pain was suggested in 1962, by the Ad Hoc Committee on Classification on Headache of the National Institute of Neurological Diseases and Blindness (Friedman et al. 1962). It was based on clinical symptoms and is not widely used.

An extraordinary effort by the International Headache Society (IHS) resulted in the classical "Classification and Diagnostic Criteria for Headache Disorders, Cranial ▶ Neuralgias and Facial Pain" (1988). It was the first time that sets of clear inclusion criteria for the different diagnoses were put together (Olesen 1988). The focus, however, was on headache, and many of the common sources for orofacial pain were grouped under its section 11: Headache or facial pain associated with

a disorder of ▶ cranium, neck, eyes, ears, nose, sinuses, teeth, mouth or other facial or cranial structures.

In order to incorporate the different subgroups of ▶ temporomandibular disorders (TMD) in the IHS-classification, the American Academy of Orofacial Pain (AAOP) provided specific inclusion and exclusion criteria (Okeson 1996). Even if clear descriptions of the different subgroups of TMD have been provided, the inclusion and exclusion criteria have been only partially operational. In the case of TMD, this has led an expert committee to focus on a subset of the most common temporomandibular disorders for which the Research Diagnostic Criteria (RDC) have been developed (Dworkin and LeResche 1992). A double axis system has been used: a somatic assessment based on primary signs and symptoms (pain and tenderness) allows classification into 3 groups (muscle problems, ▶ disc displacement and joint disorders), from which the first two are further subdivided with respect to the range of motion. In addition, a second axis examines and scores the pain severity, the psychological status of the patient and the related disability. The RDC-TMD allows for multiple diagnoses, has clear and testable inclusion and exclusion criteria, and has been operationally validated in several countries and languages.

The Task Force on Taxonomy of the IASP composed a second edition of the Classification of Chronic Pain in 1994 (Merskey and Bogduk 1994). In the section of "Relatively localised syndromes of the Head and the Neck", each pain condition has been coded, defined, specified regarding location, system involved, main clinical and technical features and diagnostic criteria.

In 1996, the AAOP expanded the original set of subdiagnoses of TMD to all conditions that could be associated with orofacial pain (Merskey and Bogduk 1994). Seven subgroups have been distinguished:

1. Intracranial pain disorders comprising tumors, hemorrhage, abscess, hematoma or edema. Due to their possible life-threatening character, they should always be ruled out expeditiously in the process of differential diagnosis.

2. The neurovascular disorders (Primary Headache disorders) include the variety of migraines, cluster headache, chronic paroxysmal hemicrania, the tension type-headaches, carotidynia and also temporal arteritis.

3. Neurogenic Pain Disorders find their etiology within the nervous system itself: the neurogenic pain may be paroxysmal (as in the typical neuralgias of the trigeminal, glossopharyngeal, nervus intermedius or superior laryngeal nerves), or continuous, comparable to deafferentation pain syndromes: peripheral neuritis, post-herpetic or posttraumatic neuralgias. The AAOP also includes in this category sympathetically maintained pain. The latter groups are characterized by their unremitting and mostly burning character.

4. Many tissues may be involved in intraoral pain: the ▶ dental pulp, the periodontium as well as the mucogingival tissues and the tongue are sources for a variety of pain conditions.

5. The group of temporomandibular disorders has been subdivided in more detail by the AAOP into masticatory muscle disorders (myofascial pain, myositis, myospasm, unclassified local myalgia, myofibrotic contracture and neoplasia), and articular disorders (congenital and developmental disorders, disc derangement disorders, dislocation of the temporomandibular joint, inflammatory disorders, noninflammatory osteoarthritis, ankylosis and fractures). Other musculoskeletal pain may be of cervical origin and referred to the orofacial area.

6. Associated structures such as the ears, eyes, nose and paranasal sinuses, the throat, salivary glands and other soft tissues may be involved in pain felt in the orofacial region. Differential diagnosis is important here, and – as in many of the other categories – correct referral to the medical discipline mostly involved in the referring area is warranted.

7. In rare cases, mental disorders are the origin of orofacial pain, e.g. somatoform disorders and pain syndromes of psychogenic origin.

As for many other classification systems, a debate, also in the orofacial area, is still going on regarding pain syndromes without a clear definition or whose underlying pathophysiology is less well understood. "Atypical facial pain" was originally used as a "waste basket" for those orofacial pain syndromes that did not correspond to any of the suggested and defined diagnoses. More recently, this term – like "atypical odontalgia" and others – has been associated with a neuropathy-like pain, with attention drawn to their similarities regarding female predominance, clinical manifestation (but in different orofacial tissues) and lack of clear underlying pathophysiology. Indeed, based on these shared characteristics, a unified concept was recently proposed to group atypical facial pain, atypical odontalgia, glossodynia (stomatodynia) and atypical facial athromyalgia (the pain component in TMD) under the heading of idiopathic facial pain, which could be expressed in the jaws, the buccal mucosa, the teeth, the masticatory muscles or the TMJ (Woda and Pionchon 1999).

This kind of discussion and "regrouping" would probably take place more often if the principles of a "mechanism-based" classification (Woolf et al. 1998) were ever implemented. In a mechanism-based classification, the subdivisions are not driven by anatomical location but merely by the underlying pathophysiological process. Grouping pain syndromes in this way could allow more general and mechanism-oriented treatment approaches, and bridge the boundaries of specific medical disciplines. At present, however, too little scientific data are available in this regard.

References

1. Dworkin SF, LeResche L (1992) Research Diagnostic Criteria for Temporomandibular Disorders. J Craniomandib Disord 6:301–355
2. Friedman AP, Finlay KH, Graham JR et al. (1962) Classification of Headache. Special Report of the Ad Hoc Committee. Arch Neurol 6:173–176
3. Merskey H, Bogduk N (1994) Classification of Chronic Pain. Descriptions of Chronic Pain Syndromes and Definitions of Pain Terms. IASP Press, Seattle, pp 59–92
4. Okeson JP (1996) Orofacial Pain: Guidelines for Assessment, Diagnosis and Management. Quintessence, Chicago, pp 45–52
5. Olesen J (1988) Classification and Diagnostic Criteria for Headache Disorders, Cranial Neuralgias and Facial Pain. Cephalalgia 8
6. Woda A, Pionchon P (1999) A Unified Concept of Idiopathic Orofacial Pain: Clinical Features. J Orofac Pain 13:172–184
7. Woolf CJ, Bennett GJ, Doherty M et al. (1998) Towards a Mechanism-Based Classification of Pain? Pain 77:227–229

Orphan G Protein-Coupled Receptor

Definition

Orphan G Protein-Coupled Receptor is deduced from nucleic acid sequence to be a G protein-coupled receptor but of unknown ligand specificity.
▶ Orphanin FQ

Orphanin FQ

DAVID K. GRANDY
Department of Physiology and Pharmacology, School of Medicine, Oregon Health and Science University, Portland, OR, USA
grandyd@ohsu.edu

Synonyms

OFQ; Nociceptin; NOC; OFQ/N; N/OFQ

Definition

OrphaninFQ, discovered in 1995, is a naturally occurring, 17 amino acid long, kappa opioid-like peptide that is evolutionarily conserved among vertebrates. The name 'orphanin' was chosen because the peptide, isolated from pig hypothalamic extracts, was found to be a potent agonist of an 'orphan' opiate receptor-like G protein-coupled receptor (now referred to as ORL-1 and NOP1). The 'FQ' was added to reflect that this peptide's N-terminal amino acid is phenylalanine (written as an 'F' in the single letter amino acid code), and its C-terminal amino acid is glutamine (Q). A peptide of identical sequence was simultaneously and independently discovered in rat brain extracts by another group of researchers, who named it 'nociceptin' based on its pronociceptive characteristics in stressed mice.

Characteristics

The cloning of the mouse delta (δ) opiate receptor cDNA quickly led to the cloning of cDNAs and genes, from a variety of vertebrate species, that code for the mu (μ)Δopiate receptor, the kappa (κ) opiate receptor, and an opiate receptor-like ▶ orphan G protein-coupled receptor (Darland et al. 1998). The latter is now referred to as both ORL-1 or NOP$_1$ (Mogil and Pasternak 2001). Based on the extensive amino acid sequence shared by ORL-1/NOP$_1$ and the 3 opiate receptor subtypes, it was predicted that this orphan opiate-like receptor would be activated by a peptide ligand resembling the opioid peptides β-endorphin, Met/Leu enkephalin and dynorphin. Furthermore, it was predicted that, when activated, this receptor would couple to second messenger systems similar, if not identical to, those modulated by the classic opiate receptors.

The search for ORL-1/NOP$_1$'s endogenous agonist culminated with the co-discovery of a dynorphin-like heptadecapeptide (PheGlyGlyPheThrGlyAlaArgLysSerAlaArgLysLeuAlaAsnGln) from pig hypothalamic and rat brain extracts that was named ▶ orphanin FQ (Reinscheid et al. 1995) and ▶ Nociceptin (Meunier et al. 1995), respectively. At the cellular level, synthetic OFQ/N inhibits cAMP production in vitro, activates inwardly rectifying potassium channels, and inhibits a variety of voltage-dependent calcium channels including the L, P, and N types (Darland et al. 1998) in tissue slices, activities shared by the classic opiate receptors. In the low nanomolar to high picomolar range, OFQ/N is a potent and selective agonist of ORL-1/NOP$_1$ receptors; however, at concentrations in the high micromolar range, the peptide can activate κ >> μ = δ opiate receptors expressed heterologously in vitro (Zhang et al. 1997).

In spite of the many physical and physiological similarities OFQ/N and ORL-1/NOP$_1$ share with the opioid peptides and their cognate receptors, respectively, the pair differ notably in that their interaction is insensitive to naloxone antagonism. Not surprisingly, this is the principle reason OFQ/N and its receptor are not generally accepted as bone fide members of the opioid peptide/opiate receptor family. Several relatively selective peptide and small molecule ORL-1/NOP$_1$ receptor antagonists have been developed recently (Mogil and Pasternak 2001), and are being used in efforts to clarify the functions of ORL-1/NOP$_1$-mediated actions of OFQ/N in vivo.

Efforts to determine the biosynthetic origin of OFQ/N led to the identification and characterization of its precursor polypeptide prepro-orphaninFQ/nociceptin (ppOFQ/N) (Mollereau et al. 1996; Nothacker et al. 1996). In this precursor polypeptide the OFQ/N sequence is flanked by paired basic amino acids that are recognized and cleaved by trypsin-like endopeptidases. Further processing of OFQ/N by a carboxypeptidase may also be important in vivo, since OFQ/N-derived peptides truncated by as many as 5 amino acid residues have been found to retain agonist activity, at least at ORL-1/NOP$_1$ receptors expressed in vitro (Butour et al. 1997; Reinscheid et al. 1996).

Analysis of ppOFQ/N amino acid sequences deduced from mus-, rattus-, and homo-derived cDNAs reveal ppOFQ/N, as is its receptor, to be evolutionarily conserved across species. Furthermore, the presence of numerous putative peptide domains flanked by endopeptidase cleavage recognition sites distributed throughout ppOFQ/N and the organization of its gene, recapitulate organizational schemes also present in the 3 opioid peptide precursors: proopiomelanocortin, preproenkephalin, and preprodynorphin (Darland et al. 1998). Taken together these features led to the prediction and eventual demonstration that ppOFQ/N codes for additional bioactive peptides; a result that suggests caution when interpreting outcomes of genetic manipulations that affect expression of the entire precursor.

Nucleic acid and antibody probes specific for ppOFQ/N and ORL-1/NOP$_1$ have been used to demonstrate the widespread, albeit unequal, distribution of both polypeptides throughout the central nervous system and periphery (Darland et al. 1998; Mogil and Pasternak 2001). Of particular note in the context of pain and nociception is the significant presence of both peptide and receptor in the periaqueductal gray (PAG), raphé nuclei, and the spinal cord (Darland et al. 1998; Mogil and Pasternak 2001).

As with the opioid peptides, early attempts to study the actions of OFQ/N in vivo were plagued by its sensitivity to proteolysis, membrane impermeability, and failure to cross the blood-brain barrier. Until recently, further complicating interpretation of in vivo studies was the lack of selective, small-molecule antagonists of the ORL1/NOP$_1$ receptor. In spite of these limitations the actions of OFQ/N in rodents and primates, have been documented.

When OFQ/N is administered intracerebroventricularly (icv), the most common observation is that it dose-dependently interferes with several opioid-mediated, naloxone-sensitive responses including antinociception. The literature also contains reports of the peptide producing hyperalgesia as well as analgesia (extensively reviewed in Mogil and Pasternak 2001). In contrast to its apparent antiopioid actions supraspinally, when administered intrathecaly OFQ/N potentiates opioid analgesia, although the gender and physiological status of the subject (e.g. pregnancy) appear to influence the peptide's effects on nociceptive sensitivity (Dawson-Basoa and Gintzler 1997). To date there are few reports describing OFQ/N's effects on nociceptive processing when administered directly into brain tissue. Microinjection of OFQ/N into the midbrain PAG region of rats produces a mild hyperalgesia (Bytner et al. 2001) while blocking the antinociceptive effects of intra-PAG administered morphine (Morgan et al. 1997). In contrast, the focal application of OFQ/N into the rostral ventral medulla produced either no effect (two studies) or analgesia (one study) (Heinricher 2003).

Although the literature contains numerous contradictory reports regarding the effects of exogenous OFQ/N on various nociceptive behaviors, the consensus emerging from recent efforts to integrate these data is that the dynorphon-like peptide OFQ/N is not "anti-opioid" or "pronociceptive." Rather, OFQ/N can be a modulator of opioid peptide/opiate alkaloid actions, exerting a potent, inhibitory effect on a wide range of cell types involved with nociceptive processing in the brain and spinal cord via the naloxone-insensitive activation of its cognate receptor. Therefore, the behavioral manifestations of exogenous OFQ/N are a reflection of the neuronal circuits present along the route of administration, as well as the species, strain, gender, and physiological status of the experimental subject (Harrison and Grandy 2000). What role, if any, endogenous OFQ/N plays in nociceptive processing remains to be established.

References

1. Bytner B, Huang YH, Yu LC et al. (2001) Nociceptin/Orphanin FQ into the Rat Periaqueductal Gray Decreases the Withdrawal Latency to Heat and Loading, an Effect Reversed by (Nphe(1))nociceptin(1-13)NH(2). Brain Res 922:118–124
2. Butour JL, Moisand C, Mazarguil H et al. (1997) Recognition and Activation of the Opioid Receptor-Like ORL 1 Receptor by Nociceptin, Nociceptin Analogs and Opioids. Eur J Pharmacol 321:97–103
3. Darland T, Heinricher MM, Grandy DK (1998) Orphanin FQ/Nociceptin: A Role in Pain and Analgesia, But So Much More. Trends Neurosci 21:215–221
4. Dawson-Basoa M, Gintzler AR (1997) Nociceptin (Orphanin FQ) Abolishes Gestational and Ovarian Sex Steroid-Induced Antinociception and Induces Hyperalgesia. Brain Res 750:48–52
5. Harrison LM, Grandy DK (2000) Opiate Modulating Properties of Nociceptin/Orphanin FQ. Peptides 21:151–172
6. Heinricher MM (2003) Orphanin FQ/Nociceptin: From Neural Circuitry to Behavior. Life Sci 73:813–822
7. Meunier JC, Mollereau C, Toll L et al. (1995) Isolation and Structure of the Endogenous Agonist of Opioid Receptor-Like ORL1 Receptor. Nature 377:532–535
8. Mogil JS, Pasternak GW (2001) The Molecular and Behavioral Pharmacology of the Orphanin FQ/Nociceptin Peptide and Receptor Family. Pharmacol Rev 53:381–415
9. Mollereau C, Simons MJ, Soularue P et al. (1996) Structure, Tissue Distribution, and Chromosomal Localization of the Prepronociceptin Gene. Proc Natl Acad Sci USA 93:8666–8670
10. Morgan MM, Grisel JE, Robbins CS et al. (1997) Antinociception Mediated by the Periaqueductal Gray is Attenuated by Orphanin FQ. Neuroreport. 8:3431–3434
11. Nothacker HP, Reinschei, RK, Mansour A et al. (1996) Primary Structure and Tissue Distribution of the Orphanin FQ Precursor. Proc Natl Acad Sci USA 93:8677–8682
12. Reinscheid RK, Nothacker HP, Bourson A et al. (1995) Orphanin FQ: A Neuropeptide that Activates an Opioid-Like G Protein-Coupled Receptor. Science 270:792–794
13. Reinscheid RK, Ardati A, Monsma FJ Jr et al. (1996) Structure-Activity Relationship Studies on the Novel Neuropeptide Orphanin FQ. J Biol Chem 271:14163–14168
14. Zhang G, Murray TF, Grandy DK (1997) Orphanin FQ has an Inhibitory Effect on the Guinea Pig Ileum and the Mouse vas Deferens. Brain Res 772:102–106

Orthodromic Activation

Definition

Electrical activity due to propagation of action potentials in the same direction to that observed when the neuron is naturally excited.
▶ Corticothalamic and Thalamocortical Interactions

Orthologues

Definition

A paralogue is an homologous member of a multigene family that may share some functional characteristics with the query sequence, whilst an orthologue is the closest relative of the query sequence in a different species, and is likely to share most or all functional characteristics with the protein encoded by the query sequence.
▶ TRPV1 Receptor, Species Variability

Orthostatic Component of Pain

Definition

Change of posture, or „intra-body"-pressure (coughing, sneezing, straining) can influence headaches due to low intracranial pressure.
▶ Headache due to Low Cerebrospinal Fluid Pressure

Orthostatic Hypotension

Definition

Orthostatic hypotension is a drop in blood pressure when standing up from a lying/sitting position.
▶ Cancer Pain Management, Anesthesiologic Interventions, Neural Blockade

Oscillations (Neuronal)

Definition

Oscillations are spike potentials that occur repeatedly at relatively fixed intervals.
▶ Thalamus, Dynamics of Nociception

Osmolysis

Definition

Osmolysis is the rupture of a cell membrane due to excessive accumulation of solvent (water), produced by an important decrease of concentration of ions inside the cell (hypoosmolarity).

▶ Post-Stroke Pain Model, Thalamic Pain (Lesion)

Osmosensitive

Definition

Sensitive to changes in the osmolarity of the surrounding medium.

▶ Mechanonociceptors

Osmotic

Definition

A chemical used in prolotherapy solutions that acts by causing an osmotic shock to cells, leading to the release of proinflammatory substances. Osmotics include concentrated solutions of glucose, glycerine and zinc sulphate.

▶ Pain Management
▶ Prolotherapy
▶ Prolotherapy Injection

Osteoarthritic Pain

Definition

Osteoarthritic pain is caused by the irritation or degeneration of the joint cartilage. When cartilage becomes worn, exposed bones can rub together and the painful symptoms of osteoarthritis may appear. Chemical messenger substances that are associated with the disease process may cause the irritation.

▶ Perireceptor Elements

Osteoarthritis

Definition

Osteoarthritis is a painful condition in which there is breakdown of the articular cartilage (the cartilage on the ends of bones which assists the smooth movement of joints). Joints may become deformed and stiff. Inflammation is generally not marked but can be severe in some patients. It has a prevalence of about 10% in western populations, and mainly afflicts elderly people.

▶ NSAIDs and their Indications

Osteoarthritis Model

▶ Arthritis Model, Osteoarthritis

Osteoblast

Definition

Osteoblasts are specialized cells that lay down osseous matrix for bone formation.

▶ Adjuvant Analgesics in Management of Cancer-Rated Bone Pain
▶ NSAIDs, Adverse Effects

Osteoblastoma

Definition

Osteoblastoma is a rare, benign, locally recurrent tumor of bone with a predilection for the spine.

▶ Chronic Back Pain and Spinal Instability

Osteoclast

Definition

A member of the macrophage-monocyte lineage of cells that is responsible for the absorption and removal of bone. Resorption is mediated by demineralization of bone by protons secreted by the osteoclast.

▶ Adjuvant Analgesics in Management of Cancer-Rated Bone Pain
▶ Cancer Pain, Animal Models
▶ NSAIDs, Adverse Effects

Osteolysis

Definition

The process of bone resorption that occurs during normal bone homeostasis, but may become pathologic in the presence of cancer cells.

► Cancer Pain, Animal Models

Osteolytic Fibrosarcoma

Definition

Osteolytic fibrosarcoma is a tumor of mesenchymal cell origin that may present as an osteolytic bone tumor. The primary tumor is comprised of malignant fibroblasts. NCTC 2472 sarcoma cells that produce osteolytic fibrosarcoma have been used to model cancer pain in mice. The clinical presentation of osteolytic fibrosarcoma features breakthrough pain as a prominent component.

► Evoked and Movement-Related Neuropathic Pain

Osteopathy

► Spinal Manipulation, Characteristics

Osteophyte

Definition

A bony excrescence or osseous outgrowth.

► Lumbar Traction

Oswestry Disability Index

OLE HAEGG
Department of Orthopedic Surgery, Sahlgren University Hospital, Goteborg, Sweden
ollehagg@hotmail.com

Synonyms

ODI; Oswestry Disability Questionnaire; Oswestry Low Back Pain Disability Questionnaire

Definition

The Oswestry Disability Index (ODI) is a self-rating condition-specific outcome measure for evaluation of low back pain ► disability. It was introduced in 1980 by Fairbank et al. (Fairbank et al. 1980), and consists of ten sections with six response alternatives describing functional impairment in a series of daily activities. There are two authorized versions, version 1.0 (Table 1) from 1980 and version 2.0 (Table 2) from 1989 (Pynsent 1993). The main difference between the versions is the construction of the section describing pain intensity.

Scoring

For each section of six statements the total score is 5; if the first statement is marked the score = 0; if the last statement is marked the score = 5. Intervening statements are scored according to rank. If more than one box is marked in each section, take the highest score. If all ten sections are completed the score is calculated as follows: Example: 16 (total score) of 50 (total possible score) $\times$ 100 = 32%. If one section is missed (or not applicable) the score is calculated as follows: Example: 16 (total score)/45 (total possible score) $\times$ 100 = 35.6%. The final score may be summarized as: (total score/(5 $\times$ number of questions answered ($\times$ 100%)). It is suggested that the total percentage is rounded to a whole number (Fairbank and Pynsent 2000). A low score = low degree of disability, a high score = high degree of disability.

Versions in Non-English Languages

The ODI is available in five validated translations (Finnish, Greek, Norwegian, Spanish, and Japanese) and another five non-validated translations (Dutch, French, German, Danish, and Swedish).

Characteristics

Validity

The ODI has been criticized for not being properly validated according to modern standards. This predicament is shared with many other outcome measures consisting of more than pure physical function, where external criteria by performance tests are available. There are no external criteria for benchmarking of outcome measures including more complex social/private activities such as personal care, sex life or social life. Validation of this type of measure is accomplished by assessing the behaviour of the outcome measure in conditions with generally accepted/established degrees of disability.

The ODI score was significantly associated with physical performance tests (Gronblad et al. 1993; Reneman et al. 2002). Radiculopathy patients had significantly greater scores than patients with low back pain (49 vs. 33) (Leclaire et al. 1997). "Normal" individuals scored lower (10) than chronic back pain (43), neurogenic claudication (37) and sciatica (45) (Fairbank and Pynsent 2000).

Reliability

Test-re-test ► reliability assessed with the Intraclass Correlation Coefficient (ICC) was 0.89 (one week, n = 32) (Pratt et al. 2002), 0.94 (two weeks, n = 37) (Holm et al. 2003), 0.84/0.92 (six weeks, n = 47/16) (Davidson and Keating 2002), 0.83 (one week, n = 20) (Gronblad et al. 1993).

O

SECTION 1 - PAIN INTENSITY
- ☐ I can tolerate the pain I have without having to use painkillers.
- ☐ The pain is bad but I manage without taking painkillers.
- ☐ Painkillers give complete relief from pain.
- ☐ Painkillers give moderate relief from pain.
- ☐ Painkillers give very little relief from pain.
- ☐ Painkillers have no effect on the pain and I do not use them.

SECTION 2 - PERSONAL CARE (washing, dressing etc.)
- ☐ I can look after myself normally, without causing extra pain.
- ☐ I can look after myself normally, but it causes extra pain.
- ☐ It is painful to look after myself and I am slow and careful.
- ☐ I need some help, but manage most of my personal care.
- ☐ I need help every day in most aspects of self-care.
- ☐ I do not get dressed, wash with difficulty and stay in bed.

SECTION 3 - LIFTING
- ☐ I can lift heavy weights without extra pain.
- ☐ I can lift heavy weights, but it gives extra pain.
- ☐ Pain prevents me from lifting heavy weights off the floor, but I can manage if they are conveniently positioned (e.g., on a table).
- ☐ Pain prevents me from lifting heavy weights but I can manage light to medium weights if they are conveniently positioned.
- ☐ I can lift only very light weights.
- ☐ I cannot lift or carry anything at all.

SECTION 4 - WALKING
- ☐ Pain does not prevent my walking any distance.
- ☐ Pain prevents me walking more than 1 mile.
- ☐ Pain prevents me walking more than ½ of mile.
- ☐ Pain prevents me walking more than ¼ mile.
- ☐ I can only walk using a stick or crutches.
- ☐ I am in bed most of the time and have to crawl to the toilet.

SECTION 5 - SITTING
- ☐ I can sit in any chair as long as I like.
- ☐ I can sit in my favourite chair as long as I like.
- ☐ Pain prevents me sitting more than 1 hour.
- ☐ Pain prevents me from sitting more than ½ an hour.
- ☐ Pain prevents me from sitting more than 10 minutes.
- ☐ Pain prevents me from sitting at all.

SECTION 6 - STANDING
- ☐ I can stand as long as I want without extra pain.
- ☐ I can stand as long as I want but it gives me extra pain.
- ☐ Pain prevents me from standing for more than 1 hour.
- ☐ Pain prevents me from standing for more than 30 minutes.
- ☐ Pain prevents me from standing for more than 10 minutes.
- ☐ Pain prevents me from standing at all.

SECTION 7 - SLEEPING
- ☐ Pain does not prevent me from sleeping well.
- ☐ I can sleep well only by using tablets.
- ☐ Even when I take tablets, I have less than 6 hours sleep.
- ☐ Even when I take tablets, I have less than 4 hours sleep.
- ☐ Even when I take tablets, I have less than 2 hours sleep.
- ☐ Pain prevents me from sleeping at all.

SECTION 8 - SEX LIFE (If applicable)
- ☐ My sex life is normal and causes no extra pain.
- ☐ My sex life is normal but causes some extra pain.
- ☐ My sex life is nearly normal but is very painful.
- ☐ My sex life is severely restricted by pain.
- ☐ My sex life is nearly absent because of pain.
- ☐ Pain prevents any sex life at all.

SECTION 9 - SOCIAL LIFE
- ☐ My social life is normal and gives me no extra pain.
- ☐ My social life is normal, but increases the degree of pain.
- ☐ Pain has no significant effect on my social life apart from limiting my more energetic interests, e.g., dancing, etc.
- ☐ Pain has restricted my social life and I do not go out as often.
- ☐ Pain has restricted my social life to my home.
- ☐ I have no social life because of pain.

SECTION 10 - TRAVELLING
- ☐ I can travel anywhere without extra pain.
- ☐ I can travel anywhere but it gives extra pain.
- ☐ Pain is bad but I manage journeys over 2 hours.
- ☐ Pain restricts me to journeys of less than 1 hour.
- ☐ Pain restricts me to short necessary journeys under 30 minutes.
- ☐ Pain prevents travel except to the doctor or hospital.

Oswestry Disability Index, Figure 1   Oswestry Disability Index Version 1.0; Patient name: File...; Date:... This questionnaire has been designed to give the doctor information as to how your back pain has affected your ability to manage in everyday life. Please answer every section and mark in each section only the ONE box that applies to you. We realize you may consider that two of the statements in any one section relate to you, but please just mark the box, which most closely describes your problem.

Responsiveness

Score changes associated with different levels of patient perceived improvement/deterioration are summarized in Table 1.

Effect Size

Patient (or combined patient/clinician) perceived improvement was associated with effect size of 0.82–0.87 (n = 970) (Walsh et al. 2003), 0.80 (n = 81) (Beurskens et al. 1996), 0.52 (n = 106) (Davidson and Keating 2002), 0.3–0.8 (n = 318) (Taylor et al. 1999) and 0.86/1.87 (n = 75/69) (Hagg et al. 2002).

Receiver Operating Characteristics (ROC)

The area below the ROC curve, as a measure of the ability to discriminate between subjects with and without back pain, was 0.76 (n = 76) (Leclaire et al. 1997), 0.78 (n = 99) (Davidson and Keating 2002), 0.78 (n = 88) (Stratford et al. 1994) and 0.72 (n = 970) (Walsh et al. 2003).

Minimal Clinically Important Difference (MCID)

Based on patient (or combined patient/clinician) perceived effect of treatment. For improvement the MCID was 10 (n = 154) and for deterioration –6 (n = 123) (Hagg et al. 2003).

SECTION 1 - PAIN INTENSITY

- ☐ I have no pain at the moment.
- ☐ The pain is very mild at the moment.
- ☐ The pain is moderate at the moment.
- ☐ The pain is fairly severe at the moment.
- ☐ The pain is very severe at the moment.
- ☐ The pain is the worst imaginable at the moment.

SECTION 2 - PERSONAL CARE (washing, dressing etc.)

- ☐ I can look after myself normally, without causing extra pain.
- ☐ I can look after myself normally, but it is very painful.
- ☐ It is painful to look after myself and I am slow and careful.
- ☐ I need some help, but manage most of my personal care.
- ☐ I need help every day in most aspects of self-care.
- ☐ I do not get dressed, wash with difficulty and stay in bed.

SECTION 3 - LIFTING

- ☐ I can lift heavy weights without extra pain.
- ☐ I can lift heavy weights, but it gives extra pain.
- ☐ Pain prevents me from lifting heavy weights off the floor, but I can manage if they are conveniently positioned (e.g., on a table).
- ☐ Pain prevents me from lifting heavy weights but I can manage light to medium weights if they are conveniently positioned.
- ☐ I can lift only very light weights.
- ☐ I cannot lift or carry anything at all.

SECTION 4 - WALKING

- ☐ Pain does not prevent me walking any distance.
- ☐ Pain prevents me walking more than 1 mile.
- ☐ Pain prevents me walking more than ½ of mile.
- ☐ Pain prevents me walking more than 100 yards.
- ☐ I can only walk using a stick or crutches.
- ☐ I am in bed most of the time and have to crawl to the toilet.

SECTION 5 - SITTING

- ☐ I can sit in any chair as long as I like.
- ☐ I can sit in my favourite chair as long as I like.
- ☐ Pain prevents me from sitting for more than 1 hour.
- ☐ Pain prevents me from sitting more than ½ an hour.
- ☐ Pain prevents me from sitting more than 10 minutes.
- ☐ Pain prevents me from sitting at all.

SECTION 6 - STANDING

- ☐ I can stand as long as I want without extra pain.
- ☐ I can stand as long as I want but it gives me extra pain.
- ☐ Pain prevents me from standing for more than 1 hour.
- ☐ Pain prevents me from standing for more than ½ an hour.
- ☐ Pain prevents me from standing for more than 10 minutes.
- ☐ Pain prevents me from standing at all.

SECTION 7 - SLEEPING

- ☐ My sleep is never disturbed by pain.
- ☐ My sleep is occasionally disturbed by pain.
- ☐ Because of pain, I have less than 6 hours of sleep.
- ☐ Because of pain, I have less than 4 hours of sleep.
- ☐ Because of pain, I have less than 2 hours of sleep.
- ☐ Pain prevents me from sleeping at all.

SECTION 8 - SEX LIFE (if applicable)

- ☐ My sex life is normal and causes no extra pain.
- ☐ My sex life is normal but causes some extra pain.
- ☐ My sex life is nearly normal but is very painful.
- ☐ My sex life is severely restricted by pain.
- ☐ My sex life is nearly absent because of pain.
- ☐ Pain prevents any sex life at all.

SECTION 9 - SOCIAL LIFE

- ☐ My social life is normal and causes me no extra pain.
- ☐ My social life is normal, but increases the degree of pain.
- ☐ Pain has no significant effect on my social life apart from limiting my more energetic interests, e.g., sports, etc.
- ☐ Pain has restricted my social life and I do not go out as often.
- ☐ Pain has restricted my social life to my home.
- ☐ I have no social life because of pain.

SECTION 10-TRAVELLING

- ☐ I can travel anywhere without pain.
- ☐ I can travel anywhere but it gives extra pain.
- ☐ Pain is bad but I manage journeys over 2 hours.
- ☐ Pain restricts me to journeys of less than 1 hour.
- ☐ Pain restricts me to short necessary journeys under 30 minutes.
- ☐ Pain prevents me from travelling except to receive treatment.

Oswestry Disability Index, Figure 2 Oswestry Disability Index 2.0; Patient name: File...; Date:... Please read instructions: Could you please complete this questionnaire? It is designed to give us information as to how your back (or leg) trouble has affected your ability to manage in everyday life. Please answer every section. Mark one box only in each section that most closely describes you today.

Error of Measurement

The ► error of measurement at repeated measurements was, with 95% tolerance interval, 10 (n = 289) (Hagg et al. 2003), and with 90% tolerance interval 11/15 (n = 16/47) (Davidson and Keating 2002).

References

1. Beurskens AJ, Vet HC de, Koke AJ (1996) Responsiveness of Functional Status in Low Back Pain: A Comparison of Different Instruments. Pain 65:71–76
2. Davidson M, Keating JL (2002) A Comparison of Five Low Back Disability Questionnaires: Reliability and Responsiveness. Phys Ther 82:8–24
3. Fairbank JC, Couper J, Davies JB et al. (1980) The Oswestry Low Back Pain Disability Questionnaire. Physiotherapy 66:271–273
4. Fairbank JC, Pynsent PB (2000) The Oswestry Disability Index. Spine 25:2940–2952
5. Gronblad M, Hupli M, Wennerstrand P et al. (1993) Intercorrelation and Test-Retest Reliability of the Pain Disability Index (PDI) and the Oswestry Disability Questionnaire (ODQ) and their Correlation with Pain Intensity in Low Back Pain Patients. Clin J Pain 9:189–195
6. Hagg O, Fritzell P, Nordwall A (2003) The Clinical Importance of Changes in Outcome Scores after Treatment for Chronic Low Back Pain. Eur Spine J 12:12–21
7. Hagg O, Fritzell P, Oden A et al. (2002) Simplifying Outcome Measurement: Evaluation of Instruments for Measuring Outcome after Fusion Surgery for Chronic Low Back Pain. Spine 27:1213–1222
8. Holm I, Friis A, Storheim K et al. (2003) Measuring Self-Reported Functional Status and Pain in Patients with Chronic Low Back Pain by Postal Questionnaires: A Reliability Study. Spine 28:828–833

O

Oswestry Disability Index, Table 1 Score changes related to different levels of patient (or combined patient/clinician) perceived treatment effect

Level of perceived effect	Reference study			
	(Beurskens et al. 1996) (n = 81)	(Davidson and Keating 2002) (n = 101)	(Taylor et al. 1999) (n = 225)	(Hagg et al. 2002) (n = 270)
Completely gone	n/a	33	n/a	n/a
Much better	n/a	16	n/a	28
Better/improved	12	9	18	10
Unchanged/non-improved	0	0	2	0
Worse	n/a	−6	−9	−6
Much worse	n/a	−4	n/a	n/a

n/a = not applicable

9. Leclaire R, Blier F, Fortin L et al. (1997) A Cross-Sectional Study Comparing the Oswestry and Roland-Morris Functional Disability Scales in Two Populations of Patients with Low Back Pain of Different Levels of Severity. Spine 22:68–71
10. Pratt RK, Fairbank JC, Virr A (2002) The Reliability of the Shuttle Walking Test, the Swiss Spinal Stenosis Questionnaire, the Oxford Spinal Stenosis Score, and the Oswestry Disability Index in the Assessment of Patients with Lumbar Spinal Stenosis. Spine 27:84–91
11. Pynsent P, Fairbank J, Carr A (1993) Outcome Measures in Orthopaedics. Butterworth-Heinemann, Oxford
12. Reneman MF, Jorritsma W, Schellekens JM et al. (2002) Concurrent Validity of Questionnaire and Performance-Based Disability Measurements in Patients with Chronic Nonspecific Low Back Pain. J Occup Rehabil 12:119–129
13. Stratford PW, Binkley J, Solomon P et al. (1994) Assessing Change Over Time in Patients with Low Back Pain. Phys Ther 74:528–533
14. Taylor SJ, Taylor AE, Foy MA et al. (1999) Responsiveness of Common Outcome Measures for Patients with Low Back Pain. Spine 24:1805–1812
15. Walsh TL, Hanscom B, Lurie JD et al. (2003) Is a Condition-Specific Instrument for Patients with Low Back Pain/Leg Symptoms Really Necessary? The Responsiveness of the Oswestry Disability Index, MODEMS, and the SF-36. Spine 28:607–615

Oswestry Disability Questionnaire

▶ Oswestry Disability Index

Oswestry Low Back Pain Disability Questionnaire

▶ Oswestry Disability Index

Outcome Measures

VICTOR WILK
Brighton Spinal Group, Brighton, VIC, Australia
vicwilk@tpg.com.au

Synonyms

Outcome Questionnaires; Outcomes Assessment Tools; pain questionnaires; Measuring Tools

Definition

An outcome measure is a feature of a patient's health status that can be quantified in order to assess the benefits of a treatment. Domains that are typically assessed include physical functioning, strength, range of movement, endurance, aerobic capacity, pain, disability, medication usage, work status, work capacity and quality of life. The term outcome measure is increasingly being used to refer to self-administered questionnaires, which seek to measure the change in status of the patient over time.

Characteristics

Principles

Self-administered questionnaires have three broad purposes. They can discriminate between subjects; predict outcome; or evaluate change over time. The outcome measure should be: reliable, valid, responsive to change, simple to administer, quick to fill out (less than 5 minutes), quick and easy to score (less than 1 minute), and low in cost. In addition to the technical and scientific issues regarding the collating of outcome measures, there are also ethical and moral issues involved in the collection of data, interpretation of data and sharing of data with others. The main domains of assessment commonly measured are:

- Physical assessment by clinician
- Functional capacity
- Pain
- Disability
- Quality of life
- Psychological measures such as depression, anxiety, fear and various personality traits.
- Utilisation of services: medical visits, hospitalisation, drugs, allied health visits, and home help
- Employment status

List of Entries

Essays are shown in bold